Clinical Textbook for Veterinary Technicians

Clinical Textbook for Veterinary Technicians

4th Edition

Dennis M. McCurnin, D.V.M., M.S.
Diplomate, American College of Veterinary Surgeons
Professor, Department of Veterinary Clinical Sciences
Associate Dean for Clinical and Public Services
Hospital Director, Veterinary Teaching Hospital and Clinics
School of Veterinary Medicine
Louisiana State University
Baton Rouge, Louisiana

W.B. SAUNDERS COMPANY
A Division of Harcourt Brace and Company
Philadelphia London Toronto Montreal Sydney Tokyo

W.B. SAUNDERS COMPANY
A Division of Harcourt Brace & Company

The Curtis Center
Independence Square West
Philadelphia, Pennsylvania 19106

Library of Congress Cataloging-in-Publication Data

Clinical textbook for veterinary technicians /
[edited by] Dennis M. McCurnin.—4th ed.

p.   cm.

ISBN 0–7216–2196–1

1. Veterinary medicine.   I. McCurnin, Dennis M.

SF745.C625 1998   636.089—dc21

DNLM/DLC   97–17014

CLINICAL TEXTBOOK FOR VETERINARY TECHNICIANS   ISBN 0–7216–2196–1

Printed in the United States of America.

Last digit is the print number: 9   8   7   6   5   4   3   2

This textbook is dedicated to the thousands of veterinary technicians who provide the technical support needed in the practice of high-quality veterinary medicine worldwide.

Dennis M. McCurnin, D.V.M., M.S.

Contributors

Marvene Augustus, B.S., Pharm.D.
Clinical Pharmacist, Veterinary Teaching
Hospital and Clinics, School of Veterinary
Medicine, Louisiana State University, Baton
Rouge, Louisiana

Pharmacology and Pharmacy

**Sandra S. Brackenridge, M.S.W., B.C.D.,
L.C.S.W.**
Assistant Professor of Social Work, Idaho
State University, Pocatello; Grief Counselor/
Consultant, Idaho Veterinary Medical
Association, Boise, Idaho

*Client Bereavement and the Grief Process;
Stress and Its Management*

**Daniel J. Burba, D.V.M., Diplomate,
American College of Veterinary Surgeons**
Associate Professor, Department of Veterinary
Clinical Sciences, Equine Surgeon, School of
Veterinary Medicine, Louisiana State
University, Baton Rouge, Louisiana

*Surgical Instruments and Aseptic Technique;
Wound Management and Bandaging*

**Christopher K. Cebra, V.M.D., M.A., M.S.,
Diplomate, American College of
Veterinary Internal Medicine**
Assistant Professor of Internal Medicine,
Department of Large Animal Clinical Sciences,
College of Veterinary Medicine, Oregon State
University, Corvallis, Oregon

Food Animal Medicine and Surgery

**Margaret L. Cebra, V.M.D., M.S.,
Diplomate, American College of
Veterinary Internal Medicine**
Consultant, Food Animal Medicine and
Surgery, Corvallis, Oregon

Food Animal Medicine and Surgery

Sharee A. Chavis, R.R.A., B.S.
Health Information Supervisor, Veterinary
Teaching Hospital and Clinics, School of
Veterinary Medicine, Louisiana State
University, Baton Rouge, Louisiana

The Medical Record

Doo-Youn Cho, D.V.M., Ph.D.
Professor, Department of Veterinary
Pathology, School of Veterinary Medicine;
Chief, Surgical Pathology and Necropsy
Service, Veterinary Teaching Hospital and
Clinics, Louisiana State University, Baton
Rouge, Louisiana

Basic Necropsy Procedures

**Janyce L. Cornick-Seahorn, D.V.M., M.S.,
Diplomate, American College of
Veterinary Anesthesiologists**
Associate Professor, Anesthesiology,

Department of Veterinary Clinical Sciences,
School of Veterinary Medicine, Louisiana State
University, Baton Rouge, Louisiana

Veterinary Anesthesia

**Stephen W. Crane, D.V.M., Diplomate,
American College of Veterinary Surgeons**
Adjunct Professor of Surgery, College of
Veterinary Medicine, North Carolina State
University, Raleigh, North Carolina; Director
of Veterinary Affairs, Hill's Pet Nutrition, Inc.,
Topeka, Kansas

Companion Animal Clinical Nutrition

**Dennis T. Crowe, Jr., D.V.M., Diplomate,
American College of Veterinary Surgeons
and American College of Veterinary
Emergency and Critical Care**
Carson Tahoe Veterinary Hospital, Carson
City, Nevada

Emergency Nursing

**Jacqueline R. Davidson, D.V.M., M.S.,
Diplomate, American College of
Veterinary Surgeons**
Assistant Professor, Companion Animal
Surgery, School of Veterinary Medicine,
Louisiana State University, Baton Rouge,
Louisiana

Surgical Instruments and Aseptic Technique

**William S. Dernell, D.V.M., M.S.,
Diplomate, American College of
Veterinary Surgeons**
Assistant Professor of Small Animal Surgery,
Department of Clinical Sciences, College of
Veterinary Medicine and Biomedical Sciences,
Colorado State University, Fort Collins,
Colorado

Veterinary Oncology

Krista Dickinson, C.V.T.
Head Oncology Nurse, Veterinary Teaching
Hospital, College of Veterinary Medicine and
Biomedical Sciences, Colorado State
University, Fort Collins, Colorado

Veterinary Oncology

**Erick L. Egger, D.V.M., Diplomate,
American College of Veterinary Surgeons**
Associate Professor of Orthopedic Surgery,
College of Veterinary Medicine and
Biomedical Sciences, Colorado State
University; Veterinary Orthopedic Consulting,
Fort Collins, Colorado

Surgical Assistance and Suture Material

**Randall Fitch, D.V.M., M.S., Diplomate,
American College of Veterinary Surgeons**
Assistant Professor, Small Animal Orthopedic
Surgery, School of Veterinary Medicine,

Louisiana State University, Baton Rouge, Louisiana

Surgical Instruments and Aseptic Technique

Marjorie S. Gill, D.V.M., M.S., Diplomate, American Board of Veterinary Practitioners
Associate Professor, Food Animal Medicine and Surgery, Department of Veterinary Clinical Sciences; Teaching Hospital and Clinics, School of Veterinary Medicine, Louisiana State University, Baton Rouge, Louisiana

Preventive Health Programs

Sheila R. Grosdidier, B.S., R.V.T.
Adjunct Professor, St. Petersburg Junior College, Pinellas Park, Florida; Senior Paraveterinary Educator, Hill's Pet Nutrition, Inc., Topeka, Kansas

Companion Animal Clinical Nutrition; Concepts in Livestock Nutrition; Professional Development

Michael G. Groves, D.V.M., M.P.H., Ph.D., Diplomate, American College of Veterinary Microbiologists and American College of Veterinary Preventive Medicine (Subspecialty of Epidemiology)
Professor and Head, Department of Epidemiology and Community Health, School of Veterinary Medicine, Louisiana State University, Baton Rouge, Louisiana

Zoonoses and Public Health

Kathleen S. Harrington, M.S.
Veterinary Laboratory Specialist II, Department of Epidemiology and Community Health, School of Veterinary Medicine, Louisiana State University, Baton Rouge, Louisiana

Zoonoses and Public Health

Suzanne Hetts, B.S., M.S., Ph.D.
Certified Applied Animal Behaviorist; President, Animal Behavior Associates, Inc., Littleton, Colorado

Animal Behavior

Richard J. Hidalgo, D.V.M., M.S., Ph.D., Diplomate, American College of Veterinary Microbiologists
Professor, Department of Veterinary Microbiology and Parasitology, School of Veterinary Medicine, Louisiana State University, Baton Rouge, Louisiana

Computer Applications in Veterinary Medicine

Robert A. Holmes, D.V.M., Ph.D.
Associate Professor of Veterinary Radiology, Department of Veterinary Clinical Sciences, School of Veterinary Medicine, Louisiana State University, Baton Rouge, Louisiana

Computer Applications in Veterinary Medicine

Giselle Hosgood, B.V.Sc., M.S., Fellow, Australian College of Veterinary Scientists; Diplomate, American College of Veterinary Surgeons
Associate Professor, Department of Veterinary Clinical Sciences, School of Veterinary Medicine, Louisiana State University, Baton Rouge, Louisiana

Wound Management and Bandaging

Johnny D. Hoskins, D.V.M., Ph.D., Diplomate, American College of Veterinary Internal Medicine
Professor Emeritus, Internal Medicine, Department of Veterinary Clinical Sciences; Internist, Veterinary Teaching Hospital and Clinics, School of Veterinary Medicine, Louisiana State University, Baton Rouge, Louisiana

Parasitology; Neonatal Care of Puppy, Kitten, and Foal; Preventive Health Programs

Judith L. Hutton, M.R.T.
Health Information Processor, Veterinary Teaching Hospital and Clinics, School of Veterinary Medicine, Louisiana State University, Baton Rouge, Louisiana

The Medical Record

Tracy J. Jaffe, B.A., B.S., D.V.M.
Associate Clinical Specialist, Veterinary Teaching Hospital and Clinics, School of Veterinary Medicine, Louisiana State University, Baton Rouge, Louisiana

Diagnostic Sampling and Treatment Techniques

Stephanie W. Johnson, B.A., M.S.W.
Counselor, Best Friend Gone Project, School of Veterinary Medicine, Louisiana State University, Baton Rouge, Louisiana

Client Bereavement and the Grief Process

Robert L. Jones, D.V.M., Ph.D., Diplomate, American College of Veterinary Microbiologists
Professor, Department of Microbiology, College of Veterinary Medicine and Biomedical Sciences, Colorado State University, Fort Collins, Colorado

Clinical Microbiology

M. Lynne Kesel, M.A., D.V.M.
Associate Professor, Department of Clinical Sciences, College of Veterinary Medicine and Biomedical Sciences, Colorado State University, Fort Collins, Colorado

Restraint and Handling of Animals

Roger L. Lukens, D.V.M.
Director and Professor of Veterinary

Technology, School of Veterinary Medicine, Purdue University, West Lafayette, Indiana

Veterinary Practice Management

Dennis M. McCurnin, D.V.M., M.S., Diplomate, American College of Veterinary Surgeons
Professor, Department of Veterinary Clinical Sciences; Associate Dean for Clinical and Public Services; Hospital Director, Veterinary Teaching Hospital and Clinics, School of Veterinary Medicine, Louisiana State University, Baton Rouge, Louisiana

Veterinary Practice Management

Diane McKelvey, B.Sc., D.V.M.
Kamloops Veterinary Clinic, Kamloops, British Columbia, Canada

Occupational Health and Safety in Veterinary Hospitals

Ellen Miller, D.V.M., Diplomate, American College of Veterinary Internal Medicine
Veterinary Internist, Animal Emergency Services of Northern Colorado, Fort Collins, Colorado

History and Physical Examination

Bonnie Rush Moore, D.V.M., M.S., Diplomate, American College of Veterinary Internal Medicine
Assistant Professor, Equine Medicine, Department of Clinical Sciences, College of Veterinary Medicine, Kansas State University, Manhattan, Kansas

Equine Medical and Surgical Nursing

Rustin M. Moore, D.V.M., Ph.D., Diplomate, American College of Veterinary Surgeons
Associate Professor, Equine Surgery, Assistant Director, Equine Veterinary Research Program, Department of Veterinary Clinical Sciences, School of Veterinary Medicine, Louisiana State University, Baton Rouge, Louisiana

Equine Medical and Surgical Nursing

T. Mark Neer, D.V.M., Diplomate, American College of Veterinary Internal Medicine
Professor of Medicine, Department of Veterinary Clinical Sciences; Small Animal Medicine Section Chief, Veterinary Teaching Hospital and Clinics, College of Veterinary Medicine, Louisiana State University, Baton Rouge, Louisiana

Small Animal Medical Nursing

David H. Neil, B.V.Sc., M.R.C.V.S.
Director Laboratory Animal Resources, University of Alberta, Edmonton, Alberta, Canada

Restraint and Handling of Animals

Ashley B. Oakes, D.V.M., Diplomate, American Veterinary Dental College
Veterinary Dentist, Tampa Bay Veterinary Dentistry, Tampa Bay Veterinary Referral, Inc., Largo, Florida

Small Animal Surgical Nursing and Dentistry

Matt G. Oakes, D.V.M., Diplomate, American College of Veterinary Surgeons
Veterinary Surgeon, Tampa Bay Veterinary Surgery, Tampa Bay Veterinary Referral, Inc., Largo, Florida

Small Animal Surgical Nursing and Dentistry

Maura G. O'Brien, D.V.M., Diplomate, American College of Veterinary Surgeons
Head, Department of Surgery, Surgical Oncologist, West Los Angeles Veterinary Medical Group, VCA West Los Angeles Animal Hospital, Los Angeles, California

Veterinary Oncology

Beth Paugh Partington, D.V.M., M.S., Diplomate, American College of Veterinary Radiology
Assistant Professor of Veterinary Radiology, Department of Veterinary Clinical Sciences, School of Veterinary Medicine, Louisiana State University, Baton Rouge, Louisiana

Diagnostic Imaging

Angel M. Rivera, A.H.T., C.V.T.
CCU Supervisor, Veterinary Medical Teaching Hospital, University of Wisconsin, Madison; Chief of Nursing Staff, Educational Coordinator, Animal Emergency Center, Veterinary Institute of Trauma, Emergency and Critical Care, Milwaukee, Wisconsin

Emergency Nursing

Ray L. Russell, B.S., D.V.M., M.A.M.
Management Faculty, University of Phoenix Graduate School, University of Phoenix; President, ExecuTrends, Executive Education; President, Employ America SW, Inc., Phoenix, Arizona

Personal Leadership

Jill E. Sackman, D.V.M., Ph.D., Diplomate, American College of Veterinary Surgeons
Principal Scientist, Ethicon Endo Surgery, Cincinnati, Ohio

Pain Management

William D. Schoenherr, M.S., Ph.D.
Principal Nutrition Scientist, Science and Technology Center, Hill's Pet Nutrition, Inc., Topeka, Kansas

Concepts in Livestock Nutrition

Tom L. Seahorn, D.V.M., M.S., Diplomate, American College of Veterinary Internal Medicine
Associate Professor of Equine Medicine, Department of Veterinary Clinical Sciences,

School of Veterinary Medicine, Louisiana State University, Baton Rouge, Louisiana

Preventive Health Programs

Deborah L. Skaggs, R.V.T.
Head Technician, Equine Surgery, Department of Clinical Sciences, College of Veterinary Medicine, Kansas State University, Manhattan, Kansas

Equine Medical and Surgical Nursing

Terry R. Spraker, D.V.M., Ph.D.
Associate Professor, Department of Pathology, College of Veterinary Medicine and Biomedical Sciences, Colorado State University College of Veterinary Medicine, Fort Collins, Colorado

Basic Necropsy Procedures

Regula Spreng, D.V.M.
Consultant in Small Animal Medicine and Surgery, Bern, Switzerland

Emergency Nursing

Cyprianna E. Swiderski, D.V.M., Ph.D., Diplomate, American College of Veterinary Internal Medicine
Department of Veterinary Microbiology and Parasitology, School of Veterinary Medicine, Louisiana State University, Baton Rouge, Louisiana

Neonatal Care of Puppy, Kitten, and Foal

Joseph Taboada, D.V.M., Diplomate, American College of Veterinary Internal Medicine
Associate Professor of Small Animal Medicine, Interim Director of Professional Instruction and Curriculum, School of Veterinary Medicine, Louisiana State University, Baton Rouge, Louisiana

Euthanasia; Client Bereavement and the Grief Process

Thomas N. Tully, Jr., D.V.M., M.S.
Associate Professor, Service Chief, Avian, Zoo, and Exotic Animal Medicine, Department of Veterinary Clinical Sciences, School of Veterinary Medicine, Louisiana State University, Baton Rouge, Louisiana

Birds, Reptiles, Ferrets, Rabbits, and Rodents

Jan L. VanSteenhouse, D.V.M., Ph.D., Diplomate, American College of Veterinary Pathologists
Associate Professor of Veterinary Clinical Pathology, Department of Veterinary Pathology, School of Veterinary Medicine, Louisiana State University, Baton Rouge, Louisiana

Clinical Pathology

Preface

As we push into the 21st century, it is appropriate to look ahead and attempt to anticipate the needs of the professional veterinary technician. With this in mind, this fourth edition has again grown in subject areas. New chapters dealing with zoonoses, concepts in livestock nutrition, personal leadership, professional development, and Occupational Safety and Health Administration standards have been added. The majority of existing chapters such as Diagnostic Imaging, Computer Applications, Clinical Nutrition, and Clinical Pathology have been extensively revised and updated. Seventeen new contributors have been used in this edition.

This textbook continues to attempt to meet the basic clinical needs of the technical student and practicing technician as their professional roles expand. A single book cannot possibly provide all the needed information; however, this book has been translated into several languages and adopted by many training programs and practices worldwide.

The fourth edition continues to be dedicated to its many loyal users, and each edition has been a labor of love for the technical and veterinary medical professionals. We all must continue to work in teams to achieve excellence in patient care and client satisfaction.

Dennis M. McCurnin, D.V.M., M.S.

Contents

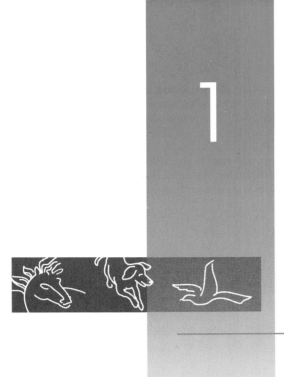

1

Restraint and Handling of Animals

M. Lynne Kesel • David H. Neil

INTRODUCTION

Most people who enter the field of veterinary medicine have had experience in handling animals, and some are even experts in handling and training certain species (e.g., dogs or horses). There is a tendency to think that if one has developed a good rapport with one species of animal the same knowledge can be transferred directly to other species. Unfortunately, handling techniques may have little transferability among different animals; sometimes the techniques are merely inefficient, and sometimes they are dangerous when applied to other animals. Few people would dream of trying to restrain a cow as they would a dog, but those unfamiliar with horses might assume that they can be handled with the same techniques used for cattle, which is not true because of their radically different personalities. Certain behavioral signs may have different meanings in different animals. For instance, a horse pawing the ground is displaying *ennui* or nervous energy, whereas a bull pawing the ground may be making an aggressive threat or may be merely flipping dirt onto his shoulders to discourage flies.

TECHNICIAN NOTE

Certain behavioral signs may have different meanings in different animals.

This chapter is intended to be a guide to the behavior, handling, and restraint of animals commonly encountered in veterinary medical practice. It is not intended to be an exhaustive text but to provide a broad range of confidence and competence. A list of recommended reading follows the text for the individual with a special interest in animal behavior or restraint of exotic animals. Restraint of exotic species has not been included. However, material on certain rodents, rabbits, and birds, which are becoming increasingly prevalent as pets (especially for people living in multiple dwellings or places in which dogs and cats are not allowed), is reviewed briefly. These small animals have their own special handling needs, which are often overlooked.

INDICATIONS FOR RESTRAINT

What are the reasons for restraining an animal? The most obvious is to control it for a procedure. Most diagnostic and therapeutic procedures that are performed on animals are unpleasant for them, and naturally they resist. The restraint itself often has aspects of unpleasantness for animals. To avoid excess discomfort for an animal, one should strive to apply the *minimum effective restraint*. It is not necessary, for instance, to "stretch" the average cat to examine its mouth; cats generally have a better attitude and cooperate more with minimal restraint. Conversely, it would be foolhardy to attempt cystocentesis on anything but a moribund cat with someone loosely cradling it. It is obvious, then, that the procedure determines the degree of restraint, and good judgment is necessary for deciding exactly how much restraint is needed.

A second important reason for effective restraint is to prevent the animal from harming itself. This is immediately evident in the use of restraining devices (e.g., Elizabethan collars, neck cradles, and so forth) to prevent self-mutilation or tearing of bandages. However, there are other ways in which animals may harm themselves while reacting to an unpleasant procedure (or

1

merely avoiding people) if they are not adequately restrained. There are environmental factors to be considered. Dogs and cats are generally examined atop tables, and scrambling off the table may result in a damaging fall. Large animals are often held in potentially hazardous environments. A barbed wire fence or protruding nails can cause cuts or punctures to a horse's skin. Horses often panic if their feet become tangled in wire and will severely cut their lower legs while thrashing around. Horses do occasionally rear, and rearing in a low barn or shed can result in severe damage to the head. Stocks and runways for cattle may have dangerously splintered boards sticking out. These are only examples—the point is that veterinary personnel must try to make the examination and treatment areas as safe as possible. The client will blame you if the animal is injured.

Animals must also be restrained so that they do not harm themselves because of the procedure itself. A simple venipuncture can result in torn vessels, hematomas, and free-flowing blood if the animal moves at the wrong time. A struggling animal might cause a rectal tear during palpation. Sutures are impossible to correctly place on a moving target.

One of the most important reasons for adequate restraint of animals is the protection of personnel. The veterinarian and the technician rely on their own functioning body parts to do their job and make their living. Relatively slight injuries may result in significant loss of income or efficiency. A badly bitten, swollen, and bruised hand cannot assist in, or perform, surgery. The use of crutches severely retards one's effectiveness around hoofed stock—especially the effectiveness of the technician, who is expected to provide the restraint. More severe injuries are generally incurred while working with large animals, which may kick, bite, or body-slam personnel. However, small animal bites may cause facial disfigurement requiring plastic surgery, or they may even cause septicemia. It should be noted that the veterinarian may be legally responsible if a client is hurt by his own animal during a veterinary procedure.

The bottom line is that effective restraint is essential for the success of the procedure and the health and safety of animals and people.

ANIMAL PERCEPTION AND BEHAVIOR

Human evolution is inextricably tied to our successful use of animals. Early humans learned enough of animal behavior and ability to prey successfully on small, then larger, animals. As time passed, certain groups of people adopted a nomadic existence in which they depended on and followed great herds of ungulates, as the Lapps follow the reindeer today. Early partnership with the dog may have been inspired by the dog's ability to flush, chase, or bring down game—useful activities for the partner hunter. True domestication of food and service animals—in which man controls all, or nearly all, aspects of the animals existence (feed, range, reproduction)—gradually arose from early, tentative uses of animals.

Humans have always been avid students of animal behavior, with the sometimes unacknowledged intent of using the knowledge so acquired to better control and maneuver animals to their own advantage. This involves an interspecies communication system, which usually is silent or, at least, nonverbal. Body language, which was "discovered" in humans a number of years ago, is in fact as old as humans and animals. The unspoken language of gesture and touch of human beings is in part the language of the silent hunter.

All of us possess an innate ability to control and manipulate animals that can be consciously developed according to interest or occupation. It is indeed gratifying, but not surprising, to see how rapidly an adequate degree of competence in manipulating animals may be attained by the majority of us. However, before you rush out to wrestle your first bull, bursting with dangerous overconfidence, remember that most of the detailed knowledge required to prevent injury to the animal or yourself during restraint and handling must be acquired through study (observing animals and reading or listening to expert advice) and extensive practice. You must learn to carefully analyze each handling and restraint situation, being concerned with the environment in which an animal is to be brought under control and the typical behavior of that species within that environment. For example, what sex are the animals, or are both sexes present? Are they young and unaccustomed to being herded? Are there young, unweaned animals still with and under the obvious protection of their mothers? As you progress through this chapter, you will see the relevance of these and additional observations. Having carefully assessed the situation, you may then apply your knowledge of species behavior, along with the appropriate equipment, to bring the animal (or animals) under control.

Perception in Domestic Animals

All animals are aware of their environment and the changes occurring in it through their five senses, particularly those of smell, sight, and hearing. One or more of the senses may be more developed in animals than in humans. Domestic and laboratory animals retain to a considerable degree the acute senses that are so important to their wild counterparts in social interaction, defense, reproduction, and the detection and selection of food. The question of how the animal senses your encroachment on its environment must be a primary consideration in approaching the various species.

Smell or Olfaction

The sense of smell, or olfaction, consists of the detection of odor molecules by the olfactory epithelium on the surface of the nasal turbinate bones. The turbinates are scrolls of bone (like loosely rolled paper) situated in the nasal cavity and covered with a vascular epithelium that provides a large warming surface for incoming air. The system is well developed in all domestic mammals but is poorly developed in domestic fowl. In the rabbit and cat, olfaction is improved by a larger area of olfactory epithelium, which covers an area 14 times greater than that found in humans.

All domestic mammals demonstrate sniffing behavior. They initially identify their own young in herds and flocks through olfaction. When an attempt is made to foster an orphaned lamb onto another ewe, one may try to render the lamb acceptable by smearing it with secretions of the ewe or her dead lamb and by temporarily bottle feeding the fostered lamb with the ewe's milk. All these measures are attempts to render the fostered lamb acceptable as judged by the ewe's sense of smell.

Smell plays an important part in the identification of places and people. This is most highly developed in the dog, which marks its territory with urine, thus creating a personal odor boundary. Tracking dogs have an exquisite sense of smell; a few seconds of exposure to a personal object will establish a tracking scent of a human. The cat marks its territory and familiar objects by rubbing scent glands on the side of its face or the pads of the feet onto outdoor marking posts and furniture in the house. Rabbits and rodents similarly mark territory by rubbing glandular skin onto objects in their environment.

Pheromones are odors secreted by animals to convey messages to other animals via the sense of smell. They are unique odors, however, in that the response of the recipient animal is unconscious or automatic. Female mice, which become anestrous when deprived of the presence of males, return to estrus at almost exactly 72 hours after being reintroduced to males or their excreta. The male horse will curl up the upper lip after smelling mare urine (Flehman response); all horses will respond to other strong odors (e.g., garlic) with a similar automatic response. Pheromones seem to be primarily associated with reproductive behavior, but the full extent of pheromone communication is not yet understood.

It is sometimes said that "animals can smell fear." Many behaviorists have pointed out that your "body language" is more likely to convey your lack of confidence and that this may be misconstrued as the "smell of fear." However, the "language" of smell clearly has a more extensive vocabulary in animals than in humans.

Hearing

Humans are deaf to the high-frequency sounds that are important in the awareness and communication of the domestic and laboratory animal. All domestic mammals have well-developed methods for collecting sound waves into the external ear. The skin-covered, cartilaginous sound collectors that most people call the ear or ear flaps are properly called *pinnae*. Domestic animals, including the rabbit, are able to move the pinnae with muscles, thus focusing on the source of the sound. The pinnae are also excellent behavioral indicators, apart from their sound-collecting function. The ears-back position in a horse signals that the animal is upset, even aggressive; a dog when dominant or actively aggressive pricks the ears forward, whereas a submissive dog wrinkles and flattens the ears.

Sounds are produced by vibration, and the greater number of vibrations or cycles per second (hz), the higher the sound or note becomes. Humans hear 20 hz at the lower end of the scale and up to 20,000 hz at the highest limit. The dog hears sounds at 40,000 hz and probably up to 60,000 hz. Incredibly, bats catch flying insects through echolocation of sounds they emit at up to 98,000 hz. The laboratory rat can hear sounds of 60,000 to 80,000 hz but not below approximately 500 hz. It has been demonstrated that social communication between rats and their young is carried out in the ultrasonic range.

Because we are unaware of the communication of animals at frequencies above our hearing capabilities, its significance at this time is in emphasizing that the sensory world of animals must not be judged by our standards.

We have used our knowledge of the perception of ultrasound by the dog to good effect. The "silent" dog whistle in fact emits a mixture of ultrasonic frequencies, which commands the animal's attention. Ultrasonic devices consisting of flat metal shapes threaded on a metal chain are commercially available. When shaken or thrown, they emit an extremely brief sound at 34,200 hz, which will rivet the attention of a dog. It elicits such

a strong orienting reaction that it is found to be extremely useful as a distractant when treating behavioral problems in dogs, especially dangerously aggressive ones.

Vision

Domestic animals (except the pig) have a reflective layer behind the sensory part of the eye (retina) that, by reflection, intensifies the perception of light entering the eye. This reflective layer, the tapetum, permits better vision at low light intensity, giving night vision that is superior to that of humans. Everyone is familiar with the way the eyes of animals reflect, in different colors depending on the animals' pigmentation, a car's headlights at night. What is visible is the tapetum, reflecting through fully dilated pupils.

Whether mammals perceive color has still not been determined. The nerve components of the retina that are responsible for color vision in humans are called *cones,* in comparison with the other components, which are called *rods*. All domestic mammals have some cones in the retina, so it is reasonable to believe that some color vision exists.

The field of vision in herbivorous domestic mammals tends to be wide, enabling them to more readily detect the encroachment of predators from various angles. This is particularly evident in the horse and rabbit, both of which enjoy almost complete all-round vision without having to move the head. The position of the eyes in the head of the rabbit is such that the only place not covered is the area immediately behind the head and a small area in front of the nose. It has a visual field of 215 degrees for each eye, overlapping in front with the blind area being immediately behind, resulting in an almost 360-degree visual field. When we describe how to approach a horse later in this chapter, we specifically warn against moving up immediately behind a horse in its blind area, and then suddenly appearing by moving out to the left or the right rear. This is a certain way to put the animal in a state of alarm and a good occasion to cause flight, a kick, or both.

The eyes of the domestic animal focus by means of muscles controlling the shape of the lens. Most animals accommodate, or focus, the eye on near objects much less readily than do humans. The horse has a particularly sluggish accommodation. What some handlers may take for fractious head raising may be nothing more than the horse attempting to visually accommodate; this particularly happens when a horse perceives a quick movement nearby.

Horses, apparently, have acute vision at middle and far distances, which is not surprising for a prey species. Many of the behavioral displays of horses are visual, and they can pick up subtle cues from human body language. Clever Hans, a 19th century equine prodigy, was thought to be able to do arithmetic problems by pawing. Instead, he was perceiving movements of his trainer, like depth of breathing, that were imperceptible to human observers. Some stories assert that Hans' trainer was unaware he was giving the cues.

The ability of the dog to discriminate form and pattern is thought to be poor compared with human ability. Despite this, there are obvious breed differences. The sight hounds (greyhounds, borzois, salukis, afghans) were bred to hunt by vision rather than by scent and are highly perceptive of movement. Herding dogs can act on human hand signals from as far away as 1.5 km.

Cats have excellent night vision, which is consonant with

their nocturnal habits. They are acutely aware of the slightest movement, which facilitates the precision of their rush after stalking their prey. Regrettably, it also facilitates the "nailing" of those who move too suddenly or find themselves in close proximity to a fearful or vengeful feline patient!

Touch

Although we tend to discount the sense of touch in the behavior of animals, contact of different body parts may be very important in the communication between animals and among animals and humans. Huddling is common in herd animals as a response to perceived threat or cold. Dogs and other pack animals may pile on each other to sleep. Mutual grooming may occur between friendly cats or between horses, which chew at each other's withers. All of these behaviors are socially solidifying in an altruistic mode.

There are also contact behaviors that appear to result from or resolve conflict. Biting, scratching, kicking, and striking may be used to resolve a hierarchy conflict. Other dominant animals may also use these, or moderations, to teach youngsters proper behavior. Canids will bite or hold the scruff of puppies' necks, hold their muzzles, or force them prone by the application of weight over the withers if their behavior is unacceptable. This is why hanging dogs or shaking them by the scruff or collar is often a potent punishment. Horses may slam a shoulder into another or kick or strike to make the point, "I'm the boss." Some people successfully use blows of the fist or knee to correct unacceptable equine behavior. However, one must carefully choose a target and possess a measure of physical strength to be effective without causing harm.

A word about how people should touch animals should be inserted here. Tentative, light touching, or patting makes many species nervous or apprehensive. A steady, firm stroke, or hearty slap (after proper introduction, of course) is reassuring to most species. Scratching and stroking the hair and skin are also relaxing to most animals.

Agonistic Behaviors

Agonistic behaviors are those associated with conflict. Many animals have to be maneuvered into a position in which restraint is possible, or they must be restrained from the outset as a safety measure. Such maneuvering is perceived by the animal as conflict, and to understand the principles of maneuvering each species, it is wise to become familiar with the predominant forms of agonistic behavior in the different species. Agonistic behaviors cover the range of response to conflict—from passive avoidance, through the assertion of dominance, to the extreme of aggression and fighting. In nature, overt aggressive attacks that lead to fights with other animals of the same or different species are not common outside sexual or predatory behavior. Dominance and submissive behavior represent the more common method of resolving disagreement over things such as territory and favors.

Flight or Fight

When an animal is approached by a stranger, the same basic principles apply whether it is a domestic or wild animal. Each species in a given environment has its own degree of response, but the factors or cues giving rise to the response are common to all animals in varying degrees. Each animal has a flight distance. If a person encroaches on that distance, which is measured visually, the animal goes into a state of alert. This has been referred to as being "adrenalinized," because the signals that travel from the brain via the sympathetic nervous system cause the secretion of adrenaline from the adrenal gland. This is what causes the pounding of one's heart and the tingling, alert sensation one feels when scared or apprehensive before competition or before speaking to a large audience. In the flight mode, the animal's muscles prepare for movement, the heart rate increases, and the available blood is routed to body parts that are essential for dealing with emergencies, namely, skeletal muscles, lungs, and brain.

Further movement toward the animal, particularly if it is unable to maintain a safe distance between itself and you, will lead to action that may take the form of avoidance or aggressive action referred to as "fight or flight."

Effects of Domestication

Domestic animals have been selected by humans for certain characteristics, such as the ability to be socialized and handled. It must have been obvious to our early ancestors that certain species of animals were more suitable for domestication than others.

The characteristics of wild species deemed suitable for domestication would be that (1) they herded or flocked easily, (2) males cohabited with females, (3) males would mate with any female in heat, (4) they easily bred and reared young, (5) they were easily approached within a relatively short flight distance, and (6) they adapted well to containment and different feedstuffs. Animals unsuitable for domestication would be those that are strongly territorial, with the males and females living separately or pair bonding, thereby requiring one male for each female. Unsuitable species would also have a strict diet, not be adaptable to a new environment, and show fear of humans by having a large flight distance.

Aggressive Behavior

Aggressive behavior is the form of agonistic or conflict behavior that leads to and includes fighting. Aggression is not the result of a single cause. The different forms of aggression are classified according to the stimuli or circumstances giving rise to ferocity.

Irritable or Pain-Induced Aggression

Inevitably, irritable or pain-induced aggression is a common problem in the veterinary hospital. Injections and certain manipulations, such as treatment of minor wounds, cause a certain degree of pain and discomfort. Even the initial injection of a local anesthetic can be most uncomfortable, no matter how skillful the anesthetist. The state of mind of the patient may have a lot to do with an aggressive outcome. If the animal is initially apprehensive and nervous, the probability for aggression is higher. It is for this reason that calming and familiarization of the patient are practiced whenever possible. Sedation may also be indicated for certain patients.

Maternal Aggression

All female domestic animals suckling their young are sensitized to interference with their offspring by strangers. The calmest, gentlest old mare in the herd may be particularly protective of her foal. The bitch can be aggressive with strangers or even less familiar family members whom she perceives to be a threat to her pups. The sow remaining in earshot of her piglets during their restraint for castration can become one of the most dangerous animals encountered. In fact, the screaming of any young pig as it is manipulated can galvanize all the sows in the farrowing house.

Predatory Aggression

Aggressive activity displayed by chasing and killing prey, which is observed in the predatory domestic animals (i.e., dog and cat), is called *predatory aggression.* It does not usually pose a threat to the animal handler, although the sight hounds or large dogs of other breeds may pull a person down to chase a cat.

Territorial Aggression

All domestic mammals are territorial in that they will protect the area over which they range from intruders, and they may exhibit territorial aggression. Separate groups of horses may share feeding sites and watering holes, but they remain apart from one another and retain control of their home range.

Dogs retain the innate characteristic of territoriality of their ancestor, the wolf. The domestic dog regards the yard as its territory, or at least the territory of its pack—its family. Thus, members of the family go about their business without hindrance, whereas strangers are treated with suspicion, which may lead to barking or even an attack. Dogs harassing mail carriers and meter readers are behaving within the norms of canine behavior. The fact that this is not socially acceptable to humans is a different matter.

The female rabbit is strongly territorial in the captive situation. If the buck rabbit is taken to her cage, she will attack him very aggressively, often causing serious injury. Thus, the doe is always taken to the buck's cage for mating. This strong female territoriality may be associated with a maternal aggression that continues even when the nesting box is empty and can be directed at humans as well as other animals. The image of an "attack rabbit" is laughable until you must reach into the cage of an obstreperous female who thumps, growls, strikes, or even bites in response.

Fear-Induced Aggression

When an animal is fearful of the environment and the people in it and it feels that it cannot avoid the situation, it will resort to aggression. Fear is a common cause of aggression in dogs in such circumstances. Fear biting is the most commonly encountered type of attack in veterinary clinics. The attack is not overtly dominant; the dog is usually giving classic signs of being intimidated, avoiding direct eye contact with head down, lips pulled back horizontally, ears flattened, and tail between the legs and perhaps emitting a low growl. If you enter the personal space of such a dog in an attempt to placate it, a sudden attack may ensue. This is fear biting, and as might be expected, this attack is usually confined to the proffered hand or forearm. Its purpose is to repel the invader.

Intermale Aggression

Aggression occurring between males, or intermale aggression, can be a problem, particularly when stud animals are being kept. Boars can be particularly vicious when confronting each other, and great care for one's own safety should be taken when dealing with them.

Sexually Induced Aggression

Sexual fighting in the presence of females in estrus is well recognized.

Dominance Aggression

The domestic dog, as we have said before, is descended from the wolf, and like the wolf it is a pack animal. The dog recognizes a hierarchy in the family and knows the pack leader. Pack leadership is established by the owner as a result of providing food, shelter, play and companionship, exercise, and authority. Certain dogs, however, establish their authority over the family, other animals, and strangers and do so quite aggressively. Alternatively, a dog may accede to dominance from one family member but attempt to assert itself aggressively with others. Such animals are a menace in the clinic, as they will not merely fear bite but also attack you. Persuasion will be of little value in handling these dogs. Forget your canine charisma and use reliable restraint from the start.

Other species housed in groups also develop hierarchies. Horse owners recognize the "pecking order" of their animals and learn to avoid being in the escape path of a submissive animal when it is challenged by an aggressively dominant one.

Typical Behavior of Domestic Animals in Aggression and Avoidance

Horses

Blatant aggressive behavior in the horse is not common. Certain horses, however, are known to be nasty, and, of course, mares with foal at foot and stallions with brood mares may be aggressive for the reasons just discussed. Aggression is characterized by lunging forward and biting, kicking with the hind legs, or striking with the forelegs. Striking is invariably accompanied by squealing. Although the field of vision for a horse is almost 360 degrees, the binocular field of vision is only 60 to 70 degrees in front. Binocular vision is essential for judging distance; therefore, vision outside the 60 to 70 degree binocular vision field will detect objects and movement and result in a change of the head position, or sometimes the body position, for further investigation.

When approaching a horse, it is obvious that one does not creep up on its blind spot from immediately behind and suddenly appear from the left or right rear. When a horse detects a new object or person in its environment, it raises its head and observes. If it is satisfied that it is a nonthreatening person or object, it will resume its previous activity. If it is anxious, it will turn its head toward the object or person, raising the neck, focusing its ears, and dilating its nostrils, thereby using its keen senses to analyze the situation. The tail is elevated, the legs are poised for flight, and, occasionally, if startled, the horse will snort, rapidly exhaling through tensed nostrils. This alarm signal will alert other horses to your approach and signal them to get ready to run from danger. A mare with a foal will usually give a warning nicker, and the foal will move in close to her side in response. If one approaches further and the horse is alarmed, it will move rapidly away to avoid the object or person. If there is more than one horse, they will move together.

Cattle

When dealing with cattle, the primary concern is with the bull, regardless of size. The smaller Channel Island dairy breed bulls are particularly unpredictable. Aggressive behavior is characterized by pawing the ground with the forefeet while holding the head with the frontal area almost vertical with the ground and snorting. A bull, after charging and knocking down a person, will make continued attempts to toss the victim, which may lead to goring if the bull has horns. In addition, he may attempt to kneel on a victim. Because little can be done to thwart a determined bull, the gory details are given merely to emphasize that bulls should *always* be treated with the utmost respect and with the appropriate means of restraint and containment. There are special handling considerations for those who work with semen donors at artificial insemination centers. Insensitive handling before and during coitus may give rise to reproductive behavior problems; suffice to say that bad handling may lead to considerable economic loss.

> ### TECHNICIAN NOTE
>
> *All* bulls must *always* be considered potentially dangerous. Those most likely to hurt people are bulls that have been hand raised; they have no fear or respect for people.

Aggressiveness in the heifer and cow seems to be directly related to breed and socialization. Dairy breed cows are generally very docile because they are handled a great deal. Beef breeds that are handled frequently are very manageable. However, the more cattle are left to themselves and the more frequently they are reared as calves with little human contact, the more aggression they will demonstrate in the situations described earlier.

The flight or fight distance for a herd of cattle will vary tremendously depending on the previous degree and type of contact with humans. There is a vast difference between handling a herd of dairy cows and herding range cattle. The flight distance for dairy cattle is very short, with the animals veering away only as their personal space is entered. The other extreme is cattle that attempt to maintain a long flight distance by gradually moving farther away. In situations in which this is no longer effective, the animals may break into a run. It is amazing how few people it can take, either on foot in a fenced situation

> ### TECHNICIAN NOTE
>
> In driving a cow, the proper position is approximately 45 degrees behind the point of the animal's shoulder, which allows her to see you yet impels her from behind. The smaller the cow's flight distance, the closer you must get to make her move.

or on horseback in a range situation, to maneuver cattle at the walk. If cattle break into a run, control is much more difficult,

if not impossible. Part of the secret to maneuvering cattle is body extension. Using a staff or stock whip when on foot is perceived by the cattle as an extension of the body. If the cattle are kept calm, such body extension is a good visual barrier to them. A person on horseback has the substantial advantage of the body extension of the horse, in addition to increased mobility.

Calves

The calf is invariably inquisitive and will become very attentive to your presence with the head stretched toward you. If you *dart* forward, the calf may panic, veer, and run away. Calves remember rough handling and, after such experiences, will be harder to approach in the future. If your approach is quiet, deliberate, and unruffled, the calf will turn slowly to avoid you. You then move to one side or the other to cut off the escape. The calf should thus be negotiated into a corner and the lower face or jaw should be grasped, with the head pulled over to one side against you. Small calves may be encouraged to move by encircling the calf from the side with one arm in front of the neck and the other arm around the hindquarters.

Adult cattle may be held by the nose, but this is too severe and inhumane for calves and may lead to handling problems later in life.

Pigs

Aggressive behavior in the domestic pig may have serious economic and physical consequences. Two strange adult boars in one another's presence will circle each other, obviously using olfaction as a principal means of perception. Threats will be made by jaw snapping and barking grunts. Fighting commences in the side-to-side, head-to-head position, with sideways pushing and slashing at one another with tusks. Such fights may, if not stopped, result in significant wounding. Only foolhardy people would use their body parts to break up a boar fight. Solid or heavyweight wire panels or plywood may be inserted between the combatants.

> ### TECHNICIAN NOTE
>
> Large numbers (more than 50) of totally unfamiliar pigs in a large enclosure adapt better than smaller numbers; there is less fighting, probably because dominance is more difficult to establish in the fluctuating social groups that result.

Pigs are mostly reared in groups, which provides opportunity for fighting. Pigs more than 2 weeks of age will fight, and hierarchies or pecking orders are established on the basis of dominance and submission. When new pigs are introduced to the group, fighting may occur, particularly if living space and trough space are limited. A sow introduced into an established group may be attacked savagely and even killed. Aggression in pigs may be reduced by allowing more space and/or diversions (e.g., playthings). Chemical manipulation (tranquilizers) may reduce initial fighting when unfamiliar swine are put together.

The fully grown sow is capable of killing a human and is

most dangerous when raising her litter. In our description of maternal aggression, we cited the sow as a prime example. We repeat, when handling unweaned pigs, always remove the sow to a secure area that is out of earshot if possible.

Avoidance behavior in young pigs in confined spaces usually involves running into corners and huddling, shoving, and even climbing over one another. When pigs are approached and some are caught, the rest may run again and huddle in another corner. This tendency continues as they get older. If kept calm, pigs in the open will move well as a herd.

Sheep

Intermale aggression in rams can lead to injury and fatal gangrenous lesions of the head from butting. An aggressive ram may be formidable to handle and, because of a willingness to challenge and butt people, should be treated with respect.

Avoidance behavior in sheep is the basis of maneuvering the flock. When sheep are approached, they will form a tight bunch and move together. This herding or flocking behavior is well understood by the sheep dog. Through breeding and training, sheep dogs have had the canine predatory behavior modified to herding. By carefully controlling their posture, speed of movement, and distance from the flock, they can use ovine avoidance behavior to maneuver the flock into an enclosure. The combined results of the observation and use of the behavior by shepherd dog and flock is undoubtedly one of the most fascinating, complex interspecies relationships in domestic animal management.

Dogs

Overt viciousness is not a common occurrence in the dog. Aggressive behavior, however, is a significant social problem. It has been estimated that there are more than 1 million dog bites in the United States annually and that close to 40% of the animals identified in biting incidents have not been vaccinated against rabies. The number of human deaths occurring as a result of dog attacks has not been accurately determined, but the number is considered to be significant, particularly among small children.

Dominance and submission are important in communication between two dogs in a conflict situation. *Dominance* is signaled by fixing the other animal in a direct stare; the ears are raised and angled forward. The front end of the body is held high, and the hackles are raised. The head is held up and lips curl to reveal the incisor and canine teeth; the tail is raised. A *submissive* role is shown by lowering the front end of the body and avoiding direct eye contact, with the tail held between the legs. The animal may squat and urinate or defecate. The backbone may adopt an **S** shape, and the animal may lie down on its side or on its back, raising the legs and exposing its undefended belly.

It should be noted that the "clinical stare" of veterinary personnel, as they examine a dog, can be taken as a dominance challenge by the dog.

When treated by a person, the dog may demonstrate potential aggression by adopting the dominantly aggressive posture already described or a submissive or intimidated stance; in this case, the dog lowers the front of the body and head. The ears are flattened back on the head, and the lips are pulled back at the corners in a "grin." The tail is held between the legs. A dog in the active or dominant aggressive posture may

attack if the threat is not removed from its fight or flight distance. The dog in the intimidated posture will bite only if you attempt to encroach on its personal or intimate distance. This, of course, is the pattern of fear biting.

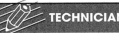

TECHNICIAN NOTE

Some dogs may show active aggression only when the owner is present, appearing to "protect" the owner. The protectiveness may actually be possessiveness, in which the dog is defending his own favored object, or territory; the lack of the owner removes the occasion of conflict.

Certain dogs do not attempt to resolve potential conflict by dominance or aggression, preferring to avoid and circumvent it completely whenever possible. Dogs that tend to face conflict situations are said to have an active defense reflex (ADR), whereas those that skillfully avoid conflict are described as having a passive defense reflex (PDR). These two major categories of canine agonistic behavior were recognized as militarily important in selecting dogs. Dogs with highly developed ADRs were selected as guard dogs, and those with strong PDRs, which would carefully avoid being captured, were selected to be message-carrying dogs.

Cats

Aggressive behavior in the cat should never be underestimated. The use of the claws of all four feet and teeth makes the cat a formidable patient in a situation of conflict. Handling cats in all moods is discussed later in this chapter. Note that the cat stalks its prey and runs short distances to pounce. It is a stealthy aggressor. The cat's true speed never becomes apparent until it is actively avoiding conflict. In the clinic, to prevent its escape, all doors and windows must be closed before an attempt is made to handle a cat.

Management Ethology

Ethology is the study of animal behavior. What we are discussing in this chapter is sometimes called "management ethology," which is the study of animal behavior as a means of determining how best to maneuver and control animals. A complete discussion on animal behavior is found in Chapter 2.

What follows is a detailed description of standard methods of approaching and handling animals that have been developed over the years. You will see that the approach and handling techniques are essentially in harmony with the behavior of the various species and the physical methods of restraint are compatible with their anatomy. The unique powers of humans to observe, and a great deal of trial and error, have brought us to the present state of the art. You must acquire that knowledge to attain competency, but nothing can substitute for keen perception, alertness, and the ability to comprehensively observe and analyze each situation. The only way to learn the art is to prepare yourself mentally and then do it, with confidence and the knowledge that you have made a sound assessment of the particular situation.

Capture and Restraint of Horses

Horses may pose interesting problems in their capture. Most horses soon learn that capture leads to work or unpleasantness and therefore practice avoidance to a greater or lesser degree. Let us begin with the horse that does not readily avoid people.

One thing that must always be kept in mind when handling horses is their innate antipathy to close confinement. Horses do not do well in "squeeze"-type situations, although most can be trained to accept them. Although most cattle will accept tight quarters for capture, this situation is liable to make a horse nervous or anxious. Close quarters may well lead to an attempt at escape and may result in injuries to the horse, people, or both.

A cardinal rule when approaching almost any animal, but *especially* a horse, is not to startle it. One should always make one's presence known by talking, calling, whistling, singing, thumping feed buckets, and so forth before entering the flight distance of the horse. For the normal domesticated horse, the flight distance is probably between 6 meters (m) and 15 m. Things that occur outside this radius are usually of little concern to the horse as threats, but once within this area sudden movements or sharp noises may easily startle it. Always be sure that the horse is observing you as you approach. If it suddenly is aware of you already inside its danger zone, it will be startled, which usually results in its jumping away from you, but it may also result in your getting kicked as an intruder.

It should be obvious to anyone that approaching a horse from the rear should be avoided if at all possible. Given the horse's zone of vision and its blind spot behind, the horse is less likely to see the person and is therefore likely to "spook" when the person's presence is discovered; in addition, the person becomes dangerously vulnerable to a kick. Horses approached from the front or side may whirl and kick, but the extra 1.5 seconds that the horse takes to turn is well used to effect a rapid retreat.

A horse's kick zone extends 1.8 to 2.5 m behind him. The furthest extension of his heels is the most dangerous and is the area of potentially fatal kicks to the head. Horses usually kick to the rear, rather than to the side as the cow kicks. Therefore, the prudent person will circle at least 3 to 3.5 m behind a horse or else directly behind and in physical contact with him. Grasping the tail as one walks around the rear of the horse may discourage a kick. Staying close to the rear end of the horse will not allow the full force of a kick and will keep the blow low on the person's body. This is not to suggest that a short-range kick is not painful or dangerous—it very well may be—but a fractured tibia is of much less importance than a fractured skull.

It should also be noted that one should never stand directly in front of a horse whether the animal is loose or on a lead. The rare horse (often a stallion or gelding) may strike with a foreleg, which can be as damaging as a kick.

The best approach to a horse is from the front and slightly to the left side. The left side is, in horseman's terminology, the "near" side, the side from which the horse is usually handled because of convention and because most people lead horses with the right hand. The horse's right side is called the "off" side. The reason for approaching somewhat from the side is to give the horse the option of turning slightly away. At the first indication of the horse turning away (the head turning away from you), you should stop or even back off a step. The horse will usually stop turning away, and your standing there talking to him will pique his curiosity. Many "shy" horses may be approached this way, in increments, with each pause assuring the horse that you do not intend to hurt him. The worst thing one can do when the horse starts to move away is to proceed toward him, because he will assume you are giving chase and will keep moving off. Once you are behind the horse and he cannot see you well, you become even more of a threat from which to flee.

The approach to a horse should be unhurried and without sudden movements. Horses may be wise to the purpose of halters or ropes, so it is often sensible to conceal these items under the clothing. One may also use a small-diameter catch rope or piece of baling twine hidden in the hand to loop around the neck before trying to halter the animal. Presenting the hands empty may help to gain the horse's confidence. Sometimes horses, especially foals, will walk right up to a person who squats on the heels. The shorter stature probably makes the figure less threatening, as well as an object of curiosity.

Once you have gotten up to a horse, it is worth a moment's attention to reward it for standing still. Most horses like to be scratched on the side of the face behind the lips. One may then work backward along the side of the jaw to the base of the neck, which is a favorite scratching spot. Some horses are "head-shy" and should be scratched on the neck first. If the horse stands quietly for these operations, it will probably accept a rope around the neck. The rope is best applied by standing on the near side about midway between head and shoulder and bringing the rope end in the left hand from under the neck on the off side, then grasping the end with the right hand, which has been slipped over the neck (Fig. 1–1). An alternate method on quiet horses is to have the right arm over the neck and pass the crown strap of the halter to the right hand. While giving the horse the impression that it is restrained by the right arm, one manipulates the halter noseband over the nose, and the crown strap is then fastened (Fig. 1–2). The type of halter that does not unfasten to go behind the ears will require that the horse be restrained by a neck rope while being haltered. This is usually best accomplished by standing on the near side and holding the neck rope with the left hand while the right

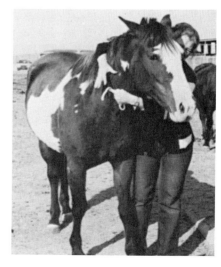

Figure 1–1. Placing the rope around the horse's neck.

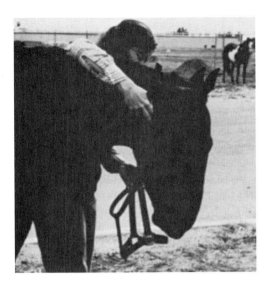

Figure 1-2. Putting the halter on the horse. Do not bump the horse's nose with the noseband.

hand glides the halter over the face and ears. The horse is usually "caught" when the crown piece is behind the ears. Some horses are gentle and good-natured and may allow someone to walk up to them and throw a rope around their necks or halter them without ceremony, but after the veterinarian's truck pulls into the yard it is more often not the case. The veterinarian's truck usually signals (whether by acute vision, memory of previous contact, medicinal smells, or a combination) the arrival of strangers who will draw blood, administer medication by stomach tube and/or injection, and so forth.

What does one do with the horse that moves off as soon as he sees a person approach? The usual answer is bribery. A handful of grain, hay or grass, or a bucket of grain may entice the horse to approach or be approached. It is best to hold the bribe in the left hand and to turn at right angles to the horse so that the neck and shoulder are within easy reach of the right hand for scratching. When confidence has been established through scratching the neck, the right hand may be placed around the neck for restraint. Some horses are cagey and cooperate up to the point of restraint with the arm, whereupon they will whirl away. These horses may be candidates for roping or trapping.

Many horses that are impossible to catch in a large field "give up" in an enclosed space. Some animals, however, may become exceptionally nervous in a small area and may be prone to kick or to try to break out in panic when approached. A pole syringe or capture gun with tranquilizer is sometimes the only answer. Luring cagey but tame animals into a corral or stall with feed may work well. It may be necessary to leave the bait inside and then sneak up and close the gate after the horse has entered.

Exciting the horse at any point is a self-defeating act. An excited horse loses its common sense and in fear can try to go over, under, around, or through whatever is containing it.

Roping the horse is impossible (except for an expert on a roping horse) unless the horse is in a reasonably small enclosure. Again, it is important to keep the horse as quiet as possible. Therefore, whirling the rope overhead is not desirable, as it will be frightening to the average horse that is unacquainted

with such cowboy tactics. Instead, one needs to cultivate a low, backhand roping technique. A loop is made that just brushes the ground when the loop and rope are held at waist level (Fig. 1–3). A generous amount of excess rope (yet not enough to touch the ground) is played out from the coils, which are held loosely in the left hand so as to peel them off with a light pull. The right hand holds the loop on the left side of the body, palm facing the body, and the roper situates himself or herself 2.5 to 3 m from a fence on his or her right side. The horse (facing the roper) is then driven past, between the roper and the fence. The roper, anticipating when the horse will go past, flips the loop backhanded for the horse to run into. The fence keeps the horse from ducking away from the movement, and strong driving from behind will force it into the loop. This technique is surprisingly successful for amateurs.

It should be stressed that one should not attempt to rope a horse without wearing gloves, for the obvious reasons. The right hand initially will be holding the rope. The coils could tighten around the left hand if they are held fast. If the horse is charging through at such a rate that it cannot be held, one should release the rope before being jerked off balance and dragged. One may always pick up the loose end of the rope after the horse has stopped running.

Horses that show signs of dangerous vices or viciousness (e.g., charging or threatening to kick) should not be given the opportunity to harm you by physical proximity. There are means of tranquilization or anesthetization that do not require being close to the horse (i.e., pole syringe, capture gun); however, they are seldom used in veterinary practice.

Capture and Restraint of Foals

Foals pose different problems of capture than do adult horses. Being without any previous knowledge of humans, newborn foals act from instinct in avoiding strange creatures and will hide behind the mother for safety.

Before approaching the foal, one must have the mare securely restrained. When her foal starts to struggle, vocalize in

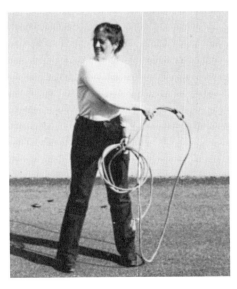

Figure 1-3. The method of holding the lariat for roping a horse.

fear, or both, a mare may try to attack whatever threatens her baby. The most docile mare may be the most protective of her foal.

When capturing a foal, one must be careful not to let it harm itself in trying to escape. The ideal situation is to crowd the foal into a corner of a stout solid fence or solid wall. The barrier must not have holes that the youngster may try to climb through and possibly hurt itself. One should never crowd a foal into a barbed wire fence or other flimsy barrier. If that is all that is available, one should use sufficient people to surround and capture the foal. Obviously, catching a foal is at least a two-person job, except when the mare and foal are in a stall in which the mare is tied.

The easiest way to catch a foal is to back the mare snugly against the wall about the length of the foal from the corner, which will form a box in the corner of the barrier. The person who is to catch the foal then enters the box at its open end and slowly approaches the foal. Almost inevitably, the foal will cower against the opposite wall with its head close to the mother's rump. The foal should be approached "amidship," with the knowledge that the nearness of hands or actually touching it will be a signal to bolt. A foal almost always bolts forward and toward its mother, and the person should be ready to catch it under the neck with one arm when this occurs, to be followed immediately by the other arm around the rump or the hand around the tail (the tail is grasped from underneath, with the palm facing the underside of the tail). Grasping the tail is the most secure way to hold the hindquarters but bear in mind that it is more uncomfortable for the foal, so it may struggle longer. Also, some owners may object to their foals being handled this way because it is a more negative experience for the foal, with long-term effects on behavior. There also is a rare chance that the tail could be injured.

If one grabs only the foal's neck, its reaction will be a rapid reverse and the foal will escape, becoming harder to catch the next time. Veterinary personnel should not contribute unduly to the negative experiences of the foal. Extra attention to scratching and getting the foal to develop trust in people is appreciated by clients and will make the youngster easier to deal with the next time.

Having grabbed the foal fore and aft, the handler may have need to push it against the fence until it stops struggling. There is a tendency to lift a foal off its feet when doing this, which is poor technique. If the foal loses its footing, it may become more frightened and struggle more vigorously, and it may severely batter your shins with its hooves.

As soon as the foal is securely caught, one should take pains to reassure it and its mother that no harm is meant. One way is to position the mare and foal so that they face each other. They should be as close as possible without the mare becoming a nuisance in whatever procedure is being carried out on the foal. It is generally a poor practice to separate mare and foal, as both will fret until they are close again.

Halter and Chain Lead

The halter is the basic restraint tool for horses, but alone it is inadequate for some tasks. Halters that have rings at the side of the nosepiece may be made more effective if a chain lead is passed from one side to the other. The lead is snapped on the side of the halter that is away from the handler after being passed through the loop near the handler, usually on the near

side. This arrangement allows finer control of the direction of the horse's nose and, if squeezed when pulled, puts some authority into the restraint because of the discomfort it causes. If at all possible, the chain lead should come in contact with the horse very lightly, or not at all, unless the horse misbehaves. Constant pressure is worrisome to the animal and does not leave any reserve.

There are three possible positions for the chain lead on the halter. The least authoritative is under the jaw, at which point it mainly causes a squeeze around the nose. Horses with very tender chins or those who are not accustomed to a chain lead may throw their heads or lunge backward when the lead is pulled. Horses that sense a squeezing of the nose as a signal to back up must be carefully retrained to respond correctly. It is often necessary to *release* pressure to allow the horse to stop its reverse. The chain over the nose is very effective (Fig. 1–4). The top of the nose is sensitive, and a pull there will make the horse drop the nose and stop forward progress. Very few stallions should be led about by a plain halter; the chain over the nose is essential. Finally, a more severe treatment would be the chain passing through the mouth; however, many stallions are hand-bred with the chain lead through the mouth, so they might associate it with breeding and become sexually excited.

Tying the Horse

There are a few simple rules to follow when a horse must be tied. First, all equipment must be strong and sound. This includes the halter, the rope, and whatever the rope will be tied to. If the halter is suspect, the rope may be passed through the nose of the halter and tied around the horse's neck with a nonslip knot, preferably a bowline. Snaps on ropes are suspect,

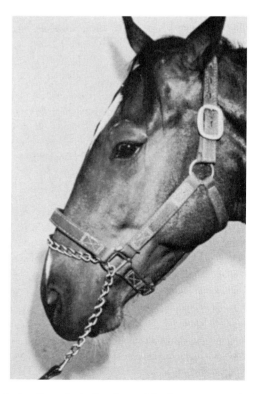

Figure 1–4. The chain lead used to increase control of the halter.

because all but the heaviest will break when a strong horse jerks back on them with all its weight. If something breaks, the horse will be free (and may learn to pull back as an escape whenever tied), but perhaps more importantly it may throw itself over backward and sustain serious harm. The second rule is that the horse be tied to something at its shoulder height or higher. There should be about only 60 centimeters (cm) of rope between the halter and the tie post (i.e., a little longer than the length of the horse's head) to prevent the horse from pawing over the rope, panicking, and pulling back. Third, there should be no hazardous objects in the tie area (i.e., children, dogs) that might spook the horse. Finally, a horse should never be left unobserved.

In general, one should be holding rather than tying horses for veterinary procedures, since horses can get into trouble while tied. It is also a general rule that the holder should stand on the same side of the horse as the veterinarian, because the head, rather than the body or hindquarters, will therefore be directed toward the practitioner if the horse should move around.

TECHNICIAN NOTE

When controlling the head, remember to stand on the same side of the horse as the person rendering treatment to the animal. If the horse begins to act up, the worse that will happen is that the body will swing away from both of you. If you were on the opposite side, the head would follow you and the body could swing into the other person, knocking him over, or the horse could swing the hindquarters into position to kick.

The Twitch

The twitch is a nerve-stimulating device that can immobilize horses and is therefore helpful in veterinary restraint. Most twitches are applied to the upper lip of the horse. The most innocuous is the so-called humane twitch, which is a hinged pair of long handles that squeeze down over the sides of the lip and may then be secured at the bottom by a thong and snapped back to the halter. The advantage of this twitch is that once applied it need not be held in place (Fig. 1–5). The disadvantage is that the pressure is fairly mild and some horses ignore it. More traditional twitches rely on a loop and a leverage device. The loop of chain or rope is placed on the lip and tightened by twisting the leverage device. The leverage may be from a piece of wood or pipe about 50 cm long. The loop needs to be seated on the lip behind the heavy gristle pad at its tip and ahead of the nostrils; on some thick-nosed horses, this area may be hard to find. Horses that have been twitched are wise and will throw their heads and tighten the lip when one attempts to apply the twitch.

To apply the twitch, place the loop over the back of three fingers and the thumb (leaving one finger, the first or second, out of the loop to keep the twitch from sliding back on the hand or wrist). Grasp the end of the horse's lip, slide the loop off your fingers, and twist the handle until the twitch is snug

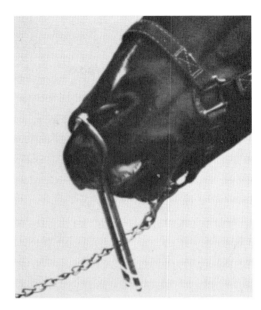

Figure 1-5. The humane twitch in place on the horse's lip.

and starts to elongate and distort the horse's lip. It is best to have someone hold the horse's halter as the twitch is applied. This will allow the second hand of the person applying the twitch to keep the handle from being flung around if the horse should throw its head. If the horse is to stand still, the twitch should be tightened until the horse responds. The average person probably cannot twist enough to damage the horse. Once the twitch has been applied, the person holding it should also be holding the halter (Fig. 1–6). To keep the long handle of the twitch from being in the way, it should be held with the cheekpiece of the halter alongside the horse's face. After removing the twitch, the horse's nose should be rubbed vigorously to counteract the discomfort and numbness that are present. This will feel good to the horse and may keep it from avoiding hands on the nose after the twitching experience. In the absence of a twitch, a person with a firm grip can hold the upper lip.

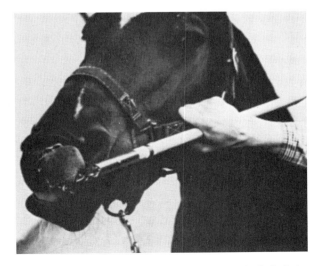

Figure 1-6. The correct way to hold the chain twitch.

TECHNICIAN NOTE

Do not begin something uncomfortable on a horse until the twitch has been in place for a few minutes. The twitch probably works through release of endogenous opioid substances, which takes time to work.

Whenever applying or holding a twitch of any kind do not stand directly in front of a horse. Sometimes twitches will encourage a horse to strike. There are people who twist horses' ears for restraint. Ear twisting is a poor practice because the supporting structures of the ear may be damaged, causing disfigurement.

Lifting the Foreleg

Some horses will stand still if a foreleg is picked up and held. When one foreleg is held up, the horse will usually leave the other three legs on the ground.

To lift up a horse's foreleg, one stands next to the horse slightly forward of the leg, facing toward the horse's rear (Fig. 1–7). It is easier to lift any leg if the horse's weight is first pushed off that leg. You may lean against the horse or push with the hand near it to effect the shifting of weight. The leg itself is grasped at the same time by running thumb and forefinger down on either side of the suspensory ligament, just behind the cannon bone. Squeezing the suspensory ligament between the cannon bone and flexor tendons is uncomfortable to the horse if it has weight on its foot, and the horse will therefore cock its knee and fetlock joint. The foot may then be picked up by the fetlock hair or by cradling the anterior aspect of the fetlock. The forefoot may then be inserted between one's legs from behind to be held between the thighs just above the knees, which frees both hands.

Lifting hind feet is almost the same as lifting forefeet; shift the horse's weight, and then grasp the leg and foot (Fig. 1–8). One stands near the horse's stifle or further anterior and lifts the foot forward to get it off the ground. Once the horse has

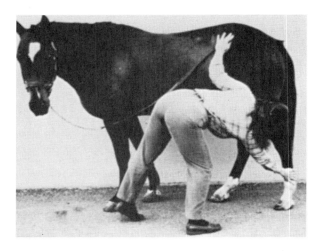

Figure 1–8. Lifting the horse's hind leg.

allowed the leg to be lifted and is holding it up, one may walk rearward with the leg, staying quite close to the horse's body and proceeding rearward until the lower leg nestles comfortably across one's upper thigh, with the hoof on the inside of the thigh, the horse's hock at about waist level, and the tibial region of its leg snug against one's side. The leg should stay braced in this position without the use of hands. The horse that threatens to kick or refuses to let its hind leg be held up may have it dragged up and forward with a scotch hobble. A foreleg may be tied up by passing a strap or rope around forearm and lower leg in a loop and doubling up the leg. A horse could fall and seriously injure the knee with a foreleg tied up. Having the hind leg pulled up with a scotch hobble (see Fig. 1–10) presents similar concerns of instability, especially if the horse is struggling. Legs should never be pulled up like this if the horse is not on a "soft" surface.

Stocks

Horses have an innate fear of being enclosed. In some horses this fear is pathological, and they will kick their way out of close situations. Therefore, the use of stocks with horses should be approached with caution, and every effort should be made to calm the horse and accustom it to the situation. The best horse stocks are heavy pipes or poles in a single row that are the height of the point of the shoulder. It is best if they have some quick-release mechanism, particularly for the piece at the rear, in case the horse should throw a fit. Horses should not be left unsupervised in stocks. Stocks are often used for rectal palpations. If no stocks are available, one might wish to stand a horse next to a wall or stout pole fence and back it up to a couple of bales of hay or straw, which might deflect or discourage kicks. Some veterinarians prefer to palpate standing unprotected tight behind the horse (especially if the veterinarian has short arms).

Tail Tie

During rectal palpations and vaginal examinations, the horse's tail may be conveniently tied out of the way with a small cord tied to the hair. The end of the rope must *never* be tied to anything but the horse itself. Tying the free end around the neck is best. If the horse gets loose with the tail tied to a

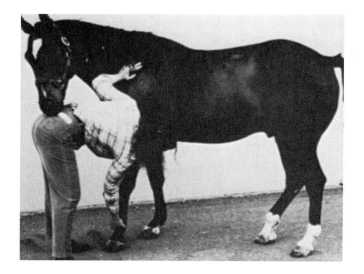

Figure 1–7. Lifting the horse's foreleg.

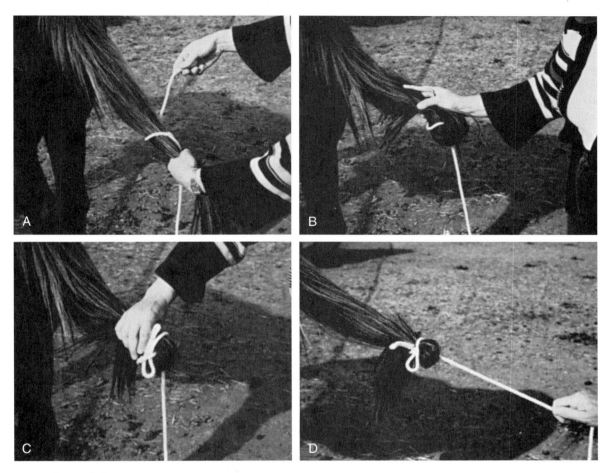

Figure 1-9. The steps in making a secure tail tie. A, The rope is placed around the tail. B, The tail is folded back on itself and on the rope. C, The short end of the rope passes over the folded tail, and a loop is pushed under the tail-encircling portion of the rope. D, Tension on the long end of the rope makes the knot snug. Pulling the short end of the rope will release the knot.

stationary object, serious injury could result. The tail tie is a simple quick-release knot using a small rope placed across the tail just below the fleshy portion (Fig. 1–9). The long end of the rope can be tied with a quick-release knot around the neck.

Hobbles

Horses are very seldom hobbled or cast (thrown to the ground) since the advent of chemical restraint. However, breeding hobbles are still used to prevent a horse from kicking effectively. These are hobbles fitted around the hocks with web or leather straps, which are tied to a neck strap or neck rope after being passed between the forelegs. They should be adjusted to snugness with the horse standing in a normal position.

The scotch hobble is a means of drawing up the hind leg (Fig. 1–10). It is often used, with or without a figure-eight on the lower leg, for holding the "up" leg for a castration procedure. A heavy rope should be used to avoid rope burn. Before the animal is anesthetized, a loop is tied with a bowline (nonslip knot) around the base of the horse's neck. Once the horse is down, a loop to catch the hindleg is passed through the neck loop and is placed behind the pastern. The leg is drawn up and forward by pulling the end of the rope, using the neck loop as a pulley. To avoid rope burn of the pastern, the leg can be pulled up by hand at the same time the rope is tightening.

Restraint of a Horse That Is Lying Down

There are times when a horse must be held lying down. Control of the head is the key, because to get up the horse must first lift its head. Therefore, sitting or kneeling on the neck near the

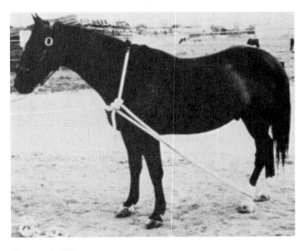

Figure 1-10. The scotch hobble on a standing horse.

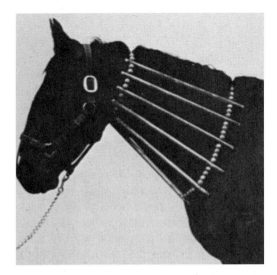

Figure 1-11. The horse wearing a neck cradle.

head will keep it down. One always climbs on the neck from the back of the horse. Any activities performed on a lying horse should be done from the back, not from the belly side, in which position a thrashing leg could strike you. In addition, to keep the horse from waggling its head and possibly damaging the down eye, one should pull the horse's nose off the ground by the nosepiece of the halter. The head can be held at almost 45 degrees to the neck. A horse that is lying down should either have its head held up or have its lateral face and eye cushioned to prevent eye and facial nerve damage. A gunny sack or coat can be folded and tucked under the halter, or an inner tube can be pushed under the head to protect the head.

Other Head and Mouth Restraints

Horses sometimes mutilate themselves or tear bandages. There are devices to restrict the movement of the head laterally; one is the cradle, a device of wooden slats that buckles over the horse's neck to brace it straight (Fig. 1–11). These devices restrict lateral movement but allow the horse to eat. A wire muzzle may be put on a horse that is to be held off feed to prevent it from eating bedding while giving it access to water.

There are at least two kinds of gags for horses' mouths. One is a simple wedge (Fig. 1–12), which is pushed up between

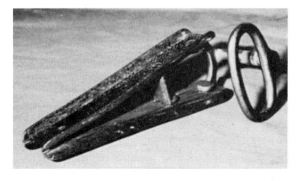

Figure 1-12. The wedge gag. The wedge is slid between upper and lower cheek teeth, and the handle comes out of the corner of the mouth.

the upper and lower cheek teeth with the handle hanging out of the side of the horse's mouth. The other, a large hinged speculum, fits over the upper and lower incisors and hangs from the halter. The mouth can be cranked open. Although this device is effective in getting the mouth open, it is, unfortunately, heavy and cumbersome. The horse's tongue may be pulled out of the side of the mouth in the interdental space and held, usually by the clinician. Some veterinarians prefer to hold the tongue to the opposite side when examining the mouth or floating the teeth, rather than using a gag.

Blindfolding a pushy horse that insists on charging around and walking all over its handler may make it reluctant or hesitant to move. A blindfold may also make the horse kick at painful or unfamiliar sensations around the hindquarters.

Chemical Restraint

Manual casting of horses has been largely replaced by chemical restraint and anesthesia. Casting has always held inherent danger for both horse and handler. One of the common injuries for the horse is damage to the knees when the forefeet are pulled out from under it. The thrashing around that tends to accompany casting can cause a variety of injuries.

The most commonly used chemical restraint for horses is xylazine hydrochloride (Rompun) in tranquilizing dosages, but many people have been dismayed by some horses that can and will kick readily under the influence of xylazine. Some practitioners use morphine with xylazine, which generally leaves horses standing stolidly in a saw-horse stance, unwilling to move. Whenever a horse has been anesthetized or tranquilized, it should be observed until it is steady on its feet. It may be necessary for several people to steady a wobbly horse so that it does not fall and hurt itself. Anesthesiology and chemical restraint are discussed in Chapter 15.

Capture and Restraint of Cattle

Cattle are less difficult to capture than are horses. Generally, except for "pet" cattle and some dairy cattle, they are not directly approachable for haltering and leading. However, they are easier to drive into chutes and stocks.

Cattle are less discriminating than horses about what (or whom) they step on or bump into. Domestic cattle have much of the natural avoidance bred out of them and are very curious. They may stand still and ogle as a person approaches, especially if there is something odd about the person (e.g., a limp or strangely shaped clothing). They will then bolt when the person gets too close. Unfortunately, they may choose to bolt over the person if there are obstacles to other routes. If cattle do not move away as they are approached within 9 to 12 m, drivers should attempt to agitate them into avoidance behavior, that is, wave arms, ropes, or other objects or jump around and shout to make them start off. There is, however, a difference between mobilizing a herd and stampeding it.

Cattle are tremendously herd oriented, so they will crowd and bunch together as they are driven, even climbing onto others' backs if they are pushed too hard from behind. Herding cattle too fast (generally they should not be herded faster than a walk or a slow jog) should be avoided because of bruising or other injuries the cattle may incur.

It must be stressed that herding cattle into weak barriers must be avoided. Most beef cattle will walk through a loose barbed wire or smooth wire fence completely unconcerned and apparently unscathed, leaving the wire somewhat looser but often still in place. Calves become adept at slipping through the lower strands of the pasture fence. Horses, in contrast, tend to see fences as psychological barriers, and the more visible fences are, the more formidable they seem as barriers.

Cattle are usually less spooky than horses about strange surroundings, but they may balk and then bolt suddenly. Generally, the balking occurs just as the cattle reach the open gate of a holding corral after being driven off an 80-acre pasture. Smart people avoid having strange things (e.g., stray dogs, raincoats flapping in the breeze) where they expect to drive the cattle.

A good cow dog is an invaluable asset in herding cattle. It is incredible how the calculated nipping at the heels and yapping of a small dog can whip a whole herd of cattle into line. It is also incredible how an undisciplined dog or two can stampede a quiet group of cattle.

Cattle, being herd animals, generally follow the leader, so a tractable animal may be used to lead them places they might ordinarily find frightening. The leaders in a herd of cattle may prove the making or unmaking of one's attempt to drive the group. If they turn around, they may either turn the whole bunch in another direction or simply mill around in the security of the group, unconcerned at the efforts to drive them from the rear. Cattle chutes are built just wide enough for one animal, to prevent the animals from turning around. A person on foot may follow cattle in a chute to drive them through but should always be cautious and ready to climb out of the way. Never enter a chute that cannot be readily evacuated.

Chutes are funneled from larger areas. They are usually arranged so that posts or boards may be slipped behind animals to prevent their moving backward. *Tailing* may be used to push a cow ahead of you; tailing is simply grasping the tail 7.0 to 15 cm from the base and pushing it up and forward over the back. This is uncomfortable and encourages the animal to move forward. A word of caution: When inside a chute, never underestimate the ability of a cow to get frightened and run backward, possibly causing serious crushing injuries. Cattle prods, sticks, or electrical shock devices have the advantage of being used from outside a chute. If chutes are not available, cattle may also be roped if they are in a small area.

A single bovid in a small stall sometimes may be haltered without resorting to a head catch or stock. It becomes a matter of maneuvering the animal until the head is between you and a wall, with the hindquarters in a corner. After loosening the chin loop of a rope halter, the crown loop can be flipped over the back of the ears with the right hand (animal facing to one's left) while the left hand guides the nosepiece over the nose; then the right hand can quickly take up the slack in the chin rope once it is under the jaw. Cattle are less head-shy than horses, and this relatively rough means of haltering does not seem to bother them.

Calves are captured much the same as are foals. One should always watch for the mother, although often she will be too frightened to charge.

Bulls are quite another story; aggression is always there, even if hidden. They should *never* be trusted. One should avoid driving bulls while afoot. Some breeding bulls (i.e., dairy bulls) can be enticed by food to a "squeeze" area, where gates and stocks may be found. They can be caught with head catches or squeeze gates or by poles with hooks for the nose ring.

Head Catch

The head catch or stock is often the final capture and restraining device for cattle (Fig. 1–13). Cattle usually will not willingly put their heads through. Most have had previous negative experiences with stocks, and unless the opening is large enough to make them think they can escape through it, they will not enter. It takes precise timing to close the head catch after the head and before the shoulders. The spring-loaded head catches in commercial stocks make capture easier but may be dangerous to personnel. Many careless people have lost teeth or have been knocked down by rapidly swinging handles. One should be absolutely certain how to operate a stock or head catch before working near it or trying to operate it.

In a suitably small enclosure, the use of a tranquilizer in a pole syringe can be attempted with an animal that is vicious and cannot be caught with a stock. Pole syringes are available commercially or may be fabricated. They discharge their contents when pressed against the animal. Capture guns are also a possibility but are seldom used with cattle. They probably should not be used by anyone who is not expert in their use or without such a person's supervision.

Restraint of the Head

The halter may be used as an adjunct to a head catch to tie an animal's head up and to the side (e.g., to expose the jugular vein for venipuncture). A strong person can grasp over the muzzle or around the lower jaw and into the mouth and effect the same restraint. The nasal septum may be pinched with thumb and forefinger in the nostrils, or nose tongs may be placed in the nose to stabilize the head. The horn or ear should be held in the other hand for leverage. The most common type of mouth gag for cattle is a block of wood approximately 15 cm long and 7.5 cm wide at the middle tapering toward the ends. There is a hole in the middle of the block to allow the passage of a tube. This gag is placed in the interdental space

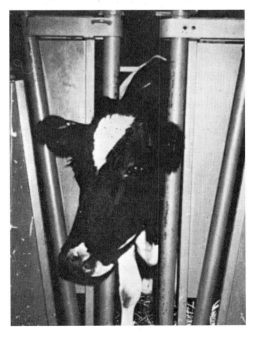

Figure 1–13. A cow in a head catch, or stock.

and is held in place by a strap behind the head. Large, metal hinged speculums may also be used for oral examinations. The tongue may be grasped and held as with the horse.

Tail

A cow's tail may be tied up just like a horse's. Again, the tail should be tied only to the animal itself or held; it should not be attached to an inanimate object. The cow's tail may also be tied up slightly differently, with the tail on one side of the cow and the tail rope passing over the back to be secured around the foreleg near the elbow on the opposite side. An annoying tail switch can also be placed under a hock hobble (see below).

Kicking Restraints

Cattle usually kick to the side and forward with a hooking action rather than to the rear. There are several devices to prevent kicking and restrain the hind legs. Milking hobbles, or hock hobbles, are flat metal hooks with a chain in between. The hooks are placed over the tendons of the hind leg just above the hock, with the open end of the hooks to the inside of the leg and the chain passing around the front of the limbs. Once the hooks are in place, the chain can be drawn up until the hocks are close together. If the brush of the tail is placed under one hook, the tail will also be restrained.

Pressure on the flank seems to discourage cows from kicking. A commercial metal device shaped like gigantic ice tongs may be squeezed over the flank, or a rope may be tied snugly around the abdomen just anterior to the udder. A hock twitch may be used to immobilize one hindleg. It is made out of heavy rope and is twist-tightened much like a tourniquet around the Achilles tendon just above the hock.

Lifting Feet

Cattle are very reluctant to lift up their feet, and to get their feet up requires an expenditure of energy. To raise a foreleg, a noose is tied around the pastern, and the end of the rope is passed over the cow's back as a pulley. The hind leg is more of a problem, as there is no portion of the cow's anatomy to use as a pulley. The limb may be tied using a beam overhead. Unfortunately, this treatment may result in injury to the cow. It is probably better if there is a strong person available to pick up and hold the hind leg much as with a horse, bearing in mind that it is simply a matter of forcing the leg up by brute force. To accomplish this feat, it helps to have the cow's head turned away from the leg by means of nose tongs.

Casting

Casting a cow is usually simple. The first point is to always tie the haltered cow to a sturdy anchor. There are several variations of the rope "harness" fashioned on the cow. The simplest technique consists of a noose around the neck, a half-hitch around the girth, and a half-hitch around the abdomen just anterior to the udder. The free end of the rope comes off the cow's back with all knots positioned dorsally. Once the rope harness is secure, a strong pull toward the rear of the cow will make her lie down. Two average-sized persons can usually easily cast a large cow.

If a cow is cast approximately 1.0 or 1.5 m from a fence and parallel to it, she may be rolled onto her back up against the fence with a bale of hay wedged beside her to hold her up.

Her legs should then be stretched to the front and rear with stout rope. To prevent bloating, cattle should be maintained on their backs or their bellies, in which positions they may continue to eructate (belch), rather than their sides. It is vital to remember that if a standing cow is in danger of going down (such as might be the case during calving), she should always be tied by the halter, never by the neck. If she goes down with a rope or chain at the neck, she may strangle and asphyxiate before she can be freed.

Small calves may be thrown by reaching over their backs to grab the forelegs and hind legs next to your body and lifting the legs up and away, letting the calves' bodies slide down your legs to the ground. Larger calves may be "flanked," which means to stand on one side and reach over the back to grab hair and skin in the lower flank and behind the elbow and then to lift and roll the calf up off its feet and drop it to the ground. A calf or cow can be restrained in lateral recumbency by placing weight on the neck.

Most bulls wear a nose ring; in addition to being captured by it, they may also be led by it. It is best not to depend entirely on the nose ring for leading, as the ring can rip through the cartilage. A bull should not be tied fast with the nose ring. Leading a cantankerous bull is at least a two-person job, with the leaders ranging to the side well out of the bull's way, keeping the ropes taut to avoid his hurting the other person. Any combination of halter ropes, ropes to the nose ring, or nose ring pole with hooks may be used to effect the leading of the bull. Bulls may be hooded or blindfolded for easier leading into areas where they do not wish to go.

Xylazine is the standard chemical restraint for cattle. It should be remembered that cattle and other ruminants are sensitive to xylazine. The dose for cattle is one tenth of the equine dosage.

Driving Sheep and Goats

Sheep and goats are also herd-conscious animals and can be driven in bunches. Dogs are an excellent adjunct to working sheep, although some goats will challenge dogs. Goats are less timid and more adventurous than sheep. Sheep and goats commingle and herd together easily, and a goat trained to follow a person or to go to a certain place can be used to lead sheep into an enclosure (the "Judas" goat). Goats and sheep seldom stand staring and then bolt as cattle may when a person approaches.

Sheep can be worked in chutes, and although they will climb on each other like cattle, they do less damage to each other because of their smaller size. Interestingly, despite their greater agility, sheep do not seem to climb on chute walls when driven (unlike cattle). Although they may spring nearly straight up into the air twice their height and well above chute walls, they seldom jump out of the chute. Temporary fencing, like slatted snow fence, may serve as effective barriers for sheep.

Kids and lambs may be acrobatic and climb or jump on fences or other structures to avoid being caught. Jumping or falling from heights can cause injury, especially leg fractures, so handlers should be alert to avoid these situations.

Goats and sheep can be caught in small enclosures in the same way as foals or calves are caught, with a hand under the neck and one under the rump. In goats that are wearing collars but that may not lead, it is probably preferable to catch the whole body rather than just the collar until they have stopped struggling.

One must never grab the wool to catch or restrain a sheep or mohair goat. The fleece itself may be damaged, or, in meat animals, a subcutaneous bruise may develop at the site.

Restraint

Sheep and goats resist being held by their horns and will only struggle if restrained this way. They can be held like foals or calves, set up on their rumps for hand restraint or held in miniature stocks. Goats may be trained to lead and tie.

Setting Up Sheep

Sheep are often set up on their rumps for several different procedures (i.e., shearing, vaccination, examinations, hoof trimming). There are several different ways to end up with the sheep on its rump with its back leaning against the holder, who is holding the forelegs (Fig. 1–14). The easiest method is for the person to begin on the sheep's left side. Reach under the base of the neck with the left hand and over the back to the right hind leg with the right hand. The sheep is gently lifted off the ground toward the right and upturned, as the right hind leg is lifted to get the animal's weight off it, after which the right hand moves to the right foreleg, the left hand moves to the left foreleg, and the sheep is held on its rump facing away from you. One person can shear a sheep or perform several other procedures unassisted with the sheep on its rump by steadying its upper torso between the arms and the lower torso between the legs as one works.

Castration and Docking

Lambs are usually docked and castrated at the same time. The method of holding the legs is the same whether one rests the

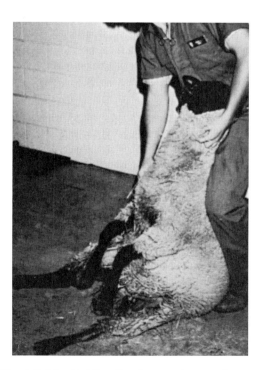

Figure 1-14. Holding the sheep set up on its rump.

torso in one's lap, on a bench, or on a fence or allows it to hang in front of one. The lamb is held head upright, with the head near the holder. The holder holds the two legs of each side together in each hand. The straightened hind legs are grasped between hock and fetlock, and the forelegs are held just below the elbows.

Drenching

Drenching, or oral administration of liquids, may be accomplished by one person. The sheep is backed into a corner, and the person straddles the sheep above its shoulders, squeezing the forequarters with the knees. With one hand, the handler lifts the head by the lower jaw, holding loosely around the muzzle, while inserting the dose syringe into the interdental space of the mouth on the opposite side with the other hand. One must be careful not to lift the jaw above a line parallel to the ground and to administer the substance slowly enough so that the sheep can swallow it. The nozzle of the syringe or gun should be inserted well back into the mouth between the cheek teeth, or the sheep will be liable to dribble the substance out of the mouth.

Goat Collars and Leading the Goat

Many of the sheep restraint techniques can be used on goats. Goats also often wear collars, which are usually leather straps with buckles. They probably should be laced closed rather than buckled to prevent the goat from rubbing the buckle loose. Goats that are trained may be led or tethered by their collars. A buck may be handled by leading him by the collar and beard, but if he does not like and respect his handler, he can be difficult.

Capture and Restraint of Swine

Catching Swine

Small piglets or pigs can be crowded into corners, and as they dart away, they can be grasped by a hind leg or two. The hind leg hold should be rapidly changed to holding in both hands around the torso for the comfort and reassurance of the pig. The technique is not applicable to full-grown swine.

TECHNICIAN NOTE

Miniature (pet) swine are more delicate than farm swine and can incur joint or ligament damage if caught by a hind leg. It is preferable to grasp the animal around the torso from the beginning.

Swine, especially boars and broody sows, can be very aggressive. One way to herd aggressive swine is to use a fence panel or large piece of plywood (at least a few inches taller and longer than a single animal) to "haze" them. Apparently, the larger barrier looks more formidable than a person and also provides some protection. When "planting" a panel to prevent animals from pushing through it, the foot should be used to steady the bottom corner, where swine will try to "root" out. Always make sure you have an escape route when entering a pen with potentially aggressive swine. Most swine can be driven by people on foot, which is to say that they avoid people getting near them. Swine are also intelligent and individualistic and may be difficult to direct in a large area. Swine tend to dart through small openings for escape. A cane may be used to tap swine on the side of the face or neck to direct them while driving. Gentle swine may also be individually directed by pushing or slapping lightly on the rump or side of the neck or face.

Swine can sometimes be enticed into a small, secure enclosure by a food trail or food placed inside. Once inside a small enclosure that they cannot break out of, swine may be caught by a snubbing rope (a lariat, in essence) or some variation of the hog snare, which is usually an adjustable metal cable loop at the end of a rigid handle (Fig. 1–15). The loop is slipped over the upper jaw of the animal from behind (usually swine will hide their heads in a corner when they are trying to get away from you), and it is tightened after it is behind the incisors. The snare has the advantage of the rigid handle for directing the snout, whereas the snubbing rope is useful only for pulling. Generally, swine brace themselves by pulling backward when caught by the snout and are immobilized but are not stifled by it. The discomfort of a snare usually results in nonstop shrieking until it is removed. Swine can be tied by a snubbing rope, which may also be combined with hobbles or ropes on the hind legs to stretch them out and hold them in a lateral reclining position. These techniques are rough and should be avoided, if possible. Some procedures can be accomplished by squeezing the pig tightly with hog panels.

Body Restraints

Pigs can be restrained on their backs in a vee trough but find it unsettling and usually complain vocally. The legs can be tied or held. A sling of canvas with holes for the legs has been used with great success in research laboratories and veterinary hospitals to cradle swine comfortably for certain procedures. The farrowing crate is essentially a restraint device for sows to keep them from lying on their pigs. The sow is restrained in a narrow corridor with areas on the sides for the young.

Pigs can be restrained for castration or vaccination by holding them off the ground by the hind legs with their backs against one's legs. Large pigs will struggle less if their forefeet

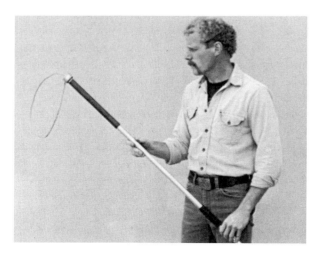

Figure 1-15. The swine snare or ``rabies'' pole for dogs.

rest on the ground. Pigs can be held for oral administration by holding them up by the forelegs and leaning their backs against one's legs while they stand on their hindlegs. Giving a sweet feed to nibble before and after a capsule will encourage them not to spit the capsule out.

Humane Restraint of Pet Swine

The reader is probably struck by the apparent (and real) brutality of some of the above-mentioned handling techniques with swine. The hog snare and the vee trough, for instance, are despised by swine. The pig is an intelligent animal that can be trained to tolerate minor discomforts and lie willingly in a sling, for instance. Unfortunately, the time involved to train swine is often "unprofitable" in agricultural animals, although it quickly pays for itself in the research or pet situation.

Miniature swine kept as individual pets are most often seen these days in small animal practices. Many of these pets are spoiled, willful creatures that run the household. Owners who allow pets to run their lives will not be impressed by rough handling, yet it is difficult to be firm and effective but not abusive. The support sling is the best method for restraint, as it causes the animal no discomfort yet provides immobilization. In the absence of a sling, they may be held like a watermelon, with one forearm under the neck, but the holder will be gouged by the hind foot nearest his body when the pig struggles. Pigs have incredibly powerful jaws and some will bite readily, especially if in pain or uncomfortable. These can be muzzled with a small rope used like gauze in a dog, but pigs will fight them, and they may be more trouble than they are worth. Muzzling, or holding the jaws closed, may be used to cut down the noise of a vocalizing pig as well.

Once a pig is restrained, its mouth can be opened by means of a gag. The gag is a U-shaped device with a handle at the bottom of the U and two bars, separated by a space, near its top. The bars are inserted into the mouth from the front to behind the canines, and the gag then is rotated to spread the jaws. Many miniature swine readily allow stomach tubing and do not bite down on a hand inserted into the mouth over the incisors to place the tube; however, fingers straying between cheek teeth are in harm's way. Never put fingers into the side of a pig's mouth.

Many pet swine are inordinately fond of having people scratch their backs, and they may even stand or lie quietly for an examination if this is done for them. Scratching the belly, especially of a gilt or sow, will often induce her to flop down on her side to expose the belly. It is always worthwhile to ask an owner if his or her pig leads on a leash, or how he or she gets it to do things. Sometimes the owner has worked out ingenious ways to make the pig do things it would not normally do willingly.

Finally, it should be mentioned that even though a miniature pig may live in the house and be trained to lead and to void and defecate outdoors, it is in the end still a pig. And one of the things pigs do most readily is to vocalize when uncomfortable or in pain or just dissatisfied with what is being done to them. Do not be surprised when that 15-kg porker emits an ear-piercing shriek as it is first picked up and continues unrelenting until it is set free. Swine can be tranquilized with acepromazine or azaparone, if necessary, but both have fairly long-lasting effects (24 to 36 hours).

Capture and Restraint of Dogs

Catching Dogs

Since most veterinarians do not make house calls for animals, the only time one usually needs to catch a dog that is not in a cage or run is if the animal has escaped. Dogs are often motivated by terror in the animal hospital, so personnel should learn to deal with fear in dogs, which results in two types of behavior. One is avoidance (running away) with abject submissiveness when cornered, and the other is avoidance until cornered and then aggression (fear biting). Unfortunately, the two types of dogs are often discriminated between only at the last moment, as one's hands approach. Almost any dog will turn around and snap if it is grabbed as it runs past, although it is difficult, if not impossible, to avoid the temptation to grab at the dog on his way to freedom.

How does one catch an elusive dog in the great outdoors? Animal control officers deal with this problem daily. Obviously, a person is not going to outrun any but the smallest and most debilitated dogs. Like horses, dogs that feel they are being chased will run. It is best to try to keep a dog in sight at a less-threatening distance until there is an opportunity to corner it or until the dog decides the pursuer is not that much of a threat. Sometimes, especially if the fugitive is male, it may help to have a canine companion to entice the dog to approach you. It never hurts to have a pocketful of bait of some sort to gain the dog's favor.

An apprehensive dog, whether it is in the examination room or in a backyard, needs reassurance that no one will harm it. Do not grab the dog's collar or try to pick it up before some reassurance is given. Most dogs respond favorably to being talked to. The higher voice usually gets better results, which may be because of the higher range of hearing and vocalization in dogs. With many dogs, it helps to "hunker down"—squat—in front of them to appear less large and overbearing. Without moving quickly or awkwardly, offer your hand for the dog to sniff at or below the level of its nose. Sometimes the point at which the hand is proffered is the first indication that the dog will bite.

> **✎ TECHNICIAN NOTE**
>
> Never confuse a wagging tail with friendliness in a dog you do not know; watch the ears, eyes, and face. Fear biters often wag submissively, and it is not unusual for an aggressive dog to hold the tail erect with a tense narrow oscillating motion before biting.

Some people say that one should offer the back of the hand to a strange dog, rather than the palm, because the palm may appear to be threatening a slap. Whether the slap notion is true or not, the fingers are a little more out of the way with a loosely cupped hand held with the palm down, and the dog will be forced to make more of an effort to bite the whole hand, possibly giving you more time to withdraw. However, a dog's bite is lightning-fast, even in the large ponderous breeds, and unless warned, you will not be able to move your hand in time.

A dog tells by body language whether it has accepted your introduction. If it is prone to think you are all right, the body will relax and the dog will actively sniff your hand. This may be followed by wagging the tail, losing interest in the hand, and approaching. If these things occur, one may begin to make friends by reaching below the ear for a scratch, starting gently and then scratching more vigorously. The next best scratching place is on the chest. Once a dog has accepted your scratching its ears or chest, it may indicate that it would just as soon have you finish the job, scratching neck, shoulders, and top of hips. It is a good idea to run the hands all over the dog in a friendly fashion before taking liberties with its body, like trying to lift it. Some dogs are naturally gregarious and trusting and require little in the way of preliminaries. There are a few dogs whose natural temperament is not so positive but that are well enough trained that they may be handled less carefully than their personalities warrant. Evaluating dogs may require evaluation of the client. Some clients have obviously been trained by their dogs rather than the reverse, and you are on your own to make your peace with the pooch. (Clients may help or hinder your efforts with dogs. Those that have no control over their animals may undermine any authority you might have with the dog by virtue of your being a stranger, so these people are best sent politely to the waiting room, if possible.)

Many times dogs may act reasonably in an initial examination with the owner present, and then, after being held in a cage or run, threaten to bite when approached. Whenever faced with a dog that will obviously bite if given the chance, the only sensible thing to do is to keep your hands out of the way. For small dogs, the answer may be heavy leather gauntlets. Sometimes these dogs will work out their aggression snapping at the gloved fingers of one hand (flesh fingers carefully withdrawn) while the other hand approaches and grabs them at the scruff of the neck. Most dogs will give up as soon as they feel restrained, but some will not.

For larger dogs that want to bite, the first step is to catch them by the neck. Always remember to keep cage doors closed as far as possible when trying to catch biters (or any other dog, for that matter), as they will be more trouble if they escape. Sometimes a lead rope with a slip knot can be tossed over a dog's head, but sometimes a rope or cable snare similar to a hog catcher is required. Most dogs will give up when caught by the neck. A few, the truly vicious or confirmed fear biters, will continue to try to bite, and even attack. In these cases, you may apply a muzzle (described later), keep the teeth a safe distance by keeping a tight grip behind the head, or use both of these methods. Sometimes vicious little dogs may be dragged out of cages snarling and snapping and can be held off the ground by the choke rope for a few moments to subdue them. There is a slight chance of permanent tracheal damage with this technique, and it is not the way to win friends. Some of these dogs are incorrigible and will hate you regardless, so there is sometimes justification in forcing them to respect you.

A truly vicious large dog is a real challenge. It should never be approached except by a snare, and even then, if it is very strong, two leads may be required (two snares or a snare and a rope) to stretch the dog between two people for leading.

A dog at large that will not allow approach may require the use of a capture gun or even a pole syringe. Animal control officers may be experienced with the capture gun and may be able to provide assistance. Inexperienced persons should not try to use capture guns. Occasionally, the darts malfunction or strike some poorly absorbing portion of the body, and the animal will not succumb in the time expected. Note that it is dangerous to repeat the dose in such an animal without knowing how much of the drug it has received. Drugs often used with capture guns include ketamine, xylazine, and nicotine.

Lifting Dogs

Dogs are generally examined on a table, and lifting them onto that table is usually the first order of business. Small dogs may be lifted by grasping on either side of the thorax behind the elbows. Medium-sized dogs are lifted by putting the arms around them, in front of the chest and behind the rump and pulling them to your chest. Unfortunately, that position places your face uncomfortably close to their teeth, but there really is no other way, except for lifting tables or prior muzzling.

Large dogs are harder to lift for at least three reasons. First, of course, is their weight, which may be prohibitive. Second, their large size makes them more awkward to lift. The third reason is that large dogs are not accustomed to being lifted, which makes them uneasy, if not downright panicky. One person may be able to lift a large dog by forklifting him, with the arms behind the forelimbs and in front of the hind legs. However, if the animal struggles it can fall forward or backward easily. Two people can lift a dog together by one person's placing the arms around the forequarters and the other person placing the arms around the hindquarters. They should both be on the same side of the dog, away from the table, of course. Some dogs, especially males, object to being lifted from under the flank area, where the male genitalia terminate. If this is the case, they will definitely need two people to lift the dog, with the person at the rear placing the arm or hand well forward of the prepuce. If a large dog is unduly nervous about being lifted or being on top of the table, it should be dealt with on the floor.

> ### TECHNICIAN NOTE
>
> Lifting a dog can result in back injury. Always use proper techniques of lifting (lift with legs, keeping back straight) and safety equipment (back braces).

Never let a dog jump down from a table. Most tables and floors have slick surfaces that invite slips and fractures. Lift the dog off the table in the same manner as it was placed there.

Injured or sick animals may pose different problems in lifting. Usually, it means providing more hands for more even support. A limb with a fracture, for example, requires separate support to prevent additional soft tissue damage and pain to the animal. An animal with a painful abdomen should not be lifted under the posterior abdomen. There are times when a stretcher may be required for lifting a badly injured dog. Lifting injured animals calls for judgment in the particular situation.

Table Restraint

The degree of restraint required for a dog on the table depends on what is being done. Regardless, however, the forequarters and hindquarters must be controlled at all times to prevent the dog from jumping or falling off the table.

The form of restraint most often used is to have the arms behind the rump and in front of the chest, pulling the dog inward, much as in lifting. In addition, one may wish to pull the head against the chest with the hand on the neck, which is adequate restraint for most dogs for examination and subcutaneous or intramuscular (thigh or forequarters) vaccinations or injections.

A rectal examination is common in male dogs, and only a slight adjustment need be made from the position just described. The holder's arm or hand should not be behind the hindquarters, as it will interfere with the examination. The arm used to restrain the hindquarters can be placed over the dog's back to stabilize lateral movement by drawing the dog's body toward the handler. A hand supporting the ventral abdomen may be required to prevent the dog from sitting down.

Whenever puppies are examined, vaccinated, have dewclaws removed, and so forth, the bitch should be out of the room. When her puppies cry, she may be inclined to attack; this is especially true when the pups are newborn. If the bitch must be in the same room, it might be worthwhile to slip her into a crate while the procedures are carried out. The pups could then be taken away from her one at a time. Dogs cannot count, and unless attention is paid when the pup is removed or the pup makes noise, she will not notice when one puppy out of several is gone.

Restraint for Venipuncture

Venipuncture, for drawing blood or administering substances, requires most exacting restraint. The animal must not be allowed to move, because movement is the most common cause of "blowing" a vessel. The resultant hematomas are painful and unsightly and obscure the vessel for future use. It should be noted that the primary reason that an animal struggles during venipuncture is anxiety. Calm, affectionate handling with lots of petting and soothing words will go far to relieve anxiety. The most painful portion of the venipuncture is usually when the vessel is pierced, although puncturing the skin and administering certain substances may also be unpleasant. At these times, restraint should be the most secure. Positioning, apart from preventing movement, is the most critical part of venipuncture because without good positioning the vessel cannot even be located.

For cephalic venipuncture, the holder must restrain the dog's body, present the forelimb, and occlude the vessel to make it fill and stand up under the skin. The animal is placed on the table near one end, facing the edge. The holder stands beside the table, facing the same direction as the dog, and nestles the animal on the table under the arm; the handler's forearm, upper arm, and elbow will exert pressure to bring the animal snugly to the person's side and down to a sternal reclining position on the table. The hand of the same arm cradles the animal's elbow with the palm and fingers while the thumb clamps down on the cephalic vein. To ensure that the vein is under the thumb and on the top (front) of the forearm, the holder grasps the limb just below the elbow with the thumb as far inside the limb as possible and then, with pressure applied, rotates the skin outward (Fig. 1–16). The fingers should rest on the table, and the dog's elbow should be pushed slightly forward to stabilize the leg. The elbow should be at or near the edge of the table to allow good access to the vein.

The free hand is used to restrain the animal's head, and

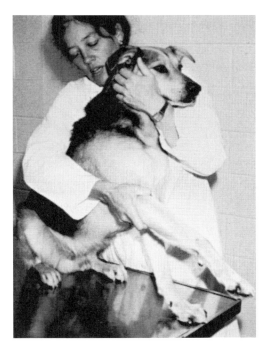

Figure 1-16. Method of holding the dog for cephalic venipuncture. This dog is being held in a sitting position rather than in a position of sternal recumbency.

for most dogs this is best accomplished by pressing the head to your chest by reaching under the neck and placing the hand behind the jaw. The hand may also go around the dog's muzzle to prevent biting, when necessary. The holder must remember to release the thumb when the other person is ready to perform the injection. Failure to release the vessel will not allow a substance to be injected into the general circulation; it may also result in the rupture of the vessel.

A large dog can be restrained on the floor for cephalic venipuncture with the handler kneeling or squatting behind the sitting dog to prevent its backward movement. Most dogs submit well to cephalic venipuncture, and their cephalic veins are large and straight enough to hit easily. However, in chondrodystrophic short-legged dogs and in certain other circumstances, the preferred site may be the jugular vein. Dogs that are gentle and phlegmatic may submit well to cephalic venipuncture while sitting up (see Fig. 1–16).

For jugular venipuncture (Fig. 1–17), the dog is placed further forward on the table, the edge of which should be just behind the forelegs. The holder stands alongside and puts the arm over the animal as in the cephalic technique, pressing the animal to the table. However, the hand of the arm over the animal is the one that restrains the head; the hand away from the table restrains the forefeet, with a finger between the feet for a secure grip. For the head restraint, the hand grasps the muzzle with the fingers under the jaw (one or two fingers may fit between the mandibles of the jaw for a more secure grip) and the thumb is over the nose. Care is taken to avoid cutting off the animal's breathing by holding the muzzle too near the nose. Also, if the fingers are too far back under the jaw, they may occlude the jugular vein so that it will not fill and therefore will not be located.

The main advantage of this position is to provide a nearly

straight plane from the angle of the dog's jaw to the forefeet for easy access to the jugular vein. The dog is somewhat "stretched" to achieve this effect. Common errors in this position are to have the dog's forelegs or shoulders too far forward, interfering with the angle of entry for the syringe, or to pull the head too far backward, stretching the skin and vessel and collapsing the vein. The dog's head should be lifted no more than slightly above 90 degrees from the neck. The head may be directed toward the handler to rest on the chest, but in this position only the vessel away from the handler is available for venipuncture. A large dog can be restrained on the floor for jugular venipuncture with the handler kneeling or squatting behind the sitting dog while steadying the chest with one hand and the muzzle with the other.

The saphenous vein, on the lateral aspect of the hind leg, is an alternate venipuncture site, for which the dog must be held in lateral recumbency. To hold a dog on its side, the handler stands behind the dog, with one forearm pressed across the animal's neck and the hand holding the forelegs (with a finger between the legs). The other forearm presses across the dog's flank, with the hind legs held in a similar manner, except that when venipuncture is being attempted, only the down leg is held; the other is stabilized by the person making the puncture.

Muzzles and Mouth Gags

Commercial muzzles are made of a variety of materials. The problem with most commercial muzzles is that they are not very adjustable, and several sizes need to be kept on hand. Therefore, one usually resorts to the gauze or rope muzzle.

Nylon rope (6.35 mm) choke leads are sometimes very handy as muzzling devices for snapping dogs. The dog must first be caught by the neck, possibly with a snare. A loop of rope, made with a single overhand knot, is positioned from

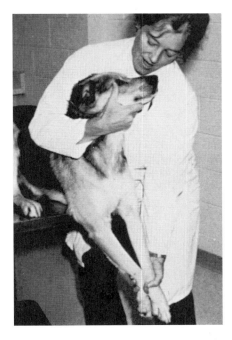

Figure 1-17. Method of holding the dog for jugular venipuncture. Note the straight line from the ramus of the mandible to the feet.

above the dog's nose until it is in place over the muzzle. Once the rope is in place, it is rapidly tightened with the knot on top of the nose. A small dog will try to push the rope loop off its nose with its forepaw. The first knot must be held snugly while a second knot is made with the ends under the nose. The second knot may be a single overhand knot or a double knot (preferably a square knot). The two free ends are then passed behind the dog's head and tied again; this knot will hold the muzzle on the dog, so it must be secure. It may be tied for fast release by using a bow knot in case the dog cannot breathe.

Gauze roll bandage (7.5 to 15 cm) may be used as a muzzle in the same fashion as the rope (Fig. 1–18). Gauze is used more often and has an advantage over rope in that it is less slick. Gauze, however, makes a less rigid loop to apply to a recalcitrant dog. For most dogs, the piece of gauze needs to be approximately 90 cm long.

Pug-nosed dogs are difficult to muzzle, and they can be determined biters. For them, the gauze bandage is tied first around the nose with the first knot tied underneath the jaw. The ends are then passed behind the head and tied with a square knot. Finally, one of the free ends of the gauze is passed over the forehead and under the loop on top of the nose and then tied back to the other side. This keeps the loop from slipping off the top of the short nose (see Fig. 1–20).

Sometimes a dog's mouth can be restrained manually by bringing the hands from the rear on both sides of the face; thumbs are placed on the forehead, and fingers are looped under the mandibles. The palms should be below the ears.

A variety of mouth gags can be used in dogs. A simple wooden dowel may be pressed to the back of the mouth, to rest between the carnassial teeth. The dowel can be tied in place behind the ears or can be handheld by the assistant. Dogs can undergo insertion of a stomach tube with the dowel in place. The commercial spring type of mouth gag has a hole on either end for the canine teeth, and it is inserted on one side of the mouth for a variety of procedures. However, this gag hangs outside the mouth, is heavy, and can fracture teeth to which it is attached. It is much better to cut off the end of an appropriately sized plastic syringe cover to place over opposing

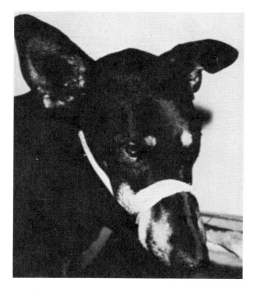

Figure 1-18. The gauze muzzle.

canine teeth. This is especially useful when a mouth gag is needed for dentistry.

Mobility-Limiting Devices

Self-mutilation and tearing of bandages can be prevented with several devices. The most common mobility-limiting devices are variations of the Elizabethan collar, which is so named because of its resemblance to the wide, stiffly starched collars popular in 17th century England. The idea is to place a stiff material extending to the tip of the dog's nose so that it cannot chew on or lick its body. Commercial plastic cone-shaped collars are available, or similar appliances can be fashioned from buckets, large bottles, or sheets of heavy plastic. It is most important with these collars to ensure that no sharp edges are present and to secure the Elizabethan collar to the neck by gauze or fasten it to the dog's neck collar. Make sure the dog knows how to eat and drink with the collar on. Commercial collars can be worn with the wide part of the cone over the body rather than over the head if the affected area is on the forequarters.

Another type of device that limits the movement of the head is made by fastening a pole along the body to a snug collar high on the neck. Usually, tape is used to keep the device from shifting.

Chemical Restraint

Drugs can be used for chemical restraint or sedation in dogs. The most common are acepromazine and xylazine. Both have tranquilizing effects that may vary from dog to dog. Dogs may still be capable of biting when tranquilized. The main reason for tranquilization is to remove anxiety, which is one of the main reasons dogs bite. More information on chemical restraint is found in Chapter 15.

Capture and Restraint of Cats [minimum restraint]

Cats are often more apprehensive than dogs with strange people and surroundings. An escaped cat will often search out a hiding place, whereas a dog that escapes will look for a route to run. This is probably because of the lower endurance that cats have for running compared with dogs and the security that cats feel in enclosed spaces. A cat that is "treed" or trapped (as in a cage) may well respond with flattened ears, hissing and scratching, and biting at an extended hand. Heavy leather gauntlet gloves may be used to subdue them as with small dogs. Grasp the scruff of the neck to lift the cat. This may be followed by a rapid "stretch" restraint by also grasping the hind legs. Certain cats are too fast and smart to succumb to the glove technique. These cats may sometimes be caught by neck rope or snare, but they react poorly to a choke compared with the scruff of the neck. Another technique worth trying may be ketamine oral spray. Although injectable ketamine can be irritating to muscle tissues, it does not seem to cause trauma to the eyes (in case some is accidentally sprayed into the eyes). The plan is to spray a syringe containing ketamine or ketamine and acepromazine into the mouth of a hissing cat, using the intramuscular tranquilizing dose. The drugs are effective orally, but of course they take longer to take effect than if injected intramuscularly or subcutaneously.

A cat may also be "lassoed" with the end of the rope passed between the cage bars, the cage rapidly closed, and the cat brought to the front of the cage with the noose. Ketamine may then be injected intramuscularly or subcutaneously into whatever body part is closest. In a similar fashion, if the tail can be hooked with a metal rod, it can be pulled between cage bars/wires until the cat's rear quarters are within reach of a syringe with ketamine. The cat will be facing away from the cage door, so it will be less likely to reach through and scratch. Finally, one of the easiest ways to catch an obstreperous cat is to force it into a box pushed into the cage. If the box is an anesthesia-induction box, the cat can be anesthetized without ever touching it. Obviously, all escapes from the box are blocked by the cage door and so forth until the cat is safely inside and the box top is closed.

Restraint for Examination

Much of the table restraint of cats is similar to that of dogs, except that cats tend to use their claws (unless declawed) as the first line of defense rather than their teeth. When there is no reason for holding them still, cats should be allowed supervised movement. Some cats are so terrified that they are best held or cuddled with the head buried under one's arm. Cats are not necessarily malicious when they climb onto a person's chest or clamp nails into a forearm. It is a good idea to wear protective gowns or laboratory coats with long sleeves when dealing with cats and not to wear knit clothing that will snag. A free nail clip at the beginning of an examination can be a practice-builder and save some scratching of personnel, especially if blood is to be drawn.

Restraint for Venipuncture

Cephalic and jugular venipuncture restraint can be applied to cats much as with dogs. Cats tend to engage their three relatively unfettered sets of claws and their teeth in an effort to get away from the hold. When they are thus inclined, they are impossible to hold like dogs, and one is forced to use other restraints. The positioning for jugular venipuncture is more appropriate for cats, as it restrains the head and forefeet more securely than in the cephalic technique. Also, wrapping the hind feet with a towel disarms all but the most persistent cat. The cat's head is held with the hand over the top of the head, and the jaw or zygomatic arch (bony arch under the eyes) is grasped with the thumb on one side and two or three fingers on the other side. This leaves the index finger free for scratching, since many cats will be thoroughly distracted from the venipuncture if the handler strokes the bridge of the nose

vigorously while talking to them. The other hand then restrains both forelimbs as in the dog.

Besides the technique described for holding dogs, there are other ways to hold cats for jugular venipuncture. They all involve the cat's being placed on its back with the holder occluding the jugular vein and the person using the syringe pushing the chin down toward the table to make the head move backward to get a straight shot at the jugular. The holder can hold all four legs (two in each hand, with a finger in between the legs) while pushing the cat down on the table and using the little finger to press on the thoracic inlet to occlude the jugular vein. A cat can also be rolled in a towel to engage its feet, or it can be placed in a cat bag for this type of jugular venipuncture. When a towel or cat bag is used, the handler need only steady the cat on its back and occlude the vessel or vessels. Some cat bags are made with zippers, so a single limb can be withdrawn and thereby used for cephalic venipuncture. The medial saphenous vein also can be used for venipuncture (see Lateral Recumbency).

Carrying Cats

Cats generally feel more secure in close quarters and seldom resist being put into a bag or rolled in a towel. They are best carried from place to place in a cat carrier or a small cardboard box with a lid. They can also be carried with one arm if they are not particularly nervous. To carry a cat, its hindquarters are placed under the elbow area and pressed securely to the holder's body with the forearm. The cat lies in a sternal position along the forearm while the forelegs are pinioned by the hand—again, with one finger between the legs. The cat may still use his hind claws to gouge the abdomen of the holder, so you should be prepared to grab the scruff of the neck and hold the cat at arm's length if it becomes wild. Also, quickly grasping the hind legs and pulling away from the scruff of the neck will effectively immobilize almost any cat. Although this is not a comfortable position for the cat, it is safer for the handler.

Lateral Recumbency

Stretching the cat from the scruff of the neck and the hind feet is generally effective for immobilizing a cat on its side (Fig. 1–19). Most cats do not seem to realize that they can use their forefeet to scratch the hand on their neck. Some cats can be restrained on their sides as with dogs, but this is generally less effective than a stretch.

A modification of the stretch allows access to the medial saphenous vein of the thigh. The holder has the scruff of the

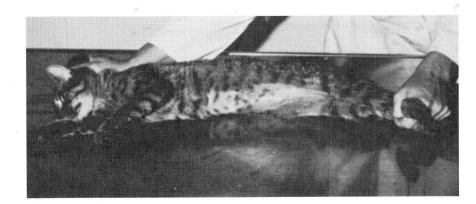

Figure 1-19. Stretching a cat on its side.

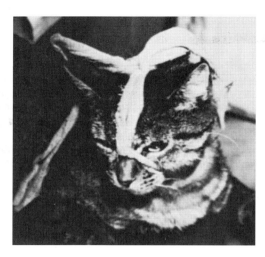

Figure 1-20. The gauze muzzle on a cat. It may also be used on a pug-nosed dog.

neck securely in one hand while the other holds the "up" rear leg flexed. The little finger can be used to hold off the vein for the venipuncturist, who stretches the "down" leg with one hand while handling the syringe with the other.

Bathing

Cats' antipathy to water is a cliché but nonetheless true. Bathing a cat may therefore be a trying experience for both the cat and the person. Most cats will try to climb up the person's arms to escape standing water or a spray. Cats should be bathed on top of a screen suspended over a tub (any metal window screen in a sturdy frame will do) and washed with a light spray of warm water. Almost always the cat will clamp all four sets of claws into the screen and stand like a statue for the entire bath.

The Muzzle

The cat may be muzzled with gauze in the same way as pug-nosed dogs (Fig. 1–20).

Chemical Restraint

The most common chemical restraint for cats is ketamine, which can be used at a tranquilizing or an anesthetic dose. The eyes of cats under the influence of ketamine should be treated with ophthalmic ointment to avoid corneal drying from the lack of blinking while the drug is in effect. Combining acepromazine with ketamine reduces the ketamine rigidity. Cats can also be given tranquilizing doses of acepromazine or xylazine alone. Both drugs can be administered intramuscularly or subcutaneously.

Restraint of Ferrets

Noncooperative ferrets are a restraint challenge. Unless the ferret is exceptionally "mellow," you are probably well advised to wear heavy gloves, as almost all ferrets will bite when frightened or hurt. Ferrets may be "stretched," in a similar manner to cats, or they may be grasped with both hands around the forequarters, using one hand on the scruff of the neck and the other to hold down the forelegs.

Ferrets are subject to "hypnosis," although it is less likely to be effective if the animal is apprehensive or in strange hands. The ferret is hung by the scruff with one hand and stroked around and the length of its torso with the other. After repeated stroking, the susceptible animal will begin to yawn and its eyelids will droop or close. The effect is not long lasting, and animals are easily startled out of the trance.

Short periods (10 to 20 minutes) of chemical restraint in ferrets can be achieved with intramuscular injection of xylazine (1 to 2 mg/kg) and ketamine (20 to 30 mg/kg).

Restraint of Rabbits

Rabbits have some peculiarities for restraint with which one should be familiar. First, rabbits have a very high muscle-to-skeleton ratio. Their bones are very small and light for animals of their size. In addition, they have tremendously powerful hind limbs. Uncontrolled kicking by a rabbit may result in too much torque in the lumbosacral area, resulting in "broken back," an imprecise lay term that means loss of neural function in the hindquarters resulting from spinal cord trauma. Not only are the rabbit's hind legs paralyzed, but also bladder and anal functions are lost. The prognosis for recovery is grim in cases of total paralysis, and although anti-inflammatory treatment, as for dachshunds with disc disease, may be undertaken, the most humane thing to do is to perform euthanasia if response is not seen within a week or two. Invariably, the rabbit traumatizes his spinal cord while being put back into his cage. He is familiar with the cage, and he will make a premature leap into it. Paralysis may be immediate or delayed until hemorrhage and edema compress the spinal cord.

How do you avoid this unhappy situation? There are essentially two ways to carry a mature rabbit: in a "hanging" carry or nestled in the arms. The nestled carry is esthetically more pleasing and probably more comfortable, but the hanging technique does not appear to be damaging or painful to even large rabbits, and *it suppresses the inclination to kick*. Although small bunnies may be safely lifted by the scruff of the neck, large, heavy rabbits are best lifted by two generous handfuls of skin over the neck and shoulders and the hindquarters (Fig. 1–21). Held this way, they usually hang quite immobile. They can be carried short distances this way without undue discomfort. Lifting by the scruff of the neck, with the second hand cradling

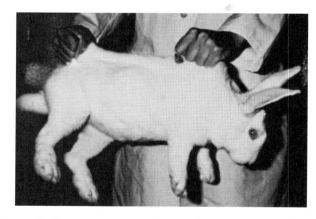

Figure 1-21. The hanging carry position for a rabbit. Even adults tend to "freeze" in this position, much like neonates while carried in the mother's mouth.

the rump (not grabbing the hind feet, which will cause resistance), is also very practical and probably more acceptable to clients. One may also grasp the rabbit about the middle to pick it up, but many rabbits readily struggle when lifted this way.

To carry rabbits longer distances, they may be set down on a table or other surface and then gathered to your body by the forearms. This snugly supports the hindquarters. Rabbits will often tuck their heads under your elbow when carried in this way. They seldom bite, and leaving the head free is therefore not a problem. The best way to replace a rabbit in a cage is by holding its skin fore and aft, placing it well inside the cage but facing outward (so that it must turn before leaping into the safety of the cage), and pressing its body down to the floor for a few moments before releasing it. One should never lift a rabbit, young or old, by its ears.

Rabbits have extremely formidable, sharp, straight nails on their rear feet, which can gouge severe scratches on your abdomen or arms if one struggles while being carried in your forearms. Although long-sleeved protective garments should always be worn, the best way to avoid being scratched is to avoid carrying rabbits for any distance in the forearms. Rabbits' nails may be trimmed easily by pressing the rabbit to the table with the forearm and chest. Hind feet are trimmed by pulling them out to the rear, as with horses' feet. Forefeet are lifted up off the table.

Rabbits do not like slick surfaces, and losing their footing on them may encourage them to struggle and kick. It is best to set them down on something on which they will have good traction, like a rubber mat, during examination or treatment.

Rabbits have sensitive whiskers and will flinch whenever the sensitive hairs of the muzzle or eyelids are touched or the mouth is approached; therefore, the head must be firmly held before attempting to examine the mouth or put something into it. To steady the head for someone to examine the mouth, the rabbit is placed facing away from the handler with the forearms pressing down on the length of the body, the thumbs behind the ears, and the fingers lifting the head from below the mandible. Incisor teeth may be trimmed with the rabbit in this position.

Rabbits may be chemically restrained with ketamine and acepromazine, and this combination may be used for induction for gas anesthesia.

Occasionally, rabbits, especially females, may be aggressive and may growl and try to scratch with the forelegs at your hand when you reach into the cage. As mentioned, rabbits seldom bite, so medium-weight gloves to prevent scratches are all that is needed to subdue them. Normally, the fight goes out of these rabbits when their forequarters are pressed to the floor and their bodies are restrained from free movement.

Rabbits may be restrained in boxes with a head-catching device, parallel sides, and some sort of rump board. The rump board should be tight against the hindquarters to push the rabbit into the head restraint. Under no circumstances should the rabbit be left with only its head restrained because it will try to back out of the box and may possibly injure itself by struggling.

Rabbits can be held for ear venipuncture by use of the same technique as described above for the oral examination.

Restraint of Hamsters and Gerbils

Hamsters and gerbils may be handled with gloves if they are wild and want to bite. Gerbils have long tails (with hair on them), so they may be caught by the tail. The tail must be grasped at its base to pick up a gerbil, not near the tip, where the hair and skin may easily be pulled off, leaving the naked flesh. A scruff-of-the-neck hold is moderately effective on gerbils and hamsters, although hamsters have a lot of redundant skin from cheek pouches, which must be gathered up in the hold. Hamsters have insignificant tails, so they must be caught in hands cupped over their bodies. This technique is also more comfortable for gerbils and should be used on them unless they are biters. These small rodents may be restricted from movement on a surface by placing the hand over them to form a cage, with the head protruding between the first and second fingers. Hamsters may be caught and restrained by "hazing" them into a small can, as they readily enter holes. Rodent restraint tunnels are available in several sizes; they are usually made of Plexiglas and have several ports available for injection.

Ketamine may be used in any of the rodent species. Light gas anesthesia may also be used for restraint, but many gerbils seem to have adverse reactions to gas anesthesia, and once they have ceased breathing, they usually die despite attempts at resuscitation.

Restraint of Guinea Pigs

The guinea pig is a docile creature that rarely bites, even when extremely fearful or when being hurt. They seldom jump, unlike most other rodents, but they scurry and dart around rapidly. They can be quite vocal during restraint. In a cage, they can be trapped in a corner or along the wall with hands, and they should be picked up by both hands encircling the body (fingers cradling underneath, thumbs on top), with one hand partially behind the other to support the entire abdomen. Pregnant guinea pigs develop enormously pendulous bellies, and they may be lifted by grasping around the thorax with one hand and placing the other hand behind and under the rump to hold them upright.

Guinea pigs can be easily held for restraint in the same fashion that they are picked up for most procedures, or the shoulder and pelvic girdles can be held in your two hands. Teeth can be clipped by holding the head with one or two hands, with the forefinger under the jaw and the thumb behind the head. The guinea pig tolerates being placed upside down in a vee trough with legs tied down much like swine.

Ketamine may be used on guinea pigs for restraint, although it is seldom necessary.

Restraint of Birds

Caged birds are captured either by hand or with a net. When using a net, one must take care not to strike the bird with the hoop or remove the bird roughly, as bones of the wings and legs are easily fractured. It is evident that the bird's wings must be restrained and that it must be prevented from biting. Small birds, like the budgerigar (parakeet), should be held with the hand cupped around the back to restrain the wings, and the thumb and forefinger should grasp the nape of the neck. The fingers should not completely encircle the body but should stay on the sides of the bird. Care should be taken to hold the head straight so that the thumb does not slip to the anterior part of the neck and occlude the trachea. A lot of the unexplained deaths of small birds while being held probably result from suffocation, since the sternum (or keel) must be able to move up and down for respiration to occur. Larger caged birds are held essentially in the same way as are the smaller ones, but heavy gloves may be required.

Predatory birds (raptors) may use their talons as defenses and therefore must be grasped first by the feet and then by the head. The movement and aggression of raptors may be curtailed by blindfolding or hooding. Wings may be wrapped.

Never release a bird in midair, as it might be disoriented, stiff, or injured and therefore fall and hurt itself. Birds should be held squatting on the ground or the floor of the cage before the hands are removed to release it. Wild birds can be given a nudge to make them move off as their heads and feet are released. You must be cautious of the possibility of being raked by the talons of raptors on their release. It may be necessary to restrain the wings of wild birds to keep them from damaging feathers in the cage. Wings and body can be encircled with adhesive tape or stockinette tube to temporarily effect this purpose.

Ketamine is the standard for chemical restraint and anesthesia in birds and is usually administered intramuscularly in the breast. Xylazine has also been used successfully in parakeets but may cause prolonged sedation. Birds may be maintained on gas anesthesia. Halothane and isoflurane are widely used.

TRANSPORTATION AND SHIPPING

Traveling with or transporting animals presents some challenges in restraint and in paperwork.

Cats are often nervous when riding in cars and usually best transported in carriers. If they are particularly nervous, they may be given one of the promazine tranquilizers, which also have an antiemetic effect. Excessive nervousness or nausea may also result in profuse salivation, which can be controlled with atropine or a similar drug. Dogs can be treated with the same drugs in appropriate doses.

Most dogs and cats do not need tranquilization when shipped on airlines, as they feel secure enough in their shipping containers if accustomed to them before the trip. Even if the animals tend to be nervous in their crates, they are probably better off untranquilized in this situation of minimal supervision.

Airlines have strict codes regarding acceptable crates for animals. Commercial shipping crates of an acceptable size for the dog or cat are useful not only for shipping but also for containment at home if needed. All animals in air freight must be accompanied by a current health certificate. Different states have different requirements for vaccination, quarantine, and so forth, and these guidelines may be found in the United States Department of Agriculture (USDA) State-Federal Health Requirements and Regulations handbook or learned by calling state veterinarian's offices (state regulations may have changed since the USDA handbook was printed, so it is a good idea to call for confirmation of regulations).

Most states require health certificates for any animal entering or traveling within their boundaries, and many people who travel by car with their small pets are not aware that they are breaking the law by not having health certificates for their cats and dogs.

Some states require negative results from a current Coggins or brucellosis test for entering horses or cattle. In addition, whenever livestock are transported, they should be accompanied by brand inspections.

Recommended Reading

Clutton-Brock J: Domesticated Animals from Early Times. The British Museum (Natural History), 1981.

Dunbar I: Dog Behavior: Why Dogs Do What They Do. Neptune, NJ, T.E.H. Publications, 1979.

Fox MW: Understanding Your Cat. New York, Bantam Books, Inc., 1974.

Fox MW: Understanding Your Dog. New York, Coward, McCann and Geogheagan, 1972.

Fowler ME: Restraint and Handling of Wild and Domestic Animals. Ames, IA, Iowa State University Press, 1978.

Fraser AF: Farm Animal Behavior. London, Balliere Tindall, 1974.

Hafez ESE: The Behavior of Domestic Animals, 3rd ed. London, Balliere Tindall, 1975.

Hart BL: Canine Behavior. Santa Barbara, Veterinary Practice Publishing Company, 1980.

Hayes MH: Illustrated Horse Training. Reprinted from 1889 edition. Hollywood, CA, Wilshire Book Co., 1973.

Kiley-Worthington M: The Behaviour of Horses in Relation to Management and Training. London, JA Allen, 1987.

Ryland LM and Bernard MS: A Clinical Guide to the Pet Ferret. Compendium for Continuing Education 5(1):1983.

2 Animal Behavior

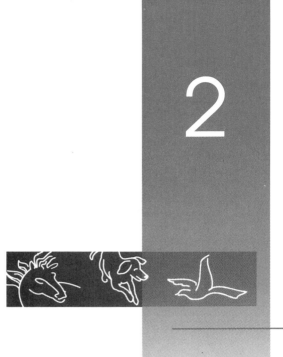

Suzanne Hetts

"My cat has started urinating outside her litterbox! How can I make her stop?"

"My dog is tearing things up and going to the bathroom in the house when I'm at work. Do you have any advice?"

Technicians and veterinarians are asked questions like these almost every day in clinical practice. These behavioral descriptions are analogous to medical symptoms; they represent manifestations of problems and not underlying causes. Before behavioral or medical problems can be treated, they must be diagnosed. Before solutions for problems such as those posed above can be suggested, detailed information must be obtained so a behavioral diagnosis can be made. Technicians must decide whether they have sufficient time and knowledge to do so or whether their role in such cases should be something other than problem solver. The goals of this chapter are to introduce the field of applied animal behavior, provide a basic understanding of principles commonly used in problem resolution, discuss a few popular solutions to behavior problems that often exacerbate rather than resolve problems, and provide guidance to assist technicians in making professional referrals and choosing their roles with behavior cases.

BRIEF HISTORY OF THE DISCIPLINE OF ANIMAL BEHAVIOR

Classic Ethology

Animal behavior is a specialized, scientific field of study. A few of the best-known classic animal behaviorists are Charles Darwin, Niko Tinbergen, and Konrad Lorenz. Classic animal behaviorists, or ethologists, observed and described behavior with four important questions in mind: (1) *causation*—what is the immediate (short-term) reason or cause for the behavior; (2) *ontogeny*—how does a particular behavior develop or change throughout the life span of the animal; (3) *evolution*—how does behavior change as species evolve and are subjected to natural (or artificial) selection; and (4) *function*—what role does the behavior play in the adaptation of the animal to its environment? Classic ethology in the early part of this century focused on describing behavior in an animal's natural habitat and comparing similar behaviors in closely related species and did not look favorably on the sole study of domestic animals.

Animal Psychology

Classic animal psychologists studied animal learning and attempted to elucidate general laws of behavior by studying species such as rats and pigeons in the laboratory under controlled experimental conditions. Important early animal psychologists include E. L. Thorndike, B. F. Skinner, and Ivan Pavlov; they and others have made enormous contributions to our understanding of how animals learn and respond to positive and negative consequences to their behavior.

Contemporary Animal Behavior

The science and study of animal behavior reflect the input from many different disciplines and a blurring of the distinctions between classic ethologists and animal psychologists. Ethologists have moved away from strictly descriptive studies and become more sophisticated in their use of the experimental method, statistical analyses, experimental controls, and theoretical models. Animal psychologists have become more aware of the narrow focus and possible distortions resulting from the study solely in the laboratory of the behavior of a limited number of species. The field of contemporary animal behavior has benefited from the contributions of many disciplines, including zoology, entomology, behavioral ecology, physiological psychology, social psychology, comparative psychology, ethology, wildlife biology, animal science, and veterinary medicine.

APPLIED ANIMAL BEHAVIOR

Applied animal behavior is the application of the body of knowledge about behavior to practical problems. Animal behavior has applications for wildlife management, endangered species, management of zoo animals, food animal production and management, welfare of laboratory animals, and other areas. The resolution of behavior problems in companion animals, often called *animal behavior counseling* or *clinical animal behavior,* is the type of applied animal behavior that is the focus of this chapter.

Animal Behavior Counseling

Animal behavior counseling can be defined as the process of working with animal owners to assist them in modifying behaviors displayed by their animals that they perceive to be problems. This definition points out it is the owner who defines the problem. A dog who jumps on people may be a problem for one owner but not another. Behaviors usually become problems when they occur in excess or in undesirable contexts or locations. Second, it is the owner who is the agent of change for the behavior. Most behavior problems are the result of an interaction among the animal, owner, and environment. Thus, the process of removing the animal from its environment and having someone else attempt to resolve the problem ignores two of the three factors that usually contribute to the problem. Last, most behavior problems represent normal animal behavior. For example, it is normal for both cats and dogs to establish surface and location preferences for elimination; this normal behavior becomes a problem if the preferences include the Persian rug in the dining room.

✎ TECHNICIAN NOTE

Animal behavior counseling can be defined as the process of working with animal owners to assist them in modifying behaviors displayed by their animals that they perceive to be problems.

Behavior counseling involves some of the same questions that classic ethologists ask, such as: (1) causation—why is this cat urinating outside the litterbox; (2) ontogeny—what are the developmental factors that may have influenced the change in this cat's pattern of elimination; (3) evolution—do the artificial selection pressures created by humans who breed cats primarily for physical characteristics predispose certain breeds of cats to be more likely to develop inappropriate elimination problems; and (4) function—how is this change of elimination patterns benefiting the cat? Behavior counseling also makes use of behavior modification techniques that were discovered by animal

psychologists. This scientific approach to the resolution of behavior problems in companion animals is clearly different from popular, anthropomorphic interpretations, such as the cat is urinating outside the litterbox because she is mad at her owner.

The following steps are used in behavior counseling. Animal behavior counseling involves determining the cause of the behavior problem, recommending techniques for resolution of the problem, and following the progress toward resolution. Whenever an animal's behavior changes, possible medical causes should first be evaluated. This is particularly true for aggressive behavior, elimination problems, stereotypies, and self-injurious behaviors such as hair pulling and excessive licking.

Diagnosis or analysis of the cause of the problem is accomplished by obtaining a detailed behavioral history and, ideally, observations of the animal and its environment. A sample of a generalized format for obtaining a behavioral history is shown in Table 2–1. The behavioral diagnosis should be clearly explained to the owner. The diagnosis will determine the behavior modification plan that needs to be implemented. The plan should then explained and, if appropriate, demonstrated to the owner, and a summary of the plan should be provided in written form.

A behavior counseling session may last from 30 minutes to 2 hours or longer, depending on the nature of the problem. The session can take place in the client's home, the clinic, the offices of the behavior consultant or, in some cases, by telephone. Advantages and disadvantages associated with each location are summarized in Table 2–2.

Follow-up visits or telephone calls are scheduled at inter-

• Table 2–1 •

FORMAT FOR A BEHAVIORAL HISTORY

(1) Signalment
Species, breed, age, gender, spayed, neutered, or intact

(2) Early History
When, where, why obtained
Behavior of sire/dam (if known)
Behavior in the litter
House-training procedures
Socialization experiences

(3) Current Environment
Time—inside/outside
Feeding—schedules/routines
Other animals/family structure
Description of "typical day"

(4) Training
Methods
Who trained
Commands to which animal responds
Methods used for punishment/discipline

(5) Presenting Problem
Owner's description
When, how it began
When, where it occurs
Developmental course
Eliciting, inhibiting stimuli
Frequency of occurrence
Owner's reactions, attempts at resolution

(6) Additional Information
Other problem behaviors
Pertinent medical history

• Table 2–2 •

SITE	ADVANTAGE	DISADVANTAGE
ADVANTAGES AND DISADVANTAGES OF SITES FOR BEHAVIOR COUNSELING		
In-home	Opportunity to observe animal in its own environment	Travel is time consuming and expensive
	Opportunity to assess potentially significant environmental factors	Scheduling problems
	May be able to interview more family members	Limited geographic area
	Direct observation of problem behavior possible	
	Convenient for owner	
In-clinic	Convenient for behaviorist	Physical environment (e.g., space, comfort) not conducive to obtaining a lengthy behavioral history
	Usually less expensive	
	Owner may be willing/able to travel when behaviorist cannot	Often prevents direct observation of important behaviors because of unfamiliar/threatening environment
Telephone	Convenient for both owner and behaviorist	No direct observation of family or owner possible, thus not allowing resolution of some problems
	When direct observation not important or possible (e.g., litterbox problem)	Liability issues in cases of aggressive behavior
	May obtain as much information as with an in-clinic visit	
	Only alternative for some clients	Increased potential for miscommunications

vals appropriate to the problem, which may range from 1 day to several weeks. Some consultants will do unlimited follow-up, and others set a maximum of several months, which is included in the fee. Animal behavior counseling requires time, energy, the use of current scientific knowledge, commitment, and effort. Behavior problems cannot be resolved in "25 words or less" or with "quick fixes" or "tips" anymore than can serious disease or illness.

TECHNICIAN NOTE

Whenever an animal's behavior changes, possible medical causes should be evaluated before behavioral counseling.

Qualifications of Animal Behavior Experts

The field of animal behavior counseling has grown significantly over the past 15 years. Some aspects of this growth have been notably positive, resulting in increases in the number of animal behavior experts, amount of research being conducted, and number of publications based on scientific knowledge. Unfortunately, there also has been an increase in the number of people who call themselves "animal behaviorists" yet have no training in animal behavior. There are no licensing requirements from a government agency for animal behaviorists; thus, anyone can legally use the term professionally. However, there are two professional certification programs for animal behaviorists.

In February 1991, professional certification for applied animal behaviorists became available through the Animal Behavior Society (ABS). The ABS was founded in 1964 and is the largest organization in North America dedicated to the study of animal behavior. The certification program evolved from a recognition that animal-related agencies and businesses, as well as the general public, often need information about animal behavior and assistance with behavior problems in companion animals. Certification provides a means for professional animal behaviorists to demonstrate they meet the minimum educational, experi-

ential, and ethical standards of a professional applied animal behaviorist as determined by the ABS. A summary of these criteria and the contact person for more information are given in Table 2–3.

In 1993, the American College of Veterinary Behaviorists was recognized by the American Veterinary Medical Association, and the first qualifying examination was administered in 1995. The primary objectives of the college are to advance veterinary behavioral science and increase the competency of those who practice in this field. Prerequisites for the examination are given in Table 2–4.

The advent of certification for applied animal behaviorists and veterinary behaviorists will aid pet owners in evaluating the credentials of individuals offering behavior counseling services. Behavior experts with formal scientific training in the field of animal behavior tend to use different types of behavior

• Table 2–3 •

CRITERIA FOR CERTIFICATION BY THE ANIMAL BEHAVIOR SOCIETY OF APPLIED ANIMAL BEHAVIORISTS

Educational
Doctoral degree in a biological or behavioral science with an emphasis on animal behavior or a doctorate in veterinary medicine plus 2 years in university-approved residency in animal behavior. A minimum of 21 semester credits in a behavioral science, including 6 in ethology, animal behavior, and/or comparative psychology and 6 in animal learning, conditioning, and/or animal psychology. Associate-level certification requires a Master's degree with the same stipulations.

Experiential
Five years of professional experience and the ability to demonstrate a thorough knowledge of the literature, scientific principles, and principles of animal behavior and original contributions to the field. Associate level requires 2 years of professional experience and the ability to perform independently and professionally in applied animal behavior.

Endorsement
Minimum of three letters of recommendation from regular ABS members

• Table 2–4 •

CRITERIA FOR BOARD CERTIFICATION BY THE AMERICAN COLLEGE OF VETERINARY BEHAVIORISTS

Prerequisites for Examination
1. Satisfactory moral and ethical standing in the profession
2. Graduate of a veterinary school or college of veterinary medicine
3. Completion of behavioral residency or nonconforming behavioral residency
4. Publication in a refereed journal
5. Three letters of recommendation from associates, one of whom must be a Diplomate of ACVB

Examination
Two-day written examination including both long and short answers and covering the basics of behavioral principles, basics of the behavior of various species, and clinical application of behavior in various species

modification plans than do those without such training. Pet owners can become very confused when trying to decide which approach is best and whose information is accurate; thus, it is important the veterinary technician be familiar with these certification programs and recognize the importance of evaluating the education and experience of individuals offering behavior services.

TECHNICIAN NOTE

It is important to evaluate the education and experience of individuals offering behavior services.

THE VETERINARY TECHNICIAN'S ROLE IN BEHAVIOR COUNSELING

Clients frequently have unrealistic expectations about what is involved in changing their animals' behavior. Veterinary technicians often find themselves in difficult positions in which clients expect accurate, simple, short, effective answers to very complex questions. The role of the technician in these situations should not necessarily be to assist in problem resolution. The previous discussion illustrated that behavior problem resolution requires specialized knowledge and sufficient time, one or both of which the technician may not have. Technicians can *educate* clients about normal animal behavior and the causes of behavior problems. In addition, technicians should be knowledgeable about behavior specialists to *assist* the client in finding the help that is needed.

Your Role as Educator

Most animal owners know little about the normal behaviors of companion animals. Much of the information they have is based on popular, nonscientific books about companion animals, the majority of which are filled with inaccurate information. In general, pet owners tend to interpret animal behavior from a human perspective and to attribute human motivations, value judgments, and reasoning processes to their animals. Some of

the reasons for this anthropomorphic outlook are discussed below. Although there is nothing ethically or morally wrong with this viewpoint, it seldom aids in resolving a behavior problem and, in fact, may create and/or maintain the problem as well as result in unfair and even cruel treatment of the animal.

Providing clients with behaviorally accurate information about possible causes for a behavior problem can change their perspective about the problem and the animal. This may result in a more tolerant and patient attitude toward the animal, and the client may be more willing to seek a solution and invest resources in resolving the problem. One of the most common interpretations that owners have, which unfortunately is often reinforced by some dog trainers, is that a behavior problem is an obedience problem. It is assumed dogs are always attempting to "take charge" of their owners and a lack of control over the dog is the basic cause of most problems. A careful analysis of behavior problems from an ethological perspective does not support this contention. For example, destructiveness or house-soiling due to separation anxiety or fear-related behavior is unrelated to obedience control. Teaching a dog obedience commands is unlikely to resolve many behavior problems.

Another common misinterpretation owners make is to believe their pet is behaving out of "spite" or "revenge." For example, a person whose dog is destructive when left alone may feel the dog is "mad" because it is "getting back" at the owner for leaving. On arriving home, the owner becomes angry at seeing the "mess" and hits or yells at the dog, only to find the next time the dog is left, it not only was destructive but also eliminated in the house! Thus, an unfortunate cycle results of more-aversive treatment and more misbehavior. However, if the owner learns that the dog's destructive and elimination behaviors are probably manifestations of separation anxiety because the animal is anxious when left alone, the anger often diminishes, and the owner stops punishing the dog and becomes more amenable to implementation of techniques to decrease the anxiety and resolve the problem.

Similarly, cat owners are convinced their cats are eliminating in various locations because they are "jealous" of a new baby or "mad" at the owner because they have not received enough attention. This can be a very strong belief when the cat is eliminating on the owner's belongings or on the bed. An ethological interpretation suggests the likelihood of a marking problem or surface preference change that can be resolved with the appropriate methods rather than having the cat leave the home.

TECHNICIAN NOTE

The first rule in behavior cases should be to ''do no harm.''

Owners need accurate information about possible causes of behavior problems, species-typical behaviors, the process of behavior counseling, animal behaviorists, and how animals learn. Information about each of these topics is included in this chapter. The importance of providing good information cannot be overemphasized. The first rule in behavior cases should be to "do no harm." Inaccurate or incomplete information has the potential to exacerbate behavior problems. In addition, it was reported that behavioral problems such as inappropriate elimination, chewing, scratching, hyperactivity, and aggression were associated with an increased risk for animals being surrendered to animal shelters (Petronek et al., 1996a and b). Just as important, advice that owners thought was not helpful or was impractical or was not tried was also associated with a greater risk of surrender. The provision of behavioral information is a task that should not be undertaken lightly.

Your Role as Facilitator

As a facilitator, you can provide clients with information about the fees and services of the resource person to whom you are referring. Have business cards from these people on hand and easily accessible. Be sure you have evaluated to the best of your ability the qualifications and competency of the persons to whom you are referring. Ask questions about their experience and training, and solicit feedback from their clients. Ask to observe a behavior counseling session. Talk to the resource person about any concerns you have with his or her methods. If the person does not seem knowledgeable or you feel uncomfortable with the techniques, find someone else. A list of certified applied animal behaviorists and board-certified veterinary behaviorists can be obtained from the sources listed (see Tables 2–3 and 2–4). Before referring a case to an animal behavior expert, all possible medical causes for the problem should be evaluated by the referring veterinarian.

TECHNICIAN NOTE

Before referring a possible behavior case, all medical causes for the problem should be evaluated by the referring veterinarian.

Provide clients with realistic expectations about what to expect from a consultation with the behavior specialist. Be familiar with the consultant's fee structure and counseling format. It can be most disappointing for clients who are merely told to "call this person for some help" and then expect to receive free assistance during a brief telephone call to find "help" actually involves several hours of their time as well as a fee.

If you are referring a client to a dog trainer, be aware that a great deal of variation exists among trainers in their knowledge of animal behavior and learning theory as well as their approach to obedience training. Observe several classes before referring clients, and obtain feedback from clients who have completed courses. Avoid trainers who rely on physically forceful, "dominant" methods; who guarantee their work; and who advocate in-kennel training. The Association of Pet Dog Trainers (APDT) seeks to promote positive, humane training methods, but membership is open to anyone and does not guarantee compliance with this philosophy. A list of helpful reading materials is provided at the end of this chapter that can be used as a basis for evaluating resource persons in your community and in a "self-help" approach if other professional assistance is not available.

THE HUMAN–COMPANION ANIMAL BOND AND BEHAVIOR PROBLEMS

Pets in the Family

Over 62 million households own one or more companion animals (dog or cat). Companion animals are playing an increasingly important role in family systems, for a number of important reasons; one is that the structure of the American family has changed significantly during the past 25 years. Extended families in which aunts, uncles, grandparents, adult siblings, cousins, and so forth live in close geographic proximity to each other are rare. The "traditional" American family consisting of mom, dad, and two children actually comprises less than 27% of contemporary family systems. Single-parent families, never-married singles, widowed elderly, and childless couples are common. In many of these families, companion animals are replacing absent family members in such roles as sibling, best friend, child, confidant, or nonjudgmental parent or grandparent. Companion animals provide nonjudgmental acceptance, a constant presence, and unconditional affection. When these types of strong attachments develop between a pet and one or more family members, the family will be more likely to want to keep the pet and be more committed to investing time, energy, and money into the resolution of behavior problems. At the same time, complex relationships between people and pets become part of the family's structure and often influence the family's ability to work together to resolve a pet's behavior problem.

Pets may be the focus of "power struggles" between family members, facilitate (or inhibit) communication between members, and be symbolic of other relationships. These factors must be taken into account when attempting to resolve behavior problems in companion animals. Although it may be obvious to the behavior professional what the best course of action would be to resolve the problem, the family may not be able or willing to implement certain techniques or to follow through with a behavior modification program. This inability may stem from beliefs, judgments, and/or fears about how such a program will change their relationship with the pet, how it will affect the pet, and how it will affect other family members.

The success of behavior counseling depends not only on the ability to correctly diagnose a problem and devise the most appropriate techniques to resolve it but also on the ability to facilitate, encourage, and convince the family to implement and follow through with the program. Because of this, training in communication skills, family systems theory, and/or basic helping skills are invaluable for anyone aiding pet owners in resolving behavior problems.

In addition to the changing nature of the American family, there are specific characteristics of our companion animals that facilitate our attachment to them and our tendency to view them in anthropomorphic ways.

Neoteny

Some breeds of dogs and cats (e.g., Pekingese, Pomeranian, Persian [Fig. 2–1]) retain infantile, or *neotenic*, characteristics into adulthood. These neotenic characteristics, which include large eyes in relation to the size of the face or head, a shortened or flattened muzzle or nose, and a sloping forehead, are what make all young animals (human infants included) appear "cute" and evoke caregiving responses from us. This phenomenon

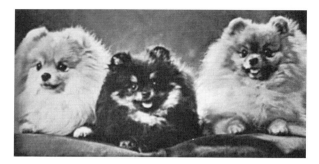

Figure 2-1. Neotenic features in Pomeranians.

makes it especially easy for a companion animal to assume the role of child in a family.

Many species of domestic animals are considered to be neotenized versions of their wild ancestors because they have retained behaviors that are more characteristic of juvenile wild animals (Coppinger and Schneider, 1995). For example, both dogs and cats are much more playful throughout their lives than are their wild counterparts. They also tend to be more vocal.

Allelomimetic Behavior

Some species of companion animals, dogs more so than cats, will at times display mimicking, or *allelomimetic*, behavior. Animals that live in groups, as do dogs and their wild ancestors, will frequently mimic the behavior of other group members (Fig. 2–2). This can be adaptive in the wild for hunting, for maintaining contact with group members, and for defense. When companion animals mimic our behavior (Fig. 2–3), it becomes easier for us to interpret their behavior from a human perspective and to view them in anthropomorphic ways. This view may interfere with an owner's ability to understand the cause of a problem and why noncontingent punishment and reinforcement are not effective in changing behavior. Implementation of appropriate techniques designed to resolve the problem may also be difficult.

Domestication History

Many of our companion animals have been domesticated for a long time. Domestication of the dog occurred between 12,000 and 15,000 years ago, the cat approximately 4,000 years ago,

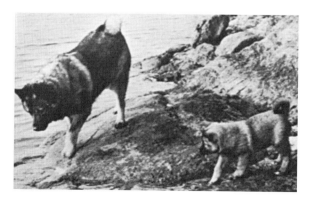

Figure 2-2. Norwegian Elkhound puppy showing allelomimetic (mimicking) behavior.

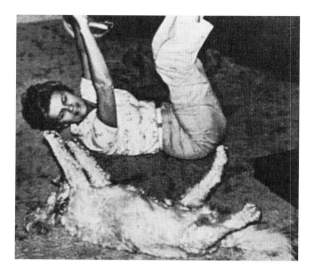

Figure 2-3. Apparent allelomimetic behavior between species.

and the horse 6,000 years ago. All of these animals have different domestication histories, which in part explains the different types of relationships we have with them and the different places they hold in society today. All of our companion animals have been under the influence of selective breeding by humans. The dog has been most affected by this process, whereas the cat has been bred selectively for only about 100 years. These selective breeding practices have resulted in companion animals with characteristics most useful for specialized functions, including hunting, protection, traveling long distances, and carrying heavy loads. However, increasingly the focus of selective breeding and the function that these animals are bred to serve is companionship rather than utilitarian functions. Thus, characteristics that facilitate this function and serve to increase our attachment to companion animals are likely to become more prominent in some breeds of these species.

 TECHNICIAN NOTE

Domestication of the dog occurred 12,000 to 15,000 years ago.

Behavior Problems as a Threat to the Bond

Data collected at the Humane Society of Denver indicated that 11% of the 8500 cats and 24% of the 6400 dogs surrendered to the shelter over a year's time were given up due to behavior problems (Hetts, unpublished data). The most common dog problem was destructive behavior (23%), followed closely by escape behavior (22%) and aggressive behavior toward people (21%). The most common cat problem, by a wide margin, was inappropriate elimination (41%, which could include spraying), followed by aggressive behavior to other animals (15%) and destructive behavior (12%). These numbers suggest that if pet owners are provided with competent, professional assistance for resolving problem behaviors, a significant number of companion animals could be kept in their homes and out of animal shelters.

Thus, the presence of a behavior problem often carries with it the threat of breaking the bond between humans and companion animals. Aggressive animals may have to be euthanatized. Some family members may refuse to tolerate house-soiling or attention-getting behaviors. Neighbors may threaten legal action against aggressive animals, barking dogs, or animals that continually escape confinement.

When owners ask for assistance with these types of problems, they may be anticipating the possible loss of their pet, which results in the experience of *anticipatory grief*. Grief of any sort produces strong emotion, physical reactions, a state of crisis, and decreased coping ability (Lagoni et al. 1994). Thus, the most appropriate response to make when this type of situation is encountered is to acknowledge and talk about the emotions and feelings involved. Intense emotion interferes with rational, objective thought. Often what clients want most is to know that someone understands their frustration and the seriousness of their situation and cares enough to listen to their fears, anger, and sense of helplessness. Crisis intervention theory holds that it is best to deal with the emotion before attempting to problem solve. Clients may often feel that their needs have been met if they feel cared about, even though the behavior problem has not been resolved. This type of approach will also decrease the pressure you may feel to help a client when there is neither the time nor the expertise to resolve the behavior problem itself.

BASIC LEARNING THEORY

Frequently used behavior modification techniques, such as counterconditioning, desensitization, aversive conditioning, shaping, and successive approximation, are based on learning theory and the consequences of a specific behavior to the animal. Resolution of problem behavior requires an understanding of these ideas. Misunderstanding or a lack of understanding about these concepts often contributes to the development and maintenance of behavior problems. Veterinary technicians must acquire a working knowledge of these techniques if they plan on assisting pet owners with or educating owners about behavior problems. These concepts are frequently misrepresented in the popular literature and as such contribute to ineffective and inappropriate problem resolution techniques.

Positive Reinforcement

Positive reinforcement is the presentation of a pleasant or rewarding stimulus immediately following a behavior that serves to increase the probability of that behavior being repeated. Positive reinforcement is most often associated with teaching or conditioning desirable behaviors. A simple example is giving a dog a tidbit of food when it places its hindquarters on the floor in response to a cue to "sit." Reinforcement must occur within 3 to 5 seconds of the desired behavior to be effective. Focusing on reinforcing acceptable behaviors rather than punishing undesirable ones results in fewer unwanted side effects and is more effective in the long term.

However, many undesirable behaviors are inadvertently encouraged through the use of inappropriate positive reinforcement. Any type of attention from the owner, including verbal scolding, may actually serve to reinforce many attention-getting behaviors even though the owner's intent was to punish the behavior. Allowing a dog to come inside when it is barking may positively reinforce the barking behavior. Examples of other behaviors that are often inadvertently reinforced include begging, stealing objects, excessive vocalizations, jumping up on people, and "pestering" behavior.

TECHNICIAN NOTE

Reinforcement must occur within 3 to 5 seconds of the desired behavior to be effective.

Fearful behavior is also often easily reinforced when the owner attempts to reassure the animal. In this case, the animal receives increased attention, petting, and what it perceives as verbal praise when it is exhibiting fearful behavior. Thus, the misuse of positive reinforcement can create, exacerbate, and/or maintain behavior problems. Conversely, positive reinforcement can be a powerful tool to elicit desirable behaviors in place of undesirable ones.

Negative Reinforcement

Negative reinforcement is usually misunderstood. It is often confused with punishment and mistakenly thought to decrease the frequency of undesirable behavior. In fact, negative reinforcement also increases the probability of a response, just as positive reinforcement does.

Negative reinforcement occurs when an animal escapes or avoids an aversive stimulus by performing a behavior. This serves to increase the probability of that behavior being repeated. Many traditional dog training methods are based on negative reinforcement. Pulling up on a leash to tighten a choke collar is one method of teaching a dog to sit. Sitting is negatively reinforced because by sitting, the dog can either escape or avoid the aversive stimulus of the constricting collar. Positively reinforcing sitting with a tidbit as described above is likely to be a more pleasant experience for both dog and owner.

Fear-motivated aggression is an example of a behavior problem that can be difficult to resolve because it is so easily negatively reinforced. For a fear-biting dog, the approach of a person is an aversive stimulus. The dog, by snapping, growling, and/or attempting to bite, drives away the approaching person. The aggression is thus negatively reinforced, as the aversive stimulus is removed. Although termination of pain and reduction of fear are powerful negative reinforcers, like punishment, they can often elicit additional fearful and aggressive behaviors.

Punishment

Punishment probably is the most overused and misused behavior modification technique performed by most pet owners. Punishment is the presentation of an aversive stimulus immediately following a behavior that serves to decrease the probability the behavior will be repeated. There are several criteria that must be met for punishment to be effective.

Be Immediate. First, punishment must immediately follow the inappropriate behavior. Learning theory research indicates if punishment is to be effective it must occur within 2 seconds after the undesirable behavior. This presents practical implementation problems as it requires owners to closely supervise the animal and be in close proximity when the undesirable behavior occurs. In contrast, punishment "after the fact" is *not* effective or fair to the animal and, in many cases, actually serves to exacerbate the problem. This is noncontingent punishment, which means the aversive event is not contingent on the animal's behavior.

Owners often have strong beliefs that animals "know they did something wrong" because they look "guilty" when they are being "punished" for earlier misbehavior (by definition, this cannot be punishment). "Guilty" looks are merely canid submissive postures that dogs display when they are threatened; these include cowering, slinking away, putting the ears back, rolling over on the back, or "grinning" (Fig. 2–4). Dogs are merely reacting to the current threat from the owner as they are being verbally or physically scolded. Using discriminative cues, dogs can sense when scolding will occur. This explains why dogs display these submissive behaviors before the owner is aware of the misbehavior. Dogs make the following discrimination: In the presence of the owner *and* a "mess" (urine, feces, household destruction), scolding follows. In the presence of only one of these factors, scolding is avoided. Thus, dogs do not look "guilty" after misbehaving when their owners are not present, nor do they appear so in their owners' presence when there is no evidence of misbehavior. By displaying these submissive postures, dogs are responding to current threats; they are not communicating that they are aware of previous misbehavior and are associating it with current scolding. Cats do not show submissive behavior and are more likely to hide or become defensive when threatened.

Be Consistent. A second criterion for effective punishment is that it be consistent. Every time the misbehavior occurs, the aversive consequence must occur. This is another practical problem with the implementation of punishment techniques, as it is unlikely the owner will be present every time the animal displays the undesirable behavior.

Be Sufficiently Aversive. Last, the punishing stimulus must be sufficiently unpleasant to quickly stop the behavior, after only a few presentations. If an owner has repeatedly attempted to punish the behavior and the behavior is still occurring at the same frequency, then by definition it has not been punished. In addition, some attempts at punishment can be perceived by the dog as positive reinforcement. If a dog is "pestering" the owner for attention and the owner is continually pushing the dog away and verbally scolding him, these acts are likely reinforcing the behavior. This is because the dog is receiving social interaction with the owner, which is exactly what he wants; thus, the "pestering" is effective and continues unabated.

Any stimulus that is sufficiently intense to quickly inhibit behavior is also highly likely to elicit fearful and/or aggressive responses. This is one of the reasons why interactive punishment (punishment delivered by the owner) is not recommended; it can result in the animal being fearful of or aggressive toward the owner. It is also difficult to precisely control the intensity and duration of aversive stimuli that are delivered by owners (leash and collar corrections, restraint, hitting, and yelling). Aversive stimuli that are too intense and/or are presented for long durations can be considered cruel. A final disadvantage of interactive punishment is that the animal learns

to inhibit a behavior in the owner's presence but not in the owner's absence. Aversive stimuli that are delivered remotely, which the animal perceives to come from the environment rather than from the owner, usually create fewer unwanted problems.

Perhaps the greatest limitation of punishment is at best it can only teach the animal to inhibit a behavior; it can never teach the animal a different, initial response. For many problems, this is crucial to the resolution of the problem. For example, if a dog growls and snaps at people who come to the door and the owner yells "no" and jerks the dog's collar, at best the dog learns not to do this when the owner is present because "bad things" will happen. The dog is still motivated to growl and snap and has not learned to display a friendly response. If the owner is not present, it is likely the dog will still behave in a threatening manner. At worst, the dog will redirect these responses to the owner when the punishment is being delivered.

TECHNICIAN NOTE

Effective punishment must be immediate, consistent, and sufficiently aversive.

Extinction

Extinction is one of the most effective behavior modification techniques but can be difficult to implement correctly. Extinction is the withholding or removal of positive reinforcement for a previously reinforced behavior. Because reinforcement is withheld, the behavior eventually ceases to occur. Several problems exist, however, when using this approach. First, it may be difficult to actually remove all the reinforcement for a behavior. Ignoring a barking dog will eliminate the attention from the owner that was reinforcing, but the act of barking itself may be enjoyable to the dog and therefore self-reinforcing. Second, when reinforcement is initially withheld, the frequency of the undesirable behavior may actually increase temporarily. If owners are not warned of this phenomenon, they may become frustrated at this point and cease to ignore the barking dog. The dog has now learned to bark longer before being reinforced. Extinction requires "outlasting" the animal. Third, when a particular behavior is no longer reinforced, the animal usually attempts to accomplish the same result by engaging in another behavior. If barking does not result in being let inside, perhaps scratching at the door will. Thus, extinction is most effective if another, acceptable response can be reinforced. Many undesirable attention-getting behaviors can be successfully eliminated using extinction procedures if the owner is able to follow through with the extinction process.

Counterconditioning and Systematic Desensitization

When correctly implemented, these two behavior modification techniques are effective in resolving a variety of behavior problems. These procedures are almost always implemented simultaneously. The process of counterconditioning can be simply defined as conditioning an animal to engage in behavior that is

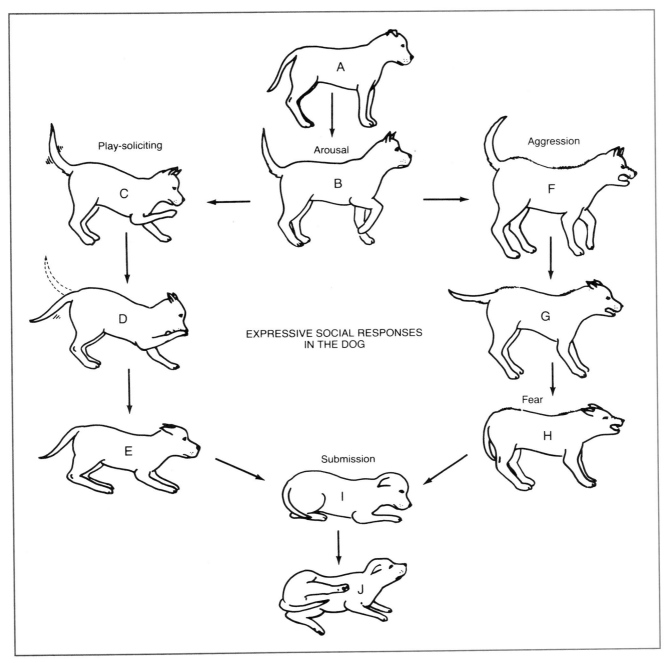

Play-soliciting

Arousal

Aggression

EXPRESSIVE SOCIAL RESPONSES
IN THE DOG

Fear

Submission

Figure 2-4. Canid body postures ranging from an alert response (A and B) to submission (E, I, and J).

counter to, and incompatible with, the undesirable behavior. Systematic desensitization is the process of exposing the animal to a gradient of stimuli, beginning at an intensity that does not evoke the undesirable response and increasing the intensity in such small increments that the stimuli eventually lose their ability to evoke the undesirable response. These procedures are most frequently used to eliminate anxiety or fear responses, as in fear-motivated aggression, separation anxiety, and bronto-phobia (fear of thunderstorms). A summary of behavior modification goals is given in Table 2–6. They can also be effective in resolving dominance aggression and some elimination problems. Correct implementation of these techniques requires care-

ful planning, determination of the correct hierarchy of stimuli, and accurate observation of the animal's response. If the procedures are incorrectly used, the behavior problem can become worse. Examples of their application are given in the following sections that describe specific problems.

COMMON BEHAVIOR PROBLEMS IN THE DOG

It would be unrealistic to assume that sufficient information could be provided about any specific behavior problem in one or two paragraphs that would enable the reader to then resolve any problem of that type. Veterinary technicians should not and cannot be expected to provide a solution to a behavior problem when queried by a client in the context of a 15-minute office call. Thus, the purpose of providing the following discussion of common behavior problems is not to offer "cookbook" solutions to complex problems but rather to provide information about possible causes of problems, what should not be done in an attempt to resolve the problem, and what general approaches can be taken to resolve the problem from a behavioral perspective. When dealing with behavior problems, the presence of organic disease must always be ruled out. A complete physical examination by the veterinarian should precede any behavioral management recommendations.

Aggression
Defining and Categorizing

Aggression is one of the most common types of behavior problems referred for behavior counseling. The term *aggression* is used very loosely and is interpreted in a variety of ways. A behavioral definition of aggression modified from several sources (Moyer, 1976; Borchelt and Voith, 1996a) that is useful to applied behaviorists is *behaviors with an intent to harm.* Many of the behaviors that we commonly refer to as aggressive, such as growling, baring of teeth, and hissing, are technically not aggression but instead threats. Behaviorists use the term *agonistic behavior* to describe these and all behaviors animals can show during social conflicts, including offensive and defensive threats, appeasement and submissive behavior, and escape behavior, as well as aggression. Because aggression is normal for most animals, it also is not technically correct to speak about "aggressive animals," as though some are aggressive and some are not. What is important is the relative threshold at which aggressive or threatening behavior is triggered in an individual animal. Some animals have very low thresholds and will respond aggressively to minor challenges, whereas others have very high thresholds and will tolerate many kinds of threats.

TECHNICIAN NOTE

Aggression is one of the most common types of behavior problems referred for behavior counseling.

Types

Aggressive behavior is categorized by the context in which it occurs and the associated body postures. Table 2–5 summarizes the common types of aggression seen in several species of companion animals. In many cases, animals display more than one type of aggression and may show both offensive and defensive behavior. Offensive body postures serve to make the animal appear large and intimidating, whereas defensive postures protect the body (see Fig. 2–4).

Intervention Procedures

The appropriate methods to resolve aggression problems are dependent on the specific type of aggression that is occurring

as well as the specific details of each individual case. Castration may be helpful with some types of aggression such as intermale, dominance, and perhaps territorial. There are no data to suggest that castration is less effective in older animals than in younger ones in decreasing the frequency of aggressive responses (Hart, 1985); however, behavior modification is almost always required in addition to castration. Drug therapy alone is rarely effective in resolving aggression problems and may actually exacerbate problems if used inappropriately. Medication should be used as part of a behavior modification program only after a specific behavioral diagnosis has been made and with a particular goal in mind—not as just a "shot in the dark" (Simpson and Simpson, 1996; Simpson, 1996).

Popular methods that focus on strong physical punishment and "dominant" techniques, such as rolling, pinning, and "scruff shaking," for aggression are inappropriate (Gibbs, 1996). Punishment severe enough to inhibit behavior often elicits aggression, which puts individuals administering such techniques at great risk. Trying to punish a dog who is displaying fear-motivated aggression will almost surely exacerbate the problem, and punishing a dominantly aggressive dog is dangerous. In addition, punishment can never teach the dog how to be friendly or nonpossessive and especially cannot make a dog less fearful.

The most effective and safest behavior modification procedures for most aggression problems are counterconditioning and desensitization, or "exposure techniques." The goal in working with aggression problems is, first, to temporarily avoid situations in which the dog is likely to be aggressive. Second, stimuli should be presented to the dog at a low enough intensity (termed *subthreshold*) that aggression is not elicited. Nonaggressive responses should be encouraged and reinforced with food, praise, and toys. How these techniques are implemented depends on the type of aggression as different eliciting stimuli will be involved in each case. Because the dog is exposed through the use of controlled, gradual procedures to situations that have previously elicited aggression, the dog may need to be muzzled during treatment to ensure the safety of others. A Gentle Leader or Promise head collar is also recommended for use with many types of aggression problems as it provides a much higher degree of control than choke or pinch collars and is definitely more humane. Summary statements of the behavior changes that need to be accomplished for common types of aggression are listed in Table 2–6.

When discussing options with owners of aggressive or threatening dogs, euthanasia should be included. It generally is not appropriate to discuss this as the first or only option because this appears to trivialize the importance of the dog's life. Owners should make their own decisions about the advisability of working with the dog or choosing euthanasia after being provided with accurate information about the nature of the problem and likelihood of resolution. Factors to keep in mind in assessing relative risk are summarized in Table 2–7. It is rarely appropriate to place a dog with an aggression problem in a new home because of the liability problems. For a more thorough discussion of euthanasia decision-making involving behavior problems, see Hetts (1996), and for a discussion involving grieving clients, see Chapter 29.

Separation Anxiety
Description

As the term implies, *separation anxiety* occurs when an animal becomes anxious and distressed when separated from the

• Table 2–5 •

EXAMPLES OF TYPES OF AGGRESSIVE BEHAVIOR IN DOGS, CATS, AND HORSES		
TYPE	**SPECIES**	**ELICITING CONDITIONS/DESCRIPTION**
Fear	Dog, cat, horse	When an animal's "personal space" is invaded and it perceives its physical safety is threatened; defensive body postures
Territorial	Dog, cat	When an animal perceives its territory is threatened and defends it; may be in reaction to other animals, people, odors, or vocalizations; often occurs when a new animal is introduced to the home, a resident animal returns after an absence, or during presence of people other than family members; territory may include more than house and yard; aggression may be offensive and/or defensive
Intermale	Dog, cat, horse	Usually involves competitive interactions with another male over important resources; interfemale aggression can also occur for similar reasons; sometimes classified as dominance or competitive aggression; offensive in nature
Dominance	Dog, horse, cat (disputed)	In reaction to body postures or behaviors from another that are perceived as threats to the animal's social status; examples in the dog include hugging, petting over the head, prolonged eye contact, and body restraint; also in reaction to competition for resources such as resting places, toys, mates, and food; thus, may overlap with possessive aggression
Possessive	Dog, cat and horse (less likely)	When an animal is in possession of food, toys, or other valued objects and does not want to relinquish them; can be offensive or defensive
Play motivated	Dog, cat, horse	Because aggression is defined as intent to harm, harm that occurs during play without intent is not considered by some to be aggression; common in young animals; associated with playful body postures
Pain elicited	Dog, cat, horse	Defensive aggression in response to physical pain or discomfort or the threat of such; sometimes classified as fear-motivated aggression; sometimes a subcategory of punishment-elicited aggression; can occur during grooming, body restraint, or medical treatment
Redirected	Dog, cat, horse	Animal directs aggression toward another animal or person who did not elicit the initial aggressive response; occurs when the animal is prevented from or inhibited about attacking the primary target; may be offensive or defensive; in cats, the redirected response may occur hours after the initiating stimulus

• Table 2–6 •

SUMMARY OF BEHAVIOR MODIFICATION GOALS FOR VARIOUS TYPES OF AGGRESSION PROBLEMS IN THE DOG

Dominance aggression
Dog is conditioned to display increasingly submissive behaviors with greater frequency and to "work" for whatever he wants. The dog becomes less likely to challenge the owner as doing so is no longer effective. Subordinate behavior brings rewards. Physical punishment is not used.

Fear-elicited aggression
Dog becomes less fearful as the result of gradual-exposure techniques in which nonfearful behavior has been elicited and reinforced. The previously feared stimuli now predict pleasant and enjoyable consequences.

Possessive aggression
On the approach of people, the dog's expectations are changed from predicting his possession will be taken away to predicting that he will receive something of even greater importance. Techniques used for dominance aggression may also be appropriate.

Protective/territorial
Unfamiliar people or other dogs are no longer viewed as territorial intruders but rather as individuals the dog either tolerates with neutral behavior or is actively friendly toward due to the outcomes of social interactions.

Redirected
The initiating stimulus must be identified and the dog's response to it modified using appropriate techniques.

These examples should not be interpreted as complete treatment programs but merely examples of the rationale for the appropriate behavior modification techniques.

• Table 2–7 •

FACTORS TO BE CONSIDERED IN ASSESSING RELATIVE RISK WITH AGGRESSIVE PROBLEMS

Duration of Problem
Has this behavior been observed from a young age or for months or years before help was sought? Has this behavior appeared relatively recently and consequently with limited frequency?

Degree of Generalization
Does the aggression/threat occur in a wide variety of contexts, and is it initiated by many different stimuli? Is the behavior confined to very narrowly defined circumstances?

Intensity of Behavior
Does the dog limit the behavior to warning growls, snaps at the air, or inhibited bites?
Does the dog bite to the point of injury?

Predictability of Behavior
Can the type of aggression be determined and the contexts in which it will occur be predicted? (This may require assistance from a behavior specialist. Although owners may describe the dog as unpredictable, a behavioral history sometimes reveals otherwise.) Does the dog become aggressive/threatening for no apparent reason?

Threshold
Is the dog easily stimulated into aggressive behavior with relatively minor challenges?
Does the dog tolerate relatively threatening stimuli and display aggression only in response to more intense stimuli?

Other Choices
When possible, does the dog attempt to escape the situation rather than display aggression? Does the dog give warnings, in the form of threats, before becoming aggressive?

owner. From a problem perspective, this anxiety is usually manifest by destructive behavior, house-soiling, escaping, and/or excessive vocalization when left alone. Occasionally, aggression is directed toward the owner when he or she attempts to leave the dog. Owners may also report their dogs neither eat nor drink when left alone, even if a special tidbit is available. Such dogs are also described as "depressed" or "pouting" but may not be presented with a behavior problem because such passive behavior generally does not present a problem for the owner.

Problem behaviors characteristically begin within the first 30 minutes of the owner's departure (Voith and Borchelt, 1996). When the owner initiates preparations to leave the house, the dog's anxiety is triggered. This anxiety generally peaks at the point of the owner's departure or within the first 30 minutes thereafter; thus, the separation anxiety behavior is displayed within this first half hour. Problem behaviors that occur randomly at any time during the owner's absence are probably not separation related. Separation behaviors also occur consistently whenever the dog is left alone rather than having an irregular pattern of manifestation. Destructive behavior due to separation anxiety is usually directed at departure points, such as doors, windows, or gates, or toward items that are saturated with the owner's scent, such as clothes, bed coverings, and couch cushions.

Behavioral Profile

Dogs with separation anxiety are more likely to have been obtained from humane societies or found as strays (McCrave, 1991). They also try to maintain close contact with their owners by following them from room to room and not wanting to be outside by themselves. Such dogs display intense and prolonged greeting behaviors and are sometimes described as "frantic" or "hyperactive" during these times. Separation anxiety behavior is usually triggered by a change in the amount of contact with the owner or other family member (Voith and Borchelt, 1996); examples include after a vacation when one or more family members have been home with the dog, a return to work after a prolonged absence, the death of another family pet to whom the dog was attached, a divorce, termination of a relationship or change in roommates, or after the dog has been boarded. A move to a new environment is also a common trigger.

Intervention

The goal of a behavior modification program is to decrease the anxiety the dog experiences when left alone. This is accomplished with counterconditioning and desensitization or habituation techniques. The overall approach is to divide the process

TECHNICIAN NOTE

The goal of behavior modification for separation anxiety is to decrease the anxiety experienced by the dog when left alone.

of preparing for departure and the subsequent absence into a series of small segments, conditioning the dog to experience these segments while not anxious, and then linking the segments back together into a normal routine.

With these procedures, the dog is initially left alone for a time period so brief (anywhere from several seconds to several minutes, depending on the dog) that separation anxiety behaviors are not triggered. The duration of these absences is gradually lengthened on a varying schedule (such as 1, 3, 5, 2, 4, 6 minutes) until the dog can tolerate at least 1 hour of separation in a nonanxious state. At this point, many dogs are able to respond favorably to much longer absences.

Because the dog's anxiety begins to increase during the owner's departure routine, the dog should concurrently be habituated to this "getting ready routine." This is accomplished by having the owner engage in discrete portions of this routine, without leaving. Examples include walking to the door, picking up keys, going to the coat closet, or activating the garage door opener. Each of these behaviors should be repeated separately over a period of days or weeks until the dog's response to them is no more than a mild interest. At that time, several of these behaviors can be chained together and practiced before, and then in conjunction with, a short absence.

Whenever counterconditioning and desensitization are used, it is always possible to make the problem worse if the procedures are implemented incorrectly. This can happen if the duration of the practice absences is consistently too long and the dog's anxiety is triggered repeatedly. Similarly, if the intervals between the repeated departure cues are too short, with insufficient time for the dog to regain a nonanxious state, the animal can actually become *sensitized* to these cues, with a resulting increase in anxiety.

During treatment, it is helpful to refrain from leaving the dog alone for long periods as this interferes with the desensitization program; perhaps the dog can be taken to doggie day care, taken to work with the owner, or left in the care of a friend or relative. Antianxiety drugs have been shown to be an effective method of managing separation anxiety problems on a short term basis, but they do not represent a long-term cure. Drugs that are most often used are tricyclic antidepressants and benzodiazepines (Voith and Borchelt, 1996; Simpson, 1996). In recent clinical trials, clomipramine has been shown to be effective (Overall, 1997). See Table 2–8 for a summary of suggested dosages.

A number of procedures are highly likely to exacerbate separation anxiety problems. Attempts to punish the unacceptable behaviors are not effective and can actually make the problem worse. If the dog is consistently scolded or hit when the owner returns home, anticipation of the return can increase the anxiety level and exacerbate the symptoms. Crate training is not recommended as a solution to a separation anxiety problem because it does not address the anxiety, which is the cause of the problem. Dogs with separation anxiety who are crated often injure themselves with frantic escape attempts. Unless the underlying anxiety is decreased, symptom substitution may occur in which one behavioral manifestation of the problem is substituted for another.

House-Soiling

Causes

House-soiling can occur because the dog is eliminating in the house or because of urine-marking behavior. Before any behav-

• Table 2–8 •

DRUG CLASS	GENERIC NAME	TRADE NAME	DOSE
Tricyclic antidepressants	Amitriptyline HCl	Elavil	1 to 2 mg/kg s.i.d. or b.i.d. 2.2 to 4.4 mg/kg s.i.d.
	Imipramine HCl	Tofranil	2.2 to 4.4 mg/kg
	Clomipramine HCl	Anafranil	1–2 mg/kg b.i.d.
Benzodiazepines	Diazepam	Valium	0.55 to 2.2 mg/kg as needed
	Clorazepate dipotassium	Tranxene	5.6 to 22.5 mg/dog s.i.d. or b.i.d.
Progestins—potential side effects require careful monitoring	Megestrol acetate	Ovaban or Megace	2.2 to 4.4 mg/kg s.i.d. for 2 weeks, then one-half dose each succeeding 2 weeks or 1 to 2 mg/kg
Phenothiazines	Acepromazine maleate	Acepromazine	No anxiolytic effects and therefore not recommended

SUGGESTED DRUGS AND DOSAGES USED CONCURRENTLY WITH BEHAVIOR MODIFICATION IN THE TREATMENT OF SEPARATION ANXIETY

See text for references.

ioral approaches are considered, possible medical causes should be thoroughly evaluated through physical examination and appropriate laboratory testing. Elimination, involving urination, defecation, or both, can occur for a variety of behavioral reasons, including (1) separation anxiety, (2) fears or phobias, (3) attention seeking, (4) submission/excitement, (5) lack of or lapse in house-training, or (6) changes in surface or location preferences. Urine-marking usually occurs in response to what the dog perceives to be threats or intrusions into his territory; males are more likely to urine-mark than females (Hart, 1985).

TECHNICIAN NOTE

The first goal in the assessment of an animal with a house-soiling problem is to differentiate, with a behavioral history, between an elimination problem and territorial urine marking.

The first goal is to differentiate, with a behavioral history, between an elimination problem and territorial urine-marking.

To do this, it is important to determine whether (1) the urination most often occurs in association with the presence of environmental changes such as new objects or visitors to the home, (2) the urination frequently occurs soon after contact with other dogs, (3) defecation is not occurring and (4) small amounts of urine in several different areas are discovered rather than one or two large "puddles." If all of the above are true, the problem is most likely urine marking rather than an elimination problem. Important factors for differentiating the underlying cause(s) for a house-soiling problem are (1) the pattern of occurrence, including when and where the behavior occurs, (2) whether the dog has ever been reliably house-trained, (3) if house-training was based primarily on punishment techniques rather than environmental management and positive reinforcement and (4) what the dog's response has been to whatever procedures the owner has attempted in order to resolve the problem. How a behavioral history differs based on the cause of the problem is summarized in Table 2–9.

Intervention

If the problem is urine-marking, castration is almost mandatory to have a reasonable chance of resolving the problem. Any other approach to the problem in intact male dogs is usually only marginally effective. Complete isolation of the dog from the stimuli that are triggering the marking would be highly effective but usually not practical. Dogs can also be counterconditioned to respond differently to the trigger stimuli, assuming the specific triggers can be identified. For example, if dogs are marking paperbags or shoes, food treats can be placed inside the objects to change the significance of the items and elicit a competing behavior. Progestins have potential side effects and are not often used. Buspirone has been shown to be effective with urine-marking in cats (Hart et al., 1993) but has not been widely used in dogs, due in part to the cost of the drug. Punishment may be partially effective if it is delivered correctly (see previous section on punishment); however, it is likely that the dog will only learn to inhibit the behavior in the owner's presence. Aversive conditioning (a process that can be used to associate an aversive stimulus with a particular physical location) can be effective in keeping the dog away from a favorite marking location. However, the dog may simply choose a new place to mark if he is still motivated to do so.

If the problem is house-soiling, intervention procedures must be based on the cause of the problem. If separation anxiety is involved, appropriate techniques described previously should be implemented. If the dog has never been reliably house-trained, puppy house-training procedures should be reestablished which are summarized in Table 2–10. If fears or phobias are involved, the source of the fear must be identified and a counterconditioning and desensitization program devised.

Submissive or excitement-motivated urination often responds to counterconditioning in which quiet, calm behaviors or nonsubmissive postures are elicited. When approaching dogs who submissively urinate, threatening postures should be avoided; these are summarized in Table 2–11 and include direct eye contact, leaning over or reaching toward the dog or over her head, and approaching her directly. Approaching people should look toward the floor, crouch down to the dog's level, let her approach, turn the side of their body toward the dog, and pet her from under the chin. Such dogs can also be distracted into more confident postures by engaging them in play.

• Table 2–9 •

DIFFERENTIAL BEHAVIORAL HISTORY FOR DOG ELIMINATION PROBLEMS	
TYPE OF PROBLEM	**DIFFERENTIAL HISTORY**
Lack of house-training	House-soiling has always been a problem, sometimes intermittently; inappropriate house-training procedures; often involves both urination and defecation
Separation anxiety	Occurs only and consistently in owner's absence, within the first 30 minutes after departure; may involve urination, defecation, or both; dog is reliably house-trained when owner is home
Fear or phobia	Dog has identifiable noise or other types of phobias; elimination correlates with presence of fear-producing stimulus; owner presence or absence not a factor; dog may have shy or timid temperament; may involve urination or defecation; reliably house-trained in absence of fearful stimulus or in different environments
Submissive urination	Occurs in what are to the dog threatening contexts; owner may rely primarily on punishment and aversive methods for managing other problems; associated with fearful body postures; occurs more often in young dogs; dog reliably house-trained in other contexts.
Excitement urination	Occurs during greetings, excited play, and other high arousal contexts; occurs more often in young dogs; dog reliably house-trained in other contexts
Urine-marking	Occurs in reaction to what the dog perceives as a threat to the integrity of his or her territory, including visitors, presence of other animals, new objects, unfamiliar odors; may be associated with conflicts between family dogs or frequent urine-markings on walks; usually small amounts, consistent locations, sometimes an area of the house not frequently used by the family; not related to opportunity to eliminate outside; seen more often in intact and neutered males than in females
Surface and location preferences	Dog prefers location or surface on which to eliminate that is not found outside; often seen in small dogs and during cold weather; sites for elimination share common characteristics

Alternatively, with excitement urination, calm quiet behavior, such as with a "sit-stay" command, can be encouraged and rewarded with the use of a tidbit. In both situations, it may be sufficient to merely ignore the dog during greetings until she is calm and/or less fearful. Many dogs will spontaneously cease the behavior as they mature, so it is important not to inadvertently reinforce the behavior or exacerbate it with punishment.

COMMON BEHAVIOR PROBLEMS IN THE CAT
House-Soiling

Elimination, urination, defecation, or both, outside the litterbox is the most frequently encountered behavior problem in cats.

• Table 2–10 •

SUMMARY OF HOUSE-TRAINING PROCEDURES FOR DOGS
Consistent Routines
This includes a regular feeding schedule as well as consistent opportunities for elimination. These should be after feeding, playing and sleeping or every 2 hours or so for young puppies, longer for older puppies and adults.
Constant Supervision
A crucial part of a good housetraining procedure is to not allow the dog to eliminate inside. This means supervision by using baby gates, etc. to keep the dog in the room with the owner at all times, tethering the dog to the owner with a leash or placing the dog in a crate for *short time periods* when she cannot be supervised. The dog should NEVER be crated for longer than she can control her bladder or bowels which means no more than about 2 hours for puppies during the day. The owner should be available to let the puppy out of the crate to eliminate at night if necessary.
Reward Desirable Behavior
When the dog eliminates outside, *immediately* praise her and even reward her with a special tidbit. This should be done while the dog is still in the elimination location *not* when she is on her way back inside or engaged in another behavior. The importance of positive reinforcement for good behavior cannot be overemphasized.
Never Punish After the Fact or Interactively
Showing the dog its "mess" is not appropriate. Unless the dog is caught in the act of eliminating, punishment will be meaningless. In addition, interactive punishment should never be part of a housetraining program as the dog should never be afraid to eliminate in front of its owner. If the dog is caught eliminating inside, she should merely be taken outside and reinforced for completing the act there.
Decrease Supervision Gradually
Most owners have unrealistic expectations about the age at which a dog should be housetrained. Some dogs are not reliably trained until 6 months or older. The dog should be allowed unsupervised access to the house only after she is reliably eliminating outdoors.

This is distinct from urine-marking, which is usually manifest as spraying, and is discussed separately. Because elimination problems have such a variety of causes, any behavior modification plan must be based on a behavioral diagnosis. A behavioral history should include detailed information about the cat's be-

• Table 2–11 •

POSTURES TO AVOID WHEN APPROACHING FEARFUL OR UNFAMILIAR DOGS	
POSTURES TO AVOID	**APPROPRIATE POSTURES**
Direct eye contact	Look at the floor, off to the side or above the dog's head
Frontal approach	Turn the side of the body toward the dog or approach at a slight angle rather than "head-on"
Reaching toward or over the dog's head or neck	Allow the dog to approach, let the dog sniff a hand held at the side of the body, pet the dog from under the chin
Leaning forward, over the dog's body	Bend at the knees, or stand straight up

havior in the litterbox; location and characteristics of the litterbox and surrounding area; important features of the cat's general environment, including the presence of and relationships with other animals; and pattern of occurrence of inappropriate elimination as well as characteristics of the soiled areas. First-hand knowledge can be extremely helpful in obtaining the necessary information; thus, an in-home visit or videotape of the cat's environment is very useful. Before an elimination problem is considered to be a behavior problem, the cat should be thoroughly evaluated by a veterinarian for any evidence of urinary tract or other disease. Even problems that at first seem to be behavioral may have a medical cause. For example, in one case, an inappropriate urination problem that developed shortly after the birth of a baby was a coincidental reoccurrence of a previous urinary tract problem and unrelated to the baby's presence.

Causes

Misconceptions abound as to the causes for litterbox problems. Many owners will cite spite, revenge, or stress as the most likely causes, when these are rarely, if ever, the cause. These are anthropomorphic interpretations of animal behavior for which there is no supporting evidence. Such interpretations are not helpful in the process of problem resolution. The most common causes for elimination outside the litterbox are surface preferences, location preferences, and/or an aversion to the litterbox or like material. A surface preference problem indicates that the cat prefers another substrate, such as carpet, over the substrate in the litterbox. Surface preferences can develop as a result of the cat's scratching a surface outside the litterbox (such as carpet) after eliminating.

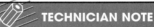

TECHNICIAN NOTE

Before attempting the management of house-soiling in the cat, the possibility of urinary tract disease must be eliminated.

A cat's surface preference can change over time for reasons not well understood. However, when offered several choices of litter material, the majority of cats prefer the soft, fine-grained clumping litter (Borchelt, 1991). Cats displaying a location preference will eliminate in a particular location, regardless of the type of surface. Location preferences often develop when the litterbox is located in a noisy or high traffic area or is not easily accessible. Changing the location of the litterbox may result in the cat's continuing to eliminate in the original location. An aversion to the litterbox can develop when the cat associates something unpleasant with the litterbox. Aversions can develop if the cat is "ambushed" there by either the owner or another household pet, if pain caused by previous disease was experienced in the litterbox during elimination, or if the cat was frightened or startled by something while eliminating. Aversion to litter *material* can develop when the box is inadequately cleaned or if the litter is scented or has an undesirable texture.

In addition to preferences and aversions, other types of problems can be manifest as inconsistent use of the litterbox. Relationship problems between cats in the family in which one cat is intimidated and cannot move freely around in the

environment results in elimination in whatever location the cat views as "safe." Any kind of fear-related problem can have the same result. In these situations, the underlying fear or relationship problem must be addressed, or the litterbox must be moved to a location within the cat's "safe" area.

Intervention Procedures

As with any behavior problem, the behavior modification plan must address the cause of the problem to be effective. Thus, making haphazard changes to the litterbox without a behavioral diagnosis is unlikely to be effective and could create additional problems. Confinement in the absence of additional procedures is seldom effective because it does nothing to address the cause of the problem. Because elimination problems are not disobedience problems, punishment is typically ineffective and often creates other problems, particularly if it is interactive. Location preferences can often be easily resolved by simply moving the litterbox to the preferred location, leaving it there for several weeks, and then *gradually* (such as several inches per day) moving it back to a location more desirable to the owner. Cats should be discouraged from eliminating in these intermediate locations as the box is moved through the placement of food or toys or aversive textures or odors. If the cat refuses to eliminate in the box when it is first moved to the preferred location, the problem is not likely to be motivated by a location preference.

Surface preference problems can be resolved by making the substrate in the litterbox more acceptable to the cat and inappropriately used areas less so. Whatever substrate is tried in the litterbox to increase its attractiveness to the cat should be similar to the texture of the soiled areas that the cat seems to prefer. For cats preferring soft textures such as carpet, clothes, or bedding, the fine-grained clumping litter can be used. For cats preferring slick surfaces such as tile, sinks, or countertops, only a thin layer of litter should be used. In some cases, cats will be attracted to an empty box or a piece of waxed paper in the bottom. If this approach attracts the cat to the box, litter can gradually be added. If cats have outdoor experience, they may prefer dirt, sand, or potting soil either alone in the box or as a layer over clay litter. If a clay litter is used, a high-quality, unscented, dust-free brand presents fewer potential problems than a generic brand or switching brands based on cost. In difficult cases, the preferred substrate can be placed in the litterbox (as a carpet remnant), but if this is done, the cat must temporarily be prevented access to the substrate in any other location. Thus, confinement may be necessary. After the cat is using the litterbox under these conditions, litter material may gradually be added and the inappropriate substrate removed.

Because of the negative association that may have developed with litterbox aversion, the problem may require providing a new box, with a different substrate, a new location, and/or counterconditioning and desensitization techniques. A behavioral diagnosis should be made before drug therapy is considered as part of a treatment plan for elimination problems. Drug treatment is generally not effective in treating surface and location preferences or litterbox aversions. It is most effective with problems based on fear or anxiety and when combined with an appropriate behavior modification plan. (See the section below on urine-marking for more information.)

Urine-Marking

Urine-marking problems are not elimination problems. Marking is usually manifest as spraying characterized by the cat assuming a standing posture, backing up against a vertical object, and releasing urine from a standing posture. Occasionally, cats will urine mark from a squatting position (Borchelt and Voith, 1996b). Spraying is easily differentiated from elimination by body posture and location of the urine. Differentiating urine-marking from a squatting posture and elimination can be very difficult. A detailed behavioral history is required, including the contexts and locations in which the behavior occurs and identification of the eliciting stimuli. The amount of urine deposited is not always diagnostic.

 TECHNICIAN NOTE

Urine-marking problems are not elimination problems.

Causes

Urine marking is a communicative behavior. It is associated with social conflict and competitive or sexual behavior. Environmental stimuli, such as the presence of other cats outdoors, conflicts between family cats, visitors to the home, or other unfamiliar stimuli, often initiate the problem. The behavior may be directed toward new furniture; visitors' belongings or bedding; shoes, purses, coats, and other items with unfamiliar odors; or the cat's territorial boundaries, such as perimeter walls, doors, or windows. Spraying occurs more frequently in intact males than in castrated males or intact or spayed females (Borchelt and Voith, 1996b). In some cases, once the behavior starts, it can become something of a "habit," even if the initiating stimuli are no longer present. Some veterinarians believe that spraying is associated with cystitis, although this has not been clinically documented.

Intervention Procedures

Spraying problems can be difficult to resolve because (1) they often occur inconsistently, (2) it may be difficult to identify the eliciting stimuli (e.g., the behavior has become a "habit"), (3) it is often difficult to remove the cat from or change his reaction to the eliciting stimuli even when they can be identified, and (4) effective behavior modification techniques may be difficult to administer in a timely fashion. Neutering is always the first recommendation.

Modifying the locations in which spraying occurs may be helpful. This can include making the areas aversive with unpleasant odors, such as muscle rubs or perfumes, or uncomfortable substrates, such as double-sided sticky tape or a vinyl carpet runner with point side up. The significance of the areas can be changed by placing food, toys, or catnip there. If the only treatment approach is to make the marked locations unattractive, it is likely the cat will continue the behavior in a different location unless the underlying cause or eliciting stimulus is also addressed.

If the problem is motivated by conflicts with other cats in the household, the relationship between the cats needs to be improved by means of counterconditioning and desensitization techniques. Indoor cats can become aroused to mark by viewing neighborhood cats through windows. The presence of outdoor cats can sometimes be discouraged with the use of motion detectors such as The Critter Getter by Amtex. Alternatively, indoor cats can be discouraged from watching outdoor cats through the windows by other "booby-traps," such as Snappy Trainers (a modified, safe mousetrap) or a windowsill Scat Mat by Comtech or by limiting the cat's view with cardboard or foil, placed on the lower part of the window.

In one clinical study the efficacy of diazepam was evaluated in the treatment of urine-marking problems, the success rate varied from 55% to 75% (Cooper and Hart, 1992). However, a small number of cats develop hepatic failure after the administration of diazepam (Center et al., 1996), so monitoring of hepatic enzymes is recommended. More recently, buspirone hydrochloride, an anxiolytic with a different mode of action than the benzodiazepines such as diazepam, was reported to stop or reduce urine-marking in 55% of 62 neutered cats (Hart et al., 1993). Because of its relative safety and inability to produce physical dependency, this may be the drug of choice for urine-marking problems (Borchelt and Voith, 1996b).

Aggression
Causes

Although an aggressive cat may not be as dangerous as an aggressive dog, a cat can still inflict significant injury by biting and scratching. Cat bites and scratches are probably more under-reported than dog bites, and so it is difficult to estimate how many cat-related injuries occur each year.

 TECHNICIAN NOTE

Cat bites and scratches are probably more under-reported than dog bites.

Many aggressive behavior problems between cats stem from the fact that cats are basically solitary, highly territorial animals. Significant variation exists in how well cats tolerate the presence of other cats in the household. It is not uncommon for a cat to show primarily affiliative behaviors toward one family cat and be aggressive and intolerant of another. The most common types of aggressive behaviors between cats are defensive, intermale, territorial, and redirected. Differentiating between these types requires a detailed behavioral history that includes the context in which the aggression occurs, body postures of the cats involved, and additional information about the daily habits of the cats and their relationship with each other. Territorial aggression is characterized by one cat chasing, stalking, and ambushing another, whereas intermale aggression involves offensive posturing, vocalizations, and threatening behavior. Redirected aggression occurs when a cat is aroused into an aggressive response by a particular individual but directs the behavior to an uninvolved target. A common example is a cat that attacks another cat in the house after becoming agitated by watching outdoor cats from the window. Aggressive behaviors to people are usually motivated by play, the poorly understood "don't-pet-me-anymore" syndrome, or redirected behaviors.

Playful aggression is common in cats less than 1 to 2 years of age. Play-motivated behavior is usually easily diagnosed by a behavior professional but often misinterpreted by owners as "mean" or "vicious" behavior. Play attacks usually involve moving targets and stalking and ambushing behavior. Some cats, more often males than females, will bite after being petted for a time. Although owners often report these attacks occur without warning, usually the cat is displaying intention movements such as quick head turns or other behaviors indicative of arousal such as dilated eyes and ear and tail flicks. Aggressive behavior can also be redirected onto people as well as other cats. Redirected aggression problems can be very difficult to diagnose because the response can occur hours after the triggering event. In one study, redirected aggression was the most frequent diagnosis in cases involving aggression toward the owner (Borchelt and Voith, 1996c). (These categories are defined and briefly explained in Table 2–6).

Intervention Procedures

As with any aggressive behavior, a behavior modification plan should be based on a behavioral diagnosis. Recommendations to resolve the problem should not be given without careful thought, consideration, and cautions to the owner. Owners should be cautioned not to handle an obviously aggressive cat. Cats that are aggressive toward each other should never be left together to "work things out." Interactive punishment should never be used with cats. Cats do not display submissive behaviors as do dogs, who can sometimes be intimidated into inhibiting their behavior (however, this is not the best way to deal with *any* problem). Attempts to use such techniques with cats will only result in the cat avoiding the owner and/or in defensive threatening or aggressive behavior. Many aggression problems can best be resolved with counterconditioning and desensitization techniques. As with dog aggression problems, the approach is to manage the environment and the interactions between cats or between the cat and humans so that aggressive behavior is not stimulated and to elicit and reward nonaggressive behavior.

If intermale or territorial aggression is occurring between cats in the same household, the goal of these behavior modification procedures is to associate the presence of the other cat with pleasant consequences, rather than with the need to attack or the threat of being attacked. The procedures must be implemented in such a way that aggression or fear is not elicited from either cat. Crates may sometimes be used, or the cats may be positioned in separate rooms on either side of a closed door. Food rewards, catnip, and/or toys can be used to elicit the desired nonaggressive response. Each cat should display a clear behavior change during limited contact with each other before they are allowed further interaction. In the meantime, it is a good idea to keep the cats separated so the opportunity for aggressive encounters does not arise. Territorial aggression does not have a good prognosis (Borchelt and Voith, 1996c). If the cats remain in the same household, one often goes into hiding, appearing only when it is unlikely to encounter the aggressor. Short-term drug therapy may be helpful in the treatment of fear-related and redirected aggression, especially when combined with behavior modification (Marder, 1991). Territorial aggression usually does not respond to drug therapy (Marder, 1991), and the potential serious physiological side effects from the use of synthetic progestins, which are sometimes helpful in the treatment of intermale aggression, are well known.

For play-motivated problems, the cat needs to be provided with consistent, ample opportunities for play. A variety of toys should be used that stimulate chasing, pouncing, and ambushing behavior. The many variations of toys on the ends of flexible rods that are available meet these behavioral needs, as do soft toys often scented with catnip that the cat can grab, hold, and claw. Owners should never play with their cats using their hands or feet as toys to be attacked. Punishment in the form of water from a squirt bottle can be used as soon as the cat initiates a playful attack. The cat's behavior should then immediately be redirected to a toy.

For reasons not well understood, many cats seem to find petting to be aversive and will bite or scratch in response. In some cats, only prolonged petting stimulates this behavior, whereas in others, it can be triggered shortly after the cat is touched. Although owners often state that the cat attacked without warning, usually these cats display subtle signals such as backward ear movements or tail twitching, which owners have not perceived, as indications of their intent to attack. In these cases, owners should be instructed to pet the cats only for relatively brief periods and to use food rewards to make petting pleasant for longer periods and delay the onset of aggression.

COMMON BEHAVIOR PROBLEMS IN THE HORSE

Experience indicates that small animal owners may be more likely to seek professional assistance with behavior problems than large animal owners. Although the horse can serve primarily a companion animal function, many horse owners may prefer to attempt to resolve behavior problems by themselves or prefer to seek advice from other horse owners. The problems selected to be discussed are ones that could also be encountered at the clinic when boarding or handling horses.

Cribbing, Wind-Sucking, and Wood-Chewing

Cribbing is a behavior in which the horse holds a section of a horizontal surface such as a trough or fence rail with its incisors, flexes its neck, and sucks in and swallows air. If a horse swallows air without grasping an object, the behavior is usually referred to as wind-sucking. Horses that display wood-chewing behavior actually ingest the wood.

Causes

The causes of cribbing and wind-sucking have been much debated. Cribbing may occur more frequently when horses are stabled or confined or are anxious or stressed. It has been suggested that the swallowing of air, which occurs in windsucking, may be pleasurable, especially if a horse is experiencing gastrointestinal pain. Cribbing, wind-sucking, and chewing may be behavioral adaptations to living in a confined environment or to other kinds of environmental stressors. Wood-chewing may also be related to dietary problems such as insufficient roughage.

Intervention Procedures

Surgical procedures and physical restraints have been used to stop cribbing and wind-sucking. These do not change the horse's motivation but simply prevent the behavior from occurring. Severing spinal nerves or neck muscles or preventing access to horizontal surfaces by the use of neck straps or by covering surfaces with metal, wire, or unpleasant-tasting substances are examples. These procedures should only be used as methods of last resort. It is much more humane to identify the causes of the stress and either remove them, such as by reducing the frequency of confinement, or to use desensitization and counterconditioning procedures to adapt the animal to the stressors.

Trailering (Loading) Problems

Causes

Many horses that are difficult to load have come to associate fear, pain, or injury with the procedures of being loaded. In addition to the horse's general neophobia (fear of new or different things), which can make loading difficult, several characteristics of the trailer itself can easily elicit fear. These include (1) interior darkness, (2) the hollow sound of hooves on the ramp, and (3) the instability of the ramp and vehicle.

Intervention Procedures

Ideally, it is much better to prevent loading problems by associating a pleasant stimulus (such as food) with the process of loading, refraining from hitting the horse during loading, and loading in a safe, cautious, and unhurried fashion so that the horse is not subjected to injury. Lighting the interior of the trailer and using more solid, stable ramps and vehicles can prevent or help to correct some loading problems. When these changes to the environment are ineffective, behavior modification such as counterconditioning and desensitization may be needed to reduce fear. These procedures reinforce the horse for loading itself by having the horse initially approach the trailer and, ultimately, enter it to eat. The food is initially placed at the bottom of the ramp and, over a period of days or weeks, gradually moved until it is at the front of the trailer. It is important that the procedure be done gradually and that the horse not be forced into the trailer. If the horse becomes fearful during the process, it should be allowed to move away until it is calm and then moved back toward the trailer later.

Because horses are herd, or social, animals, social facilitation can at times be used by encouraging a difficult horse to follow another into a trailer. If a horse must be forced into a trailer in an immediate situation, pushing by using long ropes or joining arms behind the horse is preferred over hitting. Training the horse to move in response to a touch on its body is an effective procedure that can be applied to loading problems.

Aggression

Causes

Aggressive behavior from a horse presents the threat of substantial physical injury to other horses as well as to people. Effectively resolving aggression problems requires an accurate determination of the type of aggression and consistent application of techniques based on behavioral principles. Types of aggression that are frequently encountered include pain-induced, fear-induced, intermale, dominance, possessive, playful, and redi-

rected. These categories are defined and briefly described (see Table 2–6).

TECHNICIAN NOTE

Aggressive behavior from a horse presents the threat of substantial injury.

Intervention Procedures

In most situations, the goal when encountering an aggressive horse will be to manage the animal in the current situation rather than attempting to more permanently resolve the problem. Methods of restraint are discussed in Chapter 1. Many types of aggression are most responsive to counterconditioning and desensitization techniques. The stimulus eliciting aggression should first be presented at a subthreshold level, so the aggressive response is not initiated. This can be done by keeping the stimulus at a distance or attenuating some property of the stimulus such as size, intensity or duration. This subthreshold stimulus is then paired with a pleasant stimulus, such as food, which can elicit behavior incompatible with aggression. With each succeeding trial, the stimulus level is gradually increased, dependent on the horse's response. If the procedure is done incorrectly, the aggression can actually be inadvertently reinforced. Successful implementation of the techniques results in the stimulus no longer evoking aggression because it has come to be associated with pleasurable consequences.

Punishment will only exacerbate fear-induced aggression and may also elicit pain-induced or other types of defensive aggression. Mechanical restraints (e.g., hobbles or a nose twitch) may be best if they are used correctly. It was previously thought that the twitch restrained the horse by inducing pain or focusing the horse's attention, but research indicates that the twitch may trigger endorphin release, which calms the animal (Lagerweij et al, 1984).

References

Borchelt PL: Cat elimination behavior problems. Advances in Companion Animal Behavior. Veterinary Clin North Am 21:257–264, 1991.

Borchelt PL and Voith VL: Aggressive behavior in dogs and cats. *In* Voith VL and Borchelt PL (editors): Readings in Companion Animal Behavior. Trenton, NJ, Veterinary Learning Systems, 1996a.

Borchelt PL and Voith VL: Elimination behavior problems in cats. *In* Voith VL and Borchelt PL (editors): Readings in Companion Animal Behavior. Trenton, NJ, Veterinary Learning Systems, 1996b.

Borchelt PL and Voith VL: Aggressive behavior in cats. *In* Voith VL and Borchelt PL (editors): Readings in Companion Animal Behavior. Trenton, NJ, Veterinary Learning Systems, 1996c.

Center SA, Elston TH, Rowland PH, et al: Fulminant hepatic failure associated with oral administration of diazepam in 11 cats. JAVMA 209:618–625, 1996.

Cooper L and Hart BL: Comparison of diazepam with progestins for effectiveness in suppression of urine spraying behavior in cats JAVMA 200:797–801, 1992.

Coppinger R and Schneider R: Evolution of working dogs. *In* Serpell J (editor): The Domestic Dog: Its Evolution, Behavior and Interactions with People. New York, Cambridge University Press, 1995.

Gibbs M: 'Wolfman' corrections. AKC Gazette 112:22–23, 1996.

Hart BL: The Behavior of Domestic Animals. New York, WH Freeman, 1985.

Hart BL, Eckstein RA, Powell KL, and Dodman NH: Effectiveness of buspirone on urine spraying and inappropriate urination in cats. JAVMA 203:254–258, 1993.

Hetts S: Facilitating euthanasia decisions regarding animals with behavior problems. *In* Voith VL and Borchelt PL (editors): Readings in Companion Animal Behavior. Trenton, NJ, Veterinary Learning Systems, 1996.

Lagerweij E, Nelis PC, Wiegant VM, et al: The twitch in horses: A variant of acupuncture. Science 225:1172–1174, 1984.

Lagoni L, Butler C, and Hetts S: The Human-Animal Bond and Grief. Philadelphia, WB Saunders, 1994.

Marder AR: Psychotropic drugs and behavioral therapy. Vet Clin North Am 21:329–342, 1991.

McCrave EA: Diagnostic criteria for separation anxiety in the dog. Vet Clin North Am 21:247–256, 1991.

Moyer KE: The Psychobiology of Aggression. New York, Harper & Row, 1976.

Overall K: Treatment of separation related anxiety in dogs with clomipramine: Results from a multi-center, blinded, placebo-controlled clinical trial. Paper presented at AVSAB annual meeting, Reno, July 20, 1997.

Petronek GJ, Glickman LT, Beck AM, et al: Risk factors for relinquishment of dogs to an animal shelter. JAVMA 209:572–581, 1996a.

Petronek G, Glickman LT, Beck AM, et al: Risk factors for relinquishment of cats to an animal shelter. JAVMA 209:582–588, 1996b.

Simpson BS and Simpson DM: Behavioral pharmacotherapy. *In* Voith VL and Borchelt PL (editors): Readings in Companion Animal Behavior. Trenton, NJ, Veterinary Learning Systems, 1996.

Simpson BS: Psychopharmacology for pets: Indications and side effects. *In* Convention Notes from the 133rd Annual Convention in Louisville, AVMA, Schaumburg, IL.

Voith VL and Borchelt PL: Separation anxiety in dogs. *In* Voith VL and Borchelt PL (editors): Readings in Companion Animal Behavior. Trenton, NJ, Veterinary Learning Systems, 1996.

Recommended Reading

Beaver BV: Feline Behavior: A Guide for Veterinarians. Philadelphia, WB Saunders, 1992.

Hart BL and Hart LA: Canine and Feline Behavioral Therapy. Philadelphia, Lea & Febiger, 1985.

Houpt KA: Domestic Animal Behavior for Veterinarians and Animal Scientists, 2nd edition. Ames, IA, Iowa State University Press, 1991.

Leyhausen P: Cat Behavior, New York, Garland TPM Press, 1979.

Marder A and Voith VL: Advances in companion animal behavior. Vet Clin North Am (Small Anim Pract) 21(2):203–420, 1991.

Rutherford CL and Neil DH: How to Raise a Puppy You Can Live With, 2nd edition. Loveland, CO, Alpine Pub., 1992.

Scott JP and Fuller JL: Genetics and the Social Behavior of the Dog. Chicago, University of Chicago Press, 1965.

Serpell J (editor): The Domestic Dog: Its Evolution, Behavior and Interaction with People. New York, Cambridge University Press, 1995.

Thorpe C (editor): The Waltham Book of Dog and Cat Behavior. New York, Pergamon Press, 1992.

Tortora DF: Help! This Animal Is Driving Me Crazy. Chicago, Playboy Press, 1977.

Tortora DF: Applied animal psychology: the practical implications of comparative analysis. *In* Denny MR (editor): Comparative Psychology. New York, John Wiley and Sons, 1980.

Turner DC and Barteson P (editors): The Domestic Cat: The Biology of Its Behavior. New York, Cambridge University Press, 1988.

Voith VL and Borchelt PL: Animal behavior. Vet Clin North Am (Small Anim Pract) 12(4):563–743, 1982.

Voith VL and Borchelt PL: Readings in Companion Animal Behavior. Trenton, NJ, Veterinary Learning Systems, 1996.

Waring GH: Horse Behavior: The Behavioral Traits and Adaptations of Domestic and Wild Horses, Including Ponies. Park Ridge, NJ, Noyes Pub., 1983.

Wright JC: Is Your Cat Crazy? New York, MacMillan Pub. Co., 1994.

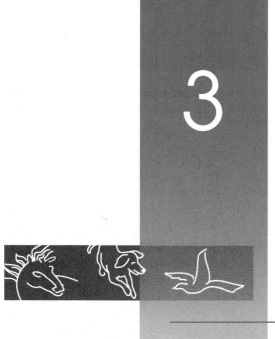

3 History and Physical Examination

Ellen Miller

OBTAINING AN ACCURATE HISTORY

Without an accurate history, even the best veterinarian may be unable to solve the problems of a particular patient. The history is the first step in reaching the ultimate diagnosis of the patient's illness. Although obtaining a history can be time consuming, information elicited from the owner may save time and effort later in the diagnostic work-up of a particular problem. For example, a common mistake is the failure to differentiate true vomiting from regurgitation; the diagnostic plans for these two problems are costly and very different. An accurate history will help the veterinarian avoid errors of this kind. In a busy practice, the technician can begin the history-taking process for the veterinarian, freeing up time for the veterinarian to later discuss the primary problem in detail with the client.

The key to history-taking is to obtain accurate information by asking the right questions. The specific questions asked will vary slightly depending on the species of animal being evaluated. In this chapter, the companion animal is the primary example.

> ✏️ **TECHNICIAN NOTE**
>
> The key to obtaining an accurate history is to ask the right questions.

Questions should be unbiased and not intended to lead the client toward a particular answer. For example, instead of asking, "Does Max drink more water than he used to?" it is preferable to ask, "Have you noticed a change in Max's water

consumption?" Many people have such a desire to please that they will, without thinking, answer your questions affirmatively. Asking a question in an unbiased fashion forces the client to think. They have to decide whether there has been a change and, if so, whether the change is positive (more water than normal) or negative (less water than normal). Sometimes, questions need to be asked two or three times but be phrased differently to ensure the owner has understood the question and is consistent with answers. In asking questions, consider the owner's ability to observe the pet. An owner may tell you that their dog does not have diarrhea when they do not normally observe their dog defecating and do not know the answer to the question. It may be better to ask, "Do you observe your dog when it defecates?" and if so, "Does your dog have diarrhea?"

Because animal patients cannot talk for themselves, the owner must be relied on to provide accurate information. The intelligence of the client and any handicaps that might interfere with the client's ability to observe his or her pet or properly understand or hear the questions must be weighed in the interpretation of answers to those questions.

Signalment of the Animal

The signalment of the animal is the age, breed, and sex, including reproductive status, of that animal. This information is vital in developing a list of the most likely rule-outs for the patient's problem. For example, a young animal is more likely to be vomiting due to an infectious agent, toxin ingestion, foreign body obstruction, or intussusception, whereas an older animal with the same complaint may be more likely to have kidney, liver, or pancreatic disease as the cause of the vomiting. Certain diseases are heritable and occur in particular breeds of dogs and cats. Knowing the breed is the first step in identifying a possible genetic defect. Knowledge of the sex of the patient and whether it is spayed or neutered obviously can help rule out disorders that affect one sex or the other.

Chief Complaint

TECHNICIAN NOTE

The chief complaint is the reason the client presented the patient for evaluation.

The chief complaint is the reason the client brought the animal to be evaluated. Discussing the chief complaint is the most important part of the history-taking process for the client. Although other problems may seem more important, failure to address the chief complaint can annoy the owner and imply that you are not listening. Be sure to spend time on the client's concerns before moving on to other questions. You may say something like, "That is important information, and I am also interested in your observations regarding. . . ."

History of the Present Illness

The purpose of this section of the history is to obtain detailed information regarding the chief complaint and any related problems. Duration, severity, progression, frequency, trigger situations, time of day, and character of the problem must be addressed if applicable. For instance, a miniature poodle that has a dry, honking cough (character) in response to excitement (trigger) two or three times daily (frequency) for more over a year (duration) without progression is likely to have a collapsing trachea at the root of the cough. All these clues will help narrow and prioritize the list of possible causes for the problem. In addition, the severity and progression will help determine the aggressiveness of the diagnostic work-up. The more severe the disease or rapid the progression, the quicker the diagnosis needs to be made.

Past Medical and Surgical History

TECHNICIAN NOTE

Past medical and surgical history can provide valuable information related to the current problem.

The past medical and surgical history can provide very important information related to the current problem in certain cases. Does the dog or cat have any medical problems or previous illnesses other than the chief complaint? Not only could the history have a bearing on the current problem, but it also may affect the approach to the new problem both diagnostically and therapeutically. For instance, knowing that a cat received megestrol acetate for a behavioral problem may pro-

vide a clue as to the reason for the increased thirst and urination the cat is experiencing. Increased thirst and urination are signs attributable to diabetes mellitus, which can be a sequela to progestogen therapy.

Has the animal ever had surgery, and if so, what type of surgery has it had? For example, a Yorkshire terrier presented with a draining tract from the medial aspect of the right stifle. The past history revealed the dog had surgery to repair a ruptured anterior cruciate ligament in the right stifle 8 months earlier. Based on the knowledge that sutures were most likely used to repair the ligament, it was probable the suture was acting as a foreign body and providing a nidus for infection. The current complaint was solved when the suture was removed. Had the history of the previous surgery not been known, an expensive work-up might have been undertaken.

Environmental History

The type of environment in which the pet lives often helps narrow the list of possible causes for a particular problem. The environment may be primarily indoor, outdoor, or a combination. The animal may live in an outdoor kennel or roam free. All these situations imply potential hazards. An animal that spends the majority of its life indoors is less likely to be traumatized, ingest poisons, or be exposed to infectious diseases (unless in a kennel or cattery situation) compared with an animal that lives outdoors or is free to roam.

Medication History

Information on any medication the animal is receiving is important for reasons that include prioritization of differential diagnoses, potential drug side effects, or drug interactions when additional drugs are prescribed. A dog receiving heartworm preventative is not likely to have heartworm disease as the cause of exercise intolerance provided the correct dose is given at the appropriate time intervals. An animal that presents with a history of increased thirst and urination while being treated with corticosteroids may not have a serious problem because these are common side effects of the drug. This knowledge can prevent an unnecessary work-up or help provide an explanation of abnormal laboratory results. An animal receiving corticosteroids for a skin disorder should not be given aspirin at the same time for an acute lameness. If the history of corticosteroid therapy was not known and aspirin was prescribed at antiinflammatory dosages, life-threatening complications, including gastrointestinal ulceration and kidney failure, may result.

Dietary History

It is important to know what type of food and how much food a patient is consuming, especially when dealing with problems of weight loss or obesity, vomiting, diarrhea, and anorexia. For instance, diet must be considered as a potential problem in a dog that has lost weight but has a good appetite. Knowledge of the diet will allow analysis of the digestibility and, therefore, the availability of the nutrients to the animal. If the diet or amount of food the dog is fed is in question, this can be addressed before a costly diagnostic work-up by feeding the dog a high-quality diet in adequate amounts for a period of time and reassessing the body weight to evaluate a response. Another situation in which dietary history is imperative is in regard to the unregulated diabetic animal. A semimoist-type diet with high quantities of simple carbohydrates will cause a postprandial rise in blood glucose, resulting in polyuria and polydipsia.

Dietary history includes questions regarding the potential for toxin, garbage, or foreign body ingestion. Again, answers to these questions may provide crucial information as to the cause of the pet's problem.

> **TECHNICIAN NOTE**
>
> A complete systems review requires that one or two questions be asked about each body system.

Systems Review

The systems review is necessary to ensure a complete history is taken. A systems review requires that one or two questions be asked regarding each body system to identify other problems that the owner may have overlooked or deemed unimportant. These problems, when put together with the chief complaint, may provide evidence to support a specific disease as the cause of the animal's illness. For example, when questioning the owner about water intake in a dog with bilaterally symmetrical, nonpruritic alopecia, you find that polyuria and polydipsia are also problems. Because this combination of clinical signs is compatible with hyperadrenocorticism, the diagnostic work-up should include a screening test for this disease. Sample questions for each system can be found in Table 3–1. For ease of remembering, major systems can be listed on a standard history form (Fig. 3–1). If a response to any of these questions is positive, then the problem should be pursued with further questions as to the duration, severity, character, and so on.

COMPONENTS OF A COMPLETE PHYSICAL EXAMINATION

General

A complete physical examination begins with a general impression of the dog or cat, including its attitude, awareness of its surroundings, gait, and general appearance (body weight, condition, and appearance of the coat). This portion of the physical examination can begin as soon as you meet the pet and lead it to the examination room. Observe the animal in its new environment. Is it curious and exploring? Is it aware of noises outside the room? Is it totally uninterested in or unable to respond to the new stimuli? Is it favoring any legs when it walks into the room? It is also appropriate to include measurement of the vital signs, including temperature, pulse, and respirations.

Systems Assessment

The systems assessment is comparable to the systems review section of the history. Each system is examined thoroughly for abnormalities. There is no particular order in which the systems are examined, but a routine pattern should be established by the individual performing the physical examination so no sys-

• Table 3–1 •

SAMPLE HISTORY QUESTIONS FOR EACH BODY SYSTEM	
SYSTEM	**QUESTION**
General	How is your pet's attitude? Is he or she interested in the family? Is your pet playful?
Integument	Is your pet scratching, licking, or biting excessively? What do you think of your pet's haircoat?
Respiratory	Is your pet coughing or sneezing? Is there any nasal discharge?
Cardiovascular	Has there been a change in your pet's activity level? Do you exercise your pet regularly, and if so, have there been any changes in the amount of exercise your pet will tolerate? Does your pet cough?
Gastrointestinal	Has there been any vomiting? How is your pet's appetite? Have there been any changes in the stool character?
Genitourinary	Has your pet ever been bred? Has there been a change in the urinating habits of your pet? Do you think your pet drinks the same amount of water as before this problem started?
Musculoskeletal	Have you noticed any lameness?
Neurologic	Does your pet seem alert and aware of his or her surroundings? Is your pet weak or unable to support weight?
Special senses	Does your pet see sufficiently well? Does your pet hear normally?

tem will be forgotten or overlooked. Some clinicians prefer to examine the animal from nose to tail, intermingling the systems together, whereas other clinicians will examine each system separately. It does not matter how it is accomplished as long as the examination is complete and thorough. A standardized physical examination form (Fig. 3–2) can provide prompting until a routine is developed. The systems can be listed and numbered at the top of the form, with boxes to check if normal or abnormal. Any abnormality can be listed in the space provided by the corresponding system number.

> **TECHNICIAN NOTE**
>
> Each of the ten body systems must be thoroughly examined during the complete physical examination.

Integument

The skin can be examined all at once or during the examination of other systems. Brush the coat with the hand in the opposite direction of the hair growth and observe for redness (erythema) or lesions such as macules, papules, pustules, or crusts. Remember to examine the skin of the extremities and check the nail beds and nails and between the toes. Is there moistness between the toes or brown discoloration indicative of excessive licking in the area? Are the foot pads normal in appearance? Are there areas of hair loss, and if so, where are they located? Is the hair loss symmetrical or patchy and random? Is the skin in areas of hair loss normal, or is it hyperpigmented,

HOSPITAL NAME

ADDRESS

OWNER INFORMATION

HISTORY

HOSPITAL REGULATION: ALL POSITIVE AS WELL AS NEGATIVE FINDINGS SHALL BE RECORDED

DATE _____ HOUR _____ | A.M. | | P.M. |

ORDER
OF
RECORDING

1. (CC) CHIEF
    COMPLAINT

2. (HPI) HISTORY
    OF PRESENT ILLNESS

3. (PH) PAST
    HISTORY
    A. MEDICAL
    B. SURGICAL
    C. TRAUMA
    D. VACCINATIONS
    E. Coggins

4. (EH) ENVIRONMENTAL
    HISTORY

5. (SR) SYSTEM
    REVIEW
    A. GENERAL
    B. SKIN
    C. HEAD/NECK
    D. (EENT) EYES-EARS-
        NOSE-THROAT
    E. RESPIRATORY
    F. CARDIOVASCULAR
    G. (GI) GASTRO-
        INTESTINAL
    H. URINARY
    I. REPRODUCTIVE
    J. MUSCULOSKELETAL
    K. NERVOUS

6. SIGNATURE

ATTENDING CLINICIAN

HISTORY

14786

Figure 3-1. A sample standard history form.

PHYSICAL EXAMINATION

(1) GENERAL APPEARANCE	☐ Normal ☐ Abnormal	(2) INTEGU-MENTARY	☐ Normal ☐ Abnormal ☐ Not examined	(3) MUSCULO-SKELETAL	☐ Normal ☐ Abnormal ☐ Not examined	(4) CIRCU-LATORY	☐ Normal ☐ Abnormal ☐ Not examined
(5) RESPIRA-TORY	☐ Normal ☐ Abnormal ☐ Not examined	(6) DIGESTIVE	☐ Normal ☐ Abnormal ☐ Not examined	(7) GENITO-URINARY	☐ Normal ☐ Abnormal ☐ Not examined	(8) EYES	☐ Normal ☐ Abnormal ☐ Not examined
(9) EARS	☐ Normal ☐ Abnormal ☐ Not examined	(10) NEURAL SYSTEM	☐ Normal ☐ Abnormal ☐ Not examined	(11) LYMPH NODES	☐ Normal ☐ Abnormal ☐ Not examined	(12) MUCOUS MEMBRANES	☐ Normal ☐ Abnormal ☐ Not examined

DESCRIBE ABNORMAL: (Use numbers above)   T _____   P _____   R _____   Wt. _____

_____

_____

_____

_____

_____

_____

_____

_____

_____

_____

_____

_____

_____

_____

_____

_____

TEMPORARY PROBLEM LIST	Initial Plan	
(1)	Dx	Rx
(2)		
(3)		
(4)		

STUDENT SIGNATURE	CLINICIAN SIGNATURE

PHYSICAL EXAMINATION

Figure 3-2. A sample standard physical examination form.

erythematous, or crusty? What is the general texture of the coat? Is it soft and fluffy like the undercoat hairs, or is it coarse like the guard hairs? Does your hand feel oily and/or dirty after touching the coat? If lumps are present, are they in the skin or under it? Are they haired or hairless? What is their overall appearance—smooth and round or irregular and cauliflower-like? Make a note of their size and location on the physical examination form. Are there areas of bruising in the skin? Is the skin excessively thin with tiny wrinkle lines and easily observed blood vessels? Are there blackheads (comedones)? All observations need to be recorded; the significance may be realized later.

Respiratory System

Examination of the respiratory system begins with the nose and throat, including the pharyngeal area. Is there a nasal discharge, and if so, is it unilateral or bilateral? What is the character of the nasal discharge? Does the animal sneeze or cough while being examined? Are the nares of normal size or stenotic as in some brachycephalic breeds? Palpate the bridge of the nose and the frontal sinus above the eyes. Are there any deformities or soft spots? In the oral cavity, examine the pharynx, tonsils, and, if possible, the edge of the soft palate and the epiglottis. Is the palate elongated? Are there any red or ulcerated areas? Are the tonsils normal and in their crypts? Use symmetry to assess for abnormalities.

Palpate the trachea and larynx. Does the animal cough easily? Are there any swellings or irregularities? Auscult over the larynx and trachea for any wheezes.

Observe the animal breathe and note the respiratory rate and pattern. Table 3–2 lists normal ranges for respiratory rates

• Table 3–2 •

NORMAL RESTING RESPIRATORY AND HEART RATES

SPECIES	RESPIRATORY RATE	HEART RATE
Cat	16–30 breaths/minute	160–240/minute
Cow	20–30 breaths/minute	50–70/minute
Dog	16–24 breaths/minute	70–180/minute (smaller breeds have higher rates; puppies can have rates up to 220/minute)
Horse	8–12 breaths/minute	36–50/minute

of four species. If the animal is having difficulty breathing, note when the problem is occurring (e.g., inspiration or expiration); this information may be important in the ultimate diagnosis of the problem. Auscult the lungs in sections or quadrants (Fig. 3–3). Normal respiratory sounds can usually be heard in a dog throughout inspiration and through the first third of expiration. The sounds are normally quiet but with exercise are louder because of the increased volume of air moving through the airways. The lung sounds of a normal cat often are heard only during inspiration. Feline lung sounds are more quiet than canine lung sounds, so if a cat's lung sounds are loud, it can be significant. If the animal is panting, all that can be heard is air moving through the large airways and the mouth noises. This is not a true representation of lung sounds, so be sure to close the animal's mouth to listen. Abnormal lung sounds are described as crackles (i.e., short, popping noises) or wheezes (i.e., longer, musical noises). Note the location and timing (expiration or inspiration) of any abnormal noises. The lack of normal respiratory sounds can also be significant and suggests a consolidated lung lobe or a lung lobe that is collapsed due to air or fluid accumulation.

Cardiovascular System

Begin with an examination of mucous membrane color and capillary refill time; blanching the color from the mucous membrane of the oral cavity over the canine tooth on the gingival mucosa or on the inner surface of the labial mucosa. It normally takes one to two seconds for the pink color to return to the area. The capillary refill time is often prolonged due to poor cardiac output as a result of dehydration or cardiac disease. Examine the jugular furrow in the neck. If the animal is standing, sitting, or lying in a sternal position, it is not normal to see a jugular pulse. Sometimes a jugular pulse can be seen in a normal animal in lateral recumbency. Palpate the femoral pulse; describe the quality as strong or weak. Does the pulse vary in intensity from pulse to pulse?

Auscult the heart over the areas as described in Figure 3–4. First, note the heart rate and rhythm. Table 3–2 lists the normal rates of four species. If the rhythm is irregular, decide whether the irregularity is related to the respiratory cycle. If the rhythm is irregularly irregular (such as no pattern at all), make a note of this. Palpate the femoral pulse while listening to the heart. Is there a pulse for every heartbeat? Next listen for any heart murmurs. Heart murmurs are described on the basis of five parameters: timing, location or point of maximal intensity, quality, grade, and radiation. Table 3–3 lists descriptions of the various murmurs. These parameters will help the veterinarian generate a list of possible differential diagnoses for the cardiac disease and give the owner some information on prognosis for their animal.

Gastrointestinal System

Examination of the gastrointestinal system begins in the oral cavity and includes the teeth, tongue, oral mucosa, and pharyn-

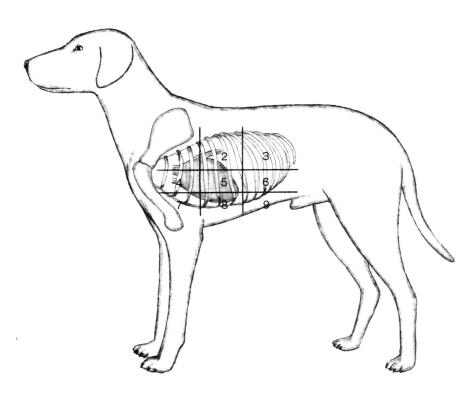

Figure 3–3. Division of the lungs into nine quadrants for auscultation and description of location of abnormal lung sounds. (From McCurnin DM and Poffenbarger EM: Small Animal Physical Diagnosis and Clinical Procedures. Philadelphia, WB Saunders, 1991.)

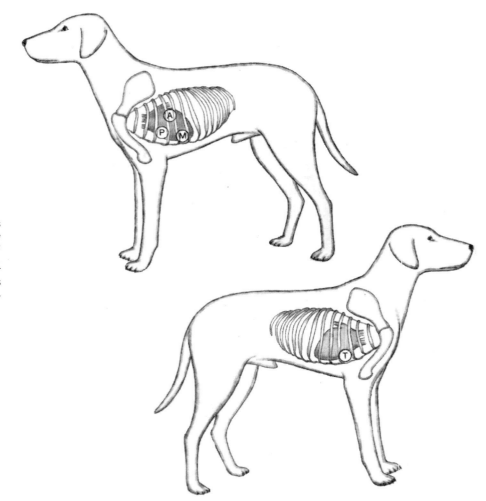

Figure 3-4. Location of heart valves as an aid in the determination of the origin of a heart murmur. P, pulmonic; A, aortic; M, mitral; and T, tricuspid. (From McCurnin DM and Poffenbarger EM: Small Animal Physical Diagnosis and Clinical Procedures. Philadelphia, WB Saunders, 1991.)

geal area. Next, palpate the neck for any esophageal masses or foreign objects.

Abdominal palpation requires practice and patience to obtain any useful information. In most dogs, a two-handed technique is the best method (Fig. 3–5). Stand on either side or to the rear of the dog. Put a hand on either side of the abdomen. The hands should be in a flat but relaxed position. Begin palpating the abdomen in the dorsal, cranial region. With gentle pressure, try to move your hands toward each other. If you move slowly, the animal usually will relax. Do not use the fingertips or the animal will tense the abdominal muscles and palpation will become very difficult. Slowly move your hands toward the ventral, cranial abdomen and feel as structures slip past your fingers. When you have reached the ventrum, move to the dorsal, central region and repeat the same steps. Finally, examine the caudal abdomen in a similar manner. Figure 3–6 illustrates the organs found in the various abdominal quadrants. In a cat or small dog, the one-handed palpation technique is often easier to use (Fig. 3–7). The thumb is placed on one side of the animal while the four fingers are placed on the other side of the abdomen. Again, using gentle pressure and a flat hand, begin palpating the dorsal, cranial region of the abdomen and move on to the other areas. Often, the four fingers can be used to trap a structure, and the thumb can be moved over its surface to get an idea of the texture, shape, and size of the structure.

With the gastrointestinal tract of a normal animal, you will not identify much except intestines slipping between your fingers. If the animal has recently consumed a meal, the stomach may be palpated behind the ribs as far caudal as the mid abdomen. Note any pain during palpation and where it is elicited. Are there any abnormal structures? If so, what is the shape, size, and consistency? Does the structure seem to have intestines coming from each end as with an intussusception, foreign body, or intestinal tumor? If the abdomen is distended and it is difficult to discern anything, make a note of that.

The perineal area should be examined for evidence of diarrhea caked on the hairs or inflammation of the surrounding skin. A rectal examination can be performed to determine whether any rectal masses, strictures, or enlargements are present. Rectal examination in the equine and bovine species is a major part of the examination to evaluate digestive and reproductive structures.

Urogenital System

The kidneys are readily palpated in the normal cat; however, due to anatomic differences, the right kidney of the normal dog is rarely palpated, and only the caudal pole of the left kidney can be palpated in a small percentage of cases. The kidneys should feel smooth on their surface. Note whether the shape is irregular or if the surface feels generally roughened. The size

• Table 3–3 •

DESCRIPTION OF HEART MURMURS

LOCATION

This is usually the valve area over which the murmur is loudest:
Aortic
Mitral
Tricuspid
Pulmonic
The location may also be described in relation to chest structures, as sternal border

TIMING

This refers to the part of the cardiac cycle during which the murmur is heard:
Systole
Diastole
Continuous

DURATION

This refers to the duration within systole or diastole in which the murmur is heard:
Early systole
Holosystolic (pansystolic)

CHARACTER

This refers to the quality of the murmur:
Plateau or regurgitant-type (same sound for the duration of the murmur)
Decrescendo, crescendo, or crescendo-decrescendo or ejection-type (intensity changes throughout the duration of the murmur)
Machinery (heard throughout systole and diastole)
Decrescendo or blowing

GRADE

1/6—Can only be heard in a quiet room after several minutes of listening
2/6—Can be heard immediately but is very soft
3/6—Low to moderate intensity
4/6—Loud but without a palpable thrill
5/6—Loud with a palpable thrill
6/6—Can be heard with the stethoscope bell slightly off the thoracic wall

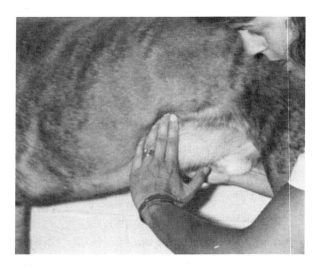

Figure 3-5. Two-handed abdominal palpation in the dog. (From McCurnin DM and Poffenbarger EM: Small Animal Physical Diagnosis and Clinical Procedures. Philadelphia, WB Saunders, 1991.)

of the kidneys varies with the size of the animal. In the average 10-lb cat, the kidney is usually 2.5 to 3.5 cm in length and spherical.

The urinary bladder can usually be palpated in the caudal ventral abdomen, depending on its degree of fullness. It will be pear shaped with the small end directed caudally in a dog, whereas it is usually spherical in a cat. It should feel fluctuant or fluid filled. Abnormalities might include a very firm bladder as occurs with chronic infection, bladder stones, or neoplasia or a gritty feel when multiple stones are present. The uterus can sometimes be palpated in the female dog if it is enlarged due to pregnancy, infection (pyometra), or neoplasia. The cervix is dorsal to the urinary bladder and can be palpated during certain stages of the estrus cycle and during pregnancy. It is a firm, tubular structure during these times. The uterine horns can be followed cranioventrally from the cervix.

The urethra can be palpated in the male or female dog rectally on the floor of the pelvis as a turgid tubular structure. In the male dog, the prostate gland can be felt as a widening in the pelvic urethra into a bilobed, firm, walnut-sized gland. Note any asymmetry, pain, or irregularities in the prostate and pelvic urethra. The male dog urethra can then be followed distally (caudally) through palpation of the perineal area on the

midline. From here it becomes surrounded by penile tissue and is impossible to make out as a separate structure. The penis should be palpated for pain and abnormal shape. Extrude the penis from its sheath and note the color and surface texture.

The testicles of the intact male dog and cat are located in the scrotum in the caudal (cat) or ventral (dog) perineal area. They should be smooth on the surface and symmetrical in shape and size. Note any pain on palpation or irregularity in size or shape.

Palpate the mammary chains of the female dog and cat for lumps. Note any pain or swelling. Milk can be expressed from the glands of lactating animals and during the last 1 or 2 weeks of gestation. Examine the milk for color changes; normal milk varies from white to a creamy yellow color.

Musculoskeletal System

Palpate the muscles of the head and limbs, and note any pain or asymmetry. Are the underlying skeletal structures more easy to palpate than normal, indicating atrophy or degeneration of the muscles?

Beginning with the toes, palpate the bones and joints of each limb. Manipulate the joints through their full range of motion, and note any pain response or crepitus (crackling). Firmly palpate the long bones and note any pain response. With your thumb, put firm but gentle pressure on the dorsal spinous process of the thoracic vertebrae one at a time, moving caudally through the lumbar region to the sacrum. Note whether the animal flinches or drops down to move away from the pressure.

Nervous System

The nervous system is technically difficult and time consuming to examine completely. Some knowledge of neuroanatomy, structure, and function is necessary to accurately assess the location and cause of a neurological problem. Therefore, a complete neurological examination is usually reserved for the patient with known or suspected neurological disease. The general appearance of the animal, including mental attitude and

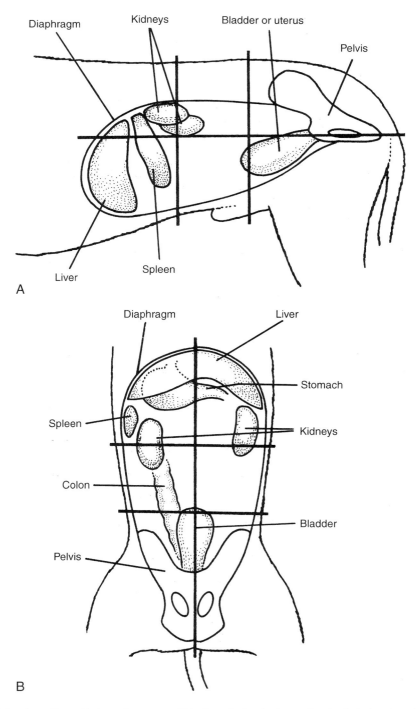

Figure 3–6. Location of internal organs within the abdominal quadrants. A, Lateral projection. B, Ventrodorsal projection. (From McCurnin DM and Poffenbarger EM: Small Animal Physical Diagnosis and Clinical Procedures. Philadelphia, WB Saunders, 1991.)

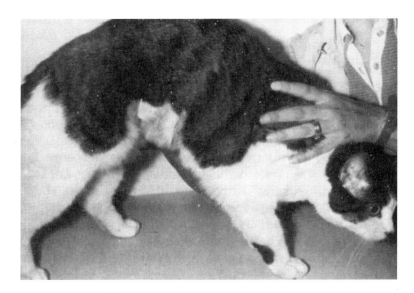

Figure 3-7. One-handed abdominal palpation in the cat. (From McCurnin DM and Poffenbarger EM: Small Animal Physical Diagnosis and Clinical Procedures. Philadelphia, WB Saunders, 1991.)

ability to ambulate, can give information regarding the need for a complete neurological examination.

The central nervous system can be divided into the brain and the spinal cord for ease of examination and localization of lesions. To assess the brain, the mental status and cranial nerves are examined. Is the animal alert and aware of its surroundings? Does it respond appropriately to stimuli, such as noises or movement? Table 3–4 lists the specific cranial nerves, tests to

assess them, and the expected outcomes in the normal and abnormal patient.

Localization and characterization of lesions within the spinal cord require assessment of spinal reflexes, postural reactions, and response to painful stimuli. Spinal reflexes are assessed by gentle but firm tapping of a tendon to note the degree of response (contraction) of the muscle. The most common reflexes assessed are the triceps in the front leg (Fig. 3–8)

• Table 3–4 •

		RESPONSE	
NERVE	**TEST**	**Normal**	**Abnormal**
I. Olfactory	Volatile substance	Sniff, recoil, nose lick	No response
II. Optic	Menace	Blink	No blink
	Pupillary light reflex	Direct, consensual responses present	No direct or consensual responses
III. Oculomotor	Pupillary light reflex	Direct, consensual responses present	No direct response, consensual intact
	Observe eye follow an object	Normal eye movement	Impaired ocular movement in ventral, dorsal, and medial directions
IV. Trochlear	Observe	Normal eye position	Dorsomedial strabismus
V. Trigeminal	Observe	Can close jaw	Jaw drop
	Palpate temporalis	Normal muscle tone	Muscle atrophy
	Corneal reflex	Eye blink	No blink
	Palpebral reflex	Eye blink	No blink
VI. Abducens	Observe	Normal eye position	Medial strabismus
VII. Facial	Observe	Facial symmetry	Lip droop
	Corneal reflex	Eye blink	No blink
	Palpebral reflex	Eye blink	No blink
	Menace	Eye blink	No blink
VIII. Acoustic	Handclap	Startle response	No response
	Move head horizontally, vertically	Normal nystagmus	No response, resting or positional nystagmus
	Observe	Normal head posture	Head tilt
	Righting response	Normal righting	Unable to right
IX. Glossopharyngeal	Gag reflex	Swallow	No response
X. Vagus	Gag reflex	Swallow	No response
	Oculocardiac reflex	Bradycardia	No response
	Laryngeal reflex	Cough	No response
XI. Accessory	Palpate neck muscles	Normal muscle tone	Muscle atrophy
XII. Hypoglossal	Tongue stretch	Retraction of tongue	No response

From McCurnin DM and Poffenbarger EM: Small Animal Physical Diagnosis and Clinical Procedures. Philadelphia, WB Saunders, 1991, p 115.

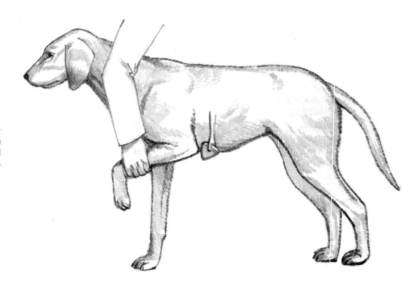

Figure 3–8. The triceps reflex can be elicited in lateral recumbency or standing, as shown. (From McCurnin DM, and Poffenbarger EM: Small Animal Physical Diagnosis and Clinical Procedures. Philadelphia, WB Saunders, 1991.)

and the quadriceps or patellar (Fig. 3–9) and gastrocnemius reflexes (Fig. 3–10) in the hind limb. The response is graded as in Table 3–5.

Postural reactions include conscious proprioception, wheel-barrowing, hemistanding and hemiwalking, and hopping. The most commonly performed test is the reaction of conscious proprioception, in which the foot is gently turned so that the animal is standing on the top of its foot. Each foot is tested individually. A normal animal will immediately right the foot. A slow or absent response is usually indicative of spinal cord disease. Wheel-barrowing is performed by holding the animal's rear legs in the air while slowly moving forward; the normal animal will move the front legs forward and maintain an upright position. Hemistanding and hemiwalking require that the front and rear legs on the same side be supported while the animal is required to stand or walk, respectively. A normal animal can stand with ease and walk with minor difficulty. Hopping responses are assessed by holding three of four legs up with the fourth allowed to touch the floor or table. The animal is slowly moved toward the side with the leg down. A normal animal will move the leg laterally to attempt to support weight and maintain balance.

Superficial and deep pain perception are assessed by pinching the skin or bone of the toe area, respectively. The normal response is withdrawal of the leg with some acknowledgment of pain, such as turning to look at the toe, dilation of

the pupils, or a growl or snap. If both responses are absent, the prognosis for recovery is poor.

The *panniculus* reflex is a simple test that aids in the localization of a spinal cord lesion. It is performed by gently pinching the skin of the back just lateral to the midline and watching for a reflex contraction of the skin. Start with the skin near the tail and slowly work forward. The lesion is approximately one vertebra caudal to the location where the first response is elicited.

Last, the anal tone and perineal reflex should be assessed. The anus should be closed and not gaping open. The perineal reflex is tested by gently stimulating the skin around the anus and watching for a "wink," or contraction, of the anal sphincter.

Peripheral Lymph Nodes

The peripheral lymph nodes that can be palpated in the normal animal include the submandibular, prescapular, and popliteal. Usually, the axillary and inguinal lymph nodes will be palpated only if enlarged. Symmetry often is a clue to any abnormalities, so palpate both sides at the same time for comparison.

The submandibular lymph nodes are located at the ventral aspect of the neck near the angle of the jaw. There usually are two on each side just cranial to the mandibular salivary gland. The trick to palpating them is to grab the extra skin of the ventral neck between the thumb and forefingers. Slowly move

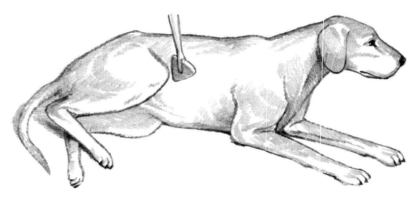

Figure 3–9. The femoral, or patellar, reflex. (From McCurnin DM and Poffenbarger EM: Small Animal Physical Diagnosis and Clinical Procedures. Philadelphia, WB Saunders, 1991.)

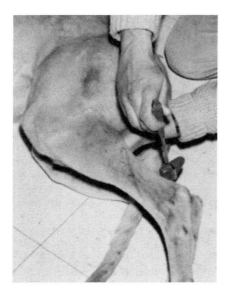

Figure 3-10. The gastrocnemius reflex. (From McCurnin DM and Poffenbarger EM: Small Animal Physical Diagnosis and Clinical Procedures. Philadelphia, WB Saunders, 1991.)

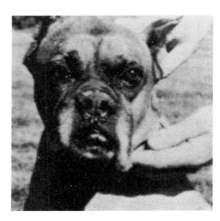

Figure 3-11. External ear and head examination showing facial nerve paralysis (note the drooped lip on the left side of the face). (From Oliver JE Jr, Hoerlein BF, Mayhew IG: Veterinary Neurology. Philadelphia, WB Saunders, 1984.)

your hands rostrally, and the nodes should slip through your fingers. In the cat, these nodes are normally pea sized, whereas in the dog, they vary from pea sized (small dogs) to small grape sized (large dogs).

The prescapular lymph nodes lie in the connective tissue just cranial and dorsal to the shoulder joint. Again, it is easiest to grab the skin and muscles and then let the lymph nodes slip through your fingers as you pull your hands cranially. These lymph nodes range from similar in size to slightly larger than the submandibular nodes.

The popliteal lymph nodes can be palpated in the fat pad just caudal to the stifle joint.

Ears

Examination of the ears involves palpation and visual examination of the pinnae, or ear flaps, as well as visual inspection of the external ear canal (Fig. 3–11). Common abnormalities of the ear flaps include hair loss, crusting margins as occurs with mange or flea-bite dermatitis, hematomas (blood-filled pockets within the pinna), and skin tumors. The external ear canal should be free of exudate, debris, or hair. If exudate is present, the character of the discharge should be noted (dark-brown and flaky as occurs with ear mites, dark brown and malodorous as occurs with yeast infections, or purulent as occurs with bacterial otitis).

If abnormalities are noted on visual inspection or ear disease is the chief complaint, an otoscopic examination should be performed. Holding the pinna up, the otoscope cone is gently inserted into the vertical ear canal. While looking through the otoscope, the otoscope is slowly advanced and rotated 90 degrees to examine the horizontal part of the ear canal. Note any redness, exudate, foreign objects, mites, polyps or tumors, or hemorrhage. The tympanic membrane or eardrum can be visualized at the end of the horizontal canal as a white translucent membrane. Note any color change or lack of translucency, which is indicative of exudate or hemorrhage in the middle ear.

Eyes

A good ocular examination includes an examination of the external ocular features (eyelids, sclera, cornea, and third eyelid [nictitating membrane]) as well as internal ocular features (anterior chamber, iris, and lens), all of which can be visualized without special equipment. First, note the character of any discharge present in or under the eyes. If present, is it watery, mucoid, purulent, or ropy? Examine the eyelid margins for small masses, aberrant eyelashes, and position. Do the eyelids seem to roll inward (entropion) so that the lashes rub on the cornea? Or do the eyelids appear to be loose and not in contact with the eye (ectropion)? Is the sclera white or red, as in the inflamed eye. Is the third eyelid in its normal position, or does it appear to be bulging or protruding across the eye? Is the cornea clear or cloudy? If cloudy, note the location of the cloudiness. Does the cornea appear wet? Are there small blood vessels present on the surface of the cornea?

The anterior chamber (portion of the eye in front of the lens and iris) should be clear, allowing easy visualization of the iris. Note any hemorrhage or purulent debris in the anterior chamber. Examine the iris and compare with the opposite side for symmetry. Are the pupil sizes equal? Are there any brown spots on the iris? Does the iris appear to be tattered? Shine a light in one eye and note the response in both eyes. Both pupils in a normal animal will constrict when a light is shined in either eye. Carefully record any deviations from normal.

Recommended Reading

McCurnin DM and Poffenbarger EM: Small Animal Physical Diagnosis and Clinical Procedures. Philadelphia, WB Saunders, 1991.

• Table 3–5 •

GRADING OF REFLEX RESPONSES	
GRADE	**DESCRIPTION**
0	No response
1	Hyporeflexia (less-than-normal response)
2	Normal response
3	Hyperreflexia (greater-than-normal response)
4	Clonus (repetitive response)

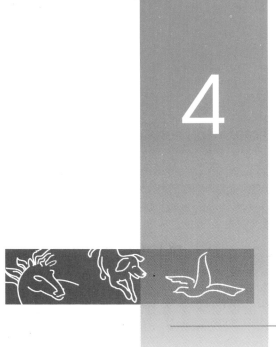

4 The Medical Record

Sharee A. Chavis • Judith L. Hutton

INTRODUCTION

The medical record is the compilation of pertinent facts about the animal patient's life and health history. It describes past and present illnesses and treatments ordered by the clinician. It serves as a basis for planning the animal's care and provides continuity in evaluating his or her condition and treatment. The combination of the history provided by the animal's owner or agent and the clinician's observations and results of any laboratory tests performed helps to determine a diagnosis and course of treatment to follow in each case.

The medical record must be compiled in a timely manner. Important medical details may be forgotten if they are not recorded quickly. The record should contain sufficient data to identify the animal, support the diagnosis, justify the treatment, and accurately document the results. The pertinent and accurate information contained therein will help the health professional diagnose and treat the animal's condition now and in the future.

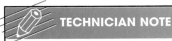

> **TECHNICIAN NOTE**
>
> Remember to stamp or write the pet's identifying information on each page in the record.

The process of ensuring that the medical record is complete and useful is a challenging and complex task. It entails a thorough knowledge of the medical record and its content, along with ancillary information concerning its purpose, ownership, value, and uses and those involved in responsibility for its maintenance.

A complete record should contain the owner's name, address, place of employment, and telephone numbers at work and home. It also includes animal identification, such as the case number, name, sex, age, color, species, and breed (Fig. 4–1). All treatment sheets, laboratory results, and electrocardiography strips should be stamped with the animal's identifying information to avoid loss of important data from the record. When the forms are not identifiable, they may be discarded and the data lost.

The comprehensive record contains but is not limited to the following sections:

1. Symptoms
2. Patient's comprehensive history
3. Vaccination status
4. Consultation/physical examination
5. Diagnosis
6. Discharge summary
7. Prognosis
8. Client education of patient's aftercare
9. Biopsy or necropsy findings if applicable
10. Client's authorization for patient's treatment
11. Financial information (mode of fee payment) such as credit card, cash, or check
12. Fee estimate (on all hospitalized cases)

OWNERSHIP OF THE RECORD

The original medical record, along with radiographic films and laboratory reports or electrodiagnostic tests, is the property of the hospital or owner of the practice providing the service. The client purchases the professional services rendered and medical

59

DATE_____   CASE NUMBER_____

COMPANION ANIMAL CLIENT/PATIENT INFORMATION FORM

Please provide the following information for our records: **PLEASE PRINT!**

OWNER INFORMATION

OWNER'S NAME Marissa Miller	SOCIAL SECURITY NUMBER 081 68 8335

STREET ADDRESS 426 Worth Main St Apt 4

CITY STATE Randolph MA	ZIP CODE 02368	PARISH OR COUNTY

TELEPHONE NUMBER(S) (Area Code, if long distance) → HOME 781-986-0935	BUSINESS 781-964-6313

DRIVER'S LICENSE NUMBER	PLACE OF EMPLOYMENT Harvard Medical School	HOW LONG?

ANIMAL INFORMATION

ANIMAL SPECIES (Dog, Cat, Other) feline	BREED DLH

ANIMAL'S NAME Spooky	SEX F	HAS ANIMAL BEEN SEXUALLY ALTERED? ☒ Yes ☐ No

COLOR Blk/wht	BIRTHDATE (Month/year, or approximate) May '99	The undersigned owner or agent certifies that the herein described animal has a maximum value of approximately $

REFERRAL INFORMATION

WERE YOU REFERRED BY A VETERINARIAN? ☐ Yes ☐ No	IF YOU WERE REFERRED BY A VETERINARIAN, PLEASE COMPLETE THE FOLLOWING:

VETERINARIAN'S NAME	PHONE

STREET ADDRESS

CITY/STATE	ZIP CODE

You will be advised of estimated cost and anticipated procedures. Please feel free to discuss the proposed treatment and its cost with the veterinarian. A minimum deposit of 50% of the initial estimated charges will be required for hospitalization of an animal patient.

STATEMENT OF OWNERSHIP AND CONSENT: I am the owner of the above described animal, or have authorization from the owner to consent to its treatment.

I hereby authorize the performance of professionally accepted diagnostic, therapeutic, anesthetic, and surgical procedures necessary for its treatment.

I accept financial responsibility for these services.

I have read the above consent and understand why the above procedures may be necessary. I also have been told of the possible complications and alternatives to the listed procedures.

PAYMENT CHOICE: ☐ Cash   ☐ Check   ☐ Bank Card

SIGNATURE (Owner/Agent)	DATE

Figure 4-1. Client/patient information form.

information but not the original record itself. The record owner (hospital or practice owner) may release any or all of the medical record information at his or her discretion, according to state law. Photocopies of part or all of the record may be released to the owner with approval of the attending veterinarian. Photocopy charges may be assessed to cover the costs in some cases.

ORDER OF THE MEDICAL RECORD

Because of the many types of forms it contains, the medical record should be put together in a consistent and timely manner. This allows the health professional to quickly and effectively locate needed information. Different colored tabs or dividers can be added to the record to speed information location.

The order of the record can be different for outpatients and inpatients. Every veterinary clinic and hospital tends to establish its own procedure for the order of records. During the patient's hospital stay, the progress notes, current laboratory results, and description of treatments performed need to be readily available. Once the patient is discharged, the diagnosis and billing information are of main concern. After patient dismissal, the record is put in permanent order. Having a uniform method of organizing the medical record will allow easy access by the professional and hospital staff.

Missing information should be readily noticed and added to the chart as soon as it becomes available. The results of laboratory tests (e.g., tissue biopsy) submitted to an outside laboratory for analysis must be added to the medical record as they are received.

The best method of organizing the medical record is the use of reverse chronological order, in which the most recent data are on top. This saves time that would otherwise be spent digging through a mountain of paperwork to find the most recent visit results.

MEDICAL RECORD FORMATS

Two formats are generally used in medical records: *conventional* and *problem oriented.*

The conventional method is source oriented. The data are entered chronologically as acquired, and this format varies in order and size. Less time is needed to complete these records, and this type of record-keeping can be easily adapted to a practice of any size. The greatest disadvantage is the lack of necessary details and documentation of procedures to maintain adequate communication and legal protection.

The problem-oriented veterinary medical record (POVMR) was adapted from the problem-oriented record that was developed in the field of human medicine. It provides an organized and detailed record for every patient. It has also proved to be a valuable teaching and research tool. In group practice, a POVMR offers improved professional communication by providing a complete compilation of the patient's problems along with any procedure or treatment that may have been performed on the patient. Although it takes more time to compile this type of record, it makes available more historical data and other information to support case planning and provide protection in the event of a legal claim.

MASTER PROBLEM LIST

A problem is anything that requires veterinary medical attention or care; it may be a symptom that the animal's owner noticed or an abnormal finding or diagnosis. The master problem list serves as a minihistory for the medical record. It lists immunizations and fecal analyses according to the dates on which they were performed and outlines problems the animal has experienced. The sheet should also include a space on which client and animal identification can be placed (Fig. 4–2).

LABORATORY DIAGNOSTICS FLOW SHEET

The laboratory diagnostics flow sheet serves as a compilation of laboratory data on individual patients. It can be used for inpatients or outpatients and shows at a glance the different values for the various laboratory tests that were performed. Specific values can be compared on different dates for blood counts, chemistry tests, blood gas, urinalysis, and coagulation (Fig. 4–3). The flow sheet is usually kept as the top sheet in the record. Some of the diagnoses for which this is particularly helpful include anemia, chronic renal failure, hepatic failure, Addison's disease, rodenticide toxicity, Cushing's disease, and diabetes. There is a blank area on the bottom of the sheet that the clinician can use to keep track of other laboratory values not specifically listed on the sheet.

DATA BASE

The history, physical examination, chief complaint, laboratory tests, and radiographic results are considered the core data base of the medical record. The hospital may have a required minimum data base. Animals admitted for either a routine visit or a hospital stay will have, for example, a complete blood count, urinalysis, and fecal analysis. The data base, however, should meet the needs of any given problem. This portion of the record will expand by the addition of data from future visits. The tests done on the first visit will be considered the original data base, and any subsequent visits should provide data for the current problems.

COMPREHENSIVE HISTORY FORM

This form is of particular importance for a new patient visit or if more than 1 year elapsed since the last visit. The comprehensive history form contains information on ownership, habitat, diet, environment, and preventative medical program. It also should include a brief systems review area, along with space for the date seen, time of appointment, and clinician examining the animal (Fig. 4–4).

PHYSICAL EXAMINATION FORM

Recorded on this form are the animal's vital signs along with other physical findings. An expanded systems review should be recorded, including the details of both normal and abnormal findings (Fig. 4–5). All 11 systems should be evaluated during each physical examination.

WORKING PROBLEM LIST

The working problem list is used in the inpatient file. It provides a comprehensive overview of the pet's problems during a particular hospitalization period. The working problem list provides a quick review of previous problems without the entire record having to be read through (Fig. 4–6).

Text continued on page 68

| HOSPITAL NAME
ADDRESS
CITY STATE ZIP CODE

MASTER PROBLEM LIST | Case Number
Client Name
Address
City State Zip Code
Species Breed Sex Birthdate
Name Color Phone |

IMMUNIZATION/PREVENTATIVE RECORD

DATE										
RABIES										
DA,PL										
PARVO										
FVR-CP										
LEUKOCELL										
FeLV										
FECAL										
KNOTTS										

PROBLEM LIST

PROBLEM	DATE ENTERED	DATE RESOLVED
1.		
2.		
3.		
4.		
5.		
6.		
7.		
8.		
9.		
10.		
11.		
12.		
13.		

Figure 4–2. Master problem list.

Hospital Name _____

Address _____

City _____ State _____ Zip Code _____

SIGNALMENT

LABORATORY DIAGNOSTICS FLOW SHEET

CHEMISTRY PANEL	DATES					HEMOGRAM	DATES				
GLUCOSE mg/dL						WBC ($\times 10^3$)/μL					
AST U/L						RBC ($\times 10^6$)/μL					
ALT U/L						HGB g/dL					
ALP U/L						HCT %					
CK U/L						MCV fl					
T. BILIRUBIN mg/dL						MCH pg					
T. PROTEIN g/dL						MCHC g/dL					
ALBUMIN g/dL						PLT ($\times 10^3$)/μL					
GLOBULIN mg/dL						PCV/TS %					
CHOLESTEROL mg/dL						SEGS ($\times 10^3$)/μL					
UREA NITROGEN mg/dL						BANDS ($\times 10^3$)/μL					
CREATININE mg/dL						LYMPHS ($\times 10^3$)/μL					
CALCIUM mg/dL						MONO ($\times 10^3$)/μL					
PHOSPHORUS mg/dL						EOS ($\times 10^3$)/μL					
SODIUM mmol/L						BASOS ($\times 10^3$)/μL					
POTASSIUM mmol/L						nRBC					
CHLORIDE mmol/L						RETIC %					
TCO_2 mmol/L						**URINALYSIS**					
ANION GAP mmol/L						COLOR					
BLOOD GAS						TURBIDITY					
pH						SPECIFIC GRAVITY					
PCO_2 mm Hg						pH					
PO_2 mm Hg						PROTEIN mg/dL					
HCO_3 mmol/L						GLUCOSE mg/dL					
TCO_2 mmol/L						KETONES					
BASE EXCESS						BILIRUBIN					
COAGULATION						HEMOGLOBIN					
ACT sec						VOLUME					
PT sec PATIENT / CONTROL						CASTS (+/−)					
PTT sec PATIENT / CONTROL						WBC					
FDP μg/mL						RBC					
BMBT (Sec)						EPITH CELLS (+/−)					
						CRYSTALS (+/−)					
						BACTERIA (+/−)					

Figure 4-3. Laboratory flow sheet with reference ranges.

Illustration continued on following page

CLINICAL PATHOLOGY REFERENCE RANGES

	units	CANINE	FELINE	EQUINE	BOVINE
Total leukocytes	(x10^3/μL)	6–17	5.5–19.5	5.5–12.5	4–12
Neutrophils	(x10^3/μL)	3–11.5	2.5–12.5	2.7–6.7	0.6–4
Bands	(x10^3/μL)	0–0.3	0–0.3	0–0.1	0–0.1
Eosinophils	(x10^3/μL)	0.1–1.2	0–1.5	0–0.9	0–2.4
Basophils	(x10^3/μL)	rare	rare	0–0.2	0–0.2
Monocytes	(x10^3/μL)	0.1–1.4	0–0.8	0–0.8	0–0.8
Lymphocytes	(x10^3/μL)	1–4.8	1.5–7	1.5–5.5	2.5–7.5
Erythrocytes	(x10^6/μL)	5–8.5	5–10	6.5–12.5	5–10
Hemoglobin	(g/dL)	12–18	9–16	11–19	8–15
Hematocrit	(%)	35–55	28–45	32–52	24–46
MCV	(fl)	60–77	39–55	34–58	40–60
MCH	(pg)	21–27	13–17	10–18	11–18
MCHC	(g/dL)	32–36	30–36	30–35	30–36
Platelets	(x10^3/μL)	200–700	200–700	100–600	100–800
Plasma Protein	(g/dL)	6–7.8	6–7.5	5.2–7.8	6–8
Fibrinogen (HPP)	(mg/dL)	–	–	100–500	100–700
Glucose	(mg/dL)	75–115	85–115	70–100	60–100
ALT	(IU/L)	<100	<90	–	–
AST	(IU/L)	<60	<40	<350	<150
CK	(IU/L)	<285	<300	<300	<300
ALP	(IU/L)	<135	<45	<300	<140
GGT	(IU/L)	–	–	<45	<45
T. Bilirubin	(mg/dL)	<0.4	<0.2	<2.0	<0.5
T. Protein	(g/dL)	5.7–7.4	6.0–8.1	6.0–8.0	6.4–8.2
Globulins	(g/dL)	2.1–4.1	2.8–4.9	2.0–4.4	2.7–4.5
Albumin	(g/dL)	2.9–4.0	2.9–3.5	3.0–4.1	3.1–4.0
BUN	(mg/dL)	6–22	15–30	14–27	10–24
Creatinine	(mg/dL)	0.4–1.5	0.6–2.2	1.2–2.5	0.7–1.8
Calcium	(mg/dL)	8.6–11.2	8.9–11.0	10–13	8.5–11.1
Phosphorus	(mg/dL)	2.5–5.5	3.1–5.8	1.9–4.7	4.0–7.2
Cholesterol	(mg/dL)	130–240	90–160	–	–
Magnesium	(mmol/L)	–	–	0.60–0.95	0.70–1.10
Amylase	(IU/L)	<900	<900	<20	–
Lipase	(IU/L)	<600	<400	<20	<50
Bile Acids, fasting	(μmol/L)	<5	<2	–	–
Bile Acids, post	(μmol/L)	<20	<20	–	–
Ammonia, fasting	(μmol/L)	<32	–	<55	–
SDH	(IU/L)	–	–	<7	<15
Sodium	(mmol/L)	140–155	140–155	130–145	135–150
Potassium	(mmol/L)	3.5–5.5	3.0–5.5	3.0–5.0	3.5–5.0
Chloride	(mmol/L)	105–120	110–125	95–110	95–110
Total CO_2	(mmol/L)	20–28	20–28	24–30	21–31
Anion Gap	(mmol/L)	8–20	8–20	6–15	6–15
pH		7.31–7.50	7.24–7.40	7.30–7.43	7.35–7.50
PCO_2	(mm Hg)	29–42	29–42	36–50	35–44
HCO_3	(mmol/L)	17–24	17–24	21–30	20–30
TCO_2	(mmol/L)	18–25	18–25	22–31	21–31

Figure 4–3 *Continued*

HOSPITAL NAME
ADDRESS
CITY STATE ZIP CODE

NUMBER

NAME _____ CASE NO.
STREET _____
CITY, STATE, ZIP _____
PHONE - BUS._____ HOME _____

SPECIES	BREED	SEX

ANIMAL'S NAME _____ DATE OF BIRTH _____
COLOR——IDENTIFYING MARKS _____

CHIEF COMPLAINT:

REFERRING VETERINARIAN:

Date:

Appt. Time:

Admitting Clinician:

ENVIRONMENTAL HISTORY:
Length of time owned: _____

Kept In:
☐ Louisiana
☐ Other _____

Obtained From: Bred ☐ Breeder ☐ Friend ☐
Pet Shop ☐ Humane Society ☐ Stray ☐ Other ☐

Environment:
Urban House ☐
Apartment ☐
Suburban ☐
Rural ☐

Confined to:
Home ☐
Outdoor pen/chain ☐
Roams ☐
Other ☐

Other Pets:
Yes ☐
No ☐
_____
_____

Diet:
Commercial Dry ☐
Semimoist ☐
Canned ☐
Table Scraps ☐
Other ☐

Frequency ___ /day
Amount: ___

PREVENTATIVE MEDICINE PROGRAM:

YES		DATE	NO	YES		DATE	NO
☐	Distemper-Hepatitis	___	☐	☐	Fecal Check	___	☐
☐	Feline Panleukopenia	___	☐	☐	Heartworm Check	___	☐
☐	FVR-calici-Panleukopenia	___	☐	☐	Heartworm Preventative	___	☐
☐	Distemper-Hep-Parainfluenza	___	☐	☐	Flea Control	___	☐
☐	Rabies	___	☐	☐	Tick Control	___	☐

MEDICAL HISTORY:
Past Medical History—prior illness, surgery, drug reactions, etc.
Current Medical History—signs, chronological course, prior therapy, system review.

System Review

Attitude
Exercise
 Tolerance
Ocular or
 Nasal
 Discharge
Sneezing
Coughing
Appetite
Vomiting
Diarrhea
P/D - P/U
Pruritus
Incoordination
Paresis
Seizures
Estrus

COMPREHENSIVE HISTORY   MEDICAL RECORDS

Figure 4-4. Example of a comprehensive history form.

HOSPITAL NAME
ADDRESS
CITY STATE ZIP CODE

NUMBER

Date: _____

Temp _____ °F   Attitude _____

Fem. Pulse _____ Charac. _____ Resp. _____

Memb. Color _____ Cap. Refill Time _____

Hydration _____ Body Weight _____

Color & Consistency of feces on Therm. _____

Body Condition — Underweight ☐   Overweight ☐   Normal ☐

NAME _____
                                              CASE NO. _____
STREET _____
CITY, STATE, ZIP _____
PHONE - BUS _____ HOME _____

| SPECIES | BREED | SEX |

ANIMAL'S NAME _____ DATE OF BIRTH _____

COLOR___ IDENTIFYING MARKS

SYSTEM REVIEW

1. Integumentary	2. Otic	3. Ophthalmic	4. Musculoskeletal
☐ Normal	☐ Normal	☐ Normal	☐ Normal
☐ Abnormal	☐ Abnormal	☐ Abnormal	☐ Abnormal

5. Nervous	6. Cardiovascular	7. Respiratory	8. Digestive
☐ Normal	☐ Normal	☐ Normal	☐ Normal
☐ Abnormal	☐ Abnormal	☐ Abnormal	☐ Abnormal

9. Lymphatic	10. Reproductive	11. Urinary
☐ Normal	☐ Normal	☐ Normal
☐ Abnormal	☐ Abnormal	☐ Abnormal

DESCRIBE ABNORMAL:

EXAMINER _____

PHYSICAL EXAMINATION   **MEDICAL RECORDS**

Figure 4-5. Example of a physical examination form.

Hospital Name _____

Address _____

City _____ State _____ Zip Code _____

WORKING PROBLEMS LIST

Case Number _____

Client Name _____

Address _____

City _____ State _____ Zip Code _____

Species _____ Breed _____ Sex _____ Birthdate _____

Name _____ Color _____ Phone _____

PROBLEM NUMBER	ACTIVE DATE	PROBLEM	DATE RESOLVED

MEDICAL RECORD

Figure 4-6. Working problem list.

PROGRESS NOTES (SOAP)

SOAP is an acronym formed by the initials of the division of the progress notes: S = subjective, O = objective, A = assessment, and P = procedure.

While an animal is hospitalized, clinical notes are kept daily or on a more-frequent basis if necessary. Each of the problems is said to be "SOAPed." Any incoming information from a referring veterinarian or an animal's owner during a current hospital stay or on a subsequent visit should also be placed in the progress notes section in chronological order. Verbal agreements made with the owner either in person or by telephone (including progress reports on the animal) should be recorded in the progress notes (Fig. 4–7); each problem is "SOAPed" separately.

Many forms compose the total record, and these can be of various sizes. What is essential for the record to be considered complete is consistency of format. This consistency will ensure that anyone taking care of the animal on a professional or paraprofessional level will readily have available all of the information on the patient. When client communication occurs in person, notes are taken and included with the progress (SOAP) sheets in chronological order, with the most recent data on top (Fig. 4–7). If client communication occurs by telephone, a telephone report form should be filled out (Fig. 4–8). This form should be placed within the progress notes if the patient is in the hospital or on top of the most recent visit if the patient has gone home.

TECHNICIAN NOTE

When writing in charts, use only approved abbreviations. Do not abbreviate the final diagnosis.

CARD FILE

To conserve space and costs, many veterinary practices use a card file system instead of maintaining medical record files on each patient. The size of the card most often used is 5 × 8 inches, with a plastic pocket attached in which to store laboratory data, radiology reports, or electrocardiograph strips. This card can be stored in a file drawer (Fig. 4–9).

Another card system involves the use of a 10 × 16-inch card, which accommodates more information on the patient. It can be folded in half and stored in a file drawer. Information contained on this type of record is brief; it must contain owner and patient information along with sufficient data to allow the proper and adequate care of the animal (Fig. 4–10). The major disadvantage of the card file system is the lack of detail for patient follow-up or legal support.

TECHNICIAN NOTE

When using the file folder format for the chart, keep all information related to each visit stapled together.

RELEASE OF INFORMATION

A signed authorization form from the animal's owner should be obtained before information is released to him or her, to another veterinarian, or to an insurance company (Fig. 4–11). The attending veterinarian should be the only person to authorize release of information contained in the record; however, there is an exception to this rule. Certain local, state, and federal agencies require the reporting of any disease that may be zoonotic (see Chapter 7). Some examples of diseases are rabies, brucellosis, and equine encephalitis. The United States Department of Agriculture has published these reporting regulations in their Animal Movement Quarantine Regulations Manual.

Inquiry may also be made by a local agency such as animal control or the humane society in the event of an animal bite to a human. The reason for the request would be to check the rabies vaccination status of the animal in question.

Medical record information to a new veterinarian should be mailed to him or her and not provided directly to the owner; the owner may not understand the terminology in the record and could be misled about his or her animal's health. A cover letter should be sent with the copy of the record in the event the new veterinarian wants to contact the previous veterinarian for additional information. A flat fee for copying of the record may be charged, or the practice may levy a fee on a page-by-page basis.

TECHNICIAN NOTE

Do not white out or scribble through mistakes in records. It is a legal document! Draw a line through the mistake once and write ''void,'' ''not error,'' plus your initials next to the mistake. Example:

COLOR CODING SYSTEMS

There are two types of color coding: *alphabetical* and *numerical*. In alphabetical color coding, a different color is assigned to each letter of the alphabet, and all names that fall within that letter group are filed behind that color in alphabetical order. Additional colors may be added, depending on the desired extent of the color coding system.

In numerical color coding, one color is assigned to each digit from 0 to 9, and the colors on the record vary according to the record number. This system is invaluable in preventing chart misfiles and as a signaling device in the search for a specific record.

Color coding may also be used to signal files to be purged or files for dead animals, bad debts, or return visits, and it can be used to mark when vaccinations are due so the client can be notified.

This system can be simple or complex, depending on the size of the practice and the personnel available to keep the system running smoothly. It is imperative constant updating of the system be undertaken, or it will become useless.

HOSPITAL NAME
ADDRESS
CITY STATE ZIP CODE

Progress Notes must be recorded at least once every 24 hours. All entries must be in the SOAP format.

Page ____ of ____

Case Number
Client Name
Address
City State Zip Code
Species Breed Sex Birthdate

DATE	TEMP:	S- Subjective Data
	PULSE	O- Objective Data
	RESP.	A- Assessment
	APPETITE	P- Procedure for diagnosis and treatment
	BOWELS	

Figure 4-7. Progress notes.

TELEPHONE REPORT

Name: _____

Species: _____ Breed: _____

Sex: _____ Animal's Name: _____

Phone #: _____ DOB: _____

Date: _____ Case Number: _____

Client History: _____

_____

_____

_____

_____

Instructions to Client: _____

_____

_____

_____

_____

_____

_____

_____

_____

_____

Prescription: _____

_____

_____

_____

_____

_____

_____

_____

Signature: _____

Figure 4-8. Telephone report.

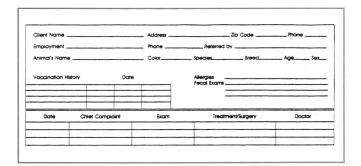

Figure 4-9. Veterinary medical record card (5 × 8 in).

FILE PURGING

Each practice or hospital will set its own rules for purging files. Generally, active records covering a 3-year period are kept in the medical records area, including files of animals that have a new veterinarian because the owner has moved. The charts of animals that have died within this period are also kept so the clinician will have them available for review or research purposes. Any inactive record that is 4 years old or older is placed in a separate storage area.

Files should be purged on a yearly basis to allow easier filing and make room available for new records. Color coding can be a big help in signaling inactive records so the entire file will not have to be checked. Recording the date of the client's last visit on the front of the file folder will allow inactive files to be easily identified and purged.

The inactive file should be in a convenient place that is easily accessible and safe, so the record can be quickly reactivated if necessary. In general, records 8 years old or older can be purged from the inactive file. They should be destroyed by shredding or burning.

LOST RECORDS

The problem of lost records in a large hospital or small practice is common. They can be lost through misfiling, incorrect spelling of names, or misplacement. At times, even after an exhaustive search, the record continues to be missing. Sometimes the loss is not discovered until the animal comes back to the practice for a return visit.

Figure 4-10. Veterinary medical record card (10 × 16 in).

It is best, in this case, to explain to the client that the record has been misplaced. A new record should be started and information requested from the client and veterinarian. In addition, copies of laboratory data, pathology reports, and radiological information should be obtained and added to reestablish the file.

Although the problem of lost records is embarrassing to the practice and inconvenient to the client, it happens with even the most elaborate record system; however, every effort possible should be made to quickly and accurately file each record after each visit. Clients place a high value on the availability of the medical record and will usually be upset if it cannot be located.

MEDICOLEGAL REQUIREMENTS

Legal requirements vary from state to state. Each state has its own guidelines on what information needs to be included, how long the records should be kept, and the requirements for release of information. It is recommended that each practice employee be familiar with these laws in the event legal questions arise.

The medical record is a legal document. Any written data contained therein must be complete, legible, and written in black ink. Any errors should not be scratched out, erased, or blotted out. A line should be drawn through the mistake and initialed. The correct information should be written and initialed next to the mistake. Any erasure or blotting out may suggest the record has been tampered with or dealt with in an unprofessional manner. This would disqualify it as a legal document. The record documents legal evidence of services and procedures performed in the event of litigation such as a malpractice suit or an insurance claim. The record is admissible as evidence in a court of law and may be subpoenaed; for this reason, the record must always be accurate and legible so it can be reviewed at any time.

> **TECHNICIAN NOTE**
>
> Use of an erasure or blotting out of information in a medical record suggests inappropriate changes.

LOGS

Logs are maintained in a veterinary facility for the purpose of recording procedures and tests performed, radiology studies, mortality and euthanasia rates, quality and inventory control, and data collection for quick retrieval and to compare or justify procedures. They also contain brief owner and pet identifying information should the need arise to look up data in this matter. Logs are kept in binders within the area of the hospital that provides that service.

Biopsy Log

The biopsy log is kept in the pathology or laboratory department. Each biopsy performed through the pathology department is recorded in the log book. It serves as a retrospective study of disease frequencies within a region, such as cancer or other diseases, and provides a review of treatment of these diseases and the outcome.

CONSENT TO DISCLOSURE OF MEDICAL RECORD

WAIVER OF CONFIDENTIALITY

BY AUTHORIZED PATIENT REPRESENTATIVE

I,_____am the_____

of _____ a_____

I understand that the information contained in _____'s

medical record is confidential. However, I specifically give my

consent for _____

to release the following specific information concerning

_____ to _____

_____

_____

_____

The above-listed information is to be disclosed for the specific

purpose of _____

_____

It is further understood that the information released is for professional
purposes only and may not be provided in whole or part to any other person
than that stated above.

_____

                                        Signature of
                                        Authorized Representative

_____

                                                 Date

Figure 4-11. Authorization form.

DATE	PATH #	SPECIES	CLINICIAN	OWNER	NEC/ BIO	DATE REC TYPE	DATE TYPED	DATE CORR.	DATE MAILED

Figure 4-12. Example of necropsy log.

Necropsy Log

The necropsy log is a compilation of data regarding animal deaths, including their cause and type of necropsy performed. The log contains the owner's name, case number, species, date, veterinarian performing the evaluation, histopathology, or special tissue submitted. It is kept in the necropsy area (Fig. 4–12).

Radiology Log

The radiology log is completed by a technician who is designated within the department to post information. The log contains date of examination, type of examination performed, owner's name, case number, animal's species and breed, exposure settings, and veterinarian's name (Fig. 4–13). This log is very useful when improved exposure technique is desired or repeat films are requested.

Surgery Log

The surgery log contains information on the procedure performed (major or minor), animal's name, case number, owner's name, date on which surgery was performed, anesthesia used, surgeon's name, duration of the surgical or anesthesia procedure, and fee. Through this log, retrospective studies are made of costs, procedures, and surgical complications (Fig. 4–14).

RADIOLOGY LOG

DATE	CASE NUMBER	OWNER	BREED	DOCTOR	EXAMINATION	EXPOSURE SETTINGS

Figure 4-13. Example of a radiology log.

SURGERY LOG

CASE NUMBER	CLIENT	SURGEON	ANESTHESIA	PROCEDURE	MAJOR	MINOR	TIME	FEE

Figure 4–14. Example of a surgery log.

THE FAX CONNECTION

The facsimile (Fax) machine plays a major role in the field of health care communication. The transmission of information in a rapid manner is of utmost importance, especially in the emergency case that occurs away from the practice usually visited for routine health care.

This method of data transmittal is also used for, but not limited to, record transfer when the animal's owner has moved to another area, information transmittal to a veterinary specialist from a referring veterinarian, or information transmittal from the specialist back to the referring veterinarian.

Although this has proved to be a convenient way to send data, confidentiality must be maintained so the integrity of the medical record is not compromised. Procedures for sending information by Fax should be established and explained to the office personnel who will carry out the transmittal procedure.

It is suggested that Fax be used only if the mail will not serve the purpose or in the event of an emergency. For information to be sent, a properly completed and authorized release of information should be obtained, to be used for that one time only. A hard copy (original form) should also be mailed to the veterinary practice to be kept as a permanent part of the record. The Fax'ed copy is kept as a part of the record until the original is received. In an emergency, the release form may not be obtainable before treatment. A policy should be developed within each practice regarding the emergency request of information. It is also recommended that Fax data be sent only when used in a patient care encounter and not for routine use.

When data are sent via Fax, a cover letter with the sender and receiver's name, address, date, telephone number, and Fax identification should be included (Fig. 4–15). It should be established beforehand whether the copies should be destroyed after having been transmitted or returned to the medical record department for their disposition. Legally, a Fax copy is as admissible in court as an original copy in the event of legal proceedings. Therefore, Fax copies must also be legible and complete so the validity of the medical record is not questioned. In all cases, the original copy of the cover letter shall be placed in the medical record for future reference. Regular mail or messenger service should cover the routine release of information by the practice. A nominal fee per page is charged for this service to help defray costs of telephone line use, paper, and time.

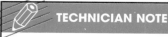

TECHNICIAN NOTE

Copying and Faxing of medical records should be done only by authorized personnel.

MORBIDITY-MORTALITY REPORT

The morbidity-mortality record includes the patient case number, clinician in charge of the case, whether surgery was performed, whether the animal was euthanatized or died of natural causes, and diagnosis at time of death. Information is entered

Hospital Name _____
Address _____
City _____ State ____ Zip Code ____

TELEFACSIMILE COVER SHEET

DATE: _____

TO: _____

DEPT. / ADDRESS: _____

_____

_____

FAX NUMBER: _____
        Country Code City Code   Area Code   Phone Number

FROM: _____

MESSAGE: _____

_____

_____

_____

_____

_____

_____

TOTAL PAGES TO BE TRANSMITTED, INCLUDING COVER: _____

Figure 4-15. Facsimile cover sheet.

daily or monthly, making this record a convenient source for compilation of statistics (Fig. 4–16).

AUTHORIZATIONS

Authorizations are not a legal requirement. Their purpose is to protect the veterinarian and to ensure each client understands

MORBIDITY – MORTALITY REPORT FOR _____ (MONTH)

CASE NUMBER:	CASE NUMBER:
CLINICIAN:	CLINICIAN:
SURGERY: YES NO	SURGERY: YES NO
DIED: EUTHANIZED:	DIED: EUTHANIZED:
DIAGNOSIS:	DIAGNOSIS:
CASE NUMBER:	CASE NUMBER:
CLINICIAN:	CLINICIAN:
SURGERY: YES NO	SURGERY: YES NO
DIED: EUTHANIZED:	DIED: EUTHANIZED:
DIAGNOSIS:	DIAGNOSIS:
CASE NUMBER:	CASE NUMBER:
CLINICIAN:	CLINICIAN:
SURGERY: YES NO	SURGERY: YES NO
DIED: EUTHANIZED:	DIED: EUTHANIZED:
DIAGNOSIS:	DIAGNOSIS:

Figure 4-16. Example of a morbidity-mortality log.

all treatments, surgical procedures, fee estimates, euthanasia approval, necropsy approval, and release of responsibility.

Several different forms may be needed to accommodate each situation. All authorizations should contain owner and animal information and become part of the permanent medical record.

The fee estimate sheet is an important form provided to the client for their approval before service. This form provides an estimate for all services the animal may need during diagnosis and treatment. A total fee estimate may be difficult to establish on admission to the hospital but must be attempted to avoid financial misunderstandings with the client. If the estimate changes during the treatment period, the client should be informed. Both the owner and veterinarian should sign the fee estimate form, and a duplicate copy should become a part of the medical record (Fig. 4–17). The euthanasia/donation authorization is critical at the time the owner is agreeing to donation and/or euthanatize an animal. Occasionally, an owner may wish to change their instructions or cancel a euthanasia. When this occurs, the completed and signed consent form is the only legal document in the medical record that authorizes such activity (Fig. 4–18).

COMPUTERS

The computer is an invaluable tool in the field of veterinary medicine. Approximately 80% of the veterinary practices have computer resources. The compilation of regular reports by the computer can provide financial statistics, case load by species, type of diagnoses and treatments, procedures performed, management reports, and herd health data. Computer-generated management information can help in planning for future practice expansion or in the retrospective evaluation of case management. Pharmacy and medical supply inventory can also be maintained through computerization. Some practices are using computerized (paperless) medical records. Computerized medical records are legally useful when the record program has been protected by security levels. If the software of the program has been secured through the transaction file, then all changes, additions, and deletions will be recorded and can be audited at any time. Computerized medical records are becoming more user friendly and efficient but must continue to develop the trust of professionals to gain common use. Additional information can be found concerning computer use in practice in Chapter 35.

VETERINARY MEDICAL DATA BASE

The Veterinary Medical Data Base (VMDB) is a national data bank located at Purdue University. It contains computerized veterinary medical data supplied by 24 veterinary schools in the United States and Canada. Each institution submits data for the VMDB on a quarterly basis to a central processing center. The data consist of abstracted data from each clinical case seen at each teaching hospital. The national data base allows allows studies of national trends in various animal diseases. It provides patient chart number, institution code, date of visit, length of stay, clinician code, sex, species, breed, discharge status, age, weight, diagnosis, and procedures for each animal. The VMDB is available for use in retrospective studies and in the evaluation of national and regional disease patterns.

HOSPITAL NAME _____			
ADDRESS_____			
CITY _____ STATE ____ ZIP CODE _____			

FEE ESTIMATE

NAME _____ CASE NO. _____
STREET _____
CITY, STATE, ZIP _____
PHONE BUS. _____ HOME _____

DATE:	TIME:

CLINICIAN:

SPECIES	BREED	SEX
ANIMAL'S NAME		DATE OF BIRTH

COLOR—IDENTIFYING MARKS

INITIAL EXAM	Routine Visit	Referral		Emergency	$
HOSPITALIZATION NO. OF DAYS	Standard	ADDITIONAL FEES FOR : Isolation		ICU	
LABORATORY Data base	Clin Path Microbiology Parasitology	LASMDL Endocrinology Histopathology		Cytology Immunology Other	
RADIOLOGY Survey Exams	Ultrasound	Other			
DIAGNOSTIC PROCEDURES Consultations	ECG EEG EMG ERG	CSF Tap Endoscopy Skin Test Biopsy		Aspirate/Washes Ultrasound Special Exams Other	
ANESTHESIA Sedation	Local	General		Other	
SURGERY O.R. Fee	Materials Supplies	Professional Service		Implants Other	
THERAPEUTICS Vaccinations Medicated Bath/Dip	In–Hosp.Trmt Fluids Transfusions	Oxygen Therapy Physical Therapy		Deworming Dentistry Other	
PHARMACY Hospital Meds	Bandage Materials	Discharge Meds		Special Diets	
OTHER	Contingencies/Comments:				

You have been advised of estimated costs and procedures. Please feel free to discuss the proposed treatment and its cost with the veterinarian. A minimum deposit of 50% of the initial charges will be required for hospitalization of an animal patient.

Amt. of Deposit $ _____ Receipt # _____ TOTAL ESTIMATE $

STATEMENT OF OWNERSHIP AND CONSENT: I am the owner of the above described animal, or have authorization from the owner to consent to its treatment.

I hereby authorize the performance of professionally accepted diagnostic, therapeutic, anesthetic, and surgical procedures necessary for its treatment.

I accept financial responsibility for these services.

I have read the above consent and understand why the above procedures may be necessary. I also have been told of the possible complications and alternatives to the listed procedures.

I will not hold _____ or its agents liable in any manner regarding the care, treatment, or safekeeping of the animal described above.

I understand that if further services are required for this animal (even if for treatment of the same condition), additional expenses will occur. Do not allow the total bill to exceed $ _____ without my authorization.

I have read and understand the above statement and have received a copy of this estimate.

_____   _____
Signature (Owner or agent)   Date

White: Client   Canary: Discharge Office   Pink: Medical records

Figure 4–17. Fee-estimation form.

HOSPITAL NAME _____

ADDRESS _____

CITY _____ STATE _____ ZIP CODE _____

NAME _____ CASE NO. _____

STREET _____

CITY, STATE, ZIP _____

PHONE BUS. _____ HOME _____

SPECIES   BREED   SEX

ANIMAL'S NAME   DATE OF BIRTH

COLOR—IDENTIFYING MARKS

EUTHANASIA – UNRESTRICTED DONATION RELEASE

Animal's Name _____ Brand, Tattoo, or ID Chip _____

Owner's Driver License #_____ Owner's Vehicle License # _____

STATE   NUMBER   STATE   NUMBER

The insurance company has been notified on _____ and has forwarded permission.

I, the undersigned, certify that I am the owner, or authorized agent of the owner of the above described animal. I hereby unconditionally release the above animal

☐   1.   To euthanatize and dispose of the animal.

☐   2.   To euthanatize and return the animal.

☐   3.   Unrestricted donation.

Special Instructions: _____

_____

_____

_____

Date: _____

Owner or Agent: _____

Witness: _____

Clinician ordering euthanasia   Date

Euthanasia was performed with _____

Drug & Amount

on _____ at _____ a.m./p.m.

Date   Time

Person performing euthanasia   Date

Figure 4–18. Euthanasia-unrestricted donation release form.

AMERICAN ANIMAL HOSPITAL ASSOCIATION

The American Animal Hospital Association (AAHA) is geared to small animal hospitals and small animal practitioners. Member hospitals are certified if they meet certain standards required by the organization. Hospital evaluations are carried out every 2, 3, or 4 years to ensure that the practice and veterinarians are complying with approved standards. A complete medical record is part of these standards. AAHA publishes a Medical Records Manual that contains the regulations for medical records, along with samples of forms that can help to develop or improve a medical record system within each practice.

It is of utmost importance to maintain a retrievable, complete, and legible medical record at all times and to make it available to anyone in the practice. A high-quality record can be developed by use of computer support along with individual record forms. This record is the only legal and tangible evidence that the veterinarian maintains.

Recommended Reading

American Animal Hospital Association: Hospital Standards and Accreditation Manual, Denver, CO, AAHA, 1996.

Hannah HW: Practice and the law. *In* McCurnin DM (editor): Veterinary Practice Management. Philadelphia, JB Lippincott, 1988.

Huffman EK: Medical Record Management. Berwyn, IL, Physician's Record Co., 1994.

Terry GR and Stallard JJ: Office Management and Control. Homewood, IL, Richard D. Irwin, Inc., 1980.

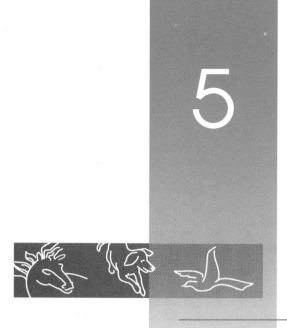

5 Clinical Pathology

Jan L. VanSteenhouse

INTRODUCTION

Accurate clinical pathology data is an invaluable component of the minimum data base used in the diagnosis of a broad spectrum of diseases of all species. Repetition of selected data also provides a means of monitoring and evaluating the success of chosen treatment regimens. Erroneous data, however, may result in misdiagnoses and be a more serious disadvantage than the lack of data.

Each practice will be faced with the decision of whether laboratory data will be generated within the clinic or be obtained from a reference laboratory. The practice's case load, availability and turnaround time of a qualified reference laboratory, and experience of the technician are important criteria used to make this determination. The competence of an individual who performs diagnostic laboratory tests can be maintained only through frequent repetition of those tests. Having clinical laboratory data available within 1 hour can be a great advantage to the veterinarian in determining the diagnosis, especially during life-threatening emergencies.

Whether samples are submitted to a reference laboratory or analyzed in the practice, the appropriately trained veterinary technician can be an invaluable asset in ensuring that valid, reliable data are obtained. In either case, the knowledge of proper sampling techniques and proper sample handling are essential. The veterinary technician should be familiar with what samples should be submitted for various tests, whether an anticoagulant should be used, volume requirements, preparation of the sample, storage requirements of the sample if it is not immediately analyzed, and how the sample should be transported.

Currently, several more affordable, "user-friendly" clinical laboratory instruments are available for veterinary practices. It is the veterinary technician's responsibility to have a thorough working knowledge of the instrument, its sample requirements, its routine maintenance procedures, and basic quality control procedures to ensure accurate laboratory results. The technician should be familiar with the care and maintenance not only of these instruments but also of all supportive laboratory equipment necessary to keep them functioning properly.

Should it be decided that a reference laboratory is more time or cost efficient for an individual practice, it is imperative that the veterinary technician communicate with the personnel of that laboratory. To avoid unnecessary delays and invalid results, the laboratory should be consulted regarding appropriate sample submission for specific tests. Most laboratories are eager to answer questions that may reduce invalid results or the need for resubmission of samples. When it is necessary to submit samples through the U.S. Postal Service, extraordinary precautions may be prudent to ensure that the samples are not damaged or destroyed in transport.

This chapter addresses the more commonly used clinical laboratory techniques and procedures in veterinary hematology, urinalysis, clinical chemistry, and cytology. Techniques and methods are emphasized rather than interpretation. The list of recommended reading will provide detailed reviews. Laboratory instrumentation and necessary quality control systems for clinical chemistry and hematology are reviewed and summarized. In addition, common errors that are made in sampling and sample handling and result in misleading values that make interpretation of laboratory data difficult are discussed.

HEMATOLOGY

The basic equipment necessary for hematological analyses includes a microscope, microhematocrit centrifuge, refractometer,

• Table 5–1 •

RECOMMENDED SAMPLE TUBES		
COLOR OF TOP	**ANTICOAGULANT**	**PURPOSE**
Purple	EDTA	CBC, platelet counts
Red	None	Chemistries
Tiger (red-black)	Separator gel	Chemistries
Green	Heparin	Electrolytes, STATs
Turquoise	Citrate	Coagulation assay

hemacytometer, and clean slides. The benefits of conscientious care and cleaning of these items cannot be overlooked. The complete blood count (CBC) provides the veterinarian with invaluable information regarding the patient's red blood cell (erythrocyte [RBC]) mass, white blood cell (leukocyte [WBC]) number and distribution, platelet number, and plasma protein. The CBC consists of a PCV (packed cell volume), WBC count, RBC count, hemoglobin determination, RBC indices, total plasma protein determination, and evaluation of the blood smear for RBC morphology and a WBC differential. Hematological procedures are performed on anticoagulated whole blood. The preferred anticoagulant is ethylenediamine tetra-acetic acid (EDTA) because it does not interfere with blood cell morphology and staining. EDTA is commercially available in purple-top Vacutainer tubes in a variety of sizes. Choosing the correct size is essential to obtain accurate results because having a small amount of blood in a large tube will alter some of the values. The various types of sample tubes available and their appropriate uses are listed in Table 5–1.

The morphology of the normal and abnormal blood cells is briefly reviewed, but it is strongly recommended that the technician have on hand and consult the appropriate references listed at the end of this chapter. Table 5–2 contains normal reference ranges for hematology values in common domestic species.

Equipment

EDTA → purple top tube used in CBC's

When choosing a microscope, the laboratory's needs must first be assessed. The fewer "extras" that are included will reduce the requirements for maintenance, service, and repairs. A good-quality binocular microscope with a mechanical stage, an adjustable substage condenser, and good-quality objective lenses will accommodate the needs of any hematology laboratory. The most important aspect, and often the cost determinant, of a good laboratory microscope is the objective lens. Planachromatic lenses are recommended because they provide a flat field of vision with superior optical properties. The entire field will be in focus, resulting in reduced eyestrain and improved microscopic image. The basic laboratory microscope should have 10×, 40× (high dry), and 100× (oil immersion) objective lenses in addition to standard 10× ocular objectives. Many microscopists find an additional 50× oil immersion objective lens useful for evaluation of both blood films and cytology specimens. The manufacturer's manual should provide directions for adjusting the light for optimal intensity (Kohler illumination), which enhances the clarity of the image.

Proper care of the microscope is essential to providing accurate results for an extended period of time. Great care should be taken to follow the manufacturer's directions for proper use, cleaning, and maintenance. The oil immersion lenses require a drop of special immersion oil on the blood film to achieve the appropriate optics. The immersion oil should be wiped from the objective after use to prevent damage to the lens. It is essential that all other objectives be kept free of oil. Lenses should be cleaned with lens paper only. A dust cover should be placed over the microscope when not in use to prevent collection of dust and hairs on the lenses and other surfaces.

TECHNICIAN NOTE

No laboratory equipment or instrument, regardless of cost, is any better than the care and maintenance it receives.

A microhematocrit centrifuge is required for determination of the packed cell volume (PCV). The centrifugal force generated by the centrifuge separates the cellular components of blood from the plasma. The manufacturer's manual should be consulted for recommended speed settings for the sample being spun. As with all laboratory equipment, the accuracy and func-

• Table 5–2 •

HEMATOLOGY VALUES				
	CANINE	**FELINE**	**EQUINE**	**BOVINE**
PCV (%)	37–55	30–45	32–48	24–46
Hemoglobin (g/dl)	12–18	8–15	10–18	8–15
Reticulocytes (%)	0–1.5	0–1.0	0	0
WBC (n/µl)	6000–17,000	5500–19,500	6000–12,000	4000–12,000
Segs (n/µl)	3000–11,400	2500–12,500	3000–6000	600–4000
Bands (n/µl)	0–300	0–300	0–100	0–120
Lymphs (n/µl)	1000–4800	1500–7000	1500–5000	2500–7500
Monos (n/µl)	150–1350	0–850	0–600	25–850
Eos (n/µl)	100–750	0–750	0–800	0–2400
Basos (n/µl)	Rare	Rare	0–300	0–200
TP (g/dl)	6.0–7.5	6.0–7.5	6.0–8.5	6.0–8.0
Fib (mg/dl)	150–300	150–300	100–400	100–600
Platelets (n/µl)	200,000–500,000	300,000–700,000	100,000–600,000	100,000–800,000

tional longevity of the centrifuge are directly related to proper care and use. Safety concerns preclude ever operating the centrifuge without the lid being closed and properly secured. Samples should always be balanced to ensure accurate separation and reduce wear on the motor. Periodic maintenance, such as lubricating the bearings and checking the commutator, should be scheduled according to the manufacturer's recommendations to extend the life of the centrifuge and ensure accurate results.

The refractometer is used to determine the plasma protein concentration by measuring the refractive index of the plasma. The refractive index of a fluid is determined by the number, charge, and mass of particles suspended in the fluid. Careful cleaning of the sample surface is imperative to prolonging the accuracy and functional life of the refractometer. There are several models available, including one designed specifically for veterinary use (Fig. 5–1). The veterinary model is less expensive, has a more shock-resistant casing, and is appropriate for use in veterinary determination of urine specific gravity. Calibration of the zero setting should be checked periodically with distilled water and adjusted according to the manufacturer's manual if necessary.

The Neubauer (recommended) hemacytometer is a small but valuable specialized counting chamber used for determining WBC and platelet counts per microliter of blood (Fig. 5–2). It has a special coverglass calibrated for accuracy; regular coverglasses cannot be substituted should it be damaged. Both the hemacytometer and coverslip must be carefully cleaned to avoid scratching the surfaces.

New, clean glass slides are essential for making usable blood films. Slides that are frosted on one end are preferred for labeling purposes.

Sample Handling

In general, EDTA is the preferred anticoagulant for hematology. Be sure to use a tube of the appropriate size for the sample being drawn. It is often difficult to obtain large samples from small dogs and cats; the 2-ml pediatric collection tube is best for a patient of this size. There are collection tubes for smaller

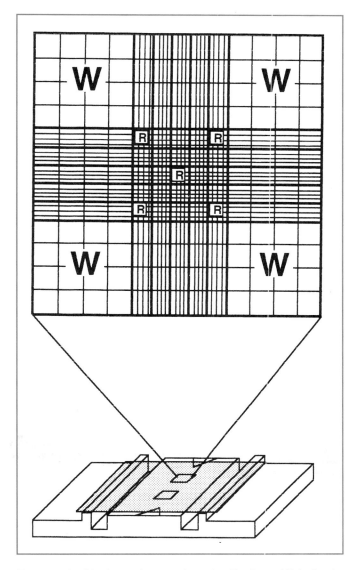

Figure 5-2. Neubauer hemacytometer. The large Ws indicate the squares that are counted for a total white blood cell count with the 1:20 dilution WBC Unopette system. The small Rs indicate the squares that are counted for a red blood cell count with the RBC Unopette system.

volumes (0.5-ml Microtainer tubes, Becton-Dickinson, Rutherford, NJ). These tubes are excellent for samples from puppies, kittens, and small exotic animal species. Excess anticoagulant in the collection tube can erroneously decrease the PCV and increase total protein determined with a refractometer.

Anticoagulated blood samples should be immediately mixed by gentle inversion of the tube. Blood films should be made from well-mixed blood within 15 minutes of obtaining the sample to decrease *in vitro* morphological changes in the blood cells. If the practice uses a reference laboratory, unstained blood films should be sent with the EDTA sample. Slides sent through the mail should be packaged in a box or tube, not sent in a flat plastic or cardboard slide holder. The flat slide holders sent in an envelope often are processed through the automated canceling machine in the post office and arrive at the laboratory in numerous small pieces. If sam-

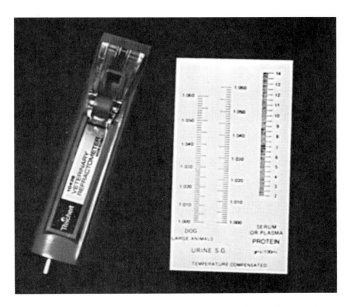

Figure 5-1. Veterinary refractometer and reading scale.

ples must be held overnight, refrigerate the whole blood but do not refrigerate the blood film. Water will condense on the surface of the blood film if it is placed in the refrigerator and cause lysis of the RBCs. In addition, the blood film should be protected from formalin vapors because they will interfere with staining.

TECHNICIAN NOTE

Blood films should always be made from fresh blood, before refrigeration, regardless of whether the CBC will be performed in the clinic or sent to a reference laboratory.

Determination of Erythrocyte Numbers

Determination of the PCV, which is the percentage of total blood volume accounted for by RBCs, is the easiest and most common means of evaluating the RBC mass. This is achieved by filling a plain microhematocrit capillary tube with anticoagulated blood, sealing one end of the tube with a specific clay, and centrifuging the sample in a microhematocrit centrifuge. The spun sample is then applied to a chart to determine the PCV. This method provides a quick and accurate measurement providing samples are spun for a standard length of time at a consistent speed. The specific time and speed are dependent on the particular centrifuge being used. Accuracy is also dependent on the care and operation of the centrifuge. Blood samples from cattle, sheep, and goats may require centrifugation for a longer time because their smaller RBCs do not pack as well as dog and cat RBCs. The plasma portion at the top of the tube should be evaluated for color and clarity and will also be used for determination of plasma protein. The *hematocrit* provides basically the same information but is obtained by calculation when an automated analyzer is used and thus may be slightly different from the measured PCV. This is most commonly seen in blood samples from collection tubes that have an inadequate volume of blood (less than 1 ml in a 5-ml tube or less than 0.5 ml in a 2-ml tube). The excess anticoagulant causes the RBCs to shrink, erroneously decreasing the PCV. When the blood is diluted by the electronic cell counter, the diluent reexpands the RBCs to their true size, providing the true value for the hematocrit.

The actual number of erythrocytes may be determined using an automated cell counter, which is primarily available in reference laboratories. Erythrocyte counts may also be performed manually but are too tedious and inaccurate to be of diagnostic value. RBC counts vary proportionately with PCV and have little to no advantage over PCV. The major advantage of automated cell counters is that they also measure hemoglobin and measure or calculate the RBC indices. Hemoglobin is the protein responsible for carrying oxygen from the lungs to the tissues.

RBC Indices

RBC indices are commonly provided when automated analyzers are used; these indices include mean corpuscular volume (MCV), mean corpuscular hemoglobin (MCH), and mean corpuscular hemoglobin concentration (MCHC). The MCH is of little value, but the MCV and MCHC are useful in evaluating and determining the cause of anemias (decreased RBC number). MCH and MCHC values calculated with an electronic cell counter will be artifactually affected by hemolysis, Heinz bodies, and lipemia and therefore cannot be interpreted for such samples.

Determination of Leukocyte Counts

The total WBC count may be determined manually using the hemacytometer or with an automated cell counter. Either way, it is important that the blood tube be well mixed before the sample is taken. Figure 5–2 diagrams the hemacytometer grid that will be seen microscopically and indicates the areas on the grid to be counted for the WBC count. The glass coverslip is one specifically designed for the hemacytometer and cannot be substituted for with regular coverslips, so it must be handled and cleaned carefully to avoid damage and should never be used for other purposes. The Unopette dilution system (Becton-Dickinson) is the most accepted method for performing manual WBC counts. There are a number of Unopette systems available for counting various cell types (Table 5–3), but the system preferred for counting leukocytes is also used for counting platelets and determining cell counts on samples such as synovial fluid. This system consists of a disposable reservoir containing diluent and an agent to lyse RBCs to accommodate the counting of leukocytes. Each Unopette system comes with detailed instructions for obtaining reliable results and a capillary pipette to draw a specific volume of blood. The interchangeable use of pipettes from another cell-counting system, such as one for RBCs, to obtain WBC counts will result in significant errors and inappropriately decreased WBC counts.

The accuracy of a manual WBC count is dependent on adherence to the directions and the proper performance of each step. Care must be taken to accurately fill the capillary tube and wipe off any excess blood on the outside of the tube without touching the tip of the pipette and drawing any of the sample out of the pipette. The blood sample must be carefully transferred to the reservoir with careful mixing to ensure complete delivery of the sample into the diluent. Blood left in the capillary tube or accidentally expelled from the top of the pipette during mixing will result in erroneous WBC counts. It will take practice and may require multiple attempts to completely and accurately fill the hemacytometer chamber. The chambers on both sides of the hemacytometer must be filled for accurate results. Counting both sides and comparing results also serves to check accuracy as the number of cells on one side should closely approximate the number of cells on the

• Table 5–3 •

UNOPETTE SYSTEMS FOR COUNTING DIFFERENT CELL TYPES			
TEST	**PIPETTE VOLUME**	**DILUTION**	**DILUENT**
Red cell count	10 μl	1:200	0.85% Saline
White cell count	20 μl	1:100	3% Acetic acid
White cell count	25 μl	1:20	3% Acetic acid
Platelet count	20 μl	1:100	1% Ammonium oxalate
Eosinophil count	25 μl	1:32	Phloxin

MCV + MCHC useful in determining causes of anemia.

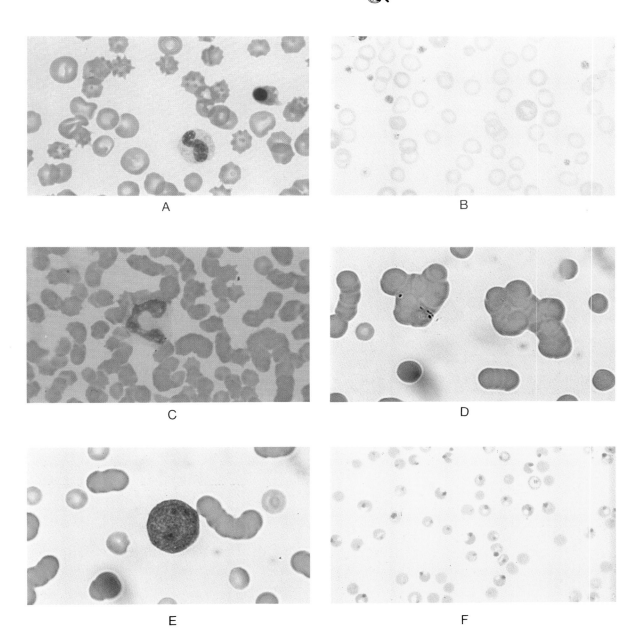

COLOR PLATE I. A, Canine blood film displaying several polychromatophilic erythrocytes and one nucleated erythrocyte. A segmented neutrophil is also present. B, Canine blood film showing hypochromic erythrocytes with increased central pallor. C, Equine blood film showing rouleau formation. D, Feline blood film showing agglutination. E, Feline blood film showing rouleau formation. F, Feline blood film, new methylene blue stain, showing dark-staining Heinz bodies on the periphery of the erythrocytes.

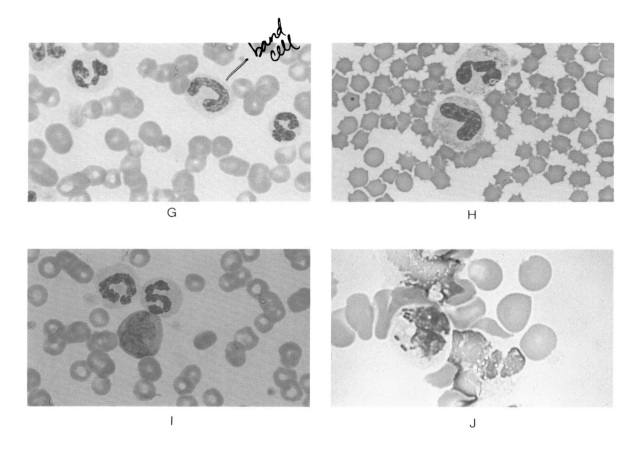

G

H

I

J

COLOR PLATE I *Continued.* G, Canine erythrocytes, segmented neutrophils, and one band neutrophil. Several platelets are also present. H, Feline blood film with two toxic neutrophils. The toxic changes evident are increased basophilia of the cytoplasm and Döhle bodies. I, Canine blood film showing two segmented neutrophils and one monocyte. J, Equine abdominal fluid showing a neutrophil with intracellular rod-shaped bacteria. Two smudged cells are also present.

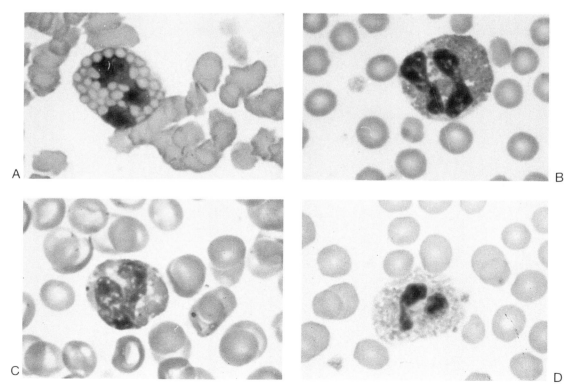

A

B

C

D

COLOR PLATE II. Species variation in eosinophil granules. A, Equine eosinophil. B, Bovine eosinophil. C, Canine eosinophil. D, Feline eosinophil.

other side. Overfilling or underfilling the chamber will cause errors in the final cell count. After charging the hemacytometer chambers, it must be allowed to sit for several minutes in a moist chamber to allow the cells to settle. WBCs will be counted using the 10× objective; lowering the condenser on the microscope will increase the contrast, making the cells more prominent and easier to identify and count accurately.

Nucleated RBCs (NRBCs) will be counted along with WBCs by either manual or automated electronic counting methods, thus giving falsely elevated WBC counts. The number of NRBCs encountered on the blood film are counted while performing the differential on 100 leukocytes. The WBC count is then corrected using the following formula if more than 10 NRBCs are counted.

$$\frac{100}{100 + \text{Number of NRBCs}} \times \text{WBC} = \text{Corrected WBC count}$$

For example, if 15 NRBCs are counted while performing the 100-cell differential and the initial WBC count is 30,000/μl, the corrected count is then calculated as:

$$\frac{100}{100 + 15} \times 30,000 = 26,087 \text{ WBCs}$$

Increased WBCs is referred to as *leukocytosis,* whereas decreased WBCs is referred to as *leukopenia*. The diagnostic significance of either leukocytosis or leukopenia cannot be appreciated without the WBC differential. The differential is performed by examining the blood film (see Blood Film Evaluation). At least 100 leukocytes are identified and counted according to cell type (as neutrophils, bands, lymphocytes, monocytes, eosinophils, or basophils). The more cells that are counted, the more accurate will be the differential. The percentages of each cell type counted are then multiplied by the total WBC count to give absolute numbers of the cell types present. These numbers are the values used for interpreting changes in the leukogram.

Avian and Reptilian Leukocyte Counts

Unlike mammals, birds and reptiles have NRBCs, which prevents determination of their WBC counts by the methods described. However, the WBC counts of these nonmammalian species may be determined indirectly using another Unopette system for eosinophil determination. This special Unopette is filled with anticoagulated blood, mixed well, and allowed to incubate for approximately 5 minutes to allow uptake of the stain by the cells. If the sample is allowed to stand for a prolonged time, it will result in all the cells taking up the stain and erroneous results. The hemacytometer is filled as for the manual WBC count described, and the red-staining cells are counted in all nine squares of the grid. With proper staining, only the eosinophils and heterophils (nonmammalian equivalent of neutrophils) will be stained. Unlike when performing the mammalian manual count, it is important to keep the microscope condenser up to decrease contrast. If the condenser is down, it will be more difficult to count the heterophils and eosinophils because of RBC interference.

The number obtained does not represent the WBC count but is used in conjunction with the differential to calculate the WBC count. When the differential is completed and the percentages of the various cell types present are known, the WBC count is calculated using the following formula:

$$\frac{\text{Cells counted on hemacytometer} \times 32}{\%\text{ Heterophils} + \text{eosinophils}} \times 100 = \text{WBC/μl}$$

For example, if 282 cells are counted on one side of the hemacytometer and you have 70% heterophils and 5% eosinophils on the differential, the total WBC count would be as follows:

$$282 \times 32 \times \frac{100}{70 + 5} = 12,032 \text{ WBC/μl}$$

Platelet Determination

Determination of platelet numbers is important because platelets play an important role in *hemostasis,* or control of blood flow. There are a number of diseases that cause decreased numbers of platelets; and these can often be diagnosed and treated before an animal develops a severe bleeding disorder. Similar to WBCs, platelets can be counted manually on a hemacytometer or with an automated cell counter. Cat platelets, in particular, have a tendency to clump, which interferes with obtaining accurate platelet counts; whether done manually or by automation, erroneously low platelet count can result. For this reason, it is important to always examine the blood film for platelet clumping. In addition, because cats often have relatively large platelets and cat RBCs are small, automated electronic counts are often inaccurate because of the inability to separate the cells by size.

Manual platelet counts can be performed using the same Unopette system and sample used for the manual WBC count. This task can be very tedious, especially if the hemacytometer and coverglass are not properly cared for. Scratches and small dust particles are very difficult to differentiate from platelets. If platelet clumps are present, the resultant count will be inaccurate. It would be best to obtain another sample with special attention given to ensure a clean venipuncture and adequate mixing of the blood with the anticoagulant. Platelets will be identified using the 40× objective and will be easier if the condenser is lowered and the light intensity is moderate. The instructions that accompany the Unopette must be followed with regard to the squares of the grid that are counted and the method of calculating the total count.

TECHNICIAN NOTE

The blood film should always be scanned for platelet clumps, especially in cats, to avoid reporting erroneously low platelet numbers.

When platelet counts are not available or to verify counts obtained manually or electronically, the number of platelets can be estimated from the blood film. While examining the appropriate area of the blood film, in which RBCs are spaced in a uniform monolayer, the average number of platelets per

100× oil immersion field in several fields (10 or more) is determined. This average number of platelets multiplied by 15,000 will provide an adequate estimation of the number of platelets per microliter.

Decreased platelet counts can have serious implications for the patient. Therefore, before reporting low platelet counts, all technical problems must be considered. The feathered edge of the blood film must be checked for platelet clumping. The tube of blood from which the sample was taken should be checked for small clots, which could deplete platelets. Either or both of these problems may occur despite the use of an anticoagulant. If neither the blood film nor the tube reveals evidence of platelet aggregation, the low platelet count should be reported as determined. If platelet clumping or clots are found, the sample should be redrawn, and the counts repeated.

Blood Film Evaluation

Examination of the stained blood smear is one of the most valuable parts of the complete blood count and cannot be overstressed. For the sake of time, many are tempted to skip this portion of the CBC, but the numbers alone can be very misleading and result in incorrect diagnoses and inappropriate treatment. Anemias cannot be classified or changes in the WBC accurately interpreted until the differential is completed and the cells are examined for morphological changes. Examination of the blood film is especially important as an internal quality control when automated electronic cell counters are used. If there appears to be a discrepancy between what the technician sees on the film and the numbers reported by the instrument, the counts should be repeated with special attention given to determining what could be causing the difference. A common cause is that the blood tube was not adequately mixed before sampling for either the count or the blood film. Another common problem is seen, particularly in leukopenic cats, with considerable platelet clumping. The platelet clumps are large enough that they are counted as WBCs in the automated system, resulting in falsely higher WBC counts made by the instrument. With time and experience, the technician will be able to scan the blood film and recognize these discrepancies between the number of leukocytes apparent on the film and the number of WBCs reported by the instrument. As a general rule of thumb, there should be approximately 20 leukocytes per 10× field in a normal canine blood sample.

There are a variety of ways to make quality blood films. New slides should always be used, and they should be handled only by the edges because oils on the slide from fingers will result in poor-quality films. (The reader is referred to Recommended Reading for examples of the different techniques.) What is most important is to try several methods, find the one that is most comfortable, and then practice repeatedly until quality films are consistently produced. A small drop of blood is placed at one end of a slide and the edge of a second slide is used to spread the drop. It is important to make the film in one even stroke and not use excessive downward pressure. Increased downward pressure on the spreader slide can cause the leukocytes to be carried to the feathered edge and may even cause the cells to rupture or become distorted. In either case, the accuracy of the differential will be lessened. The thickness of the blood film can be altered to accommodate samples from severely anemic or dehydrated animals. Increasing the angle between the two slides will concentrate the cells

when the PCV is very low. Conversely, decreasing the angle will allow greater spreading of the cells in a concentrated sample (Fig. 5–3).

Several modifications of the traditional Wright's stain are available for suitable staining of blood films for veterinary practices. Stat Stain (VWR Scientific, Philadelphia, PA), Diff-Quik (Baxter S/P, McGaw Park, IL), and CAMCO Quik Stain (Baxter S/P) are commonly used. They are relatively economical and technically easy to use and maintain. The disadvantages of these stains are few. Polychromatophilic RBCs do not stain as obviously as they do with Wright's stain, and some mast cell and eosinophil granules may be washed out.

It is best to develop a routine when evaluating a blood film and follow the same approach each time to avoid oversights and mistakes. The blood film should first be examined under low power (10×). While scanning on 10×, one can get an impression of the general distribution of nucleated cells (clumped at the edges or spread evenly throughout), estimate the total WBC count (low versus normal versus high), and examine the feathered edge of the blood film for aggregates of platelets, the larger leukocytes, neoplastic cells, and microfilaria of *Dirofilaria immitis* or *Dipetalonema recondita* (Fig. 5–4). During the low-power examination, one may identify structures or areas that need a closer look. Last, on low power, one should identify the appropriate area in which RBCs are distributed in a uniform monolayer and the leukocytes are sufficiently spread so that morphological identification on high power is possible. It is especially important to avoid being too far into the body of the blood film, where the WBCs are rounded and darkly stained. In this area, it is often difficult to differentiate the leukocytes.

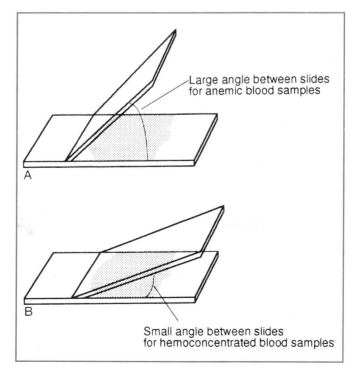

Large angle between slides for anemic blood samples

A

Small angle between slides for hemoconcentrated blood samples

B

Figure 5-3. Difference in slide angle necessary for making blood films from anemic or hemoconcentrated blood. A, Large angle for anemic blood. B, Small angle for hemoconcentrated blood.

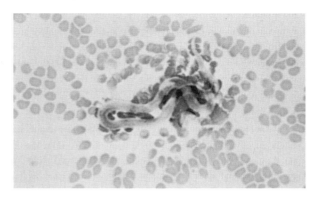

Figure 5-4. A microfilaria of *Dirofilaria immitis* at the feathered edge of a canine blood smear. The parasite is about the same width as an erythrocyte.

The blood film is then studied under high power, generally under oil immersion (100×). The WBC differential is performed at this power. Erythrocytes should be evaluated for morphological changes and parasites, and platelets should be evaluated for morphology and counted to make the estimated count. These evaluations may be made before or after the differential, but they should be done consistently as part of the routine so they are not overlooked. Platelets are cytoplasmic fragments, so they have no nucleus. They are generally round to oval or spindle shaped with purplish granules and multiple pointed projections. They may vary greatly in size, but increased numbers of large platelets may indicate an increased output from the bone marrow (Fig. 5–5). After the platelets have been evaluated, the erythrocytes should be studied.

Erythrocyte Evaluation

The erythrocytes of most mammals are disc shaped and anuclear. They appear flat with a varying degree of *central pallor* (pale area in center of cell with less hemoglobin) depending on the size. The RBCs of different domestic species differ markedly in size, with those of the dog having the largest diameter (7 μm), followed by the horse, cow, and cat (5.8 μm), the sheep (4.5 μm), and the goat (3.2 μm). Some species have RBCs that vary in size, which is termed *anisocytosis*. Cows normally have more anisocytosis than do other species. In other species, extreme anisocytosis implies either that many of the RBCs are smaller (microcytic), which may indicate iron deficiency, or that many are larger (macrocytic), which may indicate increased production and release of immature cells from the bone marrow in response to anemia. Some poodles normally have larger RBCs than do other dogs. Some Japanese Akita dogs normally have smaller RBCs. These are genetic traits and do not indicate a change in RBC dynamics.

Poikilocytosis is the general term used to indicate changes in RBC shape. *Leptocytes* are RBCs with an increased surface area that makes them highly deformable. Target cells and cells with a transverse fold are two common forms of leptocytes. Because leptocytes can occur for many reasons, they are rarely of any diagnostic significance. Immature polychromatophilic cells often appear as leptocytes.

Acanthocytes are RBCs with a membrane abnormality that causes them to develop multiple, irregularly spaced club-shaped projections from the cell surface. These must be differentiated from crenated cells, which have numerous rounded, evenly spaced projections. *Crenation* is an artifact resulting from high temperatures or slow drying of the blood film. Acanthocytes may be encountered in normal cattle, but in other species they are often associated with some neoplasms (especially visceral hemangiosarcoma) or disorders of lipid metabolism. *Schistocytes* are fragmented RBCs formed as a result of the trauma of colliding with intravascular fibrin strands; schistocytes are associated with disseminated intravascular coagulopathy, heartworm disease, and, occasionally, diseases of the spleen or liver that involve fibrin deposition within the vasculature of those organs. *Spherocytes* are RBCs that appear smaller than normal RBCs and exhibit no central pallor. Spherocytes are most commonly seen in immune hemolytic anemia and can also be seen after blood transfusions. They are more spherical because bits of their membrane have been removed, making them more rigid and unable to assume the discoid shape more typical of RBCs. They are most easily identified in canine blood, because normal canine RBCs are larger and have a distinct zone of central pallor. In the other species with smaller RBCs, which typically exhibit little or no central pallor, spherocytes are difficult to confirm. Figure 5–6 illustrates normal canine RBCs and spherocytes.

NRBCs, or *metarubricytes,* may be seen in peripheral blood films. An occasional NRBC may be found in a normal animal, but increased numbers are a significant finding and should be reported as the number of NRBCs per 100 WBCs. Care must be taken to avoid confusing NRBCs with lymphocytes. NRBCs of a size similar to small lymphocytes will have more cytoplasm relative to nuclear size and the cytoplasm will be faintly eosinophilic (reddish). Remember to correct the WBC count if more than 10 NRBCs per 100 WBCs are found (see previous discussion of determination of leukocyte counts).

The color of erythrocytes should be noted during examination of the blood film. *Polychromasia* is the term used to describe a variation in the color of RBCs. *Polychromatophilic* RBCs (Color Plate IA) are bluish, although this is not as consistently evident with Diff-Quick stain as it is with Wright's stain. Some polychromasia may be seen in normal, healthy animals, but increased polychromasia in anemias suggests the anemia is regenerative; in other words, the bone marrow is responding to a need for RBCs and releasing immature RBCs. Little or no polychromasia detected on a blood film from an anemic animal suggests the anemia is nonregenerative—the bone marrow is

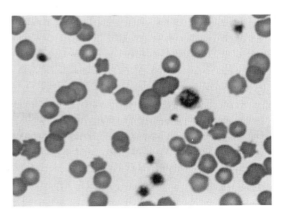

Figure 5-5. Feline erythrocytes and platelets. The platelets vary greatly in size.

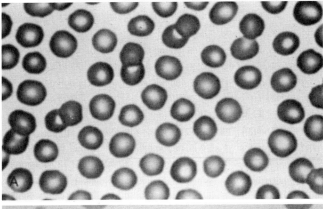

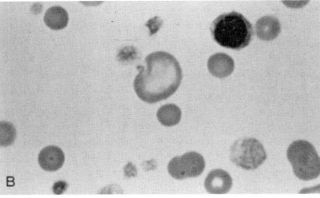

Figure 5-6. A, Normal canine red blood cells. Note the distinct central pallor. B, Blood from a dog with immune-mediated hemolytic anemia. Note the lack of central pallor in several cells, the large polychromatophilic cell, and a nucleated red blood cell.

not responding appropriately. Although the presence or absence of polychromasia may be suggestive of the bone marrow response, this should be confirmed with a reticulocyte count.

Polychromatophilic RBCs can be identified as *reticulocytes* when the blood is stained with new methylene blue (NMB). Equal amounts of blood and stain (two to five drops) are mixed in a small tube and left to stand for 5 to 10 minutes. Stain kits (Retic-Set, Curtin Matheson Scientific, Houston, TX) are available for reticulocyte counts that eliminate the need to use liquid stain; with these kits, three to five drops of whole blood are added to a stain-coated plastic tube and agitated. Whichever method is chosen, a blood film is then made from the mixed sample.

Normal RBCs appear yellowish-green with NMB. The reticulocytes will be the same color but will contain deeply basophilic (bluish) dots or strands. Cats have two types of reticulocytes. Only the reticulocytes that have prominent clumps of reticulum (aggregate reticulocytes) are counted. The RBCs with small single dots (punctate reticulocytes) are not included in the count, but their presence should be noted. A reticulocyte count is the number of reticulocytes noted in a count of 1000 RBCs expressed as a percentage (40 reticulocytes of 1000 RBCs = 4% reticulocytes). In dogs and cats, this raw reticulocyte count is then corrected relative to the patient's PCV. This is done by multiplying the raw reticulocyte count by the patient's PCV divided by the normal PCV for that species (45% for dogs

and 37% for cats). Increased reticulocytes are indicative of regenerative anemia. Horses do not release immature RBCs from the bone marrow even when they are severely anemic, so polychromasia and reticulocytosis are not seen in equine peripheral blood.

Hypochromic RBCs have an increased area of central pallor with a narrow, peripheral rim of hemoglobin resulting from an abnormally low amount of hemoglobin within the cell. The most common cause of hypochromasia is iron deficiency. Hypochromasia can be confirmed by a low MCHC provided by automated instruments. True hypochromic RBCs (Color Plate IB) must be differentiated from "punched out" RBCs, which are normochromic but have a more distinct central pallor with a thick dense rim of hemoglobinized cytoplasm. These cells are an artifact of blood film preparation, not a significant pathological change. Hyperchromasia or increased hemoglobin content in RBCs does not occur.

Rouleaux are groupings of RBCs that resemble stacked coins. Marked rouleaux formation is normal in horses (Color Plate IC) and, to a lesser extent, in cats. In dogs, rouleaux formation may occur in inflammatory or neoplastic diseases. It is important to differentiate rouleaux from true *agglutination* (clumping) of RBCs. Agglutinated RBCs tend to appear as clumps rather than as stacked coins (Color Plate ID and E). Often, agglutination of RBCs can be noted on the side of the blood tube as well as on the blood film. If there is some question in determining whether a blood sample is exhibiting rouleaux or true agglutination, a saline test can be performed. The blood cells are washed by adding one drop of blood to 5 ml of saline and centrifuging for 3 minutes. The supernatant is poured off, the RBCs are resuspended in saline, and a wet mount preparation is made. Rouleaux will disperse, but agglutinated RBCs will remain clumped.

The evaluation of erythrocytes under oil immersion should also include a search for RBC parasites, particularly in cases of anemia. *Haemobartonella felis*, the parasite responsible for feline infectious anemia, appears as small coccoid or rod-like structures on the surface of RBCs. A careful search for *H. felis* organisms should be performed on any anemic cat. These parasites may be very difficult to identify because they can be easily confused with protein and stain precipitates adhered to the cell surface. *Eperythrozoon* spp., which are found in cattle, sheep, and swine, may appear similar to *Haemobartonella felis* or may occur as ring forms on the RBCs. *Anaplasma marginale,* a parasite of bovine RBCs, appears as a small spherical body within the RBC, close to the cell margin. This parasite closely resembles Howell-Jolly bodies, but is not as apt to be distributed throughout the cell. Another RBC parasite is *Babesia* spp. which has various species that can infect any domestic animal. *Babesia* spp. are larger and lighter staining than the previously mentioned parasites, and they tend to occur as piriform structures (often paired) within the RBCs.

Other RBC morphological abnormalities associated with anemia include *Howell-Jolly bodies, basophilic stippling,* and *Heinz bodies.* Howell-Jolly bodies are small, often singular, deeply basophilic nuclear remnants that are occasionally seen on normal blood films. Increased numbers of Howell-Jolly bodies can be seen with regenerative anemias. Basophilic stippling is due to staining of small amounts of cytoplasmic RNA in RBCs. These inclusions are multiple tiny, lightly basophilic dots in the RBC cytoplasm. They can be found in markedly regenerative anemia in dogs and cats but more commonly in cattle. Baso-

basophillic stippling → lead poisoning

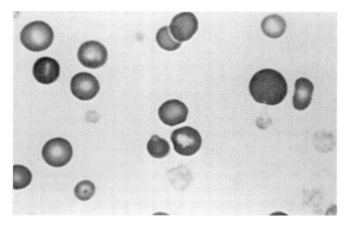

Figure 5–7. Feline blood film showing Heinz body formation. Note the small red blood cell with a distinct pale, rounded projection from its surface (Wright's stain; also see Color Plate IF).

philic stippling may also be seen occasionally in lead poisoning. The most consistent finding in lead poisoning is increased numbers of NRBCs with mild to no anemia. Heinz bodies are denatured hemoglobin that has fused to the RBC membrane and appear as refractile projections from the RBC cell membrane (Fig. 5–7). These inclusions are most readily seen with the reticulocyte (NMB) stain, when they appear as distinct darkly staining inclusions protruding from the cell surface (Color Plate IF).

Leukocyte Evaluation

The WBCs are categorized as granulocytes (*neutrophils, eosinophils,* and *basophils*) and agranulocytes (*lymphocytes* and *monocytes*). The granulocytic cells are characterized by *segmented,* or lobed, nuclei and, except for the neutrophil, distinct cytoplasmic granules. The agranulocytes are also referred to as mononuclear cells and do not have segmented nuclei.

Neutrophils. In most species, the predominant WBC is the neutrophil (Fig. 5–8). Neutrophils have phagocytic and bactericidal capabilities, which means they have an important role in

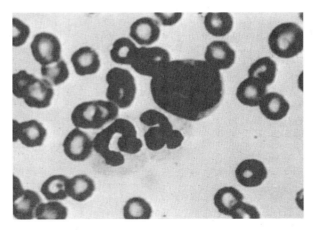

Figure 5–8. Canine blood film. Two segmented neutrophils and a monocyte are present.

inflammatory conditions. The average time spent by the neutrophil in the blood is only about 10 hours, so it is clear that neutrophil numbers can rise or fall in a matter of hours, depending on the stimuli present. Normal neutrophils have deeply staining, clumped, segmented nuclei (three to five lobes) with relatively clear cytoplasm or, at most, a very faint, almost indiscernible dusting of tiny granules. Equine neutrophils tend to have more distinct nuclear segmentation than canine neutrophils.

✎ TECHNICIAN NOTE

Extra care must be taken in differentiating monocytes from toxic band neutrophils, particularly in horses.

An important morphological change in neutrophils is the appearance of band-shaped nuclei, which indicate the release of immature neutrophils, referred to as *bands,* from the bone marrow. A band nucleus lacks the segmentation seen in the mature segmented nucleus but instead has parallel borders (Color Plate IG). Even more immature cells, with oval or bean-shaped nuclei, may be seen in cases of extreme tissue demand for neutrophils. Neutrophils, mature or immature, may also show evidence of inflammatory disease as demonstrated by certain cytoplasmic characteristics. *Toxic neutrophils* are characterized by any combination of *Döhle bodies, cytoplasmic vacuolation, basophilia,* and, rarely, cytoplasmic granulation. Cats apparently show toxic neutrophils during many kinds of illnesses (Color Plate IH), but in other species, toxic changes usually imply severe inflammatory disease. Döhle bodies are small, pale bluish-gray irregular inclusions in the cytoplasm that usually indicate mild toxemia. Generalized basophilia of the cytoplasm or cytoplasmic vacuolation are slightly more severe toxic changes. Toxic neutrophils are frequently seen with inflammatory leukograms, characterized by an increased total number of neutrophils (*neutrophilia*) and an increased number of band or other immature neutrophils. In contrast to these cytoplasmic changes, *nuclear hypersegmentation* (nuclei with five or more lobes) is a normal aging change that implies a nontoxic environment and prolonged circulation of the neutrophil. They are most frequently seen in steroid or stress leukograms, in which neutrophils remain in circulation longer than is normal.

Neutropenia, a decrease in circulating neutrophils, may occur when tissue demand is excessive as a result of severe inflammation exceeding the ability of the bone marrow to supply neutrophils. There may be an increased proportion of immature neutrophils along with the decreased number of neutrophils, which is indicative of the attempt by the bone marrow to meet tissue demands. This can be a very serious, sometimes life-threatening, situation if prolonged because neutrophils are necessary for the body to fight serious inflammation or infection.

Eosinophils. Eosinophils help to control allergic or anaphylactic hypersensitivity reactions. They are attracted to the sites of these reactions by substances released from sensitized mast cells; therefore, eosinophils tend to occur where mast cells congregate. The eosinophil is characterized by a segmented nucleus, colorless to pale-blue cytoplasm, and distinct eosinophilic (reddish-orange)–staining granules in the cytoplasm.

The morphological appearance of eosinophil granules varies from species to species, so they can be used to identify the origin of a blood sample. The eosinophils of cats contain numerous tiny rod-shaped granules that may obscure the nucleus. The eosinophil granules of dogs are less numerous and usually round but may vary considerably in size. Greyhounds often have eosinophils that have degranulated and appear vacuolated. The eosinophil granules of horses are extremely distinctive, being very large and round and a much brighter orange than those of small animals. Bovine eosinophil granules are also bright orange but are much smaller and more numerous than those of the horse and much more uniform in size than those of the dog. Color Plate II, A to D, illustrates the diversity of eosinophil granules found in various domestic species.

Basophils. Basophils are relatively rare in blood films but, when present, tend to occur in association with increased eosinophils. Classically, they have dark basophilic (blue) granules, but they also may vary considerably from species to species. Feline basophils tend to have light lavender to almost pink granules rather than the dark-purple granules seen in other species. Canine basophils may have few to no granules and must be differentiated from neutrophils on the basis of an elongated nucleus and a more basophilic cytoplasm. Equine and bovine basophils tend to have variable numbers of the more typical dark basophilic granules. Basophils are frequently confused with mast cells because of similar granules, but the basophil nucleus is segmented, and the mast cell nucleus is round or oval.

Lymphocytes. Lymphocytes are usually small to medium-sized mononuclear cells with a thin rim of light to dark-blue cytoplasm and a round, often eccentric, nucleus. Their cytoplasm may or may not contain azurophilic (red) granules. Cattle are notorious for their often large, bizarre-looking lymphocytes. In normal cattle, lymphocytes outnumber neutrophils and may be quite large, with indented (rather than round) nuclei, increased cytoplasm, and perhaps azurophilic cytoplasmic granules. During periods of antigenic stimulation in all species, some of the lymphocytes in the blood film may have extremely basophilic cytoplasm with a pale perinuclear zone (the site of the Golgi apparatus) and possibly azurophilic granules. These cells are referred to as *reactive lymphocytes.*

Monocytes. Monocytes (Color Plate II and Fig. 5–8) are derived from the bone marrow and circulate in the blood briefly before entering the tissues in which they become *macrophages.* Macrophages phagocytize (ingest) large particles and cellular debris that neutrophils cannot handle. Monocytes have gray-blue, often grainy cytoplasm and a variable-shaped nucleus. The nucleus can be round, oval, ameboid, or lobed. The monocyte is usually larger than the lymphocyte or neutrophil. The most common problem associated with the identification of monocytes is the tendency to confuse monocytes which have a bean-shaped nucleus with a band neutrophil; this is especially a problem when there is toxic change in the neutrophils. The cytoplasm of the monocyte is usually a darker blue than the band neutrophil.

Other Cells. Occasionally, evaluation of the blood film reveals abnormal circulating cell types, such as mast cells, lymphoblasts, myeloblasts, and erythroblasts. The number and type of abnormal cells should be noted because they may indicate leukemia or systemic mastocytosis. Smudge (or basket) cells are degenerated cells appearing as pale eosinophilic nuclear material lacking shape or form. These occur when excessive pressure is used in making the film or when old blood is used. A few of these are of little significance, but numerous smudge cells can affect the accuracy of the differential. Blood films with unusual or abnormal cells can be sent to a reference laboratory for evaluation.

Absolute versus Relative Numbers. The numbers obtained when doing the differential are *relative,* or percentages of the whole cell population. These numbers have no diagnostic significance but are used to calculate the absolute numbers of the various WBCs. *Absolute numbers* are the only numbers with diagnostic significance and should always be calculated and reported as such. These are obtained by multiplying the relative percentages by the total WBC count and expressed as cells per microliter.

TECHNICIAN NOTE

Only absolute numbers are significant for interpreting the differential.

Automated Cell Counters

Several instruments available for automated electronic cell counting range in price from $10,000 to $100,000. A basic understanding of the principles of electronic cell counting is useful for the veterinary technician regardless of whether the practice has an in-clinic laboratory. Many practices find it convenient to use human reference or hospital laboratories, but these instruments must be specially calibrated for use with veterinary samples due to the wide variation in blood cell size among the different species. Several instruments have been introduced specifically for veterinary medicine that are computer driven with species options and automatically change the instrument settings for multiple species use. The major advantages of electronic cell counters is their speed, accuracy, and reproducibility. In addition to providing RBC and WBC counts, most cell counters will measure hemoglobin and calculate the RBC indices.

The disadvantage of electronic cell counters is their quality control and maintenance requirements. The veterinary technician must be able to recognize when the instruments are not functioning properly and determine the problem. The manufacturer should be willing to train the technician to perform quality control and calibration procedures, keep adequate quality control records, and handle minor adjustments. In addition, the manufacturer should be available for service calls if needed. In some practices, consideration should be given to the purchase of a service contract; this should be discussed before investing in a major instrument.

The operating principle involved in electronic cell counting is based on a type of flow cytometry (the counting of particles as they flow past a detection device). This technology allows the instrument to count blood cells and measure their size. Most instruments use a simple orifice through which an electrical current passes. As particles (e.g., blood cells) move through the orifice, they disrupt the current by increasing the resistance proportional to the size of the particle. The instrument is set to detect and count only particles that produce a signal that exceeds a specific resistance or threshold. The threshold settings will determine what particles are counted, based on their size. This principle is important when an instrument is evaluated for use in veterinary medicine. Many instruments developed for human medicine do not accurately count RBCs with a volume of less than 55 femtoliters (fl). The RBCs of the cat, horse, cow, goat, and pig have mean cell volumes below this value.

WBCs from different species also have varying sizes after exposure to RBC lysing solutions. Total WBC counts on some instruments can be falsely decreased in the dog due to their small leukocytes. The reverse is true in the cat. The cat's platelets tend to form large clumps that are counted as leukocytes, thus falsely elevating the WBC count. Close inspection of the blood film will help the technician identify this problem.

Whole blood can be diluted for counting either before introducing the sample into the machine (predilution) or by the instrument as part of the sampling cycle. In the newer instruments, whole blood is aspirated and diluted for the RBC count, and a portion of the sample is lysed to remove the RBCs and allow the WBCs to be counted. The lysed sample is often used for hemoglobin determination.

Quantitative buffy coat (QBC) analysis is another automated cell-counting method that is used in many veterinary practices for measurements of PCV, total WBC count, platelet count, and a limited leukocyte differential. The QBC (IDEXX, Westbrook, ME) instrumentation consists of large-bore capillary tubes fitted with a free-floating plastic cylinder slightly smaller in diameter than the tube, a centrifuge, and a reading instrument that converts buffy coat band lengths into numerical readings. The tubes are coated with acridine orange, a dye that allows the differentiation of the granulocytes, mononuclear cells (monocytes and lymphocytes), and platelets. Figure 5–9 illustrates the expansion of the buffy coat by the plastic float and where the specific cell layers are found. The QBC instrument is relatively inexpensive compared with the electronic cell counters and provides similar information. It is important to remember, however, that the limited differential obtained should not replace the blood film examination.

✎ TECHNICIAN NOTE

The differential provided by the QBC instrument is not an adequate substitute for microscopic evaluation of the blood film.

Blood cell morphology is important in evaluating the numbers obtained in the blood cell counts. The QBC instrument cannot tell the technician whether band neutrophils, polychromatophilic RBCs, or NRBCs are present. One important advantage of the QBC instrument is improved detection of circulating microfilaria.

Plasma Protein Determination

Determination of the plasma protein concentration is another standard component of the routine CBC. The simplest method is to take the capillary tube used for measuring the PCV, break the tube at a point slightly above the *buffy coat* (cream-colored layer of WBCs and platelets just above the RBCs), and allow the plasma to run through the unbroken end onto the prism of a refractometer by capillary action. It is best not to lift the cover and tap the hematocrit tube on the prism, as this may scratch the surface of the prism. Plasma protein values obtained with a refractometer are accurate as long as the plasma is clear. If the plasma is lipemic, hemolyzed, or otherwise cloudy, the refractive index will be increased and provide an erroneously high protein measurement. Often, the lipemic samples have a very

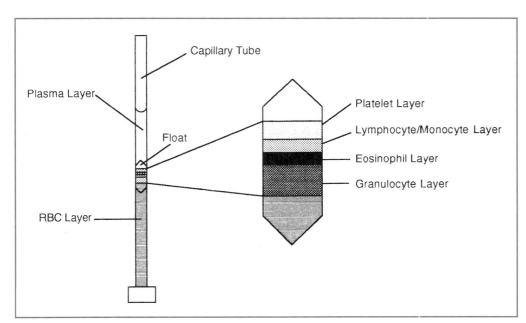

Figure 5-9. Illustration of the QBC buffy coat layers that occur through centrifugation.

Capillary Tube

Plasma Layer

Float

RBC Layer

Platelet Layer

Lymphocyte/Monocyte Layer

Eosinophil Layer

Granulocyte Layer

indistinct or unfocused line on the refractometer scale. In contrast to the dilution effect of a small blood sample in a large tube, excess anticoagulant will artifactually increase the plasma protein value obtained.

Determination of plasma *fibrinogen* levels may be useful in the detection of inflammatory processes, particularly in cattle and horses. Two capillary tubes of blood are centrifuged; one is used for the PCV and plasma protein determination, as described. The second tube is placed in a 56°C to 58°C water bath for 3 minutes to cause the precipitation of fibrinogen. The tube is then recentrifuged so the fibrinogen settles just above the buffy coat. The tube is broken above the fibrinogen, and the remaining plasma is placed on the refractometer for protein determination. The difference between protein concentration of the first tube and protein concentration of the second tube is the fibrinogen concentration.

Fibrinogen is usually expressed in milligrams per deciliter; therefore, if the first tube had a protein concentration of 7.3 g/dl and the second tube has a protein concentration of 6.9 g/dl, the plasma fibrinogen concentration is 0.4 g/dl, or 400 mg/dl. Plasma from cattle with markedly increased fibrinogen may completely coagulate during incubation; when the specimen is respun, the fibrinogen does not settle out, and a fibrinogen value cannot be determined.

Coagulation Testing

Patients will occasionally present with abnormal bleeding tendencies. *Hemostasis,* the maintenance of proper blood flow, is dependent on vascular integrity, platelet number and function, and several coagulation factors. The coagulation factors are a group of chemicals, enzymes, and cofactors that interact to stabilize a platelet plug and stem the flow of blood. Evaluation of these factors, along with a platelet count, is part of a coagulation profile.

Most of these tests require special instrumentation and are submitted to a reference laboratory; however, sample collection and submission are critical for obtaining valid results. The venipuncture must be accurate to avoid tissue injury, which will invalidate the coagulation assays. In addition to the EDTA tube for the platelet count, blood must be collected in tubes with citrate anticoagulant (turquoise top) for factor assays. Only plastic or siliconized glass should be used in handling these samples because contact with regular glass will invalidate the results. The samples should be centrifuged and the plasma tested immediately or frozen. It is recommended that the reference laboratory always be contacted for additional directions before drawing and submitting samples for coagulation testing.

URINALYSIS

Urinalysis is one clinical laboratory procedure that should be performed as a part of any minimum data base in all veterinary practices but is frequently skipped for a variety of reasons. It is an important diagnostic test that should be done on fresh urine when possible. The techniques involved are simple and require no special instrumentation. Urine samples should be collected into clean glass or plastic containers. In general, no preservatives are necessary. The best time to collect urine for urinalysis is usually first thing in the morning. Urine that accumulates during the relative inactivity of the night is less likely to be influenced by feeding or exercise. It is generally concentrated,

and therefore abnormal constituents, if present, are more easily detected.

Equipment

The equipment necessary for performing the urinalysis is minimal. A supply of clean glass or plastic collection containers, a centrifuge and conical centrifuge tubes, chemical reagent strips, clean glass slides and coverslips, a refractometer, plastic pipettes, and a microscope are all that are required.

Urine Collection

Urine may be collected by several methods. The simplest (if the animal will cooperate) is to catch a free-flow nonsterile sample as the animal voids. If this method is used, the initial stream of urine should not be caught because the first portion may contain cells and debris from the urethra and lower genital tract, resulting in contamination of the sample which may interfere with interpretation. It is better to collect a midstream sample, avoiding the very beginning or the very end of a voided urine sample.

A second method that may be used to collect urine is *cystocentesis.* This procedure involves placing a needle (with a syringe attached) through the ventral abdominal wall into the lumen of the bladder and aspirating urine. Aseptic technique must be used. By performing cystocentesis, secretions and debris of the lower urogenital tract are avoided, and interpretation of urinalysis findings is simplified. Iatrogenic hemorrhage can occur during cystocentesis; therefore, it is not unusual to have a widely varying number of RBCs in the sediment of samples obtained by this method.

Another method for collecting urine is by catheterization of the bladder. This procedure must be done as aseptically as possible to prevent introduction of bacteria into the urinary tract. Extreme care should be taken to avoid traumatizing the lining of the urethra with the catheter, or the sample may contain increased numbers of erythrocytes and epithelial cells. Additional information on cystocentesis and catheterization is found in Chapter 10.

Regardless of how the urine sample is collected, it should be analyzed as soon as possible. Many changes begin to occur immediately. Bacteria present in the urine will multiply, cells may degenerate, casts may dissolve (especially if the urine is alkaline), and bacteria that produce urease will convert urea to ammonia, causing the pH to increase. If there is to be any delay in performing the urinalysis, the sample should be refrigerated to slow these processes. However, refrigeration may cause a change in urine specific gravity and interfere with some of the chemistry reactions on the chemistry reagent strip. Before a urinalysis is performed on refrigerated urine, the specimen should be allowed to come to room temperature.

Evaluation of Physical Properties

As with all laboratory procedures, it is wise to follow the same routine protocol with every urine sample analyzed. The physical properties evaluated in most routine urinalyses include color, appearance or turbidity, and specific gravity. After making sure the sample is mixed well, the color (e.g., yellow, gold, red) and appearance (e.g., clear, hazy, flocculent) should be recorded.

Cystocentesis = "sterile" sample

Color

Normal urine is yellow to amber, depending on its concentration and constituents. Bright-red urine indicates *hematuria* (RBCs in the urine) or *hemoglobinuria* (hemoglobin in the urine). Reddish-brown urine usually suggests hemoglobinuria or *myoglobinuria* (myoglobin in the urine); note that these two pigments cannot be distinguished from one another solely on the basis of color. High concentrations of bilirubin or urobilin cause yellowish-brown urine that, when shaken, may produce yellowish foam. Whenever an unusual discoloration of the urine occurs, the history of any drug therapy should be evaluated because there are many drugs that can produce abnormally colored urine. It is important to remember urine that is markedly discolored may make it difficult or impossible to interpret color changes when evaluating chemical reagent strips.

Turbidity

Fresh urine is normally transparent, but as it cools, some salts may precipitate, causing the urine to become cloudy. Except for equine urine, fresh urine that is cloudy is often pathological, and it must be examined microscopically to identify the cause: pus, blood, mucus, bacteria, casts, or crystals. Fresh equine urine is normally cloudy because it contains mucus and calcium carbonate crystals (Fig. 5–10). Even clear urine should be examined microscopically because some abnormal constituents may be present in small amounts that may not cause urine to be visually cloudy.

Specific Gravity

Specific gravity (SG) determination is one of the most important parts of a urinalysis. It may be determined before or after centrifugation because the material that settles during centrifugation has little to no effect on SG. The SG value depends on the number and size of particles in solution and is an indicator of the ability of the kidney to concentrate urine. The SG is most accurately determined with a refractometer, which is used for determining plasma protein, and requires only one drop of urine. If the urine sample is turbid, the SG may be determined from the supernatant after centrifugation.

The normal range for SG is extremely wide: 1.001 to 1.060 in dogs and 1.001 to 1.080 in cats. The major determinant of urine SG is salt concentration because of the large number of particles involved. Protein, in contrast, has little influence on SG, because although the particles are large, they are few in number. Glucose, likewise, has relatively little effect on SG. Both of these components however, when found in large amounts in the urine, will increase the SG by about 0.001 to 0.002. SG provides a very good indication of how well the kidneys are able to function in maintaining the body's water and osmotic balance. In addition, SG is important in interpreting other tests. Because of the usual inverse relationship between SG and volume, a 2⁺ protein in dilute urine (SG <1.012) suggests a greater loss of protein than a 2⁺ protein in concentrated urine (SG >1.030).

Isosthenuria is the continued excretion of urine at the SG of glomerular filtrate (1.008 to 1.012). Isosthenuria indicates that the tubules have not attempted to concentrate urine. A single, routine urine sample with an isosthenuric SG is not necessarily abnormal because this is within the normal range and could be a chance occurrence. However, if an animal is dehydrated, azotemic, or uremic, the renal tubules are under pressure to concentrate urine, and under those circumstances, a SG lower than 1.035 in cats, 1.030 in dogs, and 1.025 in large animals indicates that the kidneys are not functioning appropriately.

Chemical Evaluation

Reagent strip chemistries should be performed on unspun urine, unless the urine is very turbid (cloudy). If it is turbid, the chemistry tests may be done after the sample has been centrifuged. Protein, glucose, ketones, blood, and bilirubin in the urine are routinely determined as well as urinary pH. The strips contain pads that are impregnated with reagents and result in a color change when the appropriate urine constituents are present. Although simple to use, proper technique and accurate timing for reading the results are critical. The strips must be properly stored, the urine must be at room temperature and well mixed, and excess urine must be shaken from the strips to obtain valid results. Significantly discolored urine may interfere with the ability to discern colors and color changes on the reagent pads.

Some commercially available strips contain reagent pads for other components, such as leukocytes. These are being evaluated for reliability but are not yet accepted as accurate.

TECHNICIAN NOTE

Refrigerated urine samples must be brought to room temperature before chemical analysis is performed.

pH

Urine pH is detected by reagent strips with chemical indicators. The symbol *pH* is used to express the hydrogen ion concentration (acidity) of a fluid. pH 7 is the neutral point. Readings above 7 are said to be alkalotic, and those below 7 are acidotic. In general, dogs and cats tend to have more acid urine than do cattle and horses. It is imperative that a fresh sample be used

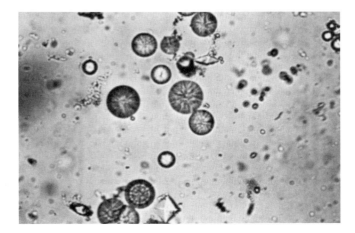

Figure 5–10. Photomicrograph of equine urine sediment showing the round calcium carbonate crystals with distinct radiating striations.

because as urine stands it loses carbon dioxide and bacteria that are present may produce ammonia, both of which result in increased alkalinity (raising the pH). The body's acid-base status may affect urine pH, but it is a mistake to use urine pH to evaluate the systemic acid-base balance. Too many other factors influence urine pH; in fact, urine pH may be completely contrary to the body's pH. For example, some cows with metabolic alkalosis have a paradoxical aciduria because the kidney attempts to maintain electrolyte balance at the expense of acid-base balance.

Protein

Most commercial urine reagent strips include a test for *protein*. It is often stated that normal urine contains no protein, but almost all urine contains a small amount of protein, which is due to normal leakage and secretion from the urinary tract lining. However, this normal amount of protein is not detected by routine methods. The strips rely on color changes in tetra-bromophenolphthalein blue to detect protein levels that are above a very small amount (>10 mg/dl) present in normal urine. The test reaction is usually graded *trace* or 1^+ through 4^+ which supposedly corresponds to various protein concentrations. As mentioned, a positive protein reaction in dilute urine implies a greater protein loss than the same level of reaction in a concentrated sample. As with most reagent strip chemistry tests, results are at best only semiquantitative and are subject to several types of error. False-positive values may occur when urine is very alkaline. Second, the strips are more sensitive to albumin than to globulins and therefore can give false-negative readings when proteinuria is caused by globulins. Because the change in color of the reagent strip pad is subjective, different technicians may make different readings on the same urine sample.

Protein loss into urine can be a significant drain on the body's protein stores. One can make a subjective evaluation of the amount being lost by comparing the results with the SG, as previously mentioned; however, a more exact method is to collect all urine produced in a 24-hour period and calculate its total protein content. The collection of 24 hours of urine output generally requires a metabolism cage and is not very practical. The ratio of urine protein to urine creatinine (P/C ratio) in any single sample is a good index of protein loss in the urine. A urine P/C ratio of less than 1.0 is considered normal; more than 2.0 indicates abnormal urinary protein loss; and from 1.0 to 2.0 is suspicious. A urine sample with a sediment that indicates inflammation (presence of WBCs) is not suitable for urine P/C ratio. The inflammation must first be successfully treated. If the patient still has proteinuria once all evidence of inflammation is gone, a urine P/C ratio can be requested. Urine P/C ratios are usually done at a reference laboratory because they require a sensitive protein determination.

In interpreting the cause for a positive urine protein test, one must also consider the results of the test for blood and the microscopic examination of sediment. These results may aid in identifying the source of urinary protein. Proteinuria without a positive blood reaction or significant cells is indicative of glomerular disease, in which defective glomeruli allow passage of albumin into the urine, often resulting in protein readings of 3^+ or 4^+. There are few extrarenal factors that may temporarily alter glomerular permeability to protein and result in proteinuria; they include fever, severe exercise, shock, cardiac or central nervous system disease, and the postcolostral period in neonates.

When excessive hemorrhage into the urinary tract occurs, the test for urine protein will be positive and erythrocytes will be seen in the sediment. Possible causes for urinary tract hemorrhage include trauma, neoplasia, and inflammation. Hemoglobin or myoglobin in the urine will cause a positive protein test as well as a positive blood test. In either of these cases, intact RBCs are not a significant part of the sediment.

When proteinuria occurs in conjunction with increased leukocytes in the urine sediment, inflammation of the urinary tract should be suspected. Inflammation rarely causes a urine protein test of more than 2^+, unless hemorrhage is associated with the inflammatory process. In some urinary tract infections, bacteria may be seen in the sediment. Determination of the location of the inflammation may be dependent on the method of collection. With testing of voided samples, the inflammation may be anywhere in the genitourinary tract, whereas if test samples were collected by cystocentesis the inflammation may be localized to the bladder or kidney.

Glucose

In addition to urine protein, a common reagent strip test for urine is the test for glucose. The reagent strips usually use glucose oxidase to detect glucose and for this reason are quite specific for glucose. However, as with all reagent strip tests, they are not quantitative. Tablets that detect glucose are available that are somewhat more quantitative but not specific. The tablets use a copper reduction method that detects many sugars and reducing agents other than glucose.

Normally, urine contains no detectable glucose. Glucose is filtered by the glomerulus, but the body preserves this energy source by reabsorbing it in the proximal renal tubules. This resorption ability is exceeded once the blood glucose level rises above 180 mg/dl in most species or above 100 mg/dl in the cow. This is the "renal threshold" for glucose, above which it will "spill" into the urine. The primary cause for *glucosuria*, therefore, is *hyperglycemia*. To confirm this, the blood glucose level should be determined at the same time as the urine glucose. Diabetes mellitus is a common cause of hyperglycemia and glucosuria.

Ketones

A test for urine ketones is included on many reagent strips; tablets are also available. Both use a nitroprusside method that detects acetone and acetoacetic acid but not beta-hydroxybutyric acid, so false-negative results are possible. Ketones will appear in the urine before they build up to a detectable level in the bloodstream, so *ketonuria* may occur before a detectable *ketonemia* occurs. Ketonuria indicates excessive fat metabolism, a deficiency in carbohydrate metabolism, or both, but is most commonly seen in conjunction with glucosuria as a complication of diabetes mellitus.

Bilirubin

There are reagent strips and tablets for detecting *bilirubinuria*, both of which use a similar reaction (diazotization), but the tablets are less subject to interference by urine color. The tablets are also highly sensitive, so a 1^+ reading, especially in concentrated urine, may not be significant. Both strips and tablets detect conjugated bilirubin and not unconjugated bilirubin. Bilirubin in urine can also be crudely detected by the *foam test*. If a yellowish foam appears when the urine sample is shaken, bilirubin is likely present. Bilirubin may be oxidized on exposure to light, so if there is much delay between obtaining the urine sample and performing the urinalysis, the sample should be protected from light to avoid false-negative results. Many normal dogs, and sometimes cattle, will exhibit bilirubinuria because the kidneys, as well as the liver, have an enzyme that can conjugate bilirubin. This, however, is lacking in cats, and any bilirubinuria is a significant abnormality in cats.

Blood

The designation "blood" is somewhat misleading because this test actually detects intact RBCs, hemoglobin, and myoglobin. Both reagent strips and tablets make use of the peroxidase property of free hemoglobin or myoglobin, which oxidizes orthotoluidine to a blue-colored derivative. If the urine is red and cloudy and erythrocytes are present in the sediment, *hematuria* is the reason for the positive blood reaction.

Hemoglobinuria (hemoglobin pigment in the urine) results in red to brown urine with a positive urine blood reaction and no erythrocytes in the sediment. A positive urine protein test may also be apparent. In contrast to hematuria, hemoglobinuria will be accompanied by *hemoglobinemia,* imparting a pink to reddish discoloration to the serum or plasma.

Myoglobinuria (myoglobin pigment in the urine) will similarly result in red to brown urine with no erythrocytes in the sediment, a positive urine blood reaction, and a positive urine protein test. However, during myoglobinuria, the blood serum or plasma generally remains clear. Myoglobin, which is derived from muscles, is a smaller molecule than hemoglobin and does not bind to serum proteins; thus, it is rapidly excreted into the urine before reaching levels sufficiently high to produce discoloration of the serum. Animals with myoglobinuria generally do not show evidence of anemia but have some type of muscle disease, such as exertional myopathy in horses ("tying up syndrome"), trauma, electrical shock, or pressure necrosis from prolonged recumbency. If it is not apparent by clinical signs, hemoglobinuria and myoglobinuria may be differentiated by electrophoresis or a more cumbersome ammonium sulfate precipitation test.

Microscopic Examination

The sediment should be prepared for microscopic examination. Urine sediment examination may reveal extremely useful diagnostic information and be crucial for correct interpretation of the chemical analyses. A few cells and a few casts may be found in normal urine, but increased numbers of various elements indicate certain diseases.

Sample Preparation

Pour a standard volume (10 ml is recommended) of urine into a conical-tip centrifuge tube. If the sample available is less than 10 ml, use all that is left after the reagent strip chemistries and SG determinations have been completed. Centrifuge the urine at a slow speed (1500 rpm) for 5 minutes. Higher speeds for centrifugation may disrupt the cells and casts that are present. Decant the supernatant, leaving the sediment in the bottom. Gently tap the tube to resuspend the sediment in the small amount of urine remaining on the sides and in the bottom of the tube. With a small pipette, transfer a drop of suspended sediment to a glass slide and place a coverslip on it. There are commercial stains (Sedi-Stain, Clay Adams, Parsippany, NJ) available for evaluating urine sediments, but with practice and experience they are not necessary.

A phase-contrast microscope is ideal for examining unstained urine sediment. A more practical and highly satisfactory alternative is to lower the condenser of the light microscope and reduce the intensity of the light (as for the manual mammalian WBC count). The slide should first be examined at 10× magnification to obtain an overall impression of how much and what type of sediment is present. The 40× or 45× power (high dry) is then used to make the final identification and count of various components. At least 10 microscopic fields must be evaluated, and the average numbers of various cells and casts per high-power field are reported. The presence and relative amounts of other components are also noted.

Epithelial Cells

Three types of epithelial cells can be found in urine sediment: squamous, transitional, and renal tubular. *Squamous epithelial cells* are very large, with angular borders and small nuclei originating from the lining of the distal urethra and vagina or prepuce and are not generally indicative of disease. *Transitional epithelial cells* are medium sized and oval, spindled, or caudate cells found lining the proximal urethra, bladder, ureters, and renal pelvis. They may occur in groups, especially if the urine was obtained by catheterization. Occasionally, if they are very large and variable, very basophilic, or in large clusters, they should be further evaluated for possible neoplasia. Renal tubular epithelial cells are small, round cells and may be indicative of tubular degeneration.

Blood Cells

Erythrocytes in unstained sediment appear colorless or yellowish and are round and slightly refractile, with no internal structure. They may be confused with fat droplets, but erythrocytes are fairly uniform in size and do not float in and out of planes of focus as do fat droplets. If there is doubt, a drop of diluted acetic acid will lyse erythrocytes, helping to differentiate them from fat droplets. In concentrated urine, erythrocytes may lose fluid and become *crenated* (shrunken and spiked). In dilute urine, they may imbibe water and swell or even lyse, becoming *ghost cells*. *Leukocytes* in urine sediment are round and granular and larger than erythrocytes but smaller than epithelial cells. The presence of more than five to eight WBCs per high-power field indicates inflammation of the urinary or urogenital tract depending on the method of collection. When this occurs, a careful check for bacteria should be made.

Casts

Casts are another prominent feature of urine sediment. They are elongated structures composed of protein from plasma and mucoprotein from the renal tubules. In general, they form in the distal tubules, in which the urine is more concentrated and acidic. Any structures that happen to be in the tubules at the time the casts form (erythrocytes, leukocytes, or epithelial cells) become embedded in the casts. The presence of increased numbers of casts helps to localize the renal disease to the tubules, but the numbers do not necessarily correlate with the severity of disease. For instance, severe chronic nephritis may be accompanied by just a few casts. There are five main types of casts. (1) *Hyaline casts* are colorless, homogeneous, and semitransparent. They may be difficult to see unless the light is reduced. They indicate mild glomerular leakage. (2) *Cellular casts* contain recognizable cells imbedded in the protein matrix. They may be epithelial cell casts that contain sloughed tubular epithelial cells, erythrocyte casts that indicate renal hemorrhage, or leukocyte casts that indicate renal inflammation or pyelonephritis. (3) *Granular casts* are derived from degenerating cells or cellular casts. They are characterized by a nonspecific granular matrix and are designated either coarsely or finely granular, depending on the degree of degeneration. They probably are the most common type of cast found in animals. (4) *Waxy casts* are wide and homogeneous, usually with distinct blunt or squared ends. They are the next stage of degeneration from granular casts and indicate a more chronic tubular lesion. (5) *Fatty casts* contain fat globules from degenerating tubular epithelial cells and are most common in cats because of the high lipid content of feline tubular epithelium.

Crystals

Crystals are another major component of urine sediment. Their precipitation and presence depend on urine pH and the solubility and concentration of the substance forming them. Crystals are common, and most are not indicative of disease. In carnivores, *phosphates, urates,* and *oxalates* are normal, whereas in herbivores, *calcium carbonate* crystals are the most common. Urine crystals that accompany pathological conditions include *ammonium biurate, monohydrate calcium oxalate, bilirubin,* and *cystine* crystals. Dihydrate calcium oxalate crystals can be found in normal urine but appear distinctly different from the monohydrate calcium oxalate crystals found with ethyleneglycol (antifreeze) toxicity. Figure 5–11 illustrates these two types of calcium oxalate crystals. Bilirubin crystals generally occur in conjunction with bilirubinuria with little to no additional significance. Ammonium biurate crystals are dark with very distinct multiple irregular protrusions and are often associated with portal caval shunts, a specific liver disorder. Cystine crystals, although sometimes seen in normal dogs, are also found in a congenital defect of cystine metabolism that leads to cysti-

nuria in dogs. Drugs, such as sulfonamides, may precipitate in the urine of animals, resulting in the formation of crystals.

Microorganisms

Bacteria in unstained urine sediment may be difficult to detect. Rods may appear singly or in chains, but cocci may be lost in brownian movement. For this reason, whenever bacteria are suspected, the sediment should be stained to examine it more thoroughly. Usually, the regular examination of the unstained sediment is completed and recorded first, and then the coverslip is removed and the underlying sediment on the slide is allowed to dry. Once dry, the slide can be stained with a Gram stain or one of the modified Wright's stains, and any bacteria present can be identified. On a Gram stain, the gram-negative rod-shaped bacteria may be difficult to see among all the pink-staining cellular debris. With the Wright stain, all bacteria stain dark purple and are relatively easy to find.

Bacteria in a voided sample often are not significant because they may be normal flora from the distal urogenital tract, especially from the prepuce or vagina. Bacteria are significant if they occur in catheterized or cystocentesis samples. Their presence should be correlated with leukocytes in urine because bacteria with no leukocyte response should raise suspicion of contamination of the sample. If bacteria are present in a urine sample, they can multiply as time passes, so this should be taken into consideration when the sample is being analyzed. Rarely, *fungal* organisms are found in urine sediment. The majority of these are insignificant contaminants, although some, such as *Blastomyces,* may be significant.

Miscellaneous

Usually insignificant components of urine sediment include mucus, fat, sperm, and parasites. Mucus appears as narrow, twisted, ribbon-like strands. It is normal in equine urine and can be seen in other species due to genital secretions or irritation of the urethra. Fat, as previously noted, takes the form of refractile, variably sized spheres in many planes of focus. Fat is rarely significant. Sperm are commonly seen in male canine urine. Parasites that can occur in urine include the ova of *Stephanurus dentatus, Dioctophyma renale,* and *Capillaria plica* and microfilaria of *Dirofilaria immitis.*

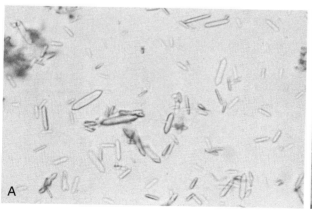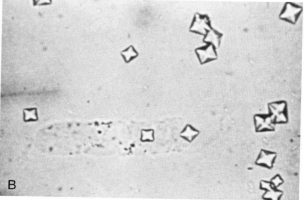

Figure 5–11. Photomicrograph of canine urine sediment showing the two forms of calcium oxalate crystals. A, Monohydrate form. B, Dihydrate form. (Courtesy of Dr. Mary Anna Thrall.)

CLINICAL CHEMISTRY

Several small relatively inexpensive clinical chemistry instruments have been developed. As with the electronic cell counters, a veterinary practice must have a demand for immediate availability of clinical laboratory data to justify the expense of these instruments. There are two general types of chemistry instrumentation: liquid reagent chemistry and dry chemistry. Instruments that use liquid reagents require more technical expertise and time in preparing reagents and monitoring their performance. The dry chemistry instruments are simpler to use and provide consistent performance. The principles of operation differ significantly between the two types of instruments, as does the extent to which specimen quality affects the measurement.

Equipment

Regardless of the decision whether to maintain and operate an in-house chemistry analyzer, veterinary practices will need a sample collection system consisting of either syringes and needles or Vacutainers, plus clean plastic or glass tubes to store or transport samples. A centrifuge and pipettes will be necessary to separate the serum or plasma from the cells.

Clinical Chemistry Instrumentation

The liquid reagent-based instruments use the principle of photometry (the measurement of light transmittance by a solution). Beer's law states that the concentration of a substance in a liquid is indirectly proportional to the amount of light that passes through the liquid. Most instruments have a spectrophotometer to measure the amount of light transmitted. A spectrophotometer consists of a light source directed through a specific path and a photosensitive detector that converts light into electrical energy. Each substance will transmit light at a specific wavelength. To increase the specificity of the measurement, filters are placed between the light source and the sample to allow only a specific wavelength to pass through the sample. The magnitude of the electrical current produced by the detector corresponds to the concentration of the substance being measured. Solutions that contain a known concentration of specific substances are called *standards* and are used to calibrate the instrument. Each instrument has specific procedures for *calibration,* which should be carefully followed to ensure optimal performance.

The instruments that use dry reagents are becoming more popular for in-clinic use. The major advantage of these instruments is the elimination of liquid reagents, which must be reconstituted or diluted before use. Dry chemistry instruments use reagent strips (similar to the strips used for urinalysis) or reagent slides. A specific amount of the patient's sample is placed on the reagent strip, and the intensity of the color that develops is measured by the principle of reflectance. Light is transmitted to the analyte slide via fiber optics, and the reflected light is conducted to a photodetector. The density of the color formed by the chemical reaction is determined and is proportional to the concentration of the substance being measured. Because this methodology does not depend on reading light transmitted through a liquid as with the spectrophotometer-based instruments, there is less interference due to lipemia or hemolysis.

Several dry chemistry instruments are available (e.g., Abbot Serolyser, Boehringer-Mannheim Reflotron, Dupont Analyzer, and Vet Test 8008). The Vet Test 8008 is designed specifically for use with veterinary samples (Fig. 5–12). Examples of chemistry tests available with this instrument are listed in Table 5–4. The primary advantage of using an instrument such as the Vet Test 8008 is the availability of predetermined reference ranges, which can be used until the laboratory can establish its own values. In many cases, especially with these instruments, little variation occurs from instrument to instrument or operator to operator. Veterinary samples can vary significantly from human samples in the concentration of particular substances. As with

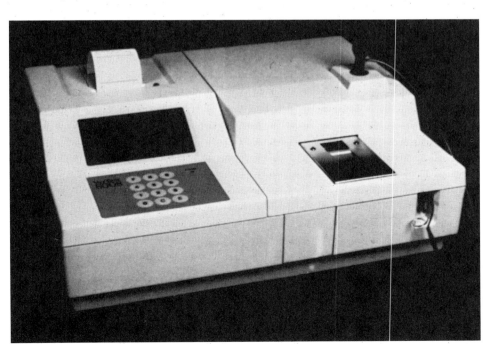

Figure 5-12. Vet Test 8008 dry chemistry analyzer (IDEXX Corp., Westbrook, ME).

• Table 5–4 •

CHEMISTRY TESTS AVAILABLE ON THE VET TEST 8008	
Urea nitrogen	Uric acid
Albumin	Creatinine
Alanine aminotransferase (ALT)	Total protein
Serum alkaline phosphatase (SAP)	Aspartate aminotransferase (AST)
Triglycerides	Cholesterol
Calcium	Glucose
Gamma-glutamyltransferase (GGT)	Creatine kinase (CK)
Amylase	Magnesium
Ammonia	Lipase
Lactate dehydrogenase (LDH)	Phosphorus
Total bilirubin	

the thresholds on the hematology instruments, the limits of the chemistry test (range of values that have a linear relationship within the methodology used) may have to be expanded to include values either above or below those seen in human samples. Good examples of this are the endocrine tests available on a few of the instruments. Thyroid hormone concentrations in dogs are much lower than those in humans, so assay procedures set up for humans will not be sufficiently sensitive to detect normal canine values.

Quality Control Programs

It is imperative that any veterinary practice that decides to establish an in-house laboratory make a commitment to quality control. Laboratory instruments will provide valid accurate results only if the samples are handled correctly, a well-maintained instrument is used, and the tests are performed correctly. The importance of routine maintenance and calibration procedures for all instruments cannot be overemphasized. However, even the most sophisticated, accurate, and well-maintained instrument cannot overcome errors in technique or poor sample quality. The technician should be familiar with the principle and limitations of all assays performed in the laboratory. Some of the more common causes for inaccurate results due to technical errors or sample quality are listed in Table 5–5. A quality control program consists of monitoring results of known *control samples* for identification of irregularities in reported values and following generally accepted laboratory procedures. Several textbooks on clinical chemistry and laboratory medicine (see Recommended Reading) provide excellent in-depth reviews of quality assurance programs. The following discussion deals primarily with the basics in monitoring an instrument to ensure the accuracy of reported data.

• Table 5–5 •

COMMON CAUSES FOR INACCURATE RESULTS
Poor-quality or outdated reagents
Failure to calibrate or run controls
Improper pipetting techniques
Improper maintenance of instrument
Lipemic or hemolyzed samples
Allowing serum to sit on clot
Use of inappropriate cuvettes
Power surges or failure

There are three levels of quality control: preanalytical procedures, analytical procedures, and analytical quality monitoring procedures. The *preanalytical procedures* deal with how the patient is prepared (fasting versus nonfasting samples), patient and specimen identification, specimen acquisition, and specimen processing. Establishment of standard procedures of each of these steps will decrease the likelihood of samples being misidentified or being of poor quality (hemolysed or lipemic). This aspect of quality control is important even in clinics that send their clinical pathology samples to a reference laboratory. *Analytical variables* include the analytical methodology, standardization and calibration procedures, documentation of analytical protocols and procedures, and monitoring of equipment while in use. This aspect of quality control is usually well defined by the manufacturer of the instrument and should be followed closely. The final level, *monitoring of analytical quality* using statistical methods and control charts, is the aspect that involves the use of control products and record-keeping. This aspect is the responsibility of the technician performing the tests.

TECHNICIAN NOTE

Valid results cannot be ensured without proper calibration and inclusion of appropriate control samples.

Controls

Control products are biological solutions, usually serum based, that have known concentrations of the various constituents or analytes that can be assayed by the instrument. These products should be stable, available in aliquots to prevent alterations due to refreezing, and have little vial-to-vial variation. Control products can be purchased from an independent source or from the company that makes the test kit or instrument. Most control products are available as normal, high abnormal, and low abnormal ranges. The control products are analyzed in a manner identical to patients' samples, and the values reported by the instrument are compared with the known values provided with the product.

Many control products are provided in a lyophilized form that requires rehydration with distilled water or a diluent provided by the manufacturer. It is essential that the solution be diluted properly to ensure the concentration of the analytes is correct. Imprecision in diluting the controls will be reflected by values that are not in concert with the known values of the product even though the instrument is working properly. It is highly recommended that volumetric or other precise pipettes be used to dilute the control products (a graduated cylinder is not acceptable).

The control values must fall within a specific acceptable range, which usually encompasses the mean ± 2 SD. This range is established by the manufacturer of the product by repeated assay of the solution. When the instrument reports a control value above or below the established range, there is a problem with the procedure, and test results for that particular sample should not be reported until the problem is identified.

A separate log of the control results should be kept and

reviewed periodically. A useful visual display of the instrument's performance for quick inspection and review is the Levy-Jennings chart. Figure 5–13 illustrates the use of the Levy-Jennings chart to keep track of quality control data. By inspection of control data over 1 month, a technician can see the control values gently drift upward or downward, indicating possible deterioration of the control product or a change in the light source intensity. Wide scatter of values outside the range on both the low and high end indicates imprecision on the part of the instrument or technician. It is best to keep the chart close to the instrument, not hidden in a file drawer. Everyone who uses the instrument must be willing to run controls and chart the results. Other useful laboratory records include calibration logs, sample logs, and maintenance logs.

Sample Handling

Sample handling is a critical step in obtaining accurate laboratory data. Several factors can interfere with analysis of a sample. The most common problems in veterinary medicine are hemolysis and lipemia. Difficulty in performing the venipuncture or excess pressure applied to the syringe during collection can cause significant hemolysis. The most common cause of lipemia is collection of a postprandial sample. There are times when both hemolysis and lipemia are unavoidable because they are the result of a disease process.

The effect hemolysis and lipemia will have on laboratory data is method dependent. There are no general rules to assist interpretation of changes due to sample quality. A good reference laboratory will provide information on how each of their tests is affected by these two changes. Manufacturers of the instruments and reagents should provide information on how interfering substances such as hemolysis and lipemia affect the methods used in their instrument. Hemolysis will commonly affect inorganic phosphorus and potassium values in horses and some Akita dogs. Lipemia will interfere with any method that depends on optical density read on a spectrophotometer. Some chemistry instruments can compensate for this change.

Again, the reference laboratory should be able to indicate which tests are affected. Errors in processing the sample can also cause artifactual changes in laboratory data. It is important to use the appropriate collection tube for the test being performed.

Samples collected for chemistry profiles can be collected in *clot tubes* (red top), which contain no anticoagulant, or in lithium heparin tubes (green top). Blood collected in clot tubes (tubes without anticoagulant) must be allowed to completely clot before the sample can be centrifuged and the serum removed; complete clot formation usually takes about 30 minutes. Clot tubes with activator gels (tiger top) will promote clotting, thus decreasing the time necessary for complete clot formation and facilitate separation of the serum from the RBCs. The sample should not be refrigerated before complete clot formation because this inhibits good serum separation. In addition, a fibrin clot forms above the RBCs if the blood is centrifuged before complete clot formation or at too fast a speed.

TECHNICIAN NOTE

Serum must be removed from the clot as soon as possible to avoid inaccurate results.

Blood collected in *lithium heparin* (green top) is excellent for emergency needs because it does not have to clot before it can be separated for analysis. Heparin may interfere with a few chemistry tests, so it is best to check with the reference laboratory before submitting heparinized plasma for chemistry panels. Lithium heparin is also excellent for emergency electrolyte panels. *EDTA* (purple top) is unacceptable for most chemistry tests because it binds calcium to prevent clot formation and thus interferes with many of the assays, particularly with those that are enzyme based. In addition, potassium EDTA will markedly increase serum potassium levels.

The necessity of separating serum from the clot as soon as

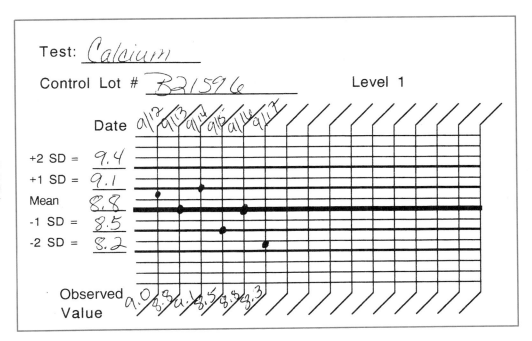

Figure 5-13. Levy-Jennings chart illustrating the common procedure used for following the performance of an individual test control serum.

possible cannot be overstressed. Prolonged exposure of serum to the cells will erroneously decrease the glucose, will increase the phosphorus, may increase potassium depending on species (especially in the horse), and may affect some enzyme activities. Do not depend on the reference laboratory courier service to get the sample to the laboratory in time to prevent these changes. It is best to take the time and responsibility to separate the serum and ensure the quality of the sample.

CYTOLOGY

Cytology is the study of cells, specifically involving the microscopic examination of individual cells that have exfoliated from a tissue or structure. Unlike histopathology, cytology is not an evaluation of the architecture of a tissue. In most instances, cytology can be used to differentiate an inflammatory lesion from a neoplastic mass. Sometimes cytological appearance reveals a very specific diagnosis, and for certain samples, such as bone marrow or mast cell tumors, it may be more helpful than histopathology. It should be emphasized that cytology is an adjunct diagnostic tool and not a replacement for histopathology.

Cytology requires a significant degree of expertise that can be acquired only through experience, especially for cytology of solid masses. Most veterinary practices prefer to send cytology samples to a reference laboratory for evaluation. For this reason, the discussion on cytology is limited to preparation of samples from solid tissues for submission to a reference laboratory and fluid analysis. Veterinary technicians interested in becoming adept at cytology should obtain specific training through continuing education workshops.

Equipment

One of the advantages of cytology is that it requires no special equipment or supplies other than those used in performing a CBC. A good microscope, clean glass slides, one or two stains (modified Wright's stain and Gram's stain), and a centrifuge for fluid samples will suffice for most cytological examinations.

Sample Preparation

Most cytology samples of solid masses are obtained through *fine needle aspiration* (FNA). Cells are aspirated from the mass with a syringe (usually 6 cc) and needle (22 to 25 gauge) inserted into the mass and the application of negative pressure. It is not necessary to aspirate so strenuously that material appears in the barrel of the syringe or even the hub of the needle. Gentle aspiration will usually pull sufficient material into the needle. The sample can then be expelled onto a glass slide. Depending on the consistency of the sample, it can be spread in a manner similar to making a blood smear or by what is referred to as the *squash prep* for more viscous samples. This is done by placing a second slide on top of the slide containing the sample. The weight of the top slide should cause the sample to spread, and then the top slide is pulled off across the bottom slide, resulting in even spreading of the cells. This method works well for many types of samples, and it may result in fewer broken cells than the traditional technique. It is important not to exert excessive pressure on the top slide or pull the slide apart too rapidly because cells are often fragile, and this will distort or "squash" the cells and make identification difficult if not impossible.

When handling excised pieces of tissue for cytological study, keep them wrapped in gauze and slightly moistened with saline so they do not dry out. Do not allow any contact with formalin, or even with formalin fumes, until after the cytological slides have been made and stained. Excised solid masses should be blotted with absorbent paper to remove blood and tissue fluid and then gently touched to a slide to make an impression slide. If the mass is of a dense consistency that does not exfoliate cells easily, it may be necessary to scrape it with a scalpel blade and then spread the material gently and thinly onto the slide. An alternative method is to cross-hatch cut the surface of the tissue with the scalpel blade and make an imprint preparation. The cross-hatching method is often gentler than the scraping method and preserves the cells better.

If the slides are to be sent to a reference laboratory, it is again recommended that the use of flat slide mailers be avoided because many will arrive shattered. Most reference laboratories prefer unstained slides, which can be stained at the laboratory by means of their standard stain protocol. If a slide has been stained and there are questions pertaining to that slide, it is a good idea to include that slide for comparison purposes.

Fluid Analysis

For fluid analysis, a refractometer and a cell-counting method (e.g., Unopettes and a hemacytometer) are also needed. Once a sample for cytology has been obtained, slides should be made as soon as possible, before the cells degenerate in the fluid. This is especially true of low-protein fluids, such as cerebrospinal fluid and tracheal washings. Many fluid samples can be prepared in the same manner as a blood film, leaving a feathered edge where the largest cells tend to migrate. If the fluid has very few cells, as is the case with cerebrospinal fluid, a direct preparation may not provide sufficient cells for a thorough examination. There are *cytocentrifuges* that are especially designed to make cytological slides from hypocellular fluids; they are gentler to cells because they spin at a slow speed and have gradual acceleration and deceleration. They also may have a special apparatus that causes cells to be deposited directly on to a slide, with filter paper taking away excess fluid. However, cytocentrifuges are probably impractical for all except the largest practices. As an alternative, these low cellularity samples can be concentrated similar to the preparation of a urine sediment. The fluid is centrifuged at slow speed, and the slide is prepared from the sediment after the supernatant is decanted or removed with a pipette. It is always advisable to make one or two direct preparations in case the techniques used to concentrate the cells result in too many ruptured cells or other artifacts.

A routine fluid analysis of samples such as abdominal, thoracic, or synovial fluid usually includes a WBC count, which is more appropriately referred to as a total nucleated cell count (TNCC), because some of the cells (mesothelial cells, synovial cells, and so forth) may not be derived directly from blood. The TNCC can be performed in the same manner as a WBC count. If there are numerous cells present, these can be counted on an automated instrument, but lower cell counts will require use of the hemacytometer as for a manual WBC count.

Total protein is another helpful parameter in fluid analysis and can be done by refractometer, generally using the supernatant portion of a centrifuged fluid sample. Total erythrocyte (RBC) count is often included in the fluid analysis if done on an automated instrument, but the RBC count alone is rarely helpful in evaluating fluid because of the frequency of peripheral blood contamination of samples. It is more important to check for *erythrophagocytosis* (phagocytosis of RBCs by macrophages) during the cytological examination because erythrophagocytosis generally implies that the RBCs were present in the fluid before sampling rather than as contaminants.

Fluid samples that have neutrophils as the predominate cell type should be closely evaluated for the presence of bacteria. Bacteria should be present within cells (intracellular) to be considered significant (Color Plate IJ). If they are only extracellular, one should consider the possibility of contamination of the sample. If no bacteria are found, it should not be assumed that they are absent. They may be in very low numbers and difficult to find.

Joint Fluid

The analysis of certain fluids includes specific tests that may add more information than routine tests. For instance, the *mucin clot test* is done on synovial fluid by mixing a diluted acetic acid solution (0.1 ml of 7N acetic acid in 4 ml of distilled water) and then adding 1 ml of synovial fluid. Normal synovial fluid contains mucin, which forms a tight white clot in the acetic acid; if the mucin has been digested by bacterial or cellular enzymes, the clot will be less distinct or may not form at all, leaving only hazy or cloudy fluid. Therefore, good mucin clot formation usually accompanies normal or noninflamed joints, whereas a poor or absent mucin clot indicates inflammation, infection, or both. The precipitation of mucin in joint fluid by acetic acid precludes the use of the WBC Unopette system because this system contains acetic acid as the diluent in the reservoir. TNCCs on joint fluid should be done using the Unopette system for both WBCs and platelets. The reservoir in this system contains ammonium oxalate, which will not precipitate mucin.

Recommended Reading

General

Duncan JR and Prasse KW: Veterinary Laboratory Medicine/Clinical Pathology. Ames, IA, Iowa State University Press, 1994.

Laboratory Equipment

Tietz NW: Fundamentals of Clinical Chemistry. 4th edition. Philadelphia, WB Saunders, 1995.

Hematology

Jain NC: Essentials of Veterinary Hematology. Philadelphia, Lea & Febiger, 1993.

Urinalysis

Osborne CA and Finco DR: Canine and Feline Nephrology and Urology. Philadelphia, Lea & Febiger, 1995.

Chemistry

Coffman JR: Equine Clinical Chemistry and Pathophysiology. Bonner Springs, KS, Veterinary Medicine Publishing Co., 1981.

Kaneko JJ (editor): Clinical Biochemistry of Domestic Animals. New York, Academic Press, 1989.

Quality Assurance Programs

Henry JB: Clinical Diagnosis and Management by Laboratory Methods. 19th edition. Philadelphia, WB Saunders, 1996.

Avian and Reptilian Hematology

Campbell TW: Avian Hematology and Cytology. Ames, IA, Iowa State University Press, 1988.

Frye FL: Biomedical and Surgical Aspects of Captive Reptile Husbandry. Edwardsville, KS, Veterinary Medicine Publishing Co., 1981.

Cytology

Cowell RL and Tyler RD: Diagnostic Cytology of the Dog and Cat. Goleta, CA, American Veterinary Publications, Inc., 1989.

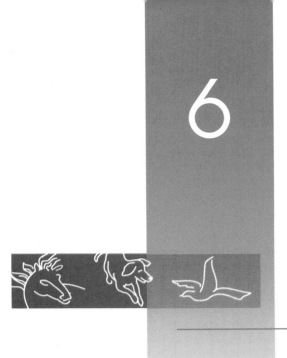

6 Parasitology

Johnny D. Hoskins

INTRODUCTION

Most parasites are capable of causing significant damage to the host. This potential may be a function of the number of parasites present in some cases; in the case of other parasites, location within the host, production of toxins, or interference with normal physiological processes produces the damage. Clinical signs associated with parasitism may include such disorders as life-threatening anemia, hypoproteinemia, diarrhea, vomiting, and intestinal obstruction, but not uncommonly the damage is more insidious, such as interference with normal weight gain or milk production. Parasitism is most severe in animals younger than 1 year, but it may affect animals of any age.

Ectoparasites (external parasites), including mites, ticks, lice, fleas, chiggers, and myiasis-inducing flies, and endoparasites (internal parasites), including protozoa, trematodes, tapeworms, and nematodes, have representative parasites on or in all animals and in every organ or tissue. Some parasites are host specific, whereas other parasites are capable of infesting or infecting a broad range of animal hosts. Modes of transmission vary considerably from simple, direct transmission to an extremely complex life cycle, involving the use of an intermediate host or transport host or specific environmental conditions. The nematode parasites have five stages in their development. Various nematodes, like the strongyle nematodes of ruminants and horses, produce an egg that passes into the environment. A first-stage larva develops within the egg. This free-living larva grows and molts (sheds the skin or cuticle) into a second-stage larva, which then grows and molts into a third-stage larva—the infective larva. The infective larva usually is ingested and develops into a fourth-stage larva and finally into a fifth-stage larva within the host.

Some nematodes have developed modifications from this life cycle. For example, hookworm larvae generally penetrate the skin and circulate in the host's tissue before completing their development in the small intestine. Others, like the roundworms and whipworms, develop into the infective stage within the egg and do not hatch until ingested by the host. Other important nematodes, like *Strongyloides,* have a first-stage larva in the egg when passed.

 TECHNICIAN NOTE

The diagnosis of parasitism is not difficult, but timing, choice of technique, and interpretation of the results are often crucial for effective treatment and control.

Treatment, including selection of the proper medication and appropriate control in the environment, always necessitates a thorough knowledge of the biology of each individual parasite.

The following sections provide discussions of specific parasites as they relate to animal host and parasite class within each host. The veterinary technician should become familiar with both the common name and the scientific name (as an example, roundworm = *Toxocara canis*) of the common parasites. Each section contains information on the life cycle, tissue location, treatment, and control for the specific parasite discussed. In addition, a section on diagnostic procedures is presented to outline the most commonly used techniques.

[handwritten notes: ingested → SI → liver → heart → lungs → cough up → ingested → SI. Hookworm → skin penetration]

ENDOPARASITES

Parasites of Dogs and Cats

Roundworms (Ascarids)

Toxocara canis, Toxocara cati, and *Toxascaris leonina* are ascarids that are thick, white to cream-colored nematodes. Mature specimens measure about 3.5 to 5 cm for males and 10 to 15 cm for females. Eggs of the *Toxocara* spp. are large, oval, and dark with a thick, rough shell. *Toxascaris leonina* is lighter in color and more egg shaped and has a thick, smooth shell (Fig. 6–1). All three species are common in most geographic regions of the United States. The larval stage develops within the egg, and the second stage is the infective larva. Eggs are highly resistant to adverse conditions and, under ideal environmental conditions, become infective in about 2 weeks. Once ingested, *Toxocara* spp. hatch in the small intestine, penetrate the mucosa, migrate through the liver, pass through the heart, and go into the lungs, in which they develop within a short period of time. Larvae are coughed, swallowed, and mature in the small intestine within 4 to 6 weeks.

Toxascaris leonina eggs hatch in the small intestine, and the larvae penetrate the intestinal mucosa to develop for about 2 to 3 months and then return to the lumen as adults. In dogs older than 5 weeks, most of the larvae leave the circulation and are stored in the somatic organs until the dog becomes pregnant. Between the 42nd and 56th days of gestation, these larvae leave the somatic tissues, cross the placenta, enter the fetal lungs, and remain there until birth. The larvae then complete the cycle already described. Consequently, a high percentage of dogs are infected by the *prenatal* or *transplacental* route. In the pregnant dog and cat, some of the activated larvae migrate to the mammary glands. These larvae are ingested by puppies and kittens when they first start to nurse. Transmammary infections are more common in cats than in dogs. The eggs of all three ascarids can be ingested by other animals (e.g., mice, chickens) and remain infective in their tissue until eaten by the appropriate host. All three species are readily diagnosed through a number of techniques, and they are amenable to treatment with a number of anthelmintics (Table 6–1). Control is difficult because the eggs are resistant, and control measures necessitate thorough cleansing of kennels, runs, yards, and so forth.

Hookworm

Ancylostoma caninum occurs in dogs, foxes, coyotes, wolves, raccoons, and badgers; *Ancylostoma braziliense* is found in dogs and cats; *Uncinaria stenocephala* occurs in dogs, cats, foxes, coyotes, and wolves; and *Ancylostoma tubaeforme* is found in cats and wild Felidae. Hookworms are all short, thick parasites, with the adult males measuring 6 to 12 mm, and the adult females measuring 6 to 20 mm. Hookworms produce a similar strongyle type of egg (Fig. 6–2). *Ancylostoma* spp. generally are found in coastal areas of high rainfall, whereas *U. stenocephala* are found in the northeastern United States. All hookworm species have a similar life cycle. Undeveloped eggs pass into the environment, develop, and hatch, releasing a first-stage larva that undergoes a free-living existence until it develops to the third-stage infective larva. Hookworms are capable of establishing in the host after ingestion, but the normal mode of infection is skin penetration. After larvae penetrate, they enter the venous circulation, going ultimately to the lungs, in which they develop for a short period of time. They are then coughed up and swallowed, and they enter the small intestine and mature. This generally occurs within 4 to 6 weeks.

> **TECHNICIAN NOTE**
>
> Hookworms are capable of establishing in the host after ingestion, but the normal mode of infection is skin penetration.

A. caninum has developed the additional modes of infection of *transplacental* or *transmammary infection.* Third-stage larvae penetrate the skin and circulate in the pregnant female host, ultimately crossing the placenta. The larvae also are stored in somatic tissues until the female host becomes pregnant. Most of the somatic larvae activated at the time of pregnancy migrate to the mammary glands of the bitch and are passed on to nursing puppies. Diagnosis is readily performed through identification of the egg by a number of techniques, and these species are amenable to treatment with a number of anthelmintics (see Table 6–1). Control is difficult, especially in warm, humid geographic regions, necessitating regular and thorough cleansing of yards, kennels, and so forth.

Intestinal Threadworm

Strongyloides stercoralis is a nematode that is a parasite of dogs, cats, foxes, humans, primates, and possibly other wild carnivores. Only the female nematode is parasitic, and she reproduces parthenogenetically (without fertilization). Parasitic females live embedded in the mucosa of the small intestine. The eggs develop in utero, and the nematode gives birth to first-stage larvae (Fig. 6–3), whose chromosome number determines whether they will develop into a free-living generation before producing larvae destined to be parasitic or become a larval stage possessing a unique chromosome and be destined to develop into third-stage infective larvae. The infective larvae are capable of establishing infection by oral ingestion, after which they penetrate the small intestine and develop there. However, the primary mode of infection is by *skin penetration.* If the larvae use skin penetration, they then penetrate the venous circulation, going ultimately to the lungs to develop for

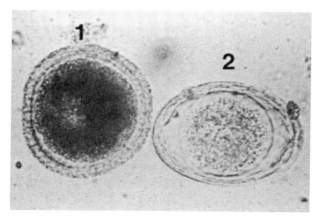

Figure 6-1. 1, *Toxocara* egg measuring approximately 66 × 42 μm. 2, *Toxascaris* egg measuring approximately 85 × 75 μm.

• Table 6–1 •

PARASITICIDES USED FOR TREATMENT AND CONTROL OF INTERNAL PARASITES IN DOGS AND CATS

DRUG; TRADE NAME	Toxocara-Toxascaris	Ancylostoma-Uncinaria	Strongyloides	Trichuris	Dirofilaria Adults	Dirofilaria Microfilariae	Taenia	Dipylidium	Giardia	Coccidia
Albendazole; Valbazen	+	+	–	+	–	–	+	–	+	–
Amprolium; Corid	–	–	–	–	–	–	–	–	–	+
Butamisole hydrochloride; Styquin	–	+	–	+	–	–	–	–	–	–
Dichlorophene; Many trade names	–	–	–	–	–	–	+	+	–	–
Dichlorophen/toluene; Many trade names	+	+	–	–	–	–	+	+	–	–
Dichlorvos; Many trade names	+	+	–	+	–	–	–	–	–	–
Diethylcarbamazine; Many trade names	+	–	–	–	–	+	–	–	–	–
Epsiprantel; Cestex	–	–	–	–	–	–	+	+	–	–
Febantel/praziquantel; Parasiticide-10	+	+	–	+	–	–	+	+	–	–
Fenbendazole; Panacur	+	+	–	+	–	–	+	–	–	–
Furazolidone; Many trade names	–	–	–	–	–	–	–	–	+	–
Ivermectin; Heartgard 30	–	–	–	–	–	+	–	–	–	–
Ivermectin; Heartgard 30 Plus	+	+	–	–	–	+	–	–	–	–
Ivermectin; Ivomec	+	+	–	+	–	+	–	–	–	–
Mebendazole; Telmintic Powder	+	+	–	+	–	–	+	–	–	–
Melarsomine dihydrochloride; Immiticide	–	–	–	–	+	–	–	–	–	–
Metronidazole; Flagyl	–	–	–	–	–	–	–	–	+	–
Milbemycin oxime; Interceptor	+	+	–	+	–	+	–	–	–	–
N-Butyl chloride; Many trade names	+	+	–	–	–	–	–	–	–	–
Nitroscanate; Lopatol	+	+	–	+	–	–	+	+	–	–
Oxibendazole/DEC; Filaribits Plus	+	+	–	+	–	+	–	–	–	–
Piperazine salts; Many trade names	+	–	–	–	–	–	–	–	–	–
Praziquantel; Droncit	–	–	–	–	–	–	+	+	–	–
Pyrantel pamoate; Nemex	+	+	–	–	–	–	–	–	–	–
Praziquantel/pyrantel pamoate; Drontal	+	+	–	–	–	–	+	+	–	–
Praziquantel/pyrantel pamoate/febantel; Drontal Plus	+	+	–	+	–	–	+	+	–	–
Quinacrine hydrochloride; Atabrine	–	–	–	–	–	–	–	–	+	+
Sulfadiazine/trimethoprim; Many trade names	–	–	–	–	–	–	–	–	–	+
Sulfadimethoxine; Many trade names	–	–	–	–	–	–	–	–	–	+
Thiabendazole; Mintezol	–	–	+	–	–	–	–	–	–	–
Thiacetarsamide sodium; Caparsolate	–	–	–	–	+	–	–	–	–	–
Tinidazole; Available in England	–	–	–	–	–	–	–	–	+	–

+, Indicated for use; –, not indicated for use.

a short period of time. Larvae are then coughed up, swallowed, and penetrate into the mucosa of the small intestine. In immunologically compromised animals, infections may be severe. *S. stercoralis* is widespread in tropical and subtropical regions, as well as in kennels and pet shops, in which environmental conditions are suitable. Diagnosis is not difficult. Frequently, a direct smear of fresh feces is suitable. Treatment is not always satisfactory, and alternate anthelmintics should be considered (see Table 6–1). Control necessitates thorough cleaning of facilities and allowing the facilities to dry.

Whipworm

Trichuris vulpis occurs in the cecum of the dog, fox, and coyote. Like all whipworms, the anterior extremity is slender, and the posterior extremity is thickened, giving them a whiplike appearance. Males and females are about the same length, measuring 45 to 75 mm. The eggs are characteristic, possessing a thick, brown-yellow shell with a clear polar plug at each end (Fig. 6–4). *T. vulpis* is widespread in temperate zones, and the incidence of infection is frequently high. The life cycle is simple and direct. The infective larva develops within the egg. When the egg is ingested, the larvae are released in the intestine, which they penetrate. Larvae develop within 8 to 10 days, return to the surface of the intestine, go to the cecum, and attach and mature in an additional 60 to 80 days. Diagnosis can be effectively accomplished by a number of procedures, but eggs are quite heavy, and interpretation of the severity of infection based on the number of eggs present is not possible. A number of treatments are available (see Table 6–1). Control is difficult be-

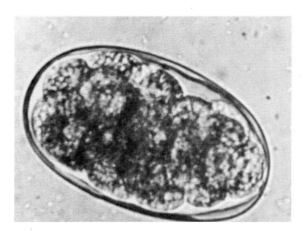

Figure 6–2. Strongyle-type egg, as seen in hookworms, measuring approximately 62 × 40μm.

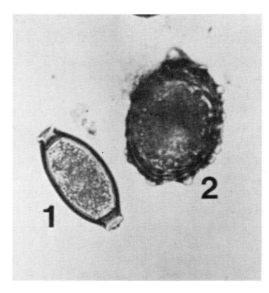

Figure 6–4. 1, Trichurid egg, as seen in whipworms, measuring approximately 80 × 36 μm. 2, Ascarid egg measuring approximately 60 × 50 μm.

cause eggs are highly resistant to environmental conditions. Sanitation, as applied for ascarids, is the best approach.

TECHNICIAN NOTE

The eggs of *Trichuris* spp. are very characteristic, possessing a thick, brown-yellow shell with a clear polar plug at each end.

Whipworm infection is uncommon in cats and wild Felidae in the United States; however, *Trichuris campanula* has been reported to occur in the United States. Occasionally, *Capillaria* spp. have been found in feces of both dogs and cats. The eggs of *Capillaria* are similar but not as dark in color and, on average, the eggs are somewhat smaller than those of whipworms.

Tapeworms

Dogs, cats, the wild Canidae, and some of the wild Felidae are susceptible to infection by a number of tapeworms. The most commonly found tapeworm species are *Dipylidium caninum*, *Taenia hydatigena*, *Taenia pisiformis*, *Taenia ovis*, *Taenia krabbei*, *Multiceps serialis*, and *Echinococcus granulosus*. Cats, and some of the wild Felidae, generally are infected with *Taenia taeniaeformis* and *Dipylidium caninum*. The species of tapeworms found in dogs and cats is dependent on their geographic location and the amount of free-ranging activity the animals are given.

TECHNICIAN NOTE

Diagnosis of *Taenia* spp. and *Dipylidium caninum* infections is normally done by finding the proglottids in the feces or around the host's anal region or hocks.

All tapeworms have an intermediate host in which the larval stage develops. *D. caninum* uses a flea, in which the larval (cysticercoid) stage develops. *T. hydatigena*, *T. ovis*, and *T. krabbei* use ruminants—usually sheep, deer, elk and moose—in which the larval stage (cysticercus) develops in the body cavity (*T. hydatigena*) or muscles (*T. ovis* and *T. krabbei*). *T. pisiformis* develops in the body cavity of rabbits, and *Taenia serialis* develops in subcutaneous areas or in the muscles of rabbits. The larval stage of *T. taeniaeformis* develops in the liver of mice, rats, and other small rodents. *E. granulosus* uses ruminants, such as sheep, deer, and elk, and humans as intermediate hosts. The larval stage is a rather large, fluid-filled bladder called a *hydatid cyst* that is easily recognized by its large size (25 to 100 mm in diameter), the presence of numerous small pieces of larval tapeworms (brood capsules) on the inner surface, and the presence of compartments within the body of the cyst in which daughter cysts have grown and fused together.

Diagnosis of *Taenia* spp. and *D. caninum* infections is

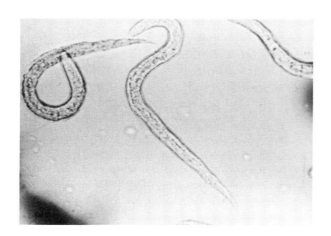

Figure 6–3. *Strongyloides* larvae from a dog. Note that the larvae are distorted in appearance because of the flotation solution.

normally done by finding the proglottids (body segments), or chain of proglottids, around the host's anal region or on their hocks. Although the eggs will float, usually they are not released to mix with the feces (Fig. 6–5). *Taenia* spp. have one genital opening per proglottid, whereas *D. caninum* has two, one on either side. Further diagnosis of *Taenia* spp. beyond the genus designation is extremely difficult, requiring morphological study of the intact parasite.

E. granulosus eggs frequently mix with the feces (unlike *Taenia* spp.), but the eggs are typical *Taenia*-type eggs, possessing a thick, striated shell. *D. caninum* eggs, if seen in feces, occur in packets contained within a thin-walled membrane. A number of treatments are available (see Table 6–1). Control is dependent on the tapeworm species. *D. caninum* obviously necessitates vigorous control of fleas. For *Taenia* spp., the dog or cat should not have access to the flesh or viscera of the intermediate host.

Heartworm and Dipetalonema → *h. ventricle + pulmonary arteries*

Dirofilaria immitis and *Dipetalonema reconditum* are the two filarial nematodes found commonly in dogs and the wild Canidae in the United States. *D. immitis* infections may also occur in cats and the wild Felidae, but it is not as common as in dogs. The heartworm, *D. immitis,* occurs primarily in the right ventricle and pulmonary arteries of the host, whereas *D. reconditum* occurs in the subcutaneous tissue. Both nematodes produce a larval form called a microfilaria, which circulates in the blood (Fig. 6–6). These filarial nematodes are found commonly in areas of the United States where the intermediate hosts occur; however, heartworm is becoming more widespread as infected dogs and cats are brought into areas where the parasite is not normally found.

D. immitis males measure 12 to 20 cm, and the females measure 25 to 31 cm long, whereas *D. reconditum* males are 9 to 17 mm long, and the females are 20 to 32 mm long. Both nematodes need an intermediate host to complete their life cycle. *D. immitis* uses several different species of mosquito, and *D. reconditum* uses the common dog and cat flea. Microfilariae, when ingested by the intermediate host, undergo reorganization and development to the third-stage infective larva. Once infective, they go into the mouthparts of the arthropod and remain there until the arthropod feeds on a susceptible

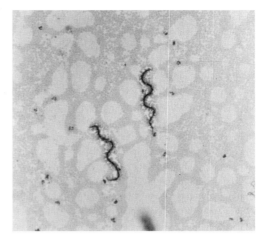

Figure 6–6. Microfilaria of *Dirofilaria immitis.*

host. *D. immitis* infective larvae enter the tissue for 85 to 120 days and develop into young adults. They then go to the heart and reach sexual maturity in another 60 to 70 days, for a total of 145 to 190 days. *D. reconditum* apparently goes directly into the subcutaneous tissues to develop to sexual maturity.

✎ TECHNICIAN NOTE

Diagnosis of heartworm disease in the dog is generally based on identification of microfilaria in the peripheral circulation.

The microfilaria of *D. immitis* is 295 to 325 μm long (average of 313 μm) and 6 to 7 μm in diameter (average of 6.9 μm), whereas the microfilaria of *D. reconditum* is somewhat shorter and more slender, measuring 250 to 288 μm long (average of 276 μm) and 4.5 to 5.5 μm in diameter (average of 4.6 μm).

Various techniques have been used to detect microfilaria, including fresh blood/saline preparation, capillary hematocrit tube, and the Knott's or filtration concentration test. Fresh blood/saline preparations are helpful in differential diagnosis of *D. immitis* and *D. reconditum* microfilaria. *D. immitis* microfilaria move in place without directional motion, whereas *D. reconditum* have a directional movement across the microscopic viewing field. Concentration tests are best used for the detection of *D. immitis* microfilaria as they are much more accurate than fresh blood/saline preparations or capillary hematocrit tube tests. Occult heartworm infections (adult heartworms without circulating microfilariae) occur in approximately 25% of dogs and 90% of cats. Several serological tests are available in commercial kits to test serum of dogs and cats for occult infection. Treatment of *D. reconditum* is unimportant because they are nonpathogenic parasites. The treatment for *D. immitis* necessitates the use of an agent effective for the adult heartworms followed by a microfilaricide (see Table 6–1). Control of *D. immitis* necessitates daily or monthly heartworm preventive therapy and mosquito control in enzootic areas.

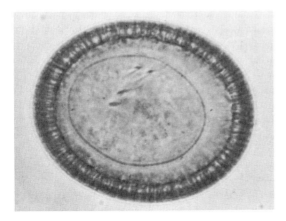

Figure 6–5. Typical *Taenia* egg measuring approximately 34 μm. *Dipylidium* eggs appear similar but are contained in packets of 1 to 20 eggs.

Giardia

Giardia spp. is a common protozoan parasite of dogs and cats in the United States. A higher incidence of infection occurs among dogs, cats, humans, and beavers than in other animals such as deer, sheep, moose, and antelope. There are two forms of *Giardia*. The motile trophozoite, which is approximately 12 to 17 μm long and 7 to 10 μm wide, is found in the small intestine. The cyst form (the infective stage) is approximately 9 to 13 μm long (Fig. 6–7). When ingested, the cyst wall is digested away in the small intestine, releasing the trophozoite, which immediately divides into two organisms. These organisms attach to the epithelial cells lining the small intestine and continue to multiply by binary fusion over the next 6 to 10 days until a large population exists. At that time, diarrhea develops, and *Giardia* begins to produce cysts. Diagnosis can be accomplished by the direct fecal/saline smear or, more effectively, the zinc sulfate centrifugal flotation technique. Treatment is available (see Table 6–1). *Giardia* is more commonly found among young dogs and cats crowded into kennels and animal shelters. The most effective control procedure is cleanliness and disinfection with quaternary ammonium compounds.

Coccidia

Dogs and cats are hosts for a number of species of *Isospora* (also called *Cystoisospora*), *Cryptosporidium*, and *Sarcocystis*, and the cat is the definitive host for *Toxoplasma gondii*. The incidence and severity of coccidial infection are dependent on the host's age and immune status, conditions in which the hosts are housed, or their diet and quality of drinking water.

The species of *Isospora* have a direct life cycle; however, some of *Isospora* spp. (*Isospora canis* and *Isospora felis*) can use an intermediate host, such as mice. The life cycle starts with an oocyst in the feces (Fig. 6–8). This oocyst must sporulate (develop into the infective form), which occurs in less than 1 week given optimum conditions of warmth and moisture. Once infective, the oocyst encloses two sporocysts, each of which encloses four small, spindle-shaped infective forms called *sporozoites* or a total of eight infective forms in each oocyst. When ingested, the oocyst and sporocyst walls are digested in the intestine, releasing sporozoites to penetrate the intestinal epithelium and enter a cell for subsequent development. Within the intestinal cell, they become spherical and begin to grow to a large size. The nucleus replicates several

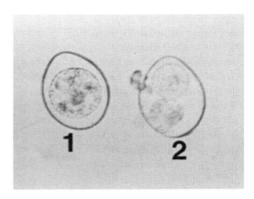

Figure 6–8. Unsporulated oocyst of *Isospora* (1) and sporulated oocyst of *Isospora* (2) measuring approximately 25 × 20 μm.

times, and ultimately thousands of small, spindle-shaped organisms called *merozoites* develop. This asexual process of reproduction is called *schizogony,* and the large structure filled with the merozoites is called a *schizont.*

Once mature, the schizont ruptures, releasing merozoites. The next step in the life cycle is species dependent, but usually they move further down the intestine, penetrate a cell, and repeat the asexual process but with smaller schizonts containing fewer merozoites. When released, the merozoites then penetrate a cell, and some of them become macrogametes (ova) and some become microgametes (sperm). Once fertilization occurs, the oocyst is produced and passes in the feces to begin the life cycle again. Although the life cycle is finite, for example, only a given number of oocysts can be produced from a single oocyst infection, the reproductive potential is great for some species.

Species of *Cryptosporidium* have essentially the same type of life cycle. *Cryptosporidium* organisms inhabit the respiratory and intestinal epithelium of many hosts, including birds, mammals, reptiles, and fish. Dogs and cats develop intestinal tract infection almost exclusively. Enteroepithelial development is limited to the luminal enterocytes; extraintestinal tissue cysts do not develop. The enteroepithelial life cycle begins with ingestion of sporulated oocysts by a suitable host. After ingestion of oocysts, four sporozoites are released from each oocyst that penetrate intestinal epithelial cells. Asexual reproduction at the intestinal surface occurs with the production of merozoites that are released and penetrate other cells. Gametogony and sporogony occur, resulting in the production of thin- and thick-walled oocysts. Sporulated thick-walled oocysts are shed in the feces of an infected host and are immediately infective to a susceptible host. Thin-walled oocysts passed into the intestinal lumen rupture, releasing the sporozoites, which penetrate additional host cells and reinitiate the developmental cycle.

Species of *Sarcocystis* have essentially the same type of life cycle, except the carnivore is the host for the sexual stages (oocyst and sporocyst), and omnivores and herbivores act as hosts for the asexual (schizogony) stage. Infected carnivores pass a thin-walled oocyst, which will rupture, that contains two small, thick-walled sporocysts in which four sporozoites have already developed and are immediately infective to the alternate host. Once ingested, the sporozoites are released and penetrate the epithelial tissue of the intestine. Generally, they enter the circulatory system and begin the first asexual (schizogony)

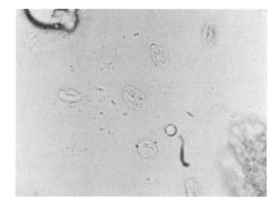

Figure 6–7. Cysts of *Giardia* sp. from a dog fecal flotation using ZnSO₄ at a specific gravity (SG) of 1.18.

phase in the kidney. The first schizont releases its small, spindle-shaped organisms, which then enter cardiac or smooth muscle, in which they develop into rather large schizonts called *sarcocysts*. When sarcocysts are ingested by a specific carnivore, and most species are specific for each carnivore-herbivore, the small, spindle-shaped organisms penetrate superficial epithelial cells of the intestine and immediately begin the sexual phase, terminating as a thin-walled oocyst about 11 to 14 days after ingestion of the infected flesh.

The life cycle of *T. gondii* is similar to that of *Sarcocystis* with the exception that most animals are suitable hosts for the development of the asexual (schizogony) stages, and only the cat is suitable as a host for the sexual stages. The typical life cycle occurs when a cat ingests the small sporulated oocyst. In the intestine, the parasite goes through two asexual stages and then into the sexual phase, producing oocysts. If, for example, a mouse should eat the oocyst, the first asexual phase occurs in this animal. When a cat eats these schizonts, the parasite goes into one asexual cycle, in the cat's intestine, followed by the sexual cycle. If the first mouse is eaten by another mouse,

Toxoplasma goes into the second asexual cycle in this mouse. When then eaten by a cat, the parasites go directly into the sexual phase. The asexual cycle can go on indefinitely as animals eat the flesh of infected animals.

Diagnosis of *Isospora, Cryptosporidium, Sarcocystis,* and *Toxoplasma* is based on recovery of the oocyst or sporocyst (for *Sarcocystis*) by a number of diagnostic procedures. Treatment is seldom administered for *Sarcocystis* or *Cryptosporidium* infection, but when clinical disease occurs, treatment is recommended for *Isospora* and *Toxoplasma* spp. (see Table 6–1). Control of *Isospora* and *Cryptosporidium* infections requires cleanliness, removal of the animal to clean premises, or both; however, these oocysts are extremely resistant to environmental conditions. Control of *Sarcocystis* is generally not practiced for the carnivore host because *Sarcocystis* is considered nonpathogenic. If control is exercised, the best approach is to prevent consumption of raw flesh from any source, including ground beef. The best control for *Toxoplasma* in cats is to prevent consumption of raw flesh and contact with feces of infected cats.

Parasites of Horses
Roundworm

The ascarid of horses (*Parascaris equorum*) is a creamy white color. The males measure about 28 cm, whereas females are about 50 cm in length. They produce a dark-brown, thick-shelled oval to spherical egg that is very resistant to environmental conditions. The larval stage develops within the egg, and the second stage is infective. Development to the infective stage requires about 2 weeks. When the egg is ingested, the larva is released in the intestine, penetrates the intestinal mucosa, enters the circulatory system, and passes through to the liver, heart, and, ultimately, the lungs, in which they develop for a period of time. Subsequently, larvae pass up the bronchial tree, enter the mouth, and are swallowed. They are passed into the small intestine and mature. This entire life cycle requires 10 to 12 weeks. Diagnosis is readily performed using a number of techniques, and these parasites are amenable to treatment by a number of anthelmintics (Table 6–2). Control is difficult because eggs are extremely resistant to environmental conditions, and the coprophagous habits of foals tend to ensure infection.

> **TECHNICIAN NOTE**
>
> The horse ascarid is common throughout the United States, and the incidence of infection, especially among younger horses, is frequently high.

Pinworm

The pinworm of horses, *Oxyuris equi,* is a white to slate gray-colored nematode with a slender, sharply pointed tail. Males are very small, measuring less than 12 mm, and females are 75 to 150 mm long. The eggs are slender and somewhat flattened along one side (Fig. 6–9). Frequently, they possess a first-stage larva when deposited. Pinworms are common in horses in the United States. The life cycle is simple and direct. Female para-

• Table 6–2 •

	PARASITE						
DRUG	*Gasterophilus*	*Ascarids*	*Strongylus vulgaris*	*Strongylus edentatus*	*Small Strongyles*	*Pinworms*	*Strongyloides*
Cambendazole Camvet	−	+	+	+	+	+	+
Dichlorvos Many trade names	+	+	+	+	+	+	−
Fenbendazole Panacur	−	+	+	+	+	+	+
Ivermectin Eqvalan	+	+	+	+	+	+	+
Oxibendazole Anthelcide EQ	−	+	+	+	+	+	+
Oxifendazole Benzelmin	−	+	+	+	+	+	+
Phenothiazine Many trade names	−	−	+	−	+	−	−
Piperazine salts Many trade names	−	+	−	−	+	+	−
Pyrantel salts Many trade names	−	+	+	+	+	−	−
Thiabendazole Many trade names	−	−	+	+	+	+	+
Thiabendazole/piperazine Equizole A	−	+	+	+	+	+	+
Thiabendazole/trichlorfon Many trade names	+	+	+	+	+	+	+
Trichlorfon Many trade names	+	+	−	−	−	+	−
Trichlorfon/phenothiazine/ piperazine Dyrex	+	+	+	−	+	+	−

PARASITICIDES USED FOR TREATMENT OF INTERNAL PARASITES IN HORSES

+, Indicated for use; −, not indicated for use.

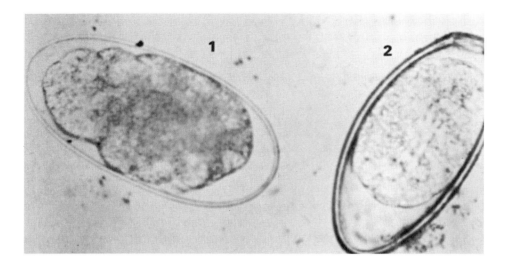

Figure 6–9. 1, Strongyle egg measuring 95 × 50 μm. 2, Egg of *Oxyuris equi* measuring 90 × 42 μm.

sites living in the cecum pass out through the anal sphincter and deposit masses of eggs on the perineum. Eggs are cemented into masses with a gelatinous material. Eggs drop off, either singly or in masses, landing on ground or feed and become infective within 3 to 5 days. Once ingested, the larvae are released in the small intestine, penetrate the intestinal mucosa, and develop for several days. Larvae then return to the mucosal surface, move to the large intestine, and reach maturity about 50 days after the initial ingestion of the egg. Diagnosis can be performed effectively only by the adhesive tape technique (see the discussion on diagnostic tests). Pinworms are amenable to treatment by a number of anthelmintics (see Table 6–2). Control is difficult because of the coprophagous habits of foals.

Small and Large Strongyles

Strongylus vulgaris, Strongylus equinus, and *Strongylus edentatus* are the three species of "large strongyles" of horses. The 40 or more species of "small strongyles" of horses, of which there are several different genera, are blood-sucking nematodes. Strongyles vary in size from less than 12 mm (small strongyles) to 38 to 47 mm (large strongyles). However, some small strongyles, like *Tridontophorous,* are nearly as large as *S. vulgaris,* the smallest of the large strongyles. All of the strongyles produce a similar thin-walled egg containing 4 to 16 brownish cells (Fig. 6–9) when deposited and are referred to collectively as *strongyle eggs,* a term that refers to the order of nematodes to which this group belongs (order Strongyloidea, the bursate nematodes).

TECHNICIAN NOTE

All equine strongyles produce a similar thin-walled egg containing 4 to 16 brownish cells.

All of the strongyles are common in horses throughout the United States, and the incidence of infection is generally high. The small strongyles that have been studied have a simple, direct life cycle. The eggs pass in feces, and a first-stage larva develops within the egg. Once developed, the larva hatches

and undergoes a free-living existence, developing and molting to a second-stage free-living larva. It then develops into a third-stage larva that does not feed and awaits ingestion. In ideal environmental conditions, development from the egg stage to the infective larva will occur in less than 1 week. Once the small strongyle is ingested, the larva goes to the cecum, penetrates the cecal mucosa, and develops for 1 to 2 weeks. The larva then returns to the mucosal surface and matures within an additional 1 to 2 weeks. All of the species in the genus *Strongylus* have very complex life cycles.

The development of the larval stages for large strongyles in the environment is the same as that for the small strongyles, and once ingested they also penetrate the mucosa of the cecum and develop within a short period of time. *S. vulgaris,* the most important of the large strongyles, leaves the mucosa and by some means goes to the cranial mesenteric artery and its branches and develops in the lumen of the arteries over the next 6 months, becoming a young adult. It then returns to the cecum and matures; the entire prepatent period (the period of time after ingestion and before eggs pass in feces) is about 180 to 200 days. *S. equinus* leaves the cecal mucosa and enters the peritoneal cavity. It then goes to the liver and develops into a young adult. The route taken back to the cecum is incompletely understood, but it may enter the pancreas. The entire prepatent period may be as long as 265 days.

S. edentatus leaves the mucosa and enters the subperitoneal tissue, particularly in the right dorsal flank. Eventually, it enters the venous circulation and goes to the liver. Supposedly, it leaves the liver and about 2 months later migrates in the mesenteries to the perirenal fat for an additional 3 months. It again migrates in the mesenteries to the large intestine, which it penetrates, and develops to maturity in the lumen of the cecum. The entire prepatent period requires 300 to 322 days. Diagnosis of the strongyles can be accomplished by a number of techniques, and they are amenable to treatment by a number of anthelmintics (see Table 6–2). Control is difficult because the parasites are prolific egg producers and development of the larva occurs rapidly. Control is best applied by a treatment and management regimen based on environmental conditions and by limiting the number of horses on the pasture.

Intestinal Threadworm

Strongyloides westeri is a common parasite of horses, principally of foals 2 weeks to 6 months of age, and is widespread across the United States. The life cycle is essentially the same as *Strongyloides stercoralis* of the dog, with the exception that the parthenogenetic female produces a thin-walled egg containing a first-stage larva when deposited (Fig. 6–10). Diagnosis can be performed by a number of techniques; however, fresh feces must be used because the eggs will hatch in older feces. Treatments recommended are given in Table 6–2. Control necessitates good hygiene, together with treatment, because the parasite can be transmitted by the transmammary route.

Tapeworms

Anoplocephala perfoliata, Anoplocephala magna, and *Paranoplocephala mamillana* are the tapeworms of horses. They are broad, thick, and white and vary in length from about 2.5 cm (*A. perfoliata*) to 75 cm (*A. magna*), although most tapeworms are about 15 cm. The eggs of all species are similar and tend to be amber or have almost no color. The eggs often have a peculiar shape, varying from almost round to somewhat square. The life cycles of all three tapeworms are similar in that the egg is ingested by a free-living mite for further development. In the mite, a small larval form, the cysticercoid, develops to the infective stage within 2 to 4 months. Once ingested by the horse, the larval stage is released from the mite and develops into an adult tapeworm within 6 to 10 weeks. Diagnosis is readily performed by a number of techniques because the eggs mix with the feces. Treatment or control is seldom practiced.

Parasites of Ruminants

Strongyles

Cattle and sheep in the United States are commonly infected by a number of species of strongyle nematodes (order Strongyloidea, the bursate nematodes). Species in the genera *Haemonchus, Ostertagia, Trichostrongylus, Cooperia,* and *Nematodirus* are the most common. These nematodes vary in size from about 6 mm (*Trichostrongylus*) to about 25 to 30 mm (*Haemonchus*). All except *Nematodirus* produce a similar "strongyle" egg, which is thin walled and contains 4 to 16 brown-colored cells when deposited (see Fig. 6–10). *Nematodirus* produces an extremely large egg (see Fig. 6–10). These

parasites are widely distributed throughout the United States, but their incidence is dependent on their ability to develop in the external environment. Some, like *Haemonchus,* need considerable warmth and moisture, whereas others, like *Ostertagia, Trichostrongylus,* and *Nematodirus,* will withstand colder, drier climates.

The life cycles, although somewhat variable among species, are similar. The first larval stage develops within the egg and hatches to undergo a free-living existence. The larval stage develops within the egg and grows and molts to the third-stage infective form in less than 2 weeks. Once ingested by the host, the larval stage generally penetrates the mucosa in the site it normally inhabits (stomach, small intestine, large intestine) and develops in a short period of time and then returns to the surface of the mucosa and matures. Diagnosis can be effectively performed by most techniques. A number of treatments are available (Table 6–3). Control is best practiced by a combination of treatment and pasture management in areas in which there is an abundance of warmth and moisture to promote survival of the larval stages on pastures.

Lungworms

The lungworms of cattle and sheep are *Dictyocaulus viviparus* (cattle) and *Dictyocaulus filaria* (sheep). They are slender, white nematodes; males are 3 to 8 cm long, whereas females are 3 to 10 cm long. Females produce an egg containing a first-stage larva that hatches in the lungs. The first-stage larva passes up the bronchial tree and is swallowed, passing with the feces. Lungworms occur in animals throughout the United States, but their distribution is discontinuous because the larval stages require a certain amount of warmth and moisture to survive. The life cycle is simple and direct. The first-stage larvae live on stored food granules, developing to the third-stage infective form within less than 1 week in optimum environmental conditions. Once ingested, they enter the intestine, penetrate the intestinal mucosa, enter the lymphatic vessels, and develop for a short period of time in lymph nodes. They go to the heart, enter the circulatory system, and then into the lungs to mature in a total of 25 to 30 days. Diagnosis is best performed by use of the Baermann funnel technique. Only a few anthelmintics are considered acceptable (see Table 6–3). Control is best exercised by proper management, ensuring that cattle and sheep do not occupy wet, swampy pastures.

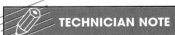

TECHNICIAN NOTE

Diagnosis of cattle and sheep lungworms is best performed by use of the Baermann funnel technique.

Tapeworms

Tapeworms in cattle and sheep are *Moniezia expansa* and *Moniezia benedeni.* In addition, *Thysanosoma actinioides* occurs in sheep. The *Moniezia* spp. reach lengths of 4 cm, whereas *Thysanosoma* is generally 25 to 30 cm long. *Moniezia* spp. are widespread across the United States, but *T. actinioides* is found only in the western regions. The life cycle of *Moniezia* spp. is the same as for the *Anoplocephala* spp. found in horses,

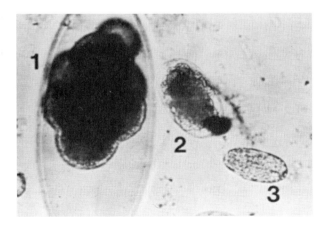

Figure 6–10. 1, Egg of *Nematodirus* measuring approximately 200 × 95μm. 2, Strongyle-type eggs measuring approximately 86 × 40 μm. 3, Egg of *Strongyloides* measuring approximately 52 × 25 μm.

• Table 6–3 •

| | PARASITE | | | | | | | | | | | | | |
| PARASITICIDES USED FOR TREATMENT OF INTERNAL PARASITES IN CATTLE, SHEEP, AND GOATS | | | | | | | | | | | | | | |
DRUG	*Haemonchus*	*Ostertagia*	*Trichostrongylus*	*Cooperia*	*Nematodirus*	*Strongyloides*	*Bunostomum*	*Trichuris*	*Oesophagostomum*	*Chabertia*	*Dictyocaulus*	*Moniezia*	*Fasciola*	*Coccidia*
Albendazole Valbazen	+	+	+	+	+	−	+	−	+	+	+	+	+	−
Amprolium Corid	−	−	−	−	−	−	−	−	−	−	−	−	−	+
Chlorsulon Curatrem	−	−	−	−	−	−	−	−	−	−	−	−	+	−
Decoquinate Deccox	−	−	−	−	−	−	−	−	−	−	−	−	−	+
Doramectin Dectomax	+	+	+	+	+	−	−	−	−	−	−	−	−	−
Fenbendazole Many trade names	+	+	+	+	+	+	+	+	+	+	+	−	−	−
Haloxon Loxon	+	+	+	+	−	−	−	−	−	−	−	−	−	−
Ivermectin Ivomec	+	+	+	+	+	+	+	−	+	+	+	−	−	−
Lasolacid Bovatec	−	−	−	−	−	−	−	−	−	−	−	−	−	+
Levamisole Many trade names	+	+	+	+	+	+	+	+	+	+	+	−	−	−
Monensin Rumensin	−	−	−	−	−	−	−	−	−	−	−	−	−	+
Morantel tartrate Rumatel	+	+	+	+	+	+	+	−	+	+	−	−	−	−
Phenothiazine Many trade names	+	+	+	−	−	−	−	−	+	−	−	−	−	−
Sulfonamides Many trade names	−	−	−	−	−	−	−	−	−	−	−	−	−	+
Thiabendazole Many trade names	+	+	+	+	+	+	+	−	+	+	−	−	−	−

+, Indicated for use; −, not indicated for use.

and they use similar free-living mites. The cycle of *T. actinioides* is not known. Diagnosis of the *Moniezia* spp. is readily accomplished by a number of acceptable techniques because the eggs mix with the feces; however, diagnosis of *T. actinioides* can be accomplished only through observation of the pearly white bell-shaped proglottid on the fecal mass. Treatment is seldom applied to *Moniezia* spp. or *T. actinioides*. Control would be difficult, necessitating control of the mites.

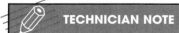

TECHNICIAN NOTE

The cattle and sheep liver fluke requires the snail as the intermediate host.

Liver Flukes

The common trematodes of cattle and sheep are *Fasciola hepatica* and *Fascioloides magna*. Both trematodes are greenish, flat, and leaf-like in shape. *F. hepatica* is about 25 mm long, and *F. magna* is about 50 to 75 mm long. The eggs of both trematodes are very similar and are large and yellow-brown with an operculum, or "lid," at one end (Fig. 6–11). *F. hepatica* and *F. magna* are widespread throughout the United States but only in

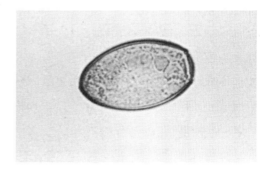

Figure 6–11. Egg of *Fasciola hepatica* measuring approximately 130 × 70 μm.

wet, swampy, or subirrigated areas that will support substantial populations of the snail intermediate hosts. The natural hosts for *F. hepatica* are cattle and sheep, but the natural hosts for *F. magna* are members of the deer family. *F. magna* cannot complete its life cycle (by passing eggs into the environment) in cattle and sheep.

The life cycles of both trematodes are similar and quite complex. Eggs passing in the feces must land in water to develop. Inside the egg, a small, ciliated miracidium develops, leaves the egg, and penetrates the tissue of a specific snail, in which it undergoes asexual replication through larval stages called *sporocysts* and *rediae,* ultimately developing into a *cercaria,* which leaves the snail to encyst on vegetation and await ingestion. Once ingested, it goes into the intestine, penetrates through to the body cavity, and penetrates the surface of the liver, in which it wanders for several weeks. *F. hepatica* eventually enters the bile ducts, whereas *F. magna* will form a cyst wall around itself with an opening into a bile duct if it infects members of the deer family. In cattle, a calcified cyst is found, whereas in sheep, the parasite continues to wander throughout the liver. The eggs are very heavy and will not float; consequently, a sedimentation procedure is used for diagnosis. Effective treatment is available (see Table 6–3). Control necessitates draining and drying wet, swampy pastures to prevent an overabundance of snails.

Coccidia

Several species of coccidia infect cattle and sheep, and all belong to the genus *Eimeria.* Coccidia are common throughout the United States, and most animals are infected with at least one of the *Eimeria* spp. The severity of the infection is dependent on the environmental condition (warmth, moisture), stocking intensity, age, and previous exposure. Oocysts of the *Eimeria* spp. sporulate in the environment and reach the infective stage in the same manner as do *Isospora* spp. *Eimeria* spp., however, develop four sporocysts, each of which contains two sporozoites, for a total of eight infective forms per oocyst. The life cycle of *Eimeria* spp. is identical to that of *Isospora* spp., with the exception that an intermediate host is not required. Diagnosis may be accomplished effectively by a number of techniques. A number of treatments are available for the clinical disease (see Table 6–3). Control is difficult because oocysts are highly resistant. Proper management for coccidiosis includes prevention of overcrowding and contamination of feed and water and the use of dry bedding.

Trichomoniasis

Trichomonas foetus is a common protozoan parasite of cattle. This small, flagellated protozoan is equipped with three anterior flagella, an undulating membrane, and a trailing flagellum. Generally, *T. foetus* is a slender, pear-shaped organism. The bull acts as a carrier, with the parasite living on the surface of the penis or in the prepuce. When transmitted by coitus to the cow, the organism develops in the vagina and uterus, causing abortion or fetal resorption. *Trichomonas* multiples by binary fission; consequently, large populations can be generated in a short period of time. The cows, given a rest through two or three estrous cycles, will usually develop partial immunity. Diagnosis and treatment are performed on the bull. Diagnosis is difficult and complex. Control necessitates resting the cows

and allowing immunity to develop, treatment or elimination of infected bulls, and purchase of virgin bulls for breeding.

Parasites of Swine
Stomach Worms

Three stomach worms occur in swine: *Hyostrongylus rubidus, Ascarops strongylina,* and *Physocephalus sexalatus. H. rubidus* is the most common and the most pathogenic of the three, usually occurring in adult pigs. Its parasitic development is similar to that of *Ostertaga* in ruminants. Diagnosis is based on finding strongyle eggs in the fecal sample, but the eggs can be confused with the eggs of *Oesophagostomum,* which also occurs in pigs. Treatment is given in Table 6–4. *Ascarops* and *Physocephalus* use beetles as their intermediate hosts and are rarely a problem in swine.

Ascarids

TECHNICIAN NOTE

Ascaris suum is the large roundworm and is by far the most common parasite encountered in pigs.

Ascaris suum is the large roundworm and is by far the most common parasite encountered in pigs. Its parasitic development is similar to that of *Parascaris* in the horse. *A. suum* is usually more common in pigs under 1 year of age. Diagnosis is based on finding ascarid eggs in fecal samples. Treatment is given in Table 6–4.

Strongyloides

Strongyloides ransomi is found in the small intestine of young swine. Its parasitic development is similar to that of *Strongyloides* in the horse. Diagnosis is based on finding embryonated eggs in fresh fecal samples. Treatment is given in Table 6–4.

Oesophagostomum

Several species of *Oesophagostomum* occur in the large intestine of pigs. Their life cycle is similar to that of *Oesophagostomum* in ruminants. Diagnosis is based on finding typical strongyle eggs in fecal samples. Again, these eggs can be confused with the eggs of *Hyostrongylus* and *Trichostrongylus.* Treatment is given in Table 6–4.

Whipworm

The whipworm of swine is *Trichuris suis.* These worms usually occur in the cecum, and their parasitic development is similar to that of *Trichuris* in dogs. Diagnosis is based on finding typical trichuris eggs in the feces. Treatment is given in Table 6–4.

Lungworm

Three species of *Metastrongylus* occur in the lungs of swine. Earthworms act as the intermediate host for the swine lungworm. Most commonly, the posteroventral part of the diaphrag-

• Table 6–4 •

PARASITICIDES USED FOR TREATMENT OF INTERNAL PARASITES IN SWINE								
	PARASITE							
DRUG	*Ascaris*	*Strongyloides*	*Oesophagostomum*	*Trichuris*	*Hyostrongylus*	*Metastrongylus*	*Stephanurus*	*Stephanurus*
Dichlorvos Atgard	+	−	+	+	+	−	−	−
Fenbendazole Many trade names	+	−	+	+	+	+	−	−
Hygromycin B Hygromix	+	−	+	+	−	−	−	−
Ivermectin Ivomec	+	+	+	−	+	+	+	−
Levamisole Many trade names	+	+	+	−	+	+	+	−
Piperazine salts Many trade names	+	−	−	−	−	−	−	−
Pyrantel tartrate Banminth	+	−	+	−	−	−	−	−
Sulfonamides Many trade names	−	−	−	−	−	−	−	+
Thiabendazole Many trade names	−	+	+	−	+	−	−	−

+, Indicated for use; −, not indicated for use.

matic lobe of the lung is involved. Diagnosis is made by finding rough-shelled, embryonated eggs in the feces. Treatment of lungworm infection in swine is given in Table 6–4.

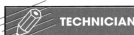

TECHNICIAN NOTE

The intermediate hosts for the swine lungworm are earthworms.

Kidney Worms

Stephanurus dentatus is the kidney worm in swine. The adult worms live in the kidneys and perirenal tissue and pass eggs into the urinary bladder. Infection in pigs occurs by ingestion of third-stage larva, ingestion of earthworms containing the third-stage larva, skin penetration, and in utero infection. Although eggs can be identified in urine, diagnosis is usually made at necropsy. Treatment is given in Table 6–4.

ECTOPARASITES

Parasites of Domesticated Animals

The ectoparasites of domesticated animals generally are members of the phylum Arthropoda. There are many different types of ectoparasites, including fleas, mites, lice, ticks, chiggers, blood-sucking flies, and myiasis-inducing flies. Some are host specific, whereas others infect any number of animals. Diagnosis generally is based on the external morphological appear-

ance, using taxonomic keys. A number of treatments are available (Tables 6–5 through 6–8). Control is often very difficult, sometimes necessitating treatment of the premises and prevention by prohibiting interaction with infected animals (e.g., fleas, ticks, and lice on companion animals).

Fleas

Ctenocephalides canis (Fig. 6–12) and *Ctenocephalides felis* are the most common fleas of dogs and cats; *C. felis* is the most common. They are not host specific and will attack other animals and humans. They are widely distributed but are much more common in warm, humid environments. When environmental conditions are favorable, the flea has a great reproductive potential. Fleas thrive at low altitudes in temperature ranges of 65°F to 80°F. Under these conditions, the flea life cycle can be completed, from hatching of an egg to the laying of the next generation of eggs, in as little as 16 days.

TECHNICIAN NOTE

The flea life cycle can be completed in as little as 16 days, making control difficult.

The female flea lays her eggs in the fur of dogs and cats. The eggs are not sticky and tend to fall out of the fur and survive in the protected places where a dog or cat sleeps or plays. The eggs will hatch into very small worm-like larvae.

• Table 6–5 •

PARASITICIDES USED FOR CONTROL OF EXTERNAL PARASITES ON DOGS AND CATS

DRUG	Fleas	Lice	Mites	Ticks
Allethrin Many trade names	+	−	−	−
Amatraz Mitaban	−	−	+	−
Carbaryl Many trade names	+	+	+	+
Chlorpyrifos Many trade names	+	+	+	+
Cythioate Proban	+	−	−	−
D-Limonene Many trade names	+	+	−	−
Diazinon Many trade names	+	+	−	+
Fenthion Pro-Spot	+	−	−	−
Fipronil Frontline	+	+	−	+
Imidacloprid Advantage	+	+	−	−
Lime-sulfur Many trade names	−	−	+	−
Lindane Many trade names	+	+	+	+
Linalool Many trade names	+	−	−	−
Lufenuron Program	+	−	−	−
Malathion Many trade names	+	+	−	+
Methylcarbamate Many trade names	+	+	−	+
Permethrin Many trade names	+	+	−	+
Phosmet Paramite	+	+	+	+
Pyrethrins Many trade names	+	+	−	+
Resmethrin Many trade names	+	+	−	−
Rotenone Many trade names	+	+	−	+

+, Indicated for use; −, not indicated for use.

• Table 6–6 •

PARASITICIDES USED FOR CONTROL OF EXTERNAL PARASITES ON HORSES

DRUG	Lice	Flies	Mites	Ticks	Maggots
Coumaphos Many trade names	+	+	−	+	+
Malathion Many trade names	+	+	+	+	−
Permethrin Many trade names	+	+	−	+	−
Pyrethrins Many trade names	+	+	−	−	−

+, Indicated for use; −, not indicated for use.

posed to insecticides used in household extermination. All effective in-house programs should take advantage of new technologies in flea control. There are insecticides that have truly long residuals (synthetic pyrethroids or microencapsulated products), and there are insect growth regulators (methoprene and fenoxycarb) marketed for preadult flea control.

Advances in outdoor environmental flea control have been less remarkable. At present, the use of insecticides (compounds that contain chlorpyrifos, malathion, or diazinon as their active ingredient) labeled for outdoor flea control is still the best and most economical approach. Such programs will have to incorporate repeated applications at 2-week intervals throughout the flea season, during which temperature and humidity are favorable for flea reproduction.

TECHNICIAN NOTE

Flea products containing lufenuron, fipronil, or imidacloprid as the active ingredient should never be administered or used on nursing animals.

The larvae feed on organic debris, especially the dried blood droppings (flea dirt) left by adult fleas. Thus, larvae depend on the dog to return time after time to the places at which the eggs dropped off. The larvae molt and form pupae that spin cocoons and then emerge as young and hungry adults in about 3 weeks. An important source of fleas to a dog and cat is these newly "hatched out" young fleas.

Once fleas have had a chance to establish the life cycle in a house and yard environment, no control program will be successful that does not emphasize environmental control. Mechanical cleaning of the house and yard environment should precede any application of insecticides. In general, the same environmental control methods may be used in households with young dogs and cats as in those with adults. Care should always be taken that animals and people are not directly ex-

All topical insecticides should only be used according to label directions because it is not legally permissible to use or recommend the use of insecticide products beyond label restrictions (see Table 6–5). In general, the use of organophosphate preparations on puppies younger than 16 weeks or on kittens younger than 6 months should be avoided. Any product containing lufenuron, fipronil, or imidacloprid as its active ingredient should never be administered or used on nursing animals. Pyrethrin-based products are generally safe for frequent application; the most effective products are synergized pyrethrin sprays or foams (see Table 6–5). Very small animals and nursing animals sprayed with alcohol-based or other volatile organic solvents may be severely chilled as the solvent evaporates. Water-based sprays are preferable, and small animals and nursing animals should never be thoroughly saturated with a spray. The safest effective products are sprays and foams with microencapsulated pyrethrins. Flea collars that are safe for

• Table 6–7 •

PARASITICIDES USED FOR CONTROL OF EXTERNAL PARASITES ON CATTLE, SHEEP, AND GOATS												
DRUG	Cattle Grub	Horn Fly	Face Fly	Other Flies	Maggots	Chewing Lice	Sucking Lice	Psoroptic Mite	Other Mites	Ear Ticks	Other Ticks	Sheep Ked
Carbaryl Many trade names	−	+	+	+	−	+	+	−	−	+	+	−
Coumaphos Many trade names	+	+	+	+	+	+	+	+	−	+	+	+
Chlorpyrifos Many trade names	−	+	−	−	−	+	+	−	−	−	−	−
Dichlorvos Many trade names	−	+	+	+	−	−	−	−	−	−	+	−
Famphur Many trade names	+	−	−	−	−	+	+	−	−	+	+	−
Doramectin Dectomax	−	−	−	−	−	+	+	−	−	−	−	−
Fenthion Many trade names	+	−	−	−	−	+	−	−	−	+	+	−
Fenvalerate Ectrin	−	+	+	−	−	−	−	−	−	+	−	−
Ivermectin Ivomec	+	−	−	−	−	−	+	+	+	+	+	−
Methoxychlor Many trade names	−	+	+	+	−	+	−	−	−	+	+	−
Permethrin Many trade names	−	+	+	−	−	−	−	−	−	+	−	−
Phosmet Many trade names	+	+	−	−	−	+	+	+	+	+	+	−
Pyrethrins Many trade names	−	+	+	+	−	−	−	−	−	−	+	−
Rotenone Many trade names	−	−	−	−	−	+	+	−	−	−	−	+
Trichlorfon Many trade names	+	+	−	−	+	+	+	−	−	+	+	−

+, Indicated for use; −, not indicated for use.

use on puppies or kittens are not effective in most environments. Topical treatments should be coordinated with in-home environmental flea control (see Table 6–5).

Rabbit Bots and Fox Maggots

Cuterebra spp., the rabbit bot, and *Wohlfahrtia* spp., the fox maggot, occasionally infest dogs, cats, rodents, rabbits, and other wildlife. *Cuterebra* spp. flies usually deposit eggs around burrows or runs. Eggs hatch, and the larvae penetrate the skin of the host, developing to the third stage in subcutaneous tissue without migrating in the host. The larvae then drop out of the host and pupate in the soil. Females of the *Wohlfahrtia* spp. deposit larvae on the skin of the host, which is usually a young animal. The larvae penetrate and develop in the subcutaneous tissues with limited migration. When they become third-stage larvae, they drop out and pupate in the soil. Diagnosis of *Cuterebra* is based on the morphological appearance of the larva, whereas *Wohlfahrtia* spp. diagnosis necessitates using the morphological appearance of the stigmatal plates and, sometimes, the morphological appearance of the cephalopharyngeal skeleton. Treatment necessitates surgical removal of the larvae and supportive wound treatment.

Bot Flies

Gasterophilus intestinalis, Gasterophilus nasalis, and *Gasterophilus hemorrhoidalis,* the bot flies of horses, are widespread and common, but *G. intestinalis* is the most common. The adult fly cements eggs to the hair of the horse. Either the eggs hatch by themselves and the larvae crawl into the mouth, or the eggs are stimulated to hatch by being licked by the horse. Once in the mouth, the larvae penetrate the mucosa and burrow down the esophagus to the stomach, in which they emerge and develop into the third stage. They usually spend about 10 months as larvae. Ultimately, the larvae pass out with the feces, burrow into the soil, pupate, and later emerge as adult flies, usually in late summer. Diagnosis is based on the type of egg and means of attachment of the spines on each segment (single row, *G. nasalis*; double row, *G. intestinalis*; double row, smaller spines, *G. hemorrhoidalis*). Treatment is generally applied in the fall with a combination of insecticides and anthelmintics or a broad-spectrum compound (see Table 6–2). Control is difficult.

Heel Flies

The heel flies of cattle, *Hypoderma lineatum* and *Hypoderma bovis*, whose larval stages are called *grubs* or *warbles*, are

• Table 6–8 •

PARASITICIDES USED FOR CONTROL OF EXTERNAL PARASITES ON SWINE				
	PARASITE			
DRUG	*Lice*	*Flies*	*Mites*	*Maggots*
Coumaphos Many trade names	+	+	−	+
Fenthion Many trade names	+	−	−	−
Ivermectin Ivomec	+	−	+	−
Malathion Many trade names	+	−	+	−
Methoxychlor Many trade names	+	−	−	−
Permethrin Many trade names	+	+	+	−
Pyrethrins Many trade names	−	+	−	−

+, Indicated for use; −, not indicated for use.

widely distributed wherever cattle are found. Emergence of these flies is dependent on environmental conditions. For example, they are active in early January in southern Texas and in early August in Montana. When both species are present, *H. bovis* emerges about 1 month later than *H. lineatum*. After emergence, *H. bovis* lays single eggs attached to hair, and *H. lineatum* lays a row of eggs just above the hooves. The larvae hatch from the egg, penetrate the skin, and wander in the subcutaneous tissue for 4 to 5 months. *H. lineatum* then goes to the esophagus for 2 months, and *H. bovis* goes to the epidural fat of the spinal cord for 2 months. Both then go to the subcutaneous tissue along the back for about 2 months. They develop, drop out, and burrow in the soil, in which they pupate for 1 to 3 months. Diagnosis is generally based on the presence of the warbles in the back of cattle; however, species can be diagnosed based on the morphological appearance of the larvae. A number of treatments are available (see Table 6–7), but they must be applied at a specific time of year.

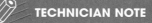

TECHNICIAN NOTE

Diagnosis of *Hypoderma* spp. of cattle is usually based on the presence of warbles in the back of cattle.

Sheep Nasal Fly

The sheep nasal fly (*Oestrus ovis*; often called the sheep nose bot) is common wherever sheep are found. Flies emerge from spring through fall and deposit first-stage larvae around the nasal opening. Larvae then enter the nasal cavity for 2 weeks to 9 months and migrate to the paranasal sinuses for a short period of time to complete their development. They leave through the nose and pupate in the soil for 15 to 60 days. The life cycle may be completed within 2 to 11 months, depending on environmental conditions. Diagnosis is based on the presence of these larvae in the nose or sinuses. There is no preferred treatment available.

Lice

Domesticated animals commonly are infested with lice of the order Anoplura (sucking lice) (Fig. 6–13) and the order Mallophaga (chewing lice). Lice live on the host continuously and infest other animals through direct contact. Lice may be a problem year round on dogs and cats but are more commonly a problem in the winter months on cattle, goats, sheep, and horses (Table 6–9). Lice deposit an egg, referred to as a *nit*, cemented to the hair or wool of the host. The eggs hatch, and the small larvae are similar to the adult (incomplete metamorphosis). They develop into nymphs and then into adults; the entire life cycle requires 3 to 5 weeks.

Diagnosis is based on the morphological appearance of the larva, nymph, or adult. Mallophaga have broad heads, and Anoplura have pointed heads. Treatment consists of dust, sprays, sponge-on dips, or shampoos, depending on the host and environmental conditions.

Mites

The mites commonly found on domesticated animals are given in Table 6–10. Most mites are host specific and even though

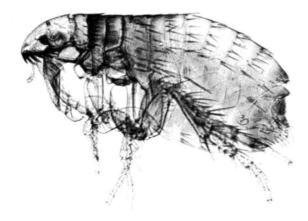

Figure 6-12. *Ctenocephalides canis,* the common dog flea.

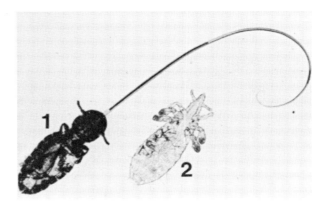

Figure 6-13. 1, Chewing louse of the order Mallophaga attached to a hair shaft. 2, Sucking louse of the order Anoplura.

• Table 6–9 •

LICE ON DOMESTIC ANIMALS
Cattle
Haematopinus eurysternus, sucking
Linognathus vituli, sucking
Solenopotes capillatus, sucking
Haematopinus quadripertussis, sucking
Damalinia bovis, chewing
Sheep
Haematopinus tuberculatus, sucking
Linognathus pedallis, sucking
Linognathus ovillus, sucking
Linognathus africanus, sucking
Damalinia ovis, chewing
Horses
Haematopinus asini, sucking
Damalinia equi, chewing
Dogs
Linognathus piliferus, sucking
Trichodectes canis, chewing
Cats
Felicola subrostratus, chewing

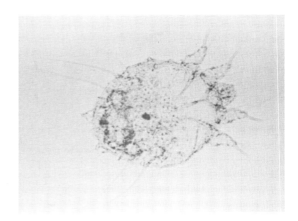

Figure 6-14. *Sarcoptes* sp. mite commonly found on dogs and swine.

TECHNICIAN NOTE

Mites are usually diagnosed by morphological appearance of the adult after a skin scraping.

---

morphologically similar, subspecies will not cross-infest other hosts. Mites live on the host continuously and infest other animals by contact. The life cycles of these mites are all slightly different because some burrow and others live on the surface of the skin. *Sarcoptes* spp. and *Notoedres cati* females burrow in the skin and deposit eggs. The eggs hatch into six-legged larvae, which develop and molt to eight-legged nymphs, which develop and molt into adults. The entire cycle requires 9 to 17 days.

Species of *Chorioptes, Psoroptes, Psorergates, Otodectes,* and *Cheyletiella* have a similar life cycle except they do not burrow to deposit eggs. *Demodex* spp. generally live in hair follicles. Their life cycle is probably direct, as in the preceding mites, but they can be found in many other tissues of the body.

Diagnosis of mites is based on the morphological appearance of the adult, and it generally requires a thorough skin scraping (Figs. 6–14 and 6–15). Sometimes mites, especially *Cheyletiella* and *Demodex,* can be diagnosed by fecal flotation in dog and cat feces. Treatment necessitates the use of dust, sprays, sponge-on dips, or shampoos (see Tables 6–5 through 6–8).

Ticks

The ticks found on domesticated animals are not host specific, although they have host preferences, and their distribution is

• Table 6–10 •

MITES ON DOMESTIC ANIMALS
Sarcoptes scabiei
Varieties are found on the body of cattle, sheep, horses, goats, swine, and dogs
Psoroptes communis
Varieties are found on the body of cattle, sheep, horses, goats, and rabbits
***Chorioptes* spp.**
Species occur on the body of cattle, sheep, goats, and rabbits
***Psorergates* spp.**
Species occur on the body of cattle and sheep
Otodectes cyanotis
Occurs in the ears of dogs, cats, and other related animals
Notoedres cati
Occurs on the head of cats
***Cheyletiella* spp.**
Occurs on the body of dogs, cats, and rabbits
***Demodex* spp.**
Occurs in hair follicles of dogs, cats, cattle, sheep, humans, and horses

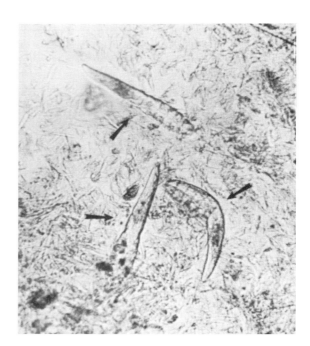

Figure 6-15. *Demodex* sp. mite commonly found on dogs.

subject to environmental conditions. The species and their host ranges are given in Table 6–11. Ticks are identified as being soft or hard. The most important soft tick is *Otobius megnini,* the spinose ear tick, which lives in the ear of its host. It attaches as a larva, enters the ear, and develops through the larval, nymphal, and adult stages. Adults mate and then drop off. The female deposits eggs and dies.

The hard ticks are generally classified into one-, two-, or three-host ticks. Some, like *Dermacentor albipictus,* are one-host ticks, attaching as a larva and developing into an adult on that host. Adults drop off, lay eggs, and then die. The three-host ticks attach as larvae, feed, drop off, and molt in the environment to nymphs; reattach to a host, feed, drop off, and molt to adults; and then as adults attach, feed, mate, and drop off to lay eggs and die. *Rhipicephalus sanguineus,* a three-host tick, uses the same host (dog) for all three stages, whereas *Dermacentor venustus* uses small rodents for the larval stage, larger rodents and rabbits for the nymphal stage, and dogs, horses, cattle, and so on for the adult stage. Three-host ticks may complete the cycle in a short period of time (*Rhipicephalus*), whereas other ticks (*Dermacentor*) require 2 years, with 1 year between each stage before reattaching to a host.

Treatment necessitates the use of dusts, sprays, sponge-on dips, or shampoos, depending on the host. Control of *R. sanguineus* requires treatment of the premises and, often, the house or kennel. Control of the other ticks is difficult at best, and the precaution of keeping animals away from infested areas can be practiced.

Myiasis-Producing Flies

Some of the myiasis-inducing flies (those developing in the tissue of animals), like *Hypoderma, Oestrus,* and *Gasterophilus,* are host specific and are discussed according to the appropriate host. Others, such as *Wohlfahrtia* spp. and *Cuterebra* spp., have a more limited host range and are discussed with the hosts usually infested. Blowflies in the genera *Lucilia, Calliphora,* and *Phormia,* the flesh flies; species of *Sarcophaga;* and the screw worm fly *Cochliomyia hominovorax* are not host specific and cause problems on several domesticated and wild animals. Blowflies and flesh flies generally deposit eggs (larvae for *Sarcophaga*) on the flesh of dead animals but can use traumatized or soiled areas. The eggs hatch, and the larvae develop through three larval stages and then drop out of the wound to pupate in the soil. Development of the larvae (maggots) is a function of temperature and varies from 2 to 19 days. Pupation lasts 3 to 7 days. The screw worm fly has essentially the same life cycle but will deposit eggs only in fresh wounds (in living tissue).

Diagnosis is based on the morphological appearance of the stigmatic plates of the third-stage larvae, except for *Cochliomyia hominovorax,* for which the presence of pigmentation of the tracheal trunks is used for diagnosis. Treatment is usually applied topically (see Tables 6–6 to 6–8). Control measures usually require that procedures such as docking and castration be performed before fly season, dead carcasses be disposed, and environmental spraying take place.

DIAGNOSTIC PROCEDURES

Fecal Flotation

The nematodes that are parasitic in animals and humans may produce undeveloped eggs, eggs containing larvae, or free

• Table 6–11 •

TICKS COMMONLY ON DOMESTIC ANIMALS
Otobius megnini: **the spinose ear tick** Most warm-blooded animals
Dermacentor albipictus: **the winter tick** One-host tick; cattle, sheep, horses, deer, elk, and moose
Dermacentor venusutus: Three-host tick; cattle, sheep, horses, wild ruminants, dogs, and humans; immature stages on rodents
Dermacentor variabilis: **the American dog tick** Three-host tick; dogs, primary host; immature stages on rodents
Dermacentor nitens: **the tropical horse tick** One-host tick; horses, donkeys, and mules
Amblyomma americanum: **the lone star tick** Three-host tick; cattle, sheep, goats, horses, dogs, cats, and wildlife; nymphs on rodents, larvae often found on birds
Amblyomma maculatum: **the Gulf coast tick** Three-host tick; cattle, sheep, goats, horses, dogs, cats, and wildlife; nymphs on rodents; larvae often found on birds
Amblyomma cajennense: **the Cayenne tick** Three-host tick; mostly horses but also cattle, sheep, goats, and wildlife
Ixodes pacificus: **the Western black-legged tick** Three-host tick; adults feed on deer, dogs, horses, and humans; immature stages found on small mammals, especially white-footed mice
Ixodes scapularis: **the black-legged tick** Three-host tick; adults feed on deer, dogs, horses, and humans; immature stages found on small mammals, especially white-footed mice
Rhipicephalus sanguineus: **the brown dog or kennel tick** Three-host tick; usually found on dogs

larvae. Consequently, special diagnostic procedures often are necessary to determine the parasite with which the animal is infected. For nematodes producing an undifferentiated egg or an egg containing a larva, fresh feces is mixed with a chemical solution of higher specific gravity than water. The chemical solutions most frequently used are sodium chloride, magnesium sulfate, zinc sulfate, sodium nitrate, and sucrose. Eggs in feces mixed with any of the preceding chemical solutions will float to the top and can be removed for examination and identification.

Direct Fecal Smear

The direct smear is best used to aid in the detection of certain protozoan trophozoites found in fecal samples, such as *Trichomonas, Giardia,* and *Balantidium.* The morphological appearance and the motility of these organisms can be seen in a direct smear. This method should not be used. The correct procedure is to mix a small quantity of fresh feces with a drop of tap water or physiological saline solution on a clean microscopic slide. Spread the sample into a thin film, place a coverslip on the slide, and examine it.

TECHNICIAN NOTE

Direct smear is not satisfactory to demonstrate eggs of tapeworms, nematodes, and coccidia.

Qualitative Fecal Examination

The Willis Technique

A qualitative fecal examination will reveal what parasites are present but not how many. There are a number of procedures for this type of examination, but the most simple technique is the Willis technique. The equipment needed is a sputum vial (or any 48-mm-deep cylinder about 24 mm in diameter), glass microscope slide, coverslip, and tongue depressor. A small amount of feces, about the size of a large pea, is placed in the vial, and sufficient flotation solution is added to cover the feces; then this is macerated and mixed. Solution is added until the vial is about half full, and the material is mixed again. The vial is filled with flotation solution until the meniscus bulges slightly, and a clean microscope slide is applied over the vial. This slide is left in place for 10 minutes and then is lifted straight up and turned over, and a coverslip is affixed. Much of the liquid will drain from the slide, but eggs remain firmly attached if the glass is clean. To determine the best level to seek eggs, focus on an air bubble. The chemical solutions most frequently used for this type of examination are sodium nitrate, magnesium sulfate, and sodium chloride.

Disposable Fecal Flotation Kits

Several commercial disposable kits are available that are modifications of the Willis technique. These kits require 1 to 2 g of fecal material, depending on the kit that is used. All of the kits have some method for preventing the large particles of fecal material from floating to the top of the vial. As in the Willis technique, a clean microscope slide is placed on top of the vial to collect the eggs that float to the top. It is recommended that the microscope slide be left on top of the flotation vial for 15 to 20 minutes.

Paper Cup Technique

One modification of the Willis technique occasionally used is to mix the chemical solution with a large amount of feces in a paper cup. After thorough maceration, the fluid is strained through several (two or three) layers of cheesecloth (gauze) into a sputum vial. The remainder of the procedure is the same as with the Willis technique. The advantages are the cup and feces can be discarded, eliminating washing containers, and cups are handy for field situations. This technique often is used for horses and sheep because of the amount of fiber in the feces. The disadvantages are the same as in the Willis technique.

The advantages of the Willis-type techniques are that they are quick and simple and will provide the observer a qualitative examination for many nematode and tapeworm eggs and some protozoan cysts. These techniques are effective for the recovery of all strongyle-type eggs, as well as eggs of ascarids, *Trichuris, Capillaria,* and *Strongyloides* (egg-producing species only); the protozoan cysts of *Eimeria, Isospora, Cryptosporidium, Sarcocystis,* and *Toxoplasma*; and all of the tapeworm eggs that mix with feces. These techniques can be used effectively in horses and ruminants when fragile cysts, larvae, or both are not suspected. However, the disadvantages inherent in these techniques are that they destroy or render unrecognizable fragile cysts and larvae. For dogs, cats, ruminants, and horses in which parasites such as lungworm (any species), *Giardia* spp., *Entamoeba* spp., and *Strongyloides stercoralis* are suspected,

another technique—the zinc sulfate centrifugal flotation technique—is recommended.

None of these techniques are suitable for trematode eggs of *Fasciola* and *Fascioloides,* because these eggs are too dense to float, but eggs of *Paragonimus* and *Nanophyetes (Troglotrema)* will float with the use of these techniques.

Zinc Sulfate Centrifugal Flotation Technique

The zinc sulfate centrifugal flotation technique is used almost exclusively for parasites of dogs, cats, and primates. It can also be used for other animals, such as exotic animals or native wild species. The reason it is used for these animals is that the technique is much more versatile, and when examining such animals, a more complete technique is necessary. The technique does not destroy fragile cysts and larvae and is just as effective in recovering the other eggs and cysts as the Willis-type techniques.

TECHNICIAN NOTE

The zinc sulfate centrifugal flotation technique is used almost exclusively for parasites of dogs, cats, and primates.

Zinc sulfate, at a specific gravity of 1.18 or 1.20, is usually employed; both specific gravities are effective, but 1.20 is probably best. A small amount of feces (about the size of a large pea) is inserted into a round-bottomed 10- or 15-ml plastic centrifuge tube. (Conical 15-ml tubes can be used and are effective, but removal of fecal matter from the tube, especially cat feces, is almost impossible). The feces should be pushed to the bottom of the tube. Five to 10 drops of Lugol's iodine solution are then added, and the mixture is quickly but thoroughly stirred. Sufficient zinc sulfate is then added to fill the tube to approximately half full, and the mixture is thoroughly macerated. Do not let the Lugol's iodine solution remain in contact with feces for more than 1 minute before dilution with zinc sulfate; otherwise, fragile protozoan cysts (e.g., *Giardia*) will distort and rupture.

Fill the tube with zinc sulfate until the meniscus bulges slightly, and then affix an 18 × 18-mm or a 22 × 22-mm glass coverslip to the top. Be certain to grasp the coverslip at the periphery because human body oils will prevent eggs and cysts from attaching. Gently press the coverslip on the tube, being certain that it makes physical contact without any fecal debris disturbing the seal; otherwise, the centrifuge will "throw" the coverslip.

Place the tube into a swinging head centrifuge and centrifuge for 3 to 5 minutes at 1000 revolutions per minute (rpm) to 1500 rpm. When the centrifuge stops, remove the coverslip, place the contents on a clean glass slide, and examine the slide microscopically. The purpose of the Lugol's solution is to stain cysts of *Giardia* and *Entamoeba*. It will also stain tapeworm eggs, larvae, some strongyle eggs, and so on, but the purpose of the stain is to facilitate recognition of the aforementioned protozoan cysts.

The zinc sulfate technique is excellent for any of the strongyle-type eggs—*Strongyloides* (both eggs and larvae), ascarids, *Trichuris, Capillaria, Physaloptera,* coccidia, *Entamoeba, Giar-*

dia, all tapeworm eggs that mix with feces, eggs of *Paragonimus* and *Nanophyetes,* and mites such as *Demodex* and *Cheyletiella.* Moreover, the lungworm larvae of dogs and cats, as well as those of ruminants and horses, will float without distortion. The technique cannot be used for *Fasciola* and *Fascioloides* because their eggs are too dense to float in any chemical solution. The technique also is not effective for the trophozoites of rumen or cecal ciliates such as *Balantidium* or the trophozoites of *Trichomonas hominis* (no cyst stage) because they are too fragile for demonstration by any technique other than direct fecal smear.

Sheather's Sugar Flotation

One modification of the zinc sulfate centrifugal flotation technique that is often employed is to use sugar instead of zinc sulfate. Sugar is somewhat less destructive than the chemical solutions used in the Willis-type techniques, but fragile cysts and larvae often are highly distorted in sugar, making diagnosis difficult; therefore, zinc sulfate is often preferred.

Formalin-Ethyl Acetate Sedimentation Technique

The formalin-ethyl acetate technique has widespread application in human parasitology and has the advantage that all eggs, cysts, and larvae form sediment and are preserved, regardless of whether they will float. This also is the inherent disadvantage: most other fecal debris likewise is sedimentable.

For this technique, you need 2% formalin (vol/vol) and ethyl acetate; the remainder of the equipment is the same as is used in the zinc sulfate technique.

In this technique, a small amount of feces (the size of a large pea) is placed into a small beaker, the beaker is half-filled (or filled) with 2% formalin, and the feces are thoroughly macerated. A two- or three-thickness layer of cheesecloth (gauze) is placed over the beaker, and the material is strained into a centrifuge tube. The resulting tube of strained material is filled with 2% formalin and centrifuged at 1000 to 1500 rpm for 1 to 2 minutes. This step is repeated until the supernatant is clear (two or three centrifugations). Approximately half of the liquid is poured off, and the fecal matter is dislodged and stirred. Ethyl acetate is added to this half-filled tube. The tube is then stoppered and shaken vigorously. The stopper is removed, and the mixture is centrifuged for 1 to 2 minutes at 1000 to 1500 rpm. When the centrifuge stops, the tube is removed, and an applicator stick is used to gently "ring" the debris at the ethyl acetate–formalin interface (the two liquids are not miscible). The purpose of the ethyl acetate is to trap the lighter debris, removing it from the sediment. Once "ringed," the supernatant is poured off, leaving the bottom 1 to 2 ml of fecal material and formalin. A small amount of this sediment or centrifugate is pipetted onto a microscope slide, a coverslip is affixed, and the material is examined for eggs, cysts, larvae, trophozoites of protozoa, and so forth. A drop of Lugol's solution is added to the periphery of the coverslip and allowed to spread beneath to stain cysts.

The advantages of this technique are that all eggs are present, including trematode eggs, fragile cysts, larvae, and trophozoites of non–cyst-forming (or even cyst-forming) protozoa.

The distinct, and often overwhelming, disadvantage of this technique is that the great majority of debris in the fecal sample (except the very low specific gravity material trapped in the ethyl acetate layer) is in the sediment, making examination extremely difficult. Moreover, the technique is time consuming.

Quantitative Fecal Examination

In many situations, especially in food-producing animals, it is not sufficient just to know whether the animal is parasitized because most food-producing animals are parasitized to some degree. The livestock producer wants to know how severely the animals are parasitized and whether deworming will increase their performance and the net return on their investment. There are several procedures used to perform a quantitative fecal examination for parasitic eggs and larvae. The most common method is described.

Stoll Dilution Technique

A special Stoll flask is available for use with this technique. The flask has two graduations: one at 56 ml and one at 60 ml. However, any 75- to 100-ml flask can be used to substitute for a Stoll flask. The method is as follows:

1. Fill the flask with decinormal caustic soda solution (0.1 N sodium hydroxide) or water to the first graduation.
2. Add feces until fluid goes to the top graduation (4-g displacement).
3. Add several glass beads, place the stop on the flask, and shake until the sample is mixed well. Samples can be stored and soaked overnight or longer in a refrigerator.
4. With a micropipette, transfer 0.15 or 0.075 ml from the thoroughly mixed sample to a clean microscope slide. Cover the fluid with a coverslip, and examine under the microscope, using low power (100×).
5. Examine the entire area under the coverslip, and count the eggs. Next, multiply by the proper dilution factor, either 100 (for 0.15 ml) or 200 (for 0.075 ml) for the eggs per gram of feces.

Stoll Centrifugation Technique

The greatest advantage to the centrifugation modification of the Stoll technique is that it is more sensitive and will detect parasitic eggs when other techniques do not. The method follows.

A regular Stoll flask or plastic vial is prepared using 56 ml of water and 4 g of feces. Fill the flask or vial with 56 ml of water to the lower mark. Add feces until the vial is filled to the upper mark (approximately 4 g of fecal material). Mix feces with the water, and when possible, allow feces to soak for 3 to 8 hours. (Mixture should be refrigerated if it stands for longer than 2 hours.) Mix thoroughly, and immediately remove 1.5 ml of mixture with a 3-ml syringe. Place the 1.5-ml sample in a 10- to 15-ml test tube, and add flotation solution until a convex meniscus forms at the top of the tube. Place tube in a swing head centrifuge and place a coverslip on top. Centrifuge at 1500 to 2000 rpm for 2 to 5 minutes. Remove coverslip, and place on a clean microscope slide. Identify and count all the eggs under the coverslip. The count made multiplied by 10 gives the number of eggs per gram. (If more than 50 eggs are seen on the first coverslip and highly accurate results are desirable, the test tube should be topped off with the chemical solution and a second coverslip added before recentrifugation.)

Interpretation of Quantitative Fecal Examination

There is no direct or positive correlation between the number of eggs or larvae found in the feces and the severity of parasitism in the animal. It must also be remembered that during the prepatent period, no eggs or cysts will be seen although the animal may have severe parasitism.

SPECIALIZED DIAGNOSTIC TESTS

Lungworm

The Baermann funnel technique (Fig. 6–16) is primarily used to recover larvae of lungworm, although it does have other uses. The funnel consists of a 12.5- to 22.5-cm-diameter plastic or glass funnel to which a short piece of rubber tubing is affixed and a centrifuge tube is attached. The funnel is filled with lukewarm tap water, and a screen, gauze, or single layer of facial tissue is lowered into the water. Feces, finely chopped tissues, or culture material is carefully added, and the system is allowed to stand for 24 hours. Larvae filter into the centrifuge tube at the bottom, and the coarse material is held back. The system should not be left for more than 24 hours because the eggs of some nematodes will hatch after this period and so

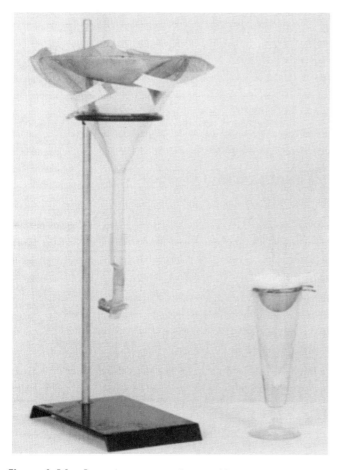

Figure 6-16. Baermann apparatus used for recovery of larvae from feces, soil, or minced tissues of an animal.

confuse the results. After 24 hours, the rubber hose is clamped, and the centrifuge tube is removed. The bottom 1 or 2 ml of fluid is examined microscopically for larvae.

Microfilaria

Filarial nematodes infect many different tissues of the body and produce an undifferentiated larva called a *microfilaria*. Depending on the species, microfilariae may be found in the blood or the dermis of their host.

Species producing microfilariae that accumulate in the dermis are diagnosed by the skin *maceration technique*. A biopsy of skin measuring at least 12 mm in diameter is finely macerated and allowed to soak for at least 6 hours in physiological saline solution at approximately 37°C or about 8 to 10 hours at room temperature (21°C). At the end of this time, the tissue is strained off, the liquid is centrifuged, and the bottom 1 or 2 ml is examined for microfilaria. Another method is histological sectioning of the skin, a procedure that is much more time consuming and not as sensitive as maceration.

For microfilaria of filarial nematodes that occur in the blood, there are a number of procedures that can be done.

Tests for Blood Microfilaria

Direct Smear. A thin film of blood is smeared on a slide and dried, and the film is stained with Wright's or Giemsa stain. This is a very poor technique and will work only if microfilariae are numerous.

Saline Preparation. A few drops of freshly drawn blood are mixed with physiological saline solution, and the resultant preparation is examined microscopically for motile microfilariae. It has the same disadvantages as the direct smear, but when used by technicians experienced in working with microfilaria, it can be very effective.

Microhematocrit Technique. The microhematocrit tube is examined for microfilariae after centrifugation. Microfilariae will be found at the plasma–blood interface (buffy coat). It has the same disadvantages as the direct smear.

Knott Technique. Add 1 ml of blood to 9 ml of 2% formalin (or 2 ml of blood in 18 ml of formalin). The mixture is then shaken until the blood hemolyses and is centrifuged at 1500 rpm for 5 minutes. The bottom 0.5 or 1 ml is examined for microfilariae. Microfilariae are preserved, lay straight, and easily measured. Measurements often are necessary to distinguish species and must be done to separate *Dirofilaria* and *Dipetalonema*. This technique is the preferred technique for identification of microfilaria.

Filter Technique. Several filter techniques are available commercially for the recovery of microfilaria from the blood. These techniques require 1 ml of blood, which is then mixed with the lysing solution (usually 9 ml) to hemolyze the red blood cells. The mixture is then passed through a plastic chamber containing a filter membrane on which the microfilariae are collected. The membrane filter is then removed and placed on a clean microscope slide. A drop of stain is placed on top of the membrane, which is covered with a coverslip for examination under the microscope.

TECHNICIAN NOTE

The two simplest and most effective techniques to detect blood microfilaria are the filter and the Knott procedures.

The two simplest and most effective techniques described here are the filter and Knott procedures. Both have advantages, depending on the host and parasite.

Pinworms

Pinworm in horses and humans must be diagnosed by a special technique called the *adhesive tape* technique. With this technique, adhesive tape is folded over a test tube or a smooth, round rod with the adhesive side out. The perianal folds are spread, the tape is applied to the skin in several places, and then the tape is placed on a clean microscope slide with the sticky side down. A few drops of xylene are allowed to seep under the tape to clear the fecal debris, and the slide is examined microscopically for typical pinworm eggs (always flat on one side).

Tapeworms

Most tapeworms occur in the small intestine of their host as adults or, as with *Thysanosoma,* have access to the intestine. All tapeworms use an intermediate host, and because swine, domestic and wild ruminants, or rabbits frequently serve in this capacity, diagnostic procedures for both adult and larval stages must be performed.

Adult Tapeworms

Some adult tapeworms, such as *Moniezia* spp. in ruminants and the anoplocephalids in horses, shed gravid proglottids that are destroyed in the intestine, releasing the eggs to mix with the feces. Any of the flotation procedures described under nematodes are satisfactory for diagnosis. However, *Thysanosoma* in ruminants and *D. caninum* and *Taenia* spp. in carnivores produce a proglottid that does not break up in the intestine. The proglottid usually passes intact when the animal defecates. Diagnosis necessitates *visual observation* of the proglottid (or chain) on the feces or around the anal region, which is frequently done by observant clients. *Echinococcus* spp. (taeniform tapeworm) in carnivores is an exception in that the eggs usually appear in the feces.

The fish tapeworms found in humans, bears, and wild carnivores shed eggs from the proglottid. Thus, the eggs mix with the feces like *Moniezia* and the anoplocephalids, but this egg is very heavy and will not float; therefore, the procedures used for diagnosis of trematodes must be applied (or the formalin-ethyl acetate technique).

Larval Tapeworms

Most species of tapeworms use arthropods, fish, or mammals as intermediate hosts (an exception is *Hymenolepis diminuta,* which can use an intermediate host but does not need one). Some tapeworms that use mammals as a host have a larva that occurs as a large bladderworm (cysticercus) on the mesenteries or the liver; others produce a small bladderworm that occurs in the muscles. The heavily exercised muscles are the preferred sites for these larvae. Diagnosis may be performed by visual observation of the small bladderworms in the heart, diaphragm, or jaw muscles; by pressing thin slices of tissue between two slides for microscopic examination; by digestion with pepsinhydrochloric acid; or by histological section. If the latter technique is used, remember that all tapeworms have small egg-shaped bodies called *calcareous corpuscles* that stain blue or purple with hematoxylin. This will identify the larva as a tapeworm, but it does not identify the species. For species identification, the specific host and the site within the host must be known.

Trematodes

Trematodes (*flukes*) occur in the bile ducts of the liver, parenchyma of the liver, rumen, lungs, small intestine, and other sites, such as skin and oviducts.

Fluke eggs (except *Troglotrema* and *Paragonimus* in the dog) are too heavy to float with the usual chemical solutions available for floating nematode and tapeworm eggs. *Troglotrema* and *Paragonimus* spp. are an exception in that they float with any of the chemical solutions listed earlier.

The diagnostic technique recommended for recovery of fluke eggs, especially liver flukes and fish tapeworm eggs, is to add a small amount of material (one fecal pellet or an equivalent amount) to a centrifuge tube and then add 0.1% detergent. Macerate the feces, shake thoroughly, and then fill with water. Allow to set 5 minutes, decant the supernatant, and repeat the procedure. Continue this until the detergent solution is clear (usually two to five times). The detergent, acting as a wetting agent, separates eggs from fecal debris and allows them to settle. Examine the bottom 1 ml of fluid microscopically for the typical operculate eggs.

Protozoa

Single-celled parasites, such as the helminths, occur in a variety of sites within the animal body. Various species occupy the circulatory system, especially the blood cells; gastrointestinal system (from mouth to anus); and reproductive system. Unfortunately, a variety of techniques must be used for correct diagnosis.

Blood Parasites

Parasites occurring in the blood of an animal, such as *Plasmodium, Haemobartonella, Cytauxzoon, Babesia, Theileria, Leucocytozoon,* or *Trypanosoma,* can be diagnosed by the direct smear technique. The slide is air dried and is then stained with Giemsa or Wright's stain. *Trypanosoma* spp. may not be demonstrable by the direct smear technique; therefore, culture in blood agar slants overlaid with liver infusion tryptose medium is the best approach.

Gastrointestinal Protozoa

Trichomonas. *Trichomonas gallinae* from the oral cavity of birds, *Trichomonas equi* from the gastrointestinal tract of horses, and *Trichomonas hominis* from dogs and humans are best demonstrated by direct smear of fresh samples. Lesions suspected of being caused by *T. gallinae* can be scraped (or swabbed), and this material can be mixed with some physiological saline solution on a clean microscope slide and examined for these typical flagellates. The presence of an undulating membrane is diagnostic. For *T. equi* of horses, a drop or two of fluid expressed from the feces can be examined. If the feces are dry, add saline solution, mix, and then examine a drop.

Hexamita meleagridis. This is the organism responsible for catarrhal enteritis of turkeys and is diagnosed by demonstration of the fast-moving flagellate in the upper part of the small intestine from freshly killed birds.

Coccidia. *Eimeria, Isospora,* and *Toxoplasma* produce an oocyst, whereas *Sarcocystis* and *Cryptosporidium* generally produce a sporulated sporocyst, all of which pass with the feces and may be easily demonstrated by either qualitative or quantitative concentration (flotation) techniques.

Sometimes, diagnosis of acute coccidiosis (in sheep or cattle) must be done at necropsy examination. In this situation, a scraping of intestinal mucosa is mixed with physiological saline solution on a clean microscope slide and examined for schizonts, oocysts, and the small, motile, tear drop–shaped merozoites.

***Giardia* spp.** *Giardia* spp. found in domestic, wild, and laboratory animals ostensibly can be diagnosed by the direct smear technique, but a more effective procedure is the zinc sulfate centrifugal flotation technique. The cysts may be stained with Lugol's solution to make the internal structures easily identifiable.

Entamoeba histolytica. The dog is sometimes a transient host for *Entamoeba histolytica* and, on occasion, will show clinical signs of infection. As with *Giardia,* the cyst form is best demonstrated by the zinc sulfate centrifugal flotation technique. Iodine will tint the cyst, facilitating identification. This is an extremely small cyst with four to eight nuclei.

***Entamoeba* spp.** This commensal ameba often is found in primates, rodents, humans, and other animals. The same techniques used for *Entamoeba histolytica* are effective. The cyst has eight nuclei.

***Balantidium* spp.** This large ciliate reportedly causes diarrhea in swine and humans, even though it is usually a commensal organism. Diagnosis is possible by direct smear, observing the large, motile trophozoite, or by the zinc sulfate centrifugal flotation technique, recovering the large cyst. Iodine will stain the sausage-shaped macronucleus as an aid in identification.

Histomonas meleagridis. This ameba forms a cyst within the egg of the nematode parasite *Heterakis gallinae,* the cecal worm of poultry. In the event of an outbreak of "blackhead" in turkeys, recovery of the eggs of *H. gallinae* from carrier birds and the presence of pathognomonic lesions in sick turkey poults are sufficient to delineate the cause of the infection as well as the source.

Trichomonas foetus. A positive diagnosis of trichomoniasis requires demonstrating the trichomonad from one or more infected animals. There is no serological or other test based on immunological reactions that has yet proved practical or specific for trichomoniasis.

Diagnosis in the bull consists of checking the breeding records and determining which bulls are probably infected. After a few days of sexual rest, these bulls should be confined, the preputial hairs clipped, the preputial orifice washed with soap and water and dried, and the bull examined. To collect the smegma sample, a dry plastic insemination pipette is attached to a 10- to 12-ml syringe. The pipette is introduced into the prepuce to its full length. A negative pressure is then created in the syringe, and the pipette is moved vigorously back and forth, scraping the glans penis and preputial membrane. In most bulls, 0.5 to 1 ml of smegma can be collected in the pipette. This material is flushed into a vial containing 2 ml of lactated Ringer's solution or physiological saline solution. The sample is then layered on Diamond's medium for culturing.

Trichomonas foetus may occur in small numbers; therefore, proper handling after collection to avoid extremes of temperature, contact with harmful chemicals, and evaporation must be avoided. It is highly desirable to examine samples within a few hours after collection. Samples should be refrigerated but not frozen if they cannot be cultured immediately. The liquid transport medium (lactated Ringer's solution) is layered on the surface of Diamond's medium and is incubated at 37°C for 48 to 72 hours.

Diamond's medium is very difficult to prepare and is not available commercially but is available from some diagnostic laboratories. Do not use other *Trichomonas* culture media because the great majority will not grow *T. foetus.*

Arthropods

Infestations with ectoparasites means the presence of mites, lice, ticks, chiggers, fleas, or the larval stages of Diptera such as screw worm flies, blowflies, *Hypoderma, Gasterophilus, Oestrus, Cuterebra, Cephenomyia* (wild ruminants), or *Wohlfahrtia.* Fortunately, except for mites, the arthropod parasites are sufficiently large that identification is not as difficult as with the other parasites. In general, the host and the site on each host are sufficient.

Mites and Chiggers

Some mites live on the surface of the skin (e.g., *Cheyletiella, Otodectes, Chorioptes, Psoroptes,* and many bird mites), whereas others are burrowing types (e.g., *Demodex, Knemidokoptes,* and *Sarcoptes*). Consequently, there is no uniform procedure for examination and recovery.

Mites and/or chiggers living under the skin, or even on the surface of the skin, are recovered by deep scraping (sufficiently deep to draw blood) at the periphery of the lesion. Suspected *Demodex* lesions, or even any suspected mite or chigger infestation, should be clipped of hair and "squeezed" at the time they are scraped to ensure adequate sample collections. This scraped material is then placed on a clean microscope slide, covered with a coverslip, and examined with a microscope.

Ticks, Fleas, and Lice

Ticks, fleas, and lice are all of a sufficient size to see with the unaided eye. Ticks and fleas are usually removed and identified. Sometimes lice are difficult to find; therefore, a careful examination for nits (louse eggs) attached to the hair may reveal their presence. Accurate louse identification often requires the service of a specialist.

Diptera

The species of *Diptera* that infest domestic and wild animals are often easily identifiable because they are host or site specific, or both (e.g., *Hypoderma, Gasterophilus, Oestrus ovis,* and *Cutere-bra*). The larval stages of other dipterous insects are not as easily identified. *Screw worm larvae* can be identified by the presence of two black, pigmented tracheal trunks leading from the spiracular openings of the body. They can be clearly seen in the living third-stage larva with the unaided eye. If a larva does not have pigmented tubules, it is one of myriad blowflies, which can be identified by the pattern of the spiracular openings at the caudal extremity of the body.

The larval stages of *Wohlfahrtia* spp. are parasitic in the very young; skin must be tender for this parasite to penetrate. Identification of the larva is based on the morphological characteristics of the spiracular plates and cephalopharyngeal skeleton of the third-stage larva.

Preserving Parasitic Samples

Ectoparasites and endoparasites may be adequately preserved in 10% formalin or 70% alcohol. Preservation of tapeworms and flukes for morphological study is best accomplished by placing the specimen in a dish of water in the refrigerator until it relaxes (overnight) and then replacing this water with cold preservative (10% cold formalin). Preservation of feces can be done with 10% formalin, but this is only satisfactory for some eggs and larvae. Eggs of ascarids, as well as oocysts, will continue to develop. Refrigeration (or even freezing) of feces often is the best approach.

PARASITOLOGY AND PUBLIC HEALTH

Many parasitic diseases can be transmitted between animals and humans (zoonoses). These diseases are always of concern to occupational groups who come into daily contact with a variety of exotic, wild, and domesticated animals. Consequently, the conditions discussed below are those personnel might encounter. Some of the more important zoonotic diseases of infectious etiology are discussed in Chapter 7 under the category of Zoonoses. Control of most parasitic diseases requires strict attention to personal hygiene and avoidance of contaminated materials.

Cryptosporidosis is caused by *Cryptosporidium* spp. The mode of infection is by direct contact with infected animals and consumption of fecal contaminated water or food. Dogs, cats, and birds are considered probable sources of infection.

Giardiasis is caused by *Giardia* spp. The mode of infection is by direct contact with infected animals and consumption of fecal contaminated water. Dogs and cats are considered probable sources of infection.

Toxoplasmosis is caused by *Toxoplasma gondii.* Infection can be acquired from sporulated oocysts in cat feces or ingestion of raw or insufficiently cooked meat.

Hydatidosis is caused by infection with the hydatid cyst of the eggs of *Echinococcus granulosis* or *Echinococcus multilocularis.*

Tapeworms are acquired by ingestion of raw or poorly cooked beef (*Taenia saginata*) or pork (*Taenia solium*).

Creeping eruption is caused by penetration of the skin by larval stages of dog and cat hookworm of the genus *Ancylostoma.*

Visceral larva migrans is caused by ingestion of the infective larvae (within the egg) of *Toxocara canis,* especially by very young children.

Strongyloidosis is caused by infection, generally by *Strongyloides stercoralis,* which infects humans, dogs, cats, and foxes.

Trichinosis is caused by infection with *Trichinella spiralis,* generally from consumption of raw or insufficiently cooked pork or bear.

Scabies include the mites that are not strictly host specific and can live for varying amounts of time on alternate hosts. Such mites include *Sarcoptes, Notoedres,* or *Cheyletiella.*

APPENDIX

Lugol's Solution

Add 10 g of potassium iodide and 5 g of iodine crystals to 1 liter of distilled water and place in a brown (amber) bottle (otherwise it will lose strength). These chemicals do not go into solution readily; heating or preparation several weeks in advance of use is necessary.

Zinc Sulfate

Zinc sulfate at an specific gravity of 1.18 is made by adding 331 g of zinc sulfate to 1 liter of distilled water (tap water will suffice). However, because zinc sulfate is hygroscopic, 331 g seldom is adequate, and a hydrometer *must* be used to adjust the specific gravity. To make a solution of specific gravity 1.20, keep adding zinc sulfate until the proper density is obtained.

Ingredients for Willis Technique

General. As indicated in the text, the simple flotation technique (Willis technique) of nematode eggs, tapeworm eggs, coccidia, and so forth, which is often used to detect gastrointestinal parasitism in animals and humans, uses concentrated sodium chloride, magnesium sulfate, sodium nitrate, or sugar solutions. All solutions are essentially equally effective, but some (sodium chloride) are more readily available and less expensive than others (sugar). The recipes for each are given below.

Sodium Chloride. Saturated sodium chloride has a specific gravity of 1.20. A saturated solution is made by adding 311 g of sodium chloride to 1 liter of water. A simple procedure is to keep adding salt to warm or hot water until no more goes into solution. Cool to room temperature. Do not decant the excess salt because this will ensure that a saturated solution is maintained.

Sodium Nitrate. This is used as a saturated solution at an specific gravity of 1.36. It is made by adding 616 g of sodium nitrate to 1 liter of water. As with sodium chloride, a simple procedure is to add sodium nitrate to warm or hot water until no more goes into solution.

Magnesium Sulfate. A saturated solution of magnesium sulfate has a specific gravity of 1.30 and is made by adding 337 g of magnesium sulfate to 1 liter of water. As with sodium chloride and sodium nitrate, it can be added to warm or hot water until no more goes into solution.

Sugar. Table sugar (cane or beet source) is used at an specific gravity of 1.2 to 1.3 and is made by adding approximately 1500 g of sugar to 1 liter of water. As in the preceding recipes, heating the water will facilitate the sugar going into solution. Between 18 and 20 ml of phenol or formaldehyde must be added as a preservative.

Baermann Funnel

The Baermann apparatus may be used for the recovery of larvae from the feces, soil, or minced tissues of an animal.

Although variable results are frequently obtained with this technique, semiquantitative results may be expected from its careful use. Identification depends on the migration of the larvae from the feces, tissues, or soil into water of a warmer temperature, which is brought into contact with the bottom of the material to be examined. Equipment consists of a glass funnel about 25 cm in diameter in which a wire gauze of 1-mm mesh (about 22.5 cm in diameter) is placed. The funnel is joined to a centrifuge tube by means of a rubber tube, the latter being provided with a pinchcock. In use, the assembled funnel is placed in a ringstand. Before use, the funnel is filled with lukewarm water to the level of the wire gauze. The material to be examined is thoroughly broken up and placed on the gauze. Usually within 10 to 15 minutes, larvae may be observed migrating into the water, and a large number may be recovered by drawing the material into the centrifuge tube by means of the pinchcock. The largest yield will be obtained by allowing the material to remain in the funnel for 24 hours before drawing off the larvae.

Recommended Reading

1. Sloss MW, Kemp RL, and Zajac AM: Veterinary Clinical Parasitology, 6th ed. Ames, IA, Iowa State University Press, 1994.
2. Thienpont D, Rochette F, and Vanparijs OFJ: Diagnosing Helminthiasis Through Coprological Examination. Washington Crossing, NJ, Pitman-Moore, 1979.
3. Williams FW, and Zajac AM: Diagnosis of Gastrointestinal Parasitism in Dogs and Cats. St. Louis, MO, Ralston Purina Co., 1980.
4. Hoskins JD, and Cupp EW: Ticks of veterinary importance. Part I. The Ixodidae family: Identification, behavior, and associated diseases. Compend Contin Educ Pract Vet 10(5):564–581, 1988.
5. Hoskins JD and Cupp EW: Ticks of veterinary importance. Part II. The Argasidae family: Identification, behavior, and associated diseases. Compend Contin Educ Pract Vet 10(6):699–709, 1988.
6. Parasitology. Compend Contin Educ Pract Vet 14(5):575–702, 1992.

7 Zoonoses and Public Health

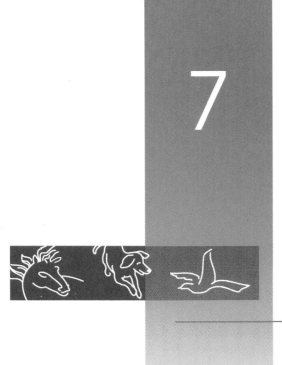

Michael G. Groves • *Kathleen S. Harrington*

INTRODUCTION

This chapter provides an overview of the major zoonotic diseases and other significant public health concerns that veterinary personnel are most likely to be exposed to in the course of their work. The focus is on the occupational exposure to these conditions, as opposed to exposure via other means. For example, some of the diseases discussed here, such as salmonellosis and brucellosis, also can be acquired by consuming contaminated food, water, or milk. Foodborne or waterborne transmission is mentioned but not described in detail; only those routes of infection that are specific to veterinary exposure are covered in depth. Likewise, outlined prevention strategies are oriented toward the veterinary profession rather than the public.

The animals listed as carriers or reservoirs of the various diseases are the ones most commonly implicated in transmission; no attempt has been made to list every host species that could possibly be associated with a given zoonosis. Finally, this chapter is not intended to be a comprehensive reference on zoonoses, but instead it presents a brief review of each disease or condition and provides suggestions for further reading. A summary of the major occupationally acquired zoonotic diseases is given in Table 7–1.

ANIMAL-ASSOCIATED INJURIES: BITE WOUNDS

There are many ways in which animals can adversely affect the health of humans, and for those who work with animals on a daily basis, the risk of sustaining an animal-associated injury is significantly higher than that of contracting a zoonotic disease.

Large animals can inflict considerable damage with their feet if they kick or step on a person, and many orthopedic surgeons regard horses as the animal most likely to cause injury.

TECHNICIAN NOTE

Animal-associated injuries most frequently sustained by veterinarians and animal care personnel are bite wounds from companion animals.

However, the animal-associated injuries most frequently sustained by veterinarians and animal care personnel are bite wounds from companion animals. A bite wound is defined as "any break in the skin caused by an animal's teeth, regardless of intention." In a recent survey of small animal practitioners, cat and dog bites accounted for more than two thirds of the injuries of veterinarians and their employees. A 3-year analysis of Workers' Compensation claims conducted for the American Veterinary Medical Association (AVMA) revealed that animal bites accounted for 49% of all reported incidents and accounted for more than $220,000 in payments to injured personnel each year.

Although cats are reported to inflict more bites in a veterinary setting than do dogs (54% versus 45% respectively), dogs are responsible for the most serious bites in both occupational and nonoccupational situations. Dog bites constitute a major public health problem. In the United States, more than 1 million dog bites are reported each year, which is equal to an annual incidence rate of 300 to 700 per 100,000 population. Probably

• Table 7-1 •

SUMMARY OF MAJOR OCCUPATIONALLY ACQUIRED ZOONOTIC DISEASES

	AGENT	SOURCE ANIMALS*	MODE OF TRANSMISSION	TYPE OF INFECTION	SEVERITY	NOTES
Bacterial Diseases						
Anthrax	*Bacillus anthracis*	**Cattle, sheep, horses, goats**				Vaccine is available for people at high risk of exposure.
Cutaneous			Cutaneous inoculation	Cutaneous lesion; may progress to septicemia	Mild (cutaneous only) to fatal (septicemia)	Early treatment prevents progression to more severe disease.
Inhalation			Inhalation of agent in contaminated dust	Mild upper respiratory symptoms progressing to acute septicemia	Usually fatal	
Brucellosis	*Brucella* spp.	**Cattle,** sheep, goats, swine	Contact with placenta or birth fluids; inhalation; injection with strain 19 vaccine	Septicemia	Severe	Convalescence is prolonged; relapses frequently occur.
Campylobacteriosis	*Campylobacter* spp.	**Dogs,** cats, cattle	Fecal-oral	Gastroenteritis, diarrhea	Mild to severe	Most patients recover without treatment.
Capnocytophaga infection	*Capnocytophaga canimorsus*	**Dogs,** cats	Bite wound	Septicemia	Severe to fatal	Asplenic and other immunocompromised people are at increased risk.
Cat scratch disease	*Bartonella henselae*	**Cats**	Bite, scratch, contact with broken skin	Influenza-like with regional lymphadenopathy	Usually mild, self-limiting	Most patients recover without treatment.
Erysipeloid	*Erysipelothrix rhusiopathiae*	**Swine,** turkeys	Cutaneous inoculation	Cutaneous lesion; rarely progresses to systemic disease	Usually mild	
Ornithosis (psittacosis)	*Chlamydia psittaci*	**Psittacine birds, turkeys**	Inhalation of agent excreted in feces	Upper respiratory illness; pneumonia	Mild to severe	Early treatment shortens duration of illness.
Pasteurellosis	*Pasteurella multocida*	**Cats,** dogs	Bite wound	Cellulitis; progression to septicemia possible	Mild to severe	Septic arthritis may develop in persons with rheumatoid arthritis
Q Fever	*Coxiella burnetii*	**Sheep,** goats, cattle	Inhalation; contact with placenta or birth fluids	Systemic, influenza-like	Mild to severe	Usually mild; in rare cases chronic disease and endocarditis develop years after initial infection

Disease	Etiologic Agent	Animals Implicated	Mode of Transmission	Clinical Signs in Humans	Severity	Comments
Rat-bite Fevers	*Streptobacillus moniliformis* and *Spirillum minus*	**Rodents**	Bite wound	Systemic, febrile, usually with polyarthritis	Mild to severe	Untreated infections may persist for weeks or months; fatalities have occurred
Salmonellosis	*Salmonella* spp.	**Reptiles**, dogs, cats, chickens, ducks	Fecal-oral	Gastroenteritis	Mild to severe	Immunocompromised people at greater risk for severe illness
Fungal Diseases						
Cryptococcosis	*Cryptococcus neoformans*	**Birds** (indirect)	Inhalation	Pneumonia; meningitis in HIV-positive people	Mild to severe	HIV-infected people at increased risk
Dermatophytosis (tinea)	*Microsporum canis, Trichophyton mentagrophytes, T. verrucosum*	Dogs, **cats, cattle**, sheep	Direct contact with infected animal or spores on hair or dander	Lesion affecting hair, skin, or nails	Usually mild	
Parasitic Diseases						
Cryptosporidiosis	*Cryptosporidium parvum*	**Cattle**	Fecal-oral	Gastroenteritis	Usually mild, self-limiting	May be life-threatening in HIV-infected people
Toxoplasmosis	*Toxoplasma gondii*	Cats	Fecal-oral	Systemic, mononucleosis-like; encephalitis	Usually subclinical in immunocompetent persons; can be life-threatening in HIV-infected people	Direct transmission from cats rare; primary infection during pregnancy can affect fetus
Viral Diseases						
Contagious ecthyma (orf)	*Parapoxvirus*	**Sheep**, goats	Direct contact with infective material	Cutaneous lesion	Usually mild, self-limiting	
Herpesvirus simiae (B-virus) infection	*Herpesvirus simiae*	**Old World monkeys**	Bite wound or other cutaneous inoculation; possible aerosol transmission	Meningoencephalitis	Usually fatal	Survivors usually have permanent neurologic sequelae.
Newcastle disease	*Paramyxovirus*	**Poultry**	Direct contact of eyes with infective material; aerosols	Conjunctivitis; occasionally systemic, influenza-like	Usually mild, self-limiting	
Rabies	*Lyssavirus*	Dogs, cats, cattle, **skunks, raccoons, foxes, bats,** etc.	Bite wound or contact with saliva	Encephalomyelitis	Fatal	All animal care personnel should receive preexposure prophylaxis.

*Boldface indicates most commonly implicated animals.

fewer than half of all bites that occur are reported, however, and some reports estimate the true number is closer to 3 million per year. Annually, more than 585,000 bite wounds in the United States require medical attention, and dogs are responsible for 80% to 90% of those.

TECHNICIAN NOTE

Zoonotic diseases that may be transmitted by dog bites include *Capnocytophaga canimorsus* infection, pasturellosis, and rabies.

In the course of their work, veterinary personnel encounter many situations that may provoke a bite, even from a dog that is not normally aggressive. Some dogs resist being placed in submissive postures or situations, such as during restraint for examination, and will attempt to bite in response to this perceived insult. Other factors that may increase the risk of bites are the stresses that an already fearful dog experiences while in unfamiliar and often uncomfortable surroundings. The unintentional inflicting of pain in the course of restraining the animal, examining it, or administering medication also can provoke a bite.

If a bite occurs, there is a possibility of serious infection developing. At particular risk are persons who are immunocompromised, which includes people who are positive for the human immunodeficiency virus (HIV) or have acquired immune deficiency syndrome (AIDS). Other at-risk persons are pregnant women, people receiving long-term corticosteroid therapy, splenectomized individuals, and others who have weakened immune systems. All immunocompromised persons should take extra precautions to avoid exposure to infection. Zoonotic diseases that may be transmitted by dog bites include *Capnocytophaga canimorsus* infection, pasturellosis, and rabies. (These diseases are detailed later in this chapter.) In addition, there is the possibility of permanent damage or disfigurement resulting from the wound.

Veterinary personnel should be alert to possible bite-provoking situations and take measures to ensure a dog does not have the opportunity to bite. In addition, people with immunosuppresive conditions should avoid handling animals that may bite.

If a bite does occur, regardless of the species of animal involved or the immune status of the person bitten, the wound should be washed immediately with soap and water and rinsed thoroughly with a strong stream of water. If the wound is severe, medical treatment should be sought as soon as possible. An immunocompromised person should consult a physician for even a minor wound because prophylactic antibiotics may be indicated. Normally healthy people with small wounds should seek medical advice if the wound penetrates a joint or the wound site becomes swollen, inflamed, or painful.

BACTERIAL ZOONOSES

Anthrax

Agent. *Bacillus anthracis* is a large, nonmotile, gram-positive rod that forms environmentally resistant endospores when exposed to air.

Reservoirs. Sheep, goats, cows, and other domestic and wild ruminants.

Occurrence. Incidence is worldwide except for the far north and some South Pacific islands, but it varies greatly by region. Anthrax in animals occurs sporadically in Eurasia, North America, and Australia but is endemic in Africa, the Middle East, India, Southeast Asia, Mexico, and parts of South America. Warm, humid areas tend to have anthrax "hot spots" because heat stress lowers animals' resistance and the climate encourages sporulation of shed organisms.

Estimates of human anthrax cases range from 20,000 to 100,000 per year, with most occurring in Africa, South America, Europe, the Middle East, and the former Soviet Union. In the United States, human anthrax is very rare, with only three cases reported between 1984 and 1993. Most cases of anthrax are occupationally acquired; people at greatest risk are veterinarians and animal care workers, abattoir workers, hide tanners, wool processors, and bonemeal producers.

Transmission. Infected animals shed the organism via hemorrhages that occur at death, thus contaminating soil with endospores that can remain viable for years. Other animals can become infected by grazing in the contaminated areas. Biting flies may be involved in mechanical transmission of the bacteria.

There are two forms of human anthrax that are occupationally associated: cutaneous and inhalation. Cutaneous anthrax is acquired when organisms enter broken skin, usually on the hands, arms, or face. Direct contact with tissues or body fluids of diseased animals and exposure to contaminated soil are the most common means of transmission. Inhalation anthrax results from inhaling viable spores that may be present in wool and processed hides of infected animals. A third form, gastrointestinal anthrax, results from eating contaminated undercooked meat and is not associated with any particular occupational exposure.

TECHNICIAN NOTE

Inhalation anthrax results from inhaling viable spores that may be present in wool and processed hides of infected animals.

Disease in Animals

Signs. Anthrax in animals manifests in three main forms: peracute, acute, and subacute to chronic. Peracute anthrax, which occurs in ruminants, is characterized by sudden death with few premonitory signs. The animal appears healthy until just before death, when there may be high fever, muscle tremors, dyspnea, and convulsions. A bloody discharge from various body orifices often occurs after death.

Both ruminants and horses can have anthrax in the acute form. In this form, signs appear up to 48 or more hours before death and may include a period of excitement followed by depression, lethargy, and anorexia. Fever, rapid respiration, and heart rate occur, and mucous membranes become hemorrhagic or congested. The tongue, throat, sternum, perineum, and flanks may become edematous and swollen.

Swine, canines, and felines that consume meat from diseased animals or other contaminated material can develop subacute to chronic anthrax. Organisms concentrate in lymph nodes in the pharyngeal region and cause swelling that obstructs the airways; death by suffocation follows. Bacteremia can also occur, and some animals may develop enteritis. Carnivores appear to be more resistant to anthrax and often recover.

Diagnosis. The organism can be cultured from blood or tissues of affected animals. A necropsy should not be performed in cases of suspected anthrax to avoid exposing any *B. anthracis* organisms to air, thus causing sporulation and contamination of the site. Since blood does not clot following death from anthrax because of toxin produced by the organism, a sample can be collected from the jugular vein using a disposable syringe. Capped syringes should be refrigerated and submitted promptly to a laboratory for culture.

Disease in Humans
Signs and Symptoms. Cutaneous anthrax accounts for more than 95% of cases. Within 1 week of inoculation a small, painless, reddish, pruritic papule forms and develops into a fluid-filled vesicle. The area surrounding the lesion becomes edematous, and secondary vesicles may form around the initial site. The typical lesion of cutaneous anthrax is a black eschar that develops after a vesicle ruptures and ulcerates. Most patients recover within 10 days of onset, but in some cases cutaneous anthrax progresses to systemic disease. Disseminated anthrax is rapidly fatal if untreated.

Inhalation anthrax is almost always fatal. It begins with mild, nonspecific upper respiratory signs, but within 3 to 5 days the patient becomes acutely ill, with fever, shock, and rapidly progressing respiratory distress. Death occurs within 24 hours of onset of the acute phase.

Diagnosis. Cutaneous anthrax is easily diagnosed if the disease is considered among the possibilities. Gram staining of the vesicular fluid often reveals large, gram-positive rods, and cultures of the fluid are usually positive for *B. anthracis* if specimens are collected before antibiotic therapy is begun.

The diagnosis of inhalation anthrax is much more difficult because early signs mimic a mild, influenza-like infection. Death usually occurs before the diagnosis is made.

TECHNICIAN NOTE

A human vaccine is available for personnel at high risk of exposure to anthrax.

Treatment. Cutaneous anthrax responds well to antibiotic treatment. Inhalation anthrax, however, is often diagnosed too late in the course of the disease for even massive doses of antibiotics to be effective.

Prevention. Laws covering the prevention of anthrax are in force in most areas. Livestock vaccines are available and effective. When an outbreak occurs, affected animals should be treated with antibiotics and survivors quarantined for 21 days after the last death has occurred. As noted above, necropsy should not be performed on any animal suspected of having died from anthrax. Carcasses should be burned at the site, if

possible, instead of buried because spores can survive for many years in soil. If an animal must be buried, there should be a deep burial, and the carcass should be covered with a layer of quick lime (anhydrous calcium oxide) before the dirt is replaced. Disposable material that must come in contact with infected animals should be burned or disinfected and buried. Contaminated surfaces and other nondisposable items should be cleaned with a disinfectant known to be effective against anthrax spores.

A human vaccine is available for personnel at high risk of exposure to anthrax, such as workers in wool- or hide-processing plants, laboratory personnel working in anthrax research, and veterinarians and veterinary technicians working in highly endemic areas. Anyone coming into contact with an animal that may have anthrax should be particularly careful about hygiene and care of any wounds.

Reporting and Surveillance. Both human and animal anthrax are reportable diseases in the United States and other developed countries. In the United States, animal cases must be reported to the appropriate state animal health agency.

Avian Chlamydiosis (Ornithosis/Psittacosis)

Agent. *Chlamydia psittaci* is an obligate intracellular gram-negative bacterium with a unique biphasic reproductive cycle, of which only one phase is infectious.

Reservoirs. Birds, especially psittacines (members of the parrot family), pigeons, and doves, and poultry, including ducks and turkeys.

Occurrence. Incidence is worldwide; it is endemic in birds and sporadic in humans. Prevalence in avian species varies widely; active chlamydiosis in wild psittacines is about 1%, whereas 50% to 95% of some feral pigeon populations may carry the disease. Humans at risk are those who own exotic pet birds, bird breeders, pigeon fanciers, poultry farm or processing plant workers, veterinarians and their technicians who treat birds, zoo keepers, avian quarantine station employees, and others who come in contact with wild, pet, or domestic birds.

Transmission. Transmission occurs through inhalation of infective particles that have become aerosolized from dried feces, ocular or nasal secretions, dust from feathers and so forth. Cleaning cages is a means of human exposure; sneezing and wing flapping by birds also spread infective material.

Disease in Animals
Signs. Birds may develop peracute, acute, or chronic disease; many are asymptomatic carriers. Clinical signs vary depending on species of host and virulence of the infecting strain, but most cases include depression, anorexia, yellowish or greenish diarrhea, conjunctivitis, nasal discharge, and respiratory difficulty. Morbidity and mortality also differ with strain virulence.

Diagnosis. Diagnosis of avian chlamydiosis can be difficult. Clinical signs can suggest the disease, but there are no pathognomonic features. Microscopic examination of impression smears or fixed sections of spleen, liver, or air sac tissue of birds that have died from the disease sometimes reveals elementary bodies, the infectious phase of *C. psittaci*. Special staining techniques are required, however, and the absence of visible elementary bodies does not rule out chlamydiosis. Serological tests, such as latex agglutination and enzyme-linked immunosorbent assay (ELISA), can be used to diagnose the disease in live birds, but results may be negative if testing is performed in the early stages of the infection. It is also possible to isolate *C. psittaci* from swabs taken from the palatine cleft, cloaca, or fresh feces, although a single negative culture should not be considered definitive because of intermittent shedding of the organism. Specimens submitted for culture attempts should be placed into a chlamydial transport medium and refrigerated until processed.

Disease in Humans

Signs and Symptoms. The incubation period for avian chlamydiosis in humans is 1 to 4 weeks. Onset can be either sudden or gradual; symptoms include fever, chills, headache, muscle aches, and upper and lower respiratory tract illness. The elderly, particularly if not treated, may develop severe disease. Complications can include encephalitis, myocarditis, hepatitis, arthritis, and thrombophlebitis. Most cases, however, are mild or moderate, with recovery in 7 to 10 days in patients receiving appropriate treatment; the case-fatality rate among such patients is less than 1%.

Diagnosis. A history of exposure to birds is suggestive. Serological tests are the means of diagnosis most frequently used, with a fourfold rise in titer between paired sera collected 2 to 3 weeks apart being considered confirmatory. The agent can be isolated from sputum or blood, but if antibiotics have been administered, the chances of recovery of the organism are reduced.

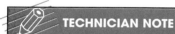

TECHNICIAN NOTE

Avian practitioners and others who work with birds should be aware of the possibility of chlamydiosis and take appropriate precautions.

Treatment. Avian chlamydiosis responds to various antibiotics, with tetracycline or doxycycline usually being the drug of choice.

Prevention. The aim of 30-day quarantine period for imported birds mandated by law in the United States is to detect birds infected with Newcastle disease virus and does not ensure that birds entering the country are free from chlamydiosis; likewise, many domestically reared birds may be carriers. Infected birds can appear healthy and still shed the organism, particularly when stressed by crowding, shipping, or other adverse conditions. Therefore, avian practitioners and others who work with birds should be aware of the possibility of chlamydiosis and take appropriate precautions. Rapid diagnosis and an effective treatment program for birds can help reduce human exposure.

If a bird is suspected of having chlamydiosis, it should be isolated, and all personnel caring for it should wear face masks and protective clothing. Cage papers should be wetted with a quaternary ammonium disinfectant before cage cleaning to minimize aerosolization of infective particles. Laboratory coats and other protective clothing should be removed and hands washed after contact with an infected bird. There is no vaccine, for either birds or humans.

Reporting and Surveillance. In the United States and many other countries, avian chlamydiosis in humans must be reported to local health authorities.

Brucellosis

Agent. *Brucella* spp. are small, gram-negative coccobacilli. Humans are susceptible to infection by *B. abortus, B. melitensis, B. suis,* and *B. canis.*

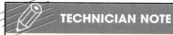

TECHNICIAN NOTE

More than 500,000 cases of human brucellosis are estimated to occur annually, with most in developing countries and most occurring due to contaminated milk.

Reservoirs. *B. abortus* is primarily carried by cattle, bison, Asian buffaloes, and North American elk; sheep, goats, horses, and other domestic livestock can maintain the infection within herds. Domestic goats and sheep are the major carriers of *B. melitensis;* cattle, camels, and dogs also are susceptible to infection with this species. *B. suis* is carried by swine, but European hares, reindeer, caribou, and some rodents are hosts for certain strains of this species. Canines, both domestic and wild, are reservoirs for *B. canis.*

Occurrence. With a worldwide incidence, more than 500,000 cases of human brucellosis are estimated to occur annually, with most in developing nations and most occurring due to contaminated milk. Countries bordering the Mediterranean and in the Middle East, India, central Asia, Mexico, and Central and South America have the highest incidence.

Human brucellosis has decreased radically in industrialized countries in which active programs to eliminate animal disease have been undertaken. In these countries, brucellosis primarily is an occupational disease among people who work with animals. In the United States, fewer than 200 cases are reported each year. Farm workers, abattoir workers, and especially veterinarians and their technicians are at the greatest risk.

Transmission. Among most animals, transmission occurs primarily through consumption of feed or other material contaminated with infected birth fluids. Although the organisms do not multiply outside a host, brucellae may survive in the environment for several months under moist, cool conditions, thus providing a source of infection for susceptible animals that may ingest contaminated material. *B. suis* and *B. canis* can be sexually transmitted.

As an occupational disease, human brucellosis is most often contracted by farmers and veterinarians via direct contact with aborted fetuses, placentas, or vaginal fluids from infected animals. The organism enters though broken skin. Accidental self-inoculation with strain 19 bovine vaccine is responsible for a small number of cases annually. Aerosol transmission is another important route of infection and can occur in farm, abattoir, and laboratory settings.

Disease in Animals

Signs. Abortion is the major sign of brucellosis, regardless of which species of animal is infected or which of the brucellae is the infective agent. *B. abortus* also can cause reduced milk production among infected cows and orchitis, seminal vesiculitis, and ampullitis among bulls; fertility of both sexes is often adversely affected. *B. suis* infections of swine cause similar clinical signs and arthritis also may occur. In sheep and goats, *B. melitensis* causes mastitis, orchitis, arthritis, and spondylitis. *B. canis* infection in dogs is characterized by bacteremia, lymphadenitis, and splenitis, in addition to reproductive tract lesions similar to those exhibited by livestock.

Diagnosis. Isolation of organisms from infective material, such as aborted fetuses and blood, is definitive, but brucellae are slow growing, and standard laboratory culture procedures may not always be effective. A variety of serological tests are available.

Disease in Humans

Signs and Symptoms. Human brucellosis is highly variable in presentation, with patients often having many vague, nonspecific symptoms. Onset may be sudden or insidious, with symptoms appearing gradually over 1 week or longer.

Most human cases are caused by *B. abortus* or *B. melitensis*. In acute systemic brucellosis caused by *B. abortus,* patients often have fever, nausea, vomiting, and other gastrointestinal complaints. In undulant fever caused by *B. melitensis,* cycles of waxing and waning fever occur. Each cycle lasts a few weeks and is followed by a brief afebrile period before another cycle begins. In both forms of the disease, osteoarticular involvement occurs in up to 60% of patients, and complications involving the male reproductive tract, such as epididymitis and orchitis, occur in up to 20% of cases. Endocarditis is a rare but significant complication and accounts for most of the fatalities associated with brucellosis (2% or fewer).

Infection with *B. suis* can produce similar clinical signs and also may result in chronic liver or splenic abscesses. *B. canis* infections are similar to those of *B. abortus* but tend to cause less severe illness and fewer complications. Some patients relapse repeatedly with febrile episodes even after successful treatment; chronic arthritis is often seen in these individuals.

Diagnosis. Definitive diagnosis is possible only when the organism is recovered from a clinical specimen. However, unless brucellosis is suspected and the laboratory is notified, routine culture procedures may not allow sufficient incubation time for the slow-growing bacteria to become detectable. Serological tests are available, but false-negative results are possible in many of these, and conventional testing does not detect antibodies to *B. canis*. DNA probes and polymerase chain reaction (PCR) techniques are new developments, but their practical application for clinical diagnosis has yet to be determined.

Treatment. Brucellosis responds best to combinations of antibiotics; treatment regimens using only one drug are not as successful. Relapses occur in some cases because of sequestered organisms; these patients require retreatment with the original combination of antibiotics.

Prevention. Control of human brucellosis is dependent on the control of brucellosis in livestock. Reservoir animals should be eliminated through testing and slaughter of infected livestock. Farmers, slaughterhouse workers, and others who come into contact with potentially infected animals should be aware of the possibility of brucellosis and should take precautions to reduce risk. Laboratory personnel working with *Brucella* spp. should be aware of the potential for aerosol spread of the organisms and handle cultures or potentially infected tissues only within biological safety cabinets.

Reporting and Surveillance. In most states and countries, both animal and human brucellosis cases must be reported to local health or veterinary authorities.

Campylobacteriosis

Agent. *Campylobacter* spp. are small, curved, gram-negative bacilli. *C. jejuni* and *C. coli* are responsible for most human clinical cases.

Reservoirs. Campylobacters are carried, often asymptomatically, in the intestinal tracts of many birds and mammals. Chickens and other commercial poultry are the main reservoirs for *C. jejuni*. Cattle and swine also carry *C. jejuni* and *C. coli,* and kittens and puppies, particularly if feral or obtained from animal shelters or other large-scale pet suppliers, often are infected with the organism.

Occurrence. Campylobacteriosis occurs worldwide in all age groups and is probably the most common cause of food- or waterborne diarrhea in the world. In the United States, incidence is estimated to be 1000 cases per 100,000 population, with an annual total exceeding 2 million cases; other industrialized nations report similar incidence rates. In developing nations, the rate of infection may be much higher.

In animals, the rate among some commercial poultry flocks approaches 100%. Up to 40% of diarrheic puppies and 10% of adult dogs with diarrhea are infected with *C. jejuni* or *coli*. The rates vary widely for other farm and companion animals.

Transmission. Although ingestion of organisms in uncooked or undercooked food is the most common means of acquiring the infection, fecal-oral transmission in a farm or veterinary environment is also an efficient means of spread. Direct contact with infected diarrheic companion or farm animals can result in human infection if the bacteria are transferred from hands to mouth. The infective dose is very small, so even a small inoculum introduced into the mouth may cause disease. In one study, it was estimated that 6.3% of cases had been acquired through exposure to diarrheic animals, mostly dogs.

Campylobacters are somewhat fragile and subject to desiccation and chemical disinfection but can survive for hours or days at room temperature in feces or other moist material.

Disease in Animals

Signs. Many animals and birds are asymptomatic carriers, shedding the organism in feces. Puppies and kittens may develop acute enterocolitis with diarrhea, vomiting, and fever. Infection in foals, calves, lambs, and kids is characterized by fever, mucoid or hemorrhagic diarrhea, depression, and dehydration.

Diagnosis. The causative organism is isolated from feces. Specimens should be collected on sterile swabs and placed in a transport medium, preferably Cary-Blair, until laboratory processing. Special culture techniques, including selective media and reduced oxygen tension, are required for *in vitro* cultivation. Incubation at 42°C enhances the likelihood of recovery of the organism from clinical samples.

Disease in Humans
Signs and Symptoms. Campylobacteriosis ranges from asymptomatic infection to severe illness. The main symptoms are acute enterocolitis, with bloody, mucoid diarrhea, abdominal pain, nausea, vomiting, and general malaise. Although most people recover without specific treatment within 2 to 5 days, adults may experience prolonged illness, and relapses are possible. Rarely, extraintestinal infections may occur, or sequelae such as reactive arthritis, meningitis, or Guillain-Barré syndrome may follow the initial enteric infection.

Diagnosis. Isolation of *Campylobacter* spp. as the sole pathogen from fecal samples is presumptive; isolation from blood culture is confirmatory. The specialized culture techniques mentioned above in the section on diagnosis of animal disease also apply here.

Treatment. Treatment is not usually necessary; in most cases, campylobacteriosis is self-limiting, and supportive care is sufficient. For prolonged or severe cases or those complicated by extraintestinal infection, erythromycin is the drug of choice.

Prevention. Strict attention to personal hygiene when handling or working around diarrheic animals or poultry can help reduce the risk of occupationally acquired campylobacteriosis.

Reporting and Surveillance. Many states require reporting of human cases to local health authorities, as do some countries. Animal infections are not reportable.

Cat Scratch Disease (*Bartonella henselae* Infection)

Agent. *Bartonella* (formerly *Rochalimaea*) *henselae* is a small, slightly curved, gram-negative bacillus.

Reservoirs. Domestic cats.

Occurrence. Incidence is worldwide. As a clinical entity, cat scratch disease (CSD) affects only humans. In the United States, about 22,000 cases of CSD are reported each year. It occurs most frequently from July through January and affects all age groups. Seropositivity rates in cats in the United States range from less than 15% in cool, dry areas to more than 90% in the warmer, humid parts of the country; overall seroprevalence approaches 30%.

Transmission. As of this writing, neither cat-to-cat nor cat-to-human transmission of *B. henselae* has been explained. However, a cat scratch or (less frequently) a bite is almost always part of the history in CSD cases. Kittens less than 1 year old are most often implicated, but the exact mode of transmission has not been determined. The presence of fleas on a cat has been linked by epidemiological evidence to increased risk of trans-

mission of CSD, and it is speculated that these parasites may in some way be involved, at least in the spread of the infection from one cat to another.

Disease in Animals
Clinical Signs. Cats infected with *B. henselae* usually do not exhibit obvious clinical signs, although one study of experimentally infected cats reported transient fever and anorexia in some of the animals. In addition, mild histopathological changes were noted in various organs. The organism does, however, cause a persistent bacteremia that may last for many months to several years despite the presence of a strong antibody response.

Diagnosis. An immunofluorescence antibody test can be used to detect *B. henselae* antibodies in serum, but this test cannot establish whether a cat has active bacteremia. Isolation of the organism from blood is definitive but specialized culture techniques must be used, and as mentioned above, several weeks are required for colony growth. In addition, experimental studies have shown that *B. henselae* is isolated intermittently from infected cats when they are monitored over time. It is unknown whether this is attributable to sporadic shedding of the organism from some internal focus of infection or whether it reflects a limitation of the microbiological procedures.

If culture is requested, blood should be collected aseptically in a 1.5-ml Wampole Isolator microbial tube (Wampole Laboratories, Cranbury, NJ), an evacuated tube containing agents that lyse erythrocytes and prevent coagulation. If this is not available, a tube containing EDTA, such as a lavender-top Vacutainer tube, may be substituted. Regardless of which type of tube is used, specimens should be frozen and thawed before culture to enhance recovery of organisms.

 TECHNICIAN NOTE

CSD usually presents as a regional lymphadenopathy 3 to 14 days after dermal inoculation of the infectious agent.

Treatment. Antibiotic therapy is not indicated for cats infected with *B. henselae*. Not only do infected cats show few or no clinical signs, but efforts to eliminate bacteremia by administration of antibiotics have met with little success.

Disease in Humans
Signs and Symptoms. Most cases of CSD are asymptomatic or so mild they are unrecognized. When clinical disease does develop, CSD usually presents as a regional lymphadenopathy 3 to 14 days after dermal inoculation of the infectious agent. Low-grade fever, myalgia, and general malaise often occur, and a papular lesion sometimes develops at the site of inoculation. Lymph nodes affected usually are those proximal to the inoculation site; often, they are very painful but rarely suppurate. In more than 90% of patients, CSD follows a mild course and resolves spontaneously, although symptoms can persist for up to 2 months. Complications are rare, and the case-fatality rate is almost nonexistent.

B. henselae infection may be much more serious in immunocompromised people. In these patients, CSD may progress to septicemia or disseminated disease affecting multiple organ systems. Very rarely, the infection may manifest as bacillary angiomatosis (BA) or bacillary peliosis (BP) instead of CSD. BA is characterized by a vasoproliferative tissue reaction that produces violaceous or colorless nodular lesions on the skin and in internal organs. In BP, blood-filled cysts develop in the parenchyma of the liver, spleen, and other reticuloendothelial structures. Both conditions are potentially life threatening and usually occur only in HIV-infected individuals.

Diagnosis. Although many physicians still diagnose CSD solely on the basis of clinical signs and a history of cat exposure, a sensitive and specific IFA test to detect antibodies against *B. henselae* is available. A titer of ≥1:64 is considered positive, and most patients show elevated antibody levels in the weeks after the onset of lymphadenopathy. The organism also can be isolated from lymph node aspirates and blood, but as in the cat, culture requires too much time to be useful as a diagnostic test.

Treatment. Antibiotic therapy generally is not indicated for CSD; in the typical patient, it does not shorten the course of the disease or lessen the discomfort of the lymphadenopathy. Surgical excision of affected lymph nodes is not recommended, but needle aspiration can be used to relieve pressure and pain in severe cases. For most CSD patients, rest, analgesics, and heat applied to swollen lymph nodes are adequate treatment. Systemic *B. henselae* infection in an immunocompromised person, however, requires immediate and aggressive antibiotic therapy.

Prevention. Common sense and careful attention to hygiene are probably the best methods of preventing CSD. Hands should always be washed after handling cats. Avoid cat bites and scratches, and thoroughly wash with soap and water any that do occur. Likewise, prevent cats from licking or coming in contact with any break in the skin; keep wounds covered until healed.

Reporting and Surveillance. CSD is not a reportable disease in the United States.

Capnocytophaga Infection

Agent. *Capnocytophaga canimorsus,* formerly known as CDC group Dysgonic Fermenter-2 (DF-2), a slow-growing, fastidious gram-negative rod.

Reservoirs. Dogs and cats.

Occurrence. Incidence is probably worldwide. Human infections with *C. canimorsus* have been reported from North America, Europe, Africa, Australia, and New Zealand. Most cases have occurred in the summer and fall, and all age groups are affected. Although only a comparatively few (fewer than 100) cases have been reported since the disease was first recognized, this is more likely attributable to the difficulty in isolating the organism from clinical specimens (making diagnoses difficult to establish) than to the true rarity of the infection.

Transmission. Dog bites or scratches are most often associated with this condition; about 65% of cases are attributable to dog-inflicted trauma. Nonbite exposure to dogs, cat bites or scratches, and other animal exposures also have been linked to

C. canimorsus infection. Even small, apparently inconsequential, dog bites have, in some cases, led to fatal disease.

Disease in Animals
Signs. There are no signs in animals. *C. canimorsus* is a commensal in the oral cavity of dogs and cats and can be isolated from the saliva of healthy animals of both species. Surveys indicate up to 24% of dogs and 17% of cats may harbor the organism.

Diagnosis. *C. canimorsus* can be isolated from gingivae, saliva, and nasal fluids. Samples should be collected using sterile cotton-tipped swabs, which should be placed in a holding medium until processed.

Disease in Humans
Signs and Symptoms. *C. canimorsus* infections can be asymptomatic or self-limiting, even in immunocompromised patients. In most known cases, however, a life-threatening illness has developed. Usually presenting initially as a nonspecific febrile illness, *C. canimorsus* infection frequently progresses to an overwhelming septicemia. Disseminated intravascular coagulation, renal failure, endocarditis, cellulitis, and gangrene may occur. In these cases, the mortality rate exceeds 30%.

TECHNICIAN NOTE

All dog bites, no matter how small, should be vigorously cleansed with a povidone-iodine solution and irrigated thoroughly with water.

Many patients have some underlying medical condition that predisposes them to infection; splenectomy is most commonly reported. Other conditions associated with increased risk include age over 50 years, alcohol abuse, steroid therapy, and chronic neoplastic, hematological, or pulmonary disease. It should be noted, however, that several otherwise healthy young people have developed fatal infections with this organism.

Diagnosis. *C. canimorsus* isolated from blood, cerebrospinal fluid, or tissues is definitive, but depending on the culture media used, mature colonies may not develop for 1 week or longer after inoculation. In bacteremic patients, a rapid, presumptive test is a Gram stain of a blood smear or buffy coat. The organism appears as elongated, filamentous gram-negative rods within polymorphonuclear cells.

Treatment. Penicillin is the usual drug of choice for this infection.

Prevention. Animal care workers should be aware of the possibility of severe or life-threatening infection with this organism. All dog bites, no matter how small, should be vigorously cleansed with a povidone-iodine solution and irrigated thoroughly with water. Likewise, an existing wound that becomes contaminated with dog saliva should be thoroughly washed. Medical evaluation should be sought; surgical debridement may be indicated. Immediate medical treatment should be sought if fever or signs of cellulitis develop after an animal bite. Delay in treatment is a risk factor for development of severe infection.

Penicillin G as prophylaxis after a dog bite often is recommended for persons with underlying conditions associated with an increased risk of *C. canimorsus* infection. Asplenic individuals probably should never handle dogs or cats.

Reporting and Surveillance. No formal reports are required.

Erysipelothrix Infection

Agent. *Erysipelothrix rhusiopathiae* is a thin, nonsporeforming gram-positive rod.

Reservoir. Domestic swine are the principal reservoirs; up to 30% of healthy animals may harbor *E. rhusiopathiae* in their tonsils and continually excrete the organism in feces.

Occurrence. Incidence of swine erysipelas is worldwide and high in parts of Europe, Asia, North and South America, and Australia. Morbidity and mortality are variable, but in some areas intensive vaccination programs are required to allow profitable swine production. Many species of wild and domestic fowl, especially turkeys, also are frequently infected. Fish and shellfish are not known to develop clinical disease, but *Erysipelothrix* frequently is present in their exterior slime.

In humans, *E. rhusiopathiae* infection is related to occupation. Persons most often affected include veterinarians and animal care workers, butchers and other meat handlers, fishermen, fish and shellfish handlers, and microbiology laboratory personnel.

Transmission. Pigs and turkeys become infected through contamination of wounds or oral exposure. The organism is resistant to many environmental influences, including direct sunlight. It can survive for long periods of time in feces, sewage, carcasses, and water. In humans, most cases occur after occupational exposure to the organism, usually via scratches, abrasions, or puncture wounds to the hands or fingers caused by knives, bone splinters, and fish hooks.

Disease in Animals
Signs. Swine erysipelas can be acute, subacute, or chronic. The acute form of the disease is septicemia that may cause sudden death. Subacute erysipelas occurs in animals that survive the initial phase of the disease; this is characterized by the appearance of raised, reddish-purple rhomboidal lesions ("diamond skin disease") that subsequently become necrotic. Chronic erysipelas may affect the joints, causing arthritis and general unthriftiness, or the heart, resulting in endocarditis and death.

Turkey erysipelas mainly affects adult male birds. In the acute, septic form, birds are depressed and somnolent, with prostration and death occurring soon after onset. Subacute erysipelas is characterized by weakness, diarrhea, and cyanosis and swelling of the snood and dewlap. As in swine, chronic infection may cause arthritis or endocarditis.

Diagnosis. The organism can be isolated from skin lesions and from blood and internal organs of animals with septicemia.

Disease in Humans
Signs and Symptoms. *Erysipelothrix* infection in humans has manifestations similar to those in animals. In humans, however, the localized cutaneous infection known as erysipeloid (to distinguish it from the human erysipelas caused by *Streptococcus* spp.) is the most frequently seen form. Erysipeloid is a cellulitis that usually develops on the fingers and hands after dermal inoculation with the organism; a raised, purplish lesion appears at the site and is accompanied by severe pain and swelling. Although erysipeloid is a self-limiting infection and usually resolves without treatment in 3 to 4 weeks, lesions may recur and last much longer in second attacks.

Systemic *Erysipelothrix* infections are uncommon and only rarely follow erysipeloid. Most patients with systemic disease develop subacute endocarditis; generalized cutaneous infection and septicemia also can occur.

Diagnosis. The organism can be isolated from biopsies taken from the edge of erysipeloid lesions. In cases of endocarditis or septicemia, routine blood cultures will allow isolation of the agent.

TECHNICIAN NOTE

The chances of contracting human erysipeloid infection by those occupationally exposed can be lessened by frequent handwashing with disinfectant soaps or detergents.

Treatment. *Erysipelothrix* is susceptible to a variety of antibiotics. Some endocarditis patients may require valve replacement.

Prevention. For swine, vaccines and bacterins are available but do not always provide lasting immunity. Good management practices, especially those involving cleanliness and sanitation, must be used as well in areas where erysipelas is endemic.

The chances of contracting human erysipeloid by those occupationally exposed can be lessened by frequent handwashing with disinfectant soaps or detergents and prompt, appropriate treatment of any wounds. No vaccine is available.

Reporting and Surveillance. *Erysipelothrix* infection, whether in animals or humans, is not reportable in the United States.

Pasteurellosis

Agent. Of the various species of *Pasteurella, P. multocida* is most commonly encountered. *P. multocida* is a small, pleomorphic, nonmotile gram-negative coccobacillus.

Reservoirs. Domestic animals, especially cats and dogs. *Pasteurella* spp., which can infect bite wounds, are found in the oropharynx of 92% and 99% of healthy dogs and cats, respectively.

Occurrence. Incidence is worldwide. Carriage of *P. multocida* is common in domestic and wild animals and birds and affects a wide variety of species. In humans, pasteurellosis occurs most frequently as a cellulitis after a cat or dog bite. Respiratory infections acquired from exposure to farm and other domestic animals also occur.

Transmission. Pasteurellae are inhabitants of the upper respiratory tract of a variety of animals. Infection can be transmitted by both bites, and aerosol routes. Among poultry, aerosol transmission is the predominant means of spread of the disease. Many people with respiratory infections caused by *Pasteurella* spp. have been exposed to cattle, fowl, or their products. Cats and dogs also may be a source of airborne infection, particularly for immunocompromised people.

Disease in Animals

Signs. Pigs, rats, rabbits, suckling mice, goats, and calves develop atrophic rhinitis after infection with certain toxin-producing strains of *P. multocida.* In sheep and swine, the infection can produce pneumonia or septicemia; in rabbits it causes coryza ("snuffles"). In Southeast Asia and Africa, certain serovars of the organism cause hemorrhagic septicemia among cattle and water buffalo. Avian pasteurellosis ("fowl cholera") is an acute septicemic disease that affects all species of domestic poultry and causes high mortality. Although dogs and cats harbor the organism in their mouths and nasopharynges with no ill effects, abscesses caused by *P. multocida* often develop after bite wounds.

Diagnosis. *Pasteurella* spp. can be cultured from the blood or internal organs of animals or birds with septicemia. The organism also can be isolated from tracheal or bronchial washings or other respiratory specimens from animals with pneumonia and from purulent drainage from wound abscesses. The gums and teeth of many healthy cats and dogs yield *P. multocida.*

Specimens for culture should be collected on sterile swabs and placed in transport media; tissues obtained at necropsy should be placed in sterile containers and kept refrigerated until processing by a microbiological laboratory.

Disease in Humans

Signs and Symptoms. *P. multocida* is the major cause of soft tissue infections of the hand after animal bites or scratches. The lower leg and face, especially in children, also may be involved. Risk factors for developing bite-associated pasteurellosis include age over 50 years, the hand being the site bitten, and puncture wounds, such as those inflicted by cats, that cannot be thoroughly cleansed. Acute inflammation, pain, swelling, serosanguineous or purulent drainage from the site, and lymphangitis develop, usually within 12 to 24 hours of the bite. In rare cases, the infection may spread into tendons, bones, or joints. In immunocompromised individuals, septicemia, endocarditis, meningoencephalitis, or other life-threatening disseminated infection may occur. *P. multocida* also can cause various respiratory infections, such as pneumonia, bronchitis, sinusitis, or tonsillitis.

Diagnosis. The acute onset of cellulitis after a cat or dog bite, as described above, is highly suggestive of pasteurellosis. Culture of the organism from the wound is definitive.

Treatment. Initial treatment should focus on immediate and thorough cleansing (preferably with a povidone-iodine solution) and rinsing of the wound, followed by professional medical evaluation. Debridement and high-pressure irrigation of the wound should be performed by a physician. As with any domestic animal bite, the rabies immunization status of the animal involved should be determined, and the patient's tetanus immunizations should be updated.

Hospitalization may be necessary if extensive cellulitis develops and there is proximal swelling of the involved limb. Most patients recover completely after treatment with topical, oral, and/or parenteral antibiotics.

Prevention. Hygienic management practices can help control pasteurellosis in animals. Bacterins and vaccines are available for some species.

Bite prevention is the single most important measure for humans. If a bite has already occurred, the major factors in development of bite-associated pasteurellosis are inadequate initial wound care and delay in seeking medical treatment. Debridement and irrigation of the wound are particularly important in preventing cellulitis. No vaccine is available for humans.

Reporting and Surveillance. Pasteurellosis is not a reportable disease in the United States.

Q Fever (Coxiellosis)

Agent. *Coxiella burnetii* is a small, obligately intracellular gram-negative bacterium. Although it has been classified as a member of the Rickettsiales, recent studies have shown that *C. burnetii* is not closely related to other members of that group and therefore should not be considered a rickettsial organism.

Reservoirs. Cattle, sheep, and goats are primary reservoirs; many other mammals, including companion animals and rodents, also may carry *C. burnetii,* as can birds, ticks, mites, and some insects.

Occurrence. Incidence is worldwide except New Zealand. All mammals and humans are susceptible to infection with *C. burnetii;* seroprevalence varies widely with geographic area. Humans at risk include ranchers, dairy farmers, abattoir and packing plant employees, veterinarians and animal care workers, and medical laboratory researchers who work with the organism.

TECHNICIAN NOTE

The primary means of transmission of Q fever is inhalation of either aerosols from infected birth fluids and ruminant placentas or dust contaminated by birth fluids or urine.

Transmission. The primary means of transmission of Q fever is inhalation of either aerosols from infected birth fluids and ruminant placentas, which can contain up to 10^9 organisms per gram of tissue or dust contaminated by birth fluids or urine. The agent also may be present in high concentrations in wool or hides or in soil in areas in which livestock are kept. *C. burnetii* is resistant to high temperatures, sunlight, and many disinfectants. Cattle and other milk-producing animals that develop chronic infection in their mammary glands continually shed the organism in milk; thus, consumption of unpasteurized milk from infected animals can lead to human infection.

Although farm animals are the most common sources of Q fever, household pets such as cats, dogs, and rabbits may also transmit the disease. Exposure to newborn or stillborn pet animals has been linked to Q fever among urban residents. *C. burnetii* is easily transmitted in a laboratory setting, with minimal exposures often resulting in disease.

Disease in Animals

Signs. Most species have only asymptomatic infection, although coxiellosis in cattle, sheep, and goats sometimes causes abortion.

Diagnosis. Various serological tests are used to diagnose coxiellosis in animals.

Disease in Humans

Signs and Symptoms. Q fever usually manifests as an acute febrile disease, often with sudden onset of fever, chills, profuse sweating, intense retro-orbital pain, and malaise 2 to 6 weeks after exposure. A maculopapular rash is common. Some patients develop atypical pneumonia and a mild cough; others may experience severe respiratory distress. Infections that occur during pregnancy may cause spontaneous abortion. Complications of acute infection may include meningoencephalitis and cardiac involvement. Most cases are mild and self-limiting; the case-fatality rate for untreated Q fever patients is less than 1% to 2.5%.

A few patients develop chronic infection, which gradually becomes apparent years after the initial illness and usually manifests as endocarditis. This form of Q fever occurs primarily in patients with a history of heart valve disease or other immunosuppressive conditions. Patients with this form of Q fever may develop hepatomegaly, splenomegaly, renal insufficiency, or stroke; progressive heart failure is common. Because of its insidious onset long after the primary episode of disease, medical care may not be sought until late in the course of the illness. Q fever endocarditis has a case fatality rate of more than 60%.

Diagnosis. Diagnosis of Q fever is easy if a physician suspects the disease; serological testing is effective in diagnosing both acute and chronic infection. Because the clinical picture of acute Q fever can mimic so many other infectious diseases, however, the illness may not be considered among differential diagnoses in areas in which Q fever does not often occur. A history of exposure to a reservoir is an important epidemiological clue. Likewise, chronic Q fever has few obvious signs but should be suspected in a patient with valvular heart disease and an unexplained infectious or inflammatory process.

Treatment. Antibiotics such as tetracycline or doxycycline are usually prescribed for both acute and chronic Q fever. The course of treatment for patients with acute disease is usually 15 to 21 days, whereas 3 or more years of antibiotic therapy may be required for cases of Q fever endocarditis.

Prevention. Avoid contact with possibly infected animals. A vaccine is available for people who work with reservoir animals.

Reporting and Surveillance. Q fever must be reported to local health authorities in the parts of the United States in which the disease is endemic. In many other countries, it is not a reportable disease.

Rat-Bite Fevers: Streptobacillosis and Spirillosis

Agents. *Streptobacillus moniliformis* is a pleomorphic, fastidious gram-negative rod that causes streptobacillosis or streptobacillary fever. Spirillosis is caused by a spiral bacterium designated *Spirillum minus,* although it probably does not belong to that genus. Because *S. minus* cannot be cultured on artificial media, its true taxonomic position has not yet been determined.

Reservoirs. Primarily rats are carriers; mice, hamsters, gerbils, guinea pigs, squirrels, and other rodents may be occasional carriers. *S. moniliformis* is part of the normal oral and upper respiratory tract flora of both wild and domestic rats and is excreted in urine. *S. minus* is found on the teeth and in the blood and conjunctival secretions of rats and other rodents. This organism has been identified in up to 48% of rats, both wild and laboratory strains, and laboratory mice.

Occurrence. Both rat-bite fevers occur sporadically worldwide, mostly in poor urban areas and among laboratory or animal care personnel who handle rodents. Spirillosis is the more common rat-bite fever in Asia, particularly Japan, where it is known as *sodoku.*

Transmission. Rat bites are the most common means of transmission of both diseases. A form of streptobacillosis known as Haverhill fever is caused by ingestion of rodent-contaminated food or water.

Disease in Animals

Signs. *S. moniliformis* generally does not cause disease in rats. However, mice, especially certain inbred laboratory strains, may be genetically more susceptible to infection. Epidemics of streptobacillosis have occurred among research colonies, causing polyarthritis and gangrene. Mortality and morbidity are high in these episodes. Streptobacillosis also may occur in turkeys that are bitten by rats. Clinical signs include purulent polyarthritis, footpad lesions, and sternal bursitis.

S. minus is not known to cause clinical disease in animals.

Diagnosis. *S. moniliformis* theoretically can be isolated from joint fluid or lesions of affected turkeys. Definitive diagnosis is difficult, however, because the organism has unusual growth requirements that routine microbiological procedures may not provide.

Disease in Humans

Signs and Symptoms. Streptobacillosis, or streptobacillary fever, usually develops within 10 days of a rat bite that has healed normally. The disease is characterized by sudden onset of headache, vomiting, malaise, fever, and chills, followed by a transient maculopapular or petechial rash that appears on the extremities. Severe pain and swelling develop in one or more joints. In untreated cases, complications can include endocarditis, myocarditis, meningitis, abscesses in various soft tissues or the brain, hepatitis, nephritis, and pneumonia; the case-fatality rate for untreated cases is about 13%. The clinical picture of

Haverhill fever is similar, although there may be more gastrointestinal and upper respiratory signs.

Spirillosis often has a longer incubation period, the onset of symptoms occurring 1 to 3 weeks or more after exposure. The wound site heals during the incubation period but later becomes swollen, painful, and discolored and develops an indurated, encrusted ulcer. A cycle of relapsing fever begins, with episodes of elevated temperature that last 1 or 2 days and recur at 3- to 9-day intervals. An exanthemous or purplish rash appears, usually on the trunk, and may spread to other areas, especially joints. Muscle aches often occur. Some patients develop various neurological symptoms, such as headache, nervousness, neuralgia, and weakness. Spirillosis can be complicated by meningoencephalitis, pneumonia, endocarditis, myocarditis, conjunctivitis, septic arthritis, and other lesions. About 10% of untreated cases are fatal, and fatalities have occurred despite antibiotic therapy.

> **TECHNICIAN NOTE**
>
> Avoiding rat bites is the most effective means of prevention of either disease.

Diagnosis. Streptobacillosis can be diagnosed on the basis of isolation of the etiological agent from blood; as noted above, specialized media and processing are required.

Spirillosis is confirmed by microscopy. Either dark-field examinations or Wright or Giemsa stains may be used to detect spiral organisms in wound exudates, lymph node aspirates, or, rarely, blood. Specimens also can be inoculated into guinea pigs or mice; spirilla can be microscopically detected in the peritoneal fluid and blood of these animals.

Both rat-bite fevers probably are underdiagnosed because the techniques required for identification of the etiological agents are not among those usually performed in a standard clinical laboratory. Unless a physician suspects streptobacillosis or spirillosis and indicates this suspicion to the laboratory, ordinary microbiological techniques and media may not be sufficient to identify either organism from clinical specimens.

Treatment. Both forms of rat-bite fever respond to antibiotic therapy.

Prevention. Avoiding rat bites is the most effective means of prevention of either disease. As with any animal bite, any wounds should be immediately and thoroughly cleansed, and medical advice should be sought.

Reporting and Surveillance. When streptobacillosis occurs epidemically in the United States, as in a foodborne or waterborne outbreak of Haverhill fever, it must be reported to health authorities. Single bite-associated cases are not reportable.

Salmonellosis

Agent. There are various serotypes of *Salmonella enteritidis,* a gram-negative rod of the family Enterobacteriaceae. These serotypes often are named for the place at which they were first isolated and are commonly referred to by genus and serotype name, such as *Salmonella arizonae,* instead of the more proper *S. enteritidis* subspecies *arizonae.* (Typhoid fever,

caused by *Salmonella typhi,* has no zoonotic occupational component and is not included in this discussion.)

Reservoirs. Salmonellae can infect a wide variety of warm- and cold-blooded animals, both domestic and wild. Reptiles, such as turtles, iguanas, and snakes, are particularly likely to be asymptomatic carriers of *Salmonella* spp.

Occurrence. Incidence is worldwide and common in both animals and humans. Human salmonellosis is mostly a foodborne or waterborne disease and a major cause of gastrointestinal illness and diarrhea. Incidence is highest among infants and young children; immunocompromised persons also are at increased risk. Occupational exposure to reptiles and other infected animals is a risk factor for veterinarians, animal care workers, zoo keepers, and pet shop employees.

Transmission. Consumption of contaminated food, particularly foods of animal origin such as poultry meat, eggs, and milk, is most often implicated in the transmission of salmonellosis. As an occupational disease, salmonellosis is transmitted via the fecal-oral route. Direct contact with infected animals, regardless of whether they show clinical signs of illness, can result in human infection if the bacteria are transferred from contaminated hands to mouth. In addition, indirect contact may be a source of infection; cages and food dishes used by infected animals may be contaminated with the bacteria, which can remain viable for months in dried feces.

> **TECHNICIAN NOTE**
>
> Consumption of contaminated food, particularly foods of animal origin such as poultry meat, eggs, and milk, is most often implicated in the transmission of salmonellosis.

Disease in Animals
Signs. Infections may be clinical, subclinical, or inapparent. In clinically affected animals, regardless of species, most exhibit weakness, recumbency, fever, and diarrhea. Young animals are more likely to show clinical signs than are adults. Chronic carrier states are common in reptiles, birds, and other animals; in some reptiles, fecal carriage rates exceed 90%.

Diagnosis. For clinically affected animals, isolation of the organism from blood or, at necropsy, from internal organs such as liver or spleen provides a definitive diagnosis. Carrier states can be detected by culturing *Salmonella* spp. from rectal or cloacal swabs or fecal samples.

Disease in Humans
Signs and Symptoms. Human salmonellosis usually manifests as an acute enterocolitis with sudden onset 12 to 36 hours after ingestion of the bacteria. Headache, abdominal pain, diarrhea, and nausea are common symptoms, and fever usually is present. Most cases are self-limiting and resolve in a few days. Salmonellosis is rarely fatal except in very young children, the elderly, and debilitated or otherwise immunocompromised people. In these groups, there is increased risk of severe complications such as meningitis or septicemia. Asymptomatic infections can occur.

Diagnosis. Salmonellosis can be diagnosed in patients with enterocolitis by isolating the agent from fecal specimens; in most cases, fecal excretion persists for several days or weeks after symptoms have resolved. For patients with septicemia, *Salmonella* spp. can be cultured from blood as well as feces.

Isolates can be sent to reference laboratories for serotyping; knowledge of the causative serotype can provide an indication of the source of infection. For example, certain exotic serotypes are rarely isolated from animals other than reptiles. When the same unusual serotype is isolated from both the patient and a suspect reptile, it can be assumed that the reptile was the source of the person's illness.

TECHNICIAN NOTE

Working with reptiles is a specific risk factor for acquiring animal-borne salmonellosis.

Treatment. Antimicrobial treatment is indicated only for those patients with severe or disseminated infections; chloramphenicol or fluroquinolones are among the drugs of choice. Uncomplicated cases of gastrointestinal salmonellosis generally should not be treated with antibiotics because there seldom is any effect on the course of the disease and because their use can prolong fecal shedding of the organism.

Prevention. Working with reptiles is a specific risk factor for acquiring animal-borne salmonellosis because touching these animals or their surroundings can result in hands becoming contaminated with *Salmonella* spp. Wild fowl also frequently carry *Salmonella* spp., and diarrheic companion animals and livestock can also be sources of infection. Careful attention to personal hygiene, especially the use of gloves and frequent handwashing, can help reduce the risk of occupationally acquired salmonellosis.

Veterinarians and technicians should advise their clients who own reptiles, baby chicks, or ducklings that these animals increase the owners' risk of acquiring *Salmonella* infection and should stress the need for thorough handwashing after handling these animals or their cages. In addition, these pets should be kept out of food preparation areas. Kitchen sinks should never be used to bathe reptiles or to wash their dishes, cages, or aquariums. Likewise, sinks or tubs in which infants and children are bathed should never be used for such purposes. The Centers for Disease Control and Prevention recommend that people at increased risk for infection or serious complications of salmonellosis, including pregnant women, children under 5 years of age, and immunocompromised individuals, avoid all contact with reptiles. Reptiles may be inappropriate pets for households with young children because some cases have been reported in which there was no known contact, direct or indirect, between the child and the reptile.

Reporting and Surveillance. In the United States, confirmed cases of human salmonellosis must be reported to local health authorities.

MYCOTIC ZOONOSES
Systemic Infections
Cryptococcosis

Agent. *Cryptococcus neoformans* is an encapsulated yeast.

Reservoirs. Although a common saprophytic organism that can be isolated from many different environmental sources such as soil and plant materials, *C. neoformans* has a particular affinity for bird excrement, especially pigeon droppings. Sites contaminated with pigeon or chicken excreta often contain much higher concentrations of *C. neoformans* than do surrounding areas; it is thought that creatinine in the droppings enhances growth of the yeast. Viable cryptococci have been recovered from an aviary that had been unused for 10 years.

Occurrence. Incidence is worldwide and in all age groups as sporadic cases, although adult males account for a majority of patients. Although many people have serological evidence of exposure, clinical cases are relatively rare and usually occur in immunocompromised individuals. In the United States, 5% to 15% of patients with AIDS develop cryptococcosis; in this group, the infection is often life threatening.

Transmission. Inhalation of the organism from environmental sources. Exposure to highly contaminated areas, such as aviaries or pigeon coops, can increase risk of disease.

TECHNICIAN NOTE

Exposure to highly contaminated areas such as aviaries or pigeon coops can increase risk of cryptococcosis

Disease in Animals
Signs. There are no apparent signs in birds, although the organism can be recovered from the feces of many avian species. Most clinically affected mammals develop a disseminated infection that includes central nervous system signs; mortality is high. In cattle, the disease often manifests as mastitis and causes abnormalities of the udder and changes in milk.

Diagnosis. *Cryptococcus* can be detected through direct microscopic examination of various clinical specimens using an India ink preparation to reveal characteristic budding yeast cells. Culture and serological testing can be used to confirm diagnoses.

Disease in Humans
Signs and Symptoms. Most immunocompetent individuals develop only subclinical infection. Among patients with AIDS, meningitis is the most common presentation of cryptococcosis. It results from hematogenous dissemination of a primary pulmonary infection that can precede nervous system involvement by months or years. Pulmonary cryptococcosis is characterized by fever, chest pain, and coughing, with expectoration of blood-tinged sputum. When the infection spreads to the brain, headache, neck stiffness, and distorted vision occur. Confusion and other personality changes may follow. Even when treated ag-

gressively, cryptococcal meningitis has a high mortality rate, and survivors often undergo relapses.

Diagnosis. As described above, direct microscopic examination of India ink–stained cerebrospinal fluid, urine, or pus can reveal cells characteristic of *C. neoformans*. Serological tests, culture, or histopathological examination provide confirmation.

Treatment. Combinations of antifungal agents are used to treat human cryptococcosis.

Prevention. For normally healthy people, no special precautions are necessary. People with immunosuppressive conditions, such as HIV infection, diabetes, or Hodgkin's disease, or who are undergoing corticosteroid therapy should avoid exposure to accumulations of pigeon or other bird droppings. Contaminated sites may be disinfected with a 5% sodium hypochlorite solution.

Reporting and Surveillance. In the United States, cases should be reported to local health authorities. Because meningeal cryptococcosis is so strongly associated with AIDS, official reports are required in some areas.

Superficial Mycoses

Dermatophytoses

Agents. Dermatophytoses, or tinea, are opportunistic fungal infections of the hair, skin, or nails. *Microsporum canis, Trichophyton mentagrophytes,* and *T. verrucosum* are the zoophilic dermatophytes most important in human infection. *M. canis* causes tinea (ringworm) in both humans and animals; in humans, this species usually affects the scalp or body (tinea capitis or tinea corporis). *T. mentagrophytes* infection in humans may appear as tinea barbae (ringworm of the beard) or tinea corporis; *T. verrucosum* usually affects the face or upper body.

Reservoirs. *M. canis* is carried by dogs and cats. Wild mice and rats are primary reservoirs of *T. mentagrophytes,* but dogs, cats, horses, sheep, rabbits, guinea pigs, and other domestic and laboratory animals frequently are infected. *T. verrucosum* is carried by cattle, sheep, and other ruminants.

Occurrence. Incidence is worldwide in both humans and a variety of domestic and wild animals. People at greatest risk are those who work with animals or who live or work in areas that may be contaminated with hairs from infected animals.

Transmission. Direct or indirect contact with infected animals or with hair from infected animals or humans.

Disease in Animals
Signs. For *M. canis,* about 90% of infected cats have no visible lesions; when present, lesions are usually on the face and paws and appear as 1- to 2-cm hairless, scaly patches. Infected dogs usually have lesions similar to those in cats; they can appear on any part of the body. For *T. mentagrophytes,* most infected animals develop 1- to 2-cm hairless, white, scaly lesions on the head or trunk. For *T. verrucosum,* young cattle are most frequently infected. Lesions can be small or extensive and begin as grayish-white, scaly patches with hair loss. The skin later thickens and becomes scabby.

Diagnosis. Examined microscopically in a wet mount of potassium hydroxide and ink, infected hairs from the inner edge of lesions of both *M. canis* and *Trichophyton* spp. may show an exterior cuff of arthrospores or mycelial elements within the hair shaft. Hairs infected with *M. canis* (but not *Trichophyton* spp.) also may fluoresce bright yellow-green when viewed under a Wood's lamp (365 nm filtered ultraviolet light), although this does not occur in all cases. Isolation of the organism from lesions is definitive. Scrapings or hairs from suspect lesions should be placed in a sterile container and submitted to a laboratory for culture.

Disease in Humans
Signs and Symptoms. For *M. canis,* tinea of the scalp produces scaly patches and temporary baldness because infected hairs are brittle and break easily. Infection of hairless parts of the body often causes formation of a *kerion,* a suppurative, boggy, raised lesion. For *T. mentagrophytes,* lesions are similar to those described for *M. canis* and usually occur on the face or upper body. Some individuals experience a highly inflammatory reaction to this infection. For *T. verrucosum,* lesions usually develop on the face, hands, arms, and upper body. The inflammatory response is severe and kerions often form; scarring is a frequent result.

Diagnosis. Same as in animal diagnoses.

 TECHNICIAN NOTE

Both oral and topical antifungal agents, often in combination, are used to treat tinea infections in both humans and domestic animals.

Treatment. Both oral and topical antifungal agents, often in combination, are used to treat tinea infections in both humans and domestic animals. If kerions are present, a keriolytic cream may be prescribed. Antibiotics may be required if a secondary bacterial infection invades the lesions. Additional measures for tinea corporis include frequent and thorough bathing with soap and water and removal of scabs and crusts; for tinea capitis or barbae, daily washing of hair and scalp with a selenium sulfide shampoo is helpful.

Prevention. Vaccines to immunize animal populations against zoophilic dermatophytoses have been developed. If the infections can be controlled in animals, prevention of human infection will become much more feasible. Whenever possible, avoid direct contact with animals that show lesions suggestive of dermatophytoses.

Reporting and Surveillance. In the United States, reporting is required for epidemic outbreaks of any dermatophytosis but not for individual cases.

Parasitic Diseases

Cryptosporidiosis

Agent. *Cryptosporidium parvum* is a coccidian protozoan parasite.

Reservoirs. Humans, cattle, and other domestic animals.

Occurrence. Incidence is worldwide. In the United States and Europe, prevalence ranges from less than 1% to 4.5%, whereas in developing nations, prevalence may be as high as 20% of the human population. People who come into contact with animals are at increased risk of contracting this infection.

Transmission. Transmission is fecal-oral, which includes human-to-human, animal-to-human, waterborne, and foodborne transmission. On reaching the intestine, the parasite infects epithelial cells and multiplies asexually via schizogony. After a sexual reproductive cycle, the organism produces infective oocysts that are passed in feces. These oocysts are resistant to many chemical disinfectants, including chlorination used in water treatment systems, and can survive in adverse environmental conditions.

Disease in Animals

Signs. Cryptosporidiosis in animals often is subclinical, particularly in adults; younger animals, especially newborns, are more likely to develop clinical signs. Those affected usually develop diarrhea that can range from mild to severe. Calves are an important source of infection to humans and other animals because they develop profuse diarrhea, during which they shed massive quantities of oocysts into the environment. The mortality rate in livestock is low. Other animals that may develop clinical cryptosporidiosis are cats with underlying feline leukemia or feline immunodeficiency virus (FIV) infection or animals undergoing prolonged therapy with corticosteroid drugs.

Diagnosis. Oocysts can be detected in feces by direct microscopy of smears, sugar or zinc sulfate flotation, or special centrifugation techniques.

Disease in Humans

Signs and Symptoms. Clinical cryptosporidiosis is characterized by profuse, watery diarrhea and cramping abdominal pain. Although symptoms may abate and recur for a time, in most otherwise healthy persons, the disease is self-limiting and resolves completely within 1 month. In immunocompromised individuals, however, the disease can be much more serious. Patients with AIDS and others who cannot clear the infection experience a severe and prolonged illness that can be fatal.

Diagnosis. Cryptosporidiosis can be difficult to diagnose unless suspected and sought. Direct identification of oocysts in fecal smears as detailed above can be successful. Likewise, various life-cycle stages can be detected by histopathological examination of intestinal biopsy specimens, but *C. parvum* is very small and easily overlooked and can be mistaken for yeast cells if the proper stains are not used. An ELISA and an immunofluorescence test have become available and are more accurate than direct microscopy.

Treatment. There is no specific effective treatment. Supportive care, mainly in the form of rehydration, is effective for normally healthy people. Any immunosuppressive drugs the patient may be taking should be reduced or stopped, if possible.

Prevention. People who are in contact with calves or other animals that have diarrhea should be especially careful about handwashing. Those with AIDS or other immunosuppressive conditions should avoid contact with diarrheic animals.

In areas in which water treatment facilities include filtration (which is standard for most cities in the United States), feces from infected animals can be discharged directly into sewers without prior disinfection. Areas contaminated with feces can be disinfected with a 10% formalin solution or 5% ammonia solution. Articles that withstand heat may be heated to 45°C for 5 to 20 minutes or to 60°C for 2 minutes.

Reporting and Surveillance. In the United States, cases of human cryptosporidiosis must be reported to local health authorities. Clusters of disease should be investigated epidemiologically to determine the source of infection.

Toxoplasmosis

TECHNICIAN NOTE

The cat is the only known host of *Toxoplasma gondii.*

Agent. *Toxoplasma gondii* is an obligate intracellular sporozoan parasite.

Reservoirs. Cats are the only known definitive host (the animal in which the parasite completes its life cycle). Sheep, goats, swine, cattle, and chickens are intermediate hosts and can carry the infective stage encysted in muscle tissue.

Occurrence. Incidence is worldwide. Up to 70% of the human adult population is seropositive, indicating exposure and probable tissue infection. Cats frequently are infected; in some countries, up to 60% of cats have serological evidence of exposure to the organism. The prevalence in livestock is related to the number of cats in pasture lands. Up to 43% of pigs and 35% of sheep have tissue cysts.

Transmission. After primary infection, cats shed oocysts in feces for only 1 to 2 weeks; subsequent intermittent shedding may occur, but this appears to be rare. *Toxoplasma* oocysts become infective 1 to 5 days after being passed; these are environmentally resistant and can survive for at least 1 year in soil in warm, humid environments. Other animals become infected when they consume soil or other material contaminated with sporulated oocysts.

In humans, toxoplasmosis may be primary or congenital. Primary toxoplasmosis is usually acquired through the ingestion of raw or undercooked meat, especially pork or mutton, in which the parasite has encysted. The mode that is of occupational importance, however, is the fecal-oral route (accidental ingestion of infective oocysts).

Congenital toxoplasmosis is acquired through transplacental infection. This occurs when a woman develops a primary infection during pregnancy; rapidly dividing tachyzoites circulate in the blood stream and can infect the fetus. The risk of serious fetal disease is highest during the first and second trimesters.

Disease in Animals

Sign. In most animals, toxoplasmosis produces only subclinical infection, with little morbidity or mortality. Toxoplasmosis in sheep, however, is an exception. In this species, the infection causes abortion or congenital disease that results in neonatal mortality; adults seldom are affected clinically. In some parts of the sheep-rearing world, economic losses from toxoplasmosis are significant. Swine are affected similarly, but the disease is not of economic importance in most areas. Outbreaks in cattle have been reported in which fever, dyspnea, and neurological signs occur. Infection in horses is usually subclinical.

Most infected cats are asymptomatic, but kittens may develop diarrhea, hepatitis, pneumonia, encephalitis, and other signs. Dogs often are seropositive, but overt disease occurs mainly in puppies weakened by other conditions.

Diagnosis. Antemortem diagnosis is difficult. Oocysts can be detected in feline feces using various flotation techniques, although definitive identification requires considerable further laboratory testing (see Chapter 6). Serological tests are available for many species but cannot be used to differentiate among active, recent, or past infections.

Disease in Humans

Signs and Symptoms. Immunocompetent adults usually have only asymptomatic infection, although toxoplasmosis occasionally causes a self-limiting, mononucleosis-like illness. After the immune response causes the initial parasitemia to wane, *T. gondii* encysts in muscle tissue; these cysts can reactivate and cause disease if the person becomes immunocompromised at some later time.

Cerebral toxoplasmosis is a common opportunistic infection among patients with AIDS, with most cases resulting from activation of latent tissue infection as the immune system deteriorates. These patients often develop subacute meningoencephalitis, diffuse encephalopathy, or a space-occupying lesion in the brain. Lymphatics, lungs, heart, joints, or eyes also may be involved. Up to 40% of patients with AIDS develop cerebral toxoplasmosis, and at least 10% die. Other immunocompromised adults (chemotherapy patients, organ transplant recipients, splenectomized people) also are at increased risk of this form of toxoplasmosis.

Congenital toxoplasmosis results from primary maternal infection during gestation. When primary toxoplasmosis occurs during the first trimester of pregnancy, 17% of fetuses become infected, and 80% of those infections are severe. For second-trimester maternal infections, 25% of fetuses become infected, and 30% of that number have severe disease; abortion or premature birth often results. Infections acquired during the third trimester produce a higher fetal infection rate but fewer cases of severe disease. Neonatal central nervous system and ocular infections are the most frequent manifestations of congenital toxoplasmosis. Some babies develop encephalitis, hydrocephalus, or chorioretinitis; blindness, mental retardation, and seizures are possible sequelae.

Diagnosis. Diagnosis is based on clinical signs and results of serological testing that support the presumption of toxoplasmosis. The organism also can be isolated from biopsy specimens or body fluids after intraperitoneal inoculation in mice; tachyzoites can be detected in mouse peritoneal fluid after 1 week, and cysts may be found in the brain after 6 weeks.

Treatment. No specific treatment is indicated for otherwise healthy people, except for pregnant women with primary infections. In these patients, spiramycin is used to prevent fetal infection; if tests indicate fetal infection has already occurred, a combination of pyrimethamine and sulfadiazine can be used. Likewise, patients with severe symptomatic disease and infants born to mothers who had a primary infection during pregnancy are treated with a combination of antitoxoplasmal drugs and folic acid.

Prevention. Pet cats are seldom the source of human infection because of their fastidious nature. They bury their feces and clean themselves immediately, so feces do not remain on their fur long enough for oocysts to sporulate. In addition, oocyst shedding generally lasts only 1 or 2 weeks after the initial infection, and repeated exposure to the organism does not cause additional shedding. Oocysts can sporulate in litterboxes, so fecal material should be removed daily and disposed of in a toilet or by incineration. Wash hands thoroughly after handling litterboxes or cat feces.

Pregnant women and immunocompromised patients who work with animals should have serological testing performed to determine whether they have a titer against toxoplasmosis. Those who are seronegative are at risk of developing primary toxoplasmosis and should avoid handling cat feces and changing litterboxes. Because most cases of toxoplasmosis are caused by consuming undercooked meat, those who are at risk also should avoid eating undercooked meat and handling raw meat, which are much more likely sources of infection than cat exposure.

> **TECHNICIAN NOTE**
>
> Wash hands thoroughly after handling litterboxes or cat feces.

Cats should not be fed meat that may contain viable oocysts. Feed only commercial cat foods or thoroughly cook or freeze any meat that is to be fed to cats. (Freezing at $-15°C$ for more than 3 days or $-20°C$ for more than 2 days kills oocysts.) Because rodents and birds can be sources of infection, cats should be kept indoors when possible to prevent hunting.

Reporting and Surveillance. Reporting is not required in most areas, but it is in some states and countries in which epidemiological studies are being conducted.

Viral Diseases

Contagious Ecthyma (Orf)

Agent. Contagious ecthyma is caused by a DNA virus of the genus *Parapoxvirus,* family Poxviridae.

Reservoirs. Domestic and wild ungulates, including sheep, goats, domestic camels, deer, reindeer, and musk oxen. The virus is hardy and can persist for long periods in the environment and on the skin and hair of animals.

Occurrence. Incidence is uncommon but worldwide wherever sheep and goats are raised; many human cases occur in New Zealand. Contagious ecthyma (orf) is an occupational disease of sheep handlers, veterinarians, and abattoir workers.

Transmission. Humans contract orf through direct contact with lesions or mucous membranes of infected animals. In addition, contaminated knives, shears, or other objects can transfer the virus from animal to human. Preparation and administration of the crude live vaccine used in some endemic areas can also be a source of human infection.

Disease in Animals

Signs. Most infections occur in young animals. Papules that progress into vesicles and pustules appear on the skin, eyelids, ears, lips, and nostrils. As lesions become confluent, they cause severe pain and often interfere with feeding. Females that nurse infected young may develop infection of teats and udders. Morbidity is often high but mortality is low, usually resulting from secondary bacterial infection or infestation by fly larvae.

Diagnosis. Clinical signs alone often are sufficient to establish diagnosis; other diseases that produce similar lesions tend to have a different course.

Disease in Humans

Signs and Symptoms. The most frequent presentation is the development of a single maculopapular or pustular lesion at the site of entry of the virus, usually on the hands, arms, or face. The papule is painful and progresses to become a firm, weeping nodule; secondary bacterial infection may cause pus formation. Most cases resolve completely in 2 to 4 weeks, but occasionally the infection is more serious. Reported complications include a widespread cutaneous eruption, ocular involvement with severe damage, and disseminated systemic disease.

Diagnosis. Demonstration of virus particles via electron microscopy of affected tissue or isolation of the virus in cell culture are definitive means of diagnosis. Serological tests are available.

Treatment. There is no specific treatment.

Prevention. Good personal hygiene, including thorough washing of skin that comes in contact with an infected animal, can help prevent human infection. Any broken skin should be kept covered and gloves should be worn when examining or treating infected sheep.

Animal housing areas should be kept clean to reduce sources of infection for susceptible lambs. In some endemic areas, a crude live vaccine is made by pulverizing scabs from infected animals and suspending the material in a glycerinated solution. Lambs are vaccinated by applying the suspension to scarified skin in the axilla. However, the efficacy of this process is variable, and as mentioned above, can cause human infection. In addition, this practice can lead to perpetuation of the virus in the farm environment.

Reporting and Surveillance. None required.

Herpesvirus simiae Infection (B-Virus)

Agent. *Herpesvirus simiae* is caused by a DNA virus of the genus *Herpesvirus,* family Herpesviridae; it is closely related to the human herpes simplex virus that causes fever blisters and mouth ulcers. It is also referred to as cercopithecine herpesvirus 1.

Reservoirs. Asian monkeys of the genus *Macaca,* especially the rhesus monkey, *M. mulatta,* are natural reservoirs; other primates in contact with infected *Macaca* spp. may acquire the virus.

Occurrence. Incidence is common in monkeys; 30% to 80% of rhesus monkeys are seropositive for this virus. In humans, B-virus infection is a rare occupational disease that has been recorded in veterinarians, animal care workers, laboratory personnel, and others in contact with Old World monkeys or monkey cell cultures.

Transmission. *H. simiae* infection is transmitted between monkeys by direct contact, bites or scratches, and saliva-contaminated food or water. Infected monkeys may or may not show any clinical signs. Humans acquire the disease when bitten by a monkey that carries the virus, when saliva from an infected monkey comes in contact with broken skin, or by conjunctival, nasal, or pharyngeal exposure to aerosols that contain the virus.

Disease in Animals

Signs. Primary B-virus infection in macaque monkeys causes sores in or around the mouth that appear similar to fever blisters in humans. The small ulcers that form heal within 1 to 2 weeks. The condition is not serious in monkeys and is rarely noticed unless lesions appear on the lips, conjunctivae, or skin. After the initial outbreak of lesions, the virus becomes latent, and the monkey is then an asymptomatic carrier. In non-macaque primates, the course of the disease is similar to that in humans and usually fatal.

Diagnosis. Serological tests used to determine B-virus infection include ELISA and radioimmunoassay. The virus can be grown in tissue culture, and identification is confirmed through the use of PCR, DNA restriction analysis, or other molecular methods.

Disease in Humans

Signs and Symptoms. B virus in humans causes a severe and usually fatal meningoencephalitis. When infection follows a monkey bite or other cutaneous inoculation of the agent, the wound becomes reddened and painful; itching and numbness can occur. Vesicles appear at the site and regional lymphadenopathy develops. After a few days to a few weeks, the disease becomes generalized, and there is sudden onset of fever, with headache, nausea, abdominal pain, and diarrhea. Various neurological signs follow, including vertigo, diaphragmatic spasms, neck stiffness, and difficulty in swallowing. In late stages of the illness, the lower extremities develop flaccid paralysis; this spreads to the upper extremities and thorax. Respiratory failure and death usually occur within 5 to 28 days of onset of clinical symptoms. More than 70% of the known cases have been fatal, and most survivors have permanent and extensive neurological damage, although recent improvements in diagnostic and therapeutic techniques offer hope for reducing fatalities and permanent sequelae.

Diagnosis. Serological tests may be useful when a patient survives long enough to produce antibodies, but most cases are diagnosed post mortem through viral isolation from brain tissue.

Treatment. Acyclovir has produced recovery in a few cases.

Prevention. Anyone who works with or comes into contact with Old World monkeys should take all precautions to prevent bites and aerosol exposure. Always wear gloves, masks, and protective clothing. Prompt treatment of any wound caused by a monkey (bite or scratch) or an object (cage or wires) that could be contaminated with monkey secretions is critical. Immediately and thoroughly scrub the wound with soap and water and disinfect it with an iodine solution. Acyclovir may be an effective prophylaxis if administered promptly. If the wound becomes painful or numb or if itching or vesicular lesions appear at or near the wound site, seek immediate expert medical advice. No vaccine is available.

TECHNICIAN NOTE

Anyone who works with or comes into contact with Old World monkeys should take all precautions to prevent bites and aerosol exposure.

Monkeys should be housed only in small groups, with a maximum of two per cage. Do not house rhesus monkeys with any other species. Quarantine all recently imported monkeys for at least 6 weeks; destroy any that have or develop lesions suggestive of *H. simiae*. Any animal responsible for a wound to a human should be observed for at least 2 weeks and tested to determine its B-virus status.

Researchers who work with tissues or body fluids from macaques should follow biosafety level 2 (BSL 2) practices. If the material is known to contain *H. simiae*, BSL 3 facilities and precautions should be used.

Reporting and Surveillance. Report any human cases to local health authorities.

Newcastle Disease

Agent. This disease is caused by an RNA virus of the genus *Paramyxovirus*, family Paramyxoviridae.

Reservoirs. Chickens.

Occurrence. Incidence is worldwide. Newcastle disease (ND) occurs in wild birds and semidomestic and domestic fowl in both epizootic and enzootic forms; it is one of the most economically important diseases affecting the poultry industry. Human disease is rare and usually occurs among poultry slaughterhouse workers, poultry vaccinators using vaccines containing live viral strains, and laboratory personnel who work with the virus.

Transmission. ND is spread from bird to bird mainly by aerosols, with the density of birds in commercial poultry farms facilitating transmission. The virus also is shed in feces. Humans become infected when the virus comes into contact with the eyes, as occurs with aerosolized vaccines.

Disease in Animals
Signs. Numerous species of birds may be affected by ND, but chickens and turkeys are especially susceptible. Signs may be respiratory, nervous, or both and usually appear throughout a flock within 2 weeks of exposure. The strain of virus determines the severity of the outbreak; lentogenic strains are the least virulent, velogenic are the most, and mesogenic strains are intermediate. In birds with respiratory involvement, there is gasping and coughing; neurological signs include drooping wings, twisted neck, depression, anorexia, and paralysis. Egg laying may cease. Some velogenic strains produce a viscerotropic syndrome, which is the most serious form of ND. Affected birds have sudden onset of watery, greenish diarrhea, tracheal discharge, and edema of the face and wattles; small hemorrhages appear in the mucosa of the proventriculus, and the intestinal mucosa becomes necrotic. There is high mortality associated with this form of ND.

Diagnosis. ND virus can be isolated from tracheal exudate, lung, or spleen tissue taken early in the outbreak. Material taken for viral isolation attempts should be placed into a sterile container and transported to the laboratory. Various serological tests also are useful.

Disease in Humans
Signs and Symptoms. In humans, ND usually causes a unilateral conjunctivitis, with excessive tear formation, pain, swelling of subconjunctival tissues, and inflammation of the lymph nodes in front of the ear. Generally, there is no systemic involvement, but some people exposed to aerosols of the virus develop an influenza-like illness that lasts for 3 to 4 days. Recovery is complete in about 1 week. Subclinical infections also occur.

Diagnosis. Isolation of ND virus is the only definitive means of diagnosis because many people do not develop a serological response. The virus can be isolated from various body fluids, including conjunctival or nasal secretions, saliva, or urine. Inoculation of embryonated chicken eggs or tissue culture techniques can be used to isolate the virus.

Treatment. Usually no treatment is necessary.

Prevention. Control of avian ND depends on maintaining good hygiene on poultry farms. Poultry houses should be separated, and all birds in a flock should be vaccinated using a live lentogenic strain vaccine. People who administer the vaccine to poultry should wear masks; laboratory personnel should avoid creating aerosols when working with the virus.

Reporting and Surveillance. The United States requires that imported live birds of any species be quarantined and prohibits imports from countries in which ND occurs.

Rabies

Agent. Rabies is caused by an RNA virus of the genus *Lyssavirus*, family Rhabdoviridae.

Reservoirs. Wild and domestic Canidae, including dogs, foxes, coyotes and wolves; wild carnivores and omnivores such as skunks, raccoons, and mongooses; and bats, including those that feed on blood (vampire bats), fruit-eaters, and insectivores.

Occurrence. Incidence is almost worldwide in animal populations; the only exceptions are parts of the Pacific and far East, including Australia, New Zealand, New Guinea, Japan, Taiwan, and most of Oceania; and some of Europe, including England, Scotland, Ireland, the Netherlands, Norway, Finland, Sweden, Spain, Portugal, and Greece. Rabies is present throughout most of the Americas except for a few Caribbean islands. In areas in which animal rabies occurs, the disease follows two cycles: urban and sylvatic. Urban rabies is transmitted by dogs and accounts for most human cases; sylvatic rabies circulates among wild carnivores and bats and causes some spillover infection of dogs, cats, and livestock. Rabies is responsible for an estimated 100,000 human deaths each year, most in developing countries.

Transmission. Rabies virus is abundant in saliva; thus, most cases are attributable to a bite inflicted by an infected animal. Aerosol transmission is possible; a few cases have occurred among field biologists working in caves in which large populations of bats roosted.

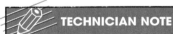

TECHNICIAN NOTE

Rabies virus is abundant in saliva; thus, most cases are attributable to a bite inflicted by an infected animal.

Disease in Animals

Signs. Rabies in dogs may be either furious or paralytic ("dumb"). In the early stages of furious rabies, the animal becomes agitated, restless, and excitable. An aggressive phase follows, with the dog attempting to bite objects, other animals, humans, and itself. Salivation is profuse because throat muscles spasm and prevent swallowing; vocal cords become affected, and the bark changes to a hoarse howl. Convulsions and paralysis occur shortly before death. In paralytic rabies, the muscles of the head and neck initially are affected, and the animal has difficulty in swallowing. Paralysis spreads to the extremities and then becomes generalized; death follows.

Rabid cats usually manifest the furious variety, whereas in cattle, rabies generally is paralytic. Furious rabies is the more common form in wild animals such as foxes, skunks, and raccoons.

Diagnosis. Behavioral changes and/or paralysis may suggest a presumptive diagnosis, particularly when rabies recently has been confirmed in the same species and geographic area. A positive direct immunofluorescence test on brain tissue is confirmatory. There are no tests available that produce satisfactory results on specimens from live animals.

Disease in Humans

Signs and Symptoms. The incubation period is variable; in most cases, onset of symptoms is within 3 to 8 weeks of exposure, but there are documented reports of disease occurring several years after a bite from a rabid animal. Rabies in humans usually begins with discomfort and irritation in the area of a previous animal bite. Vague sensory changes, apprehension, headache, low-grade fever, and malaise also may occur. As the disease progresses, salivation increases and eyes and ears become hypersensitive to light and sound. Paresis or paralysis develops, and spasmodic contractions of muscles used in swallowing cause the patient to develop an aversion to liquids ("hydrophobia") and to stop swallowing his or her own saliva. Convulsions and various mental disturbances are terminal events. Death from respiratory failure usually occurs 2 to 8 days after onset of symptoms.

Diagnosis. A presumptive diagnosis sometimes can be made by immunofluorescence staining of skin sections taken from the back of the neck. As in animals, postmortem testing of brain tissue is necessary for confirmation.

Treatment. Rabies is always fatal. Once clinical disease has developed, there is no effective treatment.

Prevention. All pet dogs and cats should be vaccinated. Cattle and horses should be vaccinated in areas where skunk rabies is endemic or vampire bats are present.

Individuals at risk, such as laboratory workers, animal control personnel, veterinarians, technicians, field zoologists, and others who come into contact with wild or unvaccinated domestic animals, should receive preexposure prophylaxis. Human diploid cell vaccine (HDCV) is the best and most effective of available vaccines, but it is expensive and may only be available in developed countries.

Local laws may vary, but in general, a dog or cat that has bitten a person should be quarantined and observed for at least 10 days. If the animal develops any sign suggestive of rabies, the animal should be killed and its brain examined by fluorescent microscopy. Any wild animal that has bitten a person should be killed immediately and tested. Any unvaccinated animal that is bitten by a rabid animal should be destroyed.

The most effective means of preventing rabies in humans is to immediately and thoroughly cleanse any animal bite or scratch wound; if used quickly, soap and water are a good means of removing rabies virus. Flush the wound with a strong stream of water, wash with soap or detergent, and rinse well. Apply a disinfectant, such as alcohol, tincture of iodine, or a quaternary ammonium compound, and seek medical attention. Bite wounds should be left unsutured, if possible, so as not to interfere with bleeding and drainage.

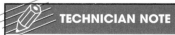

TECHNICIAN NOTE

All cases of animal and human rabies should be reported to health authorities.

For people who have not received preexposure immunization, postexposure prophylactic treatment consists of administering human rabies immune globulin (RIG) and rabies vaccine, preferably a 5-day course of HDCV. If the exposed person already has received a full course of HDCV before exposure, RIG is not considered necessary, and only two doses of HDCV are given.

Researchers who work with the virus should operate under strict biosafety level 2 (BSL 2) conditions; if aerosols are possible, BSL 3 precautions should be observed.

Reporting and Surveillance. All cases of animal and human rabies should be reported to health authorities.

Recommended Readings

General
Beran GW: Zoonoses in practice. Vet Clin North Am 23:1085–1107, 1993.

Bottone EJ, Hanna B, Hong T, et al.: Cumitech 27, Laboratory Diagnosis of Zoonotic Infections: Bacterial Infections Obtained from Companion and Laboratory Animals. Washington, DC, American Society for Microbiology, 1996.

Anthrax
Whitford HW, and Hugh-Jones ME: Anthrax. *In* Beran GW and Steele JH (editors): Handbook of Zoonoses, 2nd ed. Boca Raton, FL, CRC Press, 1994.

Avian Chlamydiosis
Koschmann JR: Avian chlamydiosis. *In* Farris R, Mahlow J, Newman E, and Nix B (editors): Health Hazards in Veterinary Practice, 3rd ed. Schaumburg, IL, American Veterinary Medical Association, 1995.

Bite Wounds and Other Injuries
August JR: Zoonosis Updates, 2nd ed. Schaumburg, IL, American Veterinary Medical Association, 1995.

Beaver BV: Animal-related injuries. *In* Farris R, Mahlow J, Newman E, and Nix B (editors). Health Hazards in Veterinary Practice, 3rd ed. Schaumburg, IL, American Veterinary Medical Association, 1995.

Weber DJ and Hansen AR: Infections resulting from animal bites. Infect Dis Clin North Am 5:663–680, 1991.

Brucellosis
Metcalf HE, Luchsinger DW, and Ray WC: Brucellosis. *In* Beran GW and Steele JH (editors): Handbook of Zoonoses, 2nd ed. Boca Raton, FL, CRC Press, 1994.

Radolf JD: Southwestern Medical Conference: Brucellosis: Don't let it get your goat! Am J Med Sci 307:64–75, 1994.

Campylobacteriosis
Benenson AS: Campylobacter enteritis. *In* Benenson AS (editor): Control of Communicable Diseases Manual. Washington, DC, American Public Health Association, 1995.

Saeed AM, Harris NV, and DiGiacomo RF: The role of exposure to animals in the etiology of Campylobacter jejuni/coli enteritis. Am J Epidemiol 137:108–114, 1993.

Capnocytophaga canimorsus Infection
Sasaki DM, Katz AR, and Middleton CR: *Capnocytophaga* and related infections. *In* Beran GW and Steele JH (editors): Handbook of Zoonoses, 2nd ed. Boca Raton, FL, CRC Press, 1994.

Cat Scratch Disease
Groves MG and Harrington KS: *Rochalimaea henselae* infections: Newly recognized zoonoses transmitted by domestic cats. J Am Vet Med Assoc 204:267–271, 1994.

Zangwill KM, Hamilton DH, Perkins BA, et al.: Cat scratch disease in Connecticut: Epidemiology, risk factors, and evaluation of a new diagnostic test. N Engl J Med 329:8–13, 1993.

Contagious Ecthyma
Acha PN and Szyfres B: Contagious ecthyma. *In* Zoonoses and Communicable Diseases Common to Man and Animals, 2nd ed. Washington, DC, Pan American Health Organization, 1987.

Benenson AS: Orf virus disease. *In* Benenson AS (editor): Control of Communicable Diseases Manual. Washington, DC, American Public Health Association, 1995.

Cryptococcosis
Benenson AS: Cryptococcosis. *In* Benenson AS (editor): Control of Communicable Diseases Manual. Washington, DC, American Public Health Association, 1995.

Levitz SM: The ecology of *Cryptococcus neoformans* and the epidemiology of cryptococcosis. Rev Infect Dis 13:1163–1169, 1991.

Cryptosporidiosis
Benenson AS: Cryptosporidiosis. *In* Benenson AS (editor): Control of Communicable Diseases Manual. Washington, DC, American Public Health Association, 1995.

Snowden KF: Cryptosporidiosis. *In* Farris R, Mahlow J, Newman E, and Nix B (editors): Health Hazards in Veterinary Practice, 3rd ed. Schaumburg, IL, American Veterinary Medical Association, 1995.

Dermatophytoses
Acha PN and Szyfres B: Dermatophytosis. *In* Zoonoses and Communicable Diseases Common to Man and Animals, 2nd ed. Washington, DC, Pan American Health Organization, 1987.

Pier AC: Superficial mycoses (dermatophytoses). *In* Beran GW and Steele JH (editors): Handbook of Zoonoses, 2nd ed. Boca Raton, FL, CRC Press, 1994.

Erysipelothrix Infections
Reboli AC and Farra WE: *Erysipelothrix rhusiopathiae:* An occupational pathogen. Clin Microbiol Rev 2:354–359, 1989.

Wood RL and Steele JH: *Erysipelothrix* infections. *In* Beran GW and Steele JH (editors): Handbook of Zoonoses, 2nd ed. Boca Raton, FL, CRC Press, 1994.

Herpesvirus simiae Infection
Acha PN and Szyfres B: *Herpesvirus simiae. In* Zoonoses and Communicable Diseases Common to Man and Animals, 2nd ed. Washington, DC, Pan American Health Organization, 1987.

Hilliard J and Lipper S: B virus. *In* Farris R, Mahlow J, Newman E, and Nix B (editors): Health Hazards in Veterinary Practice, 3rd ed. Schaumburg, IL, American Veterinary Medical Association, 1995.

Newcastle Disease
Hugh-Jones ME, Hubbert WT, and Hagstad HV: Newcastle disease. *In* Zoonoses: Recognition, Control, and Prevention. Ames, IO, Iowa State University Press, 1995.

Pasteurellosis
Acha PN and Szyfres B: Pasteurellosis. *In* Zoonoses and Communicable Diseases Common to Man and Animals, 2nd ed. Washington, DC, Pan American Health Organization, 1987.

Arons MS, Fernando L, and Polayes IM: *Pasteurella multocida*—The major cause of hand infections following domestic animal bites. J Hand Surg 7:47–52, 1982.

Q Fever
Raoult D and Marrie T: Q fever. Clin Infect Dis 20:489–496, 1995.

Williams JC and Sanchez V: Q fever and coxiellosis. *In* Beran GW and Steele JH (editors): Handbook of Zoonoses, 2nd ed., Boca Raton, FL, CRC Press, 1994.

Rabies
Benenson AS: Rabies. *In* Benenson AS (editor): Control of Communicable Diseases Manual. Washington, DC, American Public Health Association, 1995.

Clark KA: Rabies. *In* Farris R, Mahlow J, Newman E, and Nix B (editors): Health Hazards in Veterinary Practice, 3rd ed. Schaumburg, IL, American Veterinary Medical Association, 1995.

Rat-Bite Fevers
Will LA: Rat-bite fever. *In* Beran GW and Steele JH (editors): Handbook of Zoonoses, 2nd ed. Boca Raton, FL, CRC Press, 1994.

Wullenberger M: *Streptobacillus moniliformis*—A zoonotic pathogen: Taxonomic considerations, host species, diagnosis, therapy, geographical distribution. Lab Animals 29:1–15, 1995.

Salmonellosis
CDC: Reptile-associated salmonellosis—Selected states, 1994–1995. MMWR 44:347–350, 1995.

Benenson AS: Salmonellosis. *In* Benenson AS (editor): Control of Communicable Diseases Manual. Washington, DC, American Public Health Association, 1995.

Toxoplasmosis
Lappin MR: Toxoplasmosis. *In* Farris R, Mahlow J, Newman E, and Nix B (editors): Health Hazards in Veterinary Practice, 3rd ed. Schaumburg, IL, American Veterinary Medical Association, 1995.

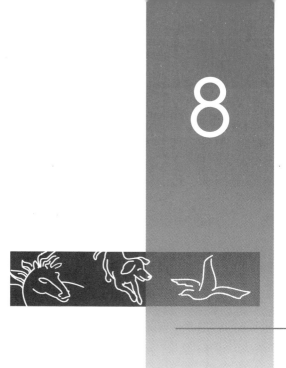

8 Clinical Microbiology

Robert L. Jones

INTRODUCTION

The purpose of the clinical microbiology laboratory is to rapidly and accurately provide the veterinarian with information concerning the presence or absence of a microbial agent that is specifically or potentially involved in an infectious disease process in a patient. This information is then used to (1) establish a diagnosis, (2) indicate the prognosis and possible complications of the disease, (3) explain the source of infection and the risk of transmission to other animals or humans, (4) aid in the prevention of infection of other animals by identifying the specific product needed for immunization, and (5) formulate specific treatment programs. Therefore, the veterinary technician who is working in or involved with the microbiology laboratory has a direct impact on the quality of patient care.

Recent advances in diagnostic techniques and increasing interest in improved patient care have made clinical microbiology services a cost-effective part of modern veterinary practice. Isolation and identification of the more common bacterial pathogens can readily be performed in the laboratories of most veterinary practices. Antimicrobial susceptibility test procedures are standardized so that reproducible results can be obtained. Limited mycology diagnostic services can be provided. The majority of viral diagnostic procedures and serological tests require special equipment and training, so they are available only through referral laboratories. However, the development of monoclonal antibody diagnostic reagents and improved immunological test methods are providing new diagnostic kits that can readily be used in small laboratories.

FUNCTION OF THE LABORATORY

Diagnostic microbiological tests are most helpful to the veterinarian when they are provided as rapidly as possible, while patient care evaluations and decisions are being made. However, the expeditious delivery of results must not be made at the expense of accuracy in the laboratory. Proper procedures must be established and carefully followed. Occasionally, specific quality assurance testing will be necessary to establish the competence of the laboratory. It is often surprising to technicians to find that the negative results they obtain are due to faulty procedures. This inadequacy in laboratory function can be identified only by obtaining known specimens for testing or sending paired specimens to a reference laboratory. When the microbiology laboratory is functioning properly, it can accurately determine the presence or absence of a specific pathogen. The laboratory services must be cost effective. The results must be useful in patient care, providing essential information, and must ultimately result in client satisfaction.

CONSIDERATIONS FOR ESTABLISHING A LOCAL LABORATORY

The sophistication of diagnostic microbiology that is undertaken in the local laboratory is dependent on the size and type of practice, cost of performing tests, and availability of a technician with appropriate diagnostic microbiology knowledge and skills. The decision to equip and operate a local laboratory must be based in part on services available through referral laboratories. When comparing the cost of services obtained from these laboratories, the packaging and shipping costs, as well as the direct charge, must be considered. The turnaround time from collection of the specimen until results are received may be unacceptable. Specimens can be submitted only on laboratory work days, whereas the specimens can be processed in a local laboratory when they are obtained, including weekends and holidays.

Shipping delays are avoided, and preliminary and final results are immediately available in the practice with its own laboratory, so waiting for communication of results from an outside laboratory is unnecessary. The overhead costs of equipment and stocking supplies are modest and acceptable to most practices. As a technician gains proficiency in the microbiology laboratory, the time commitment will be reduced. If specimens are sent out, considerable time can be spent packaging them, delivering them to shipping terminals, and calling for results. Many practices find it cost effective to operate a microbiology laboratory that is capable of processing routine bacterial cultures.

DIAGNOSTIC METHODS

The choice of methods for examining a specimen in the microbiology laboratory is dependent on the type of specimen and the pathogen sought. Traditionally, microbiologists have attempted to *isolate agents* in various types of culture systems and then use various identification schemes to characterize them. This is still the most frequently used method in bacteriology. However, there are times when the organism may be difficult to cultivate or may not be viable in the specimen presented to the laboratory. In these cases, demonstration of *specific microbial antigens* in the specimen may be more rapid and cost effective. Immunofluorescence stains have been the most commonly used method of antigen detection. Other immunological assays (e.g., enzyme immunoassays, latex particle agglutination, and protein A coagglutination procedures) are being introduced into veterinary diagnostics. In some diseases, such as botulism and mycotoxicoses, establishing the presence of a *microbial toxin* is necessary, rather than identifying the organism that produces it. Sometimes, a specific *immunological response* by the patient to an infectious agent can establish the diagnosis. Serum can be tested for the presence of specific antibodies, or skin tests can be performed. Another diagnostic method is *direct examination* of exudates and tissue biopsies. Some microorganisms present such unique morphological characteristics, host inflammatory responses, and lesions that a definitive diagnosis can be established without the need for further laboratory testing. Therefore, a direct examination is one of the most important procedures that can be performed in the clinical laboratory.

TECHNICIAN NOTE

Direct microscopic examination of stained slides (smears or impressions) prepared from specimens is one of the most important procedures performed in the clinical microbiology laboratory to provide preliminary information about the disease process and possible infectious agents.

Recent developments in biotechnology are providing new methods for direct detection of infectious agents. *Nucleic acid probes* are considered the next new wave of diagnostic tests. Direct nucleic acid hybridization probe and *gene amplification* protocols are highly specific and can be extremely sensitive.

Deoxyribonucleic acid (DNA) probe assays are particularly well suited for in situ hybridization in tissue in which the location and distribution of the organisms must be determined, identification of slow-growing or difficult-to-isolate organisms, and identification of toxicogenic strains of bacteria that cannot be differentiated from nontoxicogenic strains through the use of conventional methods. Nucleic acid amplification assays use primers and polymerase chain reaction (PCR) to provide specificity and sensitivity to detect as few as one organism or 1 to 10 copies of the specific gene sequence.

Ultimately, the goal of these molecular techniques is the direct determination of identities and antimicrobial susceptibility patterns of microorganisms in clinical specimens. As the technology for nucleic acid amplification currently stands, application of the procedure is limited to large referral laboratories and research laboratories. Partial or full automation and improved technology will begin to reduce costs and increase access to these assays. Specimen handling and preparation remain the most critical limiting step in almost all published protocols. Specimen preparation must release the nucleic acids from the target organism, prevent degradation of the free nucleic acids, remove any substances inhibitory to nucleic acid amplification or hybridization, concentrate the nucleic acids into a small volume, place the nucleic acids in amplification or hybridization buffer, and prevent false-positive results due to contaminating nucleic acids. Various samples must be processed differently for extracting the nucleic acids from their matrix. Therefore, technicians and clinicians must work closely with the laboratory to obtain useful results.

Despite their sensitivity, molecular detection procedures will not totally replace conventional culture and serological procedures because the results of nucleic acid amplification procedures and the results of culture or serology mean different things. Nucleic acid amplification procedures are used to determine whether DNA or ribonucleic acid (RNA) from a particular organism is present in the specimen; they reveal nothing about the viability of the organism (because they can detect DNA from dead organisms) or whether the organism is involved in an infectious process. Culture, on the other hand, clearly demonstrates the viability of the organism, whereas a rise in titer of antibody to a specific organism strongly suggests infection.

COLLECTION OF SPECIMENS

There is no other area in the clinical laboratory in which specimen sources and types are so diverse as in the microbiology laboratory. To compound this diversity, specimen selection, collection, and transport to the laboratory will have a major impact on results. Therefore, it is important that close communication between the technician and veterinarian be established.

Proper Specimen Collection

The goal of specimen collection is to obtain a sample from the patient that is representative of the disease process. Therefore, the culture specimen must be from the actual *infection site* (Fig. 8–1). It must be collected with a minimum of contamination from adjacent tissues or secretions. Material swabbed from superficial body surfaces (skin or mucous membranes) will usually yield a mixed growth of bacteria, often making it difficult to identify a significant pathogen. Culture specimens recovered

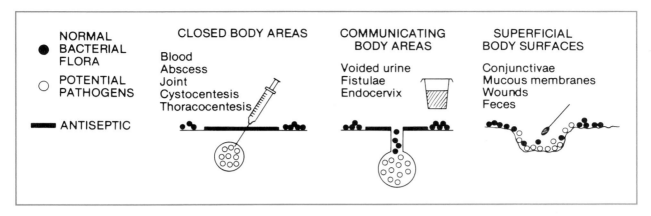

Figure 8-1. Methods used to collect bacterial culture specimens and probable sources of contamination.

from body orifices and draining tracts are frequently contaminated with normal flora. The most satisfactory specimens are those aspirated from normally sterile, closed body compartments after the surface has been aseptically prepared.

Optimal times and *sites* for specimen collection must be observed. Knowledge of the pathophysiology of infectious disease processes is important for determining the optimal specimens that will provide the best chance of recovering the agent. Infections by some viruses and mycoplasma are acute processes that are followed by secondary invasion by opportunistic bacteria; therefore, sampling must be performed early in the course of disease. Most viruses and some bacteria localize in specific tissues. Knowledge of these characteristics can be used to improve specimen selection.

Specimens obtained at necropsy for culture should be collected as soon as possible after the death of the animal (see Chapter 30). Whenever possible, culture specimens should be obtained before the administration of antimicrobials, especially if the suspected pathogen may be susceptible to the antimicrobial or the antimicrobial may be concentrated at the site of infection. However, the administration of antimicrobials does not necessarily preclude the usefulness of cultures. The antimicrobial drug may be diluted to an ineffective level in culture medium, thereby allowing the pathogen to grow. Antimicrobial-resistant or superinfecting bacteria may still be recovered. In addition, the effectiveness of therapy can be evaluated by determining the relative numbers of bacteria present.

An *adequate quantity* of material should be obtained for complete examination. All too frequently, a good specimen is collected, but only a minute amount is submitted to the laboratory on a swab for examination. Aliquots of body fluids, exudates, or pieces of tissue are always more useful than a swab. Smears can be prepared for direct examination, and multiple culture media can be inoculated when adequate material is submitted. Quantitative results can also be obtained, if needed.

Appropriate collection devices and specimen handling must be used to ensure optimal survival and recovery of significant microorganisms (Fig. 8–2). Sterile swabs are acceptable for transferring most samples from the patient to culture media. If the culture medium is not immediately inoculated, the swab must be placed in a humidified transport chamber such as the Culturette (Becton Dickinson Microbiology Systems) or into a transport medium. *Transport media* are designed to maintain

optimal conditions for survival of the suspected pathogen without allowing overgrowth by contaminating saprophytes. Semisolid transport media, such as Amies transport medium with charcoal for *aerobic bacteria* (growth in the presence of oxygen) or Port-A-Cul tubes (Becton Dickinson Microbiology Systems) for *anaerobic bacteria* (requires absence of oxygen), can preserve specimens on swabs for several days. Swabs should not be placed in nutritive broths before inoculating isolation media because an insignificant nonpathogen may overgrow and prevent recovery of the pathogen. Specimens can be collected in various sterile containers that do not contain preservatives or anticoagulants for transport. If tissues are collected for culture, each piece must be packaged separately in a leak-proof, sterile container.

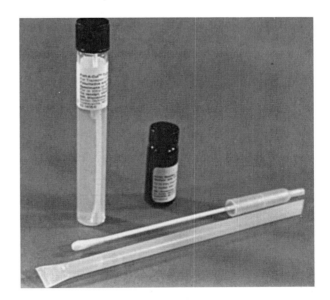

Figure 8-2. Culturette swab, tube of Amies transport medium with charcoal, and Port-A-Cul anaerobic transport tube. The Culturette swab is replaced in the plastic tube after it is inoculated, and the ampule at the bottom is crushed to provide moisture for the swab. The transport tubes are used by inserting the swab deep into the medium and breaking off the end of the swab that has been handled. The Port-A-Cul tube contains an indicator that changes color when exposed to oxygen and shows how far oxygen has diffused into the agar.

> **TECHNICIAN NOTE**
>
> Transport media can serve as excellent vehicles for submitting a bacterial isolate to a reference laboratory for further characterization. A heavily inoculated swab of the pure culture should be placed in the appropriate medium for shipping rather than submitting an inoculated growth medium.

Each culture specimen container must be *properly labeled.* Identification of the patient by name, species, case number, or owner, as appropriate, should be legibly indicated. If more than one veterinarian works in the practice, the one in charge of the case should be identified so that questions about history and preliminary reports can be communicated efficiently. The source of the specimen should also be included on the label. Nothing can be more frustrating in the laboratory than to be presented with a swab for culture and wonder if it represents conjunctiva, ear canal, skin, or endometrium. As is discussed later, the source of the specimen will be a significant factor in deciding how to set up the culture, which bacteria to identify, and how to interpret the results. If the culture specimen is to be sent to a referral laboratory, additional clinical history should be included. Results of previous culture attempts, other laboratory tests and antimicrobial treatments should be reported, as well as the major clinical manifestations and duration of illness, so laboratory personnel will be able to recognize and identify significant findings.

Special Collection and Handling Procedures

Some groups of microorganisms require special collection and handling for optimal isolation. Anaerobic bacteria must be protected from oxygen. Often, a sterile syringe with a fine-gauge needle (22- to 23-gauge) is the best collection device for aspirating exudates from an infected site. The specimen can be transported to the laboratory in the syringe if air is expressed, the needle is removed to prevent injuries, and the syringe is capped to prevent leakage. Otherwise, the specimen should be transferred to an appropriate anaerobic transport device. Survival and subsequent isolation of anaerobes are enhanced by keeping them in the reduced microenvironment in which they are found. Therefore, as stated previously, exudate and pieces of tissue are better specimens than swabs. If a swab is collected, it must be placed in an appropriate anaerobic transport device. Handling a specimen as if it contains anaerobes will not jeopardize the viability of aerobic bacteria.

In attempts to isolate fungi and mycobacteria, swabs generally are not the best specimens. These agents tend to cause chronic infections, often with small numbers of organisms present. Too few organisms may be present on a swab, or in the case of mycobacteria, they may adhere to the swab, and culture results will be negative. Exudates, biopsy material, and tissue should be submitted as quickly as possible to the microbiology laboratory.

The more fastidious groups of microorganisms, for example, *Mycoplasma, Chlamydia, Rickettsia,* and viruses, require special selective transport media. These media are usually formulated to contain antimicrobials that will inhibit the growth of other microorganisms, while preserving the viability of the desired agent. Specific transport media and instructions for proper use should be obtained from a referral laboratory that is capable of providing the desired culture service.

PROCESSING SPECIMENS

Each specimen received in the microbiology laboratory should be carefully and individually evaluated, just as each patient is individually examined, rather than being subjected to an inflexible processing scheme. Variables to be considered include anatomic source and condition of the specimen, animal family of the patient, clinical history, special requests from the veterinarian, and results of direct examination of the specimen that will collectively focus on the most likely agents.

Condition of the Specimen

Each specimen received in the microbiology laboratory should be examined to see whether it is suitable for further processing. If there is evidence that the specimen has become grossly contaminated or dried out, it is of insufficient quantity, there has been excessive delay in receipt, or any other evidence of mishandling is present, an attempt should be made to obtain a second sample. Specimens should be processed the same day they are collected, or they should be held at refrigeration temperatures if a delay is anticipated.

Clinical Information

When the microbiology laboratory receives information about the clinical history of the suspected infectious disease and the source of the specimen, the pathogen can be identified much more efficiently. Each pathogen has a preferred habitat in which it will grow and specific mechanisms for causing disease. Therefore, for a particular manifestation of disease, there will be a limited number of agents that should be considered as likely pathogens. Comparison of the clinical description of disease with the biology and pathogenicity of microorganisms will usually identify a limited number of agents that typically are involved in each type of disease process.

If the veterinarian has carefully examined the patient, the differential list of infectious agents can usually be limited to two to five microorganisms. Table 8–1 lists the most common bacterial species associated with infections of various sites in animals. If the technician can focus the search for pathogens on these most likely agents, results will often be obtained much more rapidly and with less expense.

Direct Microscopic Examination

Direct microscopic examination of exudates, impression smears from tissues or infected body fluids is the most important laboratory procedure that can be used for microbiological diagnosis. It provides immediate information on the types and numbers of microorganisms present as well as the type of host cellular inflammatory response. The likelihood of infection can be determined as can the probable type of agent (i.e., virus, bacteria or fungus), which, in turn, determines the nature of the diagnostic assays needed. Suitability of the specimen for culture can also be evaluated. The most likely pathogen (or predominant organism) may tentatively be identified. This information may

• Table 8–1 •

COMMON BACTERIAL SPECIES ASSOCIATED WITH INFECTIONS

TYPE OF INFECTION	CANINE	FELINE	EQUINE	PORCINE	RUMINANTS
Conjunctivitis	Staphylococcus Streptococcus Pseudomonas	Staphylococcus Pasteurella Chlamydia	Streptococcus Staphylococcus	Streptococcus Staphylococcus	Moroxella bovis Branhamella Streptococcus Staphylococcus Escherichia coli
Central Nervous System	Rare	Rare	Streptococcus Actinobacillus Escherichia coli	Streptococcus Escherichia coli	Haemophilus somnus Listeria Escherichia coli Pasteurella haemolytica

Gastroenteritis	Salmonella
	Clostridium
	  perfringens
	Campylobacter
		Salmonella	Salmonella
			Escherichia coli
			Actinobacillus
			Rhodococcus equi
				Salmonella
				Escherichia coli
				Serpulina
				Clostridium perfringens
					Salmonella
					Escherichia coli
					Clostridium perfringens
					Mycobacterium
					  paratuberculosis

Genital tract	Brucella canis Escherichia coli Streptococcus Staphylococcus Mycoplasma	Streptococcus Pasteurella Escherichia coli	Streptococcus Escherichia coli Klebsiella Pseudomonas	Brucella suis Streptococcus Leptospira	Brucella Listeria Actinomyces pyogenes Campylobacter Mycoplasma
Mastitis	Staphylococcus	Staphylococcus	Streptococcus	Streptococcus Staphylococcus Escherichia coli Actinobacillus Actinomyces pyogenes	Streptococcus Staphylococcus Actinomyces pyogenes Nocardia Mycobacterium Escherichia coli Klebsiella
Musculoskeletal	Staphylococcus Escherichia coli Pseudomonas Brucella canis Anaerobes	Rare	Streptococcus Actinobacillus Escherichia coli Rhodococcus equi Staphylococcus	Streptococcus Mycoplasma Escherichia coli Erysipelothrix Actinomyces pyogenes	Clostridium Actinomyces pyogenes Escherichia coli Streptococcus Erysipelothrix Haemophilus somnus Mycoplasma Chlamydia
Otitis	Staphylococcus Pseudomonas Streptococcus Clostridium perfringens	Rare	Rare	Rare Streptococcus	Rare Streptococcus Pasteurella Actinomyces pyogenes

Respiratory Upper	Bordetella
	  bronchiseptica
		Pasteurella
		  multocida
			Streptococcus equi	Bordetella
				  bronchiseptica
				Pasteurella multocida
					Haemophilus somnus
					Actinomyces pyogenes
					Fusobacterium

Pneumonia	Bordetella
	  bronchiseptica
	Pasteurella
	Klebsiella
	Escherichia coli
	Mycoplasma
	Streptococcus
	Staphylococcus
		Rare
		Pasteurella
		Chlamydia
			Streptococcus
			Actinobacillus
			Rhodococcus equi
			Pasteurella
			Staphylococcus
			Klebsiella
			Pseudomonas
			Bordetella
			  bronchiseptica
				Mycoplasma
				Haemophilus
				Pasteurella
				Streptococcus
				Actinobacillus
					Pasteurella
					Actinomyces pyogenes
					Haemophilus somnus
					Mycoplasma

Pleuritis	Fusobacterium Prevotella Porphyromonas Actinomyces	Prevotella Porphyromonas Fusobacterium Pasteurella Nocardia	Streptococcus	Actinobacillus	Pasteurella Actinomyces pyogenes

Skin wounds abscesses	Staphylococcus
	Streptococcus
	Pseudomonas
	Nocardia
	Actinomyces
	Fusobacterium
		Pasteurella
		  multocida
		Streptococcus
		Staphylococcus
		Anaerobes
			Streptococcus
			Corynebacterium
			  pseudotuberculosis
			Pseudomonas
			Dermatophilus
			Staphylococcus
				Streptococcus
				Staphylococcus
				Actinomyces pyogenes
					Actinomyces pyogenes
					Dermatophilus
					Actinomyces
					Actinobacillus
					Staphylococcus

Urinary tract	Escherichia coli Proteus Staphylococcus Streptococcus Klebsiella Pseudomonas	Staphylococcus Escherichia coli	Streptococcus Escherichia coli	Eubacterium suis Streptococcus	Corynebacterium renale Actinomyces pyogenes

be used as the basis for the interpretation of the significance of subsequent culture results.

In many situations, Gram's stain is the procedure of choice because it provides differentiation of gram-positive and gram-negative bacteria. However, some bacteria do not stain well with Gram's stain. Gram-negative bacteria may not be well differentiated from the background in exudates and tissue impression smears.

[handwritten top margin: Gt = purple   G- = pink]

Other tissue stains (i.e., Giemsa's and Wright's stains or methylene blue wet mounts) may be more useful for detecting all microorganisms present in the smear. Although these stains are more efficient in demonstrating the presence and morphology of bacteria, they do not provide differentiation of gram-positive and gram-negative bacteria. Careful direct examination may be sufficient for diagnosis without cultures, or it can narrow the diagnostic likelihood to a few bacterial species. This information helps in the selection of optimal culture conditions for identification of suspected pathogens.

Gram's Stain Procedure

The technique for preparing a Gram-stained smear is as follows:

[handwritten left margin: CV (1min) / Iodine (1min) / Alcohol / Safranin (30-60 secs)]

1. Prepare a thin smear from tissue exudates or bacterial suspension on a clean slide and allow smear to air dry.
2. Fix material to the slide so that it does not wash off during the staining procedure by passing the slide, right side up, through a flame three or four times.
3. Flood smear with crystal violet solution, and let stand for 1 minute.
4. Wash smear briefly with tap water.
5. Flood smear with Gram's iodine solution, and let stand for 1 minute.
6. Wash with tap water, and decolorize until solvent flows colorlessly from the slide. This usually requires 5 to 10 seconds.
7. Wash briefly with tap water, and flood the slide with safranin counterstain for 30 to 60 seconds.
8. Wash briefly with tap water, blot dry and examine the stained smear under the $100\times$ (oil immersion) objective of the microscope.

> **TECHNICIAN NOTE**
>
> Appearance of clinical material in Gram-stained preparations:
>
> • Gram-positive bacteria retain the crystal violet iodine complex and appear dark-blue or purple.
> • Gram-negative bacteria lose the primary complex, take up the secondary dye safranin and appear red.
> • Fungi (yeasts) appear gram-positive.
> • Inflammatory cells appear gram-negative. Epithelial cells may appear gram-positive and/or gram-negative depending on the thickness of the smear.
> • Backgrounds usually appear gram-negative but may appear gram-positive. Fibrin, mucus, and erythrocytes often stain gram-negative and may mask detection of gram-negative bacteria.

BACTERIAL ISOLATION AND IDENTIFICATION PROCEDURES

Equipment

The following is a list of equipment and supplies required for the performance of basic diagnostic bacteriology tests.

1. Binocular microscope
2. Incubator
3. Anaerobic culture system
4. Stains: Gram's stain kit, acid-fast stain kit, lactophenol cotton blue
5. Bacteriological loops, inoculating needles, and calibrated loops
6. Alcohol wick burner, Bunsen burner, or sterno burner
7. Glass slides and coverslips
8. Forceps, spatulas, and scalpels
9. Specimen-collection devices, swabs, tubes, cups, and so forth
10. Transport media: Amies, Port-A-Cul
11. Culture media (Table 8–2)
12. Antibiotic disk dispenser and disks
13. 3% Hydrogen peroxide
14. 3% Potassium hydroxide
15. Oxidase test reagent
16. Coagulase plasma
17. *Salmonella* polyvalent antiserum
18. Packaged identification system for Enterobacteriaceae (Table 8–3)
19. Kovac's reagent

The most expensive item is a good-quality binocular light microscope with a $100\times$ oil immersion objective. Dark-field and phase-contrast options are useful but not essential. Small countertop incubators are available. Important characteristics of a quality incubator include (1) insulated walls to maintain a constant temperature; (2) an adequate seal to maintain a humid atmosphere; (3) a capacity for plates, tubes, and candle jars; (4) a thermometer to check the temperature, which should not fluctuate more than $\pm2°C$; and (5) an adjustable, thermostatically controlled heating element. Storage space for media in a refrigerator is needed, as well as a convenient, clean laboratory workbench with a sink.

Culture Media

A number of different media are needed in the bacteriology laboratory for isolation of various microbial agents and for identification of these microorganisms. Both dehydrated and prepared media are readily available today. It is usually much more convenient for small laboratories to purchase prepared media than to prepare their own. In addition, the quality of purchased media will be much more consistent and usually will be quality tested before it is distributed. There are numerous distributors of prepared media throughout the United States. A few national and regional distributors are listed in Table 8–4. Names and addresses of other suppliers can be obtained from local hospitals. These microbiology supply distributors usually have a full line of prepared plates and tubes of media available, as well as the ancillary biochemical reagents, stains and miscellaneous supplies that are necessary in the laboratory (see preceding list).

Purpose of Specific Media

Solid media in plates are used for primary isolation of bacteria from clinical specimens. This type of medium allows distribution of the specimen in such a way that *isolated colonies* develop, each representing a single bacterial cell. Some primary isolation media contain inhibitory ingredients that allow them

• Table 8–2 •

BACTERIOLOGICAL PLATE AND TUBE MEDIA FOR THE PRACTITIONER'S LABORATORY

MEDIA	PURPOSE AND INOCULATION	REACTIONS AND INTERPRETATIONS
Blood agar plate (trypticase soy agar with 5% sheep blood)	Primary isolation medium for all specimens in which pathogenic bacteria are suspected. Always streak for colony isolation.	Observe growth rates, colony morphological characteristics, hemolysis. Test selected colonies for Gram reaction, catalase and oxidase. Inoculate differential tests and antimicrobial susceptibility tests from well-isolated colonies.
MacConkey agar	A primary isolation and differential plating medium for selection and recovery of Enterobacteriaceae and related gram-negative bacteria. Inoculate by streaking for isolated colonies.	Growth is usually gram-negative. Pink to red colonies (with increased redness of the medium) are lactose fermenters, e.g., species of *Escherichia, Klebsiella* and *Enterobacter.* Colorless colonies (often with a slight change of the medium to yellow) are nonlactose fermenters.
Hektoen enteric agar	A direct plating medium for fecal specimens that is highly selective for *Salmonella.* Inoculate by streaking for isolated colonies.	Disaccharide fermenters are moderately inhibited and produce bright orange to yellow to salmon to pink colonies. *Salmonella* colonies are blue-green typically with black centers from hydrogen sulfide. *Proteus* colonies may resemble *Salmonella.*
Selenite broth or Tetrathionate broth	Enrichment broth for the selective enhancement of growth by *Salmonella* from specimens containing heavy concentrations of mixed bacteria, such as feces. Inoculate relatively heavily and incubate for 18 to 24 hr.	Subculture to MacConkey agar and Hektoen enteric agar for isolation of *Salmonella.*
Triple sugar iron (TSI) agar slant	A differential medium for detection of carbohydrate (glucose, lactose, sucrose) fermentation and production of hydrogen sulfide. Inoculate by stabbing the butt once with an inoculating needle and by streaking the slant. Incubate with a loose cap.	Yellow color change indicates acidification caused by carbohydrate fermentation. In the butt, glucose fermentation is detected; in the slant, lactose and sucrose fermentation is detected (includes glucose fermentation as an intermediate product). Red color change indicates alkalinization caused by lack of carbohydrate fermentation. Black color indicates hydrogen sulfide production. Results are recorded as slant/butt; A = acid (yellow), K = alkaline (red) or NC = no change.
Christensen's urea agar slant	A differential medium for detection of urease production by an organism. Inoculate by streaking heavily over the slant.	Urease-positive bacteria produce a pink-red color change in the slant and sometimes throughout the butt. Urease-negative bacteria allow the medium to remain the original yellow color.
Motility media*	A test medium for determining if an organism is motile or nonmotile. Inoculate by stabbing the center of the tube with an inoculating needle. Incubate at 35°C for most organisms; incubate at room temperature if *Listeria* is suspected.	Motile organisms migrate from the stab line, flaring out to cause turbidity in the medium. Nonmotile organisms grow only along the stab line; the surrounding medium remains clear.
Indole test media*	A test medium for detecting the ability of bacteria to produce indole as one of the degradation products of tryptophan metabolism. Inoculate, incubate 24 to 48 hr, then add Kovac's reagent to detect indole.	Development of a red color at the interface of the reagent and the broth within seconds after adding the reagent is indicative of a positive test.

*Combination media can be purchased that provide for several tests in the same tube, such as SIM (sulfide-indole-motility), MIO or MIL (motility-indole-ornithine or motility-indole-lysine).

to be *selective* for specific groups of bacteria. MacConkey agar is selective for bacteria that can grow in the presence of bile salts, which is similar to the environment found in the intestines. A *differential* medium contains an indicator system that can distinguish different bacteria, even though both types may grow. The lactose-fermenting ability of bacteria on MacConkey agar is a differential reaction. Table 8–2 lists some of the more commonly used culture media, the indicated use of the media, and selective and differential characteristics.

Inoculation of Media

Before media are inoculated, they should be arranged on the workbench in an orderly manner and labeled. Each tube or plate should be labeled with a distinct identification and the date of inoculation. Plates should be labeled on the bottom with a waterproof marker.

Most clinical specimens that are presented for culture will be on swabs. If tissues collected postmortem are to be cultured, the surface should be seared (do not cook the tissues), and culture inoculum should be collected from deep within the specimen by using a swab. These swabs are used for direct inoculation of the primary isolation media. The same swab can be used for inoculation of several media if the least inhibitory medium is inoculated first and the most inhibitory medium is inoculated last; for example, start with blood agar and then MacConkey agar.

• Table 8–3 •

COMMERCIAL KIT SYSTEMS FOR IDENTIFICATION OF MICROORGANISMS	

Enterobacteriaceae
API 20E
  bioMérieux Vitek, Inc.
Enterotube II
  Becton Dickinson
      Microbiology Systems
Minitek Enteric Set II
  Becton Dickinson
      Microbiology Systems
Micro-ID
  Remel
 	
Staphylococcus
Minitek Gram-positive Set
  Becton Dickinson
      Microbiology Systems
API STAPH
  bioMérieux Vitek, Inc.
 	
Streptococcus
API 20 Strep
  bioMérieux Vitek, Inc.
Minitek Gram-positive Set
  Becton Dickinson
      Microbiology Systems
 	
Small Gram-positive Bacilli
API Coryne
  bioMérieux Vitek, Inc.
	Other Gram-negative Bacteria
	API 20E
	  bioMérieux Vitek, Inc.
	Minitek Nonfermenter Set
	  Becton Dickinson
	      Microbiology Systems
	OXI/FERM
	  Becton Dickinson
	      Microbiology Systems
	
	Yeast
	API 20C
	  bioMérieux Vitek, Inc.
	Minitek Yeast Set
	  Becton Dickinson
	      Microbiology Systems
	
	Anaerobic Bacteria
	API 20A
	  bioMérieux Vitek, Inc.
	Minitek Anaerobe Set II
	  Becton Dickinson
	      Microbiology Systems
	RapID-ANA II
	  Innovative Diagnostic
	      Systems, Inc.

See Table 8–4 for addresses of product manufacturers and distributors.

Between one fourth and one third of the surface of the agar plates should be inoculated with the specimen. The inoculum is then progressively diluted across the agar by successive steps of streaking with a bacteriological loop, as illustrated in Figure 8–3. There are several different streaking technique modifications, any method that yields isolated colonies is satisfactory. With the practice of a light touch to avoid tearing the agar and experience in anticipating the amount of bacterial growth that will occur, slight modifications can be made in technique from one specimen to the next to achieve the best isolation of colonies.

Media dispensed in tubes may be a broth, semisolid agar, or poured as a slant. Broth media can be inoculated with a loop or an inoculating wire by touching the side of the tube just below the surface of the medium. Depending on the purpose of the slant medium, it may require inoculation by stabbing the deep (or butt) portion of the agar (e.g. triple sugar iron [TSI] slants); the slant surface is then streaked from bottom to top (Fig. 8–4). When semisolid medium for motility testing is inoculated, it is important that the inoculating wire is inserted and removed along the same tract within the medium.

Incubation Conditions

Inoculated plates are incubated in an inverted position to prevent condensation of water on the lid. If water drops to the agar surface, it can mix the bacterial growth rather than allowing it to develop as isolated colonies. If tube media have screw tops, they should be left loose during incubation.

Temperature

Cultures should be placed in incubation at an optimal temperature as quickly as possible. The majority of specimens for isolation of pathogenic bacteria are incubated at 35°C. Although optimal growth may occur at other temperatures, in most cases alternate temperatures are more important for differentiation of bacteria than for primary isolation. However, there are exceptions that must be identified by the technician, such as specimens from cold-blooded animals, which should be incubated at room temperature or the successful isolation of pathogenic bacteria will be compromised.

• Table 8–4 •

COMMERCIAL SOURCES OF MICROBIOLOGY LABORATORY SUPPLIES
This table presents a partial listing of manufacturers and distributors of various microbiology laboratory supplies such as prepared plate and tube media, stains and reagents, susceptibility test supplies, loops, slides, swabs, incubators, microscopes, anaerobic systems, and diagnostic kits. Through consultation with other local microbiology laboratories (e.g., hospitals) other local or regional suppliers may be discovered.
Anaerobe Systems, 2200 Zanker Road, Suite C, San Jose, CA 95131, (800) 443-3108
Bacti-Lab, Inc., PO Box 1179, Mountain View, CA 94042, (800) 227-7300
Baxter Scientific Products, 1430 Waukegan Road, McGraw Park, IL 60085, (847) 689-8410
Becton Dickinson Microbiology Systems, PO Box 243, Cockeysville, MD 21030, (410) 771-0100
Becton Dickinson Vacutainer Systems, 1 Becton Drive, Franklin Lakes, NJ 07417, (201) 847-6800
Bethyl Laboratories, Inc., PO Box 850, Montgomery, TX 77356, (800) 338-9579
bioMérieVitek, Inc., 595 Anglum Drive, Hazelwood, MO 63042, (800) 638-4835
Carr-Scarborough Microbiologicals, Inc., 5342 Panola Industrial Boulevard, Decatur, GA 30035, (800) 241-0998
Centaur, Inc., PO Box 25667, Overland Park, KS 66225, (913) 236-6184
Curtin Matheson Scientific, Inc., PO Box 1546, Houston, TX 77251, (713) 878-2349
Difco Laboratories, PO Box 331058, Detroit, MI 48232, (800) 521-0851
Fisher Scientific, 2000 Park Lane, Pittsburgh, PA 15275, (800) 766-7000
IDEXX Laboratories, Inc., One IDEXX Drive, Westbrook, ME 04092, (800) 248-2483
ImmuCell Corp., 56 Evergreen Drive, Portland, ME 04103, (207) 878-2770
Innovative Diagnostic Systems, Inc., 2797 Peterson Place, Norcross, GA 30071, (800) 225-5443
Meridian Diagnostics, Inc., 3471 River Hills Drive, Cincinnati, OH 45244, (800) 543-1980
Microbio Products, Inc., 3901 Nome Street, Unit 1, Denver, CO 80239, (303) 371-4166
Unipath, 800 Proctor Avenue, Odgensburg, NY 13669, (800) 567-8378
Remel, 12076 Sante Fe Trail Drive, Lenexa, KS 66285, (800) 255-6730
Synbiotics Corp., 16420 Via Exprillo, San Diego, CA 92127, (800) 228-1725
VMRD, Inc., PO Box 502, Pullman, WA 99163, (800) 222-8673
VWR Scientific Products, 1310 Goshen Parkway, West Chester, PA 19380, (800) 932-5000

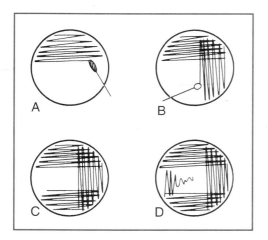

Figure 8–3. Plate inoculation and streaking method for isolation of bacterial colonies. A, Inoculate with swab, covering one fourth to one third of plate. B, Streak lightly, overlapping previous area. C, Flame loop, allow it to cool and streak next area. D, Repeat as in C.

Atmosphere

Most common pathogenic bacteria are aerobes or facultative anaerobes and will grow well in the presence of an atmosphere of air. However, there are certain bacteria, such as *Campylobacter, Brucella* and *Haemophilus* spp., that require carbon dioxide for growth. If the presence of one of these bacteria is suspected, an atmosphere with increased carbon dioxide is necessary. Microaerophilic atmosphere-generating systems are commercially available for small numbers of cultures, or carbon dioxide–enriched atmosphere incubators can be purchased. An

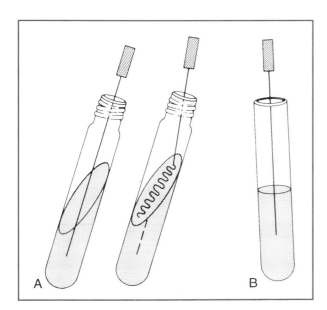

Figure 8–4. Inoculation procedure for tube medial. A, Inoculation of agar slant and butt, such as triple sugar iron (TSI). The inoculation needle is first stabbed into the butt and then removed and streaked over the agar slant surface in a back-and-forth motion. B, Inoculation of motility test media. The inoculation needle is stabbed into the medium and withdrawn along the same tract.

ideal atmosphere for growth of bacteria should have a relative humidity of about 70%. Therefore, a water reservoir, such as a pan of water on the bottom shelf of the incubator, should be provided.

Oxygen is toxic to obligate anaerobic bacteria, requiring that a special culture container from which all oxygen has been removed be used for incubation. Two excellent anaerobic systems for the small laboratory are the Bio-Bag Type A environmental chamber and the BBL Gas-Pak anaerobic system (Becton Dickinson Microbiology Systems). Each system consists of a hydrogen generator, a catalyst to facilitate the depletion of oxygen from the atmosphere by combining with the hydrogen and a sealable container to hold these components and the culture plates.

Time

All inoculated plates should be examined after 15 to 24 hours of incubation (overnight). Most cultures will have sufficient growth for evaluation and identification at this time. Culture specimens that contained bacteria on direct microscopic examination but give negative results after this time, or specimens that may be expected to contain slow-growing bacteria should be incubated up to 3 days before a final negative report is issued. Incubation of primary isolation plates beyond 3 days is rarely indicated unless there is reason to suspect an unusually slow-growing pathogen.

Routine Culture System

The majority of specimens for culture in the veterinary microbiology laboratory can be processed in a routine manner with a minimum of media. The approach presented in this section is not represented as a comprehensive culture system that will successfully isolate and identify all potentially pathogenic bacteria; rather, it is meant as a basic guideline for the veterinary technician who has the opportunity to provide a diagnostic bacteriology service within a private veterinary practice. The system is designed to be cost effective when used for routine aerobic cultures, which will usually account for 80% to 90% of culture requests. The less frequent demand for more specialized culture procedures usually does not justify the cost of maintaining an inventory of specialized media in the small laboratory. The challenge for the technician is to have the technical knowledge and ability to rapidly provide accurate culture results and the discernment to know when it is better to refer a specimen to another laboratory for more sophisticated diagnostic evaluation.

Primary Isolation Media

Blood agar, containing 5% sheep blood, is the most widely used primary isolation medium because of its ability to support growth of most pathogenic bacteria. It is also a standard medium used extensively for describing colony morphological characteristics and hemolytic patterns. MacConkey agar is also commonly used as a primary isolation medium. Although it is not always essential, it often provides significant information about bacteria and may provide presumptive identification, or at least group classification, of the isolate. If MacConkey agar is inoculated as a primary isolation medium, rather than used as a differential medium for subcultures, the identification process is often moved forward by 1 day.

In many laboratories, it is customary to include an enrichment broth as part of the primary isolation media. One of the most common broth media used for this purpose is thioglycolate. This medium can support growth of many anaerobic or facultative anaerobic bacteria that might not be recovered on primary plates incubated aerobically.

Primary growth in a broth medium is frequently difficult to interpret. It must always be compared to a direct microscopic examination because contaminating bacteria from the environment or normal flora may overgrow a pathogen in the specimen. Specimens should never be cultured solely in a broth medium for primary isolation. Further discussion of the interpretation of broth subcultures is presented later.

When specific pathogens are sought in specimens, modifications of the basic culture set-up should be incorporated into the laboratory routines. Procedures that may enhance the likelihood of recovering specific pathogens are discussed later in this chapter.

Preliminary Evaluation of Cultures

Efficient evaluation of primary cultures requires considerable skill, which is acquired only through experience in the microbiology laboratory. Clinical microbiology is probably the most subjective laboratory discipline. Decisions that must be made about isolated bacteria include their possible significance as a pathogen, which bacteria require further identification, and what additional tests are needed. As the veterinary technician gains experience in the laboratory and becomes acquainted with common bacterial pathogens, these decisions will become less difficult. One of the most important lessons to be learned is that the clinical microbiology laboratory is not a taxonomy laboratory. Clinical results, which must be obtained rapidly and accurately, must be produced at a cost economically justifiable to the client. Therefore, identification of bacteria is usually carried to the presumptive level by a few key characteristics rather than to a definitive identification. Only isolates considered to be "clinically significant" need be identified. Identification of bacterial growth that results from environmental contamination or normal flora is wasted effort.

From the initial examination of primary cultures, considerable information can be obtained to help distinguish which bacteria should be characterized in further detail. The important characteristics of primary cultures to be noted include (1) the number of different types of bacteria isolated, (2) the relative number of each type, (3) the colonial morphological characteristics of the various isolates, and (4) the changes in the media surrounding the colonies.

While making the preliminary evaluation of primary cultures, the technician must keep in mind the source of the specimen. If it was obtained from a normally sterile body site (e.g., joint fluid) and was properly handled, any growth is likely to be significant. If the specimen is from a site normally colonized by microflora (e.g., intestinal tract), interpretation becomes much more difficult. In general, if there is scant aerobic growth of three or more bacteria, the result probably reflects normal flora. Most bacterial infections, other than mixed anaerobic infections, are usually caused by only one or two agents. When a specimen from an infectious process is carefully collected, growth of a single organism in nearly pure culture will often be observed. Therefore, the most abundant colony type is usually the most important.

Some general guidelines for selection of significant isolates can be derived from colony morphological characteristics, though exceptions will always occur. Usually circular, smooth, raised, or convex opaque to gray colonies with an entire edge are more likely to be significant. Large, rough, granular, irregular, spreading, or heavily pigmented colonies are likely to be insignificant unless large numbers are recovered in nearly pure culture.

✎ TECHNICIAN NOTE

Some bacterial species characteristically produce hemolysins that can be demonstrated when the bacteria are cultured on blood agar plates, and their hemolysis affects the red blood cells (RBCs) in the zone surrounding the hemolytic colony. The following types of hemolytic activity may be observed:

- Complete hemolysis—complete lysis of RBCs in the medium resulting in a clear, colorless zone surrounding the colony. For *Streptococcus* spp., this is referred to as beta-hemolysis.
- Incomplete hemolysis—partial destruction of RBCs with some loss of hemoglobin. Due to streptococcal action on hemoglobin, a zone of greenish discoloration of the agar appears and is known as alpha-hemolysis.
- Nonhemolytic—no apparent lysis of RBCs, although there may be some discoloration of media. For *Streptococcus* spp., this is sometimes referred to as gamma-hemolysis.

Changes in the media should be carefully noted. Hemolysis in blood agar is often a good indication of a possible pathogen. Sometimes the hemolytic pattern provides adequate identification, such as the double zone of hemolysis produced by many coagulase-positive isolates of *Staphylococcus*. Pigment production can be an important characteristic to note on primary cultures. The differential features of MacConkey agar (i.e., ability to grow and lactose fermentation) are important bits of information that can aid in the identification of an isolate. Odors produced by bacteria are difficult to describe adequately, but after experience is gained, they can be another useful identifying characteristic.

The novice microbiologist may be required to rely on several differential tests for the identification of isolates. As experience is gained and confidence develops, more isolates will be recognized on the primary plates. Knowledge of the more common bacterial species to expect from a specimen (see Table 8–1) will provide a differential list of bacteria to consider so that it is not necessary to face each culture as a complete unknown.

Recording, Interpreting, and Reporting Results

Although it is impossible to devise rigid rules that provide for adequate processing of all specimens, some rigid routines are necessary for observing and recording results of cultures. A laboratory worksheet should be developed for recording all observations. It is essential that these records contain sufficient detail so that anyone who works in the laboratory can take over and complete the culture without a special briefing. A worksheet that provides adequate room for a flow chart type of illustration of culture processing and observation is easy to follow (Fig. 8–5). These work records may become part of the medical record, so care should be taken to ensure that they are complete and accurate (see Chapter 4).

As an aid to interpreting culture results, the relative abundance of growth of each type of colony should be recorded. A convenient system of recording is a scale of 1+ to 4+, in which each step on the scale represents the number of quadrants of the primary culture plate in which the colony is growing. For example, if the only colonies are in the initial streak lines in which the specimen was inoculated on the plate, growth would be rated 1+. If growth is so abundant that colonies are found in the fourth quadrant (the final streak lines), growth is rated

4+. Any bacterium isolated from broth subculture, but not on primary inoculated plates, is rated 1+, regardless of the abundance of growth on the subculture plate. Because bacterial cultures should not be evaluated empirically as positive or negative, this semiquantitative method helps the clinician to interpret the significance of the results. Specimens from most acute bacterial infections that have not been treated with antimicrobials will yield 3+ to 4+ growth. However, because of poor collection technique, mishandling the specimen, presampling antimicrobial therapy, or chronic infections, a smaller number of bacteria may be recovered. The clinician must decide whether these smaller numbers of bacteria are significant. If the culture is from a normally sterile body site, these culture results are often significant.

Normal Flora

Specimens cultured from sites with a normal flora are more difficult to interpret. Usually these cultures are insignificant if

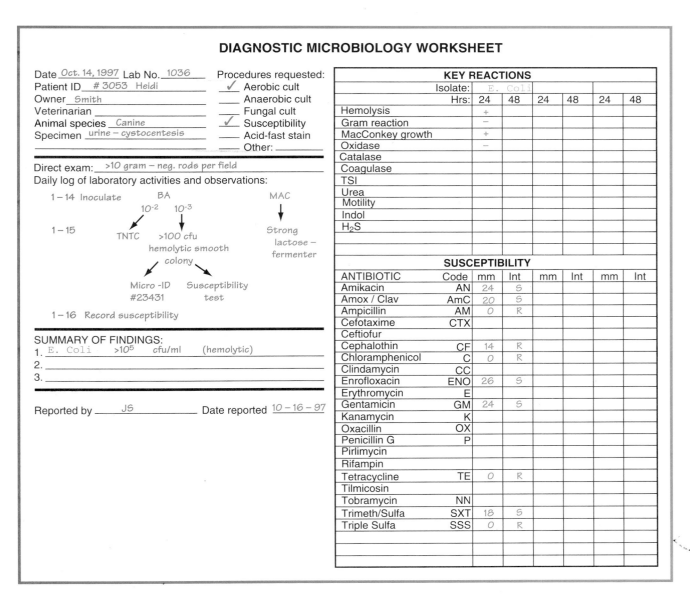

Figure 8–5. Example of a laboratory worksheet for recording results of various laboratory procedures, including microbial identification and susceptibility tests.

*Keep in mind where sample came from
↳ normal flora?
↳ sterile?

158 Chapter 8 • *Clinical Microbiology*

they result in scant growth, especially if it is a mixture of bacteria. To avoid wasting undue time precisely identifying the microflora, the technician should become familiar with flora normally found at various sites of the body (Table 8–5). Many of these bacteria are potential pathogens. If they are identified because of common recognition and are specifically reported while other, less familiar bacteria are overlooked, the report may mislead the clinician by implying undue significance.

Therefore, reporting results of cultures from sites with normal flora can be a perplexing problem. Often it is better to specify which specific pathogens have been *excluded* by careful cultural examination, such as "no *Salmonella* isolated." Between the extremes of trying to identify everything and reporting "normal flora," the technician and clinician must communicate the specific needs and most useful information expected from a given specimen. Perhaps certain potential pathogens that may be considered significant for the specimen should be carefully sought. In other situations, a predominant bacterium can be identified or groups of organisms reported (e.g., coliforms, diphtheroids, and so forth).

Identification Procedures

Rapid identification of clinically significant bacteria is best accomplished by means of a few rapid tests that can presump-

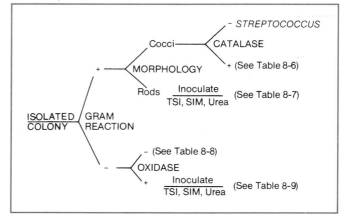

Figure 8–6. General flow chart for identification of common aerobic veterinary bacterial pathogens.

tively differentiate organisms. To one who is experienced, such characteristics as colonial morphology, hemolysis, growth on MacConkey agar, and odor may be adequate for presumptive identification. Often, additional differential tests are needed for more precise identification. Figure 8–6 presents a useful approach to identification of unknown isolates.

Gram's Reaction

The first differential characteristic that must be determined is the *Gram stain reaction*. Gram's stain can be performed on thin smears of bacteria from a single colony (see instructions for Gram's stain preparation in the section on Direct Microscopic Examination). Potassium hydroxide, 3%, may be used as an alternate and more rapid test for the Gram reaction of isolated colonies. A small drop of 3% potassium hydroxide (no larger than a colony) is dispensed on a slide, and a colony of bacteria is picked from the blood agar plate with a bacteriological loop and is mixed into the 3% potassium hydroxide. The loop is slowly and gently lifted at 5-second intervals to see whether a viscous gel is sticking to the loop. The formation of any sticky strand that can be lifted with the loop is indicative of a gram-negative bacterium. The reaction should appear within 20 to 30 seconds. Gram-positive organisms will diffusely mix in the 3% potassium hydroxide. Cellular morphological characteristics of the gram-positive bacteria are important differential characteristics that require careful examination of a stained smear.

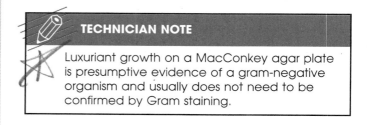

TECHNICIAN NOTE

Luxuriant growth on a MacConkey agar plate is presumptive evidence of a gram-negative organism and usually does not need to be confirmed by Gram staining.

Catalase Test

Catalase activity is an important and rapid test for differentiating *Staphylococcus* from *Streptococcus* and *Erysipelothrix* and *Actinomyces pyogenes* from other small gram-positive rods. Hydrogen peroxide (3%) is the only reagent needed and can

• Table 8–5 •

SITE	AEROBES	ANAEROBES
Skin, ear	*Staphylococcus, Micrococcus,* diphtheroids, and transient environmental and fecal contaminants	
Mouth, nasopharynx	*Micrococcus, Staphylococcus, Streptococcus* (alpha and beta), *Bacillus,* coliforms, *Proteus, Pasteurella, Actinobacillus, Haemophilus,* and *Mycoplasma*	*Bacteroides, Prevotella, Porphyromonas, Fusobacterium, Actinomyces,* spirochetes, and others
Trachea, bronchi, lungs	No residents, only transient contaminants	
Stomach, small intestine	Small numbers of alpha-*Streptococcus*	*Lactobacillus*
Large intestine	*Streptococcus, Escherichia coli, Klebsiella, Enterobacter, Proteus,* and others	*Clostridium, Fusobacterium, Bacteroides, Porphyromonas, Prevotella,* spirochetes, *Lactobacillus*
Vulva, prepuce	Diphtheroids, *Micrococcus, Staphylococcus,* and fecal organisms	
Conjunctiva, uterus, mammary glands	These areas may occasionally contain small numbers of insignificant bacteria	

NORMAL FLORA

Catalase = bacteria + hydrogen peroxide → bubbling (+)

readily be purchased from any drugstore. It should be stored in a dark bottle in the refrigerator. The *slide catalase test* is performed by picking bacteria from the center of a colony with a needle or loop and smearing the bacteria on a clean, dry slide. A drop of hydrogen peroxide is added over the bacteria and immediately observed for bubbling. Lack of bubbling is a negative test. The order of the test procedure must not be reversed or false-positive results can be obtained. If any blood agar is introduced into the test, it can also cause a false-positive result.

Oxidase Test

Cytochrome oxidase activity should be determined for all gram-negative bacteria except strong lactose fermenters, which will be negative. Commercial cytochrome oxidase test reagents are readily available and conveniently packaged for use in small laboratories. The reaction is supposed to be clearly visible within a few seconds, but with some of the reagents the reaction may be delayed for up to 2 minutes for *Pasteurella* and *Actinobacillus*. A heavy inoculum must be used for accurate testing. A wooden stick or platinum loop should be used to pick colonies for testing, because trace amounts of iron from other loops can cause false-positive results.

Presumptive Identification

When the Gram reaction, cellular morphological characteristics, and catalase and oxidase results have been determined, the bacteria can be tentatively grouped, and differential tests can be selected as indicated in Figure 8–6 for identification.

Isolates of *Streptococcus* are usually characterized by the type of hemolysis they produce. Beta-hemolytic *Streptococcus* is usually considered to be a potential pathogen. Alpha- and nonhemolytic *Streptococcus* usually originate from normal flora of skin and mucous membranes and are not considered significant unless they are isolated from normally sterile sites.

Isolates of *Staphylococcus* should be differentiated from *Micrococcus* (Table 8–6), which are considered to be nonpathogenic. Glucose-fermenting ability, determined in TSI agar slants, can be used for differentiation of these genera. If a double zone of hemolysis is observed on the blood agar plate, the bacterium can be identified as a coagulase-positive *Staphylococcus* without need for further testing. All other *Staphylococcus* isolates should be tested for coagulase activity because coagulase activ-

ity correlates with pathogenicity. Speciation of coagulase-positive and coagulase-negative *Staphylococcus* spp. may be attempted in special cases.

The small gram-positive rods can be differentiated by inoculating TSI, urea, and sulfide-indole-motility (SIM) media. The results of these tests, as well as colonial morphology and catalase activity, can identify the isolate (Table 8–7). Individual characteristics of the important pathogens in this group will be discussed later.

Most gram-negative, oxidase-negative bacteria are members of the Enterobacteriaceae family. These bacteria are reactive in biochemical tests and can be identified by one of several different systems. The most rapid and economical methods for differentiating the Enterobacteriaceae family members are the commercially available packaged multitest systems. These systems are discussed later. There are a few other organisms that may be isolated infrequently that are oxidase negative. The most common reason for nonenteric oxidase-negative results is a false-negative oxidase test result. When such results are suspected, further differentiation of oxidase-negative bacteria, as shown in Table 8–8, is necessary.

The most frequently isolated oxidase-positive, gram-negative bacteria of veterinary importance can be differentiated by using three tubes of media (TSI, urea, and SIM) as shown in Table 8–9.

• Table 8–6 •

DIFFERENTIATION OF GRAM-POSITIVE, CATALASE-POSITIVE COCCI

ORGANISM	HEMOLYSIS	HYALURONI-DASE	GLUCOSE FERMEN-TATION	COAGULASE
Staphylococcus aureus	+*	+	+	+
Staphylococcus intermedius	+*	−	+	+
Staphylococcus epidermidis	±		+	−
Micrococcus	−		−	−

*Double zones of complete and incomplete hemolysis are frequently observed.

• Table 8–7 •

DIFFERENTIATION OF SMALL, NONSPORE-FORMING GRAM-POSITIVE RODS

ORGANISM	MOTILITY (22°)	CATALASE	HYDROGEN SULFIDE IN TSI	UREASE	HEMOLYSIS	COLONY MORPHOLOGICAL CHARACTERISTICS
Listeria monocytogenes	+	+	−	−	Complete	Very small
Erysipelothrix rhusiopathiae	−	−	+	−	Slow, greenish	Very small
Actinomyces pyogenes	−	−	−	−	Complete	Very small
Corynebacterium renale	−	+	−	+	V	Medium size, entire
Corynebacterium pseudotuberculosis	−	+	−	+ (w)	V	Dry, grainy white
Rhodococcus equi	−	+	−	+ (d)		Large, mucoid, pink
Other diphtheroids	−	+	−	V	V	V

d, delayed, may require up to 2 weeks; V, variable results; w, weak.

• Table 8–8 •

DIFFERENTIATION OF GRAM-NEGATIVE, OXIDASE-NEGATIVE BACTERIA				
	GROWTH ON MACCONKEY	TSI	MOTILITY	IDENTIFICATION METHOD
Enterobacteriaceae	+	A /A, K/A	+*	Micro-ID or API 20E
Pasteurella, Actinobacillus	−	A /A, A/NC	−	See Table 8-9†
Pseudomonas	+	K/NC	+	
Acinetobacter	+ (w)	K/NC	−	

Klebsiella is nonmotile.
†Negative oxidase results are caused by very weak reactions.
w, weak; A, acid; K, alkaline; NC, no change.

Definitive Identification

The identification procedures discussed in this chapter are presumptive methods. Definitive identification of some isolates may require extensive testing. The cost of such identification in time, media and specialized techniques is usually not justifiable in a small practice laboratory. Unusual isolates should be forwarded to a referral laboratory for further identification. The isolate should be subcultured to an agar slant medium that does not contain a fermentable carbohydrate, or it should be heavily inoculated onto a swab. The swab can be transported in a transport medium such as Amies transport medium. Do not attempt to ship agar plates. Invariably, they become contaminated and overgrown, dehydrated, or broken.

Commercial Identification Kits

Commercial development of kit systems for identification of bacteria has been one of the most important advances in clinical bacteriology. These systems provide a cost-effective method for identification of bacteria in low-volume laboratories. Most kits consist of a number of test compartments arranged in a compact unit. The systems generally involve the use of microtechnique tests in various types of media systems. They may include compartments of solid agar, dehydrated broth, substrate or reagent disks, and supplementary conventional tests. All compartments are inoculated with organisms from an isolated colony

or colonies. After the specified period of incubation and the addition of required reagents, the results are recorded as positive or negative for each test. For many of the systems, these reactions have variously weighted values so that the positive results will produce a unique profile number for each combination of positive and negative results. Most systems provide profile directories or registers for identification of the isolate most likely to produce the set of observed reactions.

It is advantageous for the low-volume laboratory to use these systems because they are usually more cost effective than attempting to maintain a large inventory of conventional media. They have a reasonable shelf life (6 to 18 months) and require minimum storage space because of the compact construction. Accuracy is better than conventional media in most small laboratories, as most reactions are easy to interpret and results can be decoded more rapidly than sorting through conventional identification tables. Finally, depending on the specific system, most bacteria can be identified within 4 to 24 hours after isolation.

It is absolutely essential that the manufacturer's directions and precautions be followed implicitly or misidentification will occur. If the system is limited to oxidase-negative enteric bacteria, only those organisms should be inoculated. Other organisms can still yield a profile number, which will result in an incorrect identification. Therefore, these systems still require evaluation by a competent microbiologist who can determine

• Table 8–9 •

DIFFERENTIATION OF GRAM-NEGATIVE, OXIDASE-POSITIVE BACTERIA						
ORGANISM	GLUCOSE FERMENTATION IN TSI AGAR	GROWTH ON MACCONKEY AGAR	MOTILITY	HEMOLYSIS	UREASE	INDOLE
Aeromonas spp.	+	+	+	+	−	+
Actinobacillus spp.	+	±	−	+ (V)	+	−
Pasteurella haemolytica	+	±	−	+*	−	−
Pasteurella multocida	+	−	−	−	−	+
Pasteurella pneumotropica	+	−	−	−	+	+
Pasteurella spp.	+	−	−	−	±	−
Pseudomonas aeruginosa	−	+	+	+	±	−
Pseudomonas spp.	−	+	+	V	V	−
Bordetella bronchiseptica	−	+ (w)	+	−	+	−
Moraxella bovis	−	−	−	±	−	−
Moraxella spp.	−	−	−	±	−	−
Brucella canis	−	−	−	−	+	−

*Hemolysis under the colony.
V, variable; w, weak.

whether the results correlate with other laboratory findings and the clinical history. Problems can also arise from inoculation with an older culture, improper concentration of inoculum or mixed cultures. For the proper use of these systems, some personnel retraining may be necessary. As experience is gained, accuracy will be increased.

When selecting one of these systems, factors to consider include (1) the ease of inoculation, (2) manipulations required to add reagents, (3) the availability of interpretive charts or numerical coding devices, and (4) the data base used in development of profile registers. Often, it is difficult to discover whether significant numbers of veterinary pathogens are included in the data bases for there to be a reasonable probability of correct identification of unique veterinary pathogens.

The most beneficial use of these systems is the identification of members of the Enterobacteriaceae family (see Table 8–3). All enteric identification systems give essentially the same degree of accuracy and reliability of performance if strict attention is paid to the manufacturer's instructions. The systems that seem to have gained widest acceptance in veterinary bacteriology include API 20E, Micro-ID, and Enterotube II. The data base and accuracy of the identifications provide excellent results.

Several packaged kit systems are marketed for identification of gram-negative bacteria other than Enterobacteriaceae (see Table 8–3). These systems have limited usefulness in small veterinary laboratories. Present data bases are largely based on human pathogens rather than unique gram-negative bacteria that are host specific to various animals (*Pasteurella, Actinobacillus, Haemophilus, Moraxella,* and so forth). Presumptive identification methods outlined in this chapter are frequently more accurate and less expensive.

Identification kits are available for gram-positive cocci (see Table 8–3). Although these systems may provide more definitive identifications of some organisms, the clinical relevance and cost-effectiveness of their use has not been adequately evaluated in veterinary microbiology.

The identification kits for yeast and anaerobes are useful for large-volume laboratories, but usually the need for them in the small laboratory is not adequate to be cost effective.

Special Culture Procedures

Blood Cultures

The detection of viable bacteria in an animal's blood has considerable diagnostic and prognostic importance. Blood cultures are indicated for fever of unknown origin, suspected bacteremia associated with endocarditis, arthritis, meningitis, and neonatal septicemias. Blood cultures should be obtained from dogs that have antibodies to *Brucella canis* to aid in confirmation of the diagnosis.

Special care must be taken to avoid contaminating blood cultures with skin microflora. The venipuncture site should be decontaminated using surgical scrubbing procedures (see Chapter 16) and should not be palpated after preparation unless a sterile glove is used. Blood can be obtained by using a syringe and needle or a closed-vacuum bottle system. Often the concentration of bacteria in blood is too low to detect by direct inoculation of plate media. Therefore, inoculation of broth media is a more sensitive culture system. Ideally, a sample of 5 to 10 ml of blood should be obtained for culture. The blood should be inoculated into an approved blood culture bottle

immediately. Blood samples in anticoagulants, such as heparin and ethylenediamine-tetraacetic acid (EDTA), are not acceptable for culture because of the poor survival of some bacteria in the presence of these anticoagulants. Commercially available blood culture media bottles are recommended.

Blood culture samples should not be obtained more frequently than once per hour. If a patient in critical condition is to be started immediately on antibiotics, multiple samples should be collected from different venipuncture sites. Usually, arterial blood provides a yield that is no better than that provided by venous blood. For fever of unknown origin and subacute endocarditis, obtain two separate blood cultures on the first day and again on the second day if bacterial growth is not present in the first set of cultures.

Blood culture bottles should be incubated at 35°C to 37°C for at least 7 days and examined daily for macroscopic evidence of growth. Positive cultures can be recognized by one or more of the following characteristics, turbidity, gas bubbles, fluffy or compact colonies, and hemolysis of the blood. When growth is observed, gram-stained smears and subcultures on plate media should be prepared for examination and identification of the organism. Negative-appearing blood culture broths should be blindly subcultured before being discarded and reported as negative.

Brucella isolation from blood can be enhanced by using a biphasic system that provides an agar surface for more efficient isolation of *Brucella*. Cultures for this agent should be held for 2 to 4 weeks before being discarded as negative.

Urine Cultures → ASAP

Urine is an excellent growth medium for many bacteria because it contains electrolytes, water-soluble vitamins, residual amounts of glucose, and various nitrogenous compounds. Therefore, it is imperative that careful attention be given in proper collection and handling of urine for culture, or a small and insignificant number of bacteria can rapidly multiply to significant numbers. Urine specimens for culturing can be collected in three ways: (1) free catch, (2) catheterization, or (3) cystocentesis (see Chapter 10). The distal urethra and genitalia are colonized with microflora that contaminate free-catch and catheterization specimens. If the skin has been adequately prepared for cystocentesis specimens, and the needle does not contact any abdominal organ other than the bladder, any bacteria isolated from the specimen should be significant. To reduce overgrowth with insignificant bacteria that may contaminate urine specimens, cultures should be set up within 2 hours of collection. If cultures cannot be established within 2 hours, the sample must be refrigerated to slow the bacterial growth. Refrigeration begins to fail after 18 to 24 hours. Therefore, the best method for identifying urinary tract infections is to establish cultures as soon as possible.

The use of blood agar and MacConkey agar as selective and differential isolation media is recommended for the culture of all urine specimens. There is no need for broth medium for enrichment culturing. The bacteriological examination of urine specimens collected by methods other than cystocentesis should provide an estimate of the number of microorganisms per milliliter of urine as an aid to interpreting the results. This can be accomplished by inoculating the blood agar plate with a standard dilution loop calibrated to deliver approximately 0.001 ml, as illustrated in Figure 8–7. Each colony that grows

Cysto → if done properly, any growth is significant

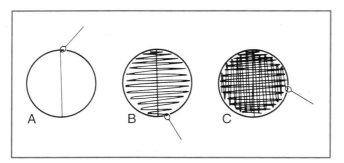

Figure 8–7. Procedure for inoculating media for semiquantitative bacterial colony counts when culturing urine. A, Primary inoculation with calibrated loop. B, Streak at right angles to primary inoculation. C, Streak at right angles to previous streak.

represents 10^3 organisms/ml in the specimen; therefore, the number of colonies is multiplied by 1000 to obtain the concentration of organisms in the specimen. The number of bacteria can also be estimated through direct microscopic examination of a gram-stained smear of uncentrifuged urine. If one or more bacteria per oil immersion field are observed, usually more than 10^5 organisms/ml should be present in cultures. If more than two types of bacteria are isolated, a second specimen should be collected and cultured to distinguish a mixed infection from contamination or mishandling of the specimen. Bacterial counts can be low because of improper handling of the specimen, dilution from forced fluid therapy, or cystocentesis samples from patients with urethritis that has not become established as a concomitant cystitis. Bacteria isolated from urine are identified as described in this chapter.

TECHNICIAN NOTE

Guidelines for interpretation of urine cultures:

- More than 10^5 bacteria/ml of a single species is indicative of significant bacteria.
- Between 10^3 and 10^5 bacteria/ml is suggestive of infection if the urine has been properly collected and neutrophils are present.
- Fewer than 10^3 bacteria/ml is suggestive of contamination or mishandling of the specimen.

If there is doubt about interpreting a colony count, the culture should be repeated with a second specimen.

COMMON BACTERIAL SPECIES

The bacterial pathogens frequently associated with many infectious processes are listed in Table 8-1. Some of the colony morphological, growth, and identifying characteristics of these bacteria are listed in Table 8–10. Additional details are given in the following discussion for special isolation and identification techniques. Clinically important characteristics are noted.

Gram-Positive Cocci

Staphylococcus

Staphylococcus spp. are catalase-positive cocci that occur in grape-like clusters. They are frequently isolated from pyogenic lesions, such as wounds, dermatitis, otitis, mastitis, cystitis, and osteomyelitis. As stated previously, they are usually divided into coagulase-positive and coagulase-negative strains. The coagulase-positive species, *S. aureus* and *S. intermedius,* are more important pathogens, and the others are usually considered to be less pathogenic. One of the most important identifying characteristics that should be noted is the development of a double zone of hemolysis (an inner zone of complete hemolysis and a second zone of incomplete hemolysis). This is a common identifying characteristic of most coagulase-positive isolates from animals. Mannitol fermentation is not a reliable correlate of coagulase activity in staphylococcal isolates from animals. Because of a high incidence of acquired antimicrobial resistance, these organisms should be tested for antimicrobial susceptibility.

Streptococcus

Streptococcus spp. are catalase-negative cocci that occur singly, in pairs, or in short chains. Chain formation is more easily demonstrated in broth cultures. *Streptococcus* is the most common bacterial pathogen of the horse and can be found to cause pyogenic infections and mastitis in all species of animals. However, the species tend to be rather host-specific. Therefore, the streptococcal pathogens of humans rarely cause infections in animals, and animals are usually not reservoirs of human pathogens. Some species cause specific diseases. *Streptococcus equi* is the cause of strangles in horses. *Streptococcus agalactiae* is an important cause of bovine mastitis. It can be identified by the CAMP test. Definitive biochemical and serological (Lancefield typing) testing is usually not clinically important. It is important to evaluate the hemolysis produced on blood agar. Beta-hemolysis (complete clearing) usually correlates well with potential pathogenicity; alpha-hemolysis (incomplete greenish discoloring) and gamma-hemolysis (nonhemolytic) are usually indications of normal flora of skin and mucous membranes. However, when isolated in nearly pure culture from normally sterile body sites, these organisms can be considered to be clinically significant. Susceptibility to antimicrobials is usually predictable, which means antimicrobial susceptibility testing may be an unnecessary expense.

The enteric group D streptococci have been reclassified as *Enterococcus* spp. Urinary tract infections are the most common presentation of these organisms; they occasionally infect wounds and cause bacteremia. They are emerging as significant nosocomial agents and are particularly troublesome because they are likely to be resistant to many antimicrobials.

Anaerobic Cocci

Anaerobic cocci belong to the genera *Peptococcus* and *Peptostreptococcus.* When isolated, these agents are usually associated with mixed anaerobic infections.

Gram-Positive Rods

Spore Formers

Bacillus spp. are the most common contaminants isolated in the laboratory. They are ubiquitous in soil, water, air, and dust.

• Table 8–10 •

IDENTIFYING CHARACTERISTICS OF COMMON VETERINARY BACTERIAL PATHOGENS			
	BLOOD AGAR	**MACCONKEY AGAR**	**OTHER CHARACTERISTICS**
Gram-positive			
Staphylococcus	Smooth, glistening white to yellow pigmented colonies.	No growth.	Catalase-positive glucose fermenter. Double-zone hemolysis usually indicates coagulase-positive. Coagulase activity is a useful differential test.
Streptococcus	Small, glistening colonies; hemolysis.	No growth except some enterococci.	Catalase-negative, usually identified by type of hemolysis. Beta-hemolytic strains more likely to be pathogens, others are often part of flora; *Streptococcus agalactiae* CAMP-positive.
Actinomyces pyogenes	Small, hemolytic strep-like colonies.	No growth.	Catalase-negative; slow growth, often requiring 48 hr for distinct colonies, growth enhanced in candle jar.
Corynebacterium pseudotuberculosis	Slow-growing, opaque, dry crumbly colonies; usually hemolytic.	No growth.	Catalase-positive; weak urease-positive.
Corynebacterium renale	Small, smooth, glistening colonies (24 hr); become opaque and dry later.	No growth.	Catalase-positive, urease-positive.
Rhodococcus equi	Small, moist, white (24 hr) become large, pink colonies, no hemolysis.	No growth.	Catalase-positive, delayed urease-positive.
Listeria monocytogenes	Small, hemolytic, glistening colonies.	No growth.	Catalase-positive, motile at room temperature.
Erysipelothrix rhusiopathiae	Small colonies after 48 hr; greenish (alpha) hemolysis.	No growth.	Catalase-negative, hydrogen sulfide-positive.
Nocardia	Slow-growing, small, dry, granular, white to orange colonies.	No growth.	Partially acid-fast, colonies tenaciously adhere to media.
Actinomyces	Slow-growing, small, rough, nodular white colonies.	No growth.	Require increased carbon dioxide or anaerobic incubation, not acid-fast.
Clostridium	Variable, round, ill-defined, irregular colonies usually hemolytic.	No growth.	Obligate anaerobes.
Bacillus	Variable, large, rough, dry or mucoid colonies.	No growth.	Usually hemolytic, large rods with endospores.
Gram-negative			
Escherichia coli	Large, gray, smooth, mucoid colonies, hemolysis variable.	Hot-pink to red colonies; red cloudiness in media.	Hemolysis frequently associated with virulence.
Klebsiella pneumoniae	Large, mucoid, sticky, whitish colonies, not hemolytic.	Large, mucoid, pink colonies.	Nonmotile, require biochemical tests to differentiate from *Enterobacter.*
Proteus	Frequently swarming without distinct colonies.	Colorless, limited swarming.	
Other enterics	Gray to white smooth, mucoid colonies.	Colorless colonies.	Biochemical tests for identification, serotyping indicated for *Salmonella.*
Pseudomonas	Irregular, spreading, grayish colonies, variable hemolysis, may show a metallic sheen.	Colorless, irregular colonies.	Oxidase-positive, fruity odor, may produce yellow-greenish soluble pigment in clear media.
Bordetella bronchiseptica	Very small, circular dewdrop colonies, variable hemolysis.	Small, colorless colonies.	May require 48 hr for distinct colonies, oxidase-positive, rapid urease-positive, citrate-positive.
Brucella canis	Very small, circular, pinpoint colonies after 48–72 hr, not hemolytic.	No growth.	Oxidase-positive, catalase-positive, urease-positive.
Moraxella	Round, translucent, grayish-white colonies, variable hemolysis.	No growth.	Oxidase- and catalase-positive, often nonreactive in routine biochemical tests. Colonies may pit media.
Actinobacillus	Round, translucent colonies, variable hemolysis.	Variable growth, colorless colonies.	Glucose fermenter, nonmotile, urease-positive. Sticky colonies.
Pasteurella haemolytica	Round, gray, smooth colonies; hemolysis under the colony.	Variable growth, colorless colonies.	Glucose fermenter in TSI, weak oxidase-positive.
Pasteurella multocida	Gray, mucoid, round to coalescing colonies, no hemolysis.	No growth.	Glucose fermenter in TSI, weak oxidase- and indole-positives.

They are large spore-forming rods that usually grow as large, rough, granular, or spreading colonies. They are usually hemolytic. Occasionally, strains of *Bacillus* will be isolated that react as if they are gram-negative and oxidase-positive. However, they can be identified by the presence of spores in stained smears. *Bacillus anthracis* (the agent that causes anthrax) is the only important pathogenic species. It is extremely virulent for humans. *Do not attempt to culture it.*

Clostridium spp. are large, spore-forming anaerobic rods. There are many nonpathogenic species of soil origin. The pathogenic species are noted for their potent toxins and extensive destruction of tissue. Infections may be accompanied by an accumulation of gas (emphysema) in the tissues. Laboratory diagnosis of the toxic diseases (tetanus, botulism, and enterotoxemia) and differentiation of the infectious diseases (blackleg, malignant edema, bacillary hemoglobinuria, and so forth) require the assistance of reference diagnostic laboratories. Often, a Gram-stained smear is a useful technique for ruling out clostridial disease or indicating it as a possibility. *Clostridium perfringens* is occasionally isolated from deep wounds with extensive tissue necrosis, such as compound fractures. The bacterium requires an anaerobic atmosphere for growth and frequently produces a double zone of hemolysis.

C. perfringens is emerging as a common agent associated with enteritis and diarrhea in dogs. The presence of enterotoxigenic strains of *C. perfringens* can be presumptively identified in fecal smears by evaluating them for the presence of increased bacterial spores because sporulation is associated with the release of enterotoxin. Spores appear as unstained, small, oval structures, usually surrounded by a halo of stained bacterial cell unless a specific spore stain is applied.

Small Rods

Corynebacterium spp. are small, club-shaped rods that tend to occur in palisades or in an angular arrangement because of their "snapping" division. Colonies are usually quite small at 24 hours but continue to enlarge and vary markedly by species. Most species are catalase positive. *Actinomyces pyogenes* (previously called *C. pyogenes*) produces a small pinpoint colony, hemolysis, and negative catalase reaction. Cellular morphological characteristics must be evaluated carefully to differentiate it from *Streptococcus*. It is the most common pyogenic agent in ruminants. *Rhodococcus equi* (also known as *Corynebacterium equi*) is a cause of pneumonia and abscesses in foals. Morphologically, individual cells are coccobacillary and larger than other *Corynebacterium* organisms. *Corynebacterium pseudotuberculosis* (formerly known as *C. ovis*) causes chronic abscesses in goats and sheep. *Corynebacterium renale* is a cause of pyelonephritis and cystitis in cows. There are many other *Corynebacterium* spp. that are nonpathogenic commensals of the skin; they are frequently referred to collectively as diphtheroids.

Listeria monocytogenes is a small, non–spore-forming rod that is catalase positive. It is the only small gram-positive rod that is motile at room temperature. It is an infrequent cause of abortion in large animals and septicemia in young animals. In ruminants, it causes an encephalitis known as circling disease. The bacteria localize in the pons and medulla (brain stem). Cultures from other parts of the brain may be negative. Isolation may require a cold enrichment technique. The brain is stored in a refrigerator and cultured weekly for up to 12 weeks before the results are considered negative.

Erysipelothrix rhusiopathiae is a pleomorphic rod, which is usually slender and small. The colony is small, and an incomplete, greenish hemolysis (alpha-like) is produced. The cellular morphological characteristics must be carefully evaluated to differentiate it from *Streptococcus* because both are catalase negative. A definitive characteristic that differentiates it from other gram-positive rods is the production of hydrogen sulfide. *Erysipelothrix* is most commonly encountered as a cause of septicemic or arthritic disease of pigs, but it is occasionally a cause of endocarditis in dogs.

Filamentous Rods

The Actinomycetaceae family contains several clinically important bacteria. Most *Actinomyces* spp. are anaerobic bacteria that may tolerate low levels of oxygen. Therefore, some species can be isolated in a candle jar, but the most efficient isolation can be achieved with an anaerobic system. *Actinomyces* spp. are usually branching, filamentous gram-positive rods. Colonies are slow to develop, requiring up to 5 days, and are usually raised and irregular in shape. When isolated, they are usually recovered from pyogranulomatous lesions of soft tissue, pyothoraces, or osteomyelitis. *Nocardia* spp. have cellular morphological characteristics similar to those of *Actinomyces*. They are partially acid-fast, which means a modified staining procedure must be used. In place of the acid-alcohol decolorizer, only an acid decolorizer is used to demonstrate acid-fastness. *Nocardia* spp. are aerobic bacteria with colonies usually appearing after 2 to 5 days of incubation. The colonies are rough and have a dry, granular texture. They adhere tenaciously to the media. *Nocardia* is occasionally isolated from pyothoraces and wounds. It may be a serious mastitis pathogen in some dairy herds. *Dermatophilus congolensis* is another branching, filamentous bacterium. It often has a beaded appearance with transverse and longitudinal divisions. It is an uncommon cause of skin infections of horses and ruminants. The organism can be demonstrated in smears of pus from under the elevated scabs containing tufts of hair. *Streptomyces* spp. are aerobic, filamentous bacteria that are not acid-fast. They are abundant in soil and may be isolated as contaminants.

Anaerobes

Anaerobic gram-positive non–spore-forming rods belong to the genera *Bifidobacterium, Eubacterium,* and *Propionibacterium*. If definitive identification of these organisms is needed, they should be sent to a reference diagnostic laboratory. They are usually isolated in mixed cultures from pyogenic lesions.

Acid-Fast Bacteria

Mycobacteria are mostly small, short rods but are occasionally pleomorphic. They stain poorly with Gram's stain but are acid-fast. These bacteria are rarely isolated in veterinary practice laboratories because special procedures and media are usually required. However, preparation of an acid-fast stained impression smear can be a useful diagnostic procedure for making a presumptive diagnosis of mycobacterial infection. Positive findings are significant; however, negative findings have limited predictive value. *Mycobacterium paratuberculosis* may be demonstrated in acid-fast stained smears prepared from intestinal mucosa or mesenteric lymph nodes of ruminants. *Mycobacterium avium* infection of birds can frequently be confirmed by examination of acid-fast smears prepared from the liver or intestinal mucosa. Occasionally, abundant acid-fast organisms can be demonstrated in the feces.

Isolation of the agents of tuberculosis, *Mycobacterium bovis* and *Mycobacterium tuberculosis,* should not be attempted in a clinic laboratory. Infrequently, a rapid-growing *Mycobacterium* may be isolated from cases of bovine mastitis. The colonies will usually appear at 3 to 5 days of incubation. These organisms should be forwarded to a reference laboratory for definitive identification.

Gram-Negative Bacteria

The Enterobacteriaceae family of bacteria is the largest group of potential pathogens and the most frequently isolated bacteria. The normal habitat of these organisms is the digestive tract and soil; therefore, they will usually grow on MacConkey agar and are frequently insignificant contaminants of specimens. They are small gram-negative rods, with some pleomorphism. Some of the common identifying characteristics include oxidase negativity, glucose fermentation and motility (except *Klebsiella*). Genus and species identification requires numerous biochemical tests, and serotyping is frequently needed to identify pathogenic strains. Acquired antimicrobial resistance from R-factors (plasmids) is common in this family of bacteria, making antimicrobial susceptibility testing a necessary clinical evaluation of isolates.

Most non-Enterobacteriaceae gram-negative bacteria are oxidase positive, and growth on MacConkey agar is variable.

Coliforms

Escherichia coli can frequently be presumptively identified by the strong lactose fermentation reaction it produces on MacConkey agar. Strains causing tissue infections and cystitis are frequently hemolytic. *Escherichia coli* is frequently associated with diarrhea in neonates (especially pigs, calves, and lambs). The pathogenic strains causing diarrhea have special surface antigens (pili) and produce enterotoxins. Identification of these characteristics requires specialized laboratory testing, such as use of the K-99 *E. coli* antigen test kit (K99 Pilitest, VMRD, Inc.). However, presumptive evidence of *E. coli* involvement in diarrhea (scours) can be obtained by Gram-staining a smear taken from small intestinal mucosa shortly after the death of the animal. If a large number (>25) of gram-negative rods are observed in each oil immersion field, it is a strong indication that *E. coli* is a cause of diarrhea.

Klebsiella spp. and *Enterobacter* spp. are occasionally involved in infections of the respiratory and urinary tracts and in mastitis. They are becoming more important in veterinary medicine as superinfecting agents after antimicrobial therapy.

Salmonella

Salmonella spp. can cause diarrhea and septicemia in all animals and in humans. When culturing feces, selective and enrichment media should be used to increase the probability of successful isolation of *Salmonella*. Hektoen enteric agar and selenite enrichment broth (see Table 8-2) are recommended. The enrichment broth should be subcultured to both MacConkey and Hektoen enteric agar. Non–lactose-fermenting colonies can rapidly be screened with *Salmonella* polyvalent O antiserum to identify them. To be able to define the epidemiology of salmonellosis outbreaks, the isolates should be forwarded to a reference laboratory for serotyping.

Proteus

Proteus spp. are frequently isolated as specimen contaminants or secondary invaders. They are important pathogens of the urinary tract. Related genera of bacteria that do not swarm on blood agar are *Morganella* and *Providencia*. The swarming *Proteus* spp. sometimes interfere with isolation of other organisms. This problem can be solved by using phenylethyl alcohol (PEA) blood agar plates. *Proteus* and other gram-negative organisms will be inhibited, providing easier isolation of gram-positive organisms.

Other Enterics

There are many other members of the Enterobacteriaceae family, including *Serratia, Citrobacter, Edwardsiella,* and *Hafnia,* that are infrequently isolated. Careful clinical evaluation is necessary to determine their significance. Often, a repeated culture helps confirm the significance of isolation.

Aeromonas

Aeromonas spp. are oxidase-positive rods that grow on MacConkey agar. They are commonly found in soil, water, and sewage and frequently infect aquatic animals. They are infrequently a cause of septicemia in terrestrial animals. Some strains grow best at room temperature.

Actinobacillus

Actinobacillus spp. are oxidase-positive, small rods that usually grow on MacConkey agar. The colony morphological characteristics are similar to those of *Pasteurella*. *Actinobacillus equuli* is the most frequently isolated species. It produces a very sticky colony. It is frequently the cause of septicemic infections in foals. It can be isolated from most horses as part of the naso-oropharyngeal flora but is generally only an opportunistic pathogen in older horses.

Pasteurella

Pasteurella spp. are usually associated with respiratory infections in most animals. In cats, they are frequently recovered from abscesses. They are small, oxidase-positive coccobacilli. Identification can be aided by noting the typically weak glucose fermentation reaction in a TSI tube. *Pasteurella* spp. tend to be nonreactive in most commercial identification kit systems and may be misidentified. All *Pasteurella* spp. are nonhemolytic except *Pasteurella haemolytica*. Its colony must be removed to observe the hemolysis that occurs directly under the colony. *Pasteurella multocida* produces a characteristic "musty" odor.

Haemophilus

Haemophilus spp. are often part of the normal flora of mucous membranes. A few species are important pathogens, usually of the respiratory system. They are small coccobacilli that require specially enriched media for growth. They may grow as satellite colonies around *Staphylococcus* on blood agar. In addition to the nutritional growth requirements, an increased concentration of carbon dioxide is necessary. These bacteria are very susceptible to antibiotics and environmental stress factors, such as drying; therefore, specimens must be collected and handled carefully or isolation will be unsuccessful.

Pseudomonas

Pseudomonas spp. are common soil and water bacteria. They are usually considered to be opportunistic pathogens of wounds and otitis. Infrequently, they are isolated from the respiratory and urinary tracts. There are many species, but *Pseudomonas aeruginosa* is the most common pathogen. It produces water-soluble yellow-green pigments that diffuse into the media, and it has a distinctive odor that aids in recognition.

Bordetella

Bordetella bronchiseptica is a small coccobacillus that is frequently recovered from respiratory infections of dogs. It is associated with atrophic rhinitis in pigs and is infrequently isolated from respiratory infections of other animals. Colonies are slow to develop and may only be pinpointed after 48 hours. Growth occurs on MacConkey agar. It is oxidase positive, urease positive (often within 4 hours), and citrate positive.

Brucella

Brucella spp. are very small coccobacilli that are usually associated with reproductive failure—abortion and infertility. Some species require increased carbon dioxide for growth: however, *Brucella canis* can be isolated in an aerobic atmosphere. Growth is slow, often requiring from 3 to 7 days for colonies to be detectable. Suspected *Brucella* isolates should be sent to a reference laboratory for definitive identification because of the economic and zoonotic importance of these agents.

Other Gram-Negative Rods

There are a large number of gram-negative bacteria that have little or undetermined clinical importance. Included are bacteria such as *Moraxella, Acinetobacter, Neisseria, Branhamella,* and related pleomorphic coccobacilli. These organisms are commonly found as part of the flora of mucous membranes and are usually secondary, opportunistic pathogens. They are relatively nonreactive in most conventional biochemical tests. Thus, identification is usually difficult, even for reference diagnostic laboratories.

Anaerobes

The gram-negative anaerobes, *Bacteroides, Porphyromonas, Prevotella,* and *Fusobacterium,* are frequently involved in mixed infections in abscesses and necrotic tissue. They are normally found in the digestive tract, so infections resulting from contamination of tissues with mucous membrane flora or intestinal contents frequently contain these organisms. Usually Gram's stain of the exudate will indicate that bacteria that do not grow aerobically are present. If obligate anaerobes are isolated, evaluation of the cellular morphological characteristics provides adequate clinical information. Species identification is rarely important. Recent taxonomic advances have resulted in the reclassification of some former *Bacteroides* spp. into the genera *Dichelobacter, Porphyromonas,* and *Prevotella.*

Spirochetes and Curved Bacteria

Leptospira spp. cause febrile infections often followed by abortion and infertility. These spirochetes are difficult to isolate and usually die within a few hours while being transported to a laboratory. Darkfield examination of urine may aid in establishing a diagnosis. Most diagnoses are made by serological testing.

Borrelia burgdorferi is a tick-transmitted spirochete that causes Lyme disease in humans and arthritis and lameness in dogs. Canine borreliosis may be accompanied by high rectal temperature and lymphadenopathy. Detection of serum antibodies to *B. burgdorferi* by indirect fluorescent antibody tests currently is the diagnostic test of choice in dogs. Isolation of *Borrelia* by culture is difficult and often nonproductive. Borreliosis appears to be a disease of emerging importance in the United States in dogs and other animals within areas infested by ticks carrying this agent.

Serpulina hyodysenteriae is a spirochete that causes dysentery in pigs. Cultural isolation is beyond the capability of most laboratories. Diagnosis of this infection may be made by examining smears of colonic mucosa for numerous large spirochetes.

Campylobacter spp. cause two different types of disease conditions. One group contains important reproductive pathogens, causing abortion and infertility. Because of special needs for enrichment and selective media and a microaerophilic atmosphere, specimens for isolation of *Campylobacter* should be sent to veterinary diagnostic laboratories specially equipped for *Campylobacter* culture. The second group is emerging as important zoonatic enteric pathogens. Most public health and hospital laboratories are equipped to isolate this group. *Campylobacter* spp. are curved gram-negative rods. They can be recognized by dark-field or phase-contrast microscopy by their darting motility.

Helicobacter spp. are helical or curved gram-negative bacteria that colonize the gastric mucosa of humans, dogs, and cats and the intestinal tract of some rodents, birds, and swine. Some species have been associated with gastritis and peptic ulceration, whereas other species are considered to be nonpathogenic flora of the gastric mucosa of animals. They can be detected and identified in histological sections, by culture in reference laboratories, and by associating strong urease activity in gastric mucus with their presence.

Mycoplasma

Mycoplasma spp. are small bacteria that lack a cell wall and, as a result, are not easily stained and observed in exudates. Arthritis and pneumonia are the most common mycoplasmal diseases. The role of *Mycoplasma* in urogenital infections is not well characterized. Special media and techniques are required for isolation and identification of *Mycoplasma*. Therefore, arrangements should be made with a reference laboratory for *Mycoplasma* transport media and specimen shipping instructions.

ANTIMICROBIAL SUSCEPTIBILITY TESTING

One of the purposes of the clinical microbiology laboratory is to provide information that can assist in the selection of appropriate therapy for infectious diseases. All antimicrobial agents have limitations in their spectra of activity. Therefore, a universal antimicrobial for all infections is not available. Some organisms are intrinsically resistant to an antimicrobial, whereas others acquire resistance. The most common mechanism for acquired resistance is the acquisition of extrachromosomal pieces of DNA (deoxyribonucleic acid) such as plasmids (R-factors) and bacteriophages. As a result, the bacteria are able to produce enzymes that modify or inactivate the antimicrobial, enable the cell to resist penetration of the drug, or alter target sites and reduce the activity of the drug. Because the acquired resistance traits are not static, the antimicrobial susceptibility pattern (*antibiogram*) is not predictable for many organisms. Therefore, susceptibility tests are necessary.

Indications for Susceptibility Testing

Susceptibility testing is indicated for most rapidly growing, aerobic and facultative anaerobic, clinically significant bacteria. Testing should be avoided for isolates representing normal flora and for those bacteria with predictable susceptibility to the antimicrobial of choice Gram-positive bacteria other than *Staphylococcus* have rather predictable antibiograms; therefore, routine testing is not needed. However, susceptibility testing may be indicated if the antimicrobial of choice cannot be safely and economically administered to the patient. *Unpredictable resistance patterns are frequently observed with the gram-negative bacteria*, thus requiring testing. Most slow-growing and anaerobic bacteria have rather predictable antibiograms, so testing is not necessary. If acquired resistance is found to be a problem in these organisms, special test methods will be necessary for testing them.

In most cases, the veterinarian will have started antimicrobial therapy before the laboratory results are available. When the test results become available, therapy can be altered or modified to provide safe, effective, least-cost therapy. In some situations, the culture specimen will be from a moribund or dead animal. Susceptibility testing may still be important because it can establish patterns of antimicrobial susceptibility for the organism when encountered in other animals in the herd or geographical region.

Susceptibility Test Methods

The simplest type of susceptibility test is one that tests for the presence of an enzyme that can inactivate an antimicrobial. Penicillin resistance by *Staphylococcus* is acquired by gaining the ability to produce beta-lactamase, an enzyme that inactivates most penicillin derivatives. Sensitive and rapid tests, such as Cefinase (Becton Dickinson Microbiology Systems), are available for detecting this enzyme. If the test is negative, penicillin or a penicillin derivative is usually the drug of choice, and no

further testing is needed. If the isolate is producing beta-lactamase, further antimicrobial susceptibility testing will be needed to select an alternative therapy. A beta-lactamase test can be a very useful part of a mastitis culture procedure to rapidly evaluate the appropriateness of penicillin therapy because it is one of the most frequently administered antimicrobials.

In most cases, tests for antimicrobial inactivating enzymes are not available. Therefore, most routine susceptibility tests measure the degree of susceptibility of the isolate to each of several antimicrobials. The broth dilution susceptibility test system is the most precise method and the reference method. This test is performed by introducing a standardized inoculum of an organism into a series of tubes (or wells in a microculture plate) containing serial dilutions of an antimicrobial in medium (Fig. 8–8). The lowest concentration of antimicrobial that macroscopically inhibits growth of the organism is the *minimal inhibitory concentration* (MIC). The MIC of an antimicrobial for a given isolate represents the degree of susceptibility to the drug. If the antimicrobial is going to be used in therapy, the MIC must be achieved at the site of infection to effectively inhibit bacterial growth. Generally, serum concentrations of antimicrobial two to four times higher than the MIC are desirable in order to overcome serum protein binding and variability in absorption and distribution.

The most commonly used method of antimicrobial susceptibility testing in small laboratories is the *agar diffusion test* using antimicrobial-impregnated paper disks that are applied to the surface of agar that has been streaked with a standardized inoculum. As the antimicrobial is absorbed from the disk into the agar, it begins diffusing in a radial pattern (Fig. 8–9). As the antimicrobial diffuses, it becomes more dilute, thereby creating a gradient effect of decreasing concentrations. The bacterial inoculum on the agar begins to grow in all areas except the places in which the antimicrobial concentration exceeds the MIC of the isolate. Zones of inhibition of growth can be observed around the disks. In carefully controlled studies, the diameters of the zones of inhibition have been correlated with MIC values. The results of the diffusion test can then be semi-quantitatively interpreted, usually as susceptible, intermediate, or resistant.

The diffusion test is easy to set up, but it requires careful attention to detail to ensure that the results are accurate. Mueller-Hinton agar has been selected as the standard culture medium so that the composition of the agar can be more

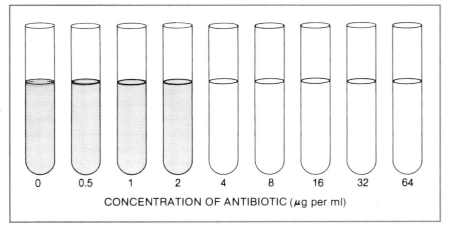

Figure 8-8. Broth dilution susceptibility test. The organism grew in broth containing 0.5, 1, and 2 μg/ml antibiotic, but growth was inhibited in the tube containing 4 μg/ml. Therefore, the minimal inhibitory concentration is 4 μg/ml.

CONCENTRATION OF ANTIBIOTIC (μg per ml)

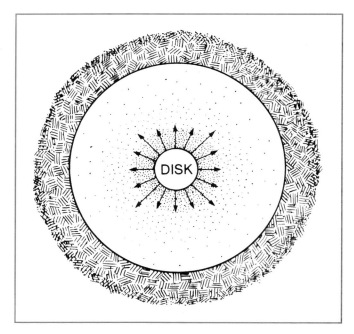

Figure 8–9. Principle of antibiotic diffusion in agar from a disk. The concentration of antibiotic is highest near the disk and logarithmically diluted as it diffuses radially into a larger area. At some point, the antibiotic is diluted below the minimal inhibitory concentration for the test organism, which allows the organism to grow. The resulting zone of inhibition is measured and interpreted with the use of Table 8–11.

uniformly controlled. However, this medium will not support growth of some of the fastidious pathogens such as *Streptococcus, Listeria, Corynebacterium, Erysipelothrix, Pasteurella,* and some other gram-negative bacteria. For these bacteria, serum or blood enrichment is necessary. Therefore, it is often more practical to use blood agar plates for susceptibility tests in low-volume laboratories. Results are usually comparable to those obtained with Mueller-Hinton agar; however, false-resistant results will often be obtained on the blood agar when testing sulfonamide activity. Fresh plates with the proper depth of agar must be used to avoid altering the kinetics of antimicrobial diffusion in a shallow or dehydrated plate.

Inoculum density must be carefully controlled. Otherwise, significant variations in zone sizes will occur, and results may be misinterpreted if the optimal ratio of bacterial cells to antimicrobial concentration is not maintained. Susceptibility tests must always be performed with a *pure culture* of bacteria. Bacteria in mixed cultures can inhibit growth of slower-growing or fastidious organisms. Therefore, if mixed cultures are tested, antimicrobial resistance of a pathogen may not be detected. Direct susceptibility testing of clinical specimens is discouraged, and, if performed, the results should always be verified by testing isolates in pure culture.

Standard antimicrobial disks should be purchased rather than attempting to prepare them from therapeutic drug solutions. It is important to make certain that the disks contain the same amount of antimicrobial as is listed in the interpretation chart (Table 8–11). Otherwise the results will not correlate with the desired MIC values. All cartridges of disks not in current use should be stored in a −20°C freezer; those currently in use should be kept in the refrigerator to avoid deterioration of the

antimicrobials. The inoculated test plate should be incubated in an aerobic atmosphere at 35°C for 18 hours. Incubation in an increased carbon dioxide atmosphere or for longer periods of time will produce spurious results.

Diffusion Test Procedure

Inoculum

Select four or five well-isolated colonies of the same morphological type from an agar plate culture. Touch the top of each colony with a wire loop, and transfer the growth to a tube containing 0.5 ml to 1 ml of saline or broth. The turbidity of the bacterial suspension should be equivalent to a MacFarland No. 0.5 standard, which is just turbid enough that a slight change in optical density of the tube is macroscopically visible. Within 15 minutes after preparing the inoculum suspension, dip a sterile nontoxic cotton swab into the suspension and rotate the swab several times with firm pressure on the inside wall of the tube to remove excess inoculum from the swab. Then inoculate the agar plate by streaking the swab over the entire agar surface. Repeat the streaking procedure two or more times, rotating the plate approximately 60 degrees each time to ensure an even distribution of inoculum.

Test Procedure

Place the appropriate antimicrobial-impregnated disks, selected from the list in Table 8-11, on the surface of the agar. Note that some disks serve as class disks for a group of related antimicrobials, thereby reducing the need for testing each drug individually. The disks should be distributed evenly on the surface of the agar so that they are no closer than 24 mm from center to center. This is best accomplished with a dispensing apparatus. With sterile forceps or needle tip, gently press each disk to the agar to ensure complete contact. Because some of the drug begins to diffuse immediately, a disk should not be moved once it has come in contact with the agar. Invert the plates, and place them in the incubator.

Measuring Zones of Inhibition

After 16 to 18 hours of incubating a properly inoculated plate, zones of inhibition around the disks should be uniformly circular with a uniformly confluent or almost completely confluent lawn of growth between zones. If only isolated colonies grow, the inoculum was too light, and the test should be repeated. The zone diameters should be carefully measured, including the diameter of the disk, and recorded to the nearest millimeter. The end point should be taken as the area showing no obvious visible growth (not including faint growth of any colonies that can be detected only with difficulty at the edge of the zone of inhibited growth). Large colonies growing within a clear zone of inhibition should be subcultured, reidentified, and retested.

Strains of *Proteus mirabilis* and *Proteus vulgaris* may swarm into areas of inhibited growth around certain antimicrobials. The zones of inhibition are usually clearly outlined, and the veil of swarming growth is ignored. With the sulfonamides, organisms may grow through several generations before they are inhibited. Slight growth (80% or more inhibition) with sulfonamides is therefore disregarded, and the margin of *heavy growth* is measured to determine the zone diameter.

• Table 8–11 •

ZONE DIAMETER (MEASURED IN MILLIMETERS) INTERPRETIVE STANDARDS FOR SUSCEPTIBILITY TESTS

ANTIMICROBIAL AGENT	DISK CONTENT	SUSCEPTIBLE	INTERMEDIATE	RESISTANT
Amikacin	30 µg	≥17	15–16	≤14
Amoxicillin/clavulanic acid (staphylococci)	20/10 µg	≥20		≤19
Amoxicillin/clavulanic acid (other organisms)	20/10 µg	≥18	14–17	≤13
Ampicillin* (gram-negative enteric organisms)	10 µg	≥17	14–16	≤13
Ampicillin* (staphylococci)	10 µg	≥29		≤28
Ampicillin* (enterococci)	10 µg	≥17		≤16
Ampicillin* (streptococci)	10 µg	≥30	22–29	≤21
Ampicillin* (*Listeria monocytogenes*)	10 µg	≥20		≤19
Cefazolin	30 µg	≥18	15–17	≤14
Cefoxitin	30 µg	≥18	15–17	≤14
Ceftiofur (respiratory pathogens only)	30 µg	≥21	18–20	≤17
Cephalothin†	30 µg	≥18	15–17	≤14
Chloramphenicol	30 µg	≥18	13–17	≤12
Clindamycin‡	2 µg	≥21	15–20	≤14
Enrofloxacin	5 µg	≥20	17–19	≤16
Erythromycin	15 µg	≥23	14–22	≤13
Gentamicin	10 µg	≥15	13–14	≤12
Kanamycin	30 µg	≥18	14–17	≤13
Oxacillin§ (staphylococci)	1 µg	≥13	11–12	≤10
Penicillin G (staphylococci)	10 units	≥29		≤28
Penicillin G (enterococci)	10 units	≥15		≤14
Penicillin G (streptococci)	10 units	≥28	20–27	≤19
Penicillin G (*Listeria monocytogenes*)	10 units	≥20		≤19
Penicillin/novobiocin‖	10 units/30 µg	≥17		≤16
Pirlimycin‖	2 µg	≥13		≤12
Rifampin	5 µg	≥20	17–19	≤16
Sulfonamides	250 or 300 µg	≥17	13–16	≤12
Tetracycline¶	30 µg	≥19	15–18	≤14
Ticarcillin (*Pseudomonas aeruginosa*)	75 µg	≥15		≤14
Ticarcillin (gram-negative enteric organisms)	75 µg	≥20	15–19	≤14
Tilmicosin	15 µg	≥15	13–14	≤12
Trimethoprim/sulfamethoxazole**	1.25/23.75 µg	≥16	11–15	≤10

*Ampicillin is used to test for susceptibility to amoxicillin and hetacillin.
†Cephalothin is used to test all first-generation cephalosporins, such as cephapirin and cefadroxil. Cefazolin should be tested separately with the gram-negative enteric organisms.
‡Clindamycin is used to test for susceptibility to clindamycin and lincomycin.
§Oxacillin is used to test for susceptibility to methicillin, nafcillin, and cloxacillin.
‖Available as an infusion product for treatment of bovine mastitis during lactation.
¶Tetracycline is used to test for susceptibility to chlortetracycline, oxytetracycline, minocycline, and doxycycline.
**Trimethoprim/sulfamethoxazole is used to test for susceptibility to trimethoprim/sulfadiazine and ormetoprim/sulfadimethoxine.
Modified from National Committee for Clinical Laboratory Standards document M31-P, Table 2, pp. 34–37, 1994.

Results

Interpret the sizes of the zones of inhibition by referring to Table 8-11, and report results for the organism as susceptible, intermediate, or resistant to each antimicrobial.

Interpretation and Limitations

It is important to understand that antimicrobial susceptibility is not an "all or none" phenomenon. Instead, bacteria have a *degree of susceptibility* as defined by the MIC value. Therefore, interpreting diffusion test results as "zone or no zone" is unacceptable. Small zones may represent organisms that can tolerate higher levels of the antimicrobial (high MIC) than can be achieved at the site of infection. The measured diameter of the inhibition zone must be compared to the standards in Table 8-11 to determine if the degree of susceptibility is comparable to the therapeutic level of the antimicrobial. The classification of "susceptible versus resistant" is a practical simplification of the

various susceptibilities of organisms in terms of expected clinical response to standard dose therapy.

Although the diffusion test has been accepted as a standard test and is used in most veterinary microbiology laboratories, there are some limitations that should be kept in mind. This test system is not applicable to slow-growing isolates or for use in special atmospheres. In many cases, the interpretative criteria (Table 8–11) are based on assumptions derived from knowledge of pharmacodynamics of antimicrobials in humans and efficacy in treating human pathogens. Dosages, absorption, and distribution of antimicrobials may be significantly different in the various species of animals. Levels of drug in tissues may significantly differ from levels in serum, such as low levels in cerebrospinal fluid. From the chart, a test may be interpreted as susceptible, but the drug may not be able to penetrate to the site of infection. Conversely, ampicillin, for example, is concentrated severalfold in the urine and may exceed the MIC value for an organism that has a small zone of inhibition. Therefore, susceptibility test results are not absolute rules for antimicrobial therapy. They should be used as guidelines in selecting therapy, in addition to clinical judgment and knowledge of the pharmacokinetics and pharmacodynamics of the antimicrobials.

Some veterinary microbiology laboratories are using microdilution tests to determine the MIC of clinical isolates. The MIC value can be compared to the levels of drug that can be obtained in the animal for final interpretion.

> **TECHNICIAN NOTE**
>
> *Susceptible* implies that infection due to the strain may be appropriately treated with the standard dosage of antimicrobial recommended for that type of infection and infecting species, unless otherwise contraindicated.
>
> *Intermediate* indicates infection due to a strain with antimicrobial agent MICs that approach usually attainable blood and tissue levels for which response rates may be lower than for susceptible isolates. This category implies clinical applicability in body sites in which the drugs are physiologically concentrated (e.g., quinolones and β-lactams in urine) or when a high dose of drug can be used (e.g., β-lactams).
>
> *Resistant* strains are not inhibited by the usually achievable systemic concentrations of the antimicrobial when normal dosage schedules are used and/or it may have MICs that fall within the range where specific, microbial resistance mechanisms are likely and clinical efficacy has not been reliable in treatment studies.

MYCOLOGY

The most frequently encountered fungal infections in veterinary medicine are the *dermatomycoses* (fungal infections of the skin). Dermatophytes can readily be cultured and identified in local laboratories. The invasive *systemic mycoses* are usually encountered less frequently. However, with the increased mobility of animals and improved intensive care procedures that prolong the life of immunocompromised patients, the geographical range and incidence of these diseases are increasing. Laboratory diagnosis of systemic mycoses often requires specialized procedures and advanced training.

Dermatophytes

The dermatophytes are keratinophilic fungi (keratin seeking) that invade hair, nails, and the superficial layers of the skin but not living tissue. They tend to cause chronic, mild inflammation rather than intense inflammation. Lesions are usually characterized by spreading areas of pruritus and accumulating crusty debris. Lesions can be single or multifocal, and hair loss is variable. Because of the peripherally expanding nature of the lesion, it is also referred to as *ringworm*. Lesions can be mark-

edly different in various species of animals, from a dry, minimally inflamed lesion without hair loss on cats to a large, wartlike crusty lesion on cattle.

Specimen Collection

Representative bits of hair, scale, or crust should be collected from the area of suspected dermatomycotic lesions. Care must be exercised to prevent heavy contamination with saprophytic fungi or bacteria, which can overgrow the culture of the desired pathogen. If the lesion is likely to be contaminated, the lesion should be cleansed gently with 70% alcohol before samples are collected. Various dermatophytes are best recovered from unique parts of the lesion, and so samples of scale, crust and hair should be selected. Pluck broken, frayed or distorted stubs of hair within the lesion area. Do not cut off hair to use as the specimen for culture. If samples are not placed directly on culture media, they should be placed in a clean, dry envelope. Do not seal them in a tube or place in transport media. When moisture is allowed to accumulate, bacteria and yeast may overgrow. Crush and separate large pieces of debris or scrape over the surface of the lesion to collect smaller pieces of scale. To culture nails suspected of having dermatophytic invasion, make fine shavings with a scalpel. Scatter the specimen over the entire surface of the culture medium. Press the hair and scale onto the agar, but do not bury it into the medium.

> **TECHNICIAN NOTE**
>
> Brush sampling is the preferred method for obtaining a dermatophyte culture specimen from asymptomatic animals, especially cats. Use a sterilized (or new) toothbrush to vigorously brush suspected lesions or brush the entire animal for 2 to 3 minutes as if grooming. Then, lightly press the brush against the surface of the culture medium several times for inoculation. Avoid pressing too firmly because the agar may tear and subsurface inoculum will not grow well.

Direct Examination

All specimens for fungal culture should be evaluated by direct microscopic examination. Direct mounts can be prepared by mixing a small portion of the material in two or three drops of 10% potassium hydroxide on a microscope slide. Addition of black India ink to the KOH solution will facilitate observation of fungal elements in the specimen. Add a coverslip over the wet mount and examine for the presence of delicate hyphae in skin scales or for the accumulation of spores on the surface of an infected hair (ectothrix). Endothrix infection does not occur with animal pathogens.

Culture Procedure

Sabouraud dextrose agar is the standard medium for isolation of fungi and can be used for the successful isolation of dermatophytes. Selective media, such as Mycosel (Becton Dickinson Microbiology Systems), are modified with antibiotics to inhibit bacteria and saprophytic fungi. A selective and differential medium (DTM—dermatophyte test medium) is probably the most convenient medium available (Synbiotics Corp. and Bacti-Lab, Inc.). The medium contains a phenol red indicator, which turns red as a dermatophyte grows and produces alkaline metabolic products. Occasionally, dermatophytes do not sporulate as well on DTM as on Sabouraud's medium, which can hinder identification. This problem can be overcome by using a supplemental medium such as Rapid Sporulation Medium (Bacti-Lab, Inc.) to enhance sporulation and identification of dermatophytes.

After the agar is inoculated, the cap should be replaced but left loose so that air exchange can occur. The culture is allowed to incubate at room temperature (22 to 25°C). It should be placed on an open shelf or counter so that it can be observed daily for up to 2 weeks for growth and color change in the medium. Dermatophytes are identified on the basis of both their gross colony characteristics and microscopic morphological characteristics. Rate of growth, texture, pattern of growth, color of the colony, and pigmentation of the reverse of the colony should be noted. Most dermatophyte colonies are white or light shades of apricot, yellow, or cream to tan. Darkly colored brown or black fungi are likely to be contaminants. The dermatophytes rapidly change the color of the DTM agar to red, even before a colony is apparent. The red color may appear as early as 3 to 5 days after inoculation and rapidly spreads to most of the agar. Nonpathogenic fungi that grow on the medium do not produce an early color change, although the medium may become red after it is heavily overgrown.

Definitive identification of a dermatophyte and speciation require microscopic examination of wet mounts prepared in *lactophenol cotton blue*. The slide is examined for microconidia, macroconidia, hyphae structures and other identifying characteristics. The distinguishing features of the common dermatophytes can be found in most clinical microbiology textbooks.

Systemic Mycoses

The three most important systemic mycoses are coccidioidomycosis, histoplasmosis, and blastomycosis. They are serious zoonotic agents; therefore, the small laboratory should not attempt to isolate them in culture systems. All culture work must be carried out in an approved biohazard safety hood. The small laboratory is limited to direct microscopic examination of clinical material. Stained smears and wet mounts are useful diagnostic tools. The size and structural characteristics of these agents in the tissue or yeast phase can serve as specific identifying criteria. If cultures are desired, the clinical material should be inoculated onto isolation media, and the inoculated tubes should be shipped to a reference laboratory. Delays in inoculation of isolation media will result in loss of viability and overgrowth of the sample by contaminating bacteria.

Sporotrichosis is a chronic infection characterized by nodular lesions of the skin or subcutaneous tissues. *Sporothrix schenckii* usually gains entrance by traumatic implantation into the tissue. Therefore, there is little danger of contagion. The agent can be observed in direct examinations of tissue and exudates or isolated and identified by routine methods.

Yeast

There are only a few clinical situations in which yeasts are significant veterinary pathogens. In general, animals seem to be much more resistant to yeast infections than are humans. If yeasts are suspected, a direct smear of exudate should be stained for microscopic examination. The best approach to the isolation of yeast is to inoculate blood agar and Sabouraud dextrose agar. The blood agar should be incubated at 35°C and the Sabouraud agar at room temperature. Media should be held at least 2 weeks before discarding it as negative. Therefore, agar slants in tubes are preferable to plates because they do not dehydrate as rapidly. Culture and identifying methods for the most common pathogenic yeasts are described.

Malassezia (Pityrosporum) pachydermatis. This yeast is frequently found in cases of external otitis. It is readily observed in gram-stained smears of exudate as an oval, budding yeast. Isolation in cultures can be difficult but is best attempted by inoculating Sabouraud dextrose agar and incubating it at 35°C in a carbon dioxide incubator.

Cryptococcus neoformans. In direct smears, this yeast may be presumptively identified by its abundant capsular material. Negative staining with India ink provides a black background that outlines the clear capsule for easier observation. It can be isolated on Sabouraud dextrose agar or blood agar. *Cryptococcus neoformans* can be differentiated from other nonpathogenic yeasts because it will grow at 35 to 37°C and is urease positive. The urease test is performed by inoculating the same urea agar slant that is used for differentiating bacteria.

Candida albicans. *Candida* is the most frequently encountered opportunistic fungal pathogen. Infections usually involve mucous membranes. In direct microscopic examinations of wet mounts, unicellular budding yeasts without a capsule are observed. Limited hyphae development may also be observed. It is readily isolated on Sabouraud dextrose agar or blood agar. Definitive identification can be made by demonstrating germ tube (pseudohyphae) development after 3 to 4 hours' incubation in rabbit serum.

Other yeasts are isolated much less frequently. It is usually not cost effective for small laboratories to attempt to identify these rare isolates. They should be forwarded to a reference laboratory for definitive identification.

VIROLOGY

Laboratory diagnosis of viral diseases depends on the examination of appropriate specimens for evidence of viral infection and then attempting to correlate infection with disease. Because of the nature of viruses and the special laboratory procedures required, most small private laboratories offer only limited viral diagnostic procedures. Viruses are obligate intracellular parasites. Therefore, they are best recovered from living tissue. Detection of viruses in dead tissues is reduced in direct proportion to the length of time since death and the extent of autolysis. Proper collection and handling of specimens are essential to obtain optimal laboratory results.

Virus Isolation

Isolation and identification of viruses depend on the inoculation of susceptible living cells for cultivation of the virus. The major methods of providing these living cells include monolayer cell cultures, embryonated hen eggs, and laboratory animal inoculation. These techniques require special laboratory facilities and up to 2 weeks for recovery of a virus. Special care must be taken to ensure that viable virus is delivered to the laboratory for isolation attempts. Therefore, specimens should be collected early in the course of infection when viruses are most numerous. At death, virus numbers in the tissues are usually reduced, and there often is extensive secondary bacterial infection. The presence of bacteria in the sample can be damaging to the cells that are being used as recovery hosts for the virus. Because many viruses are labile, and contamination by other microbes can be detrimental, specimens should be carefully collected, refrigerated, and promptly delivered to the diagnostic laboratory. Special arrangements should be made with the laboratory personnel so that they can be prepared to process the sample when it arrives. Transport media containing antibiotics and virus-stabilizing agents are often available from viral diagnostic laboratories.

Microscopic Evaluation

In some cases, viral infection can be identified by microscopic examination of infected tissues for the presence of pathognomonic changes or of body fluids for the presence of viral particles. Some viral infections produce distinct changes in host cells, such as the intranuclear inclusions of infectious canine hepatitis, which can provide a definitive diagnosis. Electron microscopic examination of body fluids and washings allows the direct visualization of viral particles. This procedure is often used for diagnosis of respiratory and enteric viral diseases because it is rapid and can detect mixed viral infections. Viruses can be detected even though cultivation methods are not available for isolation. The procedure does not require viable viruses, as long as they have retained their structural integrity. Direct electron microscopic examination is limited to cell-free viruses, such as those found in body fluids, rather than examination of infected tissue. Most diagnostic laboratories perform negative contrast-staining; therefore, virus identification is limited to morphological identification. If immunoelectron microscopy procedures are available, the type of virus within a group can be identified.

Antigen Detection

Antigen detection methods are the most frequently used viral diagnostic procedures. Advantages of antigen detection compared with viral isolation include rapid results, less expense, less technically demanding procedures, and less dependence on the presence of viable virus in the sample because most viral antigens remain intact after death of the virus. The most common methods of antigen detection are immunofluorescence staining, hemagglutination, and solid-phase immunoassays.

Immunofluorescence

Examination of selected clinical specimens using a specific antibody labeled with a fluorescent marker as a probe to identify viral antigen has been shown to be a rapid and highly reliable diagnostic method. As indicated earlier, live virus is not necessary, but autolytic or necrotic tissue samples may produce false-positive test results because of nonspecific absorption of the fluorescent-labeled antibody. Proper selection of tissue for examination is required, or false-negative results will be obtained. The two most important limitations of this procedure are the need for specific antibodies to the viral antigens and a fluorescence microscope.

A modification of this procedure that is making it practical for small laboratories is the *immunoperoxidase method*. In this assay, the specific antibody is labeled with an enzyme (usually horseradish peroxidase) instead of a fluorescent label. Attachment of the antibody to tissue sections or smears is detected using a chromogenic substrate that is deposited at the site of enzyme-antibody attachment and produces a slide similar to other differential stains. The slide can then be examined by light microscopy. Several of these assays have been developed using monoclonal antibodies to detect viral antigens in tissue, including formalin-fixed specimens.

Colloidal gold immunostaining technology is another technique that has been developed for antigen detection. This technology is currently available in the ICT Gold Test Device for canine heartworm and FeLV antigen testing (Synbiotics Corp.).

Hemagglutination

Some viruses have receptors for surface structures of cells, such as erythrocytes. The presence of these viruses in specimens can be demonstrated by mixing the specimen with erythrocytes and demonstrating hemagglutination (clumping of the erythrocytes). It is necessary to prove the specificity of this reaction by blocking or reducing the hemagglutination reaction with specific antiviral serum. Hemagglutination is a common test procedure used to detect canine parvovirus in feces.

Solid-Phase Immunoassays

The technological advancements of immunology, resulting in the development of solid-phase immunoassays and the production of monoclonal antibodies, are bringing diagnostic virology into private practice laboratories. These test systems, described in detail later in this chapter, are frequently referred to by the acronym ELISA (enzyme-linked immunosorbent assay).

Assays that have been successfully developed for detection of viral antigen include feline leukemia virus (FeLV) in blood (Virachek/FeLV, Synbiotics Corp.; SNAP FeLV, IDEXX Laboratories, Inc.), FeLV in saliva (ASSURE/FeLV, Synbiotics Corp.), canine parvovirus in feces (ASSURE/Parvo, Synbiotics Corp.; Probe and CITE Canine Parvovirus Test Kit, IDEXX Laboratories, Inc.), influenza virus in respiratory tract specimens (Directigen FluA, Becton Dickinson Microbiology Systems), and rotavirus in feces (Meritec Rota Latex Kit, Meridian Diagnostics, Inc.). Kits are also available to detect bacterial antigens (K99 Pilitest, VMRD, Inc.) and heartworm antigens (Virochek canine heartworm test kit, Synbiotics Corp., and CITE heartworm test kit, IDEXX Laboratories, Inc.).

SEROLOGY

Serological testing is an important tool in the diagnosis of infectious diseases. Serology has been used extensively in the diagnosis of viral infections and in disease surveillance programs. Serological tests for detecting a specific antibody have been developed for nearly every infectious agent. However, this indirect approach to diagnosing infection on the basis of a host immune response after exposure to an infectious agent is not always satisfactory. It is seldom as useful as isolation and identification of the etiological agent. Serological tests may vary in their sensitivity and specificity because of the type of test, immunogenicity, and cross-reactivity of the antigen and biological variation of immune responses by individual animals. Nevertheless, serological tests often remain the best diagnostic test available. In veterinary medicine, serological tests are often required by regulatory agencies to prove an animal is not infected or a carrier of a particular infectious agent.

Antibody Response to Infection

The chronology of exposure to an infectious agent and subsequent development of an antibody response are illustrated in Figure 8–10. Following exposure, there is a variable period of incubation followed by clinical illness. During the time of clinical illness the animal may be febrile, and this is when the greatest number of microorganisms are present. Therefore, it is more likely to transmit the infectious agent, and the best samples can be obtained for recovery of the agent at this time. After a variable period of time after onset of clinical signs (usually after 5 to 10 days), the animal begins to produce antibodies to the agent. Continued production of antibodies after the animal is no longer ill, referred to as the convalescent phase, will cause the titer (serum antibody level) to rise for 1 month or longer.

Interpretation of Serological Results

The presence of antibodies to a particular organism in an animal serum is not always a simple and absolute diagnosis of current or recent clinical illness caused by the organism. Therefore, detection of antibodies in a single serum sample often has limited importance unless the finding can be correlated with other clinical indications of the disease. In most situations, it is necessary to collect two samples—the first one early in the course of the illness (*acute*) and the second one (*convalescent*) at a later time—to demonstrate a change in antibody titer that would indicate recent antigenic stimulation. The change must be at least two dilution increments (usually fourfold), such as an increase from 1:4 to ≥ 1:16, to be considered diagnostically significant. This change in titer is known as a *seroconversion*.

TECHNICIAN NOTE

Sources of antibody in the serum of an animal:

- Convalescent antibody response after clinical disease or persistent infection
- Antibody response caused by exposure to an organism without clinical disease occurring
- Active immune response to vaccination
- Passive transfer of maternal antibodies to the neonate

The presence of antibody in serum may be reported quantitatively as a titer or qualitatively as positive or negative. Qualitative tests have less diagnostic value than those tests that report titers, unless the result is negative, in which case the test can exclude some agents from the differential diagnosis unless the serum was collected early in the course of disease. Most qualitative tests, such as immunodiffusion for equine infectious anemia (Coggins test) and bovine leukosis, are surveillance tests to identify animals who have been previously exposed and are possible carriers. Occasionally, a single, high-titered serum can aid in establishing a diagnosis, but it always leaves some question of whether the titer increased in association with clinical disease or is a stable, convalescent high titer.

When an animal is exposed to an organism, the first antibodies produced are usually of the IgM class with later antibody production being IgG. Some tests are designed to differentiate these antibody class responses, which can be helpful in confirming a diagnosis. If the antibody response to a virus is of the IgM type, the animal has recently been exposed. If the response is mostly IgG, it was probably exposed several weeks to months previously. Therefore, recent clinical illness was probably due to some other etiological agent. Often IgM antibodies are less specific than IgG and may cross-react, resulting in false-positive test results. To prevent this from happening, the test can be modified to exclude IgM reactions. Methods that can be used include (1) addition of 2-mercaptoethanol (2-ME), (2) addition

Figure 8–10. Antibody response to an infectious disease and optimal times for specimen collection.

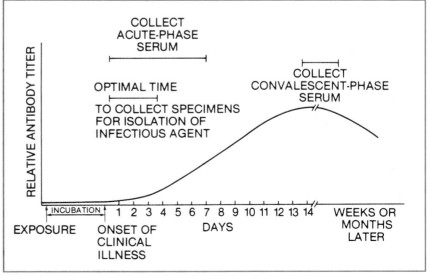

of rivanol, (3) heating the serum, and (4) acidifying the pH of the test.

Serological tests are frequently relied on as the only diagnostic procedures for abortion cases. Results are often difficult to interpret for two reasons. First, by the time abortion occurs because of infection of the fetus and its subsequent death, the dam is already in the convalescent phase of antibody production, so a seroconversion cannot be demonstrated. Second, the stress of abortion or other clinical illness may trigger reactivation of a latent viral infection. This provides an antigenic stimulus to the animal's immune system and increased antibody production. However, it is specific for the latent viral infection, not the current clinical illness.

Collection of Serum

Technicians will frequently be responsible for collecting and handling serum samples. Improper methods can render serological test results meaningless. The timing of serum collection is important (see Fig. 8–10). The first sample should be collected as soon as possible after the animal begins to show signs of clinical illness. If the sample is not collected within the first 5 to 7 days, antibody titers might have already risen. The convalescent sample should be collected at least 10 days after the acute sample. Generally, 14 to 21 days between samples is recommended, but in young animals with a less efficient immune response, up to 4 to 6 weeks may be necessary to demonstrate a seroconversion.

Serum must be collected and handled in a way that prevents any contamination. Contamination of serum can interfere in sensitive test systems, such as virus neutralization tests or ELISA assays. Excessive hemolysis of the sample is also a common problem in the serology laboratory. Improper handling of serum for complement fixation tests may cause the serum to bind complement before antigen is added to the test. These samples will be reported as anticomplementary, resulting in no test.

Blood should be collected aseptically by venipuncture with a new needle and syringe or evacuated clot tube (Vacutainer tubes and SST Sterile Serum Separation Tubes, Becton Dickinson Vacutainer Systems). Do not use recycled, washed needles, syringes or tubes. Residual detergent may cause hemolysis or may be toxic to cell cultures used in the test systems. Blood should be allowed to stand at room temperature until a clot has formed; the serum should then be removed from the clot and placed in a new, sterile tube. It may be necessary to separate the serum from the clot by centrifugation to prevent transferring cellular components of the blood. Anticoagulants should not be used to collect plasma because they can be toxic in some test systems. Avoid freezing the whole blood because that will cause hemolysis. The transfer of serum from the original blood tube must be performed aseptically. Contaminating microorganisms can grow rapidly in serum and alter the immunoglobulin molecules. Therefore, serum samples (separated from the clot and cells) should be refrigerated until testing is commenced, if within 72 hours. For longer periods of storage, serum may be preserved for extended periods by storage in a freezer ($-20°C$). Frozen serum samples should be packaged and shipped with adequate insulation and ice to prevent thawing before arrival at the laboratory. If a second sample will be collected, the first sample should be held until both can be sent to the laboratory together for valid paired testing. The technical procedures of

serological tests are difficult to duplicate exactly, therefore, results of tests performed on different days or in other laboratories should not be compared to demonstrate a seroconversion.

It is common practice to collect blood from cattle and ship it to a laboratory for brucellosis testing without removing the serum from the clot. However, this practice is not acceptable when serological tests, such as virus neutralization, are requested. Erythrocytes from most animals are more fragile and more susceptible to hemolysis than those from cattle. Therefore, all serum should be separated from the clot before sending it to a laboratory.

For shipment, the tubes of serum must be carefully labeled and packed so that they will not leak or break. When the environmental temperatures are high, refrigerant and insulating materials should be used to preserve samples during transit.

Serological Test Procedures

Only a few serological tests have been standardized and packaged for cost-effective use in veterinary practice laboratories. It is important that the directions with these tests be followed carefully. Modification of any part of the procedure can cause spurious results. A positive (or known titer) serum and a negative serum should be kept on hand and included in the test each time it is performed to verify accuracy of the results. Serology (antibody-detecting) kits are available for feline immunodeficiency virus (IDEXX Laboratories, Inc.), feline infectious peritonitis (IDEXX Laboratories, Inc.), Lyme disease (IDEXX Laboratories, Inc.) and paratuberculosis (ImmuCell Corp.)

The most frequent mistakes made when performing serological tests include the use of dirty or contaminated equipment, failure to adhere to instructions (especially incubation times), and unfamiliarity with reading results. For example, when reading agglutination results, antigen must be agglutinated throughout the test; there must not be just a few large clumps of antigen randomly distributed in the test.

ENZYME IMMUNOASSAYS

The wide use of enzyme immunoassays is based on the excellent ability of this methodology to be adapted to kits that meet practical concerns, such as minimizing reagent cost, reducing technician time required to perform the assay and simplifying the test protocol. Three typical configurations of enzyme immunoassays are illustrated in Figure 8–11. Each of the three configurations is particularly well-suited to specific applications. In the *sandwich* method, the antigen of interest reacts with antibody that is coated on the solid phase. The solid phase is then washed to remove any unbound molecules or other interfering substances. A second antibody, also specific for the antigen, that has been labeled with enzyme molecules is brought in contact with the solid phase. If any antigen is present in the original sample, it will bind to the solid phase antibody and form a bridge to the enzyme-labeled antibody. Once again, a wash step is required to remove excess unbound enzyme-labeled antibody. The solid phase is then brought into contact with an enzyme substrate solution that develops a visible color in the presence of bound enzyme. Solid phase bound enzyme activity, and thus the color observed, is directly related to the amount of antigen in the original sample. Feline leukemia virus

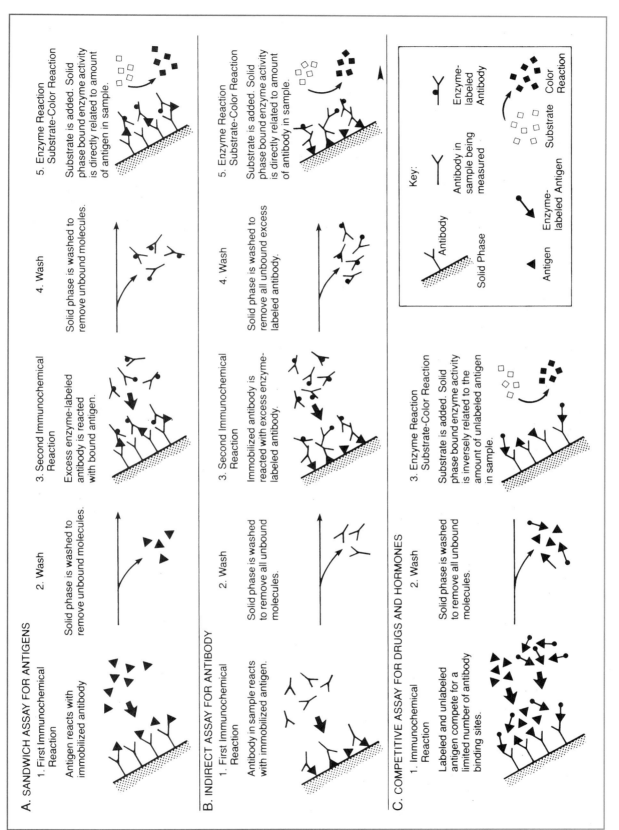

Figure 8-11. Enzyme immunoassay configurations and major steps in assay procedures. (Courtesy of E.S. Bean and E.T. Maggio, San Diego, CA.)

175

and canine heartworm antigen are detected by means of sandwich enzyme immunoassays.

The *indirect* assay method is utilized for detection of antibodies specific for a particular organism, such as antibodies to parvovirus or bovine leukemia virus. To do this, the patient sample is allowed to react with the solid phase, which has been coated with specific antigens. If the patient sample contains antibodies that recognize these specific antigens, the antibodies will attach. The solid phase is washed to remove interfering substances and unbound antibody. A second antibody, which is specific for the immunoglobulin molecules of the patient species and has been labeled with an enzyme, is added. If patient antibody has bound to antigen in the first step, the enzyme-labeled anti-immunoglobulin antibodies will bind to the unmobilized patient antibodies. The solid phase is once again washed to remove interfering substances and is placed in contact with a color developing substrate. The degree of color development will be directly related to the amount of specific antibody present in the patient sample.

A third type of immunoassay is frequently used for low-molecular-weight substances, such as drugs and hormones. Because of the small size of such molecules, it is usually not possible for two antibodies to bind simultaneously as required for a sandwich assay. As a result, low-molecular-weight substances are usually measured by the *competitive* immunoassay protocol. In competitive immunoassays, enzyme-labeled drug or hormone (labeled antigen) and the unlabeled antigen present in the patient sample are allowed to compete with a limited number of antibody molecules bound to a solid phase. Because the number of antibody-binding sites is precisely defined, and most of the antibody-binding sites are occupied with the patient antigen (if a large amount of antigen is present in the sample), very little enzyme-labeled antigen can bind to the solid phase. On the other hand, if very little antigen is present in the patient sample, more of the enzyme-labeled antigen can bind to the solid phase. In this case, the amount of enzyme bound to the solid phase is *inversely* related to the amount of antigen present in the sample. Therefore, the greater the amount of color observed, the smaller the amount of antigen present in the sample. Such a protocol is employed in enzyme immunoassays that measure the concentration of low-molecular-weight antigens, such as progesterone.

At present, there are three different solid phases commonly used in conducting enzyme immunoassays in the veterinary laboratory. The most common and least expensive solid phase for multiple tests is the microtiter well, but for individual clinical tests, dipstick and immunofiltration solid-phase assays are more efficient. The solid-phase dipstick can simplify the collection of patient sample material; for example, a dipstick coated with antibodies, which bind to feline leukemia viral antigens, can be placed directly in the cat's mouth and allowed to react with the viral antigen present in an infected cat's saliva. Both the collection of viral antigen and the first immunological reaction are thus combined into a single step. The presence of viral antigen is detected by subsequently completing the steps described above for sandwich assays. The dipstick solid phase has also proved to be particularly useful in detection of infectious disease agents in fecal samples, such as detection of K-99 pilus antigen in calf scours or detection of transmissible gastroenteritis virus (TGEV) in swine piglet scours. Immunofiltration devices, which utilize a porous membrane as the solid phase, facilitate wash steps, since solutions are poured through the solid phase and retained in an absorbent pad. Immunofiltration-type enzyme immunoassays provide rapid and simple procedures with easily read results. The internal control provided is an important aid in accurate interpretation of the test results. Immunofiltration-type enzyme immunoassay tests are well suited for in-clinic use where lower sample numbers and lower technical skill may prevail in comparison to a reference laboratory environment.

Although enzyme immunoassays are often simple to perform, they represent the incorporation of sophisticated technology into diagnostic kits. Commercial immunoassay kits are optimized to function well within a narrowly defined set of conditions established by the manufacturer. In order to guarantee reliable results, care must be taken by the user to ensure that all precautions recommended by the kit manufacturers are scrupulously observed. Alterations in the reagents or procedure not permitted by the directional insert accompanying the kit will almost always lead to a condition in which the reagents are not present in optimal ratios or amounts. For example, altering the volume of reagents, length of incubation or wash steps, temperature, or sample composition, such as using saliva when serum is specified or using serum when plasma is specified, can invalidate the test results. Extra reagents should be discarded collectively on or before the kit expiration date. It is never permissible to mix reagents from different kit lots. Complicating matters further is the potential presence of transient molecules in patient samples, such as drugs or dietary components. While the use of internal controls can help identify some problems of this nature, they are by no means foolproof. It is thus essential that the users of commercial kits follow the directions precisely and familiarize themselves with the precautions and limitations of the procedure before using the tests. Table 8–12 provides a partial list of factors that affect enzyme activity and, if altered by failure to follow the manufacturer's directions, could adversely affect performance of an enzyme immunoassay.

Immunoassay diagnostic kit manufacturers usually offer technical assistance to kit users. If you have questions about a

• Table 8–12 •

PARAMETERS AFFECTING THE PERFORMANCE OF ENZYME IMMUNOASSAYS		
STORAGE OF REAGENTS AND KITS	**PROCEDURAL DETAIL**	**SAMPLE**
Temperature	Temperature	Microbial contamination
Time	Number and intensity of washes	Improper storage
Contamination	Incubation time	Containers, diluents, additives, anticoagulants
Transfer to alternate containers		Abnormal samples (hemolysis, lipemia)
		Adulterated samples (contain drugs, unknown substances)

protocol or test result or are experiencing difficulty in conducting a test after carefully reading and following the manufacturer's instructions, call the company's technical services department and ask for assistance. Most companies provide a toll-free telephone number to facilitate this and will welcome an opportunity to assist you in using their products.

CLINICAL IMMUNOLOGY

Purpose of Evaluating Immune System Function

As the function and complexity of the immune system have been elucidated during the past two decades, an increasing need for laboratory diagnosis of dysfunction of the immune system has been recognized. Clinical immunological laboratory support has become a well-established part of the diagnostic services and patient care procedures in human medicine. Only a few of the simple clinical immunological assays are available in veterinary medicine; most of these assays require careful standardization for each species of animal. Most assays are time-consuming and often require specialized equipment. Therefore, very few tests are cost effective for practice laboratories.

Some of the simple procedures will be discussed in this section. The Recommended Reading list should be consulted for detailed and theoretical discussions of other immune system function assays.

Several types of diagnostic problems present the need for laboratory evaluation of possible immunological disorders. These disorders can be classified into four types: (1) allergies, (2) autoimmune diseases, (3) immunodeficiencies, and (4) immunoproliferative diseases. The veterinarian usually realizes the need for laboratory evaluation of immune system functions when presented with an animal suffering with (1) persistent or recurrent bacterial infections that fail to respond to routine therapy, (2) chronic inflammation of tissue in the absence of a recognized microbial pathogen, (3) persistent lymphopenia, (4) abnormal levels of immunoglobulins, (5) apparent vaccination failure, (6) spontaneous tumors, or (7) secondary diseases associated with chemotherapy. In young animals, disorders of the immune system are most frequently observed as developmental defects (sometimes inherited) or may be caused by a failure of passive transfer of maternal antibodies. However, immune function abnormalities can be observed in animals of all ages because of effects of aging, various drugs, or environmental exposure to immunomodulating toxins.

Laboratory Tests for Immunological Disorders

Allergies are usually diagnosed by physical examination, history, and response to intradermal inoculation of test antigens. Test kits for use in the clinical laboratory to screen dogs for allergies have recently become available (SNAP Allergy IgE, IDEXX Laboratories, Inc.).

Diagnosis of autoimmune disorders requires identification of the antibody specific for a particular cell or tissue. The presence of these antibodies may be detected in the patient's serum using the appropriate antigen preparation. Often these diseases can be diagnosed more efficiently by evaluating biopsied lesions. Morphological evaluation, combined with various immunohistochemical staining procedures, provides the most definitive diagnosis. It is best to consult with referral laboratories to learn which specimens they are able to analyze and how the sample should be submitted.

Immunoproliferative diseases may result in the production of abnormal amounts or unusual types of immunoglobulin proteins, referred to as *gammopathies*. The techniques of electrophoresis (usually on cellulose acetate) and immunoelectrophoresis are the laboratory tests most frequently used to diagnose these disorders. Abnormalities of routine laboratory tests, such as total protein in serum or urine and A:G ratios, frequently indicate a need for these specialized tests. Because of the infrequent demand for these tests and the cost of electrophoresis equipment, most practices request these services from referral laboratories.

Immunodeficiency or immunosuppressive disorders are the most frequently encountered immune system dysfunctions. Disorders may include defects of nonspecific immune function such as phagocytic cells and complement or specific immunity, such as cell-mediated immunity (T lymphocytes) and humoral (antibody) immunity (B lymphocytes). A long list of specific disorders that have been identified in animals could be compiled. As clinical immunology laboratory services become more readily available, additional disorders will undoubtedly be identified. Most assays of immune cell function require specialized equipment and procedures that are usually available in only a few reference laboratories. Some cellular function assays require submission of viable cells for evaluation. Recently developed assays are used to detect and quantify receptors on the surface of cells, such as CD18 deficiency in Holstein calves. Determination of immunoglobulin levels, as an indication of B-lymphocyte function, is a readily available laboratory test. Two immune disorders encountered in veterinary practices are discussed as examples of the need for evaluating the immune system of animals.

Failure of Passive Transfer

The newborn of most domestic animals are hypogammaglobulinemic (low levels of immunoglobulins). They depend on absorption of maternal antibodies from colostrum for protection from infectious diseases in the early weeks of life. Determination of the passive transfer status of foals and calves is an important evaluation that can modify patient care. Although total serum protein levels can indicate relative levels of immunoglobulins, this indirect measurement is subject to considerable variability. The reference method for quantitating serum immunoglobulins is the *radial immunodiffusion (RID) test*. The RID test consists of agar containing antisera specific for a particular antigen. In this case, the antigen is a particular immunoglobulin class such as IgG. Each test requires that quantitated standards be tested at the same time for comparison. Therefore, if single samples are being tested, the cost per sample will be greater, and it might be more cost effective to send samples to a referral laboratory. (Commercially produced RID kits for canine, bovine, llama and equine immunoglobulins are available from Bethyl Laboratories, Inc. and VMRD, Inc.)

TECHNICIAN NOTE

Failure of the neonatal animal to obtain and absorb adequate colostral immunoglobulins is frequently associated with increased morbidity and mortality from bacteremia and common neonatal diseases.

Passive transfer status of calves and foals can be evaluated rapidly and inexpensively in the practice laboratory using total serum protein concentration, zinc sulfate turbidity, sodium sulfite turbidity, radial immunodiffusion, or glutaraldehyde coagulation. The zinc sulfate turbidity test can be performed as follows (Fig. 8–12):

1. Reagent: Dissolve 208 mg of zinc sulfate ($ZnSO_4 \cdot 7H_2O$) in 1 liter of distilled water. Store in tightly closed container in refrigerator.
2. Test serum: This procedure can be used to test either foal or calf immunoglobulin levels in serum, provided there is minimal hemolysis.
3. Procedure:
   Add 0.1 ml of test serum to a clean test tube.
   Add 0.1 ml of each control serum with known concentrations of immunoglobulin to individual test tubes.
   Add 5 ml of $ZnSO_4$ reagent to each test tube and mix.
4. Interpretation: Allow 3 to 5 minutes' reaction time; then compare turbidity of test sample to known controls to estimate immunoglobulin concentration.

Note: This test is a rapid estimation of immunoglobulins. It is not an absolute quantitative measure of specific immunoglobulin classes. The reagent costs only a few cents per test, and results are available within a few minutes after the blood has clotted and the serum is collected. It is important to store the zinc sulfate reagent in a tightly stoppered bottle to prevent deterioration. Sera of known immunoglobulin quantities should be used as controls to ensure that the reagent is working properly. A negative control can be obtained by collecting serum from a newborn before it ingests any colostrum. Other sera can be collected or prepared by mixing high and low immunoglobulin concentration sera to obtain standards with the desired level of immunoglobulin. A small aliquot of the serum can be sent to a referral laboratory for RID quantitation. These reference sera can be stored in small, frozen aliquots for several years.

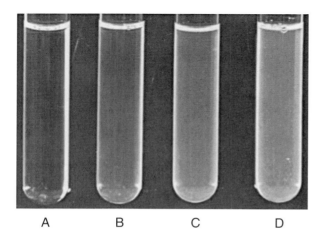

Figure 8–12. $ZnSO_4$ turbidity test for estimating immunoglobulin levels. A, Control sample (negative for immunoglobulin). B, 400 mg/dl standard. C, Unknown sample. D, 700 mg/dl standard. The relative turbidity indicates that the text sample contains more than 400 but less than 700 mg/dl immunoglobulin.

Foal IgG Test Kits

Several test kits have been developed and marketed for rapid quantification of serum IgG in foals. A semiquantitative latex agglutination test (Foal-chek, Centaur, Inc.) can be performed with either serum or whole blood. An enzyme-immunoassay test kit (CITE-Foal IgG Test, IDEXX Laboratories, Inc.) measures IgG in serum, plasma or whole blood. Both of these kits provide accurate results when performed properly and can readily be used in field or clinical laboratories for assessment of passive transfer in foals.

Combined Immunodeficiency (CID) of Arabian Foals

As implied by the name, CID of Arabian foals is a deficiency of both T lymphocytes and B lymphocytes. Therefore, the animal lacks cell-mediated immunity and the ability to produce antibodies. The disorder is inherited as a recessive trait. Therefore, accurate diagnosis is important for detection of the disease in a foal and for identifying carrier animals when they produce afflicted offspring. The foal with CID can absorb antibodies from colostrum, so it may have some resistance to disease early in its life. Also, total immunoglobulin levels (as determined by the zinc sulfate test) will not be a helpful diagnostic test. Specific quantitation of IgM, which is not passively absorbed, is necessary and is best evaluated before colostrum ingestion or treatment with any serum products. Differential white blood cell (WBC) counts and absolute lymphocyte counts are necessary. The combined evaluation of lymphocyte numbers and IgM levels can presumptively diagnose or rule out CID. The definitive diagnosis should include the histological examination of lymphoid tissues. Although some of these procedures can be performed in practice laboratories, insurance companies usually require tests to be performed in approved reference laboratories. It is important that these tests be performed accurately because other less serious immunodeficiency disorders have been identified in horses and must be differentiated.

NOSOCOMIAL INFECTIONS

An infection that results from exposure to an infectious agent while the patient is in the hospital is considered to be *nosocomial* (hospital acquired). The nosocomial infection may become clinically apparent during hospitalization or after discharge from the hospital. Infections that are incubating at the time of admission are defined as *community-acquired,* even though they become clinically apparent only during hospitalization. In veterinary practices, in addition to nosocomial infections of patients, zoonotic infections transmitted to the staff and clients can be considered part of the nosocomial problem.

The incidence of nosocomial infections in veterinary hospitals is not well documented, but it is probably similar to the incidence in human hospitals, which ranges from 3% to 5% of hospitalized patients. The incidence is known to vary with the size and type of hospital and the sophistication of infection control programs. The highest incidence rates are observed in large referral or teaching institutions. The most important institutional risk factors appear to be (1) an increased number of personnel having contact with the patient and (2) an increased mean number of hospitalization days per patient. Therefore, these infections are becoming an increasingly significant problem in teaching hospitals and large group practices in which intensive medical and surgical care is available through a large staff. These institutions also tend to care for patients with more critical and chronic disease. Because these patients have increased susceptibility to opportunistic infection, the occurrence of a nosocomial infection does not necessarily indicate negligence by the hospital staff.

TECHNICIAN NOTE

The most important vehicles for the spread of nosocomial agents are the hands of hospital personnel. Therefore, proper and frequent handwashing is the most important strategy for reducing the rate of nosocomial infections.

The microbiology laboratory has a prominent role in the recognition and control of nosocomial infections by prompt and accurate identification of etiological agents. The laboratory itself is a potential source of infectious agents; therefore, safety measures must be followed to prevent infections from laboratory materials.

The likelihood that a patient will acquire a specific nosocomial infection depends on three major factors: (1) the animal's susceptibility to infection by the agent, (2) the virulence of the agent, and (3) the nature of exposure to the agent. Because of the stressed condition of hospitalized animals, they are often more susceptible to infections than the general population. Factors that predispose an individual animal to nosocomial infection may include extremes of age (old age or neonates), debilitating disease, diagnostic or medical procedures, such as urethral catheterization, immunosuppressive therapy (corticosteroids or cytotoxic drugs), long periods of hospitalization, antimicrobial therapy, presence of other infections and presence of surgical hardware and drains. For some of the infectious diseases, such as canine distemper, the immunization status of the patient will determine its susceptibility.

Many nosocomial infections are caused by opportunistic microorganisms that infrequently cause infections in healthy animals. However, when the high-risk patient (increased susceptibility) is exposed, the agent can cause disease. Other highly virulent organisms, such as canine parvovirus and *Salmonella,* may cause disease in otherwise healthy patients.

Host susceptibility and microbial virulence are inherent characteristics that are difficult to alter. Thus, the greatest impact on the incidence of nosocomial infections can be made by understanding the sources of exposure and spread of these infectious agents. Microorganisms enter the hospital in or on people, animals, inanimate objects, air currents, and occasionally insects. Within the hospital, they are maintained in or on a variety of reservoirs, including patients with infections, healthy carriers, inanimate surfaces, solutions, food, staff, and insects. From these reservoirs, the potential pathogens may be disseminated by contact or by air to hospital personnel and patients.

Agents of Nosocomial Infections

Bacteria are the most frequent infectious agents involved in nosocomial infections, but viruses, fungi, and protozoa can also be responsible. The commonly involved bacteria tend to be somewhat environmentally resistant, and the increasing use of antibiotic therapy precedes an increased level of antibiotic resistance by nosocomial agents. Before the antibiotic era, penicillin-susceptible gram-positive cocci of the genera *Streptococcus* and *Staphylococcus* were the most common agents; then penicillin-resistant *Staphylococcus* became important. Currently, the major problems are with multiple antibiotic-resistant gram-negative bacilli such as *Escherichia coli, Salmonella, Klebsiella, Enterobacter, Serratia,* and *Pseudomonas.* Methicillin-resistant staphylococci and vancomycin-resistant enterococci are emerging as the next wave of serious nosocomial agents. Colonization (growth and establishment) of the body surfaces of the patient by these nosocomial bacterial pathogens is usually a prerequisite to infection. Therefore, the patient becomes its own major reservoir of these agents. Common reservoir sites are the lower intestinal tract and the naso-oropharyngeal area. Antimicrobial chemotherapy is the most important predisposing factor that allows the patient to become colonized because the antimicrobial suppresses normal flora and selects for resistant organisms. The most frequent locations of nosocomial bacterial infections are the urinary and respiratory systems and surgical wounds. Occasionally, infections become bacteremic. Zoonotic bacterial pathogens isolated in the laboratory that may result in accidental infection of personnel include agents of brucellosis, anthrax and salmonellosis.

Viral infections are the second most frequent group of nosocomial infections in hospitalized patients but are probably the most important nosocomial infections of outpatients. This is because some of these agents are easily transmitted and are highly infectious to susceptible but otherwise healthy animals. Diseases in this group include canine distemper, canine parvovirus, feline panleukopenia, and respiratory viral diseases of all animals (feline viral rhinotracheius, equine influenza, infectious bovine rhinotracheitis, canine tracheobronchitis, and so forth).

Other viral diseases that are not as contagious can be transmitted to susceptible patients at a veterinary hospital if adequate preventative measures are not followed. The resulting disease would be classified as a nosocomial infection. Examples include transmission of viruses of feline leukemia and equine infectious anemia in blood transfusions. Both patients and staff of veterinary hospitals are at risk of contracting rabies if exposed.

Fungi have rarely been recognized as nosocomial agents in veterinary medicine. As the awareness level of the importance of this problem is raised, no doubt more fungal infections will be identified, especially with improved intensive care of immunocompromised patients. Yeasts, such as *Candida albicans,* have occasionally been identified. The dermatophytes do not cause life-threatening infections and are usually overlooked, but they can also be transmitted as nosocomial agents to both patients and hospital staff.

Infection of animals by protozoan pathogens can be acquired in the veterinary hospital. *Cryptosporidium* spp. is relatively resistant to disinfectants and has been the cause of nosocomial enteritis. If litter pans are not properly cleaned, other animals and hospital staff could be exposed to toxoplasmosis. Hemotropic parasites (*Hemobartonella, Anaplasma, Ehrlichia, Babesia*) can be transmitted to other patients in blood transfusions or on surgical instruments that have not been washed and disinfected.

Recognition and Control of Nosocomial Infections

Since incubation periods for many infections that affect hospitalized patients are variable or even unknown, and multiple sources of exposure are possible for many patients, clinical judgment is usually required to separate community-acquired infections from nosocomial infections. The veterinarian must have excellent diagnostic microbiology laboratory support for accurate identification of infectious agents and accurate reproducible antibiograms of bacteria. An unusual number of isolations of a single pathogen or the appearance of an unusual antibiogram in hospitalized patients often provides the first indication of an outbreak of nosocomial infection.

Measures that can help reduce or control nosocomial infections include sterilization of equipment and supplies, aseptic treatment techniques, isolation practices, judicious use of antimicrobial drugs, diligent handwashing between examining patients, disposal of trash, and establishment of sound housekeeping protocols. These protocols should provide for adequate cleaning, disinfection and maintenance of patient-care equipment and environmental surfaces, such as cages, tables, floors, and walls.

The control measures that would be necessary to prevent all nosocomial infections are impractical and not economically feasible. Hospitals contain patients with increased susceptibility to infection, and short of total isolation in a controlled environment, there are few measures that are biologically guaranteed. The risk for each patient of acquiring an infection must be individually evaluated. If the risk is sufficiently great, reverse isolation procedures may be indicated to prevent the patient from being exposed to potential pathogens. If active or passive immunizing products are available, their use should be encouraged. Routine immunization programs can effectively prevent many of the viral infections that have been discussed.

Antiseptics, Disinfectants, and Sterilization

The effective use of antiseptics, disinfectants, and sterilization procedures is an important factor in preventing nosocomial infections. Although these methods are used on a daily basis, often with some interchange, the exact distinction between the three terms is extremely important if effective application is to be realized. *Sterilization* is defined as the use of physical or chemical procedures to destroy *all* microbial life, including highly resistant bacterial spores. The steam autoclave, using moist heat, is the most frequently used sterilization process. Ethylene oxide gas and some chemical compounds that are normally considered disinfectants can also be used for sterilization. *Disinfection* inactivates virtually all recognized pathogenic microorganisms but not necessarily all microbial forms, such as bacterial spores, on inanimate objects. An *antiseptic* is defined as a substance that is used on or in living tissue for the purpose of inhibiting or destroying microorganisms. Some agents may be used as both disinfectants and antiseptics, but adequacy for one purpose does not assure adequacy for the other. Many cleaning agents and detergents reduce microbial contamination by removal but have only limited germicidal activity. Consequently, these agents are neither disinfectants nor antiseptics.

Minimum standards of performance for sterilization procedures have been established and must be followed. Sterilization is not a relative procedure like disinfection. Therefore, an object is either sterile or nonsterile. However, there is a broad range of activity by disinfectants from minimal reduction in the number of contaminating microorganisms to sterility. Among factors that may have a significant effect on the results of disinfection are concentration of the chemical, length of exposure to the chemical, amount of organic matter (soil, blood, feces, and so forth) present, type, and condition (porosity, cracks, and so forth) of the material to be disinfected, ambient temperature and the nature and number of contaminating microorganisms.

Microorganisms vary widely in their susceptibility to germicidal treatments. Bacterial endospores are the most resistant type. In descending order of relative resistance after that of bacterial spores are mycobacteria, fungal spores, nonenveloped viruses, vegetative fungi, enveloped viruses, and vegetative bacterial cells. The differences in chemical resistance of various vegetative bacteria are relatively minor, except for the mycobacteria, which are relatively resistant to many disinfectants.

Selection of the most appropriate germicide for a particular situation should be made after consideration of a number of factors. These factors include (1) whether it is to be used as a disinfectant or as an antiseptic, (2) an estimation of the level of antimicrobial action needed based on the nature and number of contaminating microorganisms, and (3) the physical nature of objects to be treated. Good physical cleaning will allow better penetration of crevices and porous material. Generally, the higher the concentration of the chemical agent or the longer a process is continued, the greater its effectiveness. For temperature-based procedures, increasing temperatures will usually increase efficacy.

Product labels must always be consulted for proper mixing and diluting instructions and intended applications. Chemical incompatibilities may occur if products are mixed. Therefore, do not attempt to combine germicides or alter treatment procedures from the manufacturer's specifications.

When selecting germicidal procedures, patient-care equipment can be classified as critical, semicritical, and noncritical. Critical equipment includes those devices that are introduced directly into the body, such as surgical instruments, catheters, and implants. Sterility is essential—all contaminating microorganisms must be destroyed. Semicritical equipment includes those items that come in contact with various mucous membranes. Although sterilization is desirable, it is not essential. Disinfection of these items should inactivate vegetative bacterial cells and viruses. Semicritical equipment, such as thermometers, speculums, endotracheal tubes, and various diagnostic devices are often treated by immersion in chemical disinfectants. Noncritical patient-care equipment includes environmental surfaces, such as cages, tables, floors, walks, and so forth. Sterilization of these surfaces is impractical. Properly designed and supervised cleaning protocols are adequate. These surfaces should be cleaned periodically with a detergent and chemically disinfected.

Veterinary clinics and hospitals should restrict their use of disinfectants to Environmental Protection Agency (EPA) registered products that are labeled as a one-step cleaner-disinfectant for use in hospitals. The label should indicate that these products are effective in hard water up to 400 ppm hardness and in the presence of 5% serum. Most nonporous surfaces can be efficiently cleaned and disinfected with the newer combinations of twin chain quaternary ammonium compounds (C_8/C_{10} dimethyl ammonium chloride) and alkyl dimethyl benzyl ammonium chloride.

Biological Safety

Potential hazards in the veterinary hospital may be associated with infectious or chemical materials, physical facilities, and animal handling. Management should develop a comprehensive safety program that considers these dangers as well as preparedness for fire, accidents, and other disasters. This discussion will deal primarily with biological hazards related to infectious agents in the laboratory and hospital.

Each individual has responsibility for protecting oneself and others from accidental infection. Laboratory coats should be worn to prevent contamination of street clothes and dissemination of pathogens to homes and families. Disposable examination gloves should be worn when handling heavily contaminated materials. Good handwashing procedures should become a habit in the laboratory—between procedures if there was a chance of contamination and always before leaving the laboratory. Mouth pipetting should be prohibited in laboratories handling infectious material. Automatic or bulb pipetting devices should be used. Syringes and needles are poor substitutes for pipettes because they tend to favor creation of aerosols that may be inhaled. There is also the inherent danger of self-inoculation when handling syringes and needles. Self-inoculation must be guarded against, both in the laboratory and when inoculating animals. Modified or avirulent live vaccines are defined as nonpathogenic for a specific animal but may be much more virulent if accidentally inoculated into other animals or humans. An example is *Brucella* infection of humans inoculated with strain 19 vaccine. Centrifuge accidents, which may produce infectious aerosols, should be avoided by selecting compatible tubes, performing proper balancing, and not exceeding recommended centrifugal forces.

Good housekeeping procedures that will maintain a neat, uncluttered work area should be adopted. Eating, drinking, or smoking should not be allowed in work areas, even during break periods when there is no laboratory activity.

Immunization of personnel is recommended when they are at increased risk of infection. A minimal prophylactic immunization for all personnel employed in veterinary hospitals and laboratories should include rabies vaccine and tetanus toxoid. Other immunization products may be recommended in areas in which there is an unusually high risk of exposure to a particular infectious agent.

Primary containment equipment and laboratory design features are important factors in biological safety. Directional air flow should be from clean areas to areas of contamination and should then be exhausted from the building without recirculating. Small veterinary laboratories and hospitals usually cannot justify the cost of biological safety cabinets for diagnostic procedures. However, some infectious agents are of sufficient hazard that they must be handled only in laboratories with special design features, including biohazard cabinets. Zoonotic pathogens that small laboratories should not attempt to isolate include the agents of anthrax, brucellosis, plague, tuberculosis, tularemia, and systemic mycoses.

The clinical laboratory has a responsibility to decontaminate potentially infectious materials and wastes before they are discarded. Many states have adopted statutes and regulations that stipulate how hazardous waste materials must be handled. Clinical veterinary laboratories are required to comply with these rules as well as EPA and Occupational Safety and Health Administration (OSHA) requirements. All diagnostic specimens (swabs), inoculated media, viable cultures, glassware, instruments, and equipment should be considered to be contaminated. Decontamination methods should be applied before waste materials are discarded or reusable products are cleansed. The most practical decontamination procedure for most infectious wastes is the steam autoclave. Other methods include physical procedures (incineration, boiling, irradiation), and chemical agents (phenolics, hypochlorites, formaldehyde).

Recommended Reading

Carter CR and Chengappa MM: Microbial Diseases: A Veterinarian's Guide to the Laboratory Diagnosis. Ames, IA, Iowa State University Press, 1993.

Carter GR and Cole JR Jr: Diagnostic Procedures in Veterinary Bacteriology and Mycology, 5th ed. San Diego, Academic Press Inc., 1990.

Halliwell RE and Gorman NT: Veterinary Clinical Immunology. Philadelphia, WB Saunders, 1989.

Koneman EW, Allen SD, Dowell VR Jr, et al: Color Atlas and Textbook of Diagnostic Microbiology, 4th ed. Philadelphia, JB Lippincott, 1992.

Murray PR, Baron EJ. Pfaller MA, et al: Manual of Clinical Microbiology, 6th ed. Washington, DC, American Society for Microbiology, 1995.

National Committee for Clinical Laboratory Standards: Performance Standards for Antimicrobial Disk and Dilution Susceptibility Tests for Bacteria Isolated from Animals; Proposed Standard. NCCLS document M31-P. Villanova, PA, National Committee for Clinical Laboratory Standards. 1994.

Quinn PJ, Carter ME, Markey BK, et al.: Clinical Veterinary Microbiology. London, Mosby-Year Book Europe Limited, 1994.

Research Committee of the National Mastitis Council: Laboratory and Field Handbook on Bovine Mastitis, Fort Atkinson, WL, WD Hoard & Sons Co., 1987.

Rose NR, de Macario EC, Fahey JL, et al: Manual of Clinical Immunology, 4th ed. Washington, DC, American Society for Microbiology, 1992.

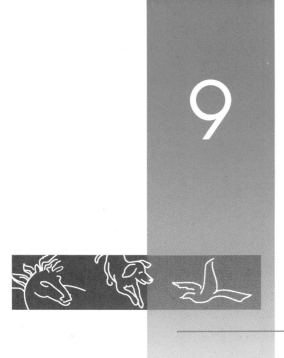

9 Diagnostic Imaging

Beth Paugh Partington

INTRODUCTION

Radiology and ultrasound are the primary diagnostic imaging techniques available to the veterinarian. However, for the veterinarian to arrive at the correct diagnosis on the basis of a radiographic or ultrasound examination, images of high quality must be available. The responsibility to provide useful diagnostic images usually falls on the shoulders of the veterinary technician.

This chapter deals with the basic, but essential, information needed to produce x-rays and sonograms of diagnostic quality. It is not the intent of this chapter to offer a course in radiation physics, ultrasound physics, and proper positioning of animals for examination. Excellent textbooks on these subjects have been written and should provide the veterinary technician with the detailed information needed; see Curry et al. (1990), Douglas et al. (1987), Han et al. (1994), Lavin (1994), Morgan (1993), and Ticer (1984). These books should be consulted when the need arises.

This chapter discusses the basic information needed to support and assist the veterinary technician in the area of radiology and diagnostic ultrasound. A short introduction into the use of nuclear imaging, computed tomography, and magnetic resonance imaging is included. Every effort is made to simplify the radiation and ultrasound physics.

RADIOLOGY

Legal Records and Film Identification

Radiographs are part of the medical record and should be clearly labeled as to which animal has been examined. The identification should include the name of the patient and owner or patient identification number, date of the examination, and name of the hospital.

TECHNICIAN NOTE

Radiographs are part of the legal medical record and must be correctly identified and carefully labeled.

Several methods of film labeling are available. The most common methods used by veterinarians are leaded numbers and letters placed on the cassette at the time of exposure (Fig. 9–1A). These show up as white markings on a finished radiograph. Also available is a special graphite-impregnated tape on which the desired information can be written or typed and placed on the cassette, or the information can be taped on a special filter as the time of exposure (Fig. 9–1B). One of the better film identification methods is a *light flasher system* (Fig. 9–2). It is simple and inexpensive. The required information is typed on a card that is placed in the imprinter. This system requires placing a small, leaded blocker in the upper lefthand corner of the intensifying screen, which will prevent exposure to that part of the film. The card is placed in the light flasher in the dark room. The unexposed, lefthand corner of the exposed radiograph is placed underneath the card, and the light is flashed through the card. The information recorded on the card is transferred to the x-ray film and will be developed when the radiograph is processed (Fig. 9–3).

One final identification method requires both a film identi-

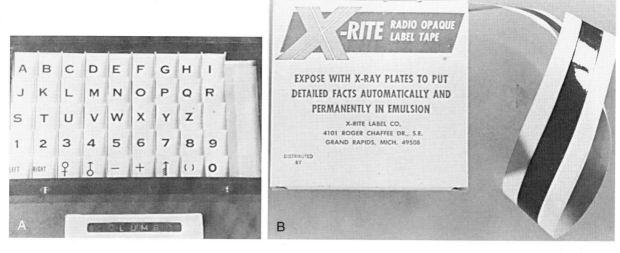

Figure 9-1. Film labeling. A, Leaded letters and numbers placed on the cassette at the time of exposure. B, Radiographic label tape.

fication camera and special windowed film cassettes. This method allows one to type the required information on a 3 × 5 card and place the card into the ID camera. The windowed corner of the cassette is then automatically opened and "flashed" by the camera, and the information is exposed on the x-ray film. The benefits of this system are that the camera will automatically identify the date and time of the examination, it can be done in daylight, and the area on the film in which the identification information is placed is constant (Fig. 9–4).

In addition to the legal identification imprinted on the film, it is necessary to identify the part radiographed at the time of exposure. Leaded right and left markers should be placed on the cassette at the time of exposure to identify the extremity radiographed or the side on which the animal is positioned for examination (i.e., right or left lateral recumbency) (Fig. 9–5). Front leg versus hind leg and medial versus lateral side identification markers are critical for proper interpretation of equine lower-extremity radiographs.

Filing of the Radiograph

Because a radiograph is part of the medical record, one must be able to retrieve it when needed. The radiographs of each examination should be placed in an x-ray envelope and filed according to the filing system used for other hospital records (i.e., by last name or case number). The following information should be recorded on the envelope: owner's address, animal identification, date, and type of examination. In addition, the radiographic technique used for the examination could be recorded on the envelope to provide an easy reference for follow-up studies.

It would be most advantageous to the veterinarian if the envelope could be coded for use as a self-teaching file. Several color tape systems have been devised to code cases for specific purposes. The system could be refined to include a combination of color to identify species, breeds, system examined, and so on. Morgan (1993) outlined an excellent color-coded system for x-ray retrieval purposes.

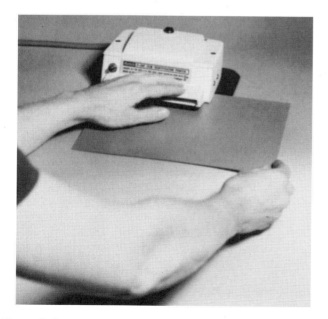

Figure 9-2. Light flasher. Patient information is printed onto a radiograph with an identification printer. (From Eastman Kodak Co.: The Fundamentals of Radiography. 12th ed. Rochester, NY, Eastman Kodak Co., Radiographic Markets Division, 1980.)

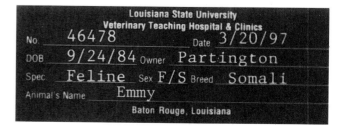

Figure 9-3. Film identification as it appears on a radiograph. The identification is flashed onto the film after x-ray exposure with a light flasher system or film identification camera.

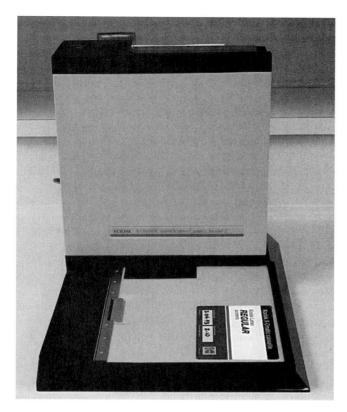

Figure 9–4. Film identification camera and special windowed x-ray cassette. Patient information is typed onto a 3 × 5-inch card and inserted into the top of the camera. The special cassette slides into the camera, which opens the window and flashes the identification onto the film.

PRODUCTION OF X-RAYS

Basic Principles

A basic understanding of x-ray production, radiological image formation, interactions of radiation with tissue, and radiation protection is essential. For those with little knowledge of physics or mathematics, the idea of having to learn basic radiation physics may be upsetting. However, the aim is not to teach radiation physics but rather to present basic concepts that are useful for those who use x-ray equipment.

X-rays can be defined as nonluminous electromagnetic radiations that are similar to visible light and to radio and television signals but are of much shorter wavelengths. The shorter the wavelenghts, the greater is the energy of the x-ray beam. The greater the energy of the x-ray beam, the greater is its penetration

X-rays are capable of penetrating opaque or solid substances, ionizing gases, and tissues through which they pass and affecting photographic plates and fluorescent screens. Because of these characteristics, x-rays are widely used in medicine for the study, diagnosis, and treatment of certain organic disorders, especially those of internal structures of the body.

Unfortunately, because of their short wavelengths, x-rays are not visible. As a consequence, many veterinarians, physicians, x-ray technologists and veterinary technicians have a tendency to become careless in the day-to-day use of x-rays by neglecting to use protective equipment or apply basic radiation safety rules.

The X-Ray Tube

Filament and Focusing Cup

The source of x-rays used in diagnostic radiology is the x-ray tube. The generators and transformers used in radiology exist only for the purpose of providing and controlling the amount of electricity reaching the x-ray tube. The x-ray tube is composed of an anode ($+$) and a cathode ($-$) enclosed in a vacuum within a glass envelope surrounded by a lead housing. The cathode contains one or two coiled wire filaments within hollowed-out wells or focusing cups. The filaments produce a source of electrons ($e-$) that are used to produce x-rays (Fig. 9–6). The filament is heated to a critical temperature, and the

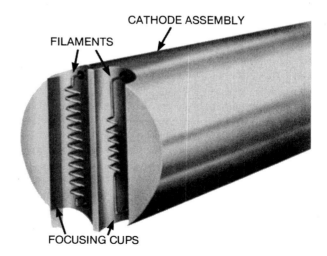

Figure 9–6. Cathode assembly showing focusing cups and filaments of two different sizes. Their arrangements produce electron beams that are focused onto narrow rectangles on the target. The smaller filament produces an electron stream of a smaller cross-sectional area and, therefore, a smaller focal spot. (From Eastman Kodak Co.: The Fundamentals of Radiography. 12th ed. Rochester, NY, Eastman Kodak Co., Radiographic Markets Division, 1980.)

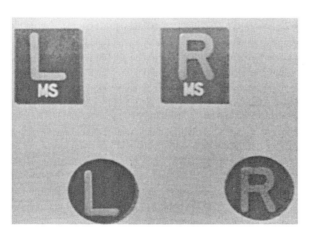

Figure 9–5. Leaded letters for film labeling. R (right) and L (left) markers are illustrated. The top markers include the initials of the technician who took the films.

electrons are boiled off and form an e− cloud within the focusing cup. The electrons are then accelerated very rapidly toward the positively charged anode. The collision of the speeding electrons into the anode results in the production of heat and x-rays. The x-rays are directed downward or vertically through the window of the tube by the angle of the anode and the lead shielding of the x-ray tube (Fig. 9–7). Two electrical circuits are present in every x-ray tube: a high-voltage, or kilovoltage (kV), circuit and a low-voltage, or milliamperage (mA), circuit. The kilovoltage circuit controls the electrical potential between the anode and cathode. This controls the speed of the electron acceleration and the energy level or penetrability of the resulting x-ray beam. The milliamperage circuit controls the electrical potential across the filament and affects the volume of electrons created and thus the number or volume of x-rays created.

The filament must produce electrons without melting. To this effect, an *alloy of tungsten* is used because it is less brittle and more efficient than pure tungsten for the production of electrons. This alloy has a high melting point and is used for the manufacture of most x-ray tube filaments.

The larger filament contains more tungsten than the small one and therefore can produce more electrons. As a result, the electron beam produced is larger and does not produce as sharp an x-ray picture as the smaller filament. Unfortunately, because of its size, the small filament may melt more rapidly than the larger one if an excess load is placed on it. As a result, the veterinarian and veterinary technician must always be aware of the limits and capabilities of the equipment when selecting which filament (focal spot) to use for a given procedure

Focal Spot

The smaller filament provides a small target region or focal spot for electrons at the anode. In general, the small filament is used to obtain images of higher quality. However, because of the limited number of electrons provided by a small filament, its use is generally restricted to lower mA·sec settings used primarily in table top (nongrid) extremity radiography. When higher tube current and shorter exposure time are desired, the larger filament must be used, although there will be a loss of detail because the focal spot will be larger.

The size of the focal spot is determined by the size of the electron beam that is accelerated within the tube when high-voltage potentials are applied between the electrodes. Thus, electrons traveling at an extremely high speed in the vacuum tube are suddenly stopped on the "target" area of the anode. As previously mentioned, the target is usually composed of an alloy of tungsten. Tungsten is used because it has special properties as a target material; these properties include the following.

1. High atomic number for the efficient production of x-rays
2. High melting point to withstand the large amount of heat generated by the electron beam
3. High capacity to transfer heat from the area in which electrons are absorbed
4. High density to absorb the electron beam in a small surface area
5. Low vapor pressure to maintain the vacuum inside the x-ray tube
6. Relatively easy machinability into the appropriate shape at a reasonable cost

Stationary Anode

In early x-ray equipment, stationary anodes were used in most x-ray tubes. This type of x-ray tube is still prevalent in some veterinary hospitals in which older equipment is used, in dental equipment, and in small portable units used extensively in large animal radiology

In x-ray tubes with stationary anodes, the target area is a small tungsten block of about 3.18 mm thick embedded in a large block of copper. The copper is used to absorb and diffuse the tremendous amount of heat generated by the interaction of the electron beam with the target areas. This type of tube is popular and effective in radiography of the extremities of horses and dogs. However, it has limited application for the abdomen and thorax. The stationary anode x-ray tube cannot produce a sufficiently powerful x-ray beam to penetrate thicker body parts. It is also limited in its ability to produce a very rapid x-ray exposure of sufficient strength for chest radiography to stop respiratory motion (see Fig. 9–7).

Rotating Anode

Rotating anodes became popular with the advent of more powerful x-ray machines and the requirement of radiologists to obtain x-ray pictures of higher quality. Rotating anode tubes can use much higher tube currents, shorter exposure times, and focal spots as small as 0.1 mm because the electrons deposit their energy over a larger target region as the anode rotates (Fig. 9–8).

The target of a rotating anode is a tungsten alloy bonded to molybdenum or graphite to help diffuse the tremendous heat generated by a high-powered x-ray machine. Rotating anodes are from 7.5 to 12.5 cm in diameter. These tubes must dissipate enormous amounts of heat. The apparatus used to rotate the anode and dissipate the heat must be of the highest quality and perfectly balanced to prevent the tube from wobbling. Any

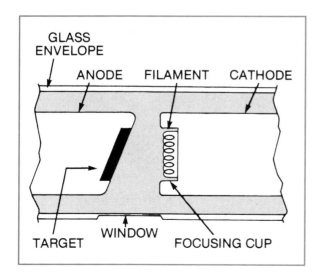

Figure 9-7. Stationary-anode x-ray tube. Diagram shows the relation of the anode and cathode. (From Eastman Kodak Co.: The Fundamentals of Radiography. 12th ed. Rochester, NY, Eastman Kodak Co., Radiographic Markets Division, 1980.)

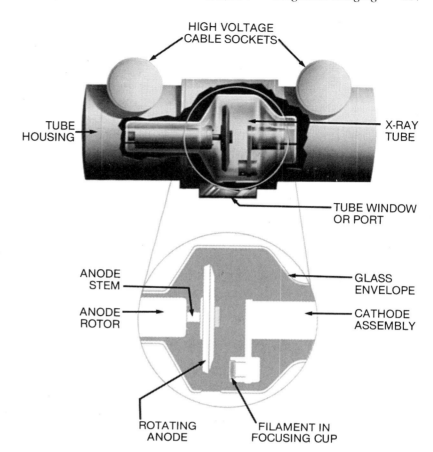

Figure 9-8. Modern rotating-anode radio graphic tube. Exploded schematic view demonstrates the relationship of the filament to the rotating target. (From Eastman Kodak Co.: The Fundamentals of Radiography. 12th ed. Rochester, NY, Eastman Kodak Co., Radiographic Markets Division, 1980.)

imbalance causes the anode to wobble, leading to loss of image quality and eventual tube destruction. Figure 9–9 represents a diagram of a rotating anode tube. Some tubes may rotate at speeds varying from 3600 revolutions per minute (rpm) to 10,000 rpm. Rotating anode x-ray machines generally have a two-step exposure switch. The first step of the switch starts the anode rotating, and the second step of the switch activates the high-voltage circuit, resulting in x-ray production. The x-rays produced at the anode are directed to the window of the x-ray tube. These x-rays form the primary x-ray beam, which, as shown later, is further modified to obtain the best possible diagnostic x-ray beam (Fig. 9–10).

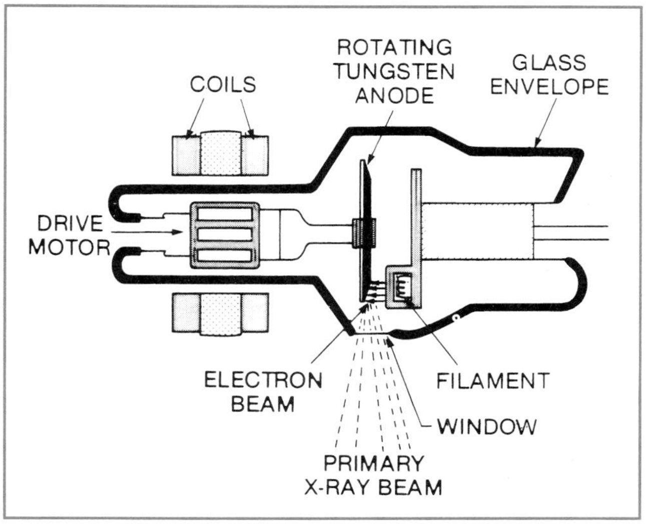

Heel Effect

When an x-ray beam leaves the tube, it has an uneven x-ray photon distribution. This phenomenon is related to the angle of the target areas and the absorption by the anode and target material. As a result of this engineering feature, the x-ray beam is more intense at the side of the cathode than in the center of the beam or on the anode side.

This feature can be used to great advantage in veterinary radiology when radiographing parts of uneven thickness. This is a common problem in thoracic and abdominal radiography of deep-chested dogs. By placing the thickest part of the patient toward the cathode side of the x-ray tube, a more uniform density can be obtained on the radiograph. This phenomenon is called the *heel effect* (Fig. 9–11).

Figure 9-9. Rotating-anode tube. Heat is better dissipated by placing the target material at the circumference of a high-speed rotating disk.

✎ **TECHNICIAN NOTE**

Always place the thickest part of the area you are radiographing toward the cathode side of the x-ray tube.

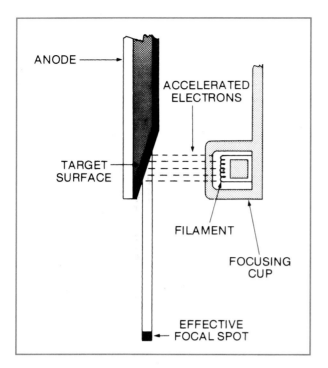

Figure 9–10. Effective focal spot. The surface area is decreased when the target area is constructed at a 20-degree angle to the electron beam.

Tube Rating Chart

A rating chart is provided by all manufacturers of x-ray tubes. The tube rating chart provides important information on the maximum safe exposure time that can be used with specific mA and kV settings. If longer-than-designated exposure times are used, tube damage may occur. The size of the anode focal spot determines the rating of the tube because size controls

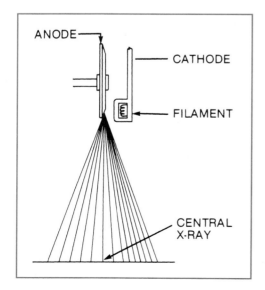

Figure 9–11. Heel effect, which is produced by the uneven intensity of the primary beam. The intensity decreases rapidly toward the anode.

the amount of energy it can absorb and convert into x-rays and heat.

The Physics of X-Ray Production

X-rays are produced when all the energy packed in extremely rapidly moving electrons comes to an abrupt stop on encountering the target in the x-ray tube. It should be mentioned at this point that most of the energy of the electrons is not converted into x-rays but is dissipated as heat. In fact, 99% of the energy dissipated in the target is lost as heat, and only 1% is converted to x-ray energy. This explains the elaborate system of heat dissipation built into the x-ray tube described in the previous section

Two events may occur when electrons approach the atoms of the target: (1) the electrons may miss the atom and its orbital electrons and go through the entire target and eventually be absorbed by the backing material of the target or the lead shielding of the x-ray tube, or (2) the incoming electrons may interact with atoms in the target material and produce x-rays by transferring their energy to these atoms. The faster the electrons travel, the greater is their energy and, therefore, the greater is the energy available for production of x-rays.

Scattered Radiations

In passing through a body of matter, an x-ray goes through attenuation; in other words, its energy decreases gradually. *Scattered radiations* are x-ray photons that have undergone a change in direction after interacting with atoms.

Scattered radiations are of concern because they decrease film quality and increase radiation exposure to the radiographer. Scattered radiations contribute to the overall film blackness or radiographic density but do not contribute to the useful image. This results in reduced subject contrast. Scattered radiations are also the primary source of radiation exposure to technicians manually restraining patients. Scattered radiations are directly increased with increases in the following three factors: (1) kilovoltage, (2) thickness of the part radiographed, and (3) size of the field (Fig. 9–12).

Careful collimation with beam-limiting devices and close attention to technical factors to avoid retakes are the best ways to decrease radiation exposure from scattered radiations. Several techniques are used to reduce scattered radiations and their effects on the radiograph. Beam-limiting devices, correct kilovolt peak (kVp) settings, and grids are a few devices that can be used to control scattered radiations. They are discussed later in this chapter.

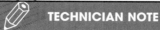
TECHNICIAN NOTE

Scattered radiations coming from the area of the patient that is exposed during radiography is the main source of radiation exposure to the veterinary technician.

X-RAY EQUIPMENT

The kind of x-ray unit encountered in a veterinary practice will vary according to the case load and type of practice. Because

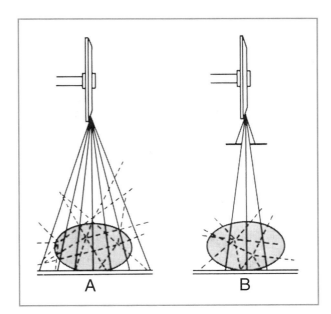

Figure 9-12. Scattered radiations. A, Scattered radiations are produced when the primary beam is not restricted by a collimator. B, Reduction in the amount of radiation produced when the primary beam is restricted by a diaphragm or collimator.

one may be working with a large or small practitioner, in a large corporate practice, or in a veterinary teaching hospital, it is necessary to be familiar with the several types of x-ray units found in such practices.

Regardless of type and model, most x-ray machines share many features. For small-animal radiology, an x-ray machine must have a table on which the animal is positioned (Fig. 9–13). For larger animals, hand-held or stationary cassette holders are most often used. All x-ray machines must have a control panel to select kilovoltage, milliamperage, and time of exposure. An x-ray machine may have numerous auxiliary meters, buttons,

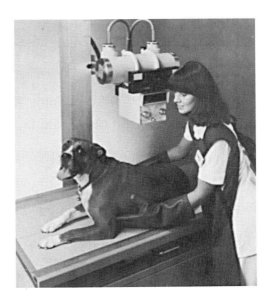

Figure 9-13. X-ray table commonly used for small animal x-ray examination.

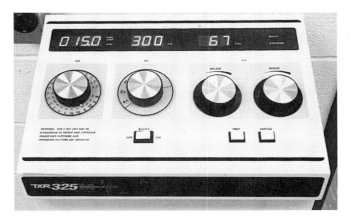

Figure 9-14. Typical instrument panel of an x-ray machine used by veterinarians showing multiple dials for selection of milliamperage, time, and kVp.

dials, or switches, but kilovoltage, milliamperage, and time of exposure are the three primary factors of x-ray production (Figs. 9–14 and 9–15). Many x-ray machines have a common selector control for milliamperage and time of exposure. This mA·sec dial or setting automatically sets the highest mA station and fastest time to give the requested mA·sec. Milliamperage × time in seconds (mA·sec) controls the volume or number of x-ray photons produced. In older machines, mA and time (in fractions of a second) must be set manually to produce a given mA·sec.

There are basically three types of x-ray machines used in veterinary practice: (1) portable unit, (2) mobile unit, and (3) stationary unit.

TECHNICIAN NOTE

Kilovoltage, milliamperage, and time of exposure are the three factors that must be set correctly to produce a properly exposed radiograph.

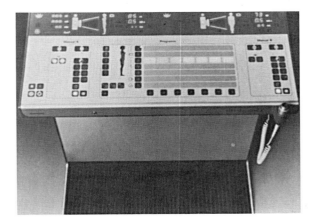

Figure 9-15. Operator control console used in some of the larger veterinary clinics and several veterinary teaching hospitals.

Portable Unit

As the name implies, portable units can be carried "easily" from one location to another. Weight varies from 6.75 to 20.25 kg or more. They are generally used on blocks or custom-made stands. From the safety aspect, these units should never be hand-held. This recommendation applies especially to lighter models that have less shielding. Hand-holding an x-ray machine not only places the operator in close proximity to the x-ray tube but also decreases film quality due to tube motion during exposure.

Common characteristics of portable units include the following:

1. A single focal spot of about 1.2 mm. stationary anode tube, and single filament, although a few models have two filaments and focal spot sizes.
2. Collimation varying from lead adaptor plate to adapt to film size to lighted collimator with adjustable field size.
3. Tube output varying up to 90 kVp at 10 mA, usually with settings at 10, 20, and 30 mA and at 70, 80, or 90 kVp.
4. Electronic timer ranging from 0.01 to 10 seconds.
5. Electrical input of 110 V with an adaptor to 220 V.

Some models may use 12 DC or operate on an automobile battery with converter (Fig. 9–16).

Mobile Unit

Mobile units are medium-powered, wheel-mounted units that can be moved around the hospital. In many small animal practices, these units are used as a fixed unit and remain in one room. They are also popular in a mixed type of practice, in

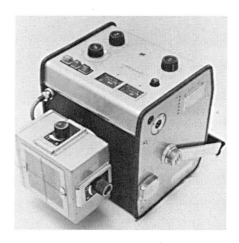

Figure 9-16. Portable x-ray unit. Such units are commonly used in large animal practices, mostly for the examination of extremities. This particular unit has a lighted collimator, which is an added safety device.

which the same unit can be used for both large and small animals.

These units are powered by 220-V or 110-V outlets. The 220-V units require more extensive electrical wiring, especially if the same units must be used at several locations. These units are equipped with a long, heavy power cord, which can be a problem when working with large animals. The 110-V units are usually lighter and therefore easier to move around, and the power cord is smaller, which can be an advantage when taking x-rays of equine extremities. However, these units are usually less powerful than the 220-V units (Fig. 9–17).

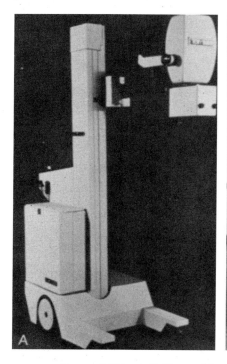
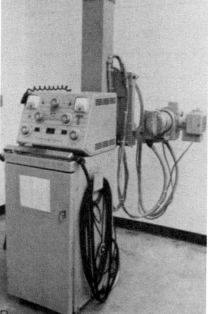
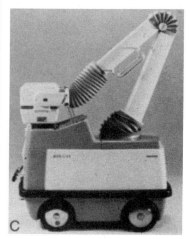

Figure 9-17. A–C, Three different types of mobile units that are used in veterinary practice. These units can be used for both large and small animal radiology in mixed practices.

Stationary Unit

Stationary units are more powerful and are found in larger small and large animal hospitals. They are common in all veterinary teaching hospitals. Some of these units are among the most powerful diagnostic x-ray units installed in the United States.

They vary in size from 300 mA, 100 kVp up to 2000 mA, 150 kVp. They can be powered by single-phase or three-phase generators. The x-ray tube may be ceiling-suspended or attached to a floor-stand support. The tube can rotate 90 degrees in all directions and usually has a heavy-duty collimator (Fig. 9–18).

The newer stationary units seen in veterinary practices are of the 300 to 500 mA type with an exposure time of 1/60 second to 1/120 second. All of these units can hold a cassette tray under the table with or without a Potter-Bucky grid. In addition, some units have an image intensifier unit for fluoroscopical study or a fixed fluoroscopical screen.

Fluoroscopy

Fluoroscopical units are more suited to the study of moving structures and dynamic processes than are x-ray films. Although films exposed close together in time provide some information about these structures and processes, an image that is continuous in time is required for maximum information. The presentation of continuous image is called *fluoroscopy,* and it involves

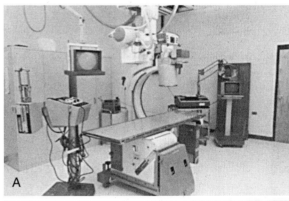

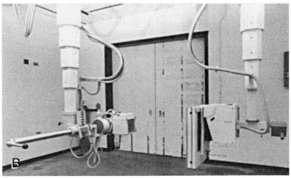

Figure 9-18. Stationary units. A, High-powered x-ray machine used for special procedures, such as angiography, in a few large and small animal hospitals and several veterinary teaching hospitals. B, High-powered stationary large animal unit that includes a ceiling-suspended x-ray unit and a Potter-Bucky suspension system. The two units can be interlocked when needed for a fixed focal spot film distance.

directing the x-ray beam through the patient and onto an x-ray–sensitive fluorescent screen. The use of fluoroscopy is usually confined to gastrointestinal studies and myelography and is essential to heart and vascular studies. It can be a very useful piece of equipment, but it is rarely used in veterinary medicine because of economic reasons. For a more extensive discussion of fluoroscopy, review the chapter discussing this subject in Curry et al. (1990), Douglas et al. (1987), Eastman Kodak Co. (1980), Lavin (1994), and Morgan (1993).

EXPOSURE FACTORS

It is the responsibility of the veterinary technician to select an x-ray technique that will provide a diagnostic x-ray film. The factors that must be selected are time of exposure, milliamperage, and kilovoltage. As previously mentioned, most recent x-ray machines have a common dial for time of exposure and milliamperage, called the mA·sec setting. The selection of each factor is based on an accurate technique chart. How to prepare a technique chart is discussed later in this chapter.

Other factors that enter into the production of a diagnostic radiograph are focal-film distance, type of intensifying screen, type of x-ray film, and tabletop versus grid technique. All these variables are discussed in greater detail.

Milliamperage

The milliamperage setting controls the quantity of electrons boiled off at the filament in the x-ray tube. It is a *quantity factor,* as it controls the amount of x-rays that will be produced at the target area. Most diagnostic units used in small animal radiology are operated at settings that vary from 50 to 300 mA. The smallest x-ray unit commonly used in large animal practices may utilize current flow as low as 10 or 20 mA, whereas the larger units used in small animal hospitals and veterinary teaching hospitals may have a current flow of 2000 mA.

Adjustments of the milliamperage setting control on an x-ray machine will control the amount of x-ray produced. When one increases the milliamperage setting, radiographic density, or film blackness, increases; conversely, when one decreases the milliamperage setting, a reduction in radiographic density, or a lighter film, results.

Exposure Time

The exposure time regulates the number of electrons that flow from the cathode to the anode per exposure. Ultimately, it regulates the quantity of x-ray reaching the film and therefore the film density By increasing the milliamperage setting, one can reduce the time of exposure for a given film density. Conversely, if a lower milliamperage setting is selected, a longer time of exposure will be needed to obtain the same film density.

As an example to illustrate this concept, an exposure made at 100 mA and 1/10 second should produce a film of equivalent density to an exposure made at 200 mA and 1/20 second. In both cases, the mA·sec factor (mA × time) is the same and is equal to 10 mA·sec. It should be remembered that shorter exposure times reduce the problem of motion, which may result in loss of detail. For this reason, a thoracic radiograph on a dog or cat should be taken at 1/20 to 1/60 second to prevent blurring of the radiograph due to respiratory motion.

Kilovoltage

Kilovoltage is a *quality factor* that regulates the energy of the x-ray beam. This setting regulates the voltage applied between the anode and cathode in the x-ray tube. The higher the voltage, the greater is the energy of the x-ray beam and therefore the greater is the amount of tissue that can be penetrated. The kilovoltage setting most often used in diagnostic radiology varies from 40,000 to 150,000 V (40 to 150 kV).

The kilovoltage setting increases the scale of contrast on a radiograph. The scale of contrast refers to the number of shades of gray that can be seen. In general, the greater the scale of contrast, the higher is the quality of the x-ray film because small differences in soft tissue density are better seen. Higher kilovoltage settings are used for soft tissue examination, such as thoracic examinations, and lower kilovoltage settings are used for bony structures. Increasing the kilovoltage will also increase radiographic density, or film blackness, because of increased patient penetration with the higher energy x-ray beam.

Focal-Film Distance

The focal-film distance refers to the distance between the target in the x-ray tube and the surface of the x-ray cassette. This factor is usually kept constant from one exposure to another. It is usually kept at a distance of 70 to 85 cm for large animal radiology and 90 to 105 cm for small animal radiology.

It is important to keep the focal-film distance constant from one exposure to the next because it has a significant influence on exposure factors. An increase in distance decreases the number of x-rays reaching the film very rapidly. If one doubles the focal-film distance, the number of x-rays reaching the film will be reduced by a factor of four. This is often referred to as the *inverse square law,* which states that the density of the x-ray beam at a given point is inversely proportional to the square of the distance from the x-ray source.

It is sometimes necessary to change the focal-film distance to obtain proper positioning. This simple calculation will help choose the proper milliampere-seconds setting when the distance is changed.

$$\text{Old pgmA·sec} \times \frac{(\text{New distance})^2}{(\text{Old distance})^2} = \text{New mA·sec setting}$$

For example, if an x-ray taken at 10 mA·sec at 100 cm must be taken at 50 cm, by using the formula given, the new milliampere-seconds setting can be calculated as.

$$10 \text{ mA·sec} \times \frac{(50)^2}{(100)^2} = 2.5 \text{ mA·sec}$$

This new mA·sec setting should produce an x-ray of similar radiographic density to the original setting of 10 mA·sec.

Technique Chart

A technique chart is an essential component for obtaining diagnostic x-ray examinations in a consistent way. A technique chart must be formulated for each x-ray machine because there are differences in output with each machine (even those made by the same manufacturer). Therefore, one should never use an x-ray chart formulated for another x-ray machine without making appropriate changes. If one selects exposure factors from a good technique chart, consistent radiographic examinations of diagnostic quality will be obtained. In addition, there will be a saving of x-ray films because waste from repeated exposures will be avoided.

There are several types of technique charts that can be formulated. Each type must be formulated with the goal of using the maximum potential of a particular x-ray machine. Perhaps the most popular type of technique chart used by veterinarians is a variable kilovoltage chart. A variable mA·sec chart is probably more appropriate for the most powerful x-ray machines. However, combination of variable kilovoltage and mA·sec technique charts is best. Such charts take into consideration the need to adapt a technique chart for different body systems, such as a thoracic and abdominal study, as well as examination involving the musculoskeletal system.

This chapter cannot discuss appropriately every type of technique chart. The principle of how to prepare a variable kilovoltage technique chart, along with an example of such a chart, is given. For a more extensive discussion of how to prepare different technique charts with examples of each, please refer to a more extensive treatment of this topic by Han et al. (1994), Lavin (1994), Morgan (1993), and Ticer (1984).

Formulation of a Technique Chart

A technique chart is formulated by a series of trial-and-error exposures. It is necessary, however, to standardize as many variable factors as possible before starting trial exposures. Factors such as the type of cassette and intensifying screen, type of x-ray film, and the focal-film distance must be constant, and a grid should be used if available. The darkroom procedures must be standardized to include fresh solution and developing time recommended by the manufacturer based on the temperature of the solution. It is most important to understand that all these factors should be constant because the technique chart will be valid only under the conditions of formulation. If, for example, cassettes and intensifying screens in a veterinary practice are of different age or speed, the film density for a given technique will be different from one study to the next, although the same factors are used.

For trial exposure, a normal dog with a lateral abdominal measurement of 8 to 10 cm should be selected. A trial exposure at a setting of 65kV at 2.5 mA·sec is suggested. Two exposures are made at this setting. In selecting the mA·sec setting, the shortest possible time of exposure for a given mA·sec setting is selected. The two films are then developed according to standard technique and are examined for proper "diagnostic" density. If the films are either overexposed or underexposed, a second series of exposures is made by halving or doubling the mA·sec setting. The films are again processed and examined for diagnostic quality. All films should be examined and compared to each other for consistent density between exposures. The best film is selected. If one of the techniques selected is completely satisfactory, a technique can be formulated starting with the factors that produced the "diagnostic" film. If, however, none of the films are totally satisfactory, a fourth series of exposures is started in which the kilovoltage setting is decreased or increased until an excellent film is obtained.

Because there is an increase in scattered radiation with an increase in thickness of a part to be radiographed, it is

• Table 9–1 •

THICKNESS (cm)	kV	mA	SECONDS	mA·sec	GRID 8:1
4	48	300	1/120	2.5	No
5	50	300	1/120	2.5	No
6	52	300	1/120	2.5	No
7	54	300	1/120	2.5	No
8	56	300	1/120	2.5	No
9	58	300	1/120	2.5	No
10	63	300	1/60	5	Yes
11	65	300	1/60	5	Yes
12	67	300	1/60	5	Yes
13	69	300	1/60	5	Yes
14	71	300	1/60	5	Yes
15	73	300	1/60	5	Yes
16	75	300	1/60	5	Yes
17	77	300	1/60	5	Yes
18	79	300	1/60	5	Yes
19	81	300	1/60	5	Yes
20	84	300	1/60	5	Yes
21	87	300	1/60	5	Yes
22	90	300	1/60	5	Yes
23	93	300	1/60	5	Yes
24	96	300	1/60	5	Yes
25	99	300	1/60	5	Yes
26	102	300	1/60	5	Yes
27	105	300	1/60	5	Yes
28	99	300	1/30	10	Yes
29	102	300	1/30	10	Yes
30	105	300	1/30	10	Yes

VARIABLE kV TECHNIQUE CHART FOR AN X-RAY MACHINE OF 300 mA, 125 kV, 1/120 SECOND TIMER WITH FFD OF 40 IN

Radiographs were taken with Kodak Lanex Regular screens and Kodak TML x-ray film.

recommended that a grid be used for thicknesses greater than 10 cm. If a grid of 5.1 ratio is used, it will necessitate a doubling of the mA·sec setting technique over the formulated technique. At this point, however, it is recommended that the accuracy of the technique chart be checked by making a few trial exposures of larger dogs using a grid.

The technique chart is formulated by subtracting 2 kV for each decrease in centimeter of thickness and adding 2kV for each increase in centimeter of thickness. One should keep in mind that a doubling of the mA·sec setting is necessary at thicknesses greater than 10 cm if a grid is used. At 80 kV and higher the increase in kilovoltage should be in steps of 3 kV for each increase in centimeter thickness until the limit of the machine is reached.

Table 9–1 illustrates a variable kilovoltage technique chart formulated for an x-ray machine of 300 mA, 125 kV, and 1/120 second minimum time of exposure. Remember, however, that this is only an illustration of how to formulate a technique chart and should not be used with any one x-ray machine without adaptation to that particular machine.

IMAGE FORMATION

When an x-ray beam penetrates a body system and reaches an x-ray film, a latent image is produced that will be revealed when the film is processed chemically. Several factors are involved in the formation of a high-quality latent image. In this section,

we discuss the factors that enter into the formation of an x-ray image.

X-Ray Cassette

Cassettes (film holders) used in veterinary medicine are of two types. The *nonscreen* type is a direct-exposure *cassette* in which the film is placed in a cardboard cassette or a plastic film holder (Fig. 9–19). The nonrigid system must be light-proof and is used when great detail is needed for an examination. The disadvantage of this type of cassette is that it will require exposure time that will be in excess of 26 times the normal exposure time of a regular par screen cassette system. Nonscreen exposures should be used only when the animal is under general anesthesia or heavy sedation to stop motion and no personnel are required for restraint in the radiology room. Nonscreen exposures are used primarily for intraoral occlusal studies of the nasal cavity and dental arches.

The second type is the more conventional *image intensifying screen,* which is placed in a *rigid cassette* (Fig 9–20). It is important that the hinges of the cassette be of the highest quality to ensure excellent and uniform contact between the x-ray film and the intensifying screen and to prevent light leakage that could fog or darken the film. Various materials are used in

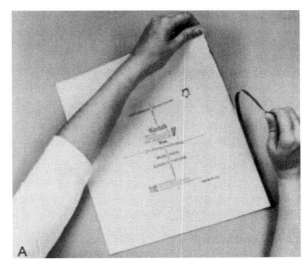

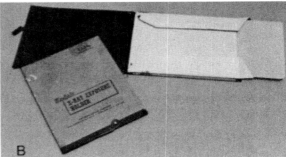

Figure 9–19. Nonscreen film. A, Ready pack film with a special emulsion for direct exposure. B, X-ray exposure holder for regular screen film. Such a cassette necessitates exposure time in excess of 26 times the normal exposure time of a regular par screen cassette system. (From Eastman Kodak Co.: The Fundamentals of Radiography. 12th ed. Rochester, NY, Eastman Kodak Co., Radiographic Markets Division, 1980.)

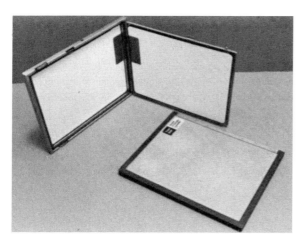

Figure 9-20. Rigid cassette with image-intensifying screens. This system is most commonly used in veterinary radiology and in human hospitals for x-ray development. The new rare earth screen system has the advantage of requiring a very short time of exposure compared with the nonscreen system.

the manufacture of x-ray cassettes. Most cassettes have a solid front made of either plastic or light metal. Recently, carbon fiber—mostly graphic—has been introduced. Such cassettes are excellent and may reduce the amount of x-rays needed to make an exposure by as much as 20%. The cassette back may be made of steel and can sustain moderate patient weight without being damaged. Sometimes, a small area of about 7 × 3 cm is shielded from the primary beam for the purpose of film identification (see Fig. 9–14).

Cassettes are expensive and should be handled with care. When dropped, they may warp, or if the cover is forced, the hinges may be damaged, resulting in a cassette that does not close properly. If the film contact is not perfect along the surface of the cassette, distortion of the x-ray image will occur. The surface of the cassette should be kept clean at all times to avoid creating film artifacts.

Intensifying Screens

Intensifying screens are layers of tiny crystals bonded together on a plastic support and covered with a protective coating.

These crystals fluoresce or emit light after exposure to x-rays. The screens are placed in the inner surfaces of the cassette, and the x-ray film is sandwiched in-between. Because film is more sensitive to light exposure than to radiation exposure, the use of fluorescent intensifying screens dramatically decreases the amount of radiation needed to produce a film of diagnostic radiographic density. Screens allow much lower mAs settings, which decrease loss of detail due to motion, decrease patient radiation exposure, and help to prolong x-ray tube life. In addition, intensifying screens increase radiographic contrast and therefore improve radiographic detail.

Intensifying screens are mounted in pairs in an x-ray cassette (Fig. 9–21). They are made of four components:

1. A backing of cardboard or plastic, most commonly mylar material
2. Reflecting layers, such as titanium dioxide, which reflect light from the active layer back toward the x-ray film
3. An active layer of light-emitting phosphor, such as calcium tungstate or rare earth material, which produces the fluorescence that exposes the film following absorption of x-rays
4. A plastic coating that reduces static electricity and provides a protective covering that can be cleaned

The screens must be cleaned on a regular basis—at least once a month or whenever screen artifacts are noted on a radiograph. It is best to use a cleaning product recommended by the manufacturer for this purpose. If this is not available, a 70% alcohol solution will work. It is essential that the surface of the screen be thoroughly dry before one inserts an x-ray film or closes the cassette; otherwise, the film will stick to the screens and permanently ruin them. Any stain on the surface of the screen will interfere with transmission of light from the screen to the film and cause an artifact. It is for this reason that emphasis is placed on the maintenance and cleanliness of screens.

Screen Speed

The speed of a screen pertains to its ability to convert absorbed x-ray energy into visible light. Screen speed is a relative term

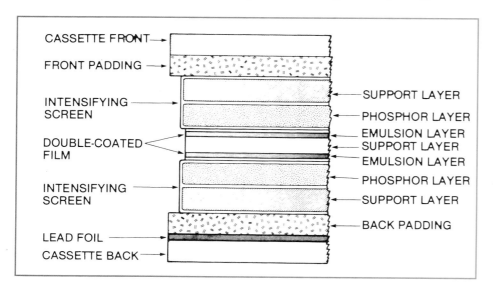

CASSETTE FRONT
FRONT PADDING
INTENSIFYING SCREEN
DOUBLE-COATED FILM
INTENSIFYING SCREEN
LEAD FOIL
CASSETTE BACK

SUPPORT LAYER
PHOSPHOR LAYER
EMULSION LAYER
SUPPORT LAYER
EMULSION LAYER
PHOSPHOR LAYER
SUPPORT LAYER
BACK PADDING

Figure 9-21. Cross section of a cassette intensifying screen system.

that refers to the amount of radiation required by that screen to produce a film of diagnostic radiographic density. A fast screen requires less radiation than a regular, medium, or par screen to produce the same degree of blackness on the radiograph. The faster the screen, the poorer is the radiographic detail or resolution. Fast screens have a thicker phosphor layer and larger crystals to increase x-ray absorption and light production. Slower or detail screens have smaller crystals and are less efficient at light conversion but produce a radiograph of greater detail and resolution. Detail screens are also called fine screens and generally require four times the amount of radiation as a medium or par screen. Regular screens are intermediate in speed between par or medium and fast screens.

The original phosphor used in intensifying screens was calcium tungstate. This phosphor produces light in the blue spectrum and is commonly found in veterinary hospitals that have acquired used cassettes and screens from local human hospitals. Improved rare earth phosphors introduced in 1975 emit light in the green spectrum and are able to produce the same degree of radiographic detail as calcium tungstate screens with less radiation exposure. Table 9–2 shows the relative speed of various calcium tungstate and rare earth screens. Rare earth screens are more efficient because they absorb more x-ray photons per crystal and produce more light per absorbed photon. These properties of rare earth screens have definite advantages in veterinary medicine and include (1) reduced exposure time; (2) reduced motion artifacts; (3) decreased tube voltage, resulting in improved contrast; (4) decreased tube current, which prolongs the life of the tube; (5) reduced production of heat in the x-ray tube; and (6) reduced patient radiation close.

TECHNICIAN NOTE

Rare earth screens are advantageous for veterinary radiography because they require fewer x-rays to produce a diagnostic radiograph. Lower exposures mean less patient and technician dose, fewer retakes due to patient motion, and longer x-ray tube life.

The main disadvantage of rare earth screens at this time is their cost, which is much greater than regular calcium tungstate screens. They have a definite place in large animal radiology because of their speed. This is an important factor when they are used with the smaller, low-capacity portable x-ray units. Table 9–3 presents an example of a technique chart that can be used with a small, portable x-ray unit in combination with the rare earth screen.

X-Ray Film

Because the recording medium for most x-ray examinations is photographic film, some basic principles of photography must be understood.

An x-ray film is prepared from a suspension of light- and x-ray–sensitive granules embedded in a gelatin emulsion coated over a polyester base. The sensitive granules are usually silver bromide crystals of different sizes. The gelatin matrix is pro-

• Table 9–2 •

RELATIVE SPEED OF CALCIUM TUNGSTATE* AND RARE EARTH† SCREENS

SCREEN TYPE	SPEED
Fine-detail calcium tungstate	30
Par calcium tungstate	100
Fine-detail rare earth	150
Regular calcium tungstate	200
Fast calcium tungstate	250
Medium rare earth	300
Regular rare earth	400
Fast rare earth	600

*Kodak X-O$_{MAT}$ with X-O$_{MAT}$ RP film.
†Kodak Lanex with T MAT L film.

tected by a thin covering called the *T coat*. Just like the image-intensifying screens, the sensitive crystals come in various sizes. Images of exceptional detail can be recorded on films containing very fine crystals. In faster films, the crystals are larger, which results in a loss of detail, which is compensated for, however, by possible shorter time of exposure. Because of the shorter time of exposure, faster films may sometimes provide better image detail because the images contain fewer motion artifacts.

X-ray film can be separated into two categories: *screen film* (Fig. 9–22) and *nonscreen*. Screen film is sensitive primarily to the wavelengths of light emitted from intensifying screens. Nonscreen films are designed for direct exposures to x-rays and are relatively insensitive to visible light from screens. Nonscreen films provide superb detail and are especially good for intraoral examination of the nasal cavity and bony extremities. Because this type of x-ray film is exposed by x-rays only, it has the disadvantage of needing very long exposure times to obtain necessary film density. Patients should be under general anesthesia and no personnel should be in the room during nonscreen film exposures.

• Table 9–3 •

TECHNIQUE CHART FOR PORTABLE X-RAY UNIT OF 10 mA AT 90 kV, 15 mA AT 80 kV AND 20 mA AT 70 kV CAPACITY USING KODAK CASSETTE WITH RARE EARTH SCREEN OF REGULAR SPEED*

EXAMINATION	SIZE	VIEW	kVp	TIME (sec)	DISTANCE (cm)
Fetlock	Foal	DP or obliques	80	0.02	60
	Large adult		80	0.04	70
Carpus	Foal	DP or obliques	80	0.02	70
	Large adult		80	0.04	70
Tarsus	Foal	L	80	0.02	70
		DP	80	0.04	70
	Adult	L	80	0.04	70
		DP	80	0.08	70
Stifle	Adult	L	80	0.1	70
		PD	90	0.25	70

*For a more complete treatment of cassette and image-intensifying screens, refer to Douglas et al. (1987) and Morgan (1993). Both give an excellent discussion of all types of screens available on the market today.
DP, dorsoplantar or dorsopalmar; PD, plantar-dorsal; L, lateral.

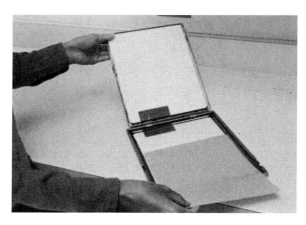

Figure 9–22. Screen film manufactured for the special purpose of being used with image-intensifying screens. The use of such film, when used with the proper combination of screen, will drastically reduce x-ray exposure time.

Screen-type films are less sensitive to direct ionizing radiation but are very sensitive to visible light. This type of film requires less exposure to produce a radiograph because of its sensitivity to the fluorescence emitted by the intensifying screens. Remember that screens produce a specific color or spectrum of light. The film used should be matched in sensitivity to the light spectrum of the screen.

Rare earth screens do need special x-ray films to produce an optimal radiograph. Every x-ray film manufacturer produces a rare earth type of x-ray film. There is great confusion because of the endless names and types of combinations of x-ray film and image-intensifying screens available on the market. Again, please refer to Douglas et al. (1987) and Morgan (1993) for a more elaborate discussion of this important topic.

 TECHNICIAN NOTE

Be sure the x-ray film you are using is maximally sensitive to the spectrum of light your screens are emitting.

Grids

When x-rays enter a patient, some pass straight through to the film cassette, but a great many are scattered or redirected along a different path before exiting the patient. The purpose of a grid is to control the scatter radiation before it reaches the x-ray cassette. A grid is constructed of a sheet of lead strips interfaced with radiolucent spacers made of plastic or aluminum. These strips are encased in an aluminum protective cover for durability. Grids come in various sizes similar to x-ray cassettes and are usually placed directly over the cassette between the animal and the cassette (Fig. 9–23).

The purpose of a grid is to allow only the primary x-ray beam to pass through and prevent scattered radiations from reaching the film. The grid is constructed in such a way as to absorb all radiations that do not pass between the lead strips. This arrangement may absorb most scattered radiations if grids of high ratios are used. However, it has the disadvantage of

absorbing part of the primary x-ray beam and therefore requires greater exposure time to obtain a given film density. Figure 9–24 illustrates how a grid absorbs scattered and secondary radiation and prevents it from reaching the film.

Grids are made of different ratios and number of strips per 2.5 cm. The ratio varies from 5:1 to 16:1 and from 60 lines (strips) per 2.5 cm to 120 lines per 2.5 cm. The higher the ratio and the number of lines per 2.5 cm, the more radiation is absorbed by the grid. The ratio of a grid refers to the relation between the height of the lead strips to the width of the radiolucent spaces. For example, if the height of the lead strip is 12 times greater than the thickness of the space, the grid ratio will be 12:1, and if it is 10 times greater, the ratio will be 10:1 and so on. The greater the ratio, the more efficiently the grid absorbs scattered radiations. Figure 9–24A illustrates the ratio of a 5:1 grid.

The grid is most useful in radiographing parts of the body in which scattering is considerable, which in practice includes all thick parts of the body (e.g., thorax, abdomen, skull) and those joints and bones in excess of 10-cm thickness. It is true that the film will show lines of the lead strips from the grid, but there will be a much improved quality of film of the part radiographed, with good detail because of the decreased scattered radiations.

Grids may be *parallel* or *focused*. A parallel grid is one constructed with strips parallel to each other. A focused grid is one in which the lead strips and spacers are gradually angulated from the center to the periphery of the grid. The distance from the point of convergence, or focal point, is referred to as its focal distance, or radius. The advantage of a focused grid is that it allows unobstructed amounts of radiation to pass through it at the center and at the edge of the grid as long as the radiations are parallel to the axis of the lead strips. Such grids can be used only at a specific focal-film distance specified by the manufacturer. If distances above or below the focal distance are used, grid cutoff will occur, which means that part of the primary beam will be absorbed by the grid.

For veterinary work, a grid with a ratio of 8:1 at 103 lines per 2.5 cm is recommended. With some minor work, a grid can be used with all sizes of cassettes if a wooden insert is constructed to fit around the smaller cassettes, always holding them at the center of the grid in a grid holder.

Cross-hatched grids are among other types of grids that

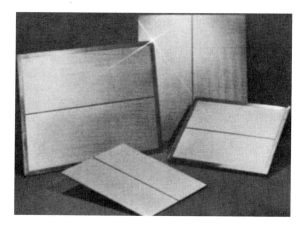

Figure 9–23. Various sizes and types of grids commonly used in veterinary radiology of large and small animals.

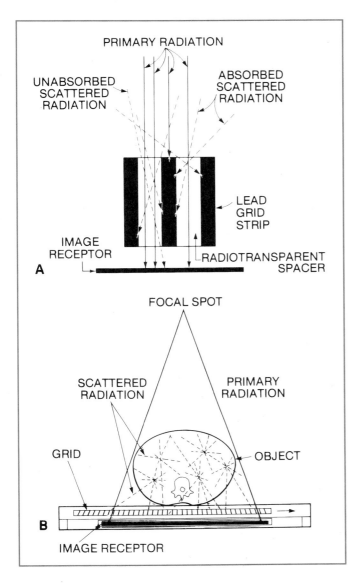

Figure 9-24. Cross section of a grid. A, Diagram of a small section of a grid showing how a large proportion of the scattered radiation is absorbed and image-forming primary radiation passes through to the image detector. B, Diagram of focused Potter-Bucky diaphragm being moved toward the right. (From Eastman Kodak Co.: The Fundamentals of Radiography. 12th ed. Rochester, NY, Eastman Kodak Co., Radiographic Markets Division, 1980.)

are used. These are stationary grids in which the lead strips crosscut others in a honeycomb pattern. The usual grid ratio of cross-hatched grids is 8:1, though a grid of 16:1 may be used with a very high kilovoltage technique. Cross-hatched grids can be obtained when necessary by placing two parallel grids at right angles to each other. There is very little need for such grids in veterinary practice because of the very high radiation exposures required with their use.

Potter-Bucky Diaphragm

One other type of grid encountered in veterinary hospitals is the *Potter-Bucky diaphragm*. This is simply a movable grid. The movement of the diaphragm is timed to suit a particular

exposure, and the grid moves across the film during the exposure so that the grid lines are not shown on the resulting film. When using a movable grid, the exposure time must be increased by a factor of four or the kilovoltage increased by about 20%. Usually, Potter-Bucky diaphragms are positioned under the table and electronically linked to the timer of the x-ray machine (Fig. 9–24B).

Another method to reduce scattered radiation is the *air gap technique*. It is a simple technique that consists of increasing the distance between the patient and the surface of the cassette. With this technique, the amount of scattered radiations produced is not reduced, but less scattered radiations reach the film because of the increased distance between patient and film. With the air gap technique, it is not necessary to increase the exposure factors, as must be done with a grid. However, this technique will decrease the sharpness of the image because of increased subject-to-film distance. It is also less effective at high kilovoltage settings, because the higher energy scatter occurs in a forward direction. This technique is used most commonly in veterinary radiology for magnification purposes and for equine thoracic radiography.

> **TECHNICIAN NOTE**
>
> Always use a grid between the patient and the film cassette when the body part you are radiographing is greater than 10 cm thick.

THE DARKROOM

The importance of the darkroom in radiography cannot be overemphasized. Radiography unquestionably begins and ends in the darkroom, in which films are loaded into cassettes ready for exposure and returned for processing into a finished radiograph. Most mistakes made in veterinary radiography are related to the processing of radiographs. It is necessary to keep the darkroom very clean and light-proof. It is also essential for the technician to have a thorough knowledge of x-ray darkroom technique and of conventional or automatic processing. The chemicals should be changed, replenished, maintained, and mixed according to the strict directions of the manufacturer.

Equipment

A darkroom need not be spacious. For most veterinary practices, a small room of about 240 × 240 cm is adequate. However, it is essential that this room be made totally dark. If there is a window in the room, there is no reason not to open it for ventilation when the room is not in use; however, the window should be light-proof when closed. It is important also that a lock be placed on the door to avoid its being opened while films are being processed. A darkroom need not be completely dark, because a safelight (a special light for darkroom use that will not expose film) can be used during film processing. It is important, however, that the safelight does not exceed the wattage recommended for the type of filter used; otherwise, the exposed films will be "fogged," or partially exposed, and the quality of the radiographs compromised. The proper type of light filter must be used in the darkroom. Orange, red, or

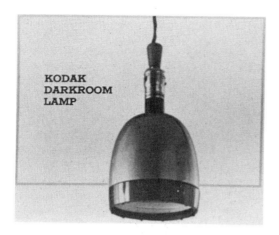

Figure 9-25. Darkroom lamp with a special filter to avoid fogging of x-ray films during loading and unloading of cassette.

yellow filters may be used with most x-ray films, but with the rare earth type of x-ray film, a special red filter must be used (Fig. 9–25). As a principle, it is important to keep in mind that no films should be exposed to the safelight any longer than necessary. It is important to work rapidly but carefully when processing x-ray films and loading and unloading films in the cassettes.

There must be a workbench in the darkroom located as far away from the processing tanks as possible so that liquid or dry chemicals will not be spilled on it. Above or below the bench there should be shelves to store film hangers and unexposed films and cassettes. It is necessary to keep x-ray film in a cool, dry place protected from extraneous x-rays.

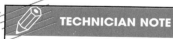

TECHNICIAN NOTE

Remember, all film and safelights are not created equal. Make sure the wavelength or color of light to which your film is sensitive is completely blocked by your safelight filter.

Hand Processing Equipment

The processing equipment should include a developing tank, rinsing tank, and fixer tank. The tanks should be big enough to accommodate several 35 × 42.5-cm films at the same time. Running water in the rinsing tank is ideal. If it is not available, the water should be changed frequently. Development and fixer solutions should be changed every 90 days regardless of use and more frequently if radiograph volume is high. The tanks should ideally be made of stainless steel for ease of cleaning (Fig. 9–26).

In certain areas of the country, it will be necessary to heat up or cool down the solutions during certain times of the year. This may be accomplished with an electric heater or a cooling device. During the heat of the summer, it may be necessary to add ice to the washing water to keep the solutions at the proper temperature. An inexpensive way to keep the solution temperature constant in processing tanks is by installing a good

quality shower-bath mixer valve. This type of valve is sufficient and economical enough to maintain the solution at a constant temperature in a low-volume practice. It is also important to have separate stirring rods made of stainless steel, plastic, or rubber and to mix the solutions thoroughly every day before starting the processing of films. Good ventilation is necessary to keep the room dry and avoid accumulation of volatile chemicals.

Automatic Film Processors

There are several makes and sizes of automatic processors on the market. In recent years, many veterinary hospitals have invested in automatic processing systems. There are small-capacity, 90-second processor units that can be installed in most darkrooms without remodeling. The larger processor units necessitate some remodeling because the input tray must be in the darkroom and the output side must be out of the darkroom. This usually necessitates some structural and plumbing modifications (Fig. 9–27).

As with manual processing tanks, it is necessary to maintain fresh solution and ensure that the solutions are flowing properly within the processor. Automatic processors may speed up and standardize film processing but require similar, if not more, maintenance compared with manual processing tanks. It is important to provide ventilation in the darkroom when automatic processors are used. Usually, a good-quality, light-tight exhaust fan installed in the ceiling is adequate.

Film Storage

X-ray films must be handled and stored properly for maximum usefulness. The film must be protected from light, x-radiations, gamma radiations, heat, moisture, and pressure. All these hazards may result in film fogging and decrease radiograph quality. As previously mentioned, the darkroom can fulfill this function if the room is kept clean and free of moisture. It may be helpful if the x-ray films are kept in their original boxes and placed in a cabinet. Special bins to store x-ray films can be purchased, but they are an unnecessary expense if proper care is used in storage (Fig. 9–28).

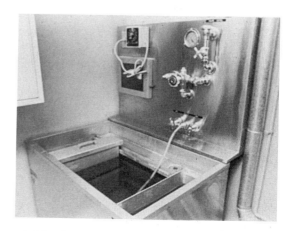

Figure 9-26. Processing tanks holding the developer (right), screening water to wash the films (middle), and the fixer (left). There is a mixing valve that maintains the solutions at a constant temperature.

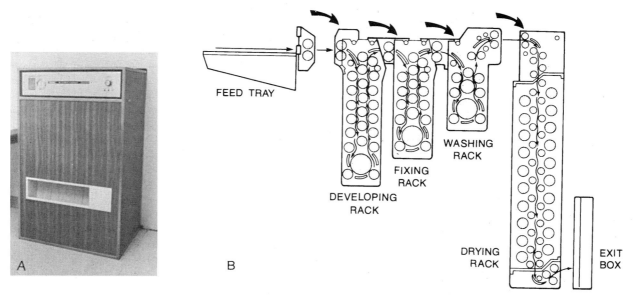

Figure 9-27. Automatic processor. A, Kodak X-OMAT processor (a 90-second processor) used in some veterinary hospitals. B, Diagram of a typical automatic x-ray processor.

Cassette Loading and Unloading

Care must be taken when transferring x-ray film from its box to the x-ray cassette to avoid static electricity, bending, creasing, or scratching. The film should be handled carefully, held only by the corners, and pulled from the box in a continuous and slow motion (Fig. 9–29). The film should be carefully placed in the cassette, making sure the edges do not extend over the edge of the film cassette. Great care should also be taken in removing x-ray film from the cassette to prevent damage or soiling of the intensifying screen.

Hanging X-Ray Film

When exposed films are placed on a film hanger after exposure, they must be handled carefully. The films should be handled

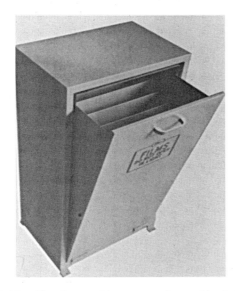

Figure 9-28. Film storage bin commonly used in darkrooms; it is designed to store open x-ray box films to load x-ray cassettes.

only by the corners and clipped to the stationary bottom clip first and then to the flexible top clip. It is most important to have dry hands when handling exposed, nonprocessed films. Any developer or fixer solution touching the film will create an artifact on the processed film (Fig 9–30).

Developing X-Ray Film

As previously mentioned, processing solutions (developer and fixer) should be stirred before inserting the film. When the film is placed in the developer, it should be agitated up and down a few times to remove air bubbles from the surface of the film. The film should be developed for 5 minutes at 20°C (68°F). If the temperature is above or below 20°C, the developing time should be adjusted according to the directions of the manufacturer. Rapid (3-minute) high-temperature film development or sight processing is not recommended due to decreased radiograph quality.

In the developing solution, the chemicals reduce the exposed silver halides in the x-ray film to metallic silver, which is black. Gradually through the developing process, the latent image is revealed. The film is then removed from the developer tank and quickly rinsed in the central water bath. It is then placed in the fixer solution, which stops the development process and preserves the film. The film should remain in the fixer for approximately twice the development time. The film is then placed in the central rinse tank for about 15 to 20 minutes. Films can be dried in a special air-circulated film dryer box or allowed to hang until dry in a well-ventilated dust-free area. For a more complete discussion of the chemistry of x-ray processing, please refer to the Kodak publication *The Fundamentals of Radiography* (1980).

Silver Recovery

In larger veterinary practices, the silver contained within the x-ray film emulsion may be removed and recovered. Most of the silver that is not exposed to x-rays is not converted to metallic

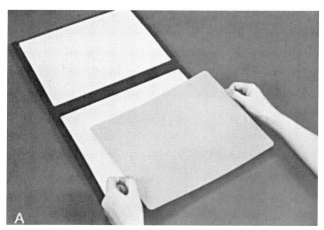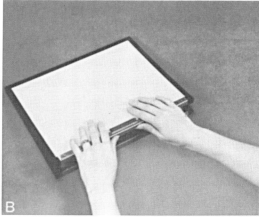

Figure 9-29.   When loading a cassette, (A) use both hands to avoid kink marks and carefully place the film into the cassette. B, The cassette must be closed and latched gently. (From Eastman Kodak Co.: The Fundamentals of Radiography. 12th ed. Rochester, NY, Eastman Kodak Co., Radiographic Markets Division, 1980.)

silver and accumulates within the fixer solution. Silver recovery units can be attached of the fixer solution to remove the silver by an electrolytic process. This, however, is only economical for the larger volume veterinary hospital. The silver can also be recovered from exposed and nonexposed x-ray film. There are a few companies that specialize in recycling x-ray film for silver recovery. This could be the source of a small "bonus" at the time an x-ray file is "purged" of the old cases on file.

RADIOGRAPHIC FILM QUALITY

It is of utmost importance to produce radiographs of excellent quality to arrive at a radiographic diagnosis. A film of good diagnostic quality should have excellent detail, correct scale of contrast, and optimal density. Each of these film characteristics is briefly discussed.

Detail

Radiographic detail refers to the degree of sharpness that defines the edge of an anatomical structure. It is the best possible

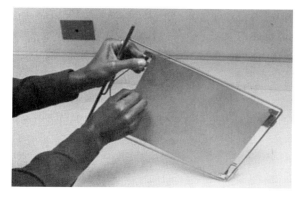

Figure 9-30.   When hanging x-ray films, they should be handled by the corners only and should be clipped first to the stationary bottom clip and then to the flexible top clip.

reproduction of an organ. Detail is influenced by every possible factor, but some are more influential than others.

The focal-film distance is one important factor in the loss of detail. If the focal spot is too close to the part radiographed, there will be magnification and lack of distinction at the margins of the structures radiographed. Therefore, it is important to keep the focal-film distance as long as possible without significantly reducing x-ray beam intensity. Most veterinary hospitals have radiographic technique charts that use a focal-film distance between 36 and 48 in. or 80 and 110 cm.

Movement in veterinary radiology is a constant problem, especially with older units that have a minimum exposure time of 1/10 second. It is difficult to produce diagnostic films of the thorax with a unit that does not have a minimum time of exposure of at least 1/30 second and ideally 1/120 second. With large animals, movement is a constant problem with a small, portable unit. This is why rare earth screens are becoming so popular in veterinary medicine; they have the advantage of requiring a much shorter exposure time.

The size of the focal spot is another important factor that regulates detail. The larger the focal spot, the poorer is the detail. Because most equipment in veterinary medicine has a rather large focal spot of 0.8 min or more, loss of detail may be significant, especially with older units that have focal spots of 1.2 to 2 min. Therefore, it is important to place the part to be radiographed as close as possible to the x-ray film. If the part is too far from the film, there will be magnification and distortion, resulting in a loss of detail. This is especially important in large animal radiology.

Other exposed factors that affect detail are poor film-screen contact and over or underexposed radiographs that often result from an improper technique chart or carelessness. Poor radiographic processing causes more ruined radiographs than all other factors combined. All processing errors affect detail. It is therefore important to standardize the developing process by following to the letter the instructions of the manufacturer.

Radiographic Contrast

Radiographic contrast refers to the density or opacity difference between two areas on a radiograph. High contrast means the opacity differences are large and there are fewer shades of gray. High-contrast radiographs are very black and white. Latitude refers to the range of different opacities on the radiograph. Long-latitude radiographs have a much larger number of shades of gray, but the difference or contrast between each shade is small. High-contrast radiographs are preferred for spine and extremity films. Long-latitude, low-contrast radiographs are preferred for thoracic films.

Kilovoltage is the factor that has the greatest influence on radiographic contrast. The higher the kilovoltage, the greater is the latitude and, therefore, the greater the number of shades of black, gray, and white. The absorption of the x-ray beam at high kilovoltage is more uniform among the various tissues in the body, resulting in less contrast. Therefore, for thoracic examinations, a high kilovoltage technique is recommended. For skeletal studies, a lower kilovoltage technique is recommended.

Other factors reducing contrast are scattered radiations (which can be markedly improved by the use of a grid), light leakage, and rapid high temperature processing techniques.

Radiographic Density

Radiographic density refers to the degree of blackness of the film. It is the result of the amount of light that was transmitted to the x-ray film after interaction of the crystals in the intensifying screens with the x-ray beam. When a film is properly exposed, the anatomic part radiographed will have good contrast with good differential absorption of the x-ray beam by the various tissue densities. Therefore, the part radiographed should be clearly seen but should not be so dark as to overexpose the anatomic structures to the degree that they are difficult to differentiate from the background film density. The thickness and density of the anatomic part radiographed do affect density. The thickest part will absorb more radiation, sometimes as much as denser tissues of lesser thickness.

The primary factor affecting density is the mA·sec setting. As you remember, the mA·sec factor is a quantity factor that regulates the amount of x-rays produced. If more x-rays reach the film, more light will be emitted by the screens, and the film will be darker. Therefore, it can be stated that *high mA·sec settings will increase film density and low mA·sec settings will reduce film density.*

Another factor that affects film density is the kilovoltage setting. At a higher kilovoltage, the x-ray tube is more efficient in producing x-rays and therefore increases the energy level of x-rays produced. If all other exposure and development factors are kept constant, increasing the kilovoltage will increase the radiographic density. This effect is more apparent at lower kilovoltage settings for a given part than at higher kilovoltage settings.

The distance from the focal spot to the surface of the film is another important factor in film density. If everything remains constant but the distance, a given examination could be markedly overexposed if the distance is reduced, or it could be underexposed if the distance is increased. This effect can be dramatic because the intensity of the radiation is reduced or increased as the square of the distance is changed. This effect was discussed in the section regarding inverse square law. It does emphasize the need for consistency and accurate measurement of the focal-film distance.

Magnification

Magnification is a technique rarely used in veterinary practices, but it is popular in veterinary teaching hospitals. Magnification is based on the principle that a larger image of an anatomic structure can be obtained if the distance between the object and the film is increased. Generally, the object to be magnified is placed halfway between the film cassette and the focal spot of the x-ray tube. This results in an x-ray image twice as large as the actual anatomic structure. However, to obtain diagnostic films, it is necessary to have a very small focal spot. A focal spot of 0.3 mm or smaller is needed for radiographic magnification. If larger focal spots are used, the advantage of direct magnification is lost because of the blurring at the margin of an organ produced by the larger focal spot. This technique would be useful to veterinarians, especially for studies of extremities in small dogs and for studies of the skull.

Technical Errors and Artifacts

Several errors can be made in handling x-ray films or in setting up a technique for an examination. In general, these errors will reduce the quality of the radiograph and in certain cases may nullify its diagnostic value. Tables 9–4, 9–5, and 9–6 are intended to help the technician identify the cause of errors and take corrective measures. Table 9-4 deals with technical errors other than those occurring as a result of film processing. Tables 9-5 and 9-6 deal with errors caused by poor film processing.

The advent of automatic processing equipment has helped tremendously in eliminating many errors made in hand tank processing techniques. It has standardized film processing and made it easier to trace the cause of processing mistakes, which are usually mechanically related. Even with automatic processors, many mistakes can be made and must be recognized and corrected to obtain the best possible radiographs.

Several other mechanical failures may occur with automatic processors. It is important to keep the processor clean at all times. It is especially important to wash the roller assembly thoroughly at least once a week. Processors are sophisticated machines that must be serviced regularly by professionals. It is unreasonable and cost-ineffective for a veterinarian to expect the technician to service the processor. However, it is the responsibility of the technician to be able to recognize processor problems and correct them when possible. It is also the technician's responsibility to keep the processor clean at all times and to ensure that fresh developer and fixer solutions are provided as needed.

RADIATION SAFETY

Since 1970, there has been a tremendous growth in the use of x-ray equipment by veterinarians. There are few diagnoses in medicine or surgery that cannot be aided by the use of diagnostic radiology. It therefore behooves one to be aware of the hazard of using x-rays or any other type of ionizing radiation.

It is the responsibility of the veterinarian to ensure that proper radiation safety measures are observed in the hospital. It is also the veterinarian's responsibility to instruct the technician in the proper use of the equipment and to ensure that the design of the x-ray room meets state regulations.

All animal tissues are sensitive to radiation; that is, absorption of radiation doses above a certain minimum roentgen value

• Table 9–4 •

TECHNICAL ERRORS

Increased Film Density
Too high mAs or kV settings
Too short focal-film distance
Wrong measurement of anatomical part
Equipment malfunction
Speed of intensifying screen too fast

Decreased Film Density
Too low mAs or kV settings
Too long focal-film distance
Wrong measurement of anatomical part
Speed of intensifying screen too slow

Black Marks or Artifacts
Film scratches
Crescent mark due to rough handling
Static electricity (linear dots or tree pattern)
Top of film black, resulting from exposure to light while still
    in box
Defective cassette that does not close properly, exposing
    margins of film to light

White Marks (Artifacts)
Dirt or debris between the film and screen
Defect or crack in screen
Contrast medium on tabletop, skin or cassette

Gray Film
Film accidentally exposed to radiation—scattered, secondary,
    or direct
Lack of grid for examination of a thick part
Outdated film
Film stored in too hot or too humid place

Distorted or Blurred Radiograph
Motion—patient, cassette, or machine
Too great focal-film distance, causing magnification and
    distortion
Poor film-screen contact
Poor centering of primary x-ray beam

Linear Artifacts
Gridlines
Grid out of focal range
Primary beam not centered
Grid upside down
Grid damage, causing distorted gridlines

Miscellaneous Artifacts
Cone cut, causing underexposed margins
Target damage, resulting in inconsistent film
    density—requires tube replacement
Double exposure
Blank film—faulty equipment, nonexposed film processed

will change or alter the tissue. The following tissues (not in order of sensitivity) are most readily affected by ionizing radiation: dermis, lymphatics, hemopoietic and leukopoietic (blood-forming tissues), breast, thyroid, bone (especially the epiphysis or growing centers), and the germinal epithelium or gonads. These tissues are sensitive to alpha, beta, gamma, or any other kind of ionizing radiation. All animal species are affected, including humans, even though there are different degrees of sensitivity among species. The more rapidly dividing tissues are affected most by radiation.

Technicians should remember that one of the best protective devices at their disposal is the ability to avoid retakes. Careful attention to patient positioning, thickness measurements, setting techniques, and film processing will decrease radiograph retakes and reduce technician and patient radiation

exposure. See Chapter 36 for additional radiation safety information.

Radiation Filtration

The x-ray beam is a composite or spectrum of x-ray photons of various energy levels. The kVp setting is the highest energy level within the beam, but there are photons of all levels from the kVp on down. The useful portion of the x-ray beam (the portion that passes through the patient to interact with the film and screens) is the upper two thirds of the energy levels. The

• Table 9–5 •

FILM PROCESSING MISTAKES IN WET TANKS

Increased Film Density
Film overdeveloped
Temperature of solution too high
Wrong concentration of developer
Defective thermometer

Decreased Film Density
Film underdeveloped
Temperature of solution too low
Exhausted developer
Contamination of developer
Developer too diluted or improperly mixed
Failure to add replenisher solution as needed
Defective thermometer

Fogged Films
Light leakage in darkroom from defective safelight, door,
    windows, around processor pipes, turning lights on in
    darkroom before film is cleared
Film exposed to radiation from any source—through wall if
    storage room adjacent to x-ray room, cassette left in x-ray
    room while exposure made
Overdeveloped film
Contaminated developer

Yellow Radiograph
Fixation time too short
Exhausted fixer solution

White Spots
Defective screens—pitted, scratched
Dust or grit on surface of film
Fixer on film before processing

Black Spots
Drops of developer solution on film before processing
Films stacked together in fixer

Air Bubbles
Film not agitated when placed in developer; air bubbles form
    on surface of film

Reticulation
Solutions have uneven temperature from bottom to top of
    tanks
Need to stir up solution to even up temperature in tanks
Weak fixer or lack of hardening solution

Brittle Radiographs
Drying temperature too high
Drying time too long

Miscellaneous Mistakes
Film wet—too short drying time
Grit on films—dirty tanks and solutions
Corner marks—wet or dirty fingers on hangers
Sticky film—film washed or dried improperly
Static electricity—low humidity and rough or too fast handling
    of films
Scratches—careless handling

• Table 9–6 •

COMMON TECHNICAL ERRORS WITH AUTOMATIC PROCESSORS

Increased Density
Temperature of developer too high
Over-replenishment
Light leak from cover or in darkroom
Speed too slow
Faulty thermostat

Decreased Density
Temperature of developer too low
Under-replenishment
Exhausted developer, necessitating thorough cleaning of tanks
    every 6 months
Faulty thermostat

Processing Streaks
Cross-over rollers dirty
Dirty wash water
Air tubes need cleaning

Scratches on Film
Guide shoes malaligned or dirty
Dryer air tubes malpositioned

Wet or Damp Film
Thermostat malfunction
Dryer temperatures too low
Insufficient air venting
Film not hardened sufficiently

Film Overlap
Film fed too rapidly into processor
Tension on rollers too high

lower third of the x-ray beam energies are too weak to pass through the patient. This radiation is called "soft radiation." It is of no use for image formation and only causes increased radiation exposure of the patient. Aluminum has a marked effect on filtration of softer (lower energy level) x-rays. Insertion of 1 or 2 mm of an aluminum filter into the path of the primary beam at the portal of the x-ray tube is essential to filter out or absorb the soft x-rays that are a component of all x-ray beams in the diagnostic range. By absorbing these soft radiations, the filter reduces the amount of radiation absorbed by the patient. Increased aluminum filtration also generally improves latitude and detail by improving the quality of the x-ray beam.

Radiation Measurement

To understand radiation safety and radiation dose units of measurement, it is necessary to define a few terms commonly used in the measurement of radiation exposure.

Roentgen. The roentgen (R) is defined as a unit of radiation exposure that will liberate a charge of 2.58×10^{-4} coulombs per kilogram of air. Roentgens are a measure of radiation exposure or x-ray machine output and are generally evaluated with an ionization chamber placed below the primary x-ray beam. As an example, a roentgen is the approximate exposure to the body surface for an anteroposterior radiograph of the abdomen for an average adult human.

Rad. The unit of absorbed dose of ionizing radiations is called a rad. It is the energy imparted by ionizing radiations to a unit mass of irradiated material and is equal to 100 ergs/g of tissue.

The number of rads deposited in tissue per roentgen of radiation exposure varies with the energy of the x-ray beam and with the composition of the absorber.

Rem. Rem is an abbreviation for rad equivalent man; it is the product of the dose in rads and the relative biological effectiveness of the radiation used. This unit of measurement makes allowance for the fact that the effect of radiation on different tissue varies with the type of radiation or relative biological effectiveness. A rem is equal to the absorbed radiation dose in rads multiplied by a quality factor.

$$Rem = rads \times quality\ factor$$

Because the quality factor for diagnostic radiation is 1, for all practical purposes in veterinary practice a rem = rad. For larger particles of radiation such as neutrons, protons, and alpha particles, the quality factor increases from 3 to 20. These larger, more dangerous particles of radiation are not emitted from diagnostic x-ray machines.

Maximum Permissible Dose. This dose should be of great interest to the veterinary technician because it is the maximum dose of radiation a person is allowed to receive during occupational exposure over a certain time. This dose is 0.1 rem average weekly dose. 3 rem over 13 weeks, 5 rem per year, and a maximum accumulated dose of 1 (N–18) rem, where N is age in years. The N–18 tells you that you should not have occupational exposure to radiation before the age of 18 years. The technician should remember that the MPD is the dose that the nuclear regulatory commission has determined should not harm the person receiving it during her or his lifetime. The MPD is maximum occupational exposure allowed by law; you should try to keep your radiation exposure as low as possible by carefully following radiation safety practices.

Personal Monitoring. To protect the staff from overexposure, the radiation that each person receives can be measured on a *film badge*. A film badge is a container that holds a special film designed to record a wide range of exposures. The film holder incorporates several different types of metal filters that permit differentiation of the type of ionizing radiation exposures. This badge should be worn outside the apron on the collar at the level of the thyroid gland. Film badges can be exposed by heat, pressure, and chemical fumes. The film badge should be taken care of and stored outside the radiology area so that the amount of radiation it detects is actually the amount to which the person was occupationally exposed.

Radiation monitoring badges come in several forms: rings, clips, and wrist badges. Several companies offer a badge service. These badges are analyzed on a monthly or quarterly basis.

Another device used to detect radiation exposure is the pocket dosimeter, which is a simple ionization chamber. Thermoluminescent dosimeters can also be used for personal monitoring; however, badges are the most common and practical means of measuring radiation exposure. Film badge readings are reported in millirem (mrem) or 1/1000 rem. The MPD equals 5000 mrem. Technicians using x-ray machines should insist that the veterinarian for whom they work provide them with a radiation monitoring device.

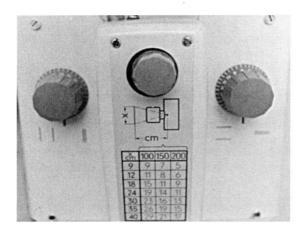

Figure 9–31. A collimator is used to limit the size of the x-ray beam to the part to be examined. By coning down on an area, the amount of scattered and secondary radiation can be drastically reduced.

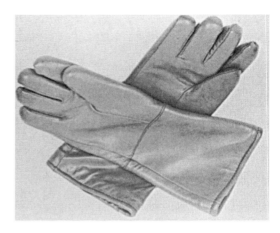

Figure 9–33. Lead gloves should have a minimum of 0.5 mm of lead equivalent; 1 mm of lead equivalent is ideal. They should always be worn when restraint is needed for examination.

Protection Practices

1. Always use a collimator and always use the smallest possible aperture that will cover the anatomic area of interest (Fig. 9–31).
2. Make sure there is an aluminum filter at the portal of the x-ray tube. This is to protect the patient, not the technician.
3. Make sure the proper exposure factors are used to avoid retakes.
4. Make sure the animal is positioned properly the first time—again to avoid retakes.
5. Never permit any part of your body to be in the path of the primary x-ray beam.
6. Always wear an apron and gloves when holding an animal or an apron alone if one has to be in the room when an exposure is made. The apron should have 0.5-mm lead equivalent minimum to ensure good protection from secondary and scattered radiations (Figs. 9–32 and 9–33).

7. Use accessory equipment designed to reduce radiation exposure, such as cassette holders, restraining devices, and positioning devices (Fig. 9–34).
8. Anesthesia and tranquilization of the patient should be used every time an animal cannot be controlled easily and adequately for a given examination.
9. Only required personnel should be in the examining room at the time of exposure. A pregnant woman should not be in the room, nor should anyone less than 18 years of age.
10. Use good, fast screens to reduce the mA settings as much as possible.
11. Higher kilovoltage techniques allow reduction of the mA·sec setting and should be used whenever possible.

> ✎ **TECHNICIAN NOTE**
>
> When working in radiology, always remember "the big three" of radiation safety: time, distance, and shielding.

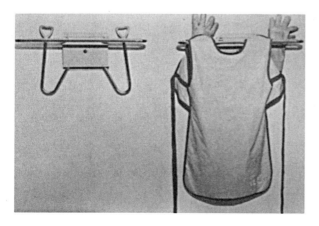

Figure 9–32. Apron and gloves on a stand. It is important to keep the apron on a stand and the gloves well aerated when not in use to increase the useful "life" of the apron and gloves. The apron should have a minimum of 0.5 mm of lead equivalent.

Radiation safety is a frame of mind. It is a habit, and it requires awareness of the danger of radiation. It is easy to become careless with radiation because it is invisible, tasteless, and odorless and produces no external stimulation at diagnostic levels. Technicians should always remember that although invisible, radiations are dangerous to one's health. X-ray effects are cumulative. The ionization that results from continued exposure to x-rays and other high-energy rays constitutes the cumulative effect. They can destroy all living tissue if the absorbed doses are high enough. Secondary radiations are less harmful than primary radiations but are still extremely harmful. Therefore, carelessness has no place in radiology. Remember "the big three" methods of radiation protection: *time, distance, and shielding*. "Time" means avoid retakes; do it right the first time. Lower your time of exposures; keep your mA as low as possible

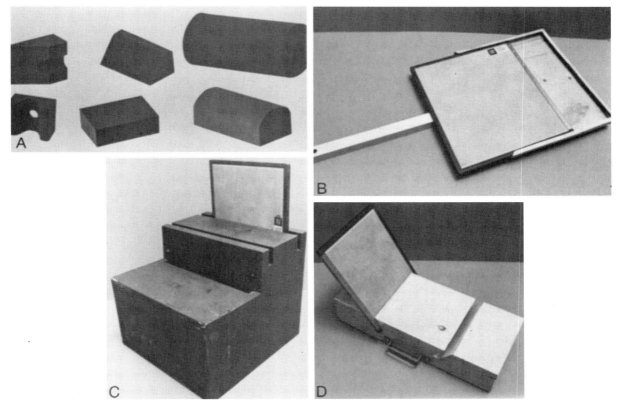

Figure 9-34. A number of commercially available positioning devices can be used to help position animals and reduce the time needed to perform the examination. A, Various foam devices used to position small animals. B, Cassette holder for large animal examinations. C, Block for examination of large animal foot. D, Block for examination of large animal fetlock and pastern joints.

and still produce diagnostic radiographs. "Distance" means stay as far away as possible from the patient and x-ray beam. "Shielding" means always wear your apron and gloves.

RADIOGRAPHIC CONTRAST AGENTS

In radiology, "contrast" means density difference. In many radiographic examinations, there is insufficient natural or inherent contrast of the anatomy to make a diagnosis; this is especially true in gastrointestinal, urogenital, and spinal cord disease. The addition of positive or negative contrast medium can increase the radiographic density difference between anatomic structures and increase the likelihood of correct image interpretation. In veterinary medicine, four types of contrast medium are used:

1. Radiolucent gases—air, nitrous oxide, carbon dioxide
2. Insoluble inert radiopaque medium—barium sulfate
3. Soluble ionic radiopaque medium—iothalamate, diatrizoate
4. Soluble nonionic radiopaque medium—iohexol, iopamidol, metrizamide

Radiolucent gases absorb very small amounts of radiation, resulting in images of greatly reduced radiographic opacity. These agents are used primarily in double-contrast gastrograms, double-contrast cystograms, and rarely, pneumoperitoneography. Contraindications for their use are primarily in patients with severe hemorrhagic cystitis, in which there is an increased likelihood for gas absorption into the circulation. Nitrous oxide and carbon dioxide are considered safer than room air because their increased solubility is less likely to cause serious air embolization.

Barium sulfate has a high atomic number and absorbs a large amount of radiation, resulting in greatly increased radiograph opacity. It is used almost exclusively for upper and lower gastrointestinal examinations. Barium sulfate is inert, nonabsorbed, and fairly soothing to the gastrointestinal tract. It coats the gastrointestinal mucosa better than organic iodides, improving visualization of the luminal surface. Barium sulfate is available in powder, paste, or liquid solutions. Micropulverized solubilized barium sulfate solutions are vastly superior to powdered barium sulfate products because of the increased uniformity in mucosal coating. Contraindications for use include patients with severe constipation or upper or lower bowel perforations. As with all oral contrast media, care should be used in patients with known aspiration pneumonia or a high likelihood of aspiration.

Soluble radiopaque ionic contrast media include iothalamate and diatrizoate. The negatively charged iothalamate and diatrizoate are benzoic acid derivatives with three iodine molecules. They are coupled with positively charged sodium or meglumine to form a soluble salt. The high atomic number of iodine increases radiation absorption and increases radiographic opacity. These products can be used orally for gastrointestinal examinations; intravascularly for venous or arterial studies and excretory urography and in the peritoneal tract, bladder, and urethra; intra–articularly and in draining wounds for fistulography and in salivary ducts for sialography. Ionic organic iodides should not be used in the respiratory tract and intrathecally for myelography. Because ionic iodides are essentially a hyperosmolar salt solution, they can result in an increase in intravascular fluid volume when used intravascularly followed by an osmotic diuresis. The hyperosmolarity can cause diarrhea when used orally. Because of these properties, these agents are contraindicated in dehydrated patients or patients with a known iodine sensitivity.

The newest class of positive contrast agents contains the nonionic organic iodines, represented by iohexol, iopamidol, iotolan, and, historically, metrizamide. These agents can be used like ionic organic iodines but have the advantage of not dissociating into positive and negatively charged ions in solution. This allows the agents to be used intrathecally (in the cerebrospinal fluid space around the spinal cord) for myelography as well as everywhere ionic iodides can be used. These contrast agents are still hyperosmolar but much less so than the ionic-organic iodides. They appear to have a lower incidence of side effects or contrast reactions but have the disadvantage of increased cost. Table 9–7 is a list of available ionic and nonionic organic iodides.

Organic iodides (both ionic and nonionic) may cause serious "contrast reactions," or side effects, when given intravenously, intra-arterially, or intrathecally. These reactions are much less likely when the agents are used orally. Contrast reactions include nausea and vomiting, hypotension, cardiac arrest, and anaphylaxis. These reactions occur very infrequently, but it is advised to have a catheter in place when using these agents and rapid access to fluids, oxygen, endotracheal tubes, and cardiovascular arrest resuscitation drugs during organic iodide contrast procedures. Do not leave these patients unattended after contrast administration. For a thorough discussion of contrast medium and contrast procedures, see Douglas et al. (1987), Han et al. (1994), Lavin (1994), Morgan (1993), and Thrall (1994).

Common Contrast Medium and Applications

Esophagus

Contrast Agents. Barium sulfate, weight/volume (w/v) suspension 100%, is used alone and diluted to evaluate an enlarged esophagus or as a thick paste if the esophagus is not enlarged. Barium mixed with food is more appropriate for diagnosis of esophageal strictures. Oral organic iodides (ionic or nonionic) are used when perforation of the esophagus is suspected.

Procedure. No special preparation is needed. Ideally, the study is done under fluoroscopy. If this is not available, the exposure must be made when the animal swallows. The barium is administered with a syringe in the buccal pouch.

Stomach and Small Bowel (Upper Gastrointestinal Studies)

Contrast Agents. Three kinds of contrast agents are used for upper gastrointestinal studies: barium sulfate 25% to 30% w/v, oral iodines, and negative contrast, including air, carbon dioxide, and nitrous oxide. Barium sulfate is the most commonly used agent for upper gastrointestinal studies when perforation is not suspected. Negative contrast media are used in combination with barium sulfate for double-contrast studies. Oral-iodin-

• Table 9–7 •

RADIOPAQUE ORGANIC IODIDE CONTRAST MEDIUM		
IONIC		
Trade Name (Manufacturer)	**Generic Formula**	**Iodine (mg/ml)**
Angio-Conray (Mallinckrodt)	Iothalamate sodium	480
Conray-30 (Mallinckrodt)	Iothalamate meglumine	141
Conray-60 (Mallinckrodt)	Iothalamate meglumine	282
Conray-400 (Mallinckrodt)	Iothalamate sodium	400
Gastrografin (Squibb)	Diatrizoate meglumine	366
Hypaque Sodium 25% (Winthrop)	Diatrizoate sodium	150
Hypaque Sodium 50% (Winthrop)	Diatrizoate sodium	300
Hypaque Meglumine 60% (Winthrop)	Diatrizoate meglumine	282
Hypaque-M 75% (Winthrop)	Diatrizoate meglumine and sodium	385
Hypaque-M 90% (Winthrop)	Diatrizoate meglumine and sodium	462
Hypaque Sodium Oral (Winthrop)	Diatrizoate sodium	249
Renovist-II (Squibb)	Diatrizoate meglumine and sodium	316
Renovist (Squibb)	Diatrizoate meglumine and sodium	372
Renografin-60 (Squibb)	Diatrizoate meglumine and sodium	288
Renografin-76 (Squibb)	Diatrizoate meglumine and sodium	370
NONIONIC		
Amipaque (Nyegaard)	Metrizamide	*
Isovue 200 (Squibb)	Iopamidol	200
Isovue 300 (Squibb)	Iopamidol	300
Omnipaque 180 (Winthrop)	Iohexol	180
Omnipaque 240 (Winthrop)	Iohexol	240
Omnipaque 300 (Winthrop)	Iohexol	300

*Metrizamide is available as a freeze-dried powder and is measured and reconstituted in sterile water. Iodine concentrations depend on measurements. Author recommends using Iohexol for myelography.

ated products are given when perforation is suspected because barium sulfate will not be resorbed once it leaks into a body cavity.

Procedure. Food should be withheld for 24 hours, and warm water enemas should be administered about 2 to 3 hours before the gastrointestinal study. Acepromazine (Ayerst Laboratories) can be used without adverse effects on the gastrointestinal motility.

Dosage. Barium sulfate, 10 ml/kg: Oral Hypaque or Gastrografin, 3 ml/kg.

Film Sequence. The survey film consists of a ventrodorsal (VD) and a lateral (L) view. Immediately after administration of contrast medium, four films should be taken to completely evaluate the stomach: a VD, a dorsoventral (DV), and both a right and left lateral. At 15 and 30 minutes and 1 hour, the film sequence consists of VD and right lateral. These same views are taken at various intervals until contrast reaches the large bowel. The timing sequence will vary with the patient and the suspected disease process.

Large Bowel (Lower Gastrointestinal Study, Barium Enema)

Contrast Agents. Barium sulfate 10% to 15% (w/v) or iodinated preparations, such as Gastrografin or Oral Hypaque, are used for the lower gastrointestinal studies.

Precautions. Barium sulfate should not be used when a perforation is suspected. A barium enema should not be performed for 48 hours after taking a biopsy of the colon or rectum.

Preparation. The preparation is similar to that for upper gastrointestinal studies. Warm water enemas must be given before the examination because it is essential that the entire large bowel be cleansed before a barium enema is performed. A Bardex (French, Bard Hospital Division, C. R. Bard, Inc.) catheter and barium container are needed for the study.

Procedure. The animal should be anesthetized. A 15% w/v barium sulfate solution is used for barium enemas. The dose is 5 to 10 ml/0.45 kg of body weight. Ideally, the study is done under fluoroscopy. Radiographic views needed are L, VD, and right and left VD oblique views. After completion, the barium is evacuated, and air is injected to obtain a double-contrast study of the large bowel.

Urinary Tract

Contrast Agents. Several kinds of contrast studies are available for study of the kidneys. However, because the *intravenous pyelogram* (IVP) is the one most used in practice, our discussion is limited to it.

An IVP, or excretory urogram, is performed by injecting contrast medium intravenously. Ionic organic iodide products are most commonly used. A meglumine diatrizoate and sodium diatrizoate preparation (Renografin, Squibb) is probably the most popular contrast product used for IVP examinations. The standard dose of contrast is 800 mg of iodine per kilogram,

which may be increased by 50% in patients with poor renal function.

Complications. The most common complications encountered with an IVP are vomiting, anaphylactoid reactions, and hypotension. Vomiting is a transient reaction of short duration and is not serious in nature. The anaphylactoid reactions are rare but must be attended to immediately. It is necessary to have epinephrine available for immediate administration whenever an IVP is done. Hypotension is rare, but when it occurs, it can be life threatening and may lead to renal failure.

Contraindications. The only serious contraindication is dehydration or iodine sensitivity.

Procedure. The animal should fast for 24 hours, but water should be available to avoid dehydration. Enemas should be given when needed, at least 2 to 3 hours before the IVP. VD and L films should be taken before the examinations. Films should be taken in the VD and L positions immediately after injection of the contrast medium and at 5 and 15 minutes after injection. When needed, follow-up studies at 20 or 25 minutes after injection may be indicated.

Urinary Bladder

Contrast Agents. Ionic organic iodide contrast materials are most desirable for retrograde cystography. Nonopaque contrast materials, such as air, carbon dioxide, and nitrous oxide, are used in addition to organic iodides for double-contrast cystography. Do not use barium sulfate.

Procedure. The colon should be cleansed. Depending on the breed and size of the animal, different catheters may be used. A Foley catheter, tomcat catheter, or soft flexible male catheter may be needed. In addition, a syringe and three-way valve are needed. Two types of cystography are commonly performed in veterinary practice: positive-contrast cystography and double-contrast cystography. Positive-contrast cystography is used to detect leaks or rupture of the lower urinary tract after trauma. Ionic organic iodide contrast at concentrations of 10% to 15% is injected retrograde into the urinary bladder at 5 to 15 ml/kg of body weight. Double-contrast cystography is used to detect all other forms of urinary bladder disease. A catheter is placed into the urinary bladder and all urine is removed. Next, 3 to 10 ml of organic iodide contrast is injected, followed by carbon dioxide or room air at 5 to 15 ml/kg of body weight. Because of the variability of urinary bladder volume, it is best to fill the bladder to palpable turgidity. Lateral and oblique VD radiographic views are most helpful.

Urethrography

Contrast Agents. Ionic organic iodide compounds at 20% concentration are best for urethrography.

Procedure. A male catheter is placed in the urethra, and 10 to 20 ml is injected while pressure is applied at the end of the urethra. A Foley catheter can also be used. The x-ray is taken during injections of the last few milliliters. An L view and two oblique (O) views should be taken during the separate injections of the contrast material.

Spinal Cord

Myelography is the contrast examination most frequently performed to localize and characterize spinal cord lesions. Myelograms are always performed with the animal under general anesthesia. Nonionic iodinated contrast medium is injected into the subarachnoid space (cerebrospinal fluid space) at the cisterna magna (skull–C1 space) or in the caudal lumbar spine area (L4–L6). Myelography is most commonly performed before surgical intervention.

Contrast Agents. Two nonionic contrast agents are currently in wide use in veterinary medicine: iopamidol (Isovue, Squibb and Sons, Princeton, NJ) and iohexol (Omnipaque, Sanofi Winthrop, New York, NY). Both of these contrast agents are superior to older myelographic contrast agents such as metrizamide (Amipaque, Winthrop, New York, NY) because they are available in sterile solution and have a decreased incidence of nausea, vomiting, and seizures. The dose of contrast medium ranges from 0.25 ml/kg for cervical evaluation with a cisternal injection to 0.45 ml/kg for cervical evaluation from a lumbar injection. The concentration of iodine should not exceed 300 mg/ml, and injection volume should not exceed 15 ml.

Contraindications. Infection of the spinal cord and meninges or when the disease is to be treated medically only are included.

Procedure. Survey films should be taken first. The site of injection should be aseptically prepared. Spinal needles of 20 to 22 gauge and 3.75 to 8.75 cm should be available because the size of the animal may vary considerably and some dogs may be so obese that even an 8.75-cm needle is short! Films are taken in the VD and L positions immediately after administration of the contrast medium.

POSITIONING

Proper positioning is essential to obtain diagnostic radiographic examinations. It is again the responsibility of the veterinary technician to properly position the animal. It is not the intent of this chapter to discuss positioning at length. Please refer to the excellent treatment of this topic by Butler et al. (1993), Douglas et al. (1987), Han et al. (1994), Lavin (1994), Morgan (1993), and Ticer (1984).

Principles of Positioning

To achieve proper positioning, it is useful for the technician to remember that two views at right angles are necessary to obtain a diagnostic study. This principle applies to all examinations in small animals and to extremities in large animals. The exceptions to this rule are thoracic examinations and spinal examinations in the horse and in cases of trauma or in debilitated animals when only lateral views can be taken without causing undue stress to the animals.

Another principle to remember is the importance of centering the primary beam on the lesion itself, when known. This is especially important in orthopedic cases in both small and large animals. For example, fracture healing may look very different when the x-ray beam is centered over the fracture line as opposed to a short distance away from it. Costly errors have been made by veterinarians who removed supporting devices before the correct time. These errors occurred because fractures may have appeared healed when the primary beam was centered away from the fracture line itself.

It is also important, when performing a radiographic examination, to use an x-ray film that is sufficiently large to completely cover the system to be examined. For example, the thorax should be included in its entirety on one film; the same applies for the abdomen. For extremities, the primary beam should be directed at the lesion. It is good to have a radiograph large enough to include the proximal and distal joint to obtain a good spatial anatomic relationship of the lesion.

These principles are basic but essential. Proper positioning is obtained through practice. These topics are well illustrated and discussed in the references mentioned. A reference textbook should be available in the radiology room of every veterinary practice.

RESTRAINT

The importance of restraint to achieve proper positioning cannot be overemphasized. It is part of radiation safety. Without proper restraint, many examinations should not be undertaken. In some cases, attempting to make examinations without restraint would be life threatening with large animals and dangerous with certain small animals.

There are many types of restraint; some are mechanical or manual, and some are chemical. For the purpose of radiation safety, manual restraint should be avoided as a routine procedure. When it is essential to be in the room with the animal, one should wear a protective lead apron and gloves, and the x-ray beam should be limited to the system to be examined by coning devices or by adjusting the collimator.

Mechanical restraint comes in various forms. A number of commercial devices designed for animal positioning are available, varying in price from a few dollars to several hundreds of dollars (see Fig. 9–34). One of the most useful and inexpensive devices to use in the dog is a simple muzzle, which often has a calming effect on an animal (see Chapter 1). Sandbags and sponges can also be used to obtain excellent positioning. When the animal is positioned properly, it is most important to take the radiograph rapidly, as one can hope for only a few seconds of restraint before the animal moves.

Chemical restraint can be achieved with tranquilizers, analgesics, or anesthesia (see Chapter 15). Chemical restraint has contributed greatly to the progress made in radiology by allowing positioning that would otherwise be impossible to achieve. For example, complete examination of the skull should not be attempted without anesthesia. Every time total immobility or relaxation is required for proper positioning, general anesthesia should be used. Most spinal examinations will prove nondiagnostic unless the examination is done with the animal under anesthesia. In several circumstances, tranquilization is adequate to control most animals. Tranquilizers are excellent to control frightened or aggressive dogs and cats. They are also most useful for controlling large animals.

Again, good positioning is essential in producing diagnostic x-ray films. It takes time to learn and become proficient at achieving every position needed for a variety of examinations in large and small animals. However, most organs can be radiographed with proper techniques, equipment, and accessory devices and the use of mechanical or chemical restraint or both.

DIAGNOSTIC ULTRASOUND

Ultrasound is the next new major diagnostic modality to enter veterinary practice. It is portable, does not require the use of ionizing radiation, and is noninvasive, well tolerated by patients, and accepted by clients. As ultrasound equipment becomes affordable, the only problem with its introduction into practice is the long learning curve associated with its use. Recent veterinary graduates are more familiar with the uses and indications for ultrasound, as veterinary schools have integrated ultrasound into the curriculum. I encourage all new veterinary technicians to familiarize themselves with the basics of diagnostic ultrasound. But remember, ultrasound is user dependent. The image and interpretation are only as good as the person doing the examination.

Ultrasound Basics

Sound is a mechanical pressure wave made up of a series of compressions and rarefactions transmitted through a medium. Sound waves are characterized by their wavelength or distance between compressions, their frequency in cycles per second, and their velocity or speed of transmission (Fig. 9–35). These characteristics are integrated by the following formula:

$$Velocity = wavelength \times frequency$$

For simplicity, we can assume the speed of sound in the body is 1540 meters per second. Therefore, as the frequency of sound increases, the wavelength decreases. Shorter sound waves produce increased image resolution but decreased patient penetration. The frequencies used in veterinary diagnostic ultrasound generally range from 2.5 to 12 megahertz (MHz). A hertz (Hz) is 1 cycle per second. Therefore, typical ultrasound frequencies will range from 2 to 12 million cycles per second, or 2.5 to 12 MHz. Audible sound will range from 20 to 20,000 Hz.

Real-time gray-scale ultrasound is based on the *pulse-echo principle*. A short pulse of sound usually 2 or 3 cycles long is produced from the transducer and transmitted into the patient. The sound wave strikes an echogenic surface and returns some of the sound to the transducer. The strength of the returning sound wave determines the brightness of the image, and the time it takes for the sound to travel into the patient and back to the transducer determines where the echo will be seen on the screen. Remember, the time it takes for a sound wave to traverse a distance and be reflected back is a function of the distance between the sender and reflector and the speed of the sound wave in that medium. For all practical purposes, the speed of sound in small animal tissues is constant at 1540 meters per second.

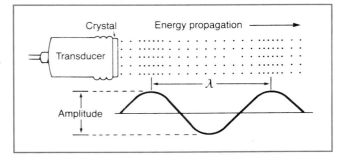

Figure 9–35. Sound wave with a wavelength = λ. Closely spaced dots, compressions. Widely spaced dots, rarefactions. The amplitude is proportional to the loudness.

Ultrasound production and reception is based on the *piezoelectric effect*. A piezoelectric crystal will change shape or thickness when subjected to a voltage pulse. Rapid pulses of electrical energy are transformed into mechanical energy or sound waves by the vibrating crystal. Returning sound waves cause the crystal to vibrate, and that mechanical energy is transmitted into electrical energy by the transducer. This electrical signal is transformed into the gray-scale image on the screen. The transducer acts as both the sound transmitter and the receiver. The operating frequency of the transducer is partially determined by the thickness of the piezoelectric crystal. The thinner the crystal, the higher is the transducer frequency. The transducer transmits sound 0.01% of the time. It receives returning sound waves 99.9% of the time.

Ultrasound Tissue Interaction

To better understand the ultrasound image, it is important to understand the interaction of ultrasound within tissue. As the sound wave proceeds through the body, it is progressively attenuated or weakened. This *attenuation* limits the depth of penetration of the sound wave and therefore limits the depth of structures that can be effectively imaged. The ultrasound beam is attenuated or weakened by absorption, reflection, scattering, refraction, and diffraction. Reflection is a redirection of the sound beam back to the transducer and is the basis of the diagnostic image. Absorption is sound energy converted to heat within the tissues. Scattering is the intertissue microreflection of sound, which is responsible for much of the echo texture of various organs. Refraction and diffraction are the bending of the sound beam as it crosses areas of differing tissue densities. Refraction attenuation is important in the generation of several ultrasound artifacts.

Sound reflection or echo production forms the basis of the ultrasound image. An echo is produced whenever the ultrasound beam crosses an acoustic interface. An acoustic interface is the boundary between two tissues of differing acoustic impedances, or Z. See the equation below.

$$Acoustic\ impedance\ (Z) = density\ (P) \\ \times\ speed\ of\ sound\ transmission\ (C)$$

$$Z = P \times C$$

If we assume the speed of sound in soft tissue to be constant at 1540 meters per second, then the main factor that influences acoustic impedance is the density or composition of tissue. The take-home message is that the more different two adjacent tissues are, the greater will be the echo reflection between them. This is why very homogeneous populations of cells (lymphoma lymph nodes, regenerative liver nodules) produce few echoes and are generally hypoechoic (darker). If the acoustic interface difference is small, only a small percentage of sound will be reflected. If the difference is large, a large portion of sound will be reflected. Most soft tissues have a Z or acoustic impedance within 1% to 2% of liver.

Interface	% Reflection
Fat-muscle	0.94
Fat-bone	49.00
Tissue-air	100.00

From looking at this list one can see the acoustic impedance (Z) between fat and muscle is very low, whereas the acoustic impedance between fat and bone and between soft tissue and air is very high. This property is why ultrasound cannot be used to image through bone or gas. Too much of the sound beam is reflected back from bone and gas interfaces because of the large change in tissue density.

Patient Preparation

Patient preparation is important because 100% of the sound is reflected when the ultrasound beam intersects air. Hair traps air, which is how it insulates the animal, but if one tries to pass ultrasound through hair, the majority of the ultrasound beam is reflected before it ever enters the animal. A careful close clip of the area to be examined, as well as removal of dirt and scales, will improve the ultrasound image. A generous volume of ultrasound gel is also beneficial to displace air and couple the transducer to the skin. Small animals are placed in a padded V-trough table on their backs for abdominal examination and in lateral or sternal recumbency for cardiac examination. Most small animals tolerate abdominal and cardiac examinations well and rarely require tranquilization. A special table with a large hole cut in it may help with cardiac examinations. The animal is placed in lateral recumbency with the chest area over the hole, which allows for better ultrasound transducer access. Large animal examinations are done in the standing tranquilized animal. Again, close clipping, especially for tendon examinations, is critical for an optimal examination.

Ultrasound Display Modes

The returning echo can be displayed in several ways. *A-mode,* or *amplitude mode,* displays the returning echoes as spikes from a baseline. The echo depth is determined by its location along the baseline. The echo intensity is displayed by the height of the spike. A-mode ultrasound machines are used predominantly in ophthalmology and would have little value in veterinary practice.

B-mode, or *brightness mode,* forms the basis for two-dimensional imaging. The returning echoes are displayed as dots. The brightness of the dot is a function of the strength of the returning echo. The placement of the dot is a function of the time it took for the echo to return to the transducer. The cross-sectional image is formed through data storage. There are two basic types of B scanners: *static* and *real-time.* With static scanners, the transducer is manually moved across the patient, and the image is held on the screen during the transducer sweep. These machines are large and cumbersome, require skill to produce an adequate image, increase the time required for an examination, and do not allow visualization of motion. These machines are readily available, generally free from hospital surplus, but are not as valuable as real-time equipment in veterinary practice. With real-time equipment, the sound beam is automatically swept across the patient while the transducer is held steady (Fig. 9–36). New images are produced rapidly, permitting direct observation of moving structures. With B-mode real-time equipment, images are displayed in gray scale. Gray scale is a technique in which the various echo strengths are displayed in numerous shades of gray from black to white.

M-mode, or *time-motion (TM) mode,* is produced by passing a narrow sound beam across a body part. Each echo interface is presented as a dot. The motion of the body part is displayed by sweeping the image across the screen or image

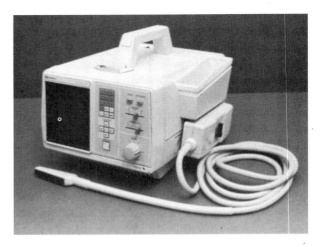

Figure 9–36. Portable real-time ultrasound unit with a linear array transducer that is used most often for large animals.

recorder. M-mode can be thought of as a very thin sector of B-mode displayed as a function of time. M-mode is primarily used for echocardiography. Ideal ultrasound equipment for veterinary practice would be a real-time B-mode scanner with M-mode capabilities (Fig. 9–37).

The selection of appropriate transducers is critical when purchasing ultrasound equipment. Transducers will vary in type, size, style, shape, and frequency. Linear array transducers are made with several piezoelectric crystals stacked side by side. The crystals are fired in rapid sequence to produce a rectangular cross-sectional image. The major drawback for linear array transducers is their large footprint or contact area. It is difficult to use these transducers for intercostal cardiac studies and for subcostal studies in the cranioabdominal area in small animals. Linear array transducers are primarily used for transrectal reproductive examinations in cattle and horses.

Sector scanners produce a triangular field (Fig. 9–38). The crystal is swept across the area by mechanical or electronic means, and the transducer generally has a small contact area.

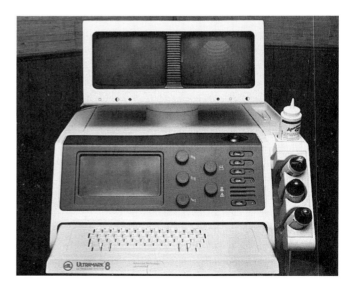

Figure 9–37. Mobile real-time ultrasound unit.

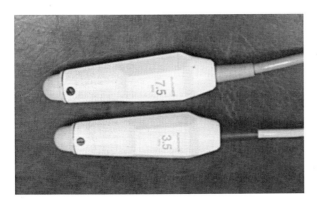

Figure 9-38. Sector transducers used with real-time ultrasound unit.

Newer, more expensive transducers may incorporate annular array and dynamic focusing technology. These transducers form the ultrasound beam by adding together many small beams from an array of small crystals. Dynamic focusing will allow the operator to place any portion within the beam into maximum resolution without having to change transducers.

Deciding what frequency of transducer to use is easy. Use as high a frequency transducer as possible to maximize resolution while still allowing penetration to the needed depth. Remember, the higher the frequency of the transducer, the shorter will be the sound wavelength and the better will be the resolution. However, as the frequency increases, the depth of sound beam penetration decreases. For abdominal ultrasound in small dogs (15 kg or less) and cats, a 7.5-MHz transducer is ideal. For middle-sized to large-breed dogs, a 5-MHz transducer works well. A guide for selecting a transducer is as follows:

High frequency: Increase resolution
Increase attenuation
Decrease penetration
Low frequency: Decrease resolution
Decrease attenuation
Increase penetration

TECHNICIAN NOTE

Use as high a frequency transducer as possible to maximize resolution while allowing penetration to the necessary depth.

The ultrasound equipment controls will vary from machine to machine, but the concept of *time-gain compensation* (TGC) is fairly universal. The echoes coming from acoustic interfaces close to the transducer are stronger than the echoes returning from farther away from the transducer. Time-gain amplification compensates for the progressive attenuation with depth in the ultrasound beam. Time-gain compensation is operator dependent and is set for the best-looking uniform image.

The Ultrasound Image

As one begins using ultrasound, the need increases to re-study anatomy. The ultrasound image is a thin cross-sectional slice through the body in a new or different orientation. It will help to use a standard image orientation, which places the head or front of the animal on the left in the sagittal or longitudinal view and the animal's right on the left of the screen on the transverse or axial view.

Ultrasound terminology is easy to remember. *Echogenicity* refers to the strength or amplitude of the returning echoes. A structure that is *sonodense* or *echogenic* (bright) produces echoes. A structure that is *anechoic* or *sonolucent* (dark) produces few or no echoes. A structure is *hyperechoic* (brighter than) if it produces more echoes than adjacent structures. A structure is *hypoechoic* (darker than) if it produces fewer echoes than surrounding structures. An *isoechoic* (same as) structure has a level of echogenicity similar to that of adjacent structures. A structure that is complexly echogenic contains multiple different echogenicities and echo textures. Mixed echogenicity refers to an organ or structure with two echogenicities. Remember that echogenicity is a relative term. We can make any structure bright by adjusting machine control settings. Compare organs at the same depth and control settings to avoid misinterpretation of relative echogenicities.

Ultrasound Artifacts

Most people fail to take the time to fully understand ultrasound artifacts. They ignore artifacts because by definition an artifact does not contribute useful image information. This is not true of ultrasound artifacts. Ultrasound artifacts provide accurate clues to what makes up the ultrasound image.

Reverberation Artifact

Reverberation is present when some of the returning sound is reflected from the transducer face or an internal interface and re-enters the patient. The second echo will have the same shape and be double the distance from the first echo. Reverberation echoes reflect from gas-filled structures and usually appear as high-amplitude parallel lines occurring at regular intervals. Each parallel line represents the distance between the transducer and the gas interface. Each reverberation is weaker than the preceding one. Reverberation artifact can also be referred to as "dirty shadowing" and "comet tails" (Fig. 9–39).

Shadowing

Shadowing artifact occurs due to inadequate sound beam penetration through a highly reflective or sound absorptive substance. Acoustic shadowing is an area of darkness or hypoechogenicity that occurs deep to very dense material, such as bone, calcium, or calculi. Very small objects cast an acoustic shadow only if they are within the focal zone or narrow portion of the ultrasound beam.

Acoustic Enhancement

If the ultrasound beam passes through an area with few tissue interfaces (low attenuation region), the emerging ultrasound beam will have more intensity than would be expected and will be brighter or more echogenic distal to the nonattenuating structure. The best example of this is the normal gallbladder surrounded by the hepatic parenchyma. The liver tissue distal or deep to the gallbladder appears brighter than adjacent hepatic tissue (Fig. 9–40). This artifact is seen deep to fluid-filled structures and is also referred to as "through transmission."

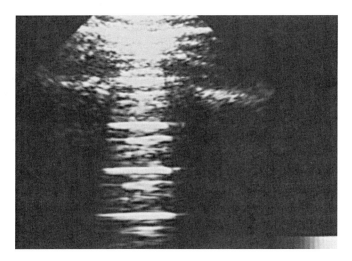

Figure 9–39. Reverberation artifact from the air-filled lung of a normal horse. The parallel, evenly spaced echogenic bands represent reverberation between the transducer and pleural surface.

Refraction or "Edge Artifact"

Refraction is a hypoechoic band or stripe at the margin of a curved structure due to the refraction or bending of the sound beam. The sound beam is deflected from its true path with an effect similar to shadowing. Edge artifact can create false hypoechoic masses in structures within its path.

Mirror-Image Artifact

The ultrasound machine places the returning echo on the viewing screen as a function of the time it took the echo to return. If the sound wave reverberates within a highly echogenic structure before returning to the transducer, the image will be duplicated on the screen distal to the original image. This is most commonly seen as a duplication of the gallbladder in mirror image.

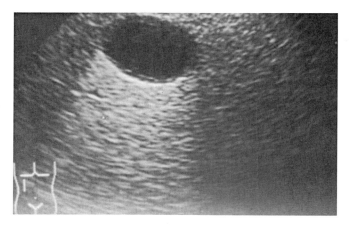

Figure 9–40. Bright echogenic band beneath the gallbladder represents acoustic enhancement. The ultrasound beam is not attenuated as much as it traverses the fluid-filled gallbladder as it is in the surrounding liver.

Slice-Thickness Artifact

If the width of the ultrasound beam cuts through both the edge of a cystic structure and solid tissue, the solid tissue may look as if it is layered within the cyst. This artifact is responsible for the erroneous appearance of debris within the urinary bladder and gallbladder, although no debris is present. The erroneous appearance is the result of volume averaging of tissue by the ultrasound machine.

The Ultrasound Examination

A complete ultrasound examination requires at least 20 to 30 minutes to perform. When ultrasound is used for a quick answer to a question such as pregnancy versus pyometra, the examination will be shorter. When using ultrasound for abdominal disease diagnosis, a complete examination should be performed every time.

It is important to have a thorough understanding of the normal appearance of the various abdominal organs before trying to identify the abnormalities associated with disease. The ranking of small animal abdominal organs from least echogenic (darkest) to most echogenic (brightest) is as follows:

Least echogenic	Renal medulla
	Liver
	Renal cortex
	Spleen
	Prostate
Most echogenic	Renal sinus fat

Remember that echogenicity is a relative term, and one must compare organs at similar control settings and similar depths to avoid misinterpretation.

Clinical Use

The clinical application of ultrasound in veterinary medicine has exploded during the past 10 years. Equipment designed for use in people is readily adaptable for use in veterinary medicine, and several companies are producing dedicated veterinary ultrasound machines. Both 5- and 7.5-mHz sector scanners are most popular for small animal and nonreproductive large animal imaging. The 3- and 5-mHz linear array transducers are extensively used for transrectal large animal reproductive ultrasonography. Traditional cardiac and solid abdominal organ examinations remain the mainstay, but ultrasound is used to answer hundreds of clinical questions in a wide variety of species. The following section is a listing of common ultrasound applications in both large and small animals.

Uses in Large and Small Animals of Ultrasound

   Tendon injury evaluation and response to surgery or
      therapy
   Diagnosis of tendon sheath infections, adhesions, and
      foreign bodies
   Evaluation of joint effusions, intra-articular injury,
      osteomyelitis, and neoplasms
   Congenital and acquired cardiac disease and response to
      therapy
   Pleural effusion, pleuritis, and pleuropneumonia

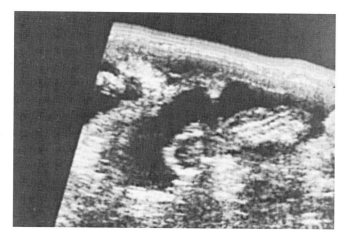

Figure 9-41. Ultrasonogram of a 52-day-old canine fetus.

Soft tissue neck, thyroid, parathyroid, tongue, and mediastinal disease

Hepatic, renal, splenic, adrenal, urinary bladder, gallbladder, and billiary disease

Abdominal and peripheral vascular malformations

Peritoneal and pleural fluid assessment and sampling

Abdominal masses of unknown origin

Intestinal foreign bodies, intussusceptions, infiltrative disease, and neoplasia

Testicular and prostate evaluation and location of retained testicles

Pregnancy diagnosis (Fig. 9–41), fetal evaluation, twin removal, and complete fertility evaluations

Soft tissue neoplasia, granulomas, abscesses, and foreign bodies

Umbilical infections and persistent and patent urachus

Ocular and orbital evaluation

Vascular thrombosis and catheter foreign body evaluation

Guidance for fine needle aspiration, drain placement, biopsy, and culture

NUCLEAR MEDICINE

Many veterinary schools and several progressive specialized veterinary practices have nuclear medicine capabilities. Nuclear medicine can be divided into therapeutic and diagnostic procedures. Currently, veterinary therapeutic nuclear medicine involves the administration of radioactive iodine (^{131}I) for the treatment of hyperthyroidism and thyroid tumors. Diagnostic nuclear medicine involves the administration of radionuclides to the animal and detection of the electromagnetic radiation emitted from the animal with a gamma scintillation camera. Radionuclides are atoms with an unstable nucleus that undergoes radioactive decay. Radioactive decay is the transformation or disintegration of an unstable nuclide by spontaneous emission of electromagnetic radiation. Electromagnetic radiations that are of nuclear origin are termed gamma rays, in contrast to diagnostic radiations (x-rays), which originate from the electron cloud that surrounds the nucleus.

Diagnostic nuclear medicine does not generate visual images equivalent to those of diagnostic radiology but detects functional or physiological, pharmacological, and kinetic data from the patient in image or numerical data form. Figure 9–42A and B shows a standard gamma scintillation camera, control panel, and nuclear medicine computer. Common clinical uses of veterinary nuclear medicine include bone scanning to detect tumor metastasis to bone and radiographically undetectable bone injury or infection, lung scanning to detect pulmonary embolism and as a pulmonary function test, renal scans to assess kidney perfusion and function, and thyroid scans for the characterization of hyperthyroid patients and to detect metastasis. Other less common nuclear medicine studies include hepatobiliary scanning, brain scans, labeled white blood cell scans

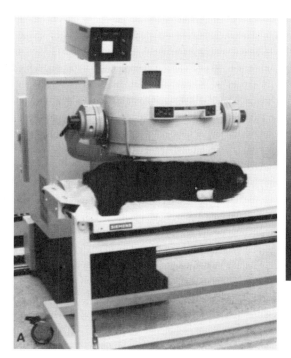

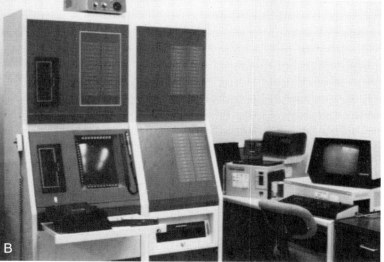

Figure 9-42. A, Gamma scintillation camera in position over a dog during a whole-body bone scan to check for metastatic neoplasia. B, Control panel monitor, nuclear medicine computer, and matrix camera.

for the detection of occult infection, lymphoscintigraphy, nuclear angiography, and scans to detect an unknown focus of blood loss.

The most commonly used radionuclide is technetium-99m (^{99m}Tc). This agent is commercially available from a disposable technetium generator. Technetium is administered in an ionic form as ^{99m}TcO$_4$ (pertechnetate) or bound to a specific organ-localizing pharmaceutical agent before administration. Technetium is the radiopharmaceutical of choice because it has a 6-hour physical half-life (T$_{1/2}$) and emits a 140-keV gamma ray, which is appropriate for most imaging studies. The radioactive or physical half-life of a radionuclide is the time required for the number of radioactive atoms to decrease by 50%.

Radiation safety practices are important with nuclear medicine. When working in a practice that uses nuclear medicine, one should insist on receiving comprehensive instruction in radiation principles and safety. This chapter is meant only as an introduction.

The primary route of radionuclide administration to veterinary patients is intravenous. Latex examination gloves should be worn and careful injection techniques should be performed to ensure the entire dose is delivered intravenously and not perivascularly. This is especially important in equine bone scans for which a large dose of radionuclide is administered. The routes of excretion of the radioactive imaging agents vary with the agent used. Technetium is primarily excreted in urine, with a lesser amount in the feces. Animals should be housed in a separate restricted area of the hospital, and their stool and urine should be carefully collected and held for decay until the levels are below exempt quantities. Always wear latex examination gloves and limit contact with patients to only that necessary for their care. Never eat or bring eating utensils (coffee cups, spoons, and so forth) into a nuclear medicine area. The dose of radiation to the patient is small, but repeated physical contact or accidental ingestion of radionuclides may be harmful to the nuclear medicine technologist. Animals should be held until they pose no radiation threat to their owners or the population at large. This is generally 3 to 10 physical half-lives of the radiopharmaceutical, depending on specific state regulations.

COMPUTED TOMOGRAPHY

In the past several years, there has been an expansion of the diagnostic imaging techniques available to veterinary patients. Most veterinary schools and several specialty practices have access to computed tomography (CT) scanning. A CT scan is obtained by passing a very thin x-ray beam transaxially through the patient and measuring the x-ray attenuation at multiple sites in a thin slice of the patient's anatomy. The computer then reconstructs the transmitted x-ray data into a cross-sectional image on a video monitor. The image can then be captured on film or video tape or stored for later use on magnetic tape. The advantage of CT over standard radiography is the greatly improved radiographic contrast, spatial resolution, and cross-sectional anatomic presentation. The most common use of CT in veterinary medicine is head and spinal examinations for neurologic disease. CT allows the veterinarian a noninvasive look inside the skull of patients (Fig. 9–43).

When a CT scan is performed, the patient is placed in VD or DV position on the long narrow movable CT table. The table then moves the patient through the circular gantry that houses the x-ray tube and detectors (Fig. 9–44). The table moves in a

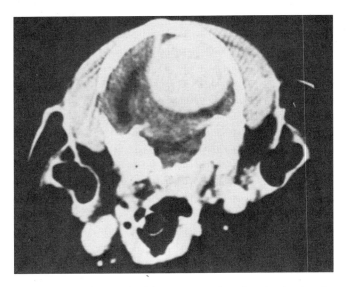

Figure 9-43. Computed tomogram of a dog brain showing a large contrast-enhancing brain tumor (meningioma) in the central cerebrum.

measured stepwise fashion. During each table step, the CT scanner obtains a single cross-sectional slice of data. The patients need to be heavily sedated or under general anesthesia to prevent any motion and must be positioned perfectly straight. Most studies are performed twice on the same animal. The first study is performed without contrast, and the second is performed after intravenous iodinated contrast administration. Urographic contrast agents are commonly administered at a dose of 800 mg of iodine per kg of body weight. Contrast will highlight vascular structures, and some neoplasms will have a characteristic contrast enhancement pattern. Besides brain studies, CT can be used to identify and characterize musculoskeletal, thoracic, and abdominal disorders.

MAGNETIC RESONANCE IMAGING

The newest imaging modality to be used in veterinary medicine is magnetic resonance imaging (MRI). MRI is similar to CT in that the image is a thin slice of cross-sectional anatomy made

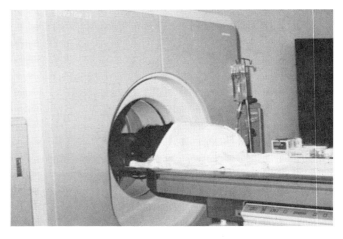

Figure 9-44. Dog in position for a head computed tomogram. The large circular gantry houses the x-ray tube and detectors.

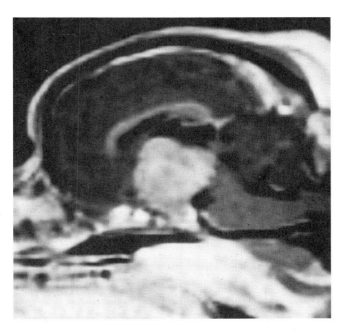

Figure 9–45. Sagittal T1 post–gadolinium contrast magnetic resonance image of a dog with a large enhancing pituitary macroadenoma.

up of a matrix of volume elements. MRI differs from CT in that it uses no ionizing radiation to create the image. Instead, the MRI represents the intensity of a radiowave signal from tissue in which hydrogen nuclei have been disturbed by a characteristic radiofrequency pulse. MRI is superior to CT in image resolution, anatomic definition, and sensitivity to tissue composition differences. Because of this, MRI is vastly superior to CT for imaging of the brain and spinal cord and is currently used primarily for head and spine evaluation. Figure 9–45 is a sagittal canine brain MRI of a patient with a large contrast-enhancing pituitary tumor.

Two general types of MRI units (also called *magnets*) are used in veterinary imaging: low field strength, or resistive, magnets and high field strength, or superconductive, magnets. Magnetic field strength is measured in tesla (T). Low field strength magnets are 0.4 T or less, and high field strength magnets are 0.6 T and above. The most typical superconducting magnet has a field strength of 1 or 1.5 T. Regardless of the type of magnet used, the technician needs to be aware of several safety measures and patient management concerns peculiar to MRI.

As with CT, almost all MRI is done off the clinic premises in an imaging center, a mobile truck–based MRI unit, or a human hospital. Only a few veterinary teaching hospitals have in-house MRI units. Therefore, everything needed to anesthetize, resuscitate, and recover a patient needs to be taken to the imaging site. Most practices that perform off-site imaging have a large tackle box or physician's bag filled with all necessary drugs, fluids, catheters, intravenous access lines, syringes, needles, tape, gauze, and endotracheal tubes. It often helps to do a mock run or pretend case before a clinical case to ensure everything is correctly packed. Imaging centers and hospitals appreciate clean, odor-free, and flea- and tick-free veterinary patients. It is a good idea to bathe the patient within 24 hours of the examination if possible and to ensure the patient's bowel and bladder are evacuated before entering the hospital or imaging center.

A serious problem with MRI is the strong magnetic field. One cannot use anything made of ferromagnetic metal in or around the magnet. The magnetic field will rapidly and forcefully pull these objects into the magnet, potentially injuring anything in its path. This generally includes the gas anesthesia machine, oxygen tank, intravenous poles, clipboards, ink pens, leashes, collars, beepers, and so forth. There are nonmagnetic products available for use during MRI, but they are generally prohibitively expensive for most veterinary hospitals. The exception is an aluminum oxygen tank. Because of this limitation, anesthesia is generally performed with injectable drugs and heavy tranquilization. Patients must be absolutely still for MRI; any motion will severely degrade the image, so they must be under fairly deep injectable anesthesia. This is sometimes complicated because it is often difficult to carefully monitor the animals during the examination due to the narrow tubular shape of some magnets and the inability to use mechanized monitoring devices. Patients that cannot tolerate deep injectable general anesthesia with minimal monitoring are not good candidates for an MRI. MRI examinations generally take 45 to 60 minutes to perform and are done with and without intravenous contrast, similar to CT examinations, but with a paramagnetic contrast agent (usually gadolinium DTPA). Organic iodide contrast will not work for MRI examinations.

Besides anesthesia and monitoring difficulties created by the high magnetic field, there are personal precautions. Credit cards and watches may be permanently damaged if carried too close to the high magnetic field. Any device that delivers a radiofrequency signal cannot be close to an MRI; these include but are not limited to televisions, radios, and pager transmitters. In addition, technicians with cardiac pacemakers, aneurysm or intracranial hemaclips, neural stimulators, metallic fragments within the orbits, hearing aids, or intrauterine devices should not be in charge of patient care during an MRI.

Recommended Reading

Butler JA, Colles DM, Dyson SJ, et al.: Clinical Radiology of the Horse. 1st ed. Oxford, Blackwell Scientific Publications, 1993.

Curry TS, Dowdey JE, Murry RC: Christensen's Introduction to the Physics of Diagnostic Radiology. 4th ed. Philadelphia, Lea & Febiger, 1990.

Douglas SW, Herrtage ME, Williamson HD: Principles of Veterinary Radiology. 4th ed. East Sussex, UK, Bailliere Tindall, 1987.

Eastman Kodak Company: The Fundamentals of Radiography. 12th ed. Rochester, NY, 1980.

Green RW: Small Animal Ultrasound. Philadelphia, Lippincott-Raven, 1996, chaps. 1, 2, and 3.

Hall EJ: Radiobiology for the Radiologist. 4th ed. Philadelphia, Lippincott-Raven, 1993.

Han CM, Hurd CD, Kurklis L: Practical Guide to Diagnostic Imaging: Radiology and Ultrasonography. Goleta, CA, Veterinary Publ. Inc., 1994.

Lavin LM: Radiography in Veterinary Technology. Philadelphia, W.B. Saunders, 1994.

Morgan JR: Techniques of Veterinary Radiography. 5th ed. Ames, IA, Iowa State University Press, 1993.

Nyland TG, Mattoon JS: Veterinary Diagnostic Ultrasound. Philadelphia, W.B. Saunders, 1995, chaps. 1, 2, 3, and 15.

Rantanen NW: Diagnostic Ultrasound. Vet Clin North Am (Equine Pract) 2:11–258, 1986.

Stashak TS: Adam's Lameness in Horses. 4th ed. Philadelphia, Lea & Febiger, 1987, chap. 4.

Thrall DE: Textbook of Veterinary Diagnostic Radiology. 2nd ed. Philadelphia, W.B. Saunders, 1994, chaps. 1 and 46.

Ticer JA: Radiographic Technique in Veterinary Practice. 2nd ed. Philadelphia, W.B. Saunders, 1984.

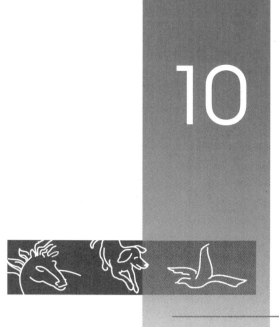

10 Diagnostic Sampling and Treatment Techniques

Tracy J. Jaffe

INTRODUCTION

The practice of veterinary medicine is becoming increasingly complex. A technician who is proficient in obtaining diagnostic samples and performing a variety of treatment techniques is a tremendous asset to a veterinary practice. Technicians should have expertise in a wide variety of procedures, such as the collection of thoracic, abdominal, and joint fluid; bone marrow; and arterial blood in addition to routine venous blood, urine, and fecal samples. It is important to be familiar with the steps involved in the placement and maintenance of venous and arterial catheters, enteral feeding tubes, intraosseous catheters, and urinary catheters. Many of the sampling and treatment methods described in this chapter can be performed by the technician under the supervision of the veterinarian.

SMALL ANIMAL SAMPLING AND TREATMENT TECHNIQUES

Blood Sample Collection

Venous Blood Sample

Blood is one of the most frequently collected samples for diagnostic purposes. Venipuncture is routinely performed to acquire blood for screening tests in healthy animals as well as in those with underlying disease processes. Only through experience does one learn to collect a blood sample quickly with a minimum of trauma to the vessel and stress and discomfort to the patient. Proper animal restraint is as integral a part of the process as the venipuncture itself.

Venipuncture is performed using either a needle and syringe or a Vacutainer (Becton Dickinson Co., Rutherford, N.J.) collection system. Which method and needle gauge is used depends on the vessel size, quantity of blood desired, and intended use of the sample. Blood from a peripheral vessel is usually obtained with a syringe and needle. When a small-gauge needle (25-gauge, 1.6-cm; or 28-gauge, 1.25-cm) is used, the amount of negative pressure applied to aspirate the blood into the syringe must not be excessive. If the syringe plunger is quickly and repeatedly pulled back to obtain the sample, the cells may become hemolyzed and yield inaccurate laboratory values. Twenty-five-gauge or 28-gauge needles are useful when only a few drops of blood are needed from a small, fragile, or repeatedly punctured vessel. Hourly sampling to establish a blood glucose curve in a cat is a situation in which use of a small-gauge needle is appropriate.

> **TECHNICIAN NOTE**
>
> Larger-gauge needles permit more rapid blood collection but cause more trauma to the vessels.

Larger-gauge needles (20-gauge, 2.5-cm; or 22-gauge, 2.5-cm) permit more rapid blood collection but cause more trauma to the vessels. The majority of venipuncture procedures in small animals are performed with 22-gauge needles. Blood collected for coagulation profiles should be drawn through a 20-gauge needle, which penetrates the vessel on the first attempt lest the clotting process start before the sample is completely collected. Regardless of which size needle is used, once the blood sample is collected inside the syringe, the needle should be removed from the syringe and the stopper taken off the collection tube before the sample is injected into the tube.

When venipuncture is performed on the jugular veins, the use of a Vacutainer collection device may make obtaining the specimen easier. A needle is twisted into the top of a plastic cylindrical holder, and a Vacutainer tube sealed with a rubber stopper is held near the base of the cylinder. The needle is placed into the vein, and the tube is inserted into the base of the holder until the stopper is punctured. Blood is automatically suctioned into the tube until it is three fourths of the way full, thereby achieving the correct ratio of anticoagulant to blood. After a sufficient volume is collected, the tube is withdrawn from the holder to break the vacuum, and the needle is removed from the vein. The tube size used is proportionate to the vessel size; the vacuum created when a large tube is used to collect blood from a narrow vessel may cause the vein to collapse.

Before venipuncture, the skin over the vessel should be saturated with 70% isopropyl alcohol; this removes superficial skin contaminants and improves visualization of the vein. It is permissible to clip the hair if the vessel is difficult to identify because of a dense hair coat. If the area over the vessel is dirty, the skin should be scrubbed with an antimicrobial cleanser and then wiped with alcohol. When a sample is being drawn for blood culture, the region on top of the vein should be shaved and aseptically prepared, and the venipuncturist should wear sterile gloves.

The most frequently used sites for canine blood collection are the cephalic, jugular, and lateral saphenous veins. The cephalic, jugular, femoral, and medial saphenous veins are readily accessible for feline venipuncture. To collect blood from the cephalic vein, the animal is restrained in sternal recumbency or a standing position. If venipuncture is to be performed on the right cephalic vein, which is located on the cranial aspect of the foreleg, the individual restraining the animal is positioned on the animal's left side. The assistant's left arm or hand is placed under the muzzle, and the animal's head is pulled toward the assistant's body. The holder's right arm is placed around the animal, and the right hand grasps the patient's right elbow and extends the foreleg. By placing the right thumb on top of the forearm and rotating it laterally, the cephalic vein becomes occluded and is more easily visualized on the dorsum of the leg. A tourniquet secured at the elbow joint can be used to occlude the vein if an assistant is not available. To prepare the site for venipuncture, the hair and skin over the vessel are wiped with 70% alcohol. The phlebotomist grasps the leg with one hand and places the thumb lateral to the vessel. This prevents the vessel from rolling to the side when the needle is introduced. The skin is pulled tautly in a distal direction to further stabilize the vein. A syringe fitted with a 22- or 25-gauge needle is held in the opposite hand. The needle penetrates the skin at a 25-degree angle just lateral to the vein and then enters the vessel. For the patient's comfort, it is important to advance the needle into the skin and vein gently and slowly; brusque, jabbing motions should be avoided. Approximately 0.5 to 1.0 cm of the needle is inserted into the vein. Once the vessel is punctured, blood will spontaneously appear in the needle hub. Slow retraction of the syringe plunger will stimulate blood to flow into the syringe (Fig. 10–1). If too much suction is applied, the vein may collapse, and blood flow into the syringe will cease. Blood flow may also be interrupted because the needle tip becomes occluded by the vessel wall. To remedy this situa-

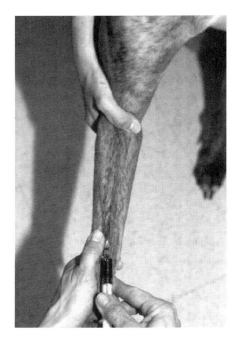

Figure 10-1. Venipuncture of the canine cephalic vein.

tion, the needle should be rotated and retracted a minimal amount. Pumping the animal's foot distal to the venipuncture site and repetitively occluding and releasing the vein may augment blood flow. After a satisfactory quantity of blood is collected in the syringe, the assistant's thumb or tourniquet is removed from the vein. The needle is then withdrawn from the vessel, and digital pressure is applied to the venipuncture site for 10 to 20 seconds. Insufficient application of pressure may result in the formation of a hematoma. If a hematoma occurs when the needle is still in the vein, the needle should be promptly removed. A gauze sponge is held firmly over the site until the bleeding subsides. When venipuncture is reattempted, the needle should be placed proximal to the initial puncture site.

The jugular vein is the preferred site for venipuncture if several milliliters of blood are needed. Help from an assistant is usually required. Animals generally resist restraint for jugular sampling more than they do for cephalic sampling. Some cats will struggle more when firmly restrained; in such situations, light restraint should be substituted. Fractious cats can be wrapped in a towel or placed in a specially designed restraint bag. Cats and small to medium–sized dogs are held in sternal recumbency on the top of an examination table. Large dogs are restrained in a seated position on the floor.

When venipuncture of the left jugular vein is to be attempted, the assistant stands on the right side of the animal. The assistant's left arm is draped around the patient's back and is used to pull the patient toward the assistant. The front legs of the animal are grasped just proximal to the elbows with the holder's left hand and extended. The front legs of the cat may be held over the edge of the table. With the right hand, the assistant holds the neck in an extended position and turns the head slightly away from the jugular vein to be sampled. The phlebotomist occludes the vein by placing pressure with the thumb lateral to the trachea at the thoracic inlet. Once distended, the jugular can be visualized or palpated as it courses

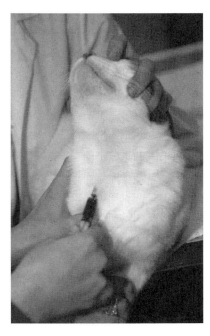

Figure 10–2. Venipuncture of the feline jugular vein.

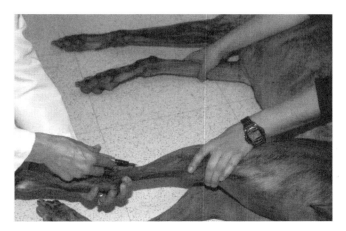

Figure 10–4. Restraint of a dog for venipuncture of the lateral saphenous vein.

from the thoracic inlet to the angle of the mandible. A 20- to 22-gauge needle on a syringe is inserted into the vein at a 25-degree angle with the bevel facing upward (Figs. 10–2 and 10–3). Bending the entire needle so the bevel side of the needle is at a 150-degree angle with the syringe before introducing it into the vein may make feline and small dog jugular venipuncture easier. After a sufficient sample enters the syringe, the digital pressure is released from the base of the vein, and the needle is removed. Pressure is applied to the puncture site for approximately 30 seconds or until the bleeding stops.

The lateral saphenous vein, which is located on the lateral aspect of the hind limb, is an ideal site for blood collection in the dog. It is often used in aggressive animals because the venipuncturist does not need to be positioned in close proximity to the dog's face. To perform venipuncture of the left lateral saphenous vein, the dog is placed in right lateral recumbency. The restrainer stands at the dog's back, places his or her right forearm on the left lateral aspect of the thorax, and grasps the medial aspect of the right front leg. With the left hand, the assistant grasps and extends the left stifle; this occludes the lateral saphenous vein and prevents the leg from being retracted. The venipuncturist grasps and extends the left tarsus and pulls the skin tautly to stabilize the vessel (Fig. 10–4). Placement of the thumb alongside the vein further limits the tendency of the vein to roll when the needle is introduced (Fig. 10–5).

The medial saphenous or femoral vein is convenient to use to obtain small quantities of blood in the feline patient. If the right vein is to be sampled, the cat is held in a stretched position in right lateral recumbency. The restrainer's left hand is used to abduct and flex the left rear leg with the palm of the hand facing the cat's inguinal region. Pressure is applied to the medial aspect of the right rear leg with the edge of the

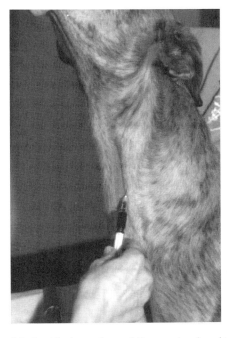

Figure 10–3. Venipuncture of the canine jugular vein.

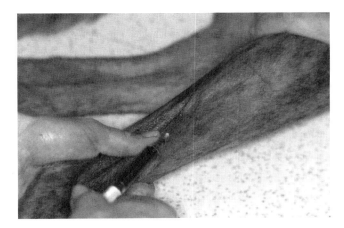

Figure 10–5. The thumb is placed alongside the lateral saphenous vein to stabilize the vessel.

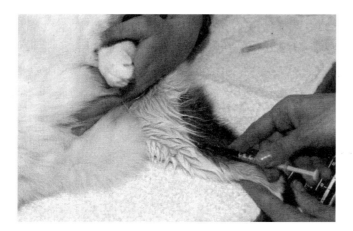

Figure 10-6. Venipuncture of the femoral vein in the cat.

restrainer's left hand, and the femoral and medial saphenous veins become distended. The individual performing the venipuncture grasps the lateral aspect of left leg at the tarsus. When the medial aspect of the leg is wiped with alcohol, the vein should be easy to identify. A 25-gauge needle on a 1- or 3-ml syringe is placed into the vein, and a blood sample is collected (Fig. 10–6). Firm pressure is applied to the puncture site for at least 60 seconds after the needle is removed because the medial saphenous and femoral veins are prone to hematoma formation.

On occasion, the technician will be required to collect a blood sample from a peripheral capillary bed to check for erythroparasitic organisms such as *Babesia* spp. or *Hemobartonella* spp. This can be accomplished by clipping the quick of a toenail or lacerating the buccal mucosa, but these methods are not highly recommended. A more desirable alternative is to collect a sample from the marginal ear vein (Fig. 10–7). The pinna of the ear is swabbed with 70% alcohol to vasodilate the marginal ear vein. A 25-gauge needle is used to puncture the ear vein. The blood is wicked up into a capillary tube, and then a drop of blood is spread on a clean microscope slide for examination.

Arterial Blood Sample

An arterial blood sample is useful to evaluate the acid-base and respiratory status of an animal. Cost-effective, easy-to-use arterial blood gas analyzers are becoming increasingly common in private veterinary practices. The technician should therefore be proficient in collecting blood from arteries. It is not necessary to occlude an artery to obtain a blood sample. Femoral and dorsal pedal arteries are used to obtain samples in conscious animals. When arterial puncture is performed in anesthetized patients, the lingual, brachial, and radial arteries may be used in addition to the femoral and dorsal pedal. Arterial blood gas samples are collected in a 1-ml or tuberculin syringe with a 25-gauge, 1.6-cm needle. The needle and syringe are coated with sodium heparin (1000 units/ml).

> **TECHNICIAN NOTE**
>
> An arterial blood sample is useful to evaluate the acid-base and respiratory status of an animal.

Femoral Artery Sample. To collect a femoral artery sample from the right leg, the patient is placed in right lateral recumbency with the right rear leg extended and the left rear leg abducted. The mammary glands or prepuce are also retracted dorsally to provide access to the femoral artery of the down leg. The inguinal region is wiped with 70% alcohol. The femoral artery pulse is palpated, and the needle is introduced into the artery at a 60-degree angle. Gentle suction is applied to the syringe, and it is advanced slightly back and forth until the artery is penetrated (Fig. 10–8). The sample will rapidly fill the syringe in a pulsatile manner, and the blood will be a brighter red color in appearance than a paired venous sample. A minimum of 0.25 ml of blood should be collected. Air bubbles are immediately expelled from the syringe and needle, and the needle is promptly capped with a rubber stopper. Bending the needle in lieu of piercing it in a rubber cork is not sufficient to maintain an anaerobic environment. Firm pressure is applied to the arterial puncture site for several minutes to prevent hematoma formation.

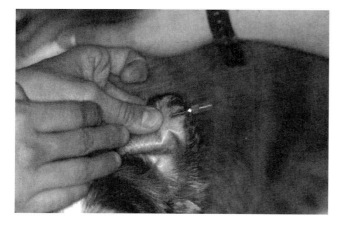

Figure 10-7. Collection of a peripheral capillary sample from the marginal ear vein in the cat.

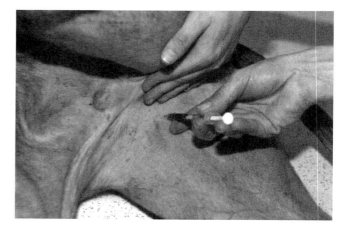

Figure 10-8. Femoral artery blood sample collection.

Dorsal Metatarsal Artery Sample. The dorsal metatarsal artery is used when the patient is obese or heavily muscled or when the femoral artery is not easily palpated or accessible. The dorsal metatarsal artery is located on the dorsal aspect of the metatarsus. The animal is placed in lateral recumbency, and the hock is extended. The dorsum of the metatarsus is clipped and aseptically prepared. The artery is isolated by palpating a pulse, and the needle is introduced into the artery at a 30-degree angle. The arterial blood sample is obtained and handled in the same manner as described for a femoral artery puncture.

Urine Sample Collection

Urine is frequently collected for analysis in veterinary practice. The technician should be familiar with the different methods used to obtain samples and understand why the veterinarian selects a specific method of collection over another. Urine samples may be collected by catching voided samples, manually expressing the bladder, catheterizing the bladder, or cystocentesis.

Voided Collection

Collection of naturally voided urine samples is the technique that is least stressful on the patient and easily performed by clients. Samples of urine collected during normal micturition are sufficient for basic screening urinalyses; however, they may be contaminated with bacteria, cells, and debris from the hair, skin, or genitourinary tract. The greatest concentration of contaminants is contained in the initial portion of the voided sample; therefore, the first portion of the urine stream should be excluded from the sample. If genitourinary tract disease is suspected, collection of an initial or end-stream sample is warranted. Urine is most easily obtained in the dog by walking it outdoors and catching a midstream sample. A collection device can be improvised by bending a loop in the end of an aluminum rod or straightened metal coat hanger. A paper cup placed in the loop serves as a urine receptacle.

Urine can be collected from a hospitalized animal by placing it on a wire grate in a clean cage. When the animal voids, the urine is collected from the cage floor with a syringe. Confinement of the animal in a metabolic cage is another means of collecting urine. Stainless steel metabolic cages consist of a grate raised above a slanted cage floor with a hole in the bottom. As natural micturition occurs, the urine flows onto the floor and through the hole. A container is placed beneath the opening to collect the urine.

Voided samples can be collected from clean, dry litter pans or pans covered with plastic bags. Specially designed plastic, nonabsorbent pellets (NoSorb, CATCO, Tifflin, OH) can be used in lieu of regular cat litter. When the cat urinates into the litter pan, the urine is simply poured out or collected with a syringe.

Bladder Expression

Urine can be collected through manual compression of the bladder. As with collection of urine from natural micturition, urine expressed from the bladder contains contaminants from the urethra, genitalia, skin, and hair. This technique may be difficult to perform in some patients, especially males, because transabdominal compression causes the pressure inside the bladder to increase but the urethral sphincter may not relax simultaneously. Pressure applied to empty the bladder should be firm and constant but not excessive. Overzealous compression is uncomfortable for the patient and may result in trauma to the bladder with subsequent hematuria. Care must be taken when attempting to express an overdistended bladder in the presence of partial or complete urethral obstruction to avoid urethral or vesicular rupture.

To express the bladder, place the animal in a standing position and place a hand on either side of the caudal abdomen. Isolate the bladder between the palmar surfaces of the fingers, and gently apply steady, firm pressure until a stream of urine is produced. It may be possible to express the bladder of cats and small dogs with only one hand. If urine is not expelled with moderate digital compression, do not continue to exert pressure. An alternative method to collect urine should be attempted.

Catheterization

Proper catheterization using an aseptic technique requires an assistant to help restrain the animal. Catheterization may induce an iatrogenic urinary tract infection, even if performed using aseptic technique. Trauma to the urinary tract during catheterization is common, so the urine samples obtained may have an increased number of red blood cells, protein, and transitional epithelial cells. Urine samples collected via a catheter may contain contaminants from the genital region and urethra but may be used when samples cannot be obtained through cystocentesis.

Male Canine. It usually is not difficult to place a urinary catheter in a male dog. A wide range of sizes and types of urinary catheters are available. A 4 to 10 Fr polypropylene urinary catheter is used. If the catheter is to remain, indwelling placement of a flexible feeding tube (Argyle, St. Louis, MO) is a more comfortable alternative to the more rigid polypropylene catheter.

The dog is placed in lateral recumbency, and the top rear leg is abducted. An assistant retracts the prepuce so the tip of the penis is exposed. The prepuce and glans penis are gently washed with warm dilute antiseptic solution and rinsed with warm sterile saline. The package containing the catheter is cut open to expose the distal 3 cm of the catheter, and sterile, water-soluble lubricant is placed on the catheter tip. If sterile gloves are used, the catheter should be removed from its package. If sterile gloves are not worn, the catheter is kept wrapped so it can be handled aseptically as it is advanced into the urethra.

To place the catheter, the lubricated tip is introduced into the urethra and slowly advanced. Resistance may be met when the catheter reaches the portion of the urethra that curves around the ischial arch. Steady gentle pressure should overcome this resistance; the catheter should never be forced through the urethra. The catheter can be guided around the flexure of the urethral canal by applying digital pressure on the perineum externally or pressing on the catheter with an index finger placed in the rectum. If the catheter cannot be passed on the first attempt, a different-size catheter should be used. When the size has been determined to be appropriate, the catheter should be slightly rotated as it is advanced the second time. Urine should flow into the catheter as it enters the bladder. A sterile 20- to 35-ml syringe is attached to the flared end of the catheter and used to gently aspirate urine from the bladder. Forceful suctioning with the syringe may traumatize the bladder or urethral mucosa by drawing the mucosa into the eyes of the catheter. The first several milliliters of urine acquired from the catheter may contain contaminants from the urogenital tract and should not be included in urine samples submitted for culture or urinalysis.

If the urinary catheter is to remain in the bladder, a butterfly bandage made out of folded waterproof tape is wrapped around the catheter at its exit from the penis. The tape is then sutured to the prepuce using 3-0 or 4-0 nylon. A urine collection system consisting of intravenous solution set tubing is connected to the flared end of the catheter, and an empty fluid bag is placed onto the other end of the solution set as a urine reservoir. Indwelling urinary catheters should occasionally be flushed with sterile 0.9% saline to ensure their patency.

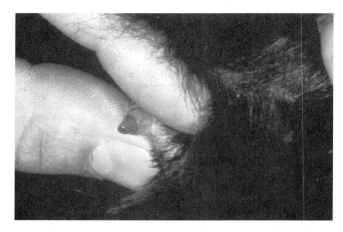

Figure 10-9. Retraction of the prepuce to expose the penis for feline urinary catheterization.

TECHNICIAN NOTE

Indwelling urinary catheters should occasionally be flushed with sterile 0.9% saline to ensure their patency.

Female Canine. Catheterization of the female dog is more challenging than that of the male due to the position of the urethral orifice. The dog is placed on a table in sternal recumbency with the hind legs dangling from the end of the table. The vulva is gently washed with a dilute, warm antiseptic solution and rinsed with warm sterile saline or water. The ventral vaginal floor is instilled with 1.0 ml of 2% lidocaine around the area of the urethral tubercle. A sterile flexible polypropylene urinary catheter is lubricated with sterile, water-soluble gel at the fenestrated end. Wearing sterile gloves, the technician places a lubricated finger into the vagina and slides it 3 to 5 cm along the ventral floor until the external urethral orifice is identified. The catheter is then introduced into the vagina and guided into the urethral orifice by the finger that is in the vestibule. It is important to avoid inadvertently passing the catheter into the clitoral fossa. The catheter is carefully advanced until it enters the bladder. If "blind catheterization" is not possible, a lighted vaginal speculum or an otoscope fitted with a large speculum is used to visualize the urethral opening.

A rigid metal catheter may be used instead of a flexible one; however, rigid catheters tend to traumatize the urethra. If the urinary catheter is to remain indwelling, a soft Foley self-retaining catheter (Jorgensen Laboratories, Loveland, CO) with a removable stylet is used. Once the Foley catheter is properly placed in the bladder, a cuff is inflated with 1 ml of water to prevent the tip of the catheter from slipping out of the bladder. The remainder of the catheter may then be taped to the tail to prevent the dog from stepping on it. A urine collection device similar to the one described for male dogs can be placed on the free end of the Foley catheter.

Male Feline. Male cats are frequently catheterized to relieve urethral obstructions. Catheterization requires the use of a short-acting anesthetic, such as a ketamine-diazepam combination or propofol, or a rapidly cleared gas anesthetic, such as isoflurane. Extra precaution should be taken when severely ill or uremic

cats are anesthetized. Catheterization performed merely to obtain a urine sample should be avoided due to the urethral inflammation that ensues.

The anesthetized male cat is placed on his back with the hind legs drawn cranial. The prepuce is retracted, and the penis is exposed (Fig. 10–9). The perineum is prepared aseptically as described for male canine catheterization. The penis is extended dorsally so the urethra is kept parallel to the vertebral column. With the use of sterile gloves, a sterile, lubricated, 3.5 Fr open-ended polyethylene tomcat catheter is passed into the urethra. The catheter is kept parallel to the vertebral column as it is advanced. If resistance is met, the catheter should be retracted and slightly rotated as it is readvanced. It should never be forced through the urethra, because a urethral obstruction may be present. Under such circumstances, a small volume of sterile water can be instilled into the catheter to flush out the material causing the obstruction so catheterization can be completed. Once a male cat is catheterized, the catheter can be secured in place by affixing a folded piece of waterproof tape around the catheter near its exit from the urethra. The tape is sutured to the prepuce with 4-0 nylon (Fig. 10–10). A urine collection system can be attached to the catheter if desired, or

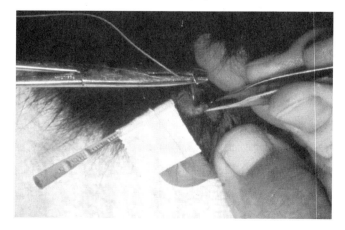

Figure 10-10. A urinary catheter is secured in place in a male cat. Tape wrapped around the catheter is sutured to the skin of the prepuce.

the catheter can be left open to drain exteriorly. The cat should be fitted with an Elizabethan collar to prevent removal of the catheter.

Female Feline. Catheterization of female cats is performed infrequently and, as with male cats, usually involves sedation. The perineal region is aseptically prepared, and the vulva is pulled caudally. A sterile, lubricated, open-ended 3.5 Fr tomcat catheter is inserted along the midline of the floor of the vagina and into the urethra. The urethral orifice may not be visualized.

Cystocentesis

Aspiration of urine directly from the bladder using a needle and syringe is termed *cystocentesis*. It is performed to collect specimens for culture and urinalysis that will be free of contamination from the distal urethra and genital tract. Cystocentesis is also used as a last resort to empty an overly distended bladder when a urethral obstruction prevents urinary catheterization. Recent surgery of the abdomen or presence of marked caudal abdominal trauma are two contraindications for cystocentesis of the bladder. When cystocentesis is performed, the majority, but not the entire quantity, of urine should be evacuated from the bladder to minimize extravasation from the puncture site once the needle is withdrawn. Removal of the entire volume of urine causes increased contact between the needle and the bladder wall, which may result in damage to the bladder.

To perform cystocentesis, the assistant restrains the animal in dorsal or lateral recumbency. When cystocentesis is performed in male dogs in dorsal recumbency, the prepuce and penis are diverted laterally, and the needle is inserted on the ventral midlne or slightly paramedian. The ventral or lateral abdominal skin is wiped with 70% alcohol. One hand is used to isolate and immobilize the bladder, and a 22-gauge, 2.5- to 3.75-cm needle attached to a 6- to 20-ml sterile syringe is inserted through the abdominal wall and into the bladder at a 45- to 75-degree angle (Fig. 10–11). If blood enters the needle hub, another attempt should be made with a different sterile needle and syringe. Excessive pressure applied to the bladder may cause urine leakage from around the needle. Do not redirect the angle of the needle within the abdominal cavity in an attempt to blindly obtain a urine sample; such a technique

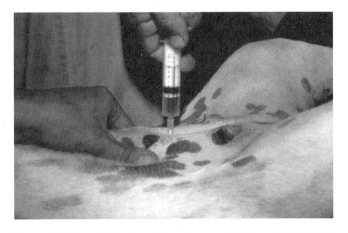

Figure 10–11. Collection of a urine sample through cystocentesis in the dog. The bladder is isolated and urine is aspirated into a syringe.

may lacerate viscera. Once a sufficient urine volume is collected, the needle is withdrawn from the abdomen. The needle is removed from the syringe before the sample is placed into a container for culture or urinalysis.

> **TECHNICIAN NOTE**
>
> Manual compression of the bladder during cystocentesis should be avoided.

Fecal Collection

Gross and microscopic examination of fecal material for intestinal parasites, blood, mucus, or fat is frequently performed in veterinary medicine. Samples are most commonly obtained by collecting them after the animal defecates. Alternatively, a lubricated fecal loop or gloved finger can be inserted into the rectum to obtain a small quantity of fecal material. The samples collected should be fresh and should be placed into an airtight container. If feces are collected for parasite examination several hours before they will be analyzed, they should be refrigerated or placed in a formalin solution. Samples for parasite examination can be refrigerated for up to 3 days.

Thoracocentesis

Thoracocentesis is a diagnostic and therapeutic procedure performed to remove air or fluid from the pleural cavity. It allows sampling of fluid from the pleural cavity for cytological analysis and culture. Thoracocentesis is often carried out when an animal is presented to the veterinarian in acute respiratory distress secondary to fluid accumulation in the pleural space or pneumothorax.

The area between the 5th and 12th ribs is clipped and surgically prepared with alternating chlorhexidine and alcohol scrubs. The seventh or eighth intercostal space is located by counting forward from the 13th rib. If fluid is expected to be removed, the site of needle introduction should be in the ventral third of the thorax. In the case of a suspected pneumothorax, the site should be more dorsal in the intercostal space. One-half milliliter of 2% lidocaine can be injected into the skin, subcutaneous tissue, and intercostal muscle to provide local anesthesia. Intercostal arteries are located just caudal to the ribs; therefore, needles are introduced just cranial to the ribs or in the middle portion of the intercostal space to avoid penetration of vessels.

To perform thoracocentesis, the animal is placed in sternal recumbency or held in a standing position. An animal with respiratory difficulties may resist being restrained in lateral recumbency. A 21-gauge butterfly catheter (E-Z Set Infusion Set, Becton Dickinson, Sandy UT) connected to a closed three-way stopcock and 60-ml syringe is directed into the intercostal space perpendicular to the body wall (Fig. 10–12). After the pleural space is penetrated, the needle is directed caudoventrally, and the stopcock is opened to the patient. Negative pressure is applied to the syringe, and the fluid or air is withdrawn from the pleural cavity. When the syringe is filled, the stopcock valve is placed in the closed position toward the patient, and the syringe contents are expelled through the third stopcock port.

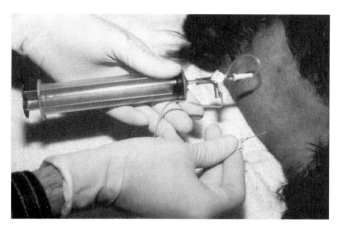

Figure 10-12. Materials used for thoracocentesis of a cat include a 21-gauge butterfly catheter attached to a three-way stopcock and 60-cc syringe.

Once a sufficient sample is obtained, the butterfly needle is withdrawn. The patient's respiratory pattern is monitored for changes for approximately 2 hours. Radiographs may be taken after the procedure to assess for iatrogenic pneumothorax or resolution of the pleural effusion.

Firm patient restraint is required so the animal does not move and cause the needle to lacerate the lung. The use of a butterfly catheter with its connected extension tubing permits manipulation of the syringe and stopcock without moving the needle; this decreases the likelihood of trauma to the lungs.

Abdominocentesis

Abdominocentesis has both a diagnostic and therapeutic purpose. It is performed to obtain a sample of fluid from the abdominal cavity for analysis or to relieve the pressure of a fluid-filled abdomen. Animals should be weighed both before and after fluid is removed. An increase in weight in the period after centesis could indicate a recurrence of fluid accumulation.

✎ TECHNICIAN NOTE

Before abdominocentesis is performed, the animal's bladder is emptied to avoid inadvertent puncture.

Before abdominocentesis is performed, the animal's bladder is emptied to avoid inadvertent puncture. A 5- to 10-cm area on the ventral abdomen between the umbilicus and bladder is clipped and aseptically prepared. The animal is restrained in a standing position. If local anesthesia is desired, 0.5 ml of 2% lidocaine is injected into the skin and underlying tissue just to the right of midline in the prepared area. An area to the right of the midline is selected to avoid tapping the spleen. An 18- to 22-gauge needle is used to penetrate the abdomen. The fluid is collected as it drips out of the needle hub, or it can be suctioned with a syringe attached to the needle. Sometimes rotating the needle or placing a second needle into the abdo-

men a few centimeters away from the first will stimulate flow of fluid from the needle. Centesis can also be performed with over-the-needle types of intravenous catheters. After the catheter and stylet puncture the abdominal cavity, the stylet is removed and a sample is collected.

Transtracheal Wash

A transtracheal wash is performed to obtain fluid samples from the lower respiratory tract for bacterial culture or cytology. Light sedation may be required in the dog, but the cough reflex should be maintained. The patient is placed in sternal recumbency or a seated position with the neck extended and head raised. The laryngeal region is clipped and aseptically prepared. A sterile gloved finger is placed on the ventral aspect of the trachea and moved in a cranial direction until of protruding cricoid cartilage is palpated. Just above the cartilage is the cricothyroid membrane, which is identified as a flattened, triangular region. From 0.5 to 1 ml of 2% lidocaine is injected through the skin and subcutaneous tissue and deep to the membrane. The needle from an 18-gauge, 20-cm through-the-needle–type catheter (I-Cath, CharterMed, Inc., Lakewood, NJ) is disengaged from the catheter. The catheter is kept in its protective sleeve, and the exposed end is placed on a sterile field. As one hand stabilizes the trachea, the needle is inserted at a 120-degree angle into the cricothyroid membrane. A burst of air accompanied by a cough occurs when the needle is successfully placed in the trachea. Placement of the needle with the bevel aimed down decreases the likelihood of laceration of the catheter as it is advanced through the needle. The catheter is reattached to the needle and advanced through the needle until it reaches the distal trachea. The needle is withdrawn from the trachea and skin, and the catheter, with stylet removed, is left in place. Alternatively, the needle can be inserted between tracheal rings in the cervical region. In large dogs, a sterile 3.5 Fr polyvinyl urinary catheter can be passed through a 14-gauge needle and advanced into the distal third of the trachea in lieu of a through-the-needle–type catheter (Fig. 10–13).

A 3-ml syringe should be attached to the catheter, and the plunger is pulled back. Air will be aspirated if the catheter is in the trachea. If only resistance is felt, the catheter should be repositioned because it is kinked, positioned against the tra-

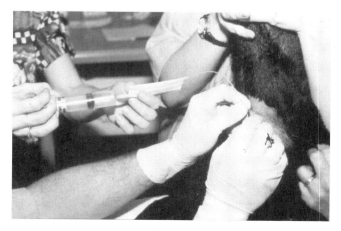

Figure 10-13. Transtracheal wash in a dog with a urinary catheter placed into the trachea.

cheal mucosa, or not in the trachea. After the catheter is properly placed in the trachea, 0.5 ml/kg of warm sterile saline is placed in a 12- to 35-ml syringe and flushed down the catheter. The patient's chest is coupaged, and when the animal coughs, negative pressure is applied to the syringe several times to aspirate a sample. Approximately 10% of the volume of fluid infused down the trachea will be reaspirated. Additional aliquots of saline are instilled into the catheter and reaspirated until a sufficient sample is obtained. Catheter position may need to be adjusted several times during the procedure. Suction is applied with the syringe as the catheter is withdrawn from the trachea. The puncture site is covered with a povidone-iodine–treated gauze sponge and bandaged. Respiration is monitored for 24 hours after the procedure.

TECHNICIAN NOTE

Approximately 10% of the volume of fluid infused down the trachea will be reaspirated.

Tracheal aspirates in the cat and very small dog are obtained in a different manner. The cat is lightly anesthetized and intubated with a sterile 3 or 4 Fr endotracheal tube. A sterile tomcat urinary catheter is threaded down the endotracheal tube to just a few centimeters above the tracheal bifurcation. From 3 to 5 ml of warm sterile saline is injected into the catheter. When the animal coughs, the sample is aspirated into a sterile 12-ml syringe. The saline injection–aspiration procedure is repeated until a sufficient sample volume is obtained.

Arthrocentesis

Aspiration of fluid from a swollen or painful joint is performed to help determine the cause of the joint problem. Synovial fluid is collected for cytological, bacterial, and biochemical analyses. An animal may not tolerate arthrocentesis of a painful joint without sedation.

Anatomy of the joint to be aspirated is reviewed to determine the appropriate site of needle insertion. For the shoulder, the needle enters from the lateral aspect and is directed medially. Aspiration of the elbow is performed from the lateral or caudal aspects and of the carpus from its dorsal surface. The coxofemoral joint is aspirated from its craniodorsal aspect. The stifle is approached from the craniolateral surface, just below the patella. A caudolateral approach is used for tarsal arthrocentesis.

To perform arthrocentesis, the skin over the joint is shaved and aseptically prepared. It is sometimes helpful to flex the joint to facilitate atraumatic insertion of the needle. A 22-gauge needle on a 3-ml syringe is inserted into the joint with the needle directed into a bone-free location (Fig. 10–14). If the needle contacts bone, it should be withdrawn slightly and redirected. After the joint is penetrated, the syringe plunger is gently retracted, and as much synovia as possible is collected. If blood is noted in the needle hub, the needle should be withdrawn. The use of needles smaller than 22 gauge will result in difficulty in aspirating inspissated joint fluid. The color, consistency, amount, and viscosity of the synovia are noted.

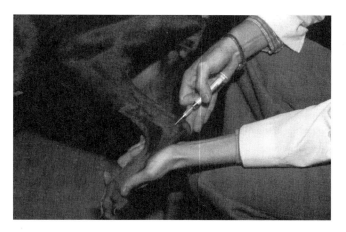

Figure 10–14. Arthrocentesis of the tibiotarsal joint through a caudolateral approach.

Normal joint fluid is clear, light yellow, and very viscous (a drop placed on a finger and stretched with another finger should be at least 10 cm long). A drop is placed on a clean microscope slide, and a smear is made for cytological analysis. A sterile sample is saved for bacterial culture and sensitivity. The remaining synovia is placed in a test tube containing an anticoagulant such as EDTA before submission for laboratory analysis.

Bone Marrow Aspiration

Bone marrow aspiration is performed to evaluate the cells present in the marrow and to check for the presence of viruses, such as feline leukemia virus. Aspirates are often obtained in anemic animals and in those with neoplasia. A blood sample of the patient is taken within 24 hours before or after the aspirate so the bone marrow aspirate sample can be interpreted. Bone marrow aspiration is an uncomfortable procedure, so sedatives of short-acting intravenous anesthetics should be used in addition to a local anesthetic.

Common sites for bone marrow aspiration include the ilial wing, femur, and humerus. The size of the patient determines which site is used. Aspirates are performed using strict aseptic technique. Hair over the site is shaved, and the skin is surgically scrubbed. Sterile gloves are worn by the person obtaining the aspirate.

TECHNICIAN NOTE

Common sites for bone marrow aspiration include the ilial wing, femur, and humerus.

Ilial Bone Marrow Aspiration

The animal is placed in lateral recumbency, and the uppermost iliac crest region is clipped and aseptically prepared. The widest part of the iliac crest is identified. From 0.5 to 1 ml of 2% lidocaine is infiltrated through a 25-gauge needle into the skin, subcutaneous tissue, and periosteum of the bone. A sterile 15- to 18-gauge Jamshidi or Rosenthal bone marrow needle (J.A.

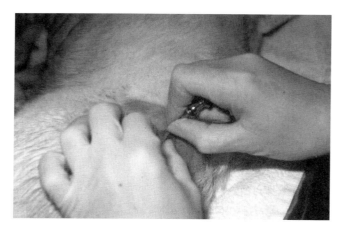

Figure 10–15. Technique for placing a bone marrow needle into the ilium of a dog.

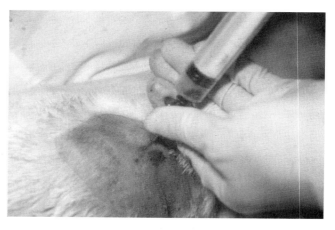

Figure 10–17. The bone marrow needle is stabilized as marrow is aspirated from the ilium.

Webster, Sterling, MA) is flushed with an anticoagulant such as dipotassium EDTA. Sterile technique should be followed for obtaining bone marrow aspirates. A No. 11 scalpel blade is used to make a 5-mm incision through the skin over the iliac crest. One hand stabilizes the ilium and the needle. With the stylet in place, the needle is introduced through the skin incision. The needle is advanced ventrocaudally until the cortex of the bone is penetrated and the marrow cavity is entered (Fig. 10–15). To penetrate the bone, significant pressure is applied to the needle. The individual placing the needle should hold the elbow flexed and stationary as the wrist is rotated in a clockwise-counterclockwise manner. The needle may slip off the bone, especially in small animals with narrow ilial wings. If this occurs, the needle is repositioned, and another attempt to penetrate the cortex is made.

When the needle is firmly seated in the bone and the tip is in the marrow cavity, the stylet is removed and placed on a sterile field (Fig. 10–16). A dipotassium EDTA–coated 12-ml syringe is attached to the end of the needle, and negative pressure is rapidly and forcefully applied. One-tenth of a milliliter of bone marrow is aspirated into the syringe (Fig. 10–17). The syringe is then detached, and drops of the sample are immediately placed onto precleaned microscope slides. Slides

are tilted to permit excess peripheral blood to trickle off the end of the slide (Fig. 10–18). A pull slide preparation is made with each sample.

The stylet may be replaced and the needle repositioned if retraction of the syringe plunger fails to provide a marrow sample. After the sample is obtained, the needle is withdrawn, and firm pressure is held on the site until hemostasis occurs. A povidone-iodine ointment–treated gauze sponge is secured over the aspirate site.

Humeral Bone Marrow Aspiration

The craniolateral aspect of the greater tubercle of the proximal humerus is another site for obtaining bone marrow aspirates (Fig. 10–19). This region has less tissue, fat, and muscle overlying the bone than the other aspirate sites. This site is advantageous for use in heavily muscled or overweight dogs when the dorsal iliac crest may be difficult to palpate or in animals with narrow ilial wings.

The animal is placed in lateral recumbency, and the proximal humerus is shaved and surgically scrubbed. To obtain marrow from the humerus, the patient's humerus is stabilized

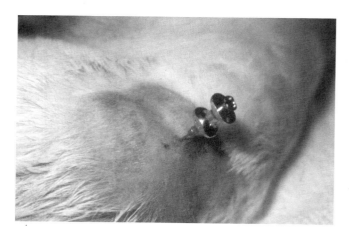

Figure 10–16. Rosenthal bone marrow needle seated in the dorsal aspect of the wing of the ilium.

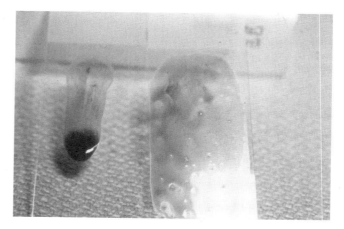

Figure 10–18. Drops of bone marrow are placed on the end of microscope slides, which are tilted to allow blood to run to the other end. A pull smear is made with the bone marrow sample.

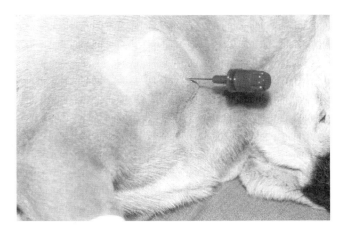

Figure 10-19. Jamshidi bone marrow needle placed into the craniolateral aspect of the proximal humerus to obtain a bone marrow aspirate.

by an assistant with the elbow flexed and the shoulder externally rotated. The needle is embedded perpendicular to the humeral shaft. The technique for site preparation, needle placement, bone marrow aspiration, and slide preparation is as previously described for ilial bone marrow aspiration.

Femoral Bone Marrow Aspiration

In small dogs and cats, the femur can be used for bone marrow aspirates. Site preparation, needle placement, marrow aspiration, and slide preparation techniques are the same as described for bone marrow aspiration from the wing of the ilium.

To obtain a sample from the right femur, the patient is placed in left lateral recumbency, and the individual who performs the aspirate stands at the dorsum of the patient. The trochanteric fossa is identified on the medial aspect of the greater trochanter of the proximal femur. The needle is introduced medial to the greater trochanter and advanced parallel to the femoral shaft. Counterpressure is applied by an assistant, who flexes the stifle, pushes the femur dorsally, and internally rotates the hip. When the needle is introduced, care is taken not to pierce the sciatic nerve, which is posteromedial to the greater trochanter.

ADMINISTRATION OF MEDICATION IN THE SMALL ANIMAL

Intravenous Administration

Many drugs are administered directly into a vein. Intravenous injection is frequently used for drugs that are tissue irritants or when a rapid onset of action is required. Certain anesthetics, chemotherapeutic agents, anticonvulsant drugs, and drugs used in cardiopulmonary resuscitation are given intravenously.

The cephalic and lateral saphenous veins are the most frequently used sites for intravenous injection in the dog. Cats are most often administered intravenous injections in the cephalic, medial saphenous, and femoral veins. Detailed venipuncture technique is previously described in this chapter. Air bubbles should be expelled from the syringe before introducing the needle into the vein. The vessel is occluded and the needle is placed into the vein. When the needle is placed in the lumen of the vein, blood should spontaneously appear in the needle

hub. Intravenous placement is further verified by slightly retracting the syringe plunger and aspirating blood into the syringe. The holder should discontinue vessel occlusion so the syringe contents can be injected into the vein. The needle is then removed, and firm pressure is placed on the venipuncture site until hemostasis occurs.

When intravenous fluids must be administered continuously, a catheter is placed in the cephalic, jugular, or saphenous vein. The technician should be familiar with catheter selection, placement, and maintenance. The three types of catheters are the butterfly catheter (E-Z Set Infusion Set, Becton Dickinson), the over-the-needle (OTN) catheter (Angiocath, Becton Dickinson), and the through-the-needle (TTN) catheters (I-Cath, CharterMed, Inc., Lakewood, NJ). If the catheter is to remain indwelling, the over- or through-the-needle types are used.

Indwelling catheters are placed using aseptic technique to minimize subsequent thrombus formation, phlebitis, and infection. The hair is clipped around the vein, and the skin surface is cleansed with an antimicrobial solution and alcohol for a minimum of three times. Ideally, the region should be scrubbed for 2 minutes. If it is necessary to palpate the skin to identify the vein, the area should be rescrubbed or the individual placing the catheter should wear sterile gloves.

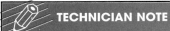

TECHNICIAN NOTE

Indwelling catheters are placed using aseptic technique to minimize subsequent thrombus formation, phlebitis, and infection.

To place an over-the-needle catheter into a peripheral vein, such as the cephalic or saphenous, the vessel is occluded using digital pressure or a tourniquet. The catheter is flushed with heparinized 0.9% sterile saline so it will not become occluded with a blood clot. With one hand, the individual placing the catheter holds the extremity with the skin pulled tautly. This minimizes vein movement as the catheter is introduced. With the stylet in place, the catheter is inserted into the vein at a 20-degree angle. When blood enters the hub of the stylet, the catheter and stylet are advanced slightly to ensure the catheter tip is well within the vessel lumen (Fig. 10–20). The catheter is then slid off the stylet and into the vein. Blood will trickle out of the end of the catheter if it is properly placed. Digital pressure is removed once the catheter enters the vein. A cap is promptly placed on the end of the catheter, and the catheter is flushed with 1 ml of heparinized saline. The saline should pass through the catheter with minimal resistance if the catheter is placed correctly in the vein. Adhesive tape in 1.3- to 2.5-cm-wide strips is placed around the circumference of the catheter and then around the leg to firmly secure the catheter to the extremity. The point of entry of the catheter into the skin is covered with a povidone-iodine–treated gauze sponge and covered with tape. Tape may be placed underneath the catheter cap to isolate it from the skin. It is important that the tape not be applied too tightly or the limb may swell. If this occurs, the catheter should be retaped or removed.

To catheterize a jugular vein, a flexible through-the-needle catheter is used. A 16- to 22-gauge 20- to 30-cm-long catheter

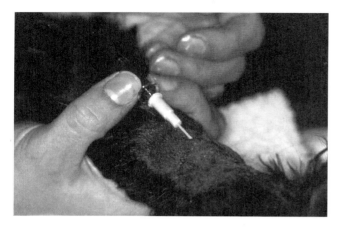

Figure 10–20. Technique for placement of an over-the-needle type of catheter into the cephalic vein of a dog.

is used, depending on the size of the animal. The ventral surface of the neck is shaved and aseptically prepared. An assistant restrains the patient in lateral recumbency with the vein to be punctured facing away from the table. The assistant holds the neck in an extended position and occludes the vein at the thoracic inlet. With the needle guard removed, the introducer needle is placed through the skin just lateral to the vein (Fig. 10–21). Once the needle is through the skin, the tip is placed against the wall of the jugular vein at a 40-degree angle. With a quick thrusting motion, the needle is inserted into the vein; several attempts may be required. Successful placement is denoted by a flashback of blood inside the catheter lumen. The angle between the needle and the skin is then decreased to 20 degrees, and the catheter is fed into the vein through a sterile protective sleeve until the catheter is inserted into the hub of the needle. If resistance is met when catheter advancement is attempted, the catheter is most likely extravascular and should be removed. Never back the catheter out through the introducer needle because the bevel may sever the catheter and create an embolus. Once the catheter has been placed in the vein, the needle is backed out of the skin and covered with the needle guard. Firm pressure is held over the site of skin entry for 30 seconds to prevent hematoma formation. Bleeding tends to

occur when the needle is withdrawn from the vein because the bore of the needle is larger than that of the catheter; a larger hole is left in the vessel than is filled by the catheter. The plastic sleeve and stylet are removed, and an extension port (T-Port, Becton Dickinson) prefilled with heparinized saline is placed on the end of the catheter. Approximately 6 ml of heparinized saline is flushed through the catheter to ensure proper placement within the vein. It should be possible to aspirate blood back through the jugular catheter if it is properly placed (Fig. 10–22). In many instances, the animal's head position may need to be adjusted to aspirate blood back through the catheter.

Once the jugular catheter is successfully placed, it should be secured to the animal. A 5-cm-wide butterfly tape is used to attach the needle guard to the needle hub. A drop of SuperGlue is placed at the junction of the catheter hub and needle to prevent the catheter from backing out of the needle. A gauze sponge with a small amount of antibiotic ointment on it is placed on top of the catheter entry site. Then, 2.5-cm-wide tape is wrapped loosely around the animal's neck on both sides of the needle guard to incorporate the gauze sponge and the butterfly. Stretch gauze bandaging material is wrapped several times around the circumference of the neck to further secure the catheter. A final layer of 5-cm-wide tape is used to cover the stretch gauze. It the patient has a history of vomiting, waterproof tape placed on top of the stretch gauze will help keep the bandage dry. Periodically check the catheter patency during the bandaging process because adjustments to the catheter may be required. Dogs with jugular catheters should be walked on a leash placed behind the front legs and not around the neck.

A long, through-the-needle catheter can be placed in a saphenous vein using the same technique as in jugular catheter placement. Saphenous catheter placement is not recommended in nonambulatory animals that are unable to stand to urinate or in animals with diarrhea or fecal incontinence. It is difficult to prevent urine and fecal contamination of the catheter in such situations.

Long, through-the-needle catheters placed in the jugular or saphenous veins are in direct communication with the vena cava. A major advantage to their placement is the ability to obtain blood samples via the catheter. To collect blood from a long catheter, the "three-syringe technique" is used. Approxi-

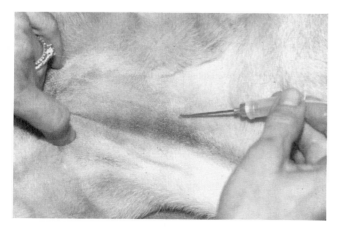

Figure 10–21. Insertion of the needle through the skin to place a through-the-needle type of intravenous catheter into the canine jugular vein.

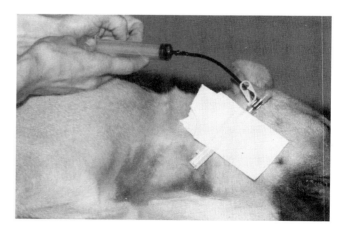

Figure 10–22. Aspiration of blood from the extension port of a through-the-needle catheter verifies placement in the jugular vein.

mately 3 to 5 ml of blood is removed from the catheter with a syringe and set aside. A second syringe is then attached to the catheter, and a blood sample is aspirated. The blood from the first syringe is injected back into the catheter, and a third syringe containing 3 to 5 ml of heparinized saline is used to flush the catheter. Extension of the animal's neck may be required to withdraw the blood sample from the catheter. Because of the large diameter of the jugular vein and the catheter placed within it, fluids can be administered at a more rapid rate than via a peripheral catheter. In addition, central venous pressure can be monitored through a catheter placed into the anterior vena cava via the jugular vein or into the caudal vena cava via the saphenous vein.

Indwelling arterial catheters are placed to allow blood pressure monitoring and collection of arterial blood samples. The 22-gauge, 2.5-cm-long, over-the-needle catheters are most frequently placed in the dorsal metatarsal artery. The method for arterial venipuncture is previously described in this chapter. Arterial catheter placement technique is similar to that of venous catheter placement except the artery is not occluded and the catheter is introduced at a more parallel angle to the vessel. Arterial catheter placement usually is more uncomfortable than venous catheter placement and may not be well tolerated in awake animals. In addition, flushing the arterial catheter may cause the patient some discomfort. ***Medications and fluids, with the exception of small boluses of heparinized saline, are never administered via an arterial catheter.***

TECHNICIAN NOTE

Indwelling arterial catheters are placed to allow blood pressure monitoring and collection of arterial blood samples.

Several important points must be made in regard to maintenance of indwelling intravenous catheters. ***Catheters should not be left in place for longer than 72 hours.*** The site must be checked frequently for pain, redness, swelling, and discharge; if any such signs are noted, the catheter should be removed. If swelling is attributed to tight application of tape and the catheter is still patent, the catheter can simply be retaped. Venous catheters should be flushed with 1 to 5 ml of heparinized saline every 4 to 6 hours to ensure patency. A catheter should be checked for patency before injecting medications and, in most instances, should be flushed with heparinized saline after drug administration. It is necessary to flush arterial catheters every 2 hours to maintain patency.

When an intravenous catheter is removed, the puncture site is covered with a gauze sponge onto which a small amount of povidone-iodine ointment has been placed. The gauze sponge is then secured with porous tape. An arterial catheter puncture site is covered with a pressure bandage for 10 minutes after the catheter is removed. After 10 minutes, the pressure wrap is replaced with a regular gauze bandage.

Intravenous Chemotherapy Administration

Chemotherapy is being used with greater frequency in small animal practices to treat a variety of neoplasias. The veterinary technician should be familiar with chemotherapy administration protocols and safety precautions (see Chapter 24). Because many chemotherapeutic agents are carcinogens, it is advisable to limit exposure as much as possible during administration. Latex gloves, safety glasses, masks, and a nonpermeable, disposable, long-sleeved gown with elastic cuffs should be worn. All materials used in the administration, including catheters, syringes, needles, and gauze sponges, should be disposed of in leak-proof containers with hazardous waste labels. An alcohol-soaked gauze pad should cover the catheter cap when the needle on the chemotherapy drug syringe is placed into or removed from the catheter. This practice decreases the amount of aerosolization of the drug.

Intravenous catheters are used to administer cytotoxic solutions, especially those that cause tissue irritation when injected extravascularly; examples of such vesicants are doxorubicin, vincristine, vinblastine, and actinomycin-D. *Intravenous catheters must be placed with extreme care.* The catheter should be placed in a peripheral vein, and the vessel must be punctured only once during placement. If a "clean stick" is not achieved on the first placement attempt, then a different vein should be used. It is permissible, but not advisable, to reattempt placement in the same vein if a more proximal site is selected and the initial site has clotted. Nonheparinized 0.9% sterile saline should be used to flush the catheter because certain drugs, such as doxorubicin, precipitate when mixed with heparin.

Catheters used for vesicant drug administration should be frequently re-evaluated for patency. The area proximal to the catheter site should be freely visible to observe for extravasation. Signs that the chemotherapeutic agent has leaked out of the vein include loss of patency of the catheter, redness or swelling at or proximal to the injection site, or vocalization or discomfort by the patient indicating pain.

If extravasation occurs, as much of the drug should be removed from the site as possible by aspirating 5 ml of blood back through the catheter. The tissue surrounding the site is infused with saline, corticosteroids, or 2% lidocaine, and either warm or cold compresses are applied depending on which chemotherapy drug is used.

When chemotherapy administration is complete, the catheter should be flushed with several milliliters of sterile nonheparinized 0.9% saline. Protective apparel should continue to be worn. A piece of alcohol-soaked gauze should cover the entire catheter as it is removed from the vein. The skin puncture is covered with an antibiotic-treated gauze and securely bandaged.

When the quantity of chemotherapeutic drug required is less than 3 ml, a 23- or 25-gauge butterfly catheter may be used. Vincristine is commonly administered through a butterfly catheter. After drug administration is complete, the tubing is crimped to prevent the drug from leaking back out of the catheter. At least 12 ml of nonheparinized 0.9% saline should be used to flush the catheter before it is removed. The needle is covered with an alcohol-soaked gauze as it is withdrawn from the skin, and the venipuncture site is bandaged.

Subcutaneous Administration

Subcutaneous injections are easily and frequently performed and allow for relatively rapid absorption of the agent injected. Absorption of drugs may be slow in obese animals due to the relatively poor vascular supply in fat. Subcutaneous injection is the most common route for administration of vaccinations. Moderate volumes of isotonic fluids can be injected under the skin to rehydrate animals if intravenous access is not available.

The most preferred site for subcutaneous injection is the dorsolateral region from the neck to the hips. The dorsal region of the neck and back should be avoided due to the difficulty in treating any abscess or hematoma that may result from the injection. The injection site is wiped with 70% isopropyl alcohol to remove superficial skin contaminants. A fold of skin is tented, and the needle is inserted at the base of the fold (Fig. 10–23). The syringe plunger is retracted slightly, and the needle hub is checked for blood before injection. If blood appears in the hub, a vessel has been penetrated, and the needle should be removed and reinserted at another location. After injection, the skin is briefly massaged to facilitate drug distribution. If more than one vaccination or medication is to be injected subcutaneously at the same time, the injection sites should be several centimeters apart. It is recommended that multiple vaccinations be administered on opposite sides of the body.

TECHNICIAN NOTE

The most preferred site for subcutaneous injection is the dorsolateral region from the neck to the hips.

Intramuscular Administration

The intramuscular route is appropriate for injection of small volumes of medication. Intramuscular injection is generally more uncomfortable for an animal than subcutaneous injection. Drugs can be administered in the lumbosacral musculature lateral to the dorsal spinous processes or in the semimembranosus or semitendinosus muscles of the rear leg. The neck is never used as a site for intramuscular injections. Deep lumbar injections in the third to fifth lumbar region are used to administer heartworm treatment (Fig. 10–24). Placement of the needle in the lumbosacral muscles is not recommended in very thin animals. If injection is made into the semimembranosus or semitendinosus muscles, the needle should enter the lateral

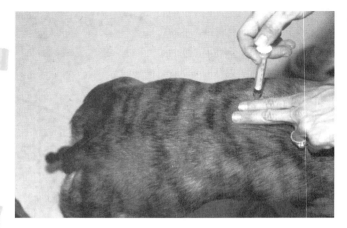

Figure 10-24. Deep intramuscular injection into the lumbar musculature of the dog.

aspect of the muscle and be directed caudally to avoid penetration of the sciatic nerve (Fig. 10–25). Contact of the needle with the sciatic nerve is painful and may result in subsequent lameness.

A 25- to 22-gauge needle should be used for intramuscular injection. The skin over the muscle is wiped with 70% isopropyl alcohol, and the muscle is isolated between the thumb and fingers. The needle is carefully embedded into the muscle. As with subcutaneous injections, the needle hub is checked for blood before administration of medication to determine that a vessel is not inadvertently penetrated. If this occurs, the needle is removed and redirected. Once proper placement within the muscle is verified, the drug is slowly injected, and the needle is then removed.

Intradermal Administration

Intradermal injections are performed primarily for allergy testing. Most animals will not tolerate skin testing unless sedated. Hair on the lateral aspect of the trunk is shaved with a No. 40 clipper blade. The skin is carefully wiped with a gauze sponge moistened with water. Vigorous scrubbing or the use of an antimicrobial cleaning solution is contraindicated because it

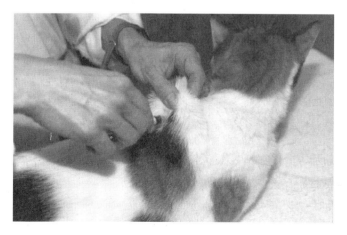

Figure 10-23. Subcutaneous injection made into the dorsolateral aspect of the neck.

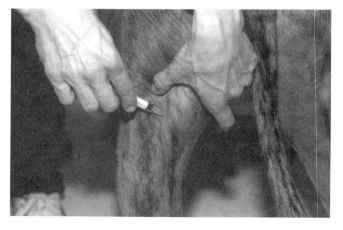

Figure 10-25. Intramuscular injection into the semimembranosus and semitendinosus muscles of the rear leg of the dog.

may irritate the skin and interfere with testing. To make an injection, a fold of skin is lifted, and a 25- to 27-gauge needle attached to a 1-ml syringe is inserted, with the bevel up, into the dermis. A 0.10-ml volume of allergen is injected at the site. The injection site will appear like a translucent lump if the injection is performed correctly. The skin is then examined for tissue reaction.

Intranasal Administration

Certain vaccines, such as those for feline infectious peritonitis and *Bordetella bronchiseptica,* are administered intranasally. The patient's muzzle is held in one hand and elevated slightly. The tip of the vaccine dispenser is placed in the nasal cavity, and the dispenser is squeezed to inject the vaccine into the nose. Animals will frequently sneeze after the liquid enters the nasal cavity.

Intratracheal Administration

In an emergency situation, such as during cardiopulmonary resuscitation, medications can be injected directly into the trachea because absorption of the drug is extremely rapid. A polypropylene urinary catheter is advanced down the trachea or the endotracheal tube, and the drug, such as epinephrine, atropine, or lidocaine, is administered as a bolus with a syringe into the urinary catheter. From 10 ml of air or 3 to 10 ml of sterile saline is injected through the urinary catheter immediately afterward to disperse the drug. If a urinary catheter is not available, the drug is sprayed down the endotracheal tube with the use of a syringe and followed with a burst of air.

TECHNICIAN NOTE

In an emergency situation, such as during cardiopulmonary resuscitation, medications can be injected directly into the trachea because absorption of the drug is extremely rapid.

Intraosseous Administration

Needles are placed directly into the bone marrow cavity to deliver fluids, drugs, and blood products when peripheral or jugular catheterization is not possible or is too time consuming. Intraosseous placement allows rapid fluid delivery to neonates, small animals, animals with circulatory collapse, and those with inaccesible peripheral vessels. Placement is contraindicated in septic patients and those with bone or skin infections or recent fractures in the site selected for catheterization.

Sites used include the proximal tibia, trochanteric fossa of the femur, ilial wing, ischium, and greater tubercle of the humerus. Needles that are used include 15- to 18-gauge bone marrow needles, specially designed Cook Intraosseous Access Needles (Cook, Bloomington, IN), 20-gauge 3.75-cm spinal needles for cats and puppies, and 18- to 22-gauge hypodermic needles for neonates.

Needle placement follows the same protocol as described for bone marrow needles. If the bone cortex is punctured in more than one site, fluid that is administered may leak into the subcutaneous tissue. If this occurs, a different bone should be used, and the initial bone site should not be used again for a minimum of 12 hours.

Once placed, the needle is secured by wrapping tape near the needle hub into a butterfly and suturing the tape to the skin. A povidone-iodine–treated gauze pad is applied to the skin entry site. A bulky, waterproof bandage is placed around the needle for stabilization. Patency of the intraosseous needle is maintained by flushing every 6 hours with 1 to 2 ml of heparinized 0.9% saline. The needle may remain in place for up to 3 days.

Topical Ophthalmic Administration

To place medication into an animal's eyes, good restraint is essential or the ophthalmic medications will be inadvertently placed on the eyelids or face. It is important not to allow the tip of the medication dispenser to make contact with any surface, or it will become contaminated. Slightly warming cold ophthalmic solutions by holding the container in the palm of the hand for a few minutes may make administration of the medication more comfortable for the patient. Liquid solutions are placed in the eye by holding the lids open with the thumb and index finger of one hand and dispensing one or two drops of medication into the eye with the other hand. It is helpful to rest the hand holding the medication on the patient's head as the drops are dispensed. Ointment is placed in the eye by holding open the lids with the thumb and index finger of one hand and squeezing a 5-mm-long strip of ointment onto the upper sclera or lower palpebral border with the remaining hand (Fig. 10–26). The ointment is dispersed across the cornea when the patient blinks.

If multiple topical medications are to be administered to the same eye, they should be added a minimum of 3 to 5 minutes apart to allow for sufficient absorption. If both a solution and an ointment are to be applied, the drop is placed in the eye at least 3 to 5 minutes before the ointment. If the ointment is placed first, it may coat the cornea and interfere with the absorption of the drop.

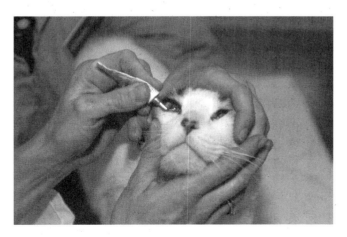

Figure 10-26. Ophthalmic ointment is placed on the lower palpebral border in a cat.

Aural Administration

Before placing medications in the ear canal, the ears should be cleared of as much debris as possible; this increases the amount of contact between the drug and epithelium and increases absorption of the medication. To place medication in the ear canal, the pinna is grasped and pulled upward and back toward the head. The tip of the medication dispenser is placed into the vertical ear canal, and the dispenser is squeezed to deliver the prescribed amount of ointment or solution. The dispenser is removed from the ear canal, and the base of the ear is gently massaged to distribute the medication into the ear canal.

Cutaneous Administration

Certain medications are applied directly to the skin of the animal and gradually absorbed. It is important for the technician to realize that topical medications will be absorbed by the individual applying the medication as well as the patient if latex gloves are not worn; nitroglycerin cream is one example. Latex gloves should be worn to smear a small quantity of ointment onto a sparsely haired region of the body. The pinna of the ear, the groin, or a shaved area on the ventral thorax are all appropriate spots to apply topical nitroglycerin. The treated area should be covered with a light bandage, if possible, so it will not be accidentally touched.

Many topical medications are dispensed by veterinarians to control ectoparasites, such as fleas and ticks. They are either sprayed over the entire body or applied to the skin between the shoulder blades. It is important to wear gloves when handling these medications and to avoid touching the treated areas for the specific length of time recommended by the drug manufacturers.

Rectal Administation

The mucosa of the large intestine is capable of absorbing medications delivered rectally. Absorption is most effective when the colon is free of fecal material. This route may be used to deliver antiemetic tablets when the animal is vomiting and cannot be administered oral medication. A gloved, lubricated finger is used to insert the tablet into the rectum a distance of at least 5 cm. The medication is then gradually absorbed. Drugs given in an emergency situation to stop a seizure, such as diazepam, can also be administered rectally if intravenous injection is difficult to perform. A small rubber feeding tube or 3.5 Fr feline urinary catheter is inserted approximately 8 to 10 cm into the rectum. The diazepam is placed into a syringe and injected into the flared end of the catheter. Several milliliters of warm water are then injected into the catheter to flush the drug into the large intestine.

Enema solutions are also delivered per rectum. Gloves should be worn and the animal should be confined in a bathtub. A single-use syringe containing the medication is lubricated and placed into the rectum. The plunger is depressed, and the enema is delivered into the large intestine. Warm soapy water enemas can be administered by placing plastic tubing into the rectum and advancing it into the large intestine. Water is then funneled into the end of the tube, which is held in an elevated position. The tube is moved back and forth and is slowly advanced up the intestinal tract as fecal material is expelled. After the feces have been cleared out of the intestinal tract, the tube is withdrawn. When a medication is placed in the enema solution and the solution must be contained in the large intestine for several minutes, a Foley urinary catheter is used. The catheter is inserted into the rectum, and the solution is injected with a syringe through the flared end. Once the desired volume has been instilled, the cuff on the catheter is inflated with 1 to 2 ml of water. The inflated cuff helps seal the rectum so the enema solution is retained. A gloved hand is used to hold the rectum closed to further retain enema solution. After the allotted time has passed, a syringe is used to deflate the cuff, and the catheter is removed. Warm water enemas are not well tolerated in cats, so sedation is usually required.

Oral Administration

An easy and frequently used route to administer medications to a dog or cat is by mouth. It is considerably easier to medicate a dog per os than a cat. Technicians should become adept at orally medicating animals and be able to demonstrate techniques to pet owners.

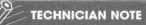

TECHNICIAN NOTE

Technicians should become adept at orally medicating animals and be able to demonstrate techniques to pet owners.

Liquids, capsules, and tablets are the three types of oral medications routinely used in veterinary medicine. Liquids are easy to administer via a dropper or syringe. Tablets can be pulverized and capsules can be opened to mix their contents with water or corn syrup. These suspensions can also be administered via a syringe. To medicate an animal with a syringe or dropper filled with fluid, the animal's lower lip is pulled out at the corner. The tip of the syringe or dropper is placed in the pouch, and small volumes of liquid are administered into the lip fold. The muzzle should be held at a neutral angle and not elevated. Hyperextension of the neck during the administration of oral liquids may result in the aspiration of the fluid into the trachea.

Tablets and capsules are most easily administered to dogs by hiding them in food such as pieces of meat, cheese, or chunks of canned pet food. Cats will rarely consume pills hidden in food; they will meticulously eat the food that surrounds the pill and leave the medication. An animal that will not consume food baited with the pill is medicated by prying open the jaws with one hand and placing the pill on the base of the tongue with the other (Fig 10–27). The jaws are immediately closed by placing a hand around the muzzle. If the tablet is not placed sufficiently far back in the pharynx, the animal will attempt to expel it. Swallowing is stimulated by rubbing under the chin, tapping on the tip of the nose, or blowing air into the nostrils. When the animal licks its nose after the tablet has been placed in the oral cavity, it can be assumed that the tablet has been swallowed. A specially designed pilling device is available to administer tablets to cats and fractious dogs. The tablet is secured into the tip of a plastic rod, which is inserted into the back of the mouth. A plunger is depressed, and the pill is propelled down the esophagus.

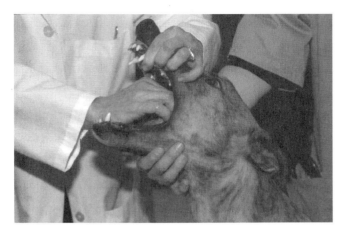

Figure 10-27. A dog's muzzle is held open as a tablet is placed into the back of the mouth.

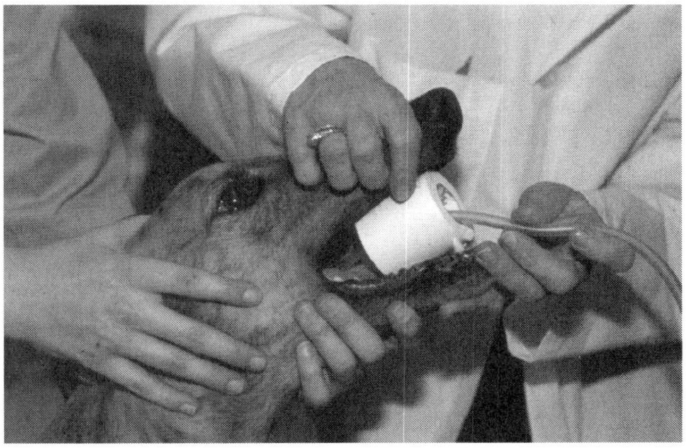

Figure 10-29. A roll of tape holds the mouth open as a stomach tube is placed into the oral cavity.

Orogastric Intubation

A tube can be placed into the stomach via the mouth to deliver fluids and medication. This technique is used to administer activated charcoal solutions for the treatment of poisoning. Dogs will permit the passage of orogastric tubes with minimal resistance. Cats, however, usually require sedation. The length of a 10 to 22 Fr plastic tube required to extend from the canine teeth to the eighth or ninth rib is measured and marked on the tube with tape or ink (Fig. 10–28). The tip of the tube is lubricated with water-soluble gel. The animal is restrained in sternal recumbency or in a standing or seated position. A roll of tape or a plastic or wooden speculum with a hole in the middle is placed behind the canine teeth to hold the mouth open. A hand is placed around the muzzle so the mouth speculum will not become dislodged. The head is placed in a normal position, not elevated. The tube is slowly passed through the speculum to enter the phyarynx (Fig. 10–29). Swallowing will be noted as the tube passes over the base of the tongue and into the esophagus. If the animal coughs during the procedure, the tube may have entered the trachea and should be promptly removed. Once the tube is in the esophagus, it is advanced to the premeasured length and enters the stomach. Correct place-ment of the tube in the gastrointestinal tract should always be determined before introducing any medications or fluids. Refer to the following section on nasoesophageal or nasogastric tubes for a detailed description of how to check tube placement. If the tube is being placed to feed an animal, then the tube is advanced only until it reaches the distal esophagus.

Liquids can be administered into the orogastric tube using several techniques. Fluid can be injected into the end of the tube via a 60-ml syringe. Large volumes can be quickly adminis-tered using a metal pump. A funnel can be placed into the flared end of the tube, and both held in an elevated position. The liquid is then poured into the funnel; gravity causes the fluid to flow into the tube. When a sufficient quantity of fluid is administered, the tube is occluded by pinching it in half and removed.

Enteral Feeding Tubes

Nutritional support of compromised animals is becoming com-monplace in veterinary medicine. Critically ill animals may have to be fed and medicated via tubes placed directly into the pharynx, esophagus, stomach, or jejunum. The technician needs to understand how the veterinarian places enteral feeding tubes and be knowledgeable about their proper maintenance. If long-term feeding is required, placement of a gastrostomy or jejunostomy tube is preferred. Food is injected into the tubes and directly enters the gastrointestinal tract. Tube diameters are narrower with nasoesophageal and nasogastric tubes than with pharyngostomy, esophagostomy, gastrostomy, and jejunostomy tubes, so a more liquified diet is required.

Nasoesophageal and Nasogastric Tubes

Nasoesophageal and nasogastric tubes are easily placed and maintained. A 3.5 to 6 Fr pediatric feeding tube is held up to the animal to determine the appropriate length that is required. For nasoesophageal placement, the distance between the nares and distal esophagus is marked on the tube with ink or tape. Likewise, for nasogastric placement, the distance from the nares to the eighth rib is measured. The patient is held in sternal recumbency, in a seated position, or in a standing position. The head is held securely with the neck slightly extended. From 0.5 to 1 ml of 2% lidocaine is infused into one nostril of the dog,

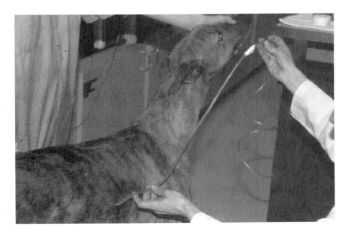

Figure 10-28. The length of stomach tube to extend from the canine teeth to the ninth rib is measured and marked with tape.

or five drops of 0.5% proparacaine is placed into one nostril of the cat. The tip of the tube is coated with xylocaine ointment and placed in the nostril dorsomedial to the alar fold. The tube is advanced into the nostril and directed ventrally. The tube then continues down the ventral meatus and into the nasopharynx. Tilting the nose downward slightly will help direct passage of the tube into the esophagus and avoid the trachea. The animal will usually swallow when the tube enters the pharynx.

The tube may be placed into the distal esophagus or stomach. To check for proper placement, a few milliliters of air are injected into the tube, and the left paralumbar fossa is simultaneously auscultated. If gurgling sounds are present, the tube has been placed in the gastointestinal tract. Alternatively, 5 ml of sterile saline may be injected into the tube; if the animal coughs, the tube is in the trachea and should be removed. A radiograph can also be taken to evaluate tube placement.

Suture or tissue adhesive is used to secure the tube to the patient. It should be sutured or glued close to its entrance to the nostril, onto the bridge of the nose, and onto the forehead. The remainder of the tube should be taped to the dorsum of the neck, and the animal should be fitted with an Elizabethan collar. A cap is placed on the end of the tube to prevent reflux.

Pharyngostomy Tube Placement

A red rubber feeding tube or silicone pharyngostomy tube ranging in size from 8 to 14 Fr for cats and small dogs and from 14 to 28 Fr for medium-sized to large dogs is used. One end of the tube is flared, and the other is fenestrated. The length of tube needed to span the distance from the angle of the mandible to the distal esophagus is measured and marked on the tube with tape or ink.

Placement of a pharyngostomy tube is performed surgically and requires general anesthesia with endotracheal intubation. The patient is placed in lateral recumbency, and a speculum is placed between the canine teeth to hold open the mouth. The lateral neck area is clipped and aseptically prepped. A gloved index finger is inserted into the mouth and placed between the hyoid apparatus and esophagus. Skin directly over the fingertip is incised with a scalpel blade. A large, curved hemostat is placed through the skin incision and used to bluntly dissect the underlying tissue, muscle, and oral mucosa. The flared end of the premeasured tube is brought into the mouth, grasped with the hemostats, and pulled exteriorly through the pharyngostomy site. The fenestrated end of the tube is then directed into the esophagus. Tube placement is checked in the same manner as described for nasoesophageal tubes.

The tube is secured by placing a butterfly tape around the proximal end and suturing the tape to the skin. Alternatively, a Chinese finger-trap suture may be placed around the tube to secure it to the skin. A povidone-iodine–treated gauze sponge should be placed around the skin-tube interface. The tube tip should either be cut so it extends a few centimeters from the skin surface or left long and bandaged over the dorsum of the neck. The exposed tube end is capped with a catheter adapter (ADDTO, Inc.) and a catheter cap (PRN Adapter, Becton Dickinson).

Esophagostomy Tube Placement

Placement of a feeding tube directly into the esophagus to provide nutritional support is a relatively new technique. Esophagostomy tubes are better tolerated by patients than are

pharyngostomy tubes because they cause less laryngeal irritation and obstruction and are less likely to induce emesis and become dislodged. As such, animals fed via esophagostomy tubes are less likely to aspirate their food than are those fed through pharyngostomy tubes. Placement requires the use of heavy sedation or short-acting anesthesia.

TECHNICIAN NOTE

Esophagostomy tubes are better tolerated by patients than are pharyngostomy tubes because they cause less laryngeal irritation and obstruction and are less likely to induce emesis and become dislodged.

A specially designed instrument is available to place esophagostomy tubes, the ELD Gastrostomy Tube Applicator (Jorgensen Laboratories, Inc., Loveland, CO). Hemostats are usually used in lieu of the ELD Applicator by most veterinarians to place esophagostomy tubes; therefore, the placement technique using hemostats is given. An instruction sheet detailing the procedure involved in using the ELD Applicator to place an esophagostomy tube is available from the manufacturer.

An esophagostomy tube is placed in the midcervical esophagus on the left side of the neck (Fig. 10–30). The animal is placed in right lateral recumbency, and the left cervical region is shaved and surgically prepared. The scapulohumeral joint and the angle of the mandible are used as guides to measure the distal and proximal limits of the cervical esophagus. The length of a 20 Fr red rubber feeding tube needed to extend from the skin in the midcervical region to the seventh rib is measured and marked on the tube with ink or tape. A pair of extra long curved hemostats is placed into the oral cavity and advanced to the left midcervical region of the esophagus. It is difficult to reach the midcervical region of the esophagus in large-breed dogs when hemostats are used instead of the longer ELD Tube Applicator. The hemostat tips should be palpable on the patient's neck. A stab incision is made with a scalpel blade

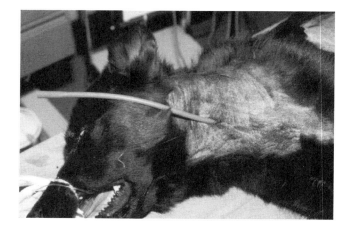

Figure 10–30. Esophagostomy tube for enteral feeding is placed into the midcervical esophagus on the left side of the neck.

through the skin and subcutaneous tissue over the tips. The scalpel blade is used to carefully dissect the subcutaneous tissue over the esophagus until the hemostats are able to bluntly penetrate the esophagus. The tips of the hemostats are then exteriorized and opened just enough to grasp the fenestrated end of the feeding tube. The hemostats with the attached feeding tube are then withdrawn back through the skin and into the esophagus toward the oral cavity. Once the fenestrated end of the tube reaches the mouth, the tube is bent and redirected back down the esophagus to the level of the seventh rib. Esophagostomy tubes are secured and maintained in the manner as described for pharyngostomy tubes. Once esophagostomy tubes are removed, healing occurs by second intention. Stricture of the esophagus at the site of tube placement is minimal after tube removal.

LARGE ANIMAL SAMPLING AND TREATMENT TECHNIQUES

Venous Blood Sample Collection

Bovine Venipuncture

Blood is collected from cattle from the jugular or coccygeal vein. Which site is used depends on the volume of blood needed and the type of restraint available. The animal should be placed in a confined area to limit movement, such as a chute or stanchion. It is easiest to collect blood using a Vacutainer collection device, but a 16- to 18-gauge, 4-cm needle and syringe can also be used.

TECHNICIAN NOTE

Blood is collected from cattle from the jugular or coccygeal vein.

When jugular venipuncture is to be performed, the head is placed in a halter. Using the halter and attached lead, the head is elevated slightly and drawn to the side opposite the jugular vein to be sampled. The restraint rope is then tied to a stationary surface. The vein is occluded with digital pressure in the jugular groove at the level of the thoracic inlet. Stroking the groove several times with an alcohol-soaked gauze sponge in a downward direction will help distend the vein. A needle is placed into the jugular at a 45-degree angle. When blood flows out of the needle, the Vacutainer tube is inserted into the needle, and a blood sample is collected (Fig. 10–31). When the desired volume has entered the tube, digital pressure is removed. The tube is withdrawn from the needle, and the needle is removed from the vein. Firm pressure is briefly applied to the site to ensure hemostasis.

Blood collection from the coccygeal vein, or "tail vein," is performed with the animal restrained in a chute. The tail is grasped in one hand and bent toward the back. The ventral surface of the tail is cleaned well with 70% isopropyl alcohol to remove fecal material. An 18- to 20-gauge, 2.5-cm-long needle is inserted between the third and forth coccygeal vertebrae perpendicular to the midline. When blood flows out of the needle hub, the syringe is attached and the sample is collected (Fig. 10–32). After venipuncture is completed, pressure is placed over the puncture site until the bleeding stops.

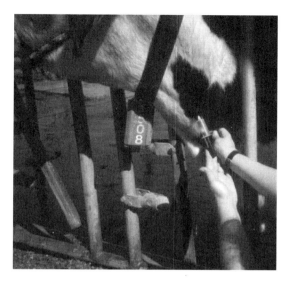

Figure 10–31. Bovine jugular venipuncture with a Vacutainer collection device.

Equine Venipuncture

The jugular vein is used to collect blood samples from the horse. Many horses can be restrained with a halter and lead rope, although some may need to be placed in a stock. The restrainer turns the head slightly in the direction opposite the vein to be sampled. Occlusion and distention of the vessel are achieved by placing pressure on the jugular groove in the lower third of the neck and stroking the vessel several times in the downward direction with an alcohol-soaked gauze sponge. The method to collect a blood sample from a horse is the same as that previously described in cattle. A 20-gauge, 2.5- to 3.75-cm needle and syringe or Vacutainer collection device is used.

TECHNICIAN NOTE

The jugular vein is used to collect blood samples from the horse.

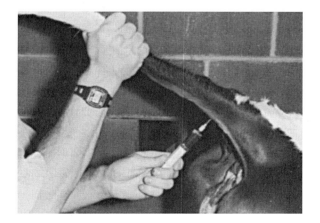

Figure 10–32. Venipuncture of the ventral coccygeal vein in the cow.

Swine Venipuncture

Anterior Vena Cava

The right anterior vena cava may be used for venipuncture in pigs. Because the phrenic nerve courses near the left exterior jugular vein, the left side of the neck should be avoided as a venipuncture site.

To obtain a blood sample from a small pig, the animal is placed on its back with the head extended and front legs crossed and caudally displaced (Fig. 10–33). An 18- to 20-gauge, 2.5- to 3.75-cm-needle is used in animals weighing less than 25 kg.

Pigs weighing more than 25 kg are restrained in a standing position with the front legs in a normal position, parallel to each other. The animal must maintain a bilaterally symmetrical position so the landmarks for venipuncture can be easily identified. A hog snare is placed around the mandible to hold the head slightly elevated in a parallel plane with the body. The individual taking the blood sample crouches in front of the right side of the pig. An 18-gauge, 5.0- to 12.5-cm needle with attached syringe is inserted into the right jugular fossa just lateral to the manubrium sterni (Fig. 10–34). It is placed at a 90-degree angle with the skin of the neck and directed at the left shoulder. An 18-gauge, 3.75-cm needle is inserted up to the hub and then slowly withdrawn as the syringe plunger is pulled back. When blood enters the syringe, the needle is held in place until a sufficient volume is collected.

Brachiocephalic or External Jugular Veins

Blood is frequently collected from the brachiocephalic or external jugular veins. Needle insertion into the vessel is near where the internal and external jugulars merge to become the brachiocephalic vein. Venipuncture is performed on the right side of the neck to avoid puncture of the phrenic nerve.

The pig is restrained in a standing position as previously described for anterior vena cava venipuncture. An imaginary

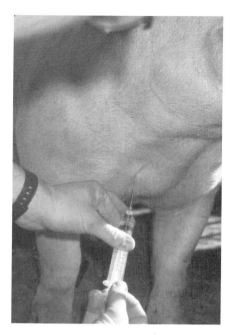

Figure 10–34. A blood sample from the anterior vena cava is taken with the needle directed into the jugular fossa just lateral to the manubrium sterni.

line parallel to the ground that passes through the shoulders and manubrium sterni is visualized. A second line is visualized that extends from the manubrium sterni to the scapula at an angle of 45 degrees with the first line. The needle is inserted at the intersection of the second visualized line with the deepest part of the right jugular fossa. For needle insertion, a 90-degree angle should be made between the needle and the skin of the neck. The needle is directed caudodorsally and should not be angled toward either scapula. Because the brachiocephalic vein is superficial, the syringe plunger should be slightly retracted as soon the needle penetrates the skin. The needle is advanced until blood is aspirated into the syringe. When a sufficient volume of blood has been collected, the needle is removed.

Auricular Vein

The auricular vein on the dorsal aspect of the pinna is a site used for collection of small volumes of blood. To perform venipuncture at this site, the pig is restrained with a hog snare around the mandible. A rubber band is placed around the base of the ear to serve as a tourniquet. The dorsal aspect of the pinna is wiped with 70% isopropyl alcohol. One hand is used to hold the ear, and a 20-gauge, 2.5-cm needle attached to a syringe is inserted into the ear vein. The sample is slowly aspirated into the syringe while carefully avoiding the application of too much suction, which might collapse the vein. When a sufficient quantity of blood has entered the syringe, the tourniquet is removed and the needle is withdrawn from the vein. Firm pressure must be applied at the venipuncture site until hemostasis occurs.

Orbital Sinus

Small quantities of blood can be collected from the venous sinus near the medial canthus of the eye. A 22-gauge needle is inserted into the medial canthus until it contacts bone. The

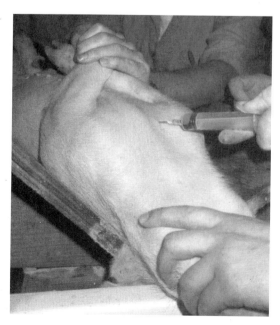

Figure 10–33. Venipuncture of the anterior vena cava in a small pig in dorsal recumbency.

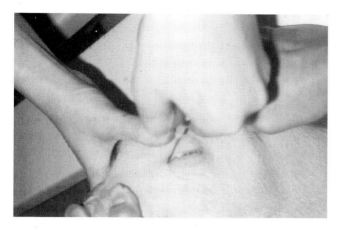

Figure 10-35. Small quantities of blood can be collected from the orbital sinus of the pig.

needle is then rotated between the fingers until blood enters the hub (Fig. 10–35). A microcapillary tube with the end broken at an angle to form a rough point can be used in lieu of a needle. When collection is complete, the needle or capillary tube is removed, and digital pressure is applied over the medial canthus with the head in an elevated position.

Ovine and Caprine Venipuncture

The most convenient site to access for venipuncture in the sheep and goat is the jugular vein. Blood collection is easiest to perform using a Vacutainer collection system, but a 20-gauge, 2.5-cm needle and syringe can be used. If the jugular vein is difficult to visualize in the sheep because of the hair coat, wool can be pulled over the jugular furrow until the vessel is identified.

Sheep become passive when tipped up on the rump. For a single-person venipuncture technique, the phlebotomist crouches or stands behind the tipped sheep and slightly moves the head in the direction opposite the vein to be used. One hand is used to occlude the jugular vein and the other hand holds the Vacutainer collection device or a 20-gauge, 2.5-cm needle and syringe. The needle is inserted into the jugular vein, and a sample is collected (Fig. 10–36).

Blood can also be collected from a sheep that is in the standing position by straddling it over the shoulders. It is sometimes helpful to back the animal into a corner to further limit its movement. The venipuncturist holds the sheep's head to the side with the arm that is used to occlude the vein and obtains the blood sample with the other hand (Fig. 10–37). This restraint and venipuncture technique can also be used in the goat.

The cephalic vein can also used to collect a blood sample in the goat. The procedure previously described for cephalic venipuncture in the dog can be applied to the goat.

Arterial Blood Sample Collection

Arterial blood samples are obtained to determine the respiratory and acid-base status of an animal. Samples are frequently obtained in horses intraoperatively when general anesthesia is used. The most frequently sampled arteries in conscious horses are the transverse facial and carotid arteries. The great metatar-

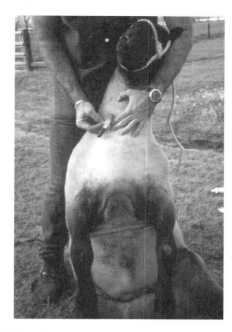

Figure 10-36. Sheep placed in a seated position to allow blood to be collected from the jugular vein.

sal artery is a site for collection in the foal; it is located on the lateral aspect of the third metatarsal bone.

The carotid artery is located on the dorsal side of the jugular grove deep to the jugular vein. The artery feels like a cord, and a pulse is not palpable. To obtain a sample from the carotid artery, the skin superficial to the artery on the lower third of the right side of the neck is cleansed with alcohol. An 18-gauge, 3.75-cm needle is directed into the artery at a 90-degree angle. Accurate placement will be noted by blood expelled under pulsatile pressure from the needle hub. Blood from a needle placed in the jugular vein will flow out at a slow,

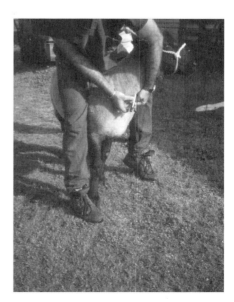

Figure 10-37. The venipuncturist straddles the sheep over the shoulders and turns the head to the side to collect blood from the jugular vein.

constant rate. As the needle in the carotid artery is stabilized with one hand, a syringe coated with sodium heparin is placed on the needle. The sample is withdrawn, and the bubbles are expelled from the needle and syringe. The needle tip is then embedded into a rubber cork. Firm pressure is held over the venipuncture site for several minutes.

The transverse facial artery is palpated just lateral to the lateral canthus of the eye. Inject 0.25 ml of 2% lidocaine subcutaneously over the vessel with a 25-gauge needle. A 21- to 23-gauge, 2.5-cm needle is introduced into the artery. The sample is collected and handled as described above.

Over-the-needle–type arterial catheters are commonly placed for intraoperative blood gas and arterial blood pressure analysis. The technique for placing and maintaining arterial catheters is previously described in the discussion of intravenous administration of medication in the small animal.

Urine Sample Collection

Bovine

Several techniques may be used to collect urine samples from cows. One method is to stimulate a cow to urinate by stroking the perineal area with straw or fingers. The tail should not be held aside because it may distract the animal. If this method fails to produce a urine sample, the lips of the vulva can be repeatedly opened and closed to stimulate urination. When micturition occurs, a midstream sample is collected in a clean, dry container. The initial portion of the stream contains the largest amount of contaminants and should not be included in the sample collected for urinalysis.

Urinary catheterization of the cow can be accomplished with a sterile flexible or rigid urinary catheter. The perineal region is scrubbed with a disinfectant and rinsed with warm water containing an antiseptic solution. A sterile-gloved, lubricated hand is inserted into the vagina. Fingers are slid along the floor of the vagina approximately 10 cm until the urethral orifice is identified. The catheter is then placed into the vagina and guided into the urethral orifice by the hand in the vagina. It is slowly advanced into the urethra until it enters the bladder. Urine will flow through the catheter when it has reached the bladder. The initial few milliliters of urine should not be included in the specimen collected for urinalysis. A midstream urine sample is collected in a dry, sterile container. Samples obtained by catheterization may have increased transitional cells, erythrocytes, and protein.

Equine

The mare can be catheterized in a manner similar to that described for the cow. The tail should be wrapped before performing catheterization to prevent the tail hair from entering the vagina, and the vulvar region is aseptically prepared. The urethral opening is approximately 10 to 12 cm from the ventral commissure of the vulvar lips. The transverse fold of the vagina overlies the opening of the urethral orifice. It is common to slide the catheter over the transverse fold of the vagina and miss the urethral orifice, which lies beneath it. Once the catheter is placed into the urethral orifice, it is advanced 7 to 10 cm until it enters the bladder. It may be necessary to aspirate urine with a syringe attached to the end of the catheter to stimulate urine flow once the catheter is in the bladder.

Urinary catheterization of the male horse requires sedation.

The administration of detomidine assists in everting the penis out of the prepuce. The prepuce and penis are cleansed with warm antibacterial solution and then rinsed with an antiseptic solution. The tip of a sterile, flexible 24 Fr, 137-cm urinary catheter is coated with sterile, water-based lubricant. Sterile gloves are worn to grasp the penis with one hand and introduce the catheter, with stylet, into the urethra with the other. The catheter is advanced approximately 60 cm into the urethra. It is usually easily advanced through the penile urethra, but resistance may be felt as it passes around the ischial arch. At this point, the stylet is gradually withdrawn as the catheter is passed over the pelvis and into the bladder. When the bladder is entered, urine may flow through the catheter. If not, a 60-ml syringe is attached onto the flared end of the catheter, and the plunger is retracted. If urine still does not appear, a small volume of air can be injected into the catheter or the catheter can be slightly repositioned.

Ovine and Caprine

A 5 to 10 Fr lubricated sterile canine urinary catheter can be used to blindly catheterize ewes and does. The technique is as described for catheterization of the canine. Urine can be collected from ewes by holding the nostrils and mouth closed. The ewe will soon struggle to breathe and will urinate at the same time. An assistant catches the voided urine sample. This technique is not routinely recommended. A much less stressful way to obtain a urine sample from sheep or goats is to wait until they stand up from a lying down position; they often urinate when they change from a lying down to a standing position.

Male goats and sheep have anatomic obstacles that make urinary catheterization extremely difficult. Urine samples are obtained primarily by free catch of voided samples as described above.

Rumen Fluid Collection

Rumen fluid is collected for analysis with the use of a stomach tube. To perform orogastric intubation of the cow, the animal is restrained in a head catch as an assistant places nose tongs into the nares to grasp the nasal septum. Pressure on the nose tongs helps control movement of the head. The individual performing the intubation stands to the side of the animal and wraps an arm around the muzzle. A speculum is inserted into the bovine's mouth. A medium-sized stomach tube is lubricated with water-based gel. Tubes with internal diameters of less than 1.5 cm have a greater likelihood of becoming blocked with ingesta and therefore are not recommended for use in rumen fluid collection.

One end of the tube is introduced into the speculum, and the other is held in the intubator's mouth. The tube is advanced to the back of the oral cavity; as the animal swallows, it is placed into the esophagus. Air is blown into one end of the tube to dilate the esophagus. This eases passage of the tube into the esophagus and down into the rumen.

Placement of the tube in the rumen is verified by one individual who auscults the area over the rumen as air is blown into the tube. If the tube is properly placed in the rumen, air will be heard bubbling through rumen contents.

Rumen fluid samples can be withdrawn through the tube with use of a dose syringe. Initial fluid portions may contain an excessive quantity of saliva, which causes an erroneously elevated pH. Because of the salivary contamination, the initial portion of fluid obtained for rumen analysis is discarded.

When rumen fluid collection is completed, the tube is occluded by bending it; it is withdrawn in a downward motion to prevent rumen contents from entering the trachea.

Abdominocentesis

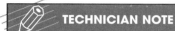

TECHNICIAN NOTE

Abdominocentesis is used as a diagnostic technique in horses with colic, chronic diarrhea, weight loss, or fever of unknown origin.

Abdominocentesis is performed to obtain samples of abdominal fluid for clinical pathological evaluation. It is often used as a diagnostic technique in horses with colic, chronic diarrhea, weight loss, or fever of unknown origin. To perform abdominocentesis in the horse, the animal is restrained in a standing position. The individual performing the tap stands close to the front legs and faces the abdomen. In this position, one avoids being kicked by the rear legs. The most dependent site of the ventral abdomen over the midline is clipped and aseptically prepared. Then, 2 ml of 2% lidocaine is infused under the skin using a 25-gauge, 15-mm needle. Wearing sterile gloves, a stab incision is made in the skin with a No. 15 blade while making certain to avoid incising any obvious vessels. The blade is then rotated to form an entrance large enough for a sterile 9-cm blunt-ended teat cannula or stainless steel canine urinary catheter to pass through. The cannula should be pushed through the center of a 4 × 4 sterile gauze sponge before being inserted into the incision (Fig. 10–38). The cannula is then inserted through the incision and into the abdomen (Fig. 10–39). The gauze prevents peripheral blood that drips down the outside of the cannula from contaminating the sample. Initial drops of fluid often contain blood or other contaminants,

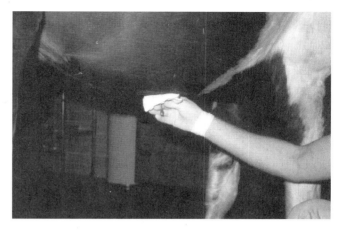

Figure 10–39. Abdominocentesis is performed in a horse by passing a teat cannula into the abdominal cavity.

so the first few milliliters of fluid to drip from the cannula are not included in the sample. The sample is collected by allowing fluid to drip into sterile tubes with and without anticoagulants. If fluid does not drain into the cannula, it may be necessary to rotate or redirect the cannula or attach a syringe to the end and apply negative pressure.

Alternatively, a spinal needle or 18-gauge, 3.75-cm needle can be used for abdominocentesis in horses and large ruminants, and a 20-gauge, 3.75-cm needle can be used in small ruminants. A local anesthetic usually is not administered if a hypodermic needle is used for centesis instead of a teat cannula. Centesis is performed as described using a teat cannula except a stab incision is not made with a blade before insertion of the needle. If fluid does not flow through the needle, 1 to 2 ml of air can be injected through the needle to dislodge any particles that are plugging it. As with the teat cannula, the needle may require rotation or redirection to obtain a sample. Sometimes, concurrent insertion of an additional needle several centimeters away from the initial one will create a vacuum and help stimulate fluid flow.

Site selection for abdominocentesis in ruminants is determined by the area at which the abdominal disorder is expected to be localized. If traumatic reticuloperitonitis is suspected, the centesis site is the ruminoreticular recess. In large ruminants, this is in the left cranial quadrant of the abdomen approximately 5 cm caudal to the xiphoid process and 5 cm to the left of midline. Centesis is performed 5 cm cranial to the udder but medial to the right flank fold when rupture of the uterus or small bowel is suspected. It is recommended that several different sites be tapped if the initial centesis does not yield fluid because peritonitis in ruminants is often highly compartmentalized. Care should be taken to avoid penetrating the large subcutaneous mammary vessels on the ventral abdomen.

Abdominocentesis in small ruminants is usually performed to evaluate for the presence of urinary tract obstruction or a ruptured bladder. To avoid puncturing the rumen, the most dependent site of the ventral abdomen is identified, and centesis is performed approximately 3 cm to the right of the midline. The procedure is performed as described for the bovine.

Complications of abdominal paracentesis in horses and ruminants are bowel laceration; introduction of bacteria at the centesis site, resulting in peritonitis or cellulitis; and damage to the xiphoid process if the centesis site chosen is too cranial.

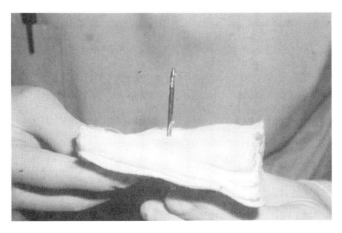

Figure 10–38. A teat cannula is pushed through sterile gauze sponges before being inserted into the abdominal cavity to prevent peripheral blood from contaminating the abdominocentesis sample.

TECHNICIAN NOTE

Abdominocentesis in small ruminants is usually performed to evaluate for the presence of urinary tract obstruction or a ruptured bladder.

Thoracocentesis

Thoracocentesis is performed in large animals to drain fluid or air from the pleural cavity. Fluid can be obtained for cytological examination and culture. In large animals, thoracocentesis is performed most commonly in the horse. A 12- or 14-gauge, 6.0- to 7.5-cm teat cannula can be used if thoracocentesis is undertaken to remove only a small quantity of fluid. If the fluid has a high fibrin content or a large volume of fluid is to be evacuated, a larger-bore cannula is used, such as a metal bitch urinary catheter or human thoracic drainage cannula.

The cutaneous region from the fifth to the ninth ribs approximately 10 cm above the level of the olecranon is clipped and surgically scrubbed. When centesis is to be performed on the right side, the sixth to seventh intercostal space is used. The eighth to ninth intercostal space is used on the left. The cranial border of the eighth rib in the ventral portion of the thorax is identified. With a 25-gauge needle, from 1 to 2 ml of 2% lidocaine is injected into the skin, subcutaneous tissue, and intercostal muscles down to the parietal pleura at the site. The lateral thoracic vein courses subcutaneously over the ventral aspect of the thorax and should be avoided. A scalpel blade is used to make a stab incision into the skin. The cannula, connected to a three-way stopcock with the valve closed toward the animal, is then inserted through the skin incision. It is carefully advanced through the underlying tissue until it penetrates the pleura. A 60-ml syringe is connected to the stopcock via extension tubing. The stopcock valve is turned to the open position toward the patient, and the syringe plunger is retracted to withdraw air or fluid from the pleural cavity. After thoracocentesis is complete, the cannula is withdrawn. Skin sutures are usually not necessary to close the incision made when the teat cannula is used; however, skin sutures are usually necessary when the human cannula or canine urinary catheter is used.

Transtracheal Wash

Transtracheal aspiration involves the collection of samples from the lower respiratory tract for cytological and microbiological analyses. The following procedure is described for equine and bovine patients. The technique for performing transtracheal aspirates in small ruminants is similar to that previously described in this chapter.

The middle tracheal region is clipped and aseptically prepared. Then, 2 ml of 2% lidocaine is injected subcutaneously over the trachea with a 25-gauge needle. Sterile gloves are worn to make a stab incision with a scalpel blade through the skin between the tracheal rings. The trachea is stabilized with one hand, and a 12- to 14-gauge needle is placed, with the bevel facing downward, through the incision and into the tracheal lumen. A burst of air will be felt as the needle penetrates the lumen. A sterile 5 or 6 Fr polyvinyl urinary catheter with the tip cut off is placed through the needle and into the trachea and advanced to the tracheal bifurcation. Once the catheter

reaches the bifurcation, a syringe is attached to the flared end of the catheter, and the plunger is retracted. Air will be aspirated without resistance if the catheter is in the trachea. If only negative pressure is felt, the catheter should be repositioned because it is either not in the trachea or is bent or the tip is occluded against the tracheal mucosa.

Once intratracheal catheter placement has been determined, the needle is withdrawn from the trachea and skin, and the catheter is left in place. Extension tubing connected to a 60-ml syringe filled with sterile saline is inserted into the flared end of the catheter. A 30- to 50-ml aliquot of sterile 0.9% saline is injected into the trachea. Saline is reaspirated, and a sample is collected. Approximately 10% of the infused volume will be reaspirated. The catheter may need to be adjusted and redirected during the procedure. The flushing-aspirating process may need to be repeated several times, with additional aliquots of saline being instilled into the catheter and reaspirated until a sufficient sample volume is obtained.

After the sample is collected, the needle and catheter are removed together. The site is covered with an antibiotic coated sterile gauze and wrapped with a bandage for 24 hours. Cellulitis at the tracheal puncture site is the most common complication. If swelling occurs, warm compresses are applied.

ADMINISTRATION OF MEDICATION IN LARGE ANIMALS

Intravenous Administration

Bovine

The jugular vein is the site most commonly used for intravenous administration of medication. The animal is restrained with a halter and placed in a chute or stanchion with the head elevated and pulled to the side opposite the jugular vein to be used. The vein is occluded by applying pressure on the jugular groove. The skin over the vein is wiped with an alcohol-soaked gauze sponge several times in a downward direction to remove superficial skin contaminants. This procedure also helps to identify the jugular vein. A 16- to 18-gauge, 3.75- to 5.0-cm needle is placed through the skin and into the vein at a 45- to 90-degree angle to the skin. The needle is adjusted until blood flows from the end of the needle; then, the needle is inserted all the way to the hub in either an upward or a downward direction. The syringe with the medication is attached to the needle. Before injection of syringe contents, the plunger is retracted slightly to ensure that blood enters the syringe. Once the needle is in the vein, the digital pressure is removed from the jugular groove, and the medication is injected. The needle is withdrawn, and pressure is placed on the venipuncture site until hemostasis occurs.

TECHNICIAN NOTE

When an animal requires repeated injections of large volumes of fluids, an intravenous catheter is placed in the jugular vein.

When an animal requires repeated injections of large volumes of fluids, an intravenous catheter is placed in the jugular vein. After the skin over the jugular vein is clipped and aseptically prepared, 1.0 ml of 2% lidocaine is instilled into the skin. A stab incision is made through the skin over the vessel with a scalpel blade or 14-gauge needle. The vein is occluded by the application of digital pressure in the jugular furrow. A 14- to 16-gauge, 13-cm over-the-needle catheter (Angiocath) is inserted through the skin incision at a 45-degree angle. The catheter is introduced into the wall of the jugular vein. Blood will appear in the catheter hub when the vessel lumen is entered. The catheter is then placed almost parallel to the vessel and is advanced with the stylet an additional 5 mm into the vein. Once it is determined that the catheter is well seated in the vessel, the pressure on the vein is released. The catheter is then slid over the stylet until it is completely inserted into the vessel. A cap or extension set is placed on the hub, and the catheter is flushed with heparinized 0.9% sterile saline. Glue, tape, or suture is used to secure the catheter to the skin. A gauze sponge soaked with a liberal amount of povidone-iodine ointment is placed at the venipuncture site. The catheter is secured with layers of adhesive tape and bandage material wrapped around the neck. Intravenous catheters should be checked several times daily for patency and monitored for signs of infection. If redness, swelling, pain, heat, or discharge is noted around the site of the catheter, it should be removed.

The ventral coccygeal vein can be used as a site for injection of small volumes of medication. Because of the proximity of the coccygeal vein to the coccygeal artery and the fecal contamination around the tail, the coccygeal vein is not recommended as an injection site.

Equine

The jugular vein is used to administer intravenous injections in the horse. The vein is large and easily palpated in the jugular groove on the neck. The right jugular vein is preferred as an injection site over the left jugular because of the presence of the esophagus in the left jugular groove.

To make an injection into the jugular vein, the vessel is occluded by placing digital pressure on the jugular groove. The area over the vein in the proximal third of the neck is wiped several times in a downward direction with a 70% isopropyl alcohol–soaked gauze sponge. The vessel should be distended and easily visualized in the jugular groove. The vessel is occluded by placing digital pressure on the jugular groove. An 18-gauge, 2.5-cm needle is embedded into the vein, up to the hub, at a 90-degree angle and then directed caudally (Fig. 10–40). If the needle inadvertently enters the carotid artery, blood will eject out of the needle hub in forceful spurts even when the jugular vein is not being compressed. Blood should trickle constantly from the needle hub if it is placed in the vein. If the needle enters the carotid, it should be removed immediately, and firm pressure should be applied for several minutes on the venipuncture site to ensure hemostasis.

TECHNICIAN NOTE

If the needle inadvertently enters the carotid artery, blood will eject out of the needle hub in forceful spurts even when the jugular vein is not being compressed.

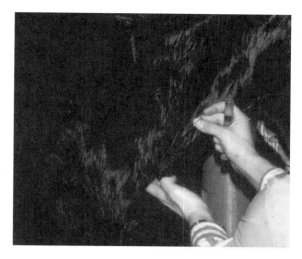

Figure 10–40. The needle is placed into the jugular vein to administer intravenous medication to the horse.

Once it is determined that the needle is placed intravenously and not intra-arterially, the syringe is placed onto the needle as one hand stabilizes the needle in the vein. The syringe plunger should be slightly withdrawn to ensure that venous blood flows back into the syringe. Digital pressure on the vein is removed, and the contents of the syringe are slowly injected.

If repeated administration of large volumes of fluid is required, an intravenous catheter is placed in the jugular vein (Fig. 10–41). Although intravenous catheters can also be placed in the cephalic and lateral thoracic veins, fluids can be administered at a more rapid rate in the larger jugular vein. The technique for placing an intravenous catheter is similar to that previously described for cattle. If a catheter is to remain indwelling for more than a few hours, it should be placed while wearing sterile gloves in addition to the routine aseptic preparation. The catheter site should be monitored for patency and signs of infection every few hours, and the catheter should be removed if any heat, swelling, redness, discharge, or pain is noted.

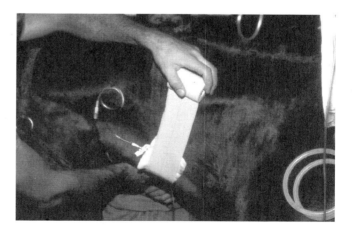

Figure 10–41. A jugular catheter is placed in a horse for intravenous fluid therapy. The catheter is secured in place by bandage material that is wrapped around the neck.

Porcine

The auricular vein, located on the dorsal aspect of the pinna, is the most commonly used vein for administration of drugs or fluids. A 19- to 21-gauge butterfly catheter or a 16- to 18-gauge over-the-needle–type catheter can be placed in the ear vein if large volumes of fluid need to be administered intravenously. A rubber band is wrapped tightly around the ear base to distend the vein. The dorsal aspect of the pinna is aseptically scrubbed. The catheter is inserted into the vein; once it is placed entirely within the lumen of the vessel, the catheter hub is affixed to the pinna with quick-setting glue. The tourniquet is removed from the base of the ear, and the catheter hub is covered with a cap. A partially used roll of 5.0-cm-wide tape is placed on the underside of the pinna, and the margins of the ear are bent around it. The tape roll serves as a wedge to support the pinna. Several strips of adhesive tape are wrapped around the ear to secure the catheter to the pinna.

TECHNICIAN NOTE

The auricular vein, which is located on the dorsal aspect of the pinna, is the most commonly used vein for administration of drugs or fluids in the pig.

Intramuscular Administration

Bovine

The only muscles recommended for intramuscular injections in cattle are those in the neck. Injection into the gluteal muscle should be avoided because this area is prone to abscessation. Intramuscular injections are performed when the animal is restrained in a stanchion or crowded into a confined area.

TECHNICIAN NOTE

The only muscles recommended for intramuscular injections in cattle are those in the neck.

The injection site is cleansed with 70% isoprophyl alcohol to remove gross skin contaminants. A 16- or 18- gauge, 3.75- to 5.0-cm needle is grasped, and a fist is formed with the same hand. The injection site is struck several times with the flat of the fist. The hand is then rotated slightly, and the animal is struck again as the needle is embedded in the skin and muscle perpendicular to the skin surface. Striking the animal in this manner distracts it and decreases its awareness of the needle insertion. The needle is not attached to a syringe until the needle is firmly embedded in muscle. After the syringe is attached to the needle, the plunger is retracted slightly, and the hub is checked for blood to ensure that a vessel has not been entered. The syringe contents are then injected, and the needle with attached syringe is withdrawn.

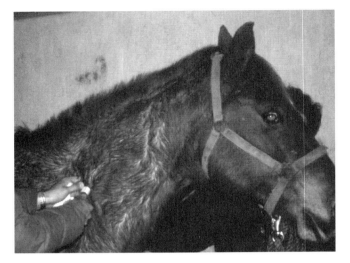

Figure 10–42. Intramuscular injection into the cervical muscles in the horse.

Equine

The areas recommended for intramuscular injection in the horse are the neck and rear legs. As in cattle, the gluteal region should be avoided because of the difficulty in treating any injection-induced abscesses. The pectoral muscles may be used, but there is an increased likelihood of inflammation at the injection site. Abscesses that may develop subsequent to injection in the pectoral region are easier to drain than are those in the gluteal muscles.

Intramuscular injections in the neck are given in the region bordered by the nuchal ligament, cervical spine, and shoulder blade (Fig. 10–42). Medication administered into the nuchal ligament is poorly absorbed. The semimembranosus and semitendinosus muscles in the caudal aspect of the rear leg are excellent injection sites, but the injector is at risk of being kicked (Fig. 10–43). The individual giving the injection should

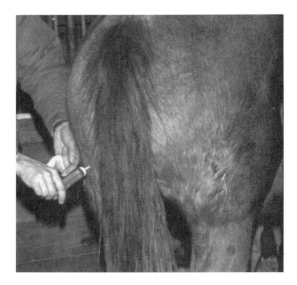

Figure 10–43. Intramuscular injection into the semimembranosus and semitendinosus muscles in the horse.

stand on one side of the horse and reach around the rear to administer the medication to the opposite leg. If the horse kicks, it will usually kick toward the side of the injection. It is best to stand as close to the horse's body as possible to avoid a kick. It is not always possible to stand on the side opposite the injection. In such a case, a restrainer should stand on the same side as the individual giving the injection and pull the horse's head toward both people. If the horse kicks, it will attempt to straighten itself and spin the rear end away from the injector and restrainer.

Equine intramuscular injections are administered using 18-gauge, 3.75-cm needles. Seventy percent isopropyl alcohol is used to clean the area over the muscle. The site is tapped with the back of the hand once or twice, and then the needle, without the syringe attached, is inserted through the skin and deep into the muscle. Once the needle is inserted to the hub, the syringe is attached. Before the medication is injected, the plunger is retracted, and the hub is checked for blood. If a vessel has been inadvertently penetrated, the needle should be removed and injection made into another location.

A maximum volume of 20 ml may be administered in one site. It is best to alternate injection sites if repeated injections are needed over a multiple-day period.

Subcutaneous Administration

Bovine and Equine

The neck is the site recommended for subcutaneous injections in horses. Any region on the lateral aspect of the neck or trunk can be used for subcutaneous injections in cattle. The site is wiped with a gauze sponge saturated with 70% isopropyl alcohol to remove superficial skin contaminants. A fold of skin is tented, and an 18- to 20-gauge, 2.5- to 3.75-cm needle with attached syringe is inserted at the base of the tented skin (Fig. 10–44). Slight negative pressure is applied by pulling back on

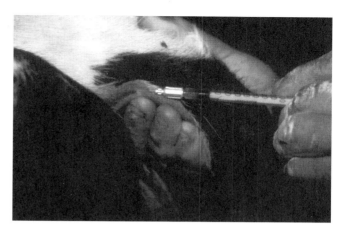

Figure 10–45. Intradermal injection is made into the caudal skin fold to test for tuberculosis in the cow.

the plunger to ensure that the needle has not entered a vessel. If placement is satisfactory, the medication is injected under the skin, and the needle is withdrawn. The area around the site can be rubbed to promote distribution of the injected substance.

Intradermal Administration

Bovine and Equine

As in small animals, intradermal injections are made primarily for the purpose of skin testing. Intradermal injection into the caudal skin fold of cattle is made to test for tuberculosis (Fig. 10–45). They are also made to inject local anesthetics before making a small skin incision to place an intravenous catheter. In addition, intradermal injections are used to treat certain nodular skin lesions and sarcoids. The technique for intradermal injection is as previously described for small animals and can be adapted to use in large animals.

Ovine and Caprine Injection Sites

The most convenient site to access for intravenous therapy in the sheep and goat is the jugular vein. To make an intravenous injection, the goat is best restrained by a handler who backs the goat into a corner, straddles it over the withers, and turns the head to the side. Restraint in sheep for intravenous injection involves either sitting the sheep up on its rump or straddling the sheep over the withers and stretching the neck laterally. These restraint techniques allow good visualization and access to the jugular vein.

Intramuscular injections in the goat and sheep are administered in the semimembranosus and semitendinosus muscles of the rear leg, triceps, neck muscles, or longissimus muscles over the lumbar region. Goats may not have sufficient muscle mass for large-volume intramuscular injections. A maximum of 5 ml should be injected at any single site. Intramuscular injections in the sheep are usually given in the semimembranosus and semitendinosus muscles; occasionally, the gluteal muscles are used.

The neck and shoulder region is frequently used for subcutaneous injections in the sheep and goat. Axillary or flank subcutaneous injections are made in show animals if the injections contain medications or vaccines, such as clostridial

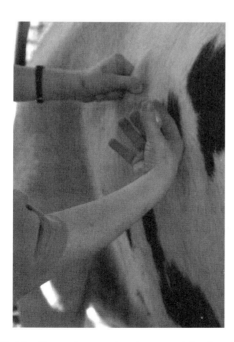

Figure 10–44. To make a subcutaneous injection in a cow, the needle is inserted into the base of a fold of skin.

vaccines, that may cause nodular swellings or abscesses. Subcutaneous masses, if located in the prescapular region, may be mistaken by show judges as caseous lymphadenitits. The back or upper flank areas should be avoided as injection sites in goats if the skin will be marketed. Sheep injections should be made when the wool is dry; they have a greater tendency toward injection site reactions if the needle is introduced into wet wool.

Intraperitoneal injections are usually used only to treat neonates with umbilical infections or hypoglycemia. The neonate is lifted by the front legs, and a 20-gauge needle with attached syringe is introduced to the left of the umbilicus to a depth of 1.0 cm. The plunger is retracted to ensure that the needle has not penetrated a vessel. Once intraperitoneal placement is confirmed, the syringe contents are injected into the peritoneal cavity.

Intramammary infusions can be made to control mastitis. They are made after aseptic preparation of the teat. If the teat is not properly cleaned before placement of the cannula, bacteria can be introduced into the udder. A sterile teat cannula or feline urinary catheter is inserted into the gland, and the teat is infused with medication.

Swine Injection Sites

Intramuscular injections are made into the cervical muscles or the semimembranosus or semitendinosus muscles of the rear leg. Lameness may occur after injection into the caudal muscles of the rear leg. The use of the muscles of the "ham" for intramuscular injections is avoided in animals for use as food because the injection may leave an undesirable mark on the muscle and downgrade the quality of the meat. Because of the tendency of pigs to store a thick layer of subcutaneous body fat, a needle that is at least 3.75 cm long is needed to penetrate to the muscle. Medications deposited in fat are absorbed much more slowly than are those deposited in the muscle, so the onset of action of the injected substances is delayed.

TECHNICIAN NOTE

The use of the muscles of the "ham" for intramuscular injections is avoided in animals intended for use as food because the injection may leave an undesirable mark on the muscle and downgrade the quality of the meat.

The skin of pigs is tight, which limits the volume of a substance that can be injected subcutaneously. Subcutaneous injections are made into the lateral side of the neck immediately posterior to the base of the ear with a 16- to 18-gauge, 2.5 to 3.75-cm needle.

In baby pigs, fluids are usually administered intraperitoneally due to the impracticality of placing an intravenous catheter for long-term fluid therapy. The site of needle introduction should be cleaned and aseptically prepared. Fluids should be warm and isotonic. To administer intraperitoneal fluids to a baby pig, the pig is grasped by the rear legs, and a 16-gauge, 1.25- to 2.5-cm needle is inserted paramedially between the

midline and flank. Intraperitoneal injection in a mature standing pig requires the insertion of a 16- to 18-gauge, 7.5-cm needle.

Oral Administration

Ovine and Caprine

Administration of tablets to adult sheep and goats can be a challenge. A balling gun is used to help perform the task. The end of the gun should be smooth and ideally made out of soft plastic. It should be inspected for sharp edges before each use. Care should be taken not to insert the balling gun too forcefully or too far back into the oral cavity. Improper use can cause trauma to the pharynx and esophagus.

To use the balling gun, the animal is backed into a corner and straddled over the shoulders by the handler. The head and neck are held in a normal position, not with the muzzle elevated. A balling gun is placed in the interdental space of the mouth and positioned over the base of the tongue. The bolus is released, and the gun is withdrawn. Observation of the animal after the pilling is required to ensure that the pill is not spit out.

Liquids are administered per os with the use of a 60-ml catheter tipped syringe, dosing bottle, or nasogastric tube. To use a dose syringe, the tip is introduced into the side of the mouth and over the base of the tongue. The liquid is then slowly injected with the head held in a normal position. If coughing occurs, administration should be ceased until the trachea is cleared of fluid.

Medication and fluids can be administered via nasogastric intubation, which is generally tolerated better than orogastric intubation (Fig. 10–46). The animal is restrained in a standing position by a handler straddling the withers. A length of flexible

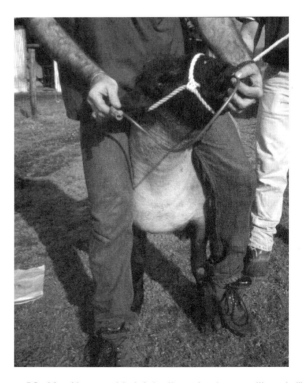

Figure 10–46. Nasogastric intubation of a sheep with a stallion urinary catheter.

plastic or rubber tube needed to extend from the nostrils to the rumen is premeasured and marked. The tube should have a smooth, rounded end and have a sufficiently small diameter to pass through the ventral nasal meatus. Instillation of 0.5 ml of 2% lidocaine can be used in one nostril to numb the nasal passage. Water-soluble lubricant or water is placed around the tube tip, and the tube is inserted into the nostril and slowly advanced into the ventral nasal meatus and nasopharynx. As the tube is further advanced, the animal should be observed swallowing the tube, and the tube may be palpated on the neck as it passes down the esophagus. If the animal coughs, the tube has entered the trachea and should be promptly removed. Once the tube has been passed to the premeasured mark, the placement should be checked to ensure that the tube is indeed in the rumen. This is performed by blowing into the end of the tube as an assistant auscults the area over the rumen to listen for air bubbling through the rumen contents. Fluids are then administered into the rumen via the tube. When completed, the tube is kinked to occlude it as it is withdrawn in a downward direction so rumen contents will not enter the trachea.

Orogastric intubation is performed by restraining the animal in a standing position. A partially used roll of tape is used as a speculum to keep the mouth open. A 9.5-mm-diameter foal tube with the length premeasured is lubricated with water or water-soluble gel. It is placed through the speculum, over the base of the tongue, and into the esophagus. The tube is then advanced until it enters the rumen. Placement of the tube in the rumen is verified before any liquids are administered. Because the diameter of the tube used for orogastric intubation is wider than that used for nasogastric intubation, fluids placed into an orogastric tube can be more viscous and can be delivered at a more rapid rate. The diameter and length of tube vary depending on the size of the animal. A 37-cm tube is passed in lambs and goats.

Bovine

A balling gun is used to administer boluses to cattle. The oral cavity should be free of food before introduction of the balling gun. The animal is confined in a head catch. The handler inserts a finger into one nostril and a thumb into the other and pulls the nose dorsally. This will cause the animal to open its mouth so the balling gun can be placed over the base of the tongue. Alternatively, a hand can be placed into the interdental space to open the mouth and insert the balling gun. The tip of the gun should always be inspected for sharp edges before it is introduced into the oral cavity.

Fluids and medications may be administered to cattle through a stomach tube passed from the nose or mouth directly into the rumen (Fig. 10–47). Refer to the discussion of rumen fluid collection for a description of the technique to perform orogastric intubation of large ruminants. The previously described technique for nasogastric intubation of the sheep and goat can be adapted for the bovine.

Equine

Oral medications are frequently administered to horses. A variety of preparations are available in paste form, including anthelmintics, vitamin-mineral supplements, antibiotics, and anti-inflammatory agents. The paste is placed in a syringe for oral administration if it is not already prepackaged. Tablets may be

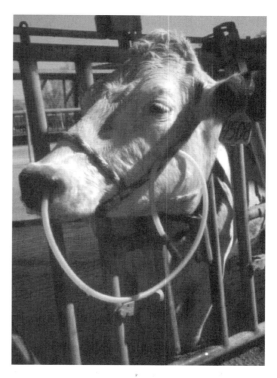

Figure 10–47. Nasogastric intubation of a bovine with a foal stomach tube.

crushed into a powder form and then combined with water and administered via a syringe or mixed with corn syrup or molasses and added to the feed.

Before oral suspensions are administered, the oral cavity should be checked to ensure that it is free of food. The head is held slightly up, and the syringe is placed into the side of the horse's mouth through the interdental space. As the plunger is depressed, the syringe contents are emptied onto the base of the tongue. The horse should be sufficiently restrained so that it does not move as the injection is made. If this occurs, the medication may trickle out of the side of the mouth. The horse should not be permitted to drink water immediately after treatment because some of the medication may be lost as the muzzle is placed in the water container. A detailed description of the technique used to pass a nasogastric tube is given in Chapter 21.

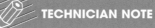

TECHNICIAN NOTE

Boluses of medication can also be delivered via nasogastric intubation. This procedure should be performed while under the direct supervision of the veterinarian.

Boluses of medication can also be delivered via nasogastric intubation. This procedure should be performed while under the direct supervision of the veterinarian. A detailed description of the technique used to pass a nasogastric tube is given in Chapter 21.

Intramammary Administration

Intramammary infusion of antibiotics is used to control mastitis. Potential exists for the introduction of organisms into the udder during the infusion process, so the procedure must be performed as aseptically as possible. After the udder is milked out, the teat is cleaned with a dip and thoroughly dried. The teat should be scrubbed with 70% isopropyl alcohol. The teats on the far side of the udder should be cleaned and disinfected before those on the near side. The infusion cannula on the syringe containing the antibiotic is partially inserted up the teat canal. The teat end is occluded by grasping it with the fingers, and the udder is massaged to help distribute the infused medication. Partial insertion of the cannula into the teat canal delivers fewer organisms into the udder than does full insertion. In addition, because antibiotic is deposited directly into the streak canal, local infection within the canal may be controlled better than when the entire volume of medication is placed in the cistern. Teats on the near side of the udder should be infused before those on the far side. After infusion, teat dip is reapplied.

ACKNOWLEDGMENTS

The author wishes to acknowledge the following faculty and staff members of the Veterinary Teaching Hospital and Clinics, School of Veterinary Medicine, Louisiana State University, who assisted in obtaining photographs for the manuscript: Dr. M. Claxton-Gill, Dr. J. Taboada, Mr. H. Cowgill, Dr. K. Wolfsheimer, Dr. D.M. McCurnin, Ms. L. Beebe, Ms. V. Dixon, Dr. R. McClure, Dr. T. Seahorn, Dr. P. Hoyt, and Ms. C. Antonellis. The author also wishes to acknowledge the work of Drs. M.J. Lucas and S.E. Lucas (Diagnostic sampling and treatment techniques. *In* McCurnin DM (editor): Clinical Textbook for Veterinary Technicians. Third ed. Philadelphia, WB Saunders, 1994).

Recommended Reading

Crowe DT: Nutritional support for the hospitalized patient: An introduction to tube feeding. Compend Contin Educ Pract Vet 12:1711–1720, 1990.

Devitt CM and Seim HB III: Clinical evaluation of tube esophagostomy in small animals. J Am Anim Hosp Assoc 33:55–60, 1997.
Ettinger SJ (editor): Textbook of Veterinary Internal Medicine. Third ed. Philadelphia, WB Saunders, 1989.
Grindem CB: Bone marrow biopsy and evaluation. Vet Clin North Am Small Anim Pract 19:669–696, 1989.
House JK, Smith BP, VanMetre DC, et al.: Ancillary tests for assessment of the ruminant digestive system. Vet Clin North Am Large Anim Pract 8:203–232, 1992.
Kirk RW, Bistner SI, and Ford RB: Handbook of Veterinary Procedures and Emergency Treatment. Fifth ed. Philadelphia, WB Saunders, 1990.
Kopcha M and Schultze AE: Peritoneal fluid. Part II. Abdominocentesis in cattle and interpretation of nonneoplastic samples. Compend Contin Educ Pract Vet 13:703–710, 1991.
Lawhorn B: A new approach for obtaining blood samples from pigs. J Am Vet Med Assoc 192:781–782, 1988.
Lucas MJ and Lucas SE: Diagnostic sampling and treatment techniques. *In* McCurnin DM (editor): Clinical Textbook for Veterinary Technicians. Third ed. Philadelphia, WB Saunders, 1994.
McCurnin DM and Poffenbarger EM (editors): Small Animal Physical Diagnosis and Clinical Procedures. Philadelphia, WB Saunders, 1991.
Moon PF and Smith LJ: General anesthetic techniques in swine. Vet Clin North Am Large Anim Pract. 12:663–691.
Osborne CA, Lees GE, and Johnston GR. *In* Kirk RW (editor): Current Veterinary Therapy. VII: Small Animal Practice. Philadelphia, WB Saunders, 1980, pp 1150–1153.
Otto CM, Kaufman GM, and Crowe DT.: Intraosseous infusion of fluids and therapeutics. Compend Contin Educ Pract Vet 11:421–430, 1989.
Raskin RE: Bone marrow. *In* Slatter D (editor): Textbook of Small Animal Surgery. Second ed. Philadelphia, WB Saunders, 1993.
Rose RJ and Hodgson DR: Manual of Equine Practice. Philadelphia, WB Saunders, 1993.
Smith MC and Sherman DM (editors): Goat Medicine. Philadelphia, Lea & Febiger, 1994.
Smith BP (editor): Large Animal Internal Medicine. Second ed. St. Louis, Mosby–Year Book, 1996.
Taylor FGR and Hillyer MH (editors): Diagnostic Techniques in Equine Medicine. Philadelphia, WB Saunders, 1997.
Tobin E and Hunt E: Supplies and technical considerations for ruminant and swine anesthesia. Vet Clin North Am Large Anim Pract 12:531–562, 1996.
Williams CSF: Routine sheep and goat procedures. Vet Clin North Am Large Anim Pract 6:737–758, 1990.

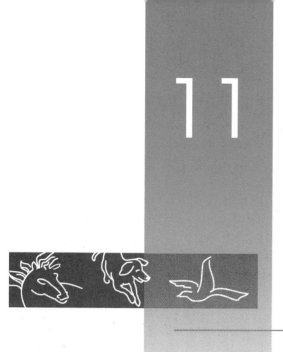

11 | Emergency Nursing

Angel M. Rivera • *Regula Spreng* • *Dennis T. Crowe, Jr.*

There can be no state of the art medicine, if there is no state of the art nursing. . . .

INTRODUCTION

The field of veterinary medicine has gone through major changes and advancements in the past four decades. Within the profession, the specialty of emergency and critical care has become an evolving, dynamic, and challenging field. Because of the uniqueness and complexity of the emergency patient, emergency nursing is evolving into a specialty field of veterinary technology.

In 1994, a group of technicians and veterinarians in the emergency and critical care field created a body that will recognize veterinary technicians in this field as a specialty. This organization will provide continuing education and evaluate the competency of veterinary technicians who work in the area of emergency and critical care. In January 1996, the North American Veterinary Technician Association (NAVTA) recognized the Academy of Veterinary Emergency and Critical Care Technicians as a specialty in veterinary technology.

Successful management of the emergency patient is dependent on several factors: the training and skills of the personnel and the readiness of the facility. The implementation of a team approach through the use of established policies, protocols, and procedures, allows a coordinated resuscitative effort. By understanding the principles of first aid (i.e., triage, primary and secondary survey, and the basic principles of assessment for shock, trauma, and hemorrhage), the technician is able to perform rapid and continuous evaluation, monitoring, and assessment of patients. The technician must have a clear understanding of his or her role in cardiopulmonary resuscitation and of the general principles of fluid and drug therapy.

The above factors (skills, protocols, and principles of pa-

tient care) require the technician understand basic anatomy, physiology, and pathophysiology. It is through knowledge and understanding of the overall organ function and disease processes that appropriate nursing assessment, monitoring, and intervention can be achieved (Table 11–1).

ELEMENTS OF EMERGENCY CARE

Personnel

Survival of the emergency patient is dependent on the collaborative effort of the veterinarian and technician (Fig. 11–1). Technicians and veterinarians should work together to resuscitate, stabilize, diagnose, and treat the emergency patient. The emergency patient requires prompt attention and rapid stabilization, which requires the technician to assume a more collaborative role with the veterinarian and other members of the team. A collaborative environment exists when there is mutual respect and understanding of the unique contributions each individual makes to the care of the patient. Improved patient care is the result of careful planning by the veterinarian and technician to identify guidelines that increase the patient's chance of survival and minimize complications.

TECHNICIAN NOTE

The emergency patient requires prompt attention and rapid stabilization.

• Table 11–1 •

RECOMMENDED SKILLS FOR THE VETERINARY TECHNICIAN PROVIDING EMERGENCY CARE

1. Scene assessment and triage skills
2. Primary and secondary survey skills
3. Vital sign data gathering and interpretation
4. Recognition of life-threatening conditions and clinical signs
5. Venipuncture of various veins
6. Ability to perform various STAT blood work as well as knowledge of expected normal values (e.g., packed cell volume [PVC], total solids [TS], activated clotting time [ACT]), buccal mucosal bleeding time, blood gases, electrolytes, and so forth
7. Placement of peripheral catheter in major veins
8. Nasal oxygen catheter placement
9. Bag-valve-mask ventilation to maintain an open airway
10. Endotracheal tube intubation
11. Basic first aid measures to include Heimlich maneuvers, rescue breathing, control of severe bleeding using applied pressure to pressure points and blood pressure cuffs, and dressing placement for wound protection

More advanced skills for the veterinary technician
1. Arterial blood sampling and arterial catheter placement
2. Nasopharyngeal, nasoesophageal, nasotracheal, and nasogastric tube placement
3. Central jugular and femoral line placement
4. Cricothyroid and tracheal oxygen delivery catheter placement
5. Mechanical ventilatory assistance to include appropriate ventilator setting, trouble shooting, and patient care
6. Calculation and preparation of continuous-rate infusion drugs such as dobutamine, dopamine, and nitroprusside
7. Knowledge of equipment needed to perform and assist the veterinarian in radiological studies such as cystography, intravenous pyelography, and arteriovenography

• Table 11–2 •

RECOMMENDED EMERGENCY EQUIPMENT	
CATEGORY	**EQUIPMENT**
Oxygen delivery devices	Portable oxygen tank or piped-in oxygen Rebreathing bags (assorted sizes) Face masks of various sizes, hood oxygen, nasal catheters, oxygen tubing, plastic bags
Resuscitation cart Airway drawer	Endotracheal tube (assorted sizes) Laryngoscope (large and small blade) Tracheostomy set: No. 10 and 15 scalpel blades, Mayo scissors, curved hemostat, Forrester forceps, tracheostomy tubes of various sizes, umbilical tape, suture material Chest tap device: 19- or 21-gauge butterfly catheter or needle, three-way stopcock, 35- to 60-ml syringe
Drug drawer	Epinephrine, lidocaine, and atropine Syringes of assorted sizes with needles
Catheter drawer	Intravenous and intraosseous catheters of various sizes, infant bone marrow cannula, spinal needle, butterfly catheters of various sizes, central catheters (jugular and femoral placement), surgical scrub, tape, heparin flush
Miscellaneous	Scissors, scalpel blades, sterile gloves, bandage materials
Fluids	Fluid pressure infuser device Fluid administration sets (macrodrips and microdrips) Infusion pumps Isotonic crystalloids and synthetic colloids Blood components, blood administration sets
Suction apparatus	Suction reservoir, suction tubing, suction tubes
Blood pressure monitoring	Doppler unit or oscillometric blood pressure unit, various size cuffs, sphygmomanometer, conduction gel
Electrocardiogaphy	ECG unit and electrode paste
Defibrillator	Internal and external paddles
Additional equipment	Chest tube pack and thoracotomy pack

Success of the team is dependent not only on the knowledge base and skill level of each member but also on the consistency of actions by the team. The predetermined delegation of specific nursing intervention in the emergency setting, such as allowing the technician to initiate basic cardiopulmonary resuscitation (CPR) or intubate a patient that has gone into respiratory arrest, fosters the efficient organization of talents and manpower, which in turn decrease the time between onset of the event or trauma causing the emergency; and the delivery of definitive care.

The technician should be skilled at placing intravenous catheters, obtaining blood samples, administering medications through various routes (IV, SC, IM), performing basic CPR, and assisting the veterinarian in advanced CPR, surgery, and administration of anesthesia. The technician should be skilled in patient monitoring based on clinical and physiological parameters and knowledgeable about the use of different types of monitoring equipment. He or she should also know how to perform various emergency laboratory tests and be familiar with their normal values.

Facility Capabilities

The receiving area of the veterinary clinic or hospital should have wide corridors with good lighting and be arranged to

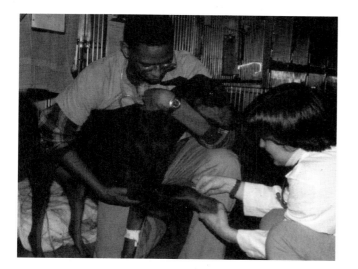

Figure 11–1. Successful delivery of emergency care is dependent on the skills, knowledge, and communication skills of all the team members.

facilitate the rapid transport of an injured animal to the emergency or centralized area of the building. Stretchers and gurneys should be easily accessible for transporting nonambulatory patients. Long boards and various sizes of plastic sheets are also recommended to be available for transport. Duct tape is needed to secure dogs to these devices with in lateral recumbency. Blankets, towels, and sheets of plastic bubble wrap can be used to provide insulation and protection.

Resuscitative equipment and drugs should be organized and readily available for use in the emergency area (Table 11–2). A portable cart should be used to store instruments and equipment if these are shared by other areas of the hospital. The anesthesia induction area is often chosen as the emergency area because key pieces of equipment, such as oxygen and endotracheal (ET) tubes, are readily accessible. The proximity of the operating room can be advantageous because some patients require immediate surgical intervention for stabilization. Clinics that lack sufficient space to equip one central area can benefit from having a tackle box that contains essential emergency materials.

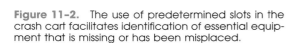

TECHNICIAN NOTE

A well-organized mobile emergency cart should be available at all times.

A well-organized mobile resuscitation cart that remains in the emergency area and has several drawers for storage is ideal. Essential equipment such as an electrocardiograph (ECG), blood pressure monitor, and suction device are placed on top. The drawers are organized into different sections, such as an airway drawer, an emergency drug drawer, and a catheter drawer. The instruments and drugs are held in place by shaping holes into foam pads that fit in the drawer; each space is labeled (Fig. 11–2). A CPR sheet is kept within the resuscitation cart for recording the cause and time of arrest, mode of ventilation, drug dosage, and route of administration.

The airway drawer should contain different sizes of ET tubes with cuff-inflating syringes that are preattached and a laryngoscope with at least two different sizes of blades. Forrester sponge forceps (for retrieval of airway foreign bodies), and tracheostomy tubes are kept in this drawer. A butterfly catheter (for small patients) and an 18-gauge, 1.5-in needle (for larger patients) three-way stopcock are set up for immediate chest tap. When a chest tube is required, having a sterile chest tube pack in the cart that is ready to open will expedite placement.

The drug drawer should contain atropine, epinephrine, and lidocaine with different sizes of syringes that are preloaded with needles. Other drugs, such as antibiotics, glucocorticoids, dopamine, or dobutamine, are kept on a nearby open shelf. A wall chart that provides drug dosages per weight and direct-current (DC) watt-second defibrillation voltages should be centrally posted for quick reference during CPR.

The catheter drawer should include all materials required for the placement of intravenous (IV) and intraosseous (IO) catheters. An additional drawer is stocked with bandage materials for use on the patient that is bleeding or has an open wound, sterile gloves for surgical interventions such as chest tube placement, and hair clippers with long extension cords.

For monitoring of cardiac rhythm and electrical activity, an ECG with alligator clips is necessary. A defibrillator with internal and external paddles is also kept on the cart ready for use in patients with ventricular fibrillation.

A suction device with different suction tips should be available. Large stiff dental suction tips work well for suctioning pharyngeal fluid; smaller pliable tips will pass through the ET tubes. Hand-held and hand-powered (by squeezing) suction units should be available if there is no electrical suction system present (Fig. 11–3). All suction units should generate up to 300 mm Hg of suction pressure within 4 to 5 seconds of the suction tip being occluded.

Basic laboratory tests used in the emergency setting include pack cell volume (PCV), total solids (TS), blood glucose (lab test strips), blood urea nitrogen (BUN; lab test strips), serum electrolytes, and urine specific gravity. Blood collection tubes, microcentrifuge tubes, a centrifuge, laboratory test strips, and a timer are part of the basic emergency laboratory equipment located in the emergency area.

To guarantee constant readiness, a checkoff list of all instruments and drugs is reviewed by each person starting a shift. The instruments should be tested for proper function (e.g., light

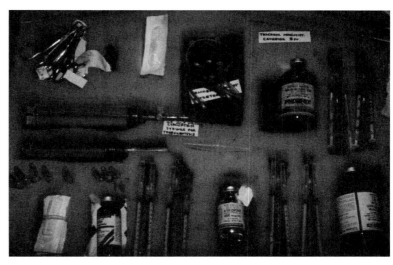

Figure 11-2. The use of predetermined slots in the crash cart facilitates identification of essential equipment that is missing or has been misplaced.

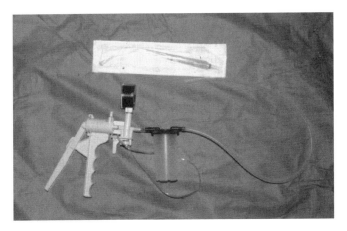

Figure 11-3. A hand-held suction device can be purchased from an auto parts shop. Yankauer suction tips (shown above suction unit) or home-made suction tips of clear plastic endotracheal tubes can be used for suctioning thick mucoid secretions.

bulb on the laryngoscope), and emergency drugs are checked for quantity, proper location, and expiration date. By reviewing the checkoff list, the technician and clinician become familiar with the materials and their location.

Policies and Procedural Protocols

Policies, procedural protocols, and guidelines provide consistency and efficiency within the organization. Policies state the organization's belief of how certain tasks should be done, at what times they are to be done, or under what conditions they are to take place. Procedural protocols mandate how to do things in a step-by-step action plan.

In the emergency setting, quick decisions and independent functions are necessary; policies and procedural protocols provide the guidance necessary to ensure acceptable response. Established policies and protocols can be used to ensure continuity of care as the patients move from one department to another. As policies and protocols evolve, the standard of care a patient receives will be consistent.

Common emergency problems that benefit from written protocols include initial stabilization of patients with gastric dilatation volvulus, head trauma, urinary tract obstruction, acute heart failure, stupor and coma, and catastrophic trauma. All team members should be familiar with the protocols, which should be discussed and reviewed at staff meetings (Table 11-3).

KEY ASPECT OF EMERGENCY NURSING

TECHNICIAN NOTE

Treatment of the emergency patient begins at the site of the accident or in the owner's home.

• Table 11-3 •

FELINE URETHRAL OBSTRUCTION PROTOCOL

1. Place IV catheter
2. Obtain database: packed cell volume (PCV), total solids (TS), blood urea nitrogen (BUN), and glucose (labsticks), electrolytes (Na^+, K^+, Cl^-, and ionized Ca^{2+})
3. Start IV fluids: Normosol-R, Plasma-Lyte, or lactated Ringer's solution at 10 ml/kg/hr initially
4. Obtain ECG: Assess for evidence of hyperkalemia
5. If hyperkalemia is sufficient to cause arrhythmias associated with poor perfusion or altered mentation:
    Give regular insulin IV 0.2 units/kg followed by 2 g of dextrose/unit of insulin. Support with 2.5% dextrose in fluids.
    or Give calcium gluconate 10% IV (slowly), at 1 ml/5 to 7 kg
    or Sodium bicarbonate IV at 1 mEq/kg
6. If sedation is required, give 5 to 10 mg/kg of ketamine IV + 0.2 mg/kg of IV diazepam + 0.05 mg/kg of atropine IV
7. Unblock urethra
    Massage penis and loosen crystal plug
    Use 5.5 Fr, open-ended tomcat catheter and saline to backflush the obstruction
    If the urethra is spasming or swollen, causing difficulty in relieving the obstruction, consider
        1 ml of 2% lidocaine diluted in 10 ml of flush solution
        Dexamethasone 0.5 mg/kg IV
8. Once the urethra is unblocked, the plastic tomcat catheter is removed, and a 3.5 Fr red rubber feeding tube is placed through the urethra into the bladder and secured into place.
9. A closed urinary collection system is attached to the catheter, and urine is totally withdrawn from the bladder. The bladder can be flushed with sterile saline to remove crystal sediment.
10. Obtain CBC and chemistry profile (specifically creatinine).
11. Once the animal is rehydrated, urine is measured hourly and must be at least 1 to 2 ml/kg/hr. Fluid input is adjusted with urinary output during diuresis phase: 2 to 5 ml/kg/hr + urine output = hourly fluid rate.
12. Monitor PCV, TS, glucose (if insulin/dextrose given), BUN (labstick), Na^+ and K^+ every 4 hours if possible.

Initial Contact and First Aid

Treatment of the critically ill or traumatized patient begins at the site of the accident or in the owner's home. Initial contact with the owner is usually made on the telephone by the receptionist or technician. The person who provides the first contact with the caller is termed a *first responder*. It is recommended that specific protocols be established on exactly what information and/or advice the first responder is to give the caller. These responses can be placed on 5 × 8-in cards and indexed according to the caller's concerns. The first responder should have some medical knowledge to properly assist the client in first aid, transport, and recognition of catastrophic emergencies (respiratory arrest, upper airway obstruction). Appropriate first aid can prevent further injury at the scene or during transport. The client should be given precise instructions for the most direct and simple route to the hospital. The telephone number for the poison control center should be readily available for reference in case of suspected toxin ingestion.

Telephone Contact, Handling, First Aid at the Scene, and Transport

It is important that on initial telephone contact, vital information be recorded such as client name and telephone number; patient species, age, and gender; presenting complaint; patient's current condition; and expected time of arrival. It is helpful to write this information on the treatment room communication board to alert the veterinary team to appropriately prepare the emergency area.

When answering a call, an immediate assessment must take place so needs can be prioritized. It is important to first determine whether a life-threatening condition exists and to instruct the client on hospital policies and guidelines. Second, it must be determined whether first aid advice is needed, and guidance should be offered according to protocols approved by the hospital administration. All other calls should be handled cautiously without diagnosis and always end with a recommendation for the caller to seek medical treatment for their pet (Table 11–4).

> ### ✎ TECHNICIAN NOTE
>
> Advise the owner to take a quiet, gentle approach while handling the injured pet.

Owners can provide significant medical assistance at the scene of the injury. The first concern is for the owner's safety. Advise the owner to take a quiet, gentle approach while handling the injured pet. He or she should use a soft and calm voice and approach very slowly so they do not startle or scare the animal. Ask that they watch for signs of aggression, snarling, or growling or any clues that they may have difficulty working with the animal.

When a dog is in pain or acting aggressively, a muzzle may be needed. A blanket will help provide the rescuer with adequate protection while attempting to handle an aggressive cat. Callers should always be cautioned that despite these preventative measures, there is a possibility of sustaining an injury.

One may be able to gain control by placing a heavy blanket over the animal while an assistant gains control of the head or places a muzzle. When placing a muzzle on the dog, a cloth strap or strip of gauze 24 in long is tied around the nose first with a simple overhand knot tied beneath the jaw. The straps are then brought around behind the neck and below the ears, where they are snugly tied together. One could improvise and use a necktie, pantyhose, or shoelace to fashion a muzzle if no other material is available. These types of muzzles are not indicated if the animal is bleeding from the nose or the nasal

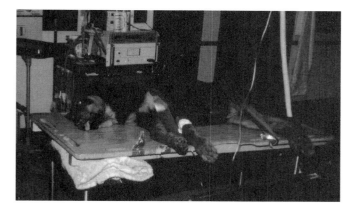

Figure 11–4. Unconscious animals should be transported from the accident site and in the veterinary facility on a firm surface such as a plastic, fiberglass, or wood board on a gurney until head and spinal injuries are ruled out.

passages appear to be occluded. Cats should be picked up slowly, with one hand supporting the chest while transporting the animal in a firm, secure manner under the arm. The front legs should be held with one hand, and the head and neck held with the other. Placing the cat into a cardboard box or pillow case is an alternative means of immobilization and transport.

To avoid further injury, care is taken to carefully transport the animal to the veterinarian. Animals with severe illness are often weak and have poor muscle coordination, putting them at a higher risk for developing injuries. Unconscious or stuporous animals are also at risk for developing injuries and are at risk of vomiting and aspirating the contents into their trachea and lower airways. Pressure should not be placed on the neck or chest because this could lead to vagal nerve–induced bradycardia, hypotension, and, in rare instances, cardiac arrest. The animal should be transported in a sternal or lateral position (Fig. 11–4).

If an injury leaves the animal unconscious or unable to walk, a spinal or cranial injury should be suspected. This animal should be immobilized to be transported laterally; it should be taped or tied down if possible on a flat wooden, cardboard, or plastic object, which is ideal for transportation as well as for x-ray examination of the neck and back without further mobilization of the pet. When sliding the animal onto a board, make certain the body remains parallel to the surface of the board to prevent excessive manipulation of the head or spine.

An animal with a chest wound may have a damaged lung on that side. When possible, animals sustaining trauma to one side of the chest should be transported with that side down to allow full expansion of the lesser traumatized lung on the opposite side. If the animal will not lie down and begins to become agitated, it is best not to use force. If the animal continues to struggle on being immobilized on its side, a respiratory problem should be suspected, and the animal should be allowed to be in a sternal position.

Fractures of the long bones below the elbow, hock, or stifle with significant displacement have potential for nerve, muscle, and skin penetration and should be supported during transport. The owner can fashion a splint from a rolled newspaper or magazine, which is then secured in place with a long piece of fabric such as a necktie or scarf. For the patient that

• Table 11–4 •

COMMON HISTORIC OR OBSERVED PROBLEMS THAT WARRANT IMMEDIATE MEDICAL ATTENTION	
Trauma	Potential snake bites
Profuse diarrhea	Heat prostration
Urethral obstruction	Open wounds: with exposure of
Labored breathing	extensive soft tissue or bones
Seizures	History of anemia
Loss of consciousness	Burns
Excessive bleeding	Dystocia
History of poisoning	Shock
Prolapse of organs	

was hit by an automobile, immobilization onto a board may be beneficial in preventing further internal bleeding.

The Veterinary Technician: Rendering First Aid

On arrival at the veterinary facility, first aid is the immediate care given to a pet that has been injured or suddenly taken ill. Knowledge of what to do will improve the pet's overall chance of recovery and possibly save its life. When using first aid, always understand one's limitations. A key principle in first aid is to seek further medical assistance in all cases of illness or injury. Do not use first aid as the only treatment.

As a first aid providers, the objectives are to:

- Care for the life-threatening condition
- Minimize further injury or complications
- Minimize the chances for further infection
- Make the pet as comfortable as possible to reduce stress
- Safely transport the pet within the veterinary hospital when required

Before You Act

Consider the following aspects when giving first aid *before* being confronted with a crisis.

Be Realistic. In certain situations, you might not be able to help; the animal may be uncooperative, the situation may be emotionally upsetting to the rescuer or others assisting in the rescue, or one's best attempts at first aid may fail.

Know Oneself. Knowledge of one's strengths and limitations, both physical and emotional, will help in the response in an urgent situation.

Be Prepared. The best way to be prepared is to receive formal training in first aid and CPR. Learn to recognize the danger signs, and familiarize yourself with potential hazards within

• Table 11–5 •

SUGGESTED ITEMS TO INCLUDE IN A FIRST AID KIT	
Blanket	Scissors and tweezers
Thermometer	Instant cold packs
Pen light	Hydrogen peroxide
Sterile 4 × 4 gauze pads	Splint material
Sterile dressing (assorted sizes)	Veterinarian's telephone number
Roll gauze	
1- and 2-in gauze	Poison control telephone number
Nonstick (Telfa) bandages	
Triangular bandage and safety pins	Glucose concentrate
	1-in adhesive tape
Plastic muzzle	Exam gloves
Stethoscope	Saline eye wash
Cloth strips	
Betadine or triple-antibiotic ointment	

From F'Aggella A: First aid, transport, and triage. Vet Clin North Am 24:998, 1994.

your environment. Learn as much as you can about how to handle different types of emergencies.

Gather Supplies. Having the appropriate instruments and knowing how to use them are essential to providing quality first aid. Owners and other potential rescuers would benefit by assembling emergency supplies before they are needed. (Table 11–5).

When first aid is properly administered, the animal's chances of recovery are greatly increased. Providers should know how to control bleeding, provide artifical ventilation and circulation assistance through CPR, and protect a pet's injuries from becoming infected. Providers should be prepared to direct the help of others who are less experienced or knowledgable in the vicinity.

When delivering first aid, one should conduct an initial assessment of the animal. It is wise to include a quick survey of the scene or area in which the animal is located. The initial response during the early moments of an emergency is critical. In addition to protecting the animal from further injury, one of the first rules involved in providing first aid is to ensure the safety of everyone providing care.

 TECHNICIAN NOTE

When first aid is properly administered the patient's chances of recovery are greatly increased.

After an evaluation of the emergency and the circumstances surrounding the event, the formation of a care plan should follow a three-step approach (AID):

A Ask for help

I Intervene

D Do no further harm

Avoiding Doing Any Further Harm

Never Block an Unconscious Animal's Airway. Unconscious animals with breathing difficulties may choke or suffocate if the airway is not protected. Never place anything, including liquids, in the mouth.

Do Not Use Force. Never force apart a conscious animal's jaws.

Never Continue a First Aid Measure if It Is Causing Severe Distress or Pain.
Never Remove an Impaled Object. The exception is an object that may be occluding the airway.

Never Move an Injured Body Part without Supporting the Injured Area. Unconscious trauma victims should be transported on a flat surface (e.g., cardboard, paneling, or a door) in case there is head or spinal injury.

Never give any medication unless instructed to do so by a veterinarian.

Initial Assessment

The initial assessment should include the standard *ABCs of emergency first aid:* (1) check for *airway* patency. (2) Is the animal *breathing*; if so, does it appear rapid, shallow, or labored, or is it normal? Is there any blood visibly associated with the respiratory system; is there blood exiting the nasal passages or the mouth? The answers to these questions will be of great benefit to the veterinary team.

(3) Next, evaluate the heart rate and *circulatory* competence. Gently feel the heartbeat by cupping the sternum in your hand midway along the rib cage. In most dogs and cats, you should be able to feel the heartbeat just behind the sternum between the fourth and sixth ribs. This is known as the *apical beat.* In large-chested animals, you may have more success feeling for a femoral pulse by using several fingers with light pressure on the inside of the thigh. One can determine the pulse rate by using the femoral pulse. When taken correctly, the absence of a femoral pulse suggests a systolic arterial blood pressure of less than 60 mm Hg (normal is more than 100 mm Hg), which can occur in shock and other low–blood volume situations (e.g., acute hemorrhage). Always follow this basic assessment through auscultation with a stethoscope to assess heart tones and breath sounds. Breath sounds should be clear and equal bilaterally, and heart sounds should be a crisp "lub-dub-lub-dub," without murmurs or additional sounds. Completion of the cardiovascular function assessment is done by noting the animal's capillary refill time (CRT), mucous membrane (MM) color, and amount of jugular vein distention.

CARDIOPULMONARY RESUSCITATION

Life-Threatening Primary Pulmonary and Cardiovascular Emergency Events

Emergency patients often present unresponsive without respirations but with a palpable pulse; this condition is termed *respiratory arrest.* However, failure to achieve effective ventilation results in a progressive acidosis and hypoxemia that may lead to cardiovascular dysfunction, hypotension, and eventual circulatory collapse.

Initially, hypoxemia enhances the peripheral chemical drive to breathe and stimulates heart rate. Profound hypoxemia, on the other hand, depresses neural function and produces bradycardia refractory to atropine. At this point, cardiovascular function is usually severely disturbed because cardiac and vascular smooth muscles function poorly under conditions of hypoxia and acidosis. In addition, there is reduced cardiac output due to decreased stroke volume and heart rate.

The heart may abruptly fail to achieve an effective output because of an arrhythmia or a suddenly impaired pump function resulting from diminished preload (volume of blood returning to the heart), excessive afterload (volume of blood being pumped by the heart), or decreased contractility. The normal heart compensates for changes in heart rate over a wide range through the Starling mechanism, which states that the more the heart is filled during diastole (within certain physiological limits), the greater is the quantity of blood it will pump. Thus, patients with dilated or stiff hearts lose this reserve and are highly sensitive to changes in heart rate. For this reason, bradycardia is poorly tolerated by patients with congestive heart failure. Animals that are sick or injured may also lose their normal ability to overcome or sympathetically override the bradycardia.

Decreases in preload sufficient to result in cardiovascular collapse are usually due to reflex veno dilation, massive hemorrhage, pericardial effusion/tamponade, or tension pneumothorax. An abrupt increase in afterload sufficient to cause catastrophic cardiovascular collapse usually affects the right ventricle and can be due to embolus in the pulmonary circuit by a blood clot or air. Cardiac muscle dysfunction can result from hypoxemia, acidosis, electrolyte imbalance, or myocardial infarction.

ABCs of Basic Life Support

The main purpose of basic life support is to maintain organ function by promoting perfusion of the two major organs: the brain and heart.

Several conditions are considered life threatening, but three in particular require immediate attention: respiratory arrest, circulatory failure, and severe bleeding. Respiratory arrest and/or circulatory failure can set off a chain of events that will lead to death. Severe uncontrolled bleeding can lead to an irreversible state of shock in which death is inevitable. Thus, first aid priorities that demand rapid and accurate assessment can be grouped as those that restrict airway, breathing, and circulation (cardiovascular to include bleeding)—after which other injuries may be addressed.

TECHNICIAN NOTE

The first priority in resuscitation is to maintain a patent airway.

Airway

Any interference with breathing produces oxygen depletion (anoxia) throughout the entire body. Therefore, the first priority is to ensure there is a patent airway and maintain its patency. A partial obstruction can become a total airway obstruction, resulting in unconsciousness and respiratory arrest. Total or partial airway obstruction may occur due to a foreign body (bone, meat chunk, ball, or stick), large blood clots, vomitus, thick saliva, or a direct blow to the larynx or trachea causing hemorrhage or spasm. During the summer, some dogs will develop laryngeal edema due to overexertion and heat-induced illness.

Signs that indicate a partially obstructed airway are difficulty breathing on inspiration, exaggerated airway sounds (usually, by this time 75% of the airway is compromised), accessory muscles of the face and neck being used, and eventually (this is a very late sign) cyanosis (blue coloration of the gums and tongue).

Partial Airway Obstruction. First aid measures in the animal with a partially obstructed airway consist of removal of any visible object from the mouth that may be causing the obstruction. Precautions should be taken not to be bitten by the animal. Remember partial obstructions can turn into total obstructions; as the animal struggles for more air, it becomes more distressed, frantic, and nonresponsive to commands, even from the owners. If the type of material causing the obstruction is known or suspected, the rescuer can attempt to dislodge the object via abdominal thrust compressions similar to those used in the Heimlich maneuver in humans. It is important that these patients be rushed to the veterinarian. If the patient is, for example, 30 minutes away and there is a closer clinic, have the owner take the victim to the nearest veterinary facility.

Signs seen in victims with total airway obstruction include no airway sounds, most often unconsciousness or near-unconsciousness, cyanosis, and no movement or expansion of the chest wall. First aid measures to consider in these patients, especially the unconscious patients, include the following:

1. Maintain the victim in a horizontal position. Elevation of the head in a hypotensive (low blood pressure) victim decreases blood flow to the brain and can precipitate a cardiopulmonary arrest.
2. Open the victim's mouth, pull the tongue forward, and extend the neck. If it is known that an obstruction is present, perform a finger sweep (insert index finger down the side of the cheeks and into the back of the throat to the base of the tongue; then, "sweep" across the back of the throat in a hooking action to dislodge the obstruction). When unsure of whether there is an obstruction or whether it is complete, attempts should be made (after the head and neck is extended) to perform rescue breathing by performing mouth-to-mouth and nose breathing or using a mask with either your mouth, an Ambu bag, or anesthetic machine with a rebreathing bag). If one is able to provide air into

the lungs, the rescue breathing should continue until a laryngoscope examination and tracheal intubation can be performed. If one is unable to inflate the lungs, the head, neck, and tongue should be reextended, with another attempt made to ventilate the patient. If ventilation still cannot be accomplished, an examination of the laryngeal opening should be performed. If a foreign body is observed, it should be removed either by a finger sweep or with the use of instruments (Fig. 11–5A & B). If instruments are not available and the foreign body cannot be removed using a finger, perform 5 to 10 abdominal (subdiaphragmatic) thrusts to aid in moving forward the object. Attempt to remove excessive saliva or secretions by using a cloth or an ear bulb suction device. Other electric suction devices that are more effective in removing saliva and secretions may need to be used.
3. Once the object has been removed, the rescuer will usually have to provide artificial (rescue) breathing. If the animal regains consciousness, it may still be necessary to provide artifical breathing because of secondary neurological dysfunction or pulmonary edema that can occur due to hypoxemia. The patient should be observed at least overnight for secondary consequences of severe airway obstruction if at all possible. A veterinarian should assess the patient to determine whether there are any conditions that developed due to anoxia or an injury that has occurred secondary to the laryngeal obstruction (e.g., lacerations or swelling due to the foreign body).

Breathing

Breathing is a function that is automatic and in which the individual (human or animal) exerts only a certain degree of control. Breathing consists of two separate acts: *inhalation*, in which the chest cavity is enlarged so air is driven into the lungs, and *exhalation*, in which the size of the chest cavity is decreased so air is driven out. The diaphragm provides most of

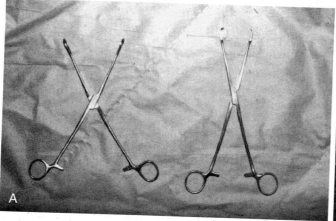 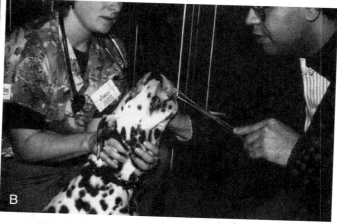

Figure 11–5. A, Forceps such as Laufe polyp forceps, which are commonly known as sponge forceps (left) and the Vulsellum forceps (right), aid in the removal of foreign bodies from the oropharyngeal area. B, Use of forceps in the removal of oropharyngeal foreign body.

the power for the act of inspiration, and exhalation is normally passive.

Providing Artificial Ventilation (Rescue Breathing). When there is absence of respiration, the rescuer should begin artificial ventilation. While extending the neck, hold the tongue out, close the jaws over the tongue (so the incisor teeth hold the tongue from moving back in the mouth and occluding the airway), and proceed to breath through both nostrils using your mouth (or place your mouth over the animal's nose and mouth in small patients) and giving 12 to 20 breaths. In brachiocephalic animals (animals with short, flat faces), it is best to hold down the upper fleshy lip over the lower jaw to aid in creating a seal. One should be able to observe the rise and fall of the chest wall with every breath. If the patient does not start breathing on its own, provide a few more breaths and assess the victim for a pulse or heartbeat. Lack of spontaneous breathing and the absence of a pulse or heart beat are indications to proceed to the "C" (circulation) of basic life support while still performing artificial ventilation. This is best achieved by recruiting another person to assist.

An animal can stop breathing for several reasons, including electrical shock, drowning, suffocation/choking, head injuries, congestive heart failure, severe hypovolemic shock, various toxicities, vagal influence, and cardiac arrhythmias. Symptoms of suffocation in the unconscious victim include dark blue (cyanotic) MM, lips, nail beds, and insides of ear flaps. The pulses may become weak and rapid initially but later become weak and slow before stopping. The pupils may become dilated over a few minutes as hypoxemia to the brain occurs. The cause of a suffocation episode is often due to an obstructed airway that prevents air from getting into the lungs; artificial ventilation is of no value until the blockage is removed.

Along with airway obstructions due to the presence of objects in the airway, suffocation may occur when a victim becomes entangled with a leash or collar. Head injuries that produce swelling of the brain and/or hemorrhage into the skull can cause breathing to be compromised.

Animals with known heart disease can develop pulmonary edema (accumulation of fluid in the lungs), which affects their ability to exchange oxygen and carbon dioxide and hinders the capability of the lung to expand. Certain abnormal heart rhythms can cause an animal to collapse and stop breathing (syncopal episodes).

Circulation/Cardiac Compression

Cardiopulmonary arrest can be defined as the cessation of functional ventilation (breathing) and effective circulation. For example, during shock, as the victim's condition progressively worsens, the brain and heart begin to decompensate. Reduced blood flow to the heart muscle (coronary blood flow) leads to damage of the heart muscle, resulting in heart failure (myocardial failure). The resulting reduced blood flow to the brain causes depression of respiratory and cardiovascular centers that control heart rate and respiratory rate. During this stage, the blood vessels dilate in the muscles, skin, and abdominal organs, causing blood to pool in these tissues. All these alterations feed a vicious cycle of changes that eventually precipitate cardiopulmonary arrest.

Signs observed in the cardiopulmonary arrest victim are absence of an auscultable or a palpable apex heartbeat, lack of palpable pulses (due to arterial hypotension), apnea (cessation of breathing) or agonal breathing (ineffective breaths taken before death), absence of bleeding even in the presence of a wound or laceration of considerable size (this will occur with blood loss of more than 40% to 55% blood volume), loss of consciousness (10 to 15 seconds after arrest), and pupillary dilatation (30 to 45 seconds after arrest).

If the animal has not responded to artificial ventilation and an apex heartbeat or pulse is not detectable, begin rhythmical chest compressions consisting of 60 to 140 compressions per minute. Chest compression should only be done *if it is determined that resuscitation is indicated.* Artificial ventilation (*rescue breathing*) should be provided at 12 to 20 breaths per minute. In cases in which significant restriction to lung expansion is observed, rescue breathing should be increased 30 to 60 breaths per minute. Ventilatory and CPR rates are dependent on the size of the animal, with the larger animal requiring slower rates.

In medium-sized to large dogs, compress the chest wall with one or two hands, depending on the size of the animal and rescuer. Place the hand or hands on the side of the chest wall where it is the widest, at or within 5 to 7 cm of the point of the elbow, or on the sternum with the dog laying on its back. Depress the rib cage 4 to 8 cm. Perform this 80 to 100 times per minute. Continue providing artificial ventilation at least 12 times per minute in large dogs if you have no help (single-rescuer technique). Chest compressions and ventilation should be coordinated to provide breaths during the compressions if this can be performed. When ventilation and compression cannot be performed together (as in larger dogs), two quick breaths should be given right after every 15 compressions.

When two rescuers are working together, artificial ventilation should be given during heart compressions with every second to fifth compression, depending on the size of the animal.

CPR should continue until:

1. The rescuer(s) becomes exhausted and cannot continue alone.
2. If out in the field, the animal is transported to a veterinary center and others can take over.
3. Spontaneous cardiac function returns; a pulse is palpable or heartbeats are felt, and they are strong and regular. In the vast majority of cases, artificial ventilation will continue to be required for a period of time, even though heart function has returned. This is due to the nervous system depression secondary to the arrest. All resuscitated animals (if not in a hospital when resuscitated) should be transported to the veterinary center for further examination and care.

When CPR is administered in the veterinary facility, intubation of the patient is considered part of basic life support. Indications for intubation include the need to gain control of the airway after arrest; the unconscious patient with excessive oral or pulmonary secretions, hypoxemia, or ventilatory failure; or when the effort of breathing contributes to the worsening of some pathophysiological process or prevents resuscitation, stabilization, and/or recovery. Before intubation with an ET tube, it is recommended that a bag-valve-mask be used to ventilate the animal. This should be attempted; giving just a few breaths will help prevent a vasovagal response and cardiac arrest.

It is recommended to use clear plastic ET tubes with inflatable cuffs that are high volume and low pressure. A clear tube allows visualization of any fluid or exudate from the trachea or lungs. A high-volume, low-pressure cuff helps reduce the incidence of pressure necrosis of the trachea when the tube is maintained for extended periods.

If the arrest is of pulmonary origin and the heart is still beating but at a very slow rate, initial ventilations may be sufficient to reestablish breathing and increase heart rate. If the patient continues to breath on its own, supplemental oxygen should be provided via nasal cannula or oxygen hood or transtracheally. It is very important to observe the patient's respiratory pattern. If it is unusually slow, shallow, or unstable, continued ventilatory support will be needed.

Patients with respiratory arrest should be intubated in lateral or dorsal recumbency to avoid manipulation of the head or neck in case of hypotension or a cervical lesion (Fig. 11–6, *A* and *B*). Using 100% oxygen, ventilate and ensure the lungs expand well. Use a stethoscope to listen for bilateral lung sounds while the patient is being ventilated. Failure to hear lung sounds bilaterally can indicate ET tube placement in one side of the main pulmonary tree or unilateral pleural space disease. If a pressure gauge is available, ventilation should achieve inspiratory pressures of 20 cm H_2O in the dog and 10 to 15 cm H_2O in the cat. Patients with suspected pleural or lung parenchymal disease will require greater inspiratory pressures. Overzealous inflation of the lungs will interfere with venous return and cause a rupture of the pulmonary tree, leading to free air in the thoracic cavity. In the absence of a pressure gauge, provide sufficient inspiratory pressure that movement of the chest wall can be visualized. When attempts to ventilate are met with increasing resistance, one should suspect a pneumothorax, and a larger needle or tube should be inserted into the pleural space to evacuate the air.

In the vast majority of cases in veterinary medicine, respiratory arrest is the principal inciting factor that leads to cardiac arrest. One exception may be the Doberman pinscher, which has been observed to have sudden onsets of ventricular fibrillation before respiratory arrest. Another exception is an animal that undergoes a vasovagal reflex with sudden stoppage of the heart due to vagus nerve stimulation. This is most commonly observed in animals after or in conjunction with micturition, defecation, vomition, or another manipulation that can stimulate parasympathetic nerve discharge in the face of ongoing sympathetic responses, such as that seen postoperatively or posttraumatically. Vasovagal reflex is more prone to occur in animals that are hypoxemic and acidemic. In very weak and older animals, a vasovagally induced arrest may also occur with insertion of the rectal thermometer to measure temperature and laryngeal manipulation, as occurs with intubation.

If the patient is deemed to have a respiratory arrest, ventilation should occur at a rate of 12 to 20 times per minute; if associated with a cardiac arrest, ventilation should be performed with every two or three chest compressions. Performing ventilation during the compression increases the airway pressures within the chest, which have been associated with improved aortic pressures generated with the chest compressions. This simultaneous compression and ventilation *cannot* be done without a cuffed ET tube in place.

Compression of the chest should be done at least 80 times per minute. Between chest compressions, one can deliver abdominal compressions (*abdominal pump*) similar to those of the chest to aid in increasing oxygen delivery, coronary blood flow, and cerebral blood flow. *Abdominal compression* should be done only with a cuffed ET tube in place.

Small animals can have chest compression done laterally over the heart to use the *cardiac pump*. However, in small animals (less than 10 kg), the chest should be compressed at the widest part of the chest. Deep-chested animals (standard poodles, Borzois, and so forth) should have chest compression

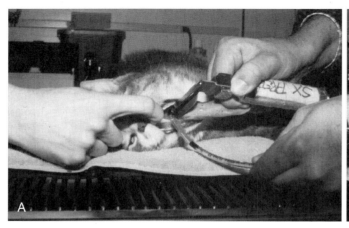
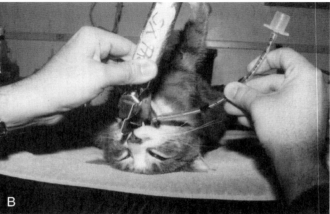

Figure 11–6.   A, Endotracheal intubation should always be done with a laryngoscope. B, Unconscious, mentally dull, or bradycardic patients exhibiting respiratory compromise or respiratory distress should be intubated while in lateral or dorsal recumbency.

applied from the sternum to the vertebral column while in dorsal recumbency. To monitor the results of compression, a Doppler flow probe should be used on the patient's eye. Blood flow generated in the external ophthalmic vessels will be detected with the Doppler probe *if flow is effectively* generated. If a Doppler probe is not available, palpation of the femoral or brachial artery for a pulse with each compression is recommended. *If no flow is detected* with basic life support skills, advanced skills that involve epinephrine delivery and, possibly, a resuscitative thoracotomy and aortic cross-clamping (encircling and occluding the thoracic aorta just distal to the arch using a feeding tube) are required.

The use of a laryngoscope with the patient in right lateral position is recommended for intubation to avoid lifting the patient's head, which could decrease blood flow to the brain, cause vomitus to migrate into the trachea, and cause a vagal response that may lead to a cardiac arrest. A laryngoscope with a good light allows actual visualization of the larynx for removal of foreign bodies or placement of an ET tube. It is recommend that an Ambu bag and reservoir be used rather than an anesthetic machine and rebreathing bag to ventilate near-arrested or arrested patients. This is because the Ambu bag does not have a pop-off valve and the compliance of the lung can be assessed more accurately with compressions of the bag. Bystanders can also be easily shown how to use the AMBU bag to assist in resuscitation attempts if this is necessary (Fig. 11–7).

Hemorrhage

Catastrophic hemorrhage is life threatening due to the massive volume of blood that may be lost (internally, externally, or both). Internal bleeding into areas that surround vital organs such as the heart and brain can create increased pressure that compromises vital organ function. Internal hemorrhage can occur in other areas, such as the chest, abdomen, and ossiofacial compartments like the pelvic area or around the humerus and femur.

Bleeding into the chest and abdomen requires the skills and assessment tools of a veterinarian. Some specific signs to observe in the animal with abdominal hemorrhage are red circular discoloration with its center at the umbilicus (caused by an accumulation of red cells under the skin) and abdominal

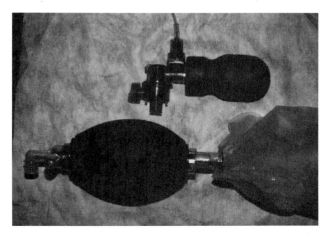

Figure 11–7. Ambu bag ventilation allows the operator to evaluate airway inflation resistance and lung compliance.

distention from blood accumulation. Abdominal distortion usually requires a blood loss of 40 ml or more of blood per kilogram of body weight. Bleeding into an ossiofacial compartment is generally due to blunt trauma; one can expect to see signs such as swelling of the area, bruises, wounds, and lacerations.

The immediate goal in any hemorrhagic event is to stop, or at least slow down, bleeding; restore volume to prevent vascular collapse (decreased volume of blood in veins and arteries); and avoid irreversible damage to organs. Shock in these patients is a result of lack of circulating blood volume, secondary to vascular collapse and hypoxia (lack of oxygen). Restoration of volume to these patients becomes a major priority and can be done only by a trained professional in a veterinary facility. These patients require rapid IV infusion of fluids consisting of crystalloid, colloids, and transfusions with blood components such as whole blood or packed red cells. Rapid restoration of blood volume is needed to maintain sufficient pressure to perfuse vital organs such as the heart, brain, and kidneys and restore red cells to serve as oxygen-carrying vehicles.

ADVANCED CPR OR ADVANCED LIFE SUPPORT

The goal of advanced cardiac life support is to intervene with appropriate pharmacological agents, restore an ECG rhythm, achieve adequate acid-base balance, and diminish neurological impairment. Advanced life support begins where basic life support stops. Chaos often surrounds initial attempts at CPR. A prompt and well-directed resuscitative effort is critical to achieve adequate cardiopulmonary and neurological function. Resuscitative equipment should be close at hand; there should be established protocols and a predetermined team. One person must be in charge of the resuscitation team. This person should integrate all pertinent information and establish priorities for response. The team leader should monitor the ECG, order medications, and direct the actions of the other team members but not be distracted from the leadership role by performing procedures.

The hallmarks of advanced CPR are (1) establishment of effective ventilation, (2) establishment of effective circulation, and monitoring to assess effectiveness, (3) preparation and administration of drugs, and (4) establishment and maintenance of intravenous access and special procedures such as internal defibrillation, direct cardiac massage, and/or aortic cross-clamping.

Ideally, at least four individuals should be involved with advanced life support attempts. The team leader makes the decisions and can be involved with invasive techniques such as thoracotomy and/or vascular access. Access is frequently done by cut-down or placement of an IO cannula. The person performing positive-pressure ventilations should also assess pupillary light responses and size and use the Doppler probe (if available) on the eye for assessment of effectiveness of compressions. The third person is the thoracic compressor and may also perform abdominal compression in small pets. The fourth person attaches the electrodes and Doppler probe, begins assessment of the present arrhythmia, and assists the team leader in securing IV access and administration of required drugs. If a fifth individual is available, this person can be the recorder and assist with procurement of items needed at the scene.

TECHNICIAN NOTE

The patient with a total upper airway obstruction should have a tracheostomy performed.

Establish Effective Ventilation

Basic support of the airway, breathing, and circulation should not be interrupted for long periods to perform adjunctive procedures. These patients require intubation by the most experienced person to achieve definitive control. Intubation attempts should not interrupt ventilation or chest compressions for more than 15 seconds. Therefore, all materials, including laryngoscope, endotracheal tubes, and suction equipment, should be assembled and tested before any attempt at intubation. When neither intubation nor effective ventilation can be accomplished because of abnormalities of the upper airway; restricted cervical motion; or patient agitation; sedation or paralysis should be considered.

The patient with a total upper airway obstruction should have a tracheostomy performed to allow effective ventilation. In the patient with a partial airway obstruction, emergency aid can be delivered by insufflation of oxygen via a large-bore needle/catheter puncture at the cricothyroid membrane, providing adequate oxygenation until a more definitive airway is established. During CPR, ventilation should normalize arterial pH and provide adequate oxygenation. The cornerstone of pH correction is adequate ventilation, not sodium bicarbonate administration. Venous blood gases can be used to assess the effectiveness of the compressions. High P_{CO_2} is seen with poor blood flow generation. End-tidal CO_2 monitoring can also be used to determine effectiveness. A value of more than 12 mm Hg has been associated with increased brain survival in experimental studies. Clinical studies in humans seem to substantiate this.

Establish Effective Circulation

Blood flow during CPR is theorized to occur via two mechanisms: cardiac pumping and thoracic pumping. The cardiac compression theory proposes that chest compressions generate positive intraventricular pressure, stimulating cardiac muscles to contract and making the heart valves function to achieve forward blood flow with each compression. Unfortunately, in most dogs more than 20 kg, the direct compression cardiac pump is not very effective due to the large size of the chest and the space taken up by lung tissue compared with humans or pigs. In animals less than 10 kg, some cardiac pumping is done, particularly if the chest can be compressed from both sides with hands or fingers plus thumb; the latter is used for very small patients.

The thoracic pump theory proposes that the heart serves as a passive conduit for blood flow. Chest compressions create a positive pressure relative to extrathoracic structures, and flow is valved at the thoracic inlet. Retrograde vena cava flow is prevented by jugular venous valves and functional compression of the inferior vena cava at the diaphragmatic hiatus.

Binding of the caudal abdomen and rear limbs using bandage materials, towels, or commercially produced MAST (military antishock trousers) can aid in decreasing blood flow to nonessential areas and increases the blood supply to the anterior portion of the body. They also can be used to splint, stabilize, and control hemorrhage of the lower extremities.

Because closed-chest CPR is only one third effective, the team should be prepared to perform open-chest CPR *if spontaneous cardiac contractions do not begin within 5 minutes.*

Electrocardiography and Drug Administration

The ECG allows characterization of any existing arrhythmia and determination of defibrillation. Five major arrhythmias are frequently associated with cardiac arrest: asystole, ventricular flutter, ventricular fibrillation, pulseless idioventricular rhythm, and electromechanical dissociation.

Asystole. Any rhythm is better than asystole, which is defined as the complete absence of electrical activity (a flat-line ECG). Therefore, the aim in CPR when encountered with this ECG reading is to stimulate electrical activity and then modify the rhythm to one with a pulse. Asystole usually indicates extended interruption of perfusion and carries a grave prognosis. An important point to remember is that low-amplitude ventricular fibrillation may go unrecognized or mistakenly be called asystole. Because of this, it is recommended that epinephrine be administered and the patient with suspected asystole be defibrillated.

Ventricular Flutter. This is a more chaotic wave than ventricular fibrillation. It represents an extreme type of ventricular tachycardia that will convert to ventricular fibrillation within a few seconds. *Lidocaine* is the first drug of choice and is used to block the excited foci. If ineffective after several boluses, defibrillation may be required.

Ventricular Fibrillation. This rhythm implies multiple foci within the ventricles firing rapidly and independently, resulting in no coordinated mechanical activity. It is an uncoordinated depolarization of the ventricle muscle that results in abrupt cessation of effective blood flow. This arrhythmia occurs only when the heart is severely damaged by ischemia, drugs, trauma, or contact with high-voltage electricity. The goal is to abruptly stop the electrical activity and allow one strong focus to take over (coarse fibrillation) rather than multiple weak foci (fine fibrillation). When fibrillation is fine, *epinephrine* is administered; if there is no change, *lidocaine* is administered before defibrillation.

Pulseless Idioventricular Rhythm. This electrical activity originates from an ectopic ventricular focus that produces insufficient pressure to generate a peripheral pulse. It is important not to suppress these slow ventricular rhythms; lidocaine is *not* to be used.

Electromechanical Dissociation. This arrhythmia is characterized by the inability to detect pulsatile activity in response to coordinated ECG complexes. When cardiac in origin, electromechanical dissociation carries a dismal prognosis because it is usually associated with massive pump destruction or free wall rupture.

In the administration of drugs during CPR, the goal is to deliver the agent to the myocardium via the coronary vessels as quickly as possible. Oxygen is the first and most important drug of CPR and should have been addressed during management of the airway and breathing. Cardiopulmonary arrest patients should be intubated and ventilated using a system such as an Ambu bag that is capable of delivering 100% oxygen.

Most CPR cases will have an ET tube placed to establish an airway. Certain drugs, such as atropine, epinephrine, and lidocaine, can be administered via an ET tube directly to the pulmonary tree, where they are rapidly absorbed and placed into the circulation. An important point to remember is that the dose of these drugs must be doubled with an equal amount of sterile saline to add sufficient volume to allow delivery of the drug at the end of the ET tube.

Other means of delivering drugs during CPR are intralingual, IO, and IV via peripheral or central lines. Administration of drugs into the venous sinuses of the tongue provides rapid drug uptake into the systemic circulation when chest compression and ventilation are used. If an IO catheter is in place before the arrest, drugs can be administered via this route. There is rapid uptake and distribution, most likely faster than the peripheral circulation.

Administration of cardiac drugs is best accomplished through a long centrally placed catheter (jugular catheter). However, most resuscitated patients also require large volumes of fluids be rapidly delivered into the intravascular space. Most central IV lines are of small diameter, limiting the amount of fluids that can be delivered.

Establishing and Maintaining IV Access

The heart simply cannot pump that which is not returned to it. In CPR, a variety of conditions produce either relative or absolute hypovolemia; therefore, provision of adequate circulating volume must be accomplished.

The choice of catheters used for fluid bolus administration is not a mundane matter. It is worth understanding that the rate of flow is directly related to the fourth power of the catheter diameter and inversely related to the length of the catheter (Poiseuille's law). Therefore, short large-bore catheters connected to a pressure device or infusion pump are preferable. In all emergency patients showing signs of shock, at least one large-bore catheter IV line (18 gauge in cats and small dogs and 14 and 16 gauge in medium-size to larger breeds) should be placed, and crystalloids, colloids, and/or blood products should administered as needed.

Several hematocrit tubes should be filled with the blood seated in the hub of the catheter. These samples can be used to obtain base-line values for PVC, TS, blood glucose, and BUN.

Special Procedures

Although the veterinary technician is not going to be performing a resuscitative thoracotomy or aortic cross-clamping to increase blood flow to the heart and brain during CPR, it is recommended that these procedures at least be understood. In some veterinary emergency centers, technicians are part of the team performing open-chest and aortic cross-clamping. They also are expected to be able to assist in the procedure and

perform cardiac compression. Other special techniques associated with CPR include defibrillation and the delivery of drugs down the airway for rapid uptake in the arrested patient that is being resuscitated.

TRIAGE, PRIMARY AND SECONDARY SURVEY

The word *triage* describes a medical decision-making process that is used in several clinical settings. Its application is widespread and ranges from the description of the initial assessment by a nurse in the emergency department to the sorting of victims at a disaster scene. *Triage* is a French term meaning *to sort* and was adopted into the English language after the Napoleonic Wars. Originally, triage described the first aid treatment on the battlefield before evaluation to hospitals behind the lines. In the emergency medical field, triage is used to screen patients into categories on the basis of severity of illness to determine their relative priority for treatment. Although its use in veterinary medicine is mostly associated with the specialty of emergency medicine, the concepts of triage, primary and secondary survey, can also be used in the critical care setting as a means of prioritization and assessment. When used correctly, the principle of triage, primary and secondary survey, guides the veterinary team in the efficient delivery of medical and patient care.

TECHNICIAN NOTE

Triage means *to sort* and was adapted from the battlefield.

The person performing triage must possess excellent assessment as well as interpersonal skills. He or she must be able to convey genuine concern, empathy, willingness to listen, and desire to help. One should approach the owner in a nonjudgmental attitude and communicate that their concerns have been taken seriously. It is important to approach the owner in a friendly, compassionate, and professional manner. Establishing trust and rapport is fundamental to providing emotional support.

During triage, a brief history is obtained from the owner that includes the nature of the emergency, the time it occurred, and any previous medical conditions or therapy. Further information can be obtained after initial assessment and resuscitation.

Patient acuity may be readily recognizable for patients with life-threatening disorders or those with low-priority, nonurgent complaints. The triage nurse or technician makes decisions regarding the degree of acuity based on chief complaint, general appearance, vital signs, past history, current medications, and patient age (Table 11–6).

Although the purpose of triage is not to diagnose, experienced triage technicians are able to recognize clinical syndromes and use this knowledge when deciding on acuity. Acuities are often determined early in assessment, especially when the presentation is classic for a given disorder. When it is determined that immediate assessment or intervention is required, the animal is moved to the ready area, and the owner

• Table 11–6 •

TRIAGE PARAMETERS		
PARAMETER	**NORMAL VALUE**	**ABNORMAL VALUE**
Heart rate, beats/min		
Cat	150–210	<150; bradycardia
		>250; tachycardia
Dog		
>25 kg	70–100	<70; bradycardia
<25 kg	90–160	>160; tachycardia
Respirations, breaths/min		
Cat	8–30	<8; bradycapnia
		>30; tachycapnia
Dog	8–20	<8; bradycapnia
		>20; tachycapnia
Mucous membrane	Pink	Pale, brown, yellow
Capillary refill time, sec	1–2	<1 or >2
Temperature, °C (°F)	38–39 (100–102)	<37 (≤99); hypothermia
		>40 (≥103); hyperthermia
Central venous pressure, cm H$_2$O		
Noncritical patient	−1 to 5	<−1 or >5
Critical patient	5 to 8	<5 or >8
Blood pressure, mm Hg		
Systolic	100–150	>160; hypertensive
Diastolic	60–110	<60; hypotensive
Mean arterial	80–120	
Urine output, ml/kg/hr	1–2	<1

*Size and breed dependent.

is assured that someone will be with them immediately. To accelerate treatment, permission for initial intervention (IV, catheter placement, fluid administration, ET intubation, oxygen supplementation) should be obtained from the owner at this time.

Triage of multiple critically ill patients involves the selection of conditions that require immediate treatment and then performing treatments that make the most efficient use of available manpower and skills. Patients deemed to have potential for compromised airway, breathing, and/or circulation (ABCs) should have their treatments and assessments done in a prioritizing manner. In other words, the condition that will kill them first should be the first priority in treatment. The assessment examination is divided into three parts: *primary survey, vital signs, and secondary survey.*

Primary Survey

Primary survey involves gathering in a capsule format information regarding what happened and then very rapidly assessing the scene for safety, gaining insight into possible mechanisms of injury, and viewing the patient's level of consciousness.

Scene safety is assessed by observing first the owner and then the patient for anything that may indicate risk. This includes an animal that is growling and not well controlled. Obvious fractious dogs should not be approached until the handler has a muzzle on the dog. If hemorrhage is observed in the pet's nose, a plastic or wire cage muzzle should be applied—*not* a wrap-a-round, tight-fitting muzzle, because this could jeopardize the animal's airway. If blood is observed on

the pet, gloves should be worn and possibly protective eyewear if blood or other chemicals could be sprayed. Animals with an unusual neurological history in rabies-endemic areas should also be suspected, and gloves and eyewear should be worn. Hand washing after the handling of each emergency patient is required. Animals having difficulty breathing should receive oxygen *first before you try to handle them*, especially cats, because handling could lead to severe bites and/or scratches by the frantic animal. In these cases, oxygen is delivered under plastic sheeting used to cover the box or container holding the animal or simply run at a high-flow stream directed to the patient's face.

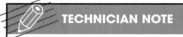

TECHNICIAN NOTE

Patients in respiratory difficulty should receive oxygen before they are moved.

During primary survey assessment, the initial management of life-threatening conditions is addressed in the following order: (1) airway maintenance, (2) breathing, (3) circulation, and (4) neurological deficit assessment. During the primary survey, neurological status can be evaluated by remembering the acronym *AVPU* (the patient is *alert*, responsive to *voice*, responsive only to *pain*, or *unresponsive*). In the patient in the intensive care unit, it is important that hypoxia; hypercapnia; metabolic derangements such as acidemia and alkalemia, hypoglycemia and hyperglycemia, hypocalcemia and hypercalcemia, and hyperammonemia; and drug effects be considered in the evaluation of a patient with altered mental status. After the primary survey, the resuscitative phase is initiated.

In many emergency centers, veterinary technicians have this initial assessment responsibility as they act as a *triage nurse* to decide the rapidity of care needed, similar to the duty of human emergency department triage nurses. Veterinarians should also perform a primary survey as they initially assess the injured pet. A suggested detailed protocol for a primary survey by the hospital staff is outlined in Table 11–7.

Primary survey and collection of vital signs then continue during triage and include but are not limited to level of consciousness (LOC), respiratory rate and effort, breathing pattern, heart rate and rhythm, and perfusion parameters such as pulse, MM, CRT, and temperature (see Table 11–6). The assessment and continuous monitoring of vital signs and parameters provide clinical signs that point to trends and developments as well as to otherwise unsuspected pitfalls and complications.

The use of the rectal thermometer is sometimes avoided so vasovagally induced cardiac arrest or near-arrest can be avoided. Arterial blood pressure (as measured with oscillometry or Doppler) and pulse oximetric data are also considered part of vital sign assessment in some hospitals.

Secondary Survey

Once the ABC areas have been addressed and resuscitation measures have been initiated, along with vital sign collection, the secondary survey is instituted. A reassessment of vital signs and a rapid, thorough examination of the entire patient from

• Table 11-7 •

RECOMMENDED PRIMARY SURVEY FOR EMERGENCY CARE PROFESSIONALS

1. Visually assess the patient from a distance, noting level of consciousness, unusual body or limb posture, presence of blood or other materials on or around the patient, and any other gross abnormalities. Note breathing effort and pattern and any airway sounds generated.
2. Approach the patient from the rostral direction, noting the patient's level of awareness and reactions to this movement. Ask questions concerning the patient's temperament to the owner, if present, in patients that are awake. Take appropriate safety precautions in "questionable" animals (muzzling, head covering, physical restraint).
3. Assess airway and breathing status by closely observing color of the oral mucous membranes (capillary refill time is also assessed at this time), listening for tracheal breath sounds (first without and then with the aid of a stethoscope), and palpating the neck, noting tracheal position and tracheal/peritracheal integrity. Injuries to the skin, subcutaneous emphysema, and blood in the nose or mouth are assessed bilaterally.
4. Continue to assess the patient's breathing status by observing, palpating, and then listening to the thorax (first without and then with the aid of a stethoscope). Lung sounds should be auscultated bilaterally (heart sounds are also assessed after lung sounds). Again, injuries to the skin over thorax and cranial abdomen, subcutaneous emphysema, and loss of chest wall (muscle, rib, and sternum) integrity are assessed bilaterally by visualization and palpation.
5. Cardiovascular assessment is completed by palpating pulses during auscultation of the heart. Pulse strength, vessel tone, and rate are easily determined in all except the very smallest animals. Assessment of heart sounds, mucous membrane color, and capillary refill time can be repeated, as well as any other part of the primary survey thus far if there are concerns.
6. The primary survey ends with very rapid observation and palpation assessment of the abdominal, flank, and pelvic regions, as well as the spinal column and limbs.

head to tail is performed. *It should be emphasized that the secondary survey is not completed until resuscitation of catastrophic emergencies is well under way.* The chest, abdomen, pelvis, and extremities are visually inspected, palpated, and auscultated where appropriate. Neurological status is repeatedly assessed. The secondary survey includes a head-to-tail tip examination, thorough history, and procurement of initial laboratory, radiographic, and other data. This is done immediately after resuscitation events are performed.

The Examination. To help prevent body areas from being missed in the examination, the following mnomonic (memory outline) was developed: *A CRASH PLAN. A,* indicates airway and breathing (nose, mouth, trachea, thoracic inlet, all lung fields); *C,* cardiovascular (MM, CRT, toe temperature, central/peripheral pulses, heart sounds); *R,* respiratory (breathing effort, chest and abdominal movement, percussion); *A,* abdomen (wounds, bruises, inguinal and retroperitoneal region; visualize, listen carefully, and percus); *S,* spine (palpate entire spine; note general movement, wounds, bruises, pain); *H,* head, eyes, ears, nose, and throat (face, skull, jaw, teeth, tongue, pharynx); *P,* pelvis (palpate ilial wings, tuber ischii, greater trochanters, rectal, genitals); *L,* legs (distal to proximal: check movement.

Feeling, function, joints, skin); *A,* arteries and veins (clip neck and examine jugular vein filling, check pulses); and *N,* nerves (assess LOC, cranial nerves, spinal function, peripheral nerves).

The History. On arrival, after a capsule history is obtained, it is recommended that the owner be given a history form to complete. This helps save time, determines the owner's ability to read and follow directions, and provides a thorough system review. It also gives the owner something to do while waiting and makes them feel they are helping. A mnemonic commonly used by paramedics and emergency medical technicians (see boxed text) can also be used to help personnel remember to ask all important historical details. In addition to mnemonic items, ask about details; for example, if the patient is a dog that was hit by an automobile, ask on which the dog was hit, what was the estimated rate of speed, whether the dog got up after he was hit, and whether he was unconscious or appeared to be dazed after the injury.

AMPEL

*A-*Allergies—Are there any known allergies to drugs, foods, and so forth?
*M-*Medications—Is the animal on any medications? If so, what type and amount?
*P-*Past history—Has the animal had any past medical problems?
*E-*Events—What is the current problem now? Provide details.
*L-*Lasts—When was the pet's last meal, bowel movement, urination, and medication dose?

Triage Classification

When dealing with more than one emergency or critically ill patient, the team can use a classification system such as the following:

Class I Patients (Catastrophic). These patients must receive treatment immediately (e.g., traumatic respiratory or cardiorespiratory arrest or failure, airway obstruction, unconsciousness). Catastrophic patients may be described as "dying before your eyes."

Class II Patients (Very Severe, Critical). These patients need attention within minutes to 1 hour (e.g., multiple injuries, shock, or bleeding but with adequate airway function).

TECHNICIAN NOTE

Evaluation of the patient through the physical examination is the gold standard of determining patient status.

Class III Patients (Serious, Urgent). These patients need action within a few hours (e.g., severe open fractures, severe open wounds or burns, penetrating wounds to abdomen without active bleeding, blunt trauma but no shock, or altered state of consciousness).

Class IV Patients (Less Serious but Still Pressing). These animals require action within 24 hours. This does not apply to most trauma patients.

VITAL SIGNS: PATHOPHYSIOLOGY, ASSESSMENT, AND INTERVENTION

Evaluation of the patient through physical findings is the *gold standard* of determining patient status. Obtaining and assessing parameters is a serial process, with the initial values acting as the baseline for the patient's data base. It is important to know what is normal for the patient and what the parameters were from the previous shift. If there is a trend of changes occurring, the technician should inform the clinician and more frequently monitor the signs. Establishing trends or comparing changes can be much more meaningful than writing down one-time values. The parameters should be evaluated in relation to the diagnosis, laboratory tests, history, and charted records.

Level of Consciousness

Pathophysiology

A declining LOC is suggestive of progressive brain pathology and worsening prognosis. The levels (in declining order) are alert and responsive, depressed, uncontrolled hyperexcitability, stupor, and coma. A mentally depressed animal is conscious but slow to respond to stimuli. An unconscious patient that responds to noxious (painful) stimuli is in a stupor. The patient that is unconscious and does not respond to any stimuli is in a coma. Coma carries the worst prognosis.

An animal can be conscious but have abnormal mental abilities. These mentation changes can include slow but appropriate responses to stimuli (severe depression), inappropriate responses to situations or stimuli (dementia), bizarre behavior (e.g., fly biting), and slow response with the animal unaware of the stimuli (mental dullness).

Etiologies for changes in LOC or mentation include metabolic problems (e.g., liver failure or shunts, hyperglycemia or hypoglycemia, hypernatremia or hyponatremia) hypoxia, hypotension, iatrogenic rapid elevation in serum osmolality (e.g., mannitol overdose, total parenteral nutrition [TPN]), trauma, toxins (e.g., ethylene glycol), primary brain pathology (e.g., tumors, infection, inflammation), and drugs (e.g., sedatives, anesthetics). Any pathology can lead to brain edema or hemorrhage and result in an increase in intracranial pressure. When this occurs, the brain tissue is compressed and malfunctions. When severe, the brain may herniate.

Stupor and coma result from an interruption in the ascending reticular activating system located in the brainstem and midbrain, terminating in the cerebral cortex. Localization of the lesion to diffuse cerebral cortex or midbrain-brainstem is important to determine prognosis and detect deterioration in clinical status. Diffuse cortical pathology generally carries a better prognosis than midbrain or brainstem pathology.

Assessment

The veterinary technician must monitor the animal's mentation and LOC. Changes in the animal's behavior, response to stimuli,

or posture may be significant. Unconscious patients should periodically be tested by toe pinch to detect their response to this painful stimuli. Any decline in the LOC suggests worsening pathology and warrants immediate neurological examination and medical or surgical intervention.

In the conscious animal with altered mentation, the cerebral cortex and diencephalon are the sites of pathology. The animal can show behavioral changes, dementia, circling to the side of the lesion, seizures, stupor, or coma. They may also have mild weakness in their limbs.

The neurological evaluation of the unconscious animal should be used to localize and determine the progression of the pathology. Pupillary size and response to light are noted. Normal, responsive pupils or equal, miotic pupils are associated with disease within the cerebral cortex or subcortical structures. Dilated or midrange fixed pupils are most commonly due to midbrain pathology and represent a grave sign. Eye position is noted, with ventral lateral strabismus (lateral gazing) indicating midbrain pathology. Nystagmus (horizontal bouncing back and forth of the eyes) is usually due to a problem in the vestibular system within either the ear or the brainstem. If there are changes in the patient's LOC along with nystagmus, the cause is central (involving the brain) versus peripheral (lesion is outside the brain encasement). Changes in posture, with the forelimbs and neck in extensor rigidity in the unconscious patient (*decerebrate rigidity*), is a grave neurological sign, indicating a midbrain lesion.

Respiratory changes in the unconscious patient imply serious pathology. A rhythmic waxing and waning of respirations (Cheyne-Stokes respiration) is due to diffuse, severe cortical pathology. Apneustic breathing (nonrhythmic waxing and waning of breathing) and uncontrolled hyperventilation are due to a brainstem lesion.

Intervention

Any change in LOC or mentation requires immediate intervention. Alert or depressed animals with a potential for decline in LOC (e.g., trauma, toxicity) require frequent neurological evaluation for any changes. Animals with uncontrolled hyperexcitability may require sedation or anesthesia and a well-padded, quiet enclosure to avoid injury. Bowls and toys are removed from the environment to prevent injury.

Efforts are required to lower intracranial pressure in the unconscious patient. The head and neck should be in a level position with the body or slightly elevated to 20 degrees. The airway is secured in patients that cannot swallow (ET tube) because salivary secretions, regurgitation, or vomiting can cause airway obstruction or aspiration pneumonia. The carbon dioxide level should be maintained between 30 and 35 mm Hg for optimal cerebral blood flow and to prevent or manage cerebral edema; this may require intubation and ventilation. The arterial oxygen must be maintained above 60 mm Hg. Oxygen supplementation may be required. Nasal oxygen should be used with caution because stimulation of a sneeze during nasal catheter placement could abruptly elevate intracranial pressure. An oxygen hood or a face mask is used only with careful monitoring to prevent carbon dioxide accumulation. These decisions are made by the veterinary team.

The tongue is kept moist with water and the eyes lubricated with an ophthalmic ointment. Jugular venipuncture is avoided. Usually, urinary catheter placement is recommended to keep the bedding and patient clean and dry. Frequent and gentle physical therapy and turning are recommended to avoid pressure sores. The unconscious patient has higher metabolic demands and requires nutritional support during treatment.

Respiration and Effort and Breathing Patterns

Pathophysiology

Respiration is the exchange of oxygen and carbon dioxide between the air and tissues. The lung, with its network of capillaries and alveoli, is the primary site of gas exchange with the blood. In addition to the lungs, the airway, larynx, pharynx, and nasal passages comprise the respiratory tract. Other functions of the respiratory tract include control of acid-base balance, defense against inhalation of foreign particles, and filtration of the circulation. The rate and pattern of breathing and the effort required to breath are controlled by the brain and respiratory muscles (intercostal muscles and diaphragm). Normally, the diaphragm is responsible for 80% to 90% of the work of breathing when the animal is resting. When increased work of breathing occurs, as might occur in pneumonia, other muscles are recruited (intercostals and diaphragm).

The rate and effort of breathing can be affected by pathology of the respiratory tract, respiratory center of the brain, or respiratory muscles. Trauma to the chest wall can hinder respiration by making it painful for the animal to breath and disrupting the mechanics of breathing (e.g., diaphragmatic rupture, pressure on the diaphragm, rib fractures, intercostal muscle damage). Metabolic changes leading to acid-base imbalance and pain are potent stimuli for abnormal breathing.

When blood carbon dioxide increases or bicarbonate decreases, the brain responds by increasing pulmonary ventilation in an effort to exhale carbon dioxide and normalize blood pH. Chemoreceptors in the carotid bodies detect increased carbon dioxide levels and stimulate the respiratory center. When carbon dioxide levels decrease, the stimulus for ventilation is removed. In addition, a decrease in blood oxygen content or pH is detected by carotid chemoreceptors and stimulates ventilation through the respiratory center.

Assessment

Clinical signs of respiratory distress change as the disease progresses. The first subtle sign of respiratory distress is an increase in respirations. This is followed by a change in respiratory pattern, which is determined by the site of pathology. As the distress progresses, the animal will assume postural positions of relief, followed by an open mouth and labored breathing. Cyanosis is a very late sign ($Pao_2 < 60$ mm Hg) that often is followed quickly by death.

Respiratory patterns guide the veterinary team to help localize the anatomic site of disease for life-saving intervention. Loud breathing or stridor (heard without the aid of a stethoscope) indicates large airway disease (nasal passages, larynx/pharynx, trachea). Inspiratory stridor directs investigation of the extrathoracic airways, especially the larynx. Expiratory stridor is usually due to intrathoracic tracheal changes. Rapid, shallow breathing is suggestive of pleural space disease (e.g., accumulation of air or fluid). Labored breathing on both inspiration and expiration is most typical of lung parenchymal disease. Distress on expiration, with a short inspiration, directs attention to the small airways.

Auscultation can help distinguish pleural disease from lung disease. Moist lung sounds suggest fluid in the lung tissues. Dry, coarse sounds on inspiration and expiration suggest fibrosis of the lung. The absence of lung sounds indicates that air or fluid in the pleural space is dampening airway noises.

As the work of breathing progresses, the animal will assume a posture to assist the efforts. Cats often sit crouched with their sternum elevated from the surface, and dogs extend their neck, abduct their elbows, and arch their back.

Respiratory rates below 8 or above 30 are considered abnormal (see Table 11–6). Low respiratory rates can be caused by trauma to the brain or spinal cord, diseases that affect respiratory drive (chronic obstructive pulmonary disease, low blood carbon dioxide level), and drugs (sedatives). Increased respiratory rates can be caused by fever, pain, anxiety, trauma to the brain or chest, metabolic alterations (alkalosis), pulmonary diseases (pneumonia or edema of the lungs), and drugs (oxymorphone).

Intervention

TECHNICIAN NOTE

Any change in breathing pattern or effort warrants immediate notification of the veterinarian.

Any change in breathing pattern or effort warrants immediate notification of the veterinarian. The veterinary technician should administer oxygen until a complete assessment can be made. If an upper airway foreign body is suspected, the technician can examine the mouth and retrieve the foreign body with a pair of sponge forceps or by performing the Heimlich maneuver. When the breathing pattern suggests pleural space disease, the technician should prepare for thoracentesis and possibly chest tube placement by the veterinary team.

When respiratory distress is severe, ET tubes and a laryngoscope should be placed by the cage. The veterinarian may need to rapidly sedate, anesthetize, or give a muscle blocker and intubate the animal or perform an awake (with the animal under lidocaine or another local anesthetic) tracheotomy to gain control of the airway, minimize the work of breathing, and provide oxygenation and ventilation. In the event that the animal stops breathing, the technician should rapidly intubate and ventilate with 100% oxygen and have equipment available for a thoracocentesis, chest tube placement, or tracheotomy as directed by the veterinarian.

Heart Rate and Rhythm

Pathophysiology

Rate. The function of the heart is to pump blood to the tissues. The amount of blood pumped by the heart is termed *cardiac output* and is dependent on the rate and force of contraction. The force of the contraction results from stretch of the myocardium from ventricular filling. The amount of blood returned to the heart (venous return) determines ventricular filling; this is also called *preload*. Heart rate and contractility are affected by stimulation of the sympathetic nerves to the heart, and the rate is controlled by parasympathetic nerves. Should the venous return be reduced due to hemorrhage or intravascular fluid loss (e.g., third spacing into the gut, uterus, peritoneum), the heart responds by increasing heart rate (tachycardia) and the force of contraction (inotropy) through sympathetic stimulation. However, sympathetically induced tachycardia can occur with stress, pain, elevated temperature, and drugs unrelated to intravascular volume loss.

An increase in heart rate (see Table 11–6) and contractility will increase the force pushing the blood to the tissues and the volume being pumped. Sinus tachycardia can be normal or associated with shock, stress, excitement, fever, and hyperthyroidism. However, when the heart rate increases above a critical level, not only does the heart muscle exhaust its energy supply, but also coronary perfusion decreases, causing myocardial hypoxia. Cardiac arrhythmias and myocardial failure can result, leading to systemic hypoxia and organ failure.

A decreased heart rate (bradycardia) can lead to decreased cardiac output. Causes of bradycardia include hypothermia, metabolic disorders (e.g., hyperkalemia, hypoglycemia, hypothyroidism), and parasympathetic (vagal) stimulation. Parasympathetic stimulation can occur with brain, pulmonary, and gastrointestinal diseases or a diseased sinoatrial node. Bradycardia can also occur with the administration of drugs that either stimulate the parasympathetic nervous system (parasympathomimetics) or decrease the sympathetic system. Heart rates that fall below a critical level can lead to tissue hypoxia, organ failure, and death.

Rhythm. The conduction system supplies the electrical stimulation for contraction of the heart. The rate at which the conduction system fires determines the heart rate, as long as the muscle responds to electrical stimulation. The rhythm of contractions is dependent on the route of electrical impulse through the nerve fibers in the heart. A normal impulse starts at the sinoatrial node in the right atrium and travels through the atria to the atrioventricular node (at the junction of the atria and ventricles) and then to the bundle of His and ventricular nerves (Purkinje fibers). This pathway provides a normal rhythm.

An *arrhythmia* is defined as an irregularity of the heartbeat, and it can be detected by simultaneously ausculting the heart and palpating a peripheral pulse. When the ventricular contraction has not been successful in forcefully propelling blood to the periphery, a pulse deficit is detected. An arrhythmia can also be defined as a heartbeat that is abnormally fast or slow. An abnormal conduction system or diseased heart muscle can cause an arrhythmia.

Not all arrhythmias are pathological. When the ECG has a P wave associated with the majority of QRS complexes and the QRS complexes are normal in width, the rhythm is termed *supraventricular*. Sinus arrhythmia is a fluctuation in the heart rate with respiration, decreasing with expiration and increasing with inspiration, and it is considered normal in the dog. When the ECG shows QRS waves that are wide and bizarre and not associated with P waves, this is termed a *ventricular rhythm*. Supraventricular and ventricular arrhythmias can be subdivided according to rate into *normal rate, bradyarrhythmic* (below normal rates), or *tachyarrhythmic* (faster than normal rates).

Assessment

The technician should listen to the heart by placing the stethoscope over the left and right side of the thorax at the 4th to 6th intercostal space while palpating the pulse (Fig. 11–8). Pericardial fluid, pleural air or fluid, severe hypovolemia, or herniated abdominal organs will cause muffled heart sounds. Tachycardia, bradycardia, muffled heart sounds, and pulse deficits require immediate attention by the veterinary team.

Intervention

When an arrhythmia is suspected, the veterinarian is alerted, and an ECG is performed. Thoracic radiographs and echocardiography may be required to better define muffled heart sounds.

Continuous ECG and blood pressure measurements may be necessary to detect changes in rate and rhythm. All vomiting animals require close monitoring because collapse may occur due to severe bradycardia from increased vagal tone. Should an arrhythmia be determined to cause impaired perfusion, oxygen supplementation is warranted while the veterinary team is treating the arrhythmia.

Perfusion Parameters

Pulse strength and quality, jugular distension, MM color, CRT, and body temperature are parameters that help evaluate how well the animal is perfusing peripheral tissues.

Pathophysiology

Pulse. Blood pumped into the aorta during ventricular contraction creates a fluid wave that travels from the heart to the peripheral arteries; this wave is called a *pulse*. The character of the pulse depends on stroke volume, heart rate, and force of ejection as well as vascular tone. Evaluation of the pulse strength is based on the difference between the systolic and diastolic pressures (*pulse pressure*). A normal pulse pressure makes the pulse easily palpated and strong. When the difference is wide, the pulse will be bounding (hyperkinetic). Causes of hyperkinetic pulses include fever, hyperthyroidism, patent ductus arteriosis, and early, compensatory stages of shock.

When the difference is small or the time to maximum systolic pressure is prolonged, the pulse feels weak (hypokinetic). Causes of hypokinetic pulses include any disease condi-

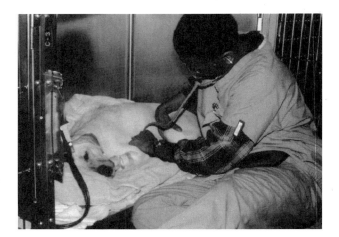

Figure 11–8. Auscultation of the heart during simultaneous assessment of femoral pulses aids the technician in determining whether there is a pulse deficit.

tions that have a decreased cardiac output (e.g., late stages of shock, heart failure, and arrhythmias).

Assessment

Pulses are palpated by lightly placing the index and middle fingers on the part of the body where an artery crosses over bone or firm tissue. The most common pulse points assessed are the femoral and dorsal pedal arteries. In cats, both femoral pulses should be assessed simultaneously to determine whether there is some degree of flow obstruction, as seen with saddle thrombus.

Intervention

Any changes in pulse quality should be reported to the veterinarian. Bounding pulses may reflect pain, fever, or early shock and will require intervention with pain medication and fluid replacement by the veterinary team. Weak pulses are cause for immediate concern and warrant aggressive measures to improve cardiac output (intravenous fluids for shock and appropriate cardiac medications for heart failure).

Jugular Vein Distention

Pathophysiology

Jugular pulse waves are related to atrial contraction and filling. Visible pulsations occur with tricuspid insufficiency, conditions causing a stiff and hypertrophied right ventricle, and arrhythmias that cause the atria to contract against closed atrioventricular valves.

Significantly increased central venous pressure may be recognized clinically by jugular venous distention (Fig. 11–9). Persistent jugular vein distention occurs with right congestive heart failure secondary to high right filling pressures, external compression of the cranial vena cava (as occurs with pericardial effusion/tamponade, tension pneumomediastinum, tension pneumothorax, or right-side heart mass), and jugular vein thrombosis.

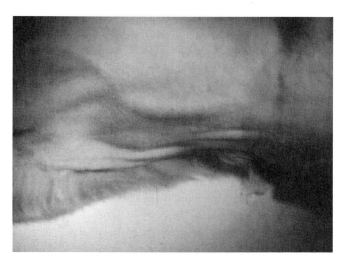

Figure 11-9. Distended jugular veins can be due to venous congestion secondary to cardiac pathology such as heart failure.

Assessment

Jugular veins should not be distended when the patient is standing with the head in a normal position, parallel to the floor. The presence of jugular pulsations higher than one third of the way up the neck is abnormal. Care must be taken to differentiate jugular pulsations from carotid pulse wave. Differentiation is done by lightly occluding the jugular vein below the area of pulsation; if the pulse disappears, it is a true jugular pulsation; if the pulse continues, it is being transmitted by the carotid artery.

Mucous Membrane Color and Capillary Refill Time

Pathophysiology

The normal pink color of the nonpigmented membranes is dependent on an appropriate blood hemoglobin concentration, tissue oxygen tension, and peripheral capillary blood flow. The CRT is a result of blood flow to the capillary beds of the membranes. This flow is dependent on cardiac output and vascular tone.

Assessment

TECHNICIAN NOTE

A CRT of more than 2 seconds suggests poor peripheral perfusion.

Although MM color is most commonly assessed by pressing the gums, the conjunctiva of the eye and membranes of the vulva and penis can also be used. The normal color of a nonpigmented membrane is pink (Table 11–8).

• Table 11–8 •

INTERPRETATION OF MUCOUS MEMBRANE COLOR		
COLOR	**INTERPRETATION**	**CAUSES**
Pink	Normal	Adequate perfusion and oxygenation at the periphery
Pale	Decreased hemoglobin concentration, poor perfusion, vasoconstriction	Anemia, shock, vasopressors
Blue	Cyanosis, inadequate oxygenation	Hypoxemia
Brick red	Hyperdynamic perfusion, vasodilatation	Early shock, sepsis, fever
Icteric	Bilirubin accumulation	Hepatic/biliary disorder, hemolysis
Brown	Methemoglobinemia	Acetaminophen toxicity
Petechia/ecchymosis	Coagulation disorder	Platelet disorder, disseminated intravascular coagulation, factor deficiencies

To obtain a CRT, pressure is applied by the index finger to a nonpigmented area of the MM and then released. The time for color to return to the blanched area is recorded as the CRT. Normal values are 1 to 2 seconds. A prolonged CRT (more than 2 seconds) suggests poor peripheral perfusion (as found in the late stage of shock, severe vasodilation or vasoconstriction, pericardial effusion, heart failure). A rapid CRT (less than 1 second) can be due to anxiety, compensatory shock, fever, and pain.

Intervention

Abnormal MM color or CRT should be immediately brought to the attention of the veterinarian. Pale gums with prolonged CRT necessitates oxygen administration and a rapid search for the underlying cause. The veterinary technician should be prepared to measure the blood pressure, measure the central venous pressure, perform an ECG, or determine the PCV while recording the data. Aggressive fluid resuscitation might be required, and the technician should be prepared for rapid intervention.

Temperature

Pathophysiology

The body maintains temperature homeostasis by balancing heat production with heat loss through a thermostatic feedback mechanism in the hypothalamus of the brain. During illness or a central nervous system disorder, this mechanism may be altered. Chemical substances released in the disease state can reset the thermoregulatory center, increasing the metabolic rate, producing and conserving heat, and elevating body temperature. These chemicals may be pyrogens secreted by bacteria or cytokines associated with inflammation. Primary brain disease (e.g., cerebral edema, brain trauma, or tumors) can reset the thermostat to a higher level.

Hyperthermia creates increased tissue oxygen requirements. The body responds by increasing ventilation to release body heat. Should the Pco_2 decrease to a low level, cerebral vasoconstriction and brain hypoxia can result. Cardiac work load and oxygen demands increased. Peripheral vasodilation occurs in an effort to release heat. Damage to vascular cells can lead to disseminated intravascular coagulation (DIC), sloughing of gastrointestinal mucosa, bacterial translocation, and significant intravascular volume deficits.

Hypothermia results in a reduced metabolic rate and enzyme functions. There is a decrease in oxygen consumption and a decrease in the ability of hemoglobin to release oxygen to tissues. Hypothermia affects the cardiovascular system by causing peripheral vasoconstriction, decreased heart rate, and hypotension. Gastrointestinal motility is decreased, and ileus may occur.

Assessment

Emergency patients should have the temperature monitored several times daily. Patients with infections, excessive panting, or hyperactivity and postoperative patients should have their temperature checked more frequently. Ideally, temperatures are monitored from the same site, usually rectally. Other sites of monitoring include the axillary and inguinal regions. These areas usually are 1 to 2 degrees lower than rectal temperature.

Ear temperatures can be obtained using a ear probe. Serial temperatures taken from the same area are more important than single values.

Intervention

Any abnormal temperature must be reported to the veterinarian, who will determine what aggressive methods are required to cool hyperthermic and warm hypothermic patients. Hyperthermic patients may benefit from being placed in front of a low current of air (blowing from a fan), being laid on the metal surface of the cage or a grate without bedding or with cool towels, having cool compresses placed in the inguinal and axillary regions, having a cool bath, having alcohol on the pads, and receiving cool intravenous fluids and enemas. Cooling measures should cease when the rectal temperature reaches 40°C (103°F) to prevent overcooling.

Hypothermic patients can be treated by covering them with a warm blanket and warm water bottles. The patient can be placed under a heating lamp, but strict monitoring is essential to prevent burns. Circulating warm water blankets are preferred over heating blankets and lamps because there is less chance of accidental thermal burns. No surface heat should be provided without volume replacement because vasodilation from the heat may exacerbate the condition. Severe or prolonged hypothermia may require more aggressive approaches such as active core warming with warmed IV fluids, warm peritoneal lavage, or intracolonic lavage with warm isotonic fluids. The recumbent patient should be turned every 2 to 4 hours to avoid thermal injury. Heating should be discontinued after the rectal temperature is low normal (38°C/100°F).

PHYSIOLOGICAL PARAMETERS ASSESSED IN THE EMERGENCY PATIENT

Urine Output

Pathophysiology

The main function of the kidneys is to excrete metabolic wastes and reabsorb vital electrolytes and water. The volume and contents of the urine produced are a result of the function of the population of nephrons, made up of the glomerulus and renal tubules. The volume of urine produced is dependent on the glomerular filtration rate (GFR) and the ability of the renal tubules to reabsorb sodium and water. Factors governing the GFR are the size of the glomerular capillary bed, permeability of the capillaries, and hydrostatic and oncotic pressure gradients across the capillary walls. Factors governing the function of the tubular cells include oxygen utilization, glucose availability, and integrity of the cellular enzyme systems. Variations in these factors have predictable results. For example, should the mean arterial blood pressure fall below 60 mm Hg, the hydrostatic pressure gradient declines across the glomerular capillary beds and glomerular filtration almost stops (*oliguria*). Severe prolonged hypoxia can cause the dysfunction or death of the glomerular and tubular cells, leading to inadequate urine production. In addition, interruption of the tubular cells' ability to reabsorb sodium results in high urine sodium and an increased urine production.

Procedure

Accurate and frequent measurement of urine output requires bladder catheterization. A sterile soft red rubber or polyurethane feeding tube is used in the male dog, and a Foley catheter is used in the female dog. Open-ended tomcat catheters or 3.5 Fr soft red rubber feeding tubes are used in cats. The use of aseptic technique, with sterile gloves, minimizes iatrogenic urinary tract infections. The catheter is lubricated and advanced slowly through the urethra into the neck of the urinary bladder and sutured to the vulva or prepuce. A closed urinary collection system with a sterile collection bag and IV line is attached with the bag, which is maintained off the floor and below the level of the catheter. The bladder is immediately emptied, and the time is recorded as time zero (start of collection). The frequency of measuring urine output (UO) is determined by the rate of onset and severity of the disease. In general, UO is measured every 2 hours. Daily examination of urine sediment is performed to monitor for infection. Urinary catheters should be flushed with sterile saline and inspected for kinks and clots in the line at least every 8 hours or if there is a sudden decline in collected urine.

An indirect method of estimating UO is to place diaper sheets (under pads) in the patient's cage to collect the urine. The weight of a dry diaper is subtracted from the weight of a urine-soaked diaper. Each 1-mg increase in weight equals 1 ml of urine. An alternate method is to place the animal on a grate elevated off the cage floor (metabolic cage). Urine is then collected and measured.

Fluid input and UO are recorded, including any fluids administered via the enteral or parental route. Quantities of fluid lost through vomiting and diarrhea are estimated and recorded.

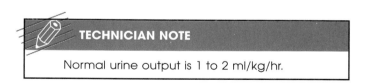

TECHNICIAN NOTE

Normal urine output is 1 to 2 ml/kg/hr.

Assessment

Normal UO is 1 to 2 ml/kg/hr. Oliguria is defined as UO of <0.27 ml/kg/hr, and *anuria* defined as <0.08 ml/kg/hr. However, as urine falls below 1 ml/kg/hr, oliguria is anticipated. Oliguria can result from prerenal, renal, or postrenal causes. Prerenal conditions such as hypovolemia, cardiac failure, hypotension, excessive vasoconstriction, or hypercalcemia can lead to reduced GFR. Dehydration and hypotension will decrease UO (prerenal) until adequate intravascular volume has been restored. Renal changes affect the glomeruli and/or tubular cell function, and potential etiologies include sepsis, trauma, toxins (e.g., aminoglycosides, amphotericin), radiocontrast agents, and infections (e.g., pyelonephritis). Postrenal problems cause interruption of the flow of urine through the ureters, bladder, or urethra and include renal calculi, blood clots, neoplasia, or trauma.

True oliguria in an animal receiving IV fluids will result in a decreased PCV and TS due to hemodilution. The central venous pressure (CVP) will increase, and harsh or wet lung sounds may develop. The body weight will increase rapidly as fluid accumulates. Increasing blood levels of urea nitrogen, creatinine, and potassium suggest renal failure or postrenal obstruction and warrant immediate veterinary attention.

Excessive urine production is called *polyuria* and can be due to IV fluid overload or impaired renal tubular absorption of sodium and water. Other conditions such as medullary washout, postobstructive diuresis, and sepsis can causes polyuria and require large amounts of IV fluids.

Intervention

The technician must evaluate the UO in relation to the hematocrit, TS, CVP, blood pressure, heart rate, and body weight. Any decrease in UO in an adequately hydrated and perfused animal warrants immediate notification of the veterinarian. The IV fluid rate is reduced, and the urinary collection system is examined for postrenal causes of urine outflow obstruction. If the origin of the condition is determined to be renal, the veterinarian will administer *mannitol* or *furosemide* and *dopamine* to stimulate urine production.

A polyuric animal will require a greater quantity of IV fluids for maintenance of normal hydration. Medullary washout often occurs and requires a slow tapering from IV fluids to oral fluids to avoid significant dehydration. Potassium is commonly low in these animals and requires aggressive supplementation.

Blood Pressure

Pathophysiology

Arterial blood pressure is a product of cardiac output (heart rate and stroke volume) and peripheral vascular resistance. Systolic pressure is the pressure exerted by the blood as a result of contraction of the left ventricle. Diastolic pressure is the pressure exerted by the blood within the vessel when the ventricle is at rest. The difference between diastolic and systolic pressures is called the pulse pressure. Mean arterial pressure (MAP) is the diastolic pressure plus one third of the pulse pressure. Any factor that alters cardiac output or peripheral vascular resistance will alter the blood pressure.

Procedure

Blood pressure can be measured directly or indirectly. Direct (invasive) blood pressure measurement requires the insertion of a catheter into an artery (e.g., femoral or dorsal pedal artery) and connecting a transducer linked to a monitor. The direct arterial pressure is demonstrated in waveform on an oscilloscope with the high point being the systolic pressure and the low point being the diastolic pressure. Although direct measurement provides the most accurate pressure values, expensive and sophisticated monitoring equipment is required. A surgical approach is often necessary for arterial catheter placement in hypotensive or obese animals.

Indirect (noninvasive) blood pressure measurements, although less accurate, are more easily obtained with affordable equipment. Blood pressure cuffs can be placed around the distal portion of a leg or around the tail. The two most common methods used for indirect blood pressure instruments in veterinary medicine are oscillometry and Doppler. Systolic pressure should be above 100 mm Hg. Systolic pressure below 80 mm Hg is significant, and pressure below 60 mm Hg may be associated with poor renal perfusion and oliguria. Cerebral circulation is compromised when systolic pressure falls below 50 mm Hg, with brain ischemia occurring when systolic pressures are below 30 to 35 mm Hg for 2 hours. Coronary perfusion is best maintained when systolic pressures are higher than 70 mm Hg. Hypertension with systolic pressures above 200 mm Hg can be associated with a hyperdynamic stage of shock, excessive endogenous production of renin, chronic renal failure, and excessive sympathetic stimulation.

Oscillometric measurement involves the use of a microprocessor and cuff that determines systolic and diastolic pressures from oscillations detected from the blood vessel as the cuff is automatically inflated and deflated. The optimal width of the cuff bladder is 40% to 60% of the circumference of the extremity to which it is applied. It is important when using an automated oscillometric unit to obtain five consecutive readings; discard the lowest and highest values and average the remaining three.

The Doppler flow probe emits ultrasonic signals and detects these signals as they are reflected from the moving column of blood in the vessel. The reflected wave is shifted slightly from the transmitted wave, and the difference is converted into an audible signal. The frequency varies directly with blood velocity. The flow probe is lubricated with ultrasonic gel and secured to the shaved skin over an artery (e.g., the digital or dorsal metatarsal artery). The flow probe is attached to an amplifier that produces the sound of blood moving through the vessel.

A blood pressure cuff with sphygmomanometer is secured to the limb proximal to the probe. The optimal width of the cuff bladder is 40% to 60% of the circumference of the extremity to which it is applied. The cuff is inflated until the swishing sound is not heard. The valve on the manometer is gradually opened to slowly allow the cuff to deflate. The point at which the swishing sound is first heard again is the systolic pressure. The point at which the swishing sound changes from its short pulsatile character to a more continuous swishing, longer-lasting sound is the approximate diastolic pressure.

Assessment

The normal blood pressure in the dog and cat averages 120 mm Hg systolic and 80 mm Hg diastolic. The mean arterial pressure is normally 80 to 90 mm Hg. Increases in blood pressure can be caused by any condition that increases cardiac output, such as fever, exercise, and septic shock. Decreases in blood pressure can be caused by cardiac failure, hypovolemic shock, drugs (e.g., sedatives, opioids, anesthetics). Blood pressure should be evaluated together with the animal's perfusion parameters, UO, and disease state. As with any other monitoring parameter, repeated measurements are needed to detect a trend in change. Renal perfusion over the short term is considered adequate if blood pressure is maintained above 60 mm Hg.

Shivering, trembling, struggling, vasoconstriction, and inappropriate cuff size are common causes of erroneous measurements when using the oscillometric method. There also is a decreased reliability when attached to animals weighing less than 15 lb. Erroneous results can occur with the Doppler method due to malpositioning of transducer, inappropriate cuff size, poor contact with coupling gel, and flexion of the limb.

Intervention

Any blood pressure outside the normal value must be reported to the veterinarian. Intervention by the veterinary team is performed after complete patient assessment, including LOC, CVP, perfusion, and UO. Hypotension may be treated by hemostasis, crystalloid or colloid infusion, and potentially positive inotropes or vasopressors. Hypertension can be treated by pain relievers, diuretics, or, possibly, vasodilators.

Central Venous Pressure

Pathophysiology

CVP is a function of four independent forces: volume and flow of blood in the vena cava, distensibility and contractility of the right chambers during filling, venomotor activity in the vena cava, and intrathoracic pressure. When right heart function and intrathoracic pressure are normal, CVP can be used as a reflection of intravascular volume. Changes in blood volume will result in pressure changes in the vena cava and are reflected by the CVP.

Procedure

Central Venous Pressure Monitoring Set-up (Fig. 11–10). CVP measurement requires placement of a central catheter into the cranial vena cava (through the jugular vein), with the tip lying near the base of the heart (right atrium). The catheter is attached to IV extension tubing, which is connected at right angles to a water manometer by a three-way stopcock. Across from the IV extension tubing on the stopcock is an IV line and fluids. The zero on the water manometer should be at the level of the right atrium. A horizontal line drawn between the thoracic inlet and the manometer establishes the zero reference level.

The stopcock is off to the manometer when the patient is receiving IV fluids. To measure CVP, the manometer is filled with fluid from the IV bag and the stopcock is turned off to the bag, leaving a column of fluid within the manometer. The stopcock is then opened toward the patient, allowing fluid in the manometer to reach the patient. The fluid level in the manometer is allowed to equilibrate with the pressure in the jugular vein. The fluid level may oscillate a few millimeters with each respiration or heart beat. Three values or readings are obtained to ensure consistent readings.

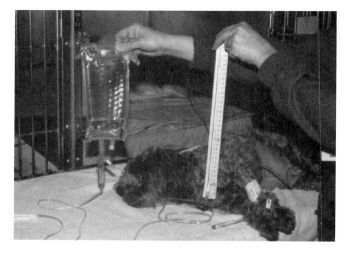

Figure 11–10. Emergency patients require large amounts of fluids during their resuscitation. Monitoring of central venous pressure allows assessment of the ability of the heart to handle large volumes of fluids.

Assessment

Normal CVP measurements are reported as −1 to 5 cm H_2O. However, critical animals are resuscitated to supranormal values, and the CVP is optimally maintained between 5 and 8 cm H_2O. Values of less than 5 cm H_2O are suggestive of insufficient intravascular volume. Values of more than 14 cm H_2O are of concern for right heart failure or significant volume overload. Factors unrelated to right heart function and volume overload (e.g., pleural, pericardial, or mediastinal pressure and increases in pulmonary hypertension) can also raise the CVP.

If readings do not fluctuate with respiration, the readings are inaccurate. Note the side on which the animal is positioned; future readings should be made with the animal laying on the same side. Always use the same zero point reference (thoracic inlet) so readings are comparable. Always obtain three or five consecutive readings at a time. Each reading should be approximately close in measurement. Huge discrepancies in readings should alert the technician to troubleshoot the CVP setup for kinks, clogs, or changes in catheter or patient position.

Intervention

The CVP can be used to guide aggressive intravascular fluid resuscitation. When the CVP is low in a hypotensive animal, crystalloids and colloids are rapidly administered until the CVP is between 5 and 8 cm H_2O. At that time, if hypotension persists, positive anatropes or pressor agents are administered.

High CVP measurements warrant examination of the system for occlusion of the catheter. If the system is patent, then fluid overload or right heart failure is suspected. The fluid rate is lowered, and the veterinarian will opt to administer diuretics or drugs specific for the cardiac condition. Any CVP measurements outside of the target values set by the veterinary team should be reported to the attending veterinarian.

Pulse Oximetry

Pathophysiology

Pulse oximetry is a quick and reliable noninvasive method of measuring arterial oxygen saturation (SaO_2) (Fig. 11–11). SaO_2 is the percentage of hemoglobin sites that are chemically combined with oxygen. SaO_2 and pulse rate are determined by passing two wavelengths of light, one red and one infrared, through body tissue to a photodetector. The signal strength resulting from each light source determines the SaO_2. Pulse oximetry can be affected by the color and thickness of body tissues, probe placement, intensity of the light source, and absorption of arterial and venous blood in the body tissue.

> **TECHNICIAN NOTE**
>
> The use of pulse oximetry can provide an early warning of pulmonary or cardiovascular deterioration.

Procedure

There are several types of probes that can be placed. Probes that are clamps can be placed on the tongue or on a shaved,

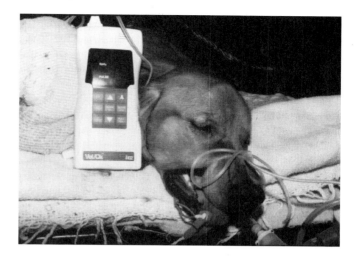

Figure 11-11. Pulse oximetry is used to noninvasively measure arterial oxygen saturation and is routinely used to monitor patients during and after surgery.

nonpigmented skin surface. The rectal probe is placed against the rectal mucosa, which has been cleared of feces. The oximeter is turned on, and SaO_2 and pulse rate are digitally reported.

Assessment

Animals requiring oxygen therapy or under anesthesia should have their SaO_2 monitored as well as physical signs of hypoxia (e.g., decreased LOC, tachycardia, arrhythmias, restlessness, altered blood pressure, increased respiratory rate, and changes in MM color). The use of pulse oximetry for monitoring SaO_2 and pulse rate can provide early warning of pulmonary or cardiovascular deterioration before it is clinically apparent. Normal SaO_2 is 98%. Values below 90% are correlated with PO_2 of less than 60 mm Hg, and cyanosis is eminent. It is of the greatest value when the arterial SaO_2 is between 90% and 95%.

Limitations of pulse oximetry include its inability to differentiate carboxyhemoglobin (seen with carbon monoxide poisoning) from hemoglobin. The pulse oximeter cannot distinguish a declining PaO_2 that is above 100 mm Hg (e.g., a fall from 330 to 100 mm Hg will still generate a report of an SaO_2 of 100%) or the presence of methemoglobin. Results can be erroneous in animals with poor peripheral perfusion, heavily pigmented skin, hypothermia, icterus, and anemia.

Intervention

Any sudden decrease in SaO_2 with proper probe placement requires immediate notification of the veterinarian and rapid assessment of the animal's cardiopulmonary function. The oxygen concentration may need to be increased or the method of ventilation improved.

SHOCK: PATHOPHYSIOLOGY, CLINICAL SIGNS, AND THERAPY

Shock may accompany many emergency situations, so an understanding of its pathophysiology, assessment, and therapy is essential for those providing emergency care. *Shock* can be defined as ineffective circulation and failure to provide adequate oxygen-rich blood to organs throughout the body. Shock is usually due to a failure of the patient's circulatory system to function properly, causing a deficit known as *inadequate tissue perfusion.*

Circulation depends on a proper balance of the following: adequate blood volume, efficient heart pump (effective cardiac output), and healthy vascular bed (vascular resistance). The vascular bed maintains the peripheral resistance necessary to distribute blood and maintain venous return. The vascular bed is composed of a network of arteries, veins, and capillaries or microcirculation (composed of arterioles and venules). All of these anatomic structures normally work together in a state of dynamic equilibrium. However, the heart, arteries, and veins function somewhat independent of the microcirculation. Impulses from the sinoatrial node induce myocardial contraction. The heart, arteries, and veins are also subject to direct stimulation of the sympathetic nervous system.

The *microcirculation* is primarily responsive to local tissue needs. It delivers body fluids and solutes such as nutrients, electrolytes, and oxygen to the tissue cells and removes waste. It also helps regulate total blood volume and adjust and direct blood flow by constricting and relaxing precapillary sphincters. The ability of some vessels in the capillary network to dilate and constrict permits the microcirculation to selectively supply undernourished tissue while temporarily bypassing tissues with no immediate need. The microcirculation includes more than 90% of the body's blood vessels, and at any given time only 6% to 7% of capillary vessels are perfused with blood. If too many capillary bed vessels dilate and fill with blood, the remainder of the circulatory system becomes depleted, and blood pressure drops precipitously.

At the Cellular Level

Shock can be due to various causes, but the overall effect of cellular damage or death is the same regardless of the precipitating factor. Shock is a progressive process, with an initial systemic compensatory reaction, but if adequate intervention is not instituted at this time, decompensation and eventually an irreversible stage of shock will ensue. Regardless of the type or cause, shock produces circulatory insufficiency that reduces blood flow through the microcirculation.

Inside the cell, the mitochondria are responsible for producing the energy supply of the cells. By oxidizing glucose and other nutrients, the mitochondria manufacture adenosine triphosphate (ATP), fuel for all cellular activity. The mitochondria use 90% of all oxygen entering the cell to make ATP; this process is called *aerobic metabolism.*

Eventually, tissue cells supplied by the microcirculation become so deprived of oxygen that they can no longer maintain aerobic metabolism and other normal activities. The cell mitochondria adopt an anaerobic metabolism (metabolism without oxygen). This process permits the cell to continue manufacturing ATP but far less efficiently. As a result, the cell uses up ATP faster than it can replenish the supply and eventually runs out of fuel for other cell functions, such as membrane maintenance.

Anaerobic metabolism also produces lactic acid. Normally, only muscle tissue produces lactic acid, which is then metabolized by the heart and liver. However, in shock, lactic acid pours out through the debilitated cell membranes of hypoxic cells in other tissues. The liver and heart cannot accommodate

this excess, which then accumulates in the blood, resulting in a metabolic acidosis.

Alterations in the cellular metabolism and oxidative energy production of ATP eventually lead to failure of the sodium-potassium pump, causing redistribution of cellular ions and fluid shifts. It is important to remember that the cell is surrounded by the interstitial fluid compartment. The cell membrane, by means of passive and active transport, moves oxygen and nutrients into the cells and moves out waste products.

In passive transport, osmosis and diffusion move substances (water and oxygen) through the cell membrane without any energy expenditure by the cell. *Diffusion* is the tendency of molecules and particles to spread throughout a medium until molecule and particle concentrations are equal throughout. *Osmosis* maintains a balance between fluid and dissolved particles inside and outside of the cells.

Active transport requires energy expenditure by the cell. This transport mechanism handles molecules and particles (glucose, potassium, sodium) that cannot easily pass through the pores of the cell. Hypoxia, which is a key finding that accompanies shock, debilitates the cell membrane, causing these transport mechanism to malfunction.

Increased amounts of sodium and fluid enter the cell; the cell becomes swollen, and eventually blebs or blisters develop on the cell surface. Potassium exits from the intracellular compartment into the extracellular spaces, leading to hyperkalemia. Calcium within the cellular mitochondria contract the mitochondrial compartment, changing the cell shape. This leads to mitochondrial membrane damage. Lysosomes (cytoplasmic organelles containing proteolytic enzymes) deteriorate and release enzymes into the cytoplasma of the cell. Cellular acidosis enhances their activity, and they begin to digest the cytoplasma.

If the cycle is not interrupted, cellular hypoxia (oxygen deficiency) leads to cell and tissue death, the final stage in the progression of shock. As more cells are compromised or destroyed, the tissues and organs they constitute begin to fail. In most instances, oxygen restoration within several minutes can return cell function and energy production to normal.

In conclusion, decompensatory stages of shock ensue as a result of unequal tissue oxygen supply compared with oxygen demand at the cellular level, resulting in a oxygen debt. In shock, the cellular oxygen debt, along with cellular damage and poor removal of waste products, occurs due to inadequate perfusion or inadequate oxygen delivery to tissue structures.

Clinical Characteristics of Shock

Clinical signs of shock develop in a specific order. Patients in shock will demonstrate different clinical signs depending on the stage of shock they are experiencing at the time of the assessment. The stage of shock also determines the patient's acuity level.

Decompensatory Stage of Shock. Clinical signs include cyanotic, ashen, white MM; cold skin; decreased rectal temperature; absent or weak femoral pulses; oliguria (due to pressure of less than 60 mm Hg), prolonged or absent CRT; and unconsciousness, stupor, or semiconsciousness. During substantial hemorrhage, the animal may have had seizures due to low blood pressure. These patients are categorized as class I, or *catastrophic* (multiple injuries, shock, or bleeding but with adequate airway function).

Mild Stage of Shock. Clinical signs include pale or ashen MM, cool skin, low rectal temperature, weak femoral pulses, tachycardia, decreased UO, prolonged CRT, and altered mental status (depression, seizures, uncontrolled hyperexcitability). Hemorrhage may be active or a slow trickle. These patients are categorized as class II, or *very severe or critical.*

Compensatory Stage of Shock (False Stability). Clinical signs include slightly rapid or labored breathing or normal respiration, red or pale MM, normal skin and rectal temperature, normal or bounding pulses, tachycardia, normal UO and CRT less than 1 second or normal. The animal is mentally alert/conscious (aware of surroundings, mildly depressed to excited). Hemorrhage may be slight to absent. These are termed class III, or *serious or urgent.*

Early Compensatory Shock. Class IV patients are less serious, but the condition is still pressing and requires action within 24 hours. Clinical signs consist of breathing pattern that is outwardly normal, normal perfusion or early compensatory shock, red or pink MM, normal skin and rectal temperature, normal or bounding pulses, normal or rapid heart rate, normal UO, normal or rapid CRT, and normal or excited mental state.

TECHNICIAN NOTE

The major goal of shock therapy is to restore and maintain tissue perfusion by expanding intravascular volume.

Therapy in Shock

The main goal of therapy is to restore and maintain tissue perfusion and correct the underlying physiological abnormality. This is accomplished by replacing intravascular volume with a combination of crystalloids (lactated Ringer's, Plasmacyte), colloids (albumin, dextran, or hetastarch), and blood. Initially, the lost volume is replaced quickly through more than one peripheral catheter until the state of shock is corrected, as demonstrated by the achievement of predetermined end points in heart rate, arterial blood pressure, lactate clearance, and UO.

Crystalloid solutions are used most of the time as the primary fluid for acute intravascular volume expansion. When care is taken to titrate the total amount of fluid infusion volume needed to reach the physiologic end point, resuscitation can be successful, without the development of pulmonary edema. A concern with the use of isotonic fluids is the large volume often required for resuscitation. This may result in peripheral and pulmonary edema. Intravenous colloid solutions have in common the presence of large molecules that are relatively impermeable to the capillary membrane.

After an acute massive blood loss, red blood cell transfusions are indicated for restoration of the oxygen-carrying capacity of the blood. The development of blood component therapy has made it possible to reduce the number of whole blood transfusions. Component therapy consists of fractionation of whole blood at the time of collection into red blood cells (packed red blood cell unit), platelets (platelet-rich plasma), and plasma.

Autotransfusion, which is the collection of the patient's blood from a body cavity (abdomen or thorax) and its readministration, is an accepted resuscitative measure in trauma and emergency patients. Antishock garments (to apply pressure to the lower body) may also be used for patients in profound states of shock as a means of increasing venous return.

Pharmacological agents such as vasoactive drugs are frequently required because of either myocardial depression or persistent hypotension after fluid resuscitation efforts. Dobutamine is a $beta_1$/$beta_2$-adrenergic agent that has inotropic and vasodilatory properties and is used to augment cardiac output when persistent evidence of hypotension exists. Dopamine administered at low dosages improves renal blood flow in patients receiving other pressors. At higher dosages, dopamine improves contractility and increases cardiac output and peripheral vascular resistance, causing renal and mesenteric arterial vasoconstriction.

SUMMARY

Emergency nursing is an integral and important part of the veterinary medicine team activities. Should the technician or veterinarian be inadequate or incompetent, the effectiveness of the team diminishes or fails, resulting in the patient experiencing unnecessary complications or death. Once the responsibility of providing emergency care is accepted, we personnel must constantly prepare, educate, and train to be ready. Without highly skilled and trained emergency technicians, the emergency veterinary service cannot serve its patients in a way that both the patient and owners have a right to expect from the profession.

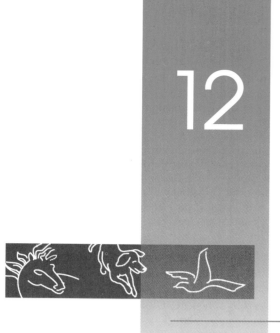

12 Small Animal Medical Nursing

T. Mark Neer

INTRODUCTION

Small animal medical nursing consists of attending to the total needs of a medical illness. The nursing process can be viewed as a traditional exercise in problem solving. Problem solving can be divided into several components: data collection, data interpretation, implementation of a plan, and evaluation of the response to the plan. The veterinary technician should apply each of these steps to small animal medical nursing.

The cornerstone of data collection for the technician is *observation*. Effective observation requires an understanding that many clinical problems are dynamic processes that are capable of rapid change. If change is to be recognized, careful, detailed, and systematic observation is required. The precise system and nature of patient monitoring will vary depending on the specific clinical situation; however, the evaluation of all patients should take place according to a regular and reliable schedule. An important part of any system of observation is to establish an accurate baseline for whatever parameters are being serially monitored.

Observations by the veterinary technician are invaluable in providing optimal medical care for the ill animal. In many instances, the technician has observed the patient for longer periods of time than has the veterinarian. Thus, the technician may be able to recognize changes that are not readily apparent to the veterinarian during routine daily physical examination. Also, the manifestations of certain significant medical problems, such as pain, can be subtle. Dogs may manifest pain by being restless or uneasy without displaying any other sign of discomfort.

Data interpretation by the veterinary technician consists of recognizing and correctly interpreting the observations that have been made. Stated differently, the technician must recognize and define clinical problems. A clinical problem is anything that interferes with the well-being of the animal patient or anything that requires treatment or further diagnostic evaluation. Examples of clinical problems that might be recognized by the technician include diarrhea, vomiting, anorexia, and respiratory distress.

It is important to document that a problem exists before implementing a diagnostic or therapeutic plan. For example, the technician may suspect increased water consumption, but before an extensive evaluation is initiated it may be wise to accurately measure the water consumed over a 24-hour period. In certain instances, documentation of a problem may simply consist of repeating a clinical determination or measurement.

Formulation, organization, and implementation of a diagnostic or therapeutic plan constitute the next step in the total nursing process. Usually, this occurs after consultation with the attending veterinarian. For nursing to be optimally effective, a mechanism should exist for the ready exchange of information between technician and veterinarian. A team approach to animal health care is the ultimate goal, with veterinarian and technician each contributing their unique skills and abilities to the task of returning the patient to health.

The need for thorough observation does not end once the diagnostic or therapeutic plan has been initiated. Frequently, the plan is modified because of a changing clinical situation or because of the response to the specific plan.

When implementing any diagnostic or therapeutic plan, it is important to remember that the quantity and nature of nursing care should always be individualized. One patient may readily accept a specific procedure, whereas another will resist to the point that the intended benefit is lost. Although excessive intervention may be detrimental to certain animals, this should not be construed as an excuse for medical neglect. The fundamental principle is that if a patient is not meeting a requirement for survival, the technician must promptly intervene. Certain animals require tremendous amounts of attention and affection from the technician simply to maintain the will to live during periods of separation from the owner.

Each technician and the head of every animal hospital should establish and maintain consistent standards of nursing care. Veterinary technicians have a professional and moral obligation to every animal patient to provide the following basic necessities:

1. A clean, comfortable environment, as free of stress as possible
2. Food and water at all times unless restricted for medical reasons
3. Adequate exercise and grooming care unless restricted for medical reasons
4. Suffering to be relieved promptly and humanely
5. Every patient to be treated humanely and with dignity at all times

GENERAL CARE

Grooming and bathing are aspects of the general care of the animal patient that are important for several reasons. First, a clean and well-groomed animal has an enhanced sense of well-being and potentially will recover from an illness more rapidly. Second, a clean animal is much less likely to develop severe contact dermatitis from urine scalding and fecal soiling of the skin, which, if it does occur, becomes another clinical problem to manage. Third, grooming and medicated baths are recommended for the prevention or treatment of many dermatological problems. Bathing with shampoo that contains an insecticide is a useful adjunct in the control of ectoparasites. Finally, the cleanliness of the patient at the time of discharge is an indication to the owner of the overall quality of the health care provided.

Every animal hospital should have an adequate collection of grooming and bathing equipment and supplies, that is, combs, brushes, scissors, towels for drying, electrical dryers, and a selection of shampoos appropriate for different situations. Care must be taken to prevent the spread of infectious problems, such as dermatomycosis, from one animal to another via grooming instruments. These instruments should be thoroughly cleansed in an appropriate disinfectant solution after each use.

When clipping or removing hair from an animal for medical reasons, it is important to obtain the owner's permission, whenever possible. This is particularly important in animals used for show purposes. In certain breeds, such as the Afghan hound, regrowth of hair is extremely slow.

Bathing

The basic technique for bathing dogs and cats is self-evident; however, the following points warrant emphasis. The eyes should be protected from chemical injury by instilling a drop of mineral oil or a small amount of boric acid ophthalmic ointment before the bath. Care should be exercised to prevent water from entering the external ear canal; this can be accomplished by placing a small piece of cotton in each ear. Remember to remove the cotton when the bath has been completed.

Thermal injury from excessively hot water can be prevented by constantly monitoring the water temperature. Thorough rinsing with clean water prevents irritation of the skin from residual shampoo. The axillary and scrotal regions of long-haired dogs are particularly vulnerable to residual shampoo irritation. If a cage dryer is used, caution must be exercised to prevent overheating (hyperthermia). Shampoos containing insecticides should be used only with the approval of the attending veterinarian because of the possibility of cumulative toxicity or drug interactions. If insecticidal dips are used, correct dilutions are necessary to avoid toxic reactions. If a complete immersion bath is contraindicated, localized soiling of the animal may be handled with a sponge bath.

Exercise

Moderate exercise is beneficial for the general care of the animal patient. Exercise should take place in a secure, controlled, and safe environment so that injury or loss of the animal does not occur. Contraindications to exercise include many, but not all, respiratory, cardiovascular, and musculoskeletal problems. The decision whether to restrict exercise should be made after consultation with the attending veterinarian. Moderate exercise can be considered the simplest and most basic form of physical therapy and can be a useful means of reducing peripheral edema and improving muscle tone and strength.

Feeding

The animal health technician plays a particularly pivotal role in ensuring that each patient remains in a positive energy balance, in which caloric intake exceeds metabolic requirements. As stated earlier, the technician is in an excellent position to observe complete or partial anorexia (loss of appetite) and to take appropriate action to rectify the situation. In certain instances, merely substituting a more palatable food will solve the problem. Familiarity with the home feeding regimen will aid in the selection of palatable alternative diets. In certain instances, it may even be advisable for the owner to prepare food at home and bring it to the hospital. It is helpful to stock a variety of types of food, such as canned, semimoist, and dry, in a variety of flavors to satisfy even the most discriminating patient. Although not suitable for long-term nutritional maintenance, meat-flavored baby food may be used to stimulate an animal's appetite. In other instances, personalized attention at the time of feeding will increase food intake. Hand feeding will usually be sufficient, but forced feeding may be required in selected cases. Forced feeding consists of manually placing boluses of food in the caudal pharynx to stimulate the swallowing reflex. High-calorie density supplements, such as Nutrical (Evsco), may facilitate meeting the caloric requirements of the patient but by no means will meet the animal's daily requirements by themselves. In many animals requiring forced feeding for an extended period, gastric gavage is preferred because it is less stressful (both to the patient and to the veterinary technician). The technique for gastric gavage (stomach tubing) is discussed in Chapter 10. Other methods of enteral nutrition are being used with increased frequency; these include feeding by way of nasogastric, pharyngostomy, gastrostomy, and jejunostomy tubes. Specially tailored complete diets may be administered through these routes to ensure adequate nutrition in a variety of disease states, such as hepatic lipidosis in cats and renal

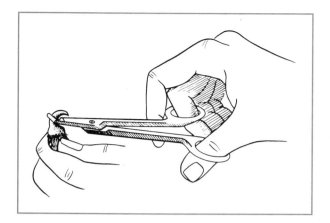

Figure 12-1. Schematic diagram depicting pedicure technique in the cat.

failure. One such complete diet, which can be forced through a 60 ml syringe, is Prescription Diet A/D (Hills).

Nail Trimming

Nail trimming (pedicure) is an important general care technique. Excessive nail length results in altered gait and the potential accentuation of lameness problems. Excessively long nails are more likely to be traumatically avulsed. Finally, untrimmed nails can become ingrown (usually into the footpads), resulting in cellulitis or abscess formation.

A sturdy, durable nail trimmer is required for this procedure. Two common types are available (Resco and Whites nail trim). To avoid cutting pigmented (black) nails too short in the dog, the cutting surface of the nail trimmer should be held parallel to the palmar (plantar) surface of the digital foot pads, and the nail is cut in this plane. In cats, the nails can be exposed by grasping the paw between the thumb and index finger and sliding the skin on the dorsum of the paw away from the nails (Fig. 12–1). Once exposed, the nails can be trimmed as described for the dog. Because certain animals vehemently resent handling of their feet for nail trimming, it is a good practice to routinely give a pedicure to any animal anesthetized or tranquilized for any procedure. If the blood vessel in the nail is inadvertently severed ("the quick is cut"), silver nitrate sticks can be used to stop the hemorrhage by means of chemical cautery. If the owner is receptive, it is desirable to provide instructions in the proper technique of nail trimming so this routine task can be accomplished at home.

Ear Cleaning

The external ear canal may accumulate cerumen, exudate, or cellular debris as a sequela to otitis externa or a foreign body (e.g., grass awn), which then requires cleaning. Certain breeds, notably poodles, Bedlington terriers, and Kerry blue terriers, also may accumulate excessive hair in the external ear canal. The initial and essential step in the treatment of any external ear problem is complete and thorough cleaning of the entire ear canal. Frequently, satisfactory cleaning requires the administration of a short-acting general anesthetic or heavy tranquilization. The first step is to remove any hair that is present and, if excessive wax is present, a ceruminolytic agent (i.e., dioctyl

sodium succinate [Cerusol, Burns-Biotech Labs]) can be instilled to soften the wax. Caution should be used when instilling ceruminolytics into an ear canal when the integrity of the tympanum is not known. If this is the situation, one may elect to use normal saline as the initial cleansing agent. Excessive wax and debris can then be removed by using a soft rubber bulb syringe and a dilute disinfectant solution to lavage the external ear canal. Balls of cotton and cotton applicator sticks can be used to gently wipe the wax from the external ear canal. Some of this debris should be suspended in mineral oil and smeared on a microscope slide to be examined under low power for the presence of *Otodectes* (ear mites). Cleaning the horizontal ear canal should be done gently and with extreme caution to prevent damage to the tympanic membrane or the packing of debris deep into the horizontal canal (Fig. 12–2). If the ear canal contains purulent debris, a sample should be obtained for cytological evaluation (smear) and bacterial culture before instrumentation and cleaning. If bacterial growth is observed, antibiotic sensitivity should be evaluated *in vitro* (see Chapter 6). If the cytological preparation reveals the presence of yeast (*Malassezia*), appropriate therapy should be initiated. Some practitioners advocate the use of pulsating streams of water from a dental hygiene apparatus (Water Pik, Teledyne Inc.) to clean the external ear canal. Approximately 5 ml of povidone-iodine (Betadine, Purdue-Frederick) or Nolvasan solution (Fort Dodge Laboratories) is added to approximately 236 to 384 ml

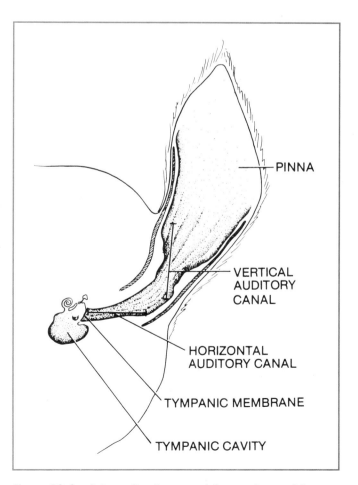

Figure 12-2. Schematic diagram of the anatomy of the canine ear.

of warm water. The stream of water should be applied in a rotating motion and directed parallel to the external ear canal. The excess water and debris can be caught in an ear irrigation basin or similar vessel. An inexpensive alternative is the use of a rubber bulb syringe to manually loosen debris and aid in flushing the ear canal. This technique is not recommended if the tympanic membrane is not intact.

TECHNICIAN NOTE

Ceruminolytics and disinfecting solutions should be used with caution if the integrity of the tympanic membrane is not known. Cleansing with warm normal saline should be attempted first.

Regardless of the technique employed to clean the external ear canal, a second otoscopic examination should be performed to evaluate the completeness of the ear cleaning. Once the ear canal is sufficiently clean, the canal should be carefully dried with clean cotton swabs, and the initial dose of prescribed otic preparation instilled.

Anal Sacs

The anal sacs are reservoirs for the secretions produced by the anal glands. The anal glands line the walls of the anal sacs and produce a foul-smelling fluid that varies from serous to pasty in consistency and is brown to off-white. The anal sacs are paired structures, approximately 1 cm in diameter, that lie between the internal and external anal sphincter muscles on either side of the anal canal. Each sac opens into the lateral margin of the anus by a single duct, at approximately the four and eight o'clock positions of the anus.

Clinical signs associated with impacted anal sacs include excessive licking of the perineum; "scooting," or dragging the perineum on the floor; abnormal carriage of the tail; and vague indications of pain or discomfort in the perineal region.

The anal sacs are best expressed by inserting a lubricated, gloved forefinger into the rectum. The distended sacs are immobilized between the forefinger and the thumb, which remains external to the anus. The sacs are generally found in a ventrolateral location. Gentle pressure is applied until the secretions are forced through the ducts. Because the ducts as well as the sac are occasionally compressed with this technique, if the sac cannot be expressed with gentle pressure, the finger and thumb are repositioned and pressure is reapplied. Paper toweling or cotton placed over the anus can be used to prevent the extremely unpleasant liquid from soiling the patient, environment, or technician!

Bedding

The optimal means of keeping an ambulatory dog clean is by the appropriate use of bedding and exercise runs. Several types of bedding are routinely used in small animal practice; they include newspaper, other types of paper products, blankets, and towels. It is important that the bedding material selected be either disposable or readily and effectively cleaned between uses. Because occasionally dogs will ingest their bedding, it is also important that the material be safe and nontoxic. Most dogs are extremely reluctant to urinate or defecate in their cage; therefore, keeping the cage and patient clean is facilitated by the regular use of exercise runs. Specifically, dogs should be placed in the runs several times a day for an adequate period of time. Dogs should be run individually to prevent fight injuries, and the run should be inspected periodically to be certain that it is secure and free of sharp edges.

Generally, cats are easier to keep clean than dogs during periods of hospitalization. Cats will use litter pans and groom and clean themselves unless they are seriously ill. Litter should be changed daily, and pans or trays should be either disposable or constructed of materials that will allow thorough cleaning and disinfection between uses. It is unnecessary to place cats in exercise runs unless the hospital stay is unusually long.

Decubital Sores

Keeping the nonambulatory patient clean and free of associated problems is far more challenging. Prevention and management of *decubital sores* (bedsores) and urine scald are extremely important aspects of the care of recumbent patients. Animals with various neurological or orthopedic problems can be recumbent for prolonged periods and require special care. Urine and fecal soiling can cause serious problems that can complicate recovery from the underlying condition. Scalding due to urine or diarrhea can be prevented by a light topical application of a protective compound, such as Aquaphor (Beiersdorf, Inc., Norwalk, CT) or petrolatum (e.g., Vaseline) to susceptible perineal or inguinal areas.

Decubital sores not only complicate recovery but also can be a source of sepsis, which can lead to the demise of the patient. The best treatment for decubital sores is *prevention.* Decubital sores develop over bony prominences as the result of continuous pressure and damage to the overlying skin. Various types of bedding have been advocated to reduce the frequency and severity of decubital sores; they include the use of air or water mattresses, foam padding, synthetic fleeces, grids or grates, and straw. The material should either be disposable or have an impermeable surface that does not retain moisture or microorganisms and can be thoroughly cleaned. A potential problem with impermeable surfaces is that urine and moisture tend to remain in contact with the skin and can exacerbate the problem. Therefore, care should be taken to keep the skin surface as dry as possible. This is why, for long-term management, straw is beneficial since adequate cushioning is available for the animal and urine drains through the straw away from the patient.

Other routine measures that help to prevent decubital sores include frequent turning of the patient from side to side, intermittent use of slings or carts to prevent continuous pressure over the bony prominences, and frequent baths to keep the skin clean.

Once decubital sores have developed, they should be thoroughly cleaned with a surgical scrub. Surgical debridement of necrotic tissue may be necessary. After cleaning, the area should be completely dried. Soaking the affected area two to four times daily with a mild astringent will aid in keeping the decubital sore dry. A 1:40 astringent solution of aluminum acetate (Burow's solution) may be made by dissolving one packet

(Domeboro solution, Dome Laboratories) per pint of warm water. Ideally, the area of the decubital sore should be padded to prevent further pressure injury; however, the sore itself should remain exposed to the air to prevent retention of moisture. One way of accomplishing this is to fashion a "donut" from foam rubber and to fix this to the skin by means of adhesive tape. Unfortunately, it is difficult to maintain these pads in the proper location for long periods of time.

Topical antimicrobial agents should be applied judiciously because many contain ointment or cream bases that form an occlusive dressing that will retain moisture. Furthermore, it is questionable how beneficial they are in controlling an infected decubital sore.

Routine Immunization Program for Dogs and Cats

One of the greatest areas of advancement in veterinary medicine in the past 50 years is in the prevention of infectious diseases. The purpose of any vaccination program is to prevent clinical disease by preventing or limiting infection (Schultz, 1982). The vaccination program can also be the foundation of a complete well-animal health maintenance program. At the time of vaccination, owners should be counseled regarding nutrition, parasite control, and matters regarding reproduction. Chapter 14 provides a complete overview of canine and feline preventive health programs and vaccination recommendations.

A physical examination by the veterinarian at the time of vaccination is extremely important because a number of conditions will potentially influence the immunization procedure, such as pregnancy, debilitation, and fever.

Numerous factors influence the patient's ability to respond to vaccination. Factors that are of practical significance include colostral antibodies, vaccine type, route of administration, age of the patient, nutritional status of the patient, and concurrent infection or drug therapy.

Colostral Antibodies

In puppies and kittens, approximately 95% of the circulating immunoglobulins come from absorption of *colostrum* (first milk) shortly after birth. These circulating immunoglobulins provide essential temporary protection, but they also have the ability to interfere with more permanent protection. Interference occurs because the vaccine does not reach the appropriate cells to stimulate the active immunity process. Consequently, it is necessary for the level of circulating immunoglobulins derived from the colostrum to be reduced before successful vaccination is possible. In puppies born to bitches that have received vaccinations against canine distemper and infectious canine hepatitis, this period of uncertain response to vaccination may extend to 14 weeks of age. Thus, the last dose of vaccine should be administered at 14 to 16 weeks of age to optimize the success of the vaccination program. Colostral immunoglobulins to canine parvovirus may last for at least 16 weeks in puppies; therefore, the last dose of vaccine for parvovirus should be given no earlier than 16 weeks of age. In the Rottweiler and Doberman breeds, it is suggested that the last dose of parvovirus vaccine be given at 18 weeks of age.

An alternative technique to prevent or reduce the blocking effect of colostral antibodies on canine distemper vaccination is to use measles virus vaccine. Approximately 50% of puppies at 6 weeks of age will not respond to canine distemper virus vaccination, whereas the vast majority will respond to measles virus vaccine. Measles virus vaccine prevents clinical disease but does not prevent infection. Measles virus vaccine should be considered a temporary method of preventing canine distemper until the dog can respond to the canine distemper vaccine. There is no reason to use vaccines containing measles virus in dogs older than 16 weeks of age. There are no known public health dangers associated with the use of measles virus–containing vaccines. Measles virus vaccine does not provide protection against infectious canine hepatitis.

Methods of overcoming the effects of colostral (maternal) antibodies are not absolute. Therefore, research is continuing in this area. Although colostral antibodies interfere with the immunization process, colostrum is extremely important for the protection of the neonate against a number of potentially harmful microorganisms. Puppies and kittens should never be deliberately deprived of colostrum.

Type of Vaccine

The type of vaccine is very important in formulating a successful vaccination program. Viral vaccines can be either *inactivated* or *modified live* virus vaccines. Because live virus vaccines depend on viral replication in the recipient animal to provide protection, the vaccine must be handled strictly according to the instructions supplied by the manufacturer. Inactivated vaccines are less labile; however, in general they must be administered several times to get an adequate protective response. It is impossible to state that one type of vaccine is categorically better than another; in the future, both inactivated and modified live virus types of vaccine will continue to be used.

To achieve the optimal response, the entire dose of vaccine should be given as recommended; the dose should not be split and given to more than one animal. Different vaccine products should not be mixed in the same syringe prior to administration. Frequently, vaccines contain preservatives that will interfere with another vaccine.

Route of Administration

The route of administration specified in the manufacturer's instructions should be followed. With certain viruses, significant differences in response occur, depending on the route of administration. For example, with measles virus and some rabies virus vaccines, the intramuscular route is much more effective than the subcutaneous route. The manufacturer's recommendations must be understood and followed for all vaccines.

With certain viruses—for example, feline viral rhinotracheitis, calicivirus, and feline infectious peritonitis—vaccines that produce local immunity have been developed. These vaccines are given by the intranasal and intraocular routes. An example of a bacterial disease for which an intranasal vaccine has been developed is *Bordetella bronchiseptica*. The basis for this approach is the concept that if the vaccine is administered by the same route that natural infection takes, greater protection will be achieved. Unfortunately, these vaccines can produce mild clinical disease.

Age of Patient

The age of the animal is important, not only because of the persistence of colostral antibodies but also because of the relative immaturity of the immune response in the puppy and kitten during the first 2 weeks of life. This phenomenon is at least partially due to the hypothermia that exists during this period. Optimal functioning of the cells of the immune system depends on a normal body temperature.

Orphaned pups should not be vaccinated during the first 2 weeks of life. Instead of being vaccinated, pups and kittens should be given *immune serum*, either by parenteral injection or by mouth. The immune serum can be mixed with artificial milk replacer.

Age of vaccination is also important in older patients. It has been shown that certain older dogs (more than 7 years of age) do not respond as well to vaccination as do younger animals. Consequently, annual revaccination is particularly important in these patients to ensure adequate protection.

Nutritional Status

An animal in poor nutritional condition may not respond adequately to vaccination. Generally, caution should be exercised in giving modified live virus vaccines to debilitated animals. However, a debilitated animal should be vaccinated if it is to be hospitalized. Although there is a chance the animal may not respond to the vaccination, it is also possible that the animal will be protected from infection with a virulent organism. If a debilitated dog or cat is vaccinated, vaccination should be repeated when the patient's nutritional status has improved so that immunity is more certain. Every veterinary hospital should establish a specific vaccination policy and protocol and adhere to it at all times. This will prevent errors of omission that could result if the vaccination policy is not clearly defined.

Concurrent Disease or Therapy

Occasionally, dogs and cats presented for vaccination are incubating an infectious disease. A detailed history of possible exposure to infected animals as well as a complete physical examination may suggest this situation. However, it is impossible to definitively diagnose most infections in the incubation stage. If there is a history of exposure to an infected animal, the owner should be informed that there is a risk of their animal developing disease despite vaccination.

Certain infections and diseases may be associated with alteration of the immune system and may interfere with successful response to vaccination; examples include dogs infected with demodectic mange and cats infected with feline leukemia virus or feline immunodeficiency virus.

It has been suggested that certain virus vaccines may increase the susceptibility of the recipient animal to other agents or may alter the natural history of infection with other agents. These interactions have been proposed for canine distemper virus vaccine and canine parvovirus as well as canine adenovirus type 1 (CAV-1) vaccine and the canine distemper virus.

Modified live virus vaccines are not recommended in dogs and cats receiving immunosuppressive agents. Drugs that suppress the immune system are frequently given to animals with cancer or autoimmune diseases, such as immune-mediated hemolytic anemia. Commonly used immunosuppressive agents include cyclophosphamide, azathioprine, methotrexate, and corticosteroids. When corticosteroids are used at anti-inflammatory dose levels (less than 2 mg/kg of body weight), the response to virus vaccines is not altered. Other drugs that are not used exclusively as immunosuppressive agents (i.e., levamisole) may also alter the response to vaccination.

Program Guidelines

When all of the clinical factors discussed are considered, along with economic factors, it is safe to conclude that there is no single perfect vaccination program. Nonetheless, certain general guidelines are possible. Usually, the first vaccination should be administered when the animal is between 6 and 8 weeks of age. Animals should be revaccinated at 10, 12, and 16 to 18 weeks of age. Revaccination should occur annually for the entire life of the animal. Although annual revaccination is probably unnecessary for certain viral diseases, for others it is of critical importance.

Geriatric Nursing

With improved veterinary care, pets are enjoying an increased life span; consequently, the number of geriatric patients seen in small animal practices is increasing. The geriatric patient can be presented with a number of problems that directly influence the nursing process. These problems are generally related to or are secondary to degenerative diseases and other geriatric changes, such as arthritis, deafness, and blindness.

Dogs with arthritis or other degenerative diseases of the musculoskeletal system may be suffering from chronic pain. These animals are likely to react aggressively when an affected body part is touched or manipulated. Dogs suffering from central nervous system disorders (e.g., a brain tumor or cerebral infarction) may also display aggressive behavior.

Deafness is another disorder that frequently accompanies old age. It is easy to surprise or startle a deaf, older dog, and certain dogs will instinctively respond by biting. When approaching a deaf dog, it is important that the patient be able to see you before you attempt to handle it or perform a procedure.

Blindness can occur in older dogs from cataracts, retinal degeneration, glaucoma, and other diseases. As is the case with deaf dogs, blind dogs should be approached cautiously. It is best to move slowly and speak as you approach the dog. Generally, elderly dogs and cats show less response to external stimuli. They appear to be less interested in their surroundings and frequently remain inactive for prolonged periods. In fact, they tend to resent any interference and react aggressively when disturbed. Some dogs forget previous training and may fail to respond to basic commands. Finally, the geriatric dog or cat is resistant to changes in daily routine. The stress of hospitalization alone can sometimes cause rapid deterioration. Obviously, it is impossible to correct or reverse many of the changes associated with aging; however, a willingness to provide gentle, compassionate nursing care is of paramount importance.

Pediatric Nursing

The clinical situation that best illustrates the skills required in pediatric nursing is the hand-rearing of orphaned puppies or kittens. The first step is to determine the caloric requirements of the puppy or kitten. During the first week of life, these requirements are approximately 27 calories/kg/day, 32 to 36 calories/kg/day during the second week, 36 to 41 calories/kg/

day during the third week; and 41 to 45 calories kg day during the fourth week. A number of artificial milk replacers (Esbilac, Borden; Unilac, Upjohn) are available for use in puppies. These products provide approximately 30 to 40 calories per approximately 29.5 ml. KMR (Borden) is an artificial replacement for queen's milk (see Table 12–1 for formula dosage). The following formula can be used as a short-term emergency supplement in puppies: 8 ounces of cow's milk mixed with 2 egg yolks and 1 teaspoon of corn oil. For an emergency formula in kittens, 4 ounces of cow's milk can be mixed with 2 egg yolks and 1 drop of multivitamins. Once the total daily requirement has been calculated, this amount can be divided into four equal feedings. Frequent feedings are necessary to prevent overdistention of the stomach and subsequent emesis and aspiration pneumonia. Generally, it is faster and easier to use gavage via an orogastric tube than to bottle feed.

The technique for gavage is to use a soft rubber feeding tube (Fr. 8 to 16). The tube is marked with a marking pen or tape at a point equal to the distance between the tip of the nose and the eighth rib. The tube is advanced into the pharynx and down the esophagus to the level of the midthorax. A syringe can be used to inject the artificial milk replacer slowly. The stomach capacity of puppies and kittens can be calculated at 9 ml/kg of body weight, and this amount should not be exceeded in a single feeding.

If the puppies or kittens are vigorous nursers, an alternative technique would be to use Pet Nursettes (Borden) or human premature baby bottle nipples. This technique is slower but may satisfy the pups and kittens more, so the incidence of littermate nursing on each other will be reduced.

The neonatal puppy is essentially poikilothermic (body temperature varies with ambient temperature); therefore, it is imperative that the ambient temperature of the whelping box be maintained between 30°C and 33°C. If hypothermia occurs, it will reduce feeding by the neonate and may enhance the pathogenicity of certain viruses, such as canine herpes. To detect hypothermia in neonates, it is desirable to use a low-reading clinical rectal thermometer.

Ideally, puppies and kittens should nurse during the first 24 hours of life to ensure maximal transfer of protective immunoglobulins. If the neonate has not nursed, it is recommended that between 1 and 5 ml of serum be obtained from the dam and either injected subcutaneously or mixed with milk replacer and administered orally.

A highly effective monitoring technique during the neonatal period is to weigh the neonates frequently. Puppies should gain approximately 10% to 20% of their birth weight daily for the first week of life. Postage or food scales should be used to weigh each animal two or three times daily, especially during the first 2 weeks of life. Weight loss or failure to gain weight each day may be the first sign of illness.

PRACTICAL NURSING PROCEDURES

In many veterinary practices, it is the responsibility of the veterinary technician to monitor the patient's vital signs (i.e., temperature, pulse, and respirations).

Temperature

One routine method for determining the body temperature of a small animal is to use a standard mercury-in-glass clinical rectal thermometer. Veterinary thermometers differ from those used in humans in that the storage reservoir for the mercury is short and spherical rather than elongated. Human thermometers can be used in dogs and cats without difficulty. Thermometers can be calibrated in Fahrenheit or Celsius degrees. A Fahrenheit reading can be converted to Celsius by using the formula degrees C = degrees F − 32 × $\frac{5}{9}$.

When taking the patient's temperature, one should first shake the thermometer so that the mercury is below the constriction in the glass tube. The thermometer is well lubricated with petrolatum, mineral oil, or a mild soap and inserted into the rectum with a gentle twisting motion. The thermometer is advanced into the rectum beyond the bulb and is held in place for the minimum period of time stated on the thermometer. The patient is restrained to prevent the thermometer from being broken. The thermometer is withdrawn, and the bulb and stem are wiped clean with an alcohol-soaked cotton swab. The thermometer is held horizontally and rotated until the magnified scale is clearly visible. Because of the constriction in the glass tube, the level of the mercury does not fall until it is shaken down. Finally, the thermometer should be stored in an antiseptic solution (e.g., benzalkonium chloride). Hot water should not be used for cleaning thermometers.

Certain diseases that produce fever display a diurnal pattern (i.e., the temperature fluctuates) during the day. If the patient's temperature is taken just once per day, the periods of fever may not be recognized. If this situation is suspected, a temperature chart may be kept by taking and recording the temperature at regular intervals, for example, every 4 hours.

The normal rectal temperature in the dog is 38.9°C. The normal rectal temperature in the cat is 38.6°C. Excitement or activity can elevate the temperature above these limits. In rare clinical situations (i.e., rectal laceration or rectal prolapse), it may not be possible to measure the rectal temperature. In these situations, the temperature may be taken in either the axilla or external ear canal. The temperature recorded in these sites will be significantly lower than the simultaneous rectal temperature. In general, 2°C can be added to an axillary or ear canal temperature to approximate rectal temperature. These alternative techniques for determining the body temperature are useful when the same site is used serially in an individual patient, and the results are compared. The temperature is taken by placing the bulb of the thermometer deep in the axilla or ear canal for several minutes.

Recently, electronic thermometers and thermocouples have come into widespread clinical use (Fig. 12–3). These devices allow continual monitoring of the body temperature in critically

• Table 12–1 •

ORPHAN FORMULA DOSAGE FOR PUPPIES AND KITTENS	
AGE (WEEKS)	DOSAGE* (ml/100 g BODY WEIGHT/DAY)
1	13
2	17
3†	20
4	22

* Divide and feed four times daily.
† Begin to feed solid food.

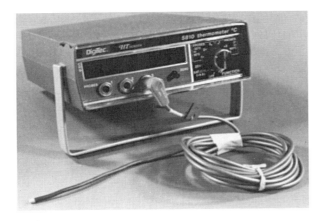

Figure 12-3. Digital electronic thermometer.

ill animals. An infrared thermometer has been developed that records accurate body core temperatures by focusing the infrared beam upon the tympanic membrane. This thermometer is helpful in those patients with very low rectal temperatures or in those for which taking a rectal temperature is contraindicated (Exergen Veterinary Infrared Tympanic Temperature Scanner, Newton, MA).

Pulse

The rate and character of the pulse are valuable means of assessing the cardiovascular status of the patient. The pulse can be palpated in any artery located close to the body surface. The pulse is most commonly felt in the femoral artery. The femoral artery is usually palpated on the medial aspect of the thigh, proximal to the stifle. Palpation of the femoral pulse requires practice and can be difficult in a trembling patient or in a patient with short, heavily muscled legs. Alternate sites for taking the pulse are the palmar aspect of the carpus and the ventral aspect of the base of the tail. The *normal pulse rate* in adult dogs is 60 to 160 beats per minute, up to 180 beats per minute in toy breeds and 220 beats per minute for puppies. The maximum rate in cats is 240 beats per minute.

The heart rate can be counted by palpation or auscultation at the point of maximal intensity of the heart beat. The point of maximal intensity is located at the sternal border between the left fourth and sixth intercostal spaces. If the pulse rate is taken at the same time as the heart rate and the pulse rate is less, it is called a *pulse deficit*. A pulse deficit generally indicates a cardiac dysrhythmia.

The dog can have heart and pulse rates that are "regularly irregular." Characteristically, the heart and pulse rates increase with inspiration and decrease with expiration. This normal variation is called *sinus arrhythmia*.

In addition to taking the pulse rate, it is beneficial to evaluate the pulse pressure and character of the pulse. Decreased pulse pressure may indicate systemic hypotension (drop in blood pressure) secondary to a process such as hypovolemic shock. Instrumentation has been developed for the noninvasive measurement of blood pressure in the dog and cat (Dinamap 8300, Critikon, Tampa, FL) (Fig. 12-4).

Respiration

The respiratory rate should be counted when the animal is at rest but not sleeping. Respiration involves both an inspiratory

and expiratory phase. When counting the respiratory rate, it is necessary to count either inspirations or expirations but not both. The normal rate in the dog is between 15 and 30 breaths per minute. Smaller breeds tend to have a more rapid rate of respiration than larger breeds. The rate in cats is between 20 and 30 breaths per minute. In addition to determining the rate, it is important to characterize the respiratory status of the patient by inspection.

Several terms are used to describe respiratory function. *Tachypnea* refers to very rapid breathing. *Hyperpnea* indicates a condition in which the respiration is deeper and more rapid than normal. *Depth of respiration* indicates the volume of air inspired with each breath. Increased depth of respiration indicates a greater demand for oxygen. Shallow respiration can be due to either metabolic derangement (e.g., acidosis) or mechanical injuries (e.g., fractured ribs). *Dyspnea* is a term used to indicate the subjective impression of increased difficulty or distress in breathing.

All hospitalized patients should have their vital signs monitored at least once per day. Depending on the underlying problem and the status of the patient, it may be necessary to monitor the patient more frequently. The temperature, pulse, and respiration rate should be recorded in the medical record every time they are taken. This will facilitate recognition of abnormalities as early as possible. Furthermore, serial observations will permit recognition of clinical trends.

Administration of Medications

It is important for the animal health technician to be familiar with several basic principles of clinical pharmacology. These principles are important when considering the route of administration of various drugs. Drugs can be administered parenterally (e.g., by injection), orally, or topically. The parenteral techniques routinely used in veterinary medicine include the intravenous, intramuscular, and subcutaneous routes. The specific techniques used to administer drugs by these various routes are

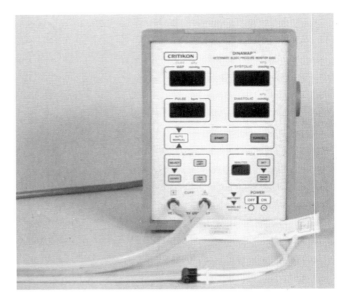

Figure 12-4. Dinamap 8300 (Critikon, Tampa, FL) instrument for noninvasive measurement of blood pressure.

discussed in Chapter 10. This discussion is concerned with the selection of an appropriate route in various clinical situations.

In choosing the route of administration, a variety of factors must be considered. First, the pharmacological properties of the drug should be considered. Certain drugs are not adequately absorbed when given by a certain route (e.g., gentamicin is poorly absorbed from the gastrointestinal tract). Similarly, insulin must be given by injection because it is destroyed in the gastrointestinal tract. Other drugs cannot be given by a certain route because they produce severe tissue reactions (e.g., thiamylal sodium causes sloughing of the skin if it is given subcutaneously). Another pharmacological factor to consider is the rate of absorption. If an animal is critically ill, the route of administration that will provide the earliest onset of action is preferred. For example, an animal with a severe, overwhelming infection should receive an antibiotic intravenously rather than orally.

It is also important to consider the patient when considering the route of administration. For example, it is generally inadvisable to administer oral medications to a vomiting patient or to an animal with severe respiratory embarrassment. The temperament of the patient should also be considered. In a fractious animal, it may be impossible to administer drugs topically, orally, or intravenously. Subcutaneous or intramuscular injections may be the only feasible routes of administration. Finally, convenience and compliance of the client will influence therapeutic decision. Obviously, the topical and oral routes are preferred for treatment at home.

The principal advantages of the oral route are convenience and reduced risk of infection or abscess caused by faulty injection technique. Disadvantages of the oral route include the potential for inhalation of liquid medications and the potential for animals to spit out the medication so the prescribed dose is not absorbed.

Advantages of parenteral injections include, in general, more rapid absorption and greater assurance that the prescribed dose is accurately delivered.

The major advantage to topical medication is that systemic effects are reduced and safety is thus increased. The major disadvantage is that most systemic illnesses do not respond to topical medication alone.

Whenever any drug is administered, it is essential to record the treatment (drug, dose, time) and route of administration completely and accurately in the medical record. The notation should be made immediately after administering the medication. If this procedure is consistently followed, patient care will improve because it is less likely that treatments will be omitted or inadvertently repeated. In addition to improving the level of patient care, it should be remembered that this policy is important because the medical record is a legal document, and every treatment should be recorded in case of subsequent litigation.

It is also of utmost importance that all medications, either those used in the hospital or those dispensed for use at home, be labeled correctly. The dispensing label information should include the complete name of the drug, size or concentration of the drug, number of tablets or capsules or milliliters of drug dispensed, dose and frequency of administration, name of the client, and name of the hospital. If potentially toxic drugs are dispensed, child-proof containers should be used, as determined by state and federal regulations.

Fluid Therapy

The veterinary technician generally will not be called on to formulate a fluid order in a hospitalized patient without supervision of the attending veterinarian. However, familiarity with certain fundamental points will allow the technician to participate actively in this essential process.

The total volume of fluid required to treat an animal can be approximated by considering the volume of fluid needed to rehydrate the patient, volume of fluid needed for maintenance requirements, and volume of fluid needed to correct ongoing losses:

1. Dehydration deficit—estimate as percentage from chart found in Table 12–2
2. Maintenance requirement—60 ml/kg of body weight per day
3. Contemporary (ongoing losses)—estimated volume lost in diarrhea or vomitus in milliliters

Sensible losses are roughly equivalent to urine output. *Insensible losses* represent the fluid lost in the feces and during respiration. *Contemporary losses* are due to ongoing problems (i.e., vomiting and diarrhea).

The hydration status, and thus the rehydration requirement, can be assessed by the following physical examination criteria: skin turgor, dryness of the mucous membranes, capillary refill time, and degree of sinkage of the eyes into the bony orbit. Several laboratory criteria are beneficial, particularly if they are followed serially; these include the hematocrit, total protein determination, and urine specific gravity (SG). Finally, serial body weights can be valuable in determining changes in hydration status. One pound of body weight is equivalent to 1 pint or 480 ml of fluid.

By using the physical examination findings mentioned, the degree of dehydration is estimated as a percentage of body weight (see Table 12–2). Thus, an animal that shows only a slight alteration in skin turgor is approximately 5% to 6% dehydrated. Skin turgor is evaluated by pinching a fold of the skin and subjectively assessing the rate at which it returns to its normal position. An animal that is 10% to 12% dehydrated will display pronounced changes in skin turgor; dry, tacky mucous membranes; prolonged capillary refill time; and eyes that are sunken into the orbits. The physical alterations associated with dehydration are a continuum so an animal that is 8% dehydrated should have abnormalities midway between the end points described. It should be stressed that physical examination findings are at best very crude indicators of the degree

• Table 12–2 •

DIAGNOSIS OF DEHYDRATION: PHYSICAL EXAMINATION FINDINGS	
PERCENT DEHYDRATION	**CLINICAL SIGNS**
<5%	Undetectable
5–6%	Skin slightly doughy, inelastic consistency
6–8%	Skin definitely inelastic; eyes very slightly sunken in orbits
10–12%	Increased skin turgor; eyes sunken in orbits, prolonged refill time, dry mucous membranes
12–15%	Shock and imminent death

of dehydration. The quantitative value of these parameters is improved if they are carefully and critically assessed over time.

The laboratory criteria used to assess the degree of dehydration evaluate the extent of hemoconcentration. Thus, the higher the hematocrit and the total protein determination, the more hemoconcentrated and thus dehydrated is the patient. These laboratory tests are useful in detecting relative changes and do not necessarily measure the absolute hydration status of the patient. If the concentrating ability of the kidneys is normal, a urine SG of more than 1.035 in the dog and 1.040 in the cat provides further evidence that the patient may be dehydrated.

Because changes in body weight over short periods are caused by changes in fluid balance rather than by the loss or gain of body mass, an accurate daily weight can also be helpful in assessing changes in the hydration status of the patient.

The most reliable means of establishing the degree of dehydration is to make a collective judgment based on as many of the criteria mentioned as possible.

Once the degree of dehydration has been estimated, it can be used in calculating the volume of fluids needed to rehydrate the patient. The percent dehydration is multiplied by the body weight in kilograms and then by 1000. This is the number of milliliters needed to rehydrate the patient.

Generally, the volume required to rehydrate the animal is not replaced immediately. One procedure is to administer approximately 80% of this volume over the first 24 hours and the remaining 20% over the next 24 hours. In addition to the volume required for rehydration, the maintenance requirement must be incorporated in the calculation of the daily fluid order. The maintenance requirement consists of estimates of both sensible and insensible losses.

As mentioned, sensible losses refer to the urine output. Insensible losses represent the fluid lost from the body via the gastrointestinal and respiratory tracts. Although sensible and insensible losses will vary somewhat depending on the clinical setting, a useful clinical approximation is 60 ml/kg/day. If the animal is not taking any liquids by mouth, a volume equivalent to the sensible and insensible losses (e.g., the maintenance requirement) should be included in the daily fluid order.

Most animals with problems requiring fluid therapy do not resolve these problems immediately on initiation of fluid therapy. Therefore, contemporary or ongoing losses must also be considered in determining the daily fluid order. For example, if a patient has gastroenteritis, the volume of fluid lost with each episode of vomiting and diarrhea should be estimated and added to the rehydration and maintenance volumes. The volume of diarrhea and vomitus is frequently underestimated; therefore, it has been recommended that the visual estimate be *doubled* to more accurately reflect the actual volume lost.

Routes of Fluid Administration

Oral fluid administration is the preferred method because of reduced expense, ease of administration, and safety. Contraindications to oral fluid administration include vomiting and severe, life-threatening fluid imbalances that require immediate correction.

Many conditions respond well to subcutaneous administration of fluids. Fluids given subcutaneously should be warmed to body temperature and must be isotonic with extracellular fluid. Isotonic fluids have an osmotic pressure approximately equal to that of extracellular fluid. Never give subcutaneously dextrose solutions with a concentration of more than 2.5%; sloughing of skin and abscess formation are common sequelae. The volume and rate of subcutaneous fluids that can be given will vary from patient to patient. A rough guideline for total daily volume is approximately 60 ml/kg. Absorption of subcutaneous fluids will occur over 6 to 8 hours; therefore, this total daily dose can be divided and given every 6 to 8 hours. It is necessary and desirable to administer this divided dose in as many sites as possible. Subcutaneous fluid administration is safe and easy; however, it is not the recommended route of administration when prompt correction of severe deficits is required.

The intraperitoneal route of fluid administration is not recommended. Peritonitis and intra-abdominal abscess formation may result from this form of fluid therapy. The rate of absorption of intraperitoneal fluids is roughly equivalent to the rate of absorption of subcutaneous fluids.

Signs of volume overload include restlessness, hyperpnea (increased respiratory rate), serous (watery) nasal discharge, chemosis (edema of the ocular conjunctiva), and pitting edema. Volume overload can be due to either an excessive total volume or an excessive rate of fluid administration. Decreased cardiac function or decreased plasma protein can predispose to a volume overload state. If volume overload is suspected, the lungs should be auscultated for evidence of pulmonary edema, and the central venous pressure should be determined. Before the development of pulmonary edema or elevated central venous pressure, weight gain may be seen. Therefore, it is advisable to weigh the animal three times daily while intravenous fluid therapy is being used, especially in those patients who are less able to handle a fluid load (e.g., patients with cardiac or renal disease).

Fluid therapy is a dynamic process that must be reassessed at frequent intervals and adjusted to obtain the maximum results. The technician's role in clinically assessing the patient is important in making appropriate adjustments.

Central Venous Pressure

The measurement of central venous pressure is a useful aid in evaluating the fluid status of a patient. When used and interpreted properly, it can substantially reduce the likelihood of excessive fluid administration. Measurement of the central venous pressure is a simple technique that can be performed in all veterinary practices.

To measure the central venous pressure, an indwelling intravenous catheter is placed in the cranial vena cava via the external jugular vein. It is very important that the catheter tip be located in the cranial vena cava at the level of the right atrium. If the intravenous catheter is properly placed, a 2- to 5-mm fluctuation in central venous pressure will be noted with each respiration.

Next, a sterile three-way stopcock is attached to the intravenous catheter. The open line of the three-way stopcock is connected to the intravenous fluid source. The intravenous fluids are used to prime the manometer, that is, the manometer is filled to overflowing with the intravenous fluids. With the patient in lateral recumbency, the zero point of the manometer is positioned at the level of the sternum (Fig. 12–5). The central venous pressure is equal to the level of intravenous fluid in the manometer once equilibrium has been established. To improve

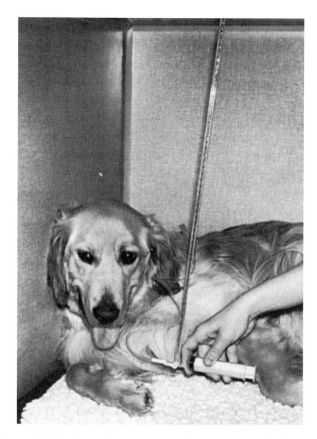

Figure 12-5. Use of a manometer to measure central venous pressure in a dog.

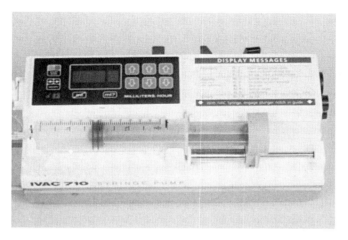

Figure 12-6. IVAC 710 Syringe Pump (IVAC, San Diego, CA) fluid pump used for the administration of small volumes and slow rates of fluid to the cat and small dog.

accuracy, this determination should be repeated a total of three times. If the pressure is high, prevent blood from entering the manometer because a blood clot may alter the measurements.

The following points are important considerations when measuring and interpreting central venous pressure measurements: Serial measurements should be performed with the same zero point and the patient in the same position. If the catheter is obstructed because of blood clots or kinking, the central venous pressure will be falsely elevated. Obstruction should be suspected if the level of the manometer does not fluctuate with respiration. Because continuous recording is not possible, pressure measurements are made intermittently. If intravenous fluids are not being administered between central venous pressure measurements, the catheter should be flushed with heparinized saline. Heparinized saline is prepared by adding 5 U of heparin per ml of saline. When evaluating the central venous pressure, it is better to evaluate trends rather than single measurements. Usually, changes of less than 3 cm of water are not significant. Using the sternum as the zero point, normal central venous pressure in the dog and cat varies between 0 and 5 cm of intravenous fluid. If the central venous pressure is consistently more than 8 to 10 cm of intravenous fluid, volume overload is suspected and fluid administration should be slowed or stopped.

The chance of inadvertent fluid overload can be reduced by using indwelling intravenous catheters and administering fluids over prolonged periods of time rather than using rapid bolus techniques. In addition, Minidrip (Travenol Laboratories,

Inc.) and Buretrol (Travenol Laboratories, Inc.) administration sets can be used in cats and small dogs. Also, syringe pumps are useful in administering fluids to cats and very small dogs (IVAC 710 Syringe Pump, San Diego, CA) (Fig. 12–6).

Several basic types of fluid are routinely used in small animal practice. They include physiological (0.9%) saline, 5% dextrose in water, and extracellular fluid replacement solutions such as lactated Ringer's solution or Ringer's solution. Combinations of these basic fluid types are also used. These basic parenteral fluid types can be supplemented with concentrated solutions of electrolytes and dextrose to produce the desired fluid composition appropriate for the specific clinical situation (Table 12–3).

Frequently, antimicrobials are added to intravenous fluids for administration. A number of the commonly used antimicrobials are incompatible with certain fluids (Table 12–4). The physical incompatibilities include precipitation of the drug out of solution and chemical inactivation. In addition to these incompatibilities, it has been noted that when certain drugs are mixed in infusion solutions, inactivation occurs. For example, when carbenicillin is added to a solution containing gentamicin, the gentamicin is inactivated. As a general rule, it is undesirable to mix multiple drugs in a syringe or intravenous fluids. Frequently, the interaction is visible on mixing, but other times it will not be observed before administration.

• Table 12–3 •

BASIC FLUIDS						
	FLUID COMPOSITION PER LITER					
FLUID TYPE	Na+	Cl-	K+	Ca2+	Lactate	Kcal
Lactated Ringer's solution	130	109	4	3	28	9
Ringer's solution	147	156	4	5	0	0
0.9% Saline	154	154	0	0	0	0
2.5% Dextrose in ½ normal saline	77	77	0	0	0	85
5% Dextrose in lactated Ringer's solution	130	109	4	3	28	179
5% Dextrose in water	0	0	0	0	0	179

• Table 12–4 •

PHYSICAL INCOMPATIBILITIES OF ANTIMICROBIALS IN INTRAVENOUS SOLUTIONS	
ANTIMICROBIAL	**INCOMPATIBLE WITH**
Amphotericin B	Normal saline
Cephalothin sodium	Lactated Ringer's solution, calcium gluconate, calcium chloride
Chloramphenicol sodium succinate	Vitamin B complex with vitamin C
Chlortetracycline hydrochloride, oxytetracycline hydrochloride, tetracycline hydrochloride	Lactated Ringer's solution, sodium bicarbonate, and calcium chloride
Penicillins	Dextrose-containing solutions with pH greater than 8 (i.e., added sodium bicarbonate)
Penicillin G potassium	Vitamin B complex with vitamin C

Blood Transfusion

Blood transfusion is an effective method of fluid replacement but a potentially hazardous form of treatment. Clear indications for its use must be present. The effectiveness of transfusion is temporary. Consequently, every effort must be made to identify and correct underlying problems.

Severe blood loss is an indication for transfusion therapy. Massive hemorrhage can occur after trauma or surgery. Measurement of the packed cell volume (PCV) can be misleading immediately after acute blood loss because of compensatory vasoconstriction, and splenic contraction. The PCV may remain normal for as long as 6 hours after an acute bleeding episode, but the total protein will decrease soon after the bleeding episode and therefore can be used as an early indicator of blood loss. As the intravascular volume is restored by the redistribution of body fluids, the PCV will drop. Collectively, the following clinical parameters are better indicators of acute hemorrhage than the PCV: total protein, pulse pressure, depth and rate of respiration, mucous membrane color, capillary refill time, urine production, central venous pressure, and arterial blood gases.

In the treatment of chronic anemia, blood is used primarily for its oxygen-carrying capabilities and should not be considered definitive therapy. The decision to transfuse should be based on clinical signs (e.g., respiratory distress and weakness) rather than an arbitrarily determined PCV or hemoglobin concentration. Some animals with chronic anemia have been shown to be able to increase oxygen delivery at the tissue level by means of biochemical changes within the red cells. Thus, one dog with a PCV of 12 may be well compensated, whereas another with the same PCV will be severely compromised and will require a transfusion.

Transfusions may be indicated to stop or prevent bleeding resulting from decreased number of platelets or abnormal platelet function, but large quantities of blood are needed to significantly raise the platelet count; therefore, platelet-rich plasma is the preferred method to replace platelets. Because platelets survive for less than 12 hours in stored blood, freshly drawn blood should be used. Transfusion therapy is also useful in the treatment of hereditary or acquired bleeding disorders, such as hemophilia or disseminated intravascular coagulation (DIC). As with platelets, some coagulation factors are labile, so transfused blood should be less than 12 hours old. The basis for this use is to provide adequate concentrations of the deficient coagulation factor at the bleeding site.

Transfusion of blood is indicated in autoimmune hemolytic anemia only in life-threatening situations. Transfusion of a patient with autoimmune hemolytic anemia can initiate or accelerate a hemolytic crisis and increase production of antibodies directed against red blood cells (RBCs). If transfusion is necessary as a life-saving measure, only the absolute minimum number of RBCs should be administered. An initial replacement volume of not more than 12 ml/kg of body weight would be acceptable in this situation.

Transfusions to correct leukopenia (low white blood cell [WBC] count) or hypoproteinemia (low serum protein) are of equivocal long-term benefit and require such large volumes to effect a significant rise in these parameters that they are impractical for this use.

There are eight canine blood groups. Blood groups are designated by the presence of specific *canine erythrocyte antigens* (e.g., CEA-1, CEA-2, CEA-3, and so forth). Any of these erythrocyte antigens can stimulate antibody production if it is transfused into a recipient that is negative for that particular antigen. CEA-1 is the most powerful stimulus for such antibody production. Reactions to CEA-2 are less pronounced; however, they can still be of clinical significance. Reactions to the other canine erythrocyte antigens are generally clinically insignificant. Antibodies directed against CEA-1 and CEA-2 do not occur naturally; consequently, clinically significant adverse reactions do not occur on initial transfusion.

Because 60% of dogs have either CEA-1 or CEA-2 antigens, transfusion with blood from a random donor (i.e., untyped donor) has a 24% chance of stimulating CEA-1 or CEA-2 antibody production. On subsequent repeated random transfusions, the incidence of transfusion reactions is about 15%. Besides the possibility of transfusion reactions, other problems associated with the transfusion of untyped blood include decreased survival of transfused cells in the recipient and hemolytic disease of newborn pups born to dams sensitized by transfusion.

Unfortunately, blood typing sera are not readily available. Therefore, in many veterinary practices it is necessary to use untyped blood. If multiple blood transfusions are required, cross-matching should be performed to detect donor-recipient incompatibility. A major cross-match is performed by combining two drops of a 4% suspension of the donor's RBCs suspended in the donor's serum with two drops of the recipient's serum and incubated in a test tube at room temperature for 15 minutes. The tube is centrifuged at 1000 revolutions per minute (rpm) for 1 minute, and the contents are examined for hemolysis. If hemolysis is present, the transfusion is incompatible, and that donor blood should not be used.

Although blood groups have been reported in the cat, most cats appear to belong to the same blood group. Transfusion reactions caused by blood group incompatibility are rarely observed in practice.

Blood Donors

Canine blood donors should not have CEA-1 or CEA-2 and should be negative for heartworms, *Ehrlichia canis,* and *Babe-*

sia canis. Donor cats are not routinely typed; however, they should not have feline leukemia virus, feline immunodeficiency virus, or *Haemobartonella.* In large blood donor programs, each animal should be permanently identified and have a permanent medical record.

TECHNICIAN NOTE

Canine blood donors should be group A blood type negative and also be negative for heartworms, *Babesia canis,* and *Ehrlichia canis* with serological testing.

Routine periodic laboratory evaluation, that is, a complete blood count (CBC), biochemistry panel, urinalysis, and fecal flotation, will help to assess the health status of the donors. Routine immunizations should be performed as required. The donors should be fed a good commercial diet and receive a hematinic (vitamin and iron supplement).

The ideal canine donor is an 18- to 27-kg, medium-build dog in good health and of good temperament. Approximately 10 to 20 ml of blood per kg of body weight may be drawn every 3 weeks without excessively stressing the canine donor. In the cat, approximately 60 ml can be drawn every 3 weeks without excessive stress to the donor.

Blood Collection

The actual method of collection will vary, depending on the specific situation. The donor that is to be sacrificed at the end of the collection is first anesthetized, and a surgical preparation of the collection site is performed. Possible collection sites in the dog include the jugular vein, heart, or femoral artery. In the cat, the jugular vein and heart are possible sites. In permanent donors, the jugular vein is the preferred site. Blood collection should be performed rapidly and without interruption, using a single site to avoid excessive activation of the clotting cascade and damage to the RBCs. If acid citrate dextrose (ACD Evacuated Blood Collection Bottle, Diamond Laboratories, Inc.) is being used, a separate collection set should be used. If citrate phosphate dextrose (CPD) plastic Blood Pack Units (with Integral Donor Tube, Fenwall Laboratories, Inc.) are used, the attached needle should be used. If the vacuum bottles are used, care should be taken not to lose the vacuum at the time of venipuncture.

In the cat, a 19-gauge butterfly needle (Travenol Laboratories) and a large syringe containing the desired anticoagulant can be used.

Several anticoagulants are available for routine collection of blood. Blood drawn in heparin must be used within 24 to 48 hours because of the marked increase in pH and the subsequent decrease in red cell adenosine triphosphate observed when heparin is used as an anticoagulant. These chemical changes result in rigid red cells that do not deform and thus are rapidly removed from the recipient's circulation.

If blood is to be stored for longer than 48 hours, either acid citrate dextrose (ACD Evacuated Blood Collection Bottle) or citrate phosphate dextrose (CPD Blood Pack Units with Integral Donor Tube) must be used as the anticoagulant and

the blood stored at 1°C to 6°C. The temperature cannot vary by more than 2°C, and if the blood is out of refrigeration long enough to warm to 10°C (approximately 30 minutes), it must be used immediately. During storage, the blood should be gently mixed periodically. When collected and stored as described, blood drawn in ACD has an effective storage life of approximately 14 days, and blood drawn in CPD has an effective storage life of approximately 21 days. Blood stored beyond these limits will have reduced post-transfusion survival. The CPD plastic packs generally require the use of a vacuum collection device. This device provides negative-powered pressure for quick, efficient filling as well as a means of gently mixing the blood with the anticoagulant. Each pack or bottle should be immediately labeled with the donor's name, expiration date, and blood type.

Blood should be gradually warmed to approximately 37°C before administration. Refrigerated blood can be warmed by passing it through a coiled tube in a 40°C water bath or by other appropriate means. Care should be exercised to prevent excessive warming (more than 50°C). Excessive warming will cause hemolysis.

It is essential that strict asepsis be maintained during collection, storage, and administration of blood and blood products. Once a blood storage container has been entered, the stored blood should be used within 24 hours.

Blood should be administered through a sterile blood administration kit (Blood Administration Set, Diamond Laboratories, Inc.). A micropore filter is suggested to reduce the transfusion of microemboli found in stored blood.

If the practice has a frequent demand for transfusion therapy, it is desirable to make optimal use of the available donors by separating blood into its components and administering only the needed component. Packed red cells can be produced by either centrifugation or by sedimentation of whole blood. Sedimented packed red cells are separated from plasma by gravity. The recovery of plasma is less efficient by this method; however, a centrifuge is not necessary. If collected in glass vacuum bottles, approximately 25% to 30% of the blood volume separates into plasma by 7 to 9 days, and 45% of the blood volume is available as plasma after 14 to 16 days. Plasma is harvested from the glass collection bottles with a sterile 17.5-cm needle and a sterile syringe. Blood in plastic packs separates more rapidly than blood in glass bottles. Plasma can be collected from plastic packs by means of either a sterile needle and syringe or a plasma transfer pack (Plasma Transfer Sets, Fenwall Laboratories) and a plasma extractor (Plasma Extractor, Fenwall Laboratories). The plasma transfer packs have attached tubing and adaptors as well as sealable entry ports. Thus, the plasma can be collected in a closed, sterile system. If the plasma is to be stored at refrigerator temperatures (1°C to 6°C) for longer than 24 hours, a closed system is essential. Plasma frozen at less than −20°C has a storage life of longer than 1 year. If frozen plasma is to be used to treat bleeding disorders, it should be frozen within a few hours of collection.

If the major indication for transfusion is decreased oxygen-carrying capability, the patient should receive packed red cells. Packed red cells can be administered rapidly with less risk of creating volume overload in a patient with compromised cardiovascular function. The use of packed red cells will also reduce the frequency of transfusion reactions caused by plasma protein incompatibility.

Plasma transfusions are used primarily to expand the extracellular fluid volume. Plasma is also used for its transient benefit in the management of hypoproteinemia. Fresh frozen plasma is a source of coagulation factors V and VIII.

Transfusion Reactions

Complications of blood transfusion can be both immunological and nonimmunological in origin. Immunological reactions can result from the transfusion of incompatible blood. Incompatible RBCs in a previously unsensitized recipient will be destroyed 7 to 10 days after transfusion. If the recipient is subsequently exposed to incompatible blood, a more acute hemolytic reaction may occur. Clinical consequences of hemolytic transfusion reactions include the rapid development of tachycardia, hypotension, vomiting, salivation, and muscle tremors. Laboratory changes associated with significant acute hemolysis include hemoglobinemia, hemoglobinuria, and possible acquired coagulation disorders.

Delayed hemolytic reactions will sometimes occur following multiple transfusions. Delayed hemolysis should be suspected if the PCV drops unexpectedly 2 to 21 days after transfusion. The clinical and laboratory signs of acute hemolysis mentioned may not be detected in delayed hemolytic reactions. Transfusion reactions may also be caused by immunological reactions due to leukocyte, platelet, or plasma protein incompatibilities. Reactions between antigens and antibodies may activate the complement system and thus release vasoactive substances that may be responsible for trembling, vomiting, and urticaria (hives). Prior transfusion is not required for these reactions to occur. Some authorities have advocated the use of antihistamines (diphenhydramine hydrochloride) approximately 30 minutes before transfusion to reduce these reactions.

Transfusion-induced fever is due to the response of the donor to foreign proteins. The initial step in controlling transfusion-induced fever is to slow the rate of transfusion. If no response is noted when the rate is reduced, antipyretics, such as aspirin, should be administered. Bacterial contamination of the transfused blood will also produce fever.

Nonimmunological transfusion reactions are principally due to vascular overload. Signs of vascular overload include a dry cough, respiratory distress, and vomiting. If there is evidence of preexisting cardiac dysfunction, the rate of administration of blood should be reduced to approximately 1 ml/kg/hr. Because vomiting is a potential adverse reaction to transfusion, food and water should be withheld from the patient during the transfusion.

Physical Therapy

Physical therapy can be defined as the use of cold, heat, water, electrical impulses, and therapeutic exercise to treat an injury or disease. When used appropriately, these techniques can either prevent permanent dysfunction or hasten the return of normal function. Physical therapy is especially useful in treating diseases of the musculoskeletal and neuromuscular systems.

Physical therapy can be of tremendous value in reducing muscle spasm, relieving pain, resolving peripheral edema, improving blood supply to a specific site, improving muscle tone, and increasing the range of motion of a joint.

In veterinary practice basically five treatment modalities are employed: (1) superficial heat, (2) cold, (3) massage, (4) active exercise, and (5) electrical stimulation. All of these forms of treatment will influence blood supply and edema.

Superficial heat increases the temperature of local tissues, which results in increased metabolism, improved blood supply and mild analgesia. In contrast, deep heat (e.g., *diathermy*) can potentially increase peripheral edema by increasing capillary hydrostatic pressure. Superficial heat can be applied by means of whirlpool baths, hot packs, or infrared radiation. Moist heat is preferred to dry heat because of its greater action in reducing pain and muscle spasms. Use of a whirlpool bath provides superficial heat as well as buoyancy to support the affected body part (Fig. 12–7). The jet streams of warm water can also stimulate peripheral nerves and cleanse soiled areas. The technique for applying hot packs is to soak a towel or cloth in water as hot as the technician can comfortably stand, wring lightly, and apply to the affected part. As the temperature of the towel decreases, the towel can be rinsed with hot water and reapplied. Twenty minutes is an adequate period of time for this form of heat treatment.

In most traumatic injuries, *early* application of cold will reduce swelling and muscle spasm. Towels or cloths soaked in either cold water or ice water and wrung lightly are a means of applying cold to an animal patient. Alternatively, commercial cold packs or ice packs can be used; however, they should be used with caution in order to prevent cold-induced injury. Fifteen to 20 minutes are usually required for treatment.

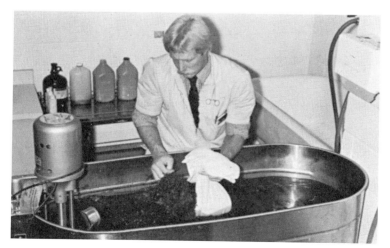

Figure 12-7. Patient receiving a whirlpool bath while being supported with a towel.

If peripheral edema is present, massage may be beneficial. The technique for therapeutic massage consists of gentle stroking and light kneading of the involved area. An attempt should be made to direct the peripheral edema from the involved area toward the heart. This will enhance venous return of the edematous fluid.

Active movement should be encouraged as soon as it can be accomplished safely and without pain. Active movement can be accomplished by swimming the patient in a whirlpool or bathtub. Most animals will swim with encouragement and then actively exercise a body part that otherwise would not be exercised. A towel or sling can be used for support and to keep the animal upright. When appropriate, therapeutic exercise can occur on any nonslippery surface. If the patient is not able to ambulate without assistance, a towel or sling can provide the necessary support. Active therapeutic exercise is of greater benefit than passive exercise.

Although not widely used in veterinary practice, electrical stimulation is beneficial in the treatment of some neuromuscular diseases and neurogenic atrophy.

Owners of animals that would benefit from physical therapy are usually willing to perform physical therapy at home. However, the owner must be carefully instructed on how to perform the treatments and why it will be beneficial to the patient. The technician is usually the best person in the practice to demonstrate the proper technique.

Oxygen Therapy

The primary indication for oxygen therapy is *hypoxia,* which refers to a deficiency of oxygen at the tissue level. Tissue hypoxia may be due to a reduction in perfusion (reduced blood flow) or a reduction in oxygen content of the blood. Hypoxia is probably more common than is recognized in veterinary medicine because a caged animal at rest will not show signs until the oxygen content of the blood is severely reduced.

Hypoxia can be manifested in a variety of ways, and the veterinary technician must be alert to identify these changes. Abnormalities that may be noted in the cardiovascular system include tachycardia or dysrhythmias. An increased respiratory rate, open-mouthed breathing and dyspnea may also be noted. *Dyspnea* is the term used to indicate subjective difficulty or distress in breathing. With severe hypoxia, central nervous system changes may be noted and include drowsiness, altered motor abilities, or increased excitability. Finally, cold extremities may indicate an inadequate supply of oxygen at the tissue level. *Cyanosis* is not a reliable indicator of hypoxia, especially if the animal is anemic. Cyanosis refers to dark bluish or purplish discoloration of the skin and mucous membranes.

Although the basic defect in hypoxia is decreased oxygen availability at the tissue level, it can occur by a variety of mechanisms. For example, it can result from lung disease, decreased cardiac output, or severe anemia.

In small animal practice, oxygen therapy is used primarily in the following clinical situations: pulmonary edema, severe bronchopneumonia, upper airway disease in brachycephalic breeds such as English bulldog and Boston terrier, pulmonary trauma, atelectasis of lung lobes, and shock.

Methods of oxygen therapy include oxygen cages, human pediatric incubators, masks, nasal catheters, endotracheal tubes, and intratracheal catheters.

Oxygen Cage

Oxygen cages for veterinary use are sold commercially. These cages permit control of not only the oxygen concentration but also temperature and humidity (Fig. 12–8). These cages are useful in animals able to ventilate without assistance. However, they are expensive and consume large amounts of oxygen. Surplus human pediatric incubators are a less expensive means of providing similar therapy to small dogs, cats, or exotic animal. Oxygen cages and incubators should be flushed (filled) with oxygen after they have been opened. Some units are equipped with entry ports that allow access to the patient without excessive loss of oxygen.

Mask Induction

In certain circumstances, masks can be used to administer oxygen. Masks are available in a variety of sizes and shapes suitable for use in dogs and cats. If an oxygen mask is used, it is important to provide a high oxygen flow rate to prevent excessive accumulation of carbon dioxide. Administration of oxygen via a mask is suitable for short periods of time only and only in selected patients. Some patients will resist the use of an oxygen mask, and the resultant stress will negate any beneficial effect of the oxygen.

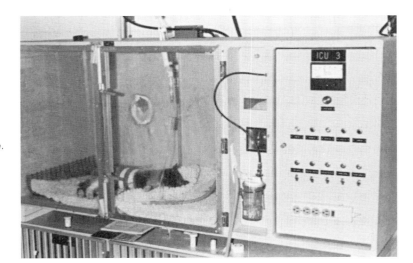

Figure 12-8. Small animal oxygen cage.

Intratracheal Catheter Induction

An alternative means of oxygen administration that is both inexpensive and effective is the intratracheal catheter. This technique is reserved for critically ill patients. The skin is aseptically prepared, and a local anesthetic is administered over the trachea in the midcervical area. An intravenous catheter (14, 16, or 18 gauge) is introduced into the trachea and advanced to a point craniad to the bifurcation of the trachea. The delivered oxygen should be humidified and administered at a flow rate of 0.5 to 4 L/min. The flow rate should be adjusted, depending on the size of the animal.

Nasal Catheter Induction

Nasal catheters can also be used to administer oxygen for brief periods to severely depressed animals. In this technique, a small (5 to 8 Fr) soft rubber feeding tube or urinary catheter is inserted through the external nares to the level of the caudal nasopharynx. The catheter can be coated with a topical anesthetic cream, or topical anesthetic drops can be instilled in the nostril to facilitate passage. Adhesive tape is attached to the catheter, and the tape is sutured to the forehead. An Elizabethan collar should be used to prevent the patient from dislodging the catheter.

An inspired oxygen concentration of 30% to 40% is adequate for animals requiring oxygen therapy. Excessively high oxygen concentrations can result in oxygen toxicity. Neonatal kittens appear to be particularly susceptible to retinal changes induced by oxygen toxicity.

Respiratory Physical Therapy

Physical therapy of the respiratory system is a valuable adjunct to other forms of therapy for diseases of the lungs and airways. Appropriate physical therapy is also useful as a preventative measure in patients at high risk for the development of pulmonary disease. Secondary bronchopneumonia is a common complication in patients with atelectasis. Stimulation of the cough reflex by compressing the trachea will expand the lungs maximally and prevent atelectasis. Regular turning of recumbent patients will enhance drainage and circulation and thus prevent hypostatic congestion.

Percussion (coupage), also known as *tapping* or *clapping*, is a technique of striking the animal's chest to loosen bronchial secretion and thus facilitate drainage. The chest is struck with the hand held slightly cupped with fingers and thumb closed so a cushion of air is trapped between the technician's hand and the chest wall. Best results come from using both hands alternately in rapid sequence for several seconds, moving from ventral to dorsal on the lung fields. When done properly, this is a noisy procedure; however, it is not painful to the patient. An electric hand vibrator can be used to set up fine vibration that will also aid the drainage of secretions. If the animal is ambulatory, a brief walk after coupage will aid in mobilization of respiratory secretions.

Whenever possible, animals with pulmonary problems should be maintained in an upright position (i.e., sternal recumbency). If necessary, slings or supports should be used to maintain this posture. This position will decrease the amount of hypostatic congestion that develops.

Topical Therapy

Topical therapy plays an important role in the treatment of dermatological disease. It can be used to treat a specific disease, such as sarcoptic mange. More frequently, however, topical therapy is used either in conjunction with systemic medications or as a form of symptomatic therapy when the diagnosis is unknown.

Plain tap water is one of the most effective topical agents. Depending on how water is used, it can either hydrate or dehydrate the skin. Frequent wetting of the skin will stimulate evaporation from the skin and thus cause dehydration. This approach can be useful in managing any acute moist dermatitis ("hot spot"). In contrast, if a film of oil (e.g., Alpha Keri, Westwood Pharmaceuticals, Inc.) is applied immediately after soaking with water, evaporation is slowed or stopped, and the skin remains moist.

Soaks

Soaks are an effective means of handling localized acute eruptions. Soaks can be applied with moist towels or by placing the animal in a water-filled basin or tub. Soaks for local acute dermatosis should be applied for 10 to 15 minutes three or more times daily. The involved area should be kept constantly moist, and the warm temperature of the soak should be maintained by adding hot water as needed. Some of the solutions commonly used for soaks in veterinary medicine include water, aluminum acetate (Burow's solution, Domeboro solution, Dome Laboratories) and magnesium sulfate (1:65 solution in water, 1 tablespoonful per 1000 ml of water).

Astringents

Astringents precipitate proteins on the surface of an area of acute damage and form a beneficial covering. These agents do not penetrate deeply. Aluminum acetate is an excellent mild astringent. Another effective astringent is tannic acid. Tannic acid is combined with salicylic acid and alcohol in several products to form a potent astringent. These combination products are especially useful as part of the management of localized acute moist dermatitis; however, this agent should be applied only once to an involved area.

Baths

Cleansing baths are an important part of topical dermatological therapy. Baths aid in the removal of dirt, debris, and scale. A variety of effective mild cleansing soaps or detergents are available. Mild dishwashing detergents or soaps (e.g., Joy and Palmolive liquid) are effective and inexpensive. If a milder, less irritating product is desired, a balanced pH soap, such as Johnson's Baby Shampoo (Johnson & Johnson), can be used. If an even milder product is needed, vegetable oil soaps (coconut oil) are the most bland. Regardless of how mild the soap or detergent, it should always be thoroughly rinsed out of the coat with copious volumes of clean water.

A medicated bath can be applied as a shampoo or as a rinse applied to the animal after a routine cleansing bath. Medicated baths contain ingredients that enhance the actions of routine cleansing shampoos. Medicated shampoos should be lathered into the coat for 10 to 15 minutes. This allows the medicated component of the shampoo time for effect or limited absorption. Types of medicated baths used in small animal practice include colloidal oatmeal, tar-sulfur, sulfur-salicylic, and benzoyl peroxide products. Colloidal oatmeal (Aveeno, Cooper Care, Inc., and Epi-Soothe cream rinse, Allerderm, Inc.) baths are used for their soothing and antipruritic properties. Tar-sulfur shampoos (Lytar, Dermatologics for Veterinary Medicine, Inc., and Allerseb-T, Allerderm, Inc.) are used in the management of oily, flaky seborrheic conditions. Sulfur and salicylic shampoos (Sebalyte, Dermatologics for Veterinary Medicine, Inc., and Sebolux, Allerderm, Inc.) are used in the management of dry, flaky seborrheic conditions, and benzoyl peroxide shampoos (Oxydex, Dermatologics for Veterinary Medicine, Inc., and Pyoben, Allerderm, Inc.) are useful in the treatment of superficial pyoderma (bacterial skin infection), excessive crusting and debris problems and oily seborrheic conditions. The underlying condition and the individual response to the medicated bath determine the required frequency of application.

Dips and Rinses

Dips or rinses use water as a means of delivering various antifungal or antiparasitic agents to the skin. Although applied to the skin, some of these agents have the potential to cause systemic toxicities. Clipping the hair and using cleansing baths help to obtain greater penetration in animals with excessive scale or crust. Dips that are useful in the treatment of dermatophytosis (ringworm) include dilute sodium hypochlorite solution, dilute Nolvasan solution (Fort Dodge Laboratories), dilute iodine solutions, or lime-sulfur solutions. Antiparasitic products used as dips or rinses include chlorpyrifos (Dursban), pyrethrins, pyrethroids, organophosphates (malathion), and carbamates. Amitraz (Mitaban, Upjohn Co.) is useful in the treatment of generalized demodectic mange.

Before using any topical agent the label should be checked to be sure it is safe to use in dogs, cats, puppies, and kittens. The age of young animals should be noted as some products are not recommended in the very young.

Powders

Powders are occasionally used in veterinary medicine as drying agents and vehicles for parasiticides and to reduce friction and irritation. When used as a drying agent, powders may be in the form of true powders, shake lotions, or pastes. Components that improve the drying action of various powdered products include talc, zinc oxide, cornstarch, and tannic acid. Carbaryl powders are a valuable part of flea control programs in the dog and cat. Labels should be checked carefully to be certain that the specific product is safe for dogs and cats. The powder must be worked down into the hair coat to increase the parasiticidal effect. This can be accomplished by rubbing the hair coat against the grain as the powder is applied. The powder should be applied to the entire body, excluding the face. Fractious or frightened cats can be treated by wrapping them in a thick bath towel and medicating small sections until the entire animal has been covered. Flea sprays can be used similarly.

Creams and Ointments

Creams and ointments are also used in the topical treatment of dermatological problems. The area of treatment should be clipped, if not hairless, and protected from immediate removal by licking. For practical and economic reasons, the area to be treated should be relatively small. Ointments are thicker than creams and leave a greasy feeling when applied to the skin. Ointments and creams soften, lubricate and protect the skin, and aid in the removal of scale and crusts. Ointments and creams form an occlusive covering and therefore are not indicated for moist or oozing skin lesions.

Topical creams and ointments can be used to treat localized dermatophytosis (ringworm). They can be used as the sole type of therapy or as an adjunct to oral therapy or topical rinses. Creams and ointments must be restricted to small lesions because of expense and convenience. Effective topical fungicidal products used in veterinary medicine contain miconazole and thiabendazole. Because the use of ointments and creams alone is often insufficient to clear the infection or prevent reinfection, rinses or dips are important.

Otic Preparations

Most topical otic preparations contain various combinations of antibiotic, anti-inflammatory, fungicidal, and parasiticidal agents. Topical antimicrobial agents are indicated whenever infection is present. Chloramphenicol, neomycin, polymyxin, and gentamicin are the commonly used antibiotics in these combination otic preparations. Neomycin and gentamicin have been reported to cause ototoxicity when used for prolonged periods in dogs with ruptured eardrums. (Gentamicin is inactivated by pus; therefore, the ears must be thoroughly cleaned before use.)

Corticosteroids are used in these combination products because they decrease inflammation and the build-up of discharge and, consequently, decrease self-trauma by the animal. The antifungals are useful in treating dermatophytes and yeast organisms such as *Malassezia pachydermitis* (*Pityrosporon*). Thiabendazole and miconazole are effective topical antifungal agents.

Certain drugs owe their efficacy to their ability to alter the pH in the ear canal. Acetic acid (dilute vinegar solution) and Domeboro Otic (Dome Laboratories) are specific examples. Remember not to use products that lower the pH with gentamicin because the effectiveness of gentamicin is significantly reduced in an acid environment.

Products that contain rotenone in oil or thiabendazole are used to treat ear mites. It is essential that treatment for ear mites be continued for at least 3 weeks and that all animals in the household be treated. Otic instillation of ivermectin, as a one-time application (on occasion, two to four treatments may be needed), has also been shown to be effective in the treatment of ear mites.

INFECTIOUS DISEASES

This section will discuss a number of common medical problems of dogs and cats. It is not intended to be a comprehensive review of internal medicine; rather, a number of specific problems have been selected that illustrate or emphasize important aspects of medical nursing.

Canine Respiratory Disease Complex

Synonyms for canine upper respiratory disease complex include kennel cough and infectious tracheobronchitis. This complex is composed of a number of different disease processes. Causative factors include viral and bacterial agents as well as predisposing environmental factors. These factors may occur singly or in combination. The diagnosis of this complex is usually based on historical and physical examination findings rather than on laboratory tests. This problem is most often self-limiting, and the duration of signs generally is no more than 2 weeks.

Treatment involves nursing care and the correction of any environmental factors that may have predisposed to the illness. The dog should be kept in a warm space that is well ventilated and free of drafts and should be fed a highly palatable diet. Appetite will be enhanced if eyes and nose are kept free of accumulated discharge. If anorectic, the patient should be hand or force fed. Intravenous or subcutaneous fluid therapy is occasionally necessary. Steam or vaporizer therapy may provide symptomatic relief. Steam therapy can be performed by placing the dog in a steam-filled bathroom several times a day. Alternatively, cold mist vaporizers can be used several times a day.

The decision to use antitussive (cough suppressant) therapy should be based upon the frequency of coughing and how prolonged the episodes are. If codeine-derivative cough suppressants are used to excess, depression and anorexia will result.

Treatment with antibiotics usually is not indicated unless there is evidence of lower respiratory or systemic involvement—for example, fever. If antibiotic therapy is instituted, a complete regimen of 10 to 14 days at full therapeutic doses should be completed. The selection of an antibiotic would ideally be based on the results of culture and sensitivity testing of a transtracheal wash. If these are not available, chloramphenicol, trimethoprim-sulfonamide combination, or tetracyclines are usually effective. The use of systemic products containing both antibiotics and corticosteroids is not indicated. Likewise, the intratracheal injection of any product is inappropriate therapy.

Due to the highly contagious nature of the causative organisms, an infected dog should be isolated from other hospitalized patients. If possible, hospitalization should be avoided. Once an outbreak occurs in a kennel or veterinary hospital, control is difficult. Ideally, the area should be kept vacant for approximately 2 weeks, and appropriate preventative measures should be instituted, consisting of the implementation of an effective vaccination protocol for every hospitalized patient. All dogs should preferably be vaccinated at least 10 days before exposure. Yearly revaccination of all patients should be a consistent hospital policy. Although parenteral immunization is widely used, studies suggest that intranasal vaccines are more efficacious in preventing infection. Vaccination is recommended more often than yearly for animals at high risk of exposure to the causative agents (e.g., frequent boarding or dog shows). The commonly used disinfectants, such as chlorhexidine (Novalsan) and benzalkonium (Roccal), effectively kill the causative bacteria and viruses.

Feline Respiratory Disease Complex

The principal components of the feline respiratory disease complex are feline viral rhinotracheitis and feline calicivirus. Less frequently incriminated agents include feline reovirus, feline pneumonitis (*Chlamydia psittaci*), *Mycoplasma*, and various bacteria.

Clinical signs of this complex include fever, cough, paroxysms of sneezing, and hypersalivation. As the infection progresses, mucopurulent ocular and nasal discharge, lacrimation, and open-mouthed breathing can be seen. Ulceration of the tongue, hard palate, and nasal pad has been reported with feline calicivirus. The severity of signs and the mortality rate are greatest in young (less than 1 year of age), nonvaccinated cats and kittens. The severity of the clinical signs will vary widely from patient to patient. The variability results from a number of interacting factors, which include the virulence of the virus, infecting dose of virus, and general health and immune status of the infected cat.

Diagnosis is based primarily on history and clinical signs rather than on laboratory findings. Occasionally, laboratory confirmation of the diagnosis by means of virus isolation or the demonstration of serum antibodies is indicated. The additional expense of laboratory confirmation is justified only when dealing with groups of cats having a chronic history of feline respiratory disease complex.

Treatment will vary, depending on the severity of signs. Some cats will show only mild, transient signs, and they require no treatment. Secondary bacterial infection will occasionally be a sequela to the feline respiratory disease complex, and therefore a broad-spectrum antibiotic may be indicated in the very young kitten (<12 weeks of age).

General nursing care is of much greater importance than antibiotics in typical cases. Whenever possible, infected cats should be treated at home rather than in the hospital.

A vital part of nursing care is to gently clean away accumulated ocular or nasal discharge. If the nostrils are kept patent, the cat is more likely to continue eating. To ensure that this happens, the owner should indulge the pet and provide highly palatable foods. Strongly flavored or odorous foods are more likely to stimulate the appetite of an anorectic cat. Steam therapy is frequently useful and can be achieved by placing the cat in a steam-filled bathroom or by using a vaporizer.

In cats that become completely anorectic, subcutaneous or intravenous fluids may be required until the appetite returns to normal. Force feeding or repeated syringe feedings may be attempted; however, in certain cats, the associated stress may negate any beneficial effect. Alternatives that appear to be better tolerated include nasogastric or pharyngostomy tubes. These procedures should be reserved for severely cachectic cats.

Proper care of the eyes is required to prevent serious injury and subsequent blindness. In most instances, a broad-spectrum antibiotic ophthalmic ointment is preferred. If pneumonitis is suspected, tetracycline ophthalmic ointment is the treatment of choice. Corticosteroids should not be used under any circumstance if feline respiratory disease complex is suspected. Specific antiviral and mucolytic ophthalmic preparations may be indicated in cases with corneal ulceration.

The virus is usually transmitted through direct contact with an infected cat. Sneezing with subsequent aerosolization of the virus will spread the virus a distance of approximately 15 to 20 cm. Fomite transmission via hands, clothing, litter boxes, and food and water dishes is a more significant means of transmission than aerosolization in veterinary hospitals. The agents responsible for the feline respiratory disease complex are sensitive to hypochlorite disinfection.

The best way to prevent outbreaks of feline respiratory disease complex in hospitalized cats is to have an effective immunization protocol. Adequate ventilation will reduce the likelihood that infection will spread within the hospital. The humidity should be maintained between 30% and 50%. Disposable food trays and litter pans and autoclavable water dishes should be used. Cats should not be moved from one cage to another unless absolutely necessary during an outbreak. Cages should be thoroughly cleansed with a dilute hypochlorite solution. Finally, because the infection can be spread via hands and clothing, meticulous hygiene on the part of all hospital personnel is essential. It is important to understand that up to 80% of the cats that go through this respiratory complex remain lifelong carriers of the organism(s). They can pose a risk to other cats or can experience a recrudescence of the complex in stressful situations.

Canine Distemper

Canine distemper is an important viral disease of dogs because of the ubiquitous nature of the virus and the mortality associated with infection. The severity of signs will vary from a transient, subclinical infection to a severe fatal disease that involves several different organ systems. This variability is due to the differing virulence of various virus strains and differences in host immunity.

The initial phase of the infection is associated with fever, transient anorexia, lethargy, and a mild serous ocular discharge after an approximate 9- to 14-day incubation period. Obviously, these signs are not specific for canine distemper. Later, as the virus spreads to the respiratory and gastrointestinal systems, mucopurulent ocular and nasal discharge, coughing, diarrhea, and, occasionally, vomiting are noted. Many dogs are anorectic at this point and become severely dehydrated. Involvement of the central nervous system may occur and can be the only signs manifested by some dogs. These dogs may develop seizures or other evidence of neurological disease. Some dogs will seemingly recover from the severe respiratory and gastrointestinal signs, but weeks or months later they develop neurological signs that either are fatal or require euthanasia because of their severity.

Although the virus may survive in the environment for weeks at near-freezing temperatures (0° to 4°C), it is susceptible to heat, drying, and ultraviolet light. Routine disinfection is usually effective in destroying the virus in a hospital or kennel.

Feline Panleukopenia

Feline panleukopenia is a potentially severe, highly contagious parvoviral disease of cats. Synonyms are feline distemper and infectious enteritis.

The typical clinical signs associated with feline panleukopenia include lethargy, anorexia, vomiting, and diarrhea after a 7-day incubation period. Characteristically, the feces are yellowish, semiformed to fluid in consistency, and may be blood-tinged. Severe dehydration may be present. Cats will occasionally hang their heads over water bowls but will not drink. The temperature may be elevated or subnormal. Feline panleukopenia can be an acute disease. Rarely, development of signs is so rapid that the owner may suspect malicious poisoning. Kittens and young cats appear to be more severely affected.

Diagnosis of feline panleukopenia is based on the presence of the clinical signs described above in the presence of a low total leukocyte count (less than 2000 WBCs/mm³). The low total count is primarily due to low numbers of neutrophils. The diagnosis of feline panleukopenia can be confirmed by virus isolation and serological and histopathological characteristics.

Treatment is primarily supportive because specific antiviral drugs are not available. The cornerstone of successful therapy is the correction of fluid and electrolyte imbalances and prevention of sepsis by the use of broad-spectrum antibiotics. Symptomatic control of vomiting and diarrhea is usually indicated. Another complication the technician should be alert to is the development of hypoglycemia (low blood glucose). This may be manifested by the development of extreme weakness, seizure activity, or both.

The prognosis for recovery is good if the cat survives the initial 3 to 6 days of severe clinical signs. The prognosis for kittens and young cats is guarded. A rising WBC count indicates a more favorable prognosis. During the recovery phase, the WBC count may exceed 50,000/mm³ and reveal a significant leftward shift. This should not be confused with the development of another infection, because this can be a normal response.

If the queen is infected during pregnancy, fetal death or congenital defects in the kitten may result. The fetus is susceptible to the virus because most tissues have high cell-proliferation rates. If the fetus is infected just before or immediately after birth, the development of the cerebellum may be affected. These kittens show balance and coordination problems beginning at about 3 to 4 weeks of age.

Fortunately, because of the availability of excellent vaccines, feline panleukopenia is currently an infrequent clinical problem.

Feline Leukemia Virus and Feline Immunodeficiency Virus Infection

These two distinct retroviral infections in cats may cause similar clinical signs. Feline leukemia virus (FeLV) has been recognized for many years and may cause immunosuppression, neoplasia, or both. Lymphosarcoma and bone marrow disorders are the more common disorders associated with FeLV. The virus is transmitted between cats by direct contact through grooming, sharing food dishes, and fighting. The virus is easily killed in the environment, and isolation of an infected cat is adequate to prevent transmission to susceptible cats. Although most cats that are exposed to the virus successfully eliminate the infection, 1% to 3% of cats in single-cat households and up to 30% of cats in multi-cat households will become persistently infected with the virus. These infected cats are then at risk for the development of the plethora of FeLV-related diseases. FeLV infection can be identified by an in-hospital test. There are many such in-hospital tests on the market and available to the practicing veterinarian. There are several vaccines available for the prevention of FeLV, and as many as 70% of cats will be protected with a successful immunization program.

Feline immunodeficiency virus (FIV), also called T-lymphotrophic T cell lentivirus (FTLV), is a recently identified virus of cats that causes primarily immunosuppression. Common clinical signs of infection with this virus include gingivitis, chronic diarrhea, generalized lymphadenopathy, fever, conjunctivitis, rhinitis, and dermatitis. It is notable that all of these signs may be seen in cats infected with FeLV. FIV is found nationwide and, indeed, worldwide. Most cats infected with this virus will not become immune, which differs from FeLV infection. The disease is spread by inoculation of the virus through cat bites. Transmission of the virus by direct contact through grooming, sharing of food dishes, and close contact is less than that seen with FeLV. No treatment or vaccine is available for this disease. Commercial kits detecting antibodies to this virus are available for in-hospital testing.

TECHNICIAN NOTE

FeLV infection is spread by direct and repeated close contact such as grooming or sharing of food and water dishes, whereas FIV infection is transmitted by inoculation of the virus through cat bites.

Pet-Associated Zoonoses

A zoonosis is a disease of animals that is transmissible to humans under natural conditions. The technician is frequently questioned by clients about the public health significance of animal diseases. Hospitalized animals may represent potential sources of zoonotic infection; thus, these infections may be considered occupational diseases.

It is beyond the scope of this section to discuss all the pet-associated zoonoses, but several of the more important infections are described. It is important to stress that when questions about human medical care arise, a physician should be consulted.

Canine brucellosis rarely occurs in humans. Transmission from an infected dog to a human can occur by contact with blood, urine, semen, milk, and infected tissues. Vaginal discharges, aborted fetuses, and placental material after abortion contain large numbers of bacteria. Infection in humans can be an insidious, chronic disease that resembles infection with other strains of *Brucella*, or it can result in relatively mild flu-like symptoms.

Toxoplasmosis can be acquired by human exposure to cat feces containing infective oocysts. Cats are an obligate host in the life cycle of *Toxoplasma*. *Toxoplasma* oocysts can remain viable in the environment for as long as 6 months under ideal conditions. The following recommendations to reduce the exposure hazard from toxoplasmosis-infected cats should be followed: Plastic gloves should be worn when cleaning litter pans or handling potentially contaminated soil. Children's sandboxes should be covered and basic principles of sanitation should be followed. Immunodeficient people and women of child-bearing age should exercise extreme caution to reduce the risk of exposure. Women contemplating pregnancy should have their antibody status determined by a physician. Those with a significant titer against toxoplasmosis are probably protected from reinfection. Antibody titers in cats are of little value because they do not indicate which cats are actively shedding infective oocysts. A recently developed enzyme-linked immunosorbent assay (ELISA), currently available through the University of Georgia and Colorado State University Veterinary Schools, identifies IgM and IgG antibodies in a cat's serum and may provide evidence for an acute or a recent infection in a cat. It should be stressed to the concerned client that eating raw or improperly cooked meat probably is the most common source of human toxoplasmosis.

Campylobacter and *Salmonella* are bacteria that can produce pet-associated zoonosis. Pets appear to be relatively infrequent sources of *Campylobacter*. When pets are incriminated, it is usually a stray or recently adopted puppy or kitten that has had recent diarrhea. The incidence of *Salmonella* infection acquired from pets is unknown. Animals can be asymptomatic shedders of this organism for an average of 6 weeks. Because the route of transmission is the fecal-oral route, good sanitation is important.

Reports of human leptospirosis attributed to vaccinated pets have appeared in medical literature. The *Leptospira* bacteria that are used for routine immunization may not protect against subclinical infection and shedding of the organisms in the urine. Because transmission is via infected urine, good sanitation is essential.

Visceral and cutaneous larval migrans are due to the migration of animal parasite larvae in human hosts. The technician plays an important role in prevention by educating clients about the risks posed by pets infected with intestinal parasites. Treatment of infected animals and reducing environmental contamination will reduce the incidence of these problems.

Plague is an infectious disease of animals that is transmitted to humans by the bite of an infected ectoparasite, usually the flea. Although the majority of cases in humans result from exposure to infected wild rodents, domestic cats have been associated with a number of infections in humans. Infections have been reported in persons employed in veterinary hospitals. Cats with suppurative lymphadenitis (infected draining lymph nodes) should be considered plague suspects, and caution should be exercised by the veterinary technician when handling exudates or treating draining wounds.

Cat-scratch disease is a disease of humans that usually is associated with cat scratches or close contact with cats. Rarely, exposure to cats has not occurred and other injuries are incriminated, such as splinters, thorns, dog scratches, and so on. The causative agent is *Bartonella henselae*. It is presumed that cats simply act as vectors for the disease because they are not ill. Multiple cases in the same household have occurred over a period of months or even years. In immunocompromised patients (e.g., humans infected with the human immunodeficiency virus), the disease can cause severe problems and therefore may pose a significant risk to these individuals. Usually, the disease in people is a mild self-limiting problem.

Rabies is an acute, fatal viral disease of the central nervous system that affects all mammals. Rabies is transmitted by infected secretions, usually saliva. In the United States, the skunk and bat are the most important sources of human exposure. However, raccoons, foxes, and unimmunized dogs and cats may also represent a hazard. In most areas of the world, the dog is the most important vector of rabies.

If human exposure to rabies is suspected, a physician or public health official should be consulted immediately. Technicians should be familiar with local laws governing the handling of animals who have bitten humans.

Animal bites can cause serious infectious complications, including cellulitis, lymphangitis, soft tissue abscesses, osteomyelitis, meningitis, and bacteremia. Humans who have undergone splenectomy are at particular risk of bacteremia and possibly death if the organism known as DF-2, isolated from the nasal and oral secretions of healthy dogs, is inoculated into tissues by a bite.

OPHTHALMOLOGY

Glaucoma

Glaucoma is defined as an increase in intraocular pressure. Glaucoma may cause blindness, and there are certain breeds predisposed to primary glaucoma (Table 12–5).

• Table 12–5 •

BREEDS PREDISPOSED TO THE DEVELOPMENT OF GLAUCOMA	
Afghan	Fox terriers
American cocker spaniel	Great Dane
Basset hound	Malamute
Beagle	Norwegian elkhound
Bedlington terrier	Saluki
Brittany spaniel	Samoyed
Dachshund	Sealyham terrier
Dalmatian	Siberian husky
English cocker spaniel	Toy and miniature poodles
English springer spaniel	

The signs in early glaucoma are often subtle and can be variable. Acute glaucoma is a painful process; signs include tearing, sensitivity to bright light, and pawing at the eye. Inspection of the eye may reveal congested episcleral blood vessels, a dilated nonresponsive pupil, and a cloudy cornea. In chronic glaucoma, the major finding is an enlarged globe.

The diagnosis is made by documenting an increased intraocular pressure. Several methods are used to measure intraocular pressure. Tonometers are the most accurate, but some are expensive. The Schiøtz tonometer is useful and costs approximately $300 to $400, which is well within the means of most veterinary practices (Fig. 12–9).

Glaucoma is considered a medical emergency because delay in treatment may result in permanent damage to the eye. A number of drugs are available to treat glaucoma, all of which work by either reducing aqueous production or increasing the opening at the drainage angle.

Cataracts

A cataract is a focal or diffuse opacity within the lens and its capsule. Cataracts may be hereditary or nonhereditary. They should be differentiated from nuclear sclerosis, which is a normal aging change that decreases the clarity of the nucleus of the lens.

Inherited cataracts occur in many breeds and may be associated with other eye abnormalities. Different modes of inheritance have been reported in different breeds. Breeds reported to have inherited cataracts include the beagle, German shepherd, golden retriever, labrador retriever, Afghan hound, American cocker spaniel, Boston terrier, poodle, and miniature schnauzer. Inherited cataracts have not been reported in the cat.

Cataracts can be due to metabolic abnormalities—for example, diabetes mellitus, inflammation, or trauma. Inflammatory diseases associated with cataracts include feline infectious peritonitis, feline leukemia virus, leptospirosis, and systemic mycoses.

There is no successful medical treatment for cataracts, but any associated inflammation should be treated. Medications that dilate the pupil may be helpful in improving vision in cases of immature or hypermature cataracts. Currently, the only effective therapy for cataracts is surgical removal of the lens.

Corneal Ulcers

Superficial corneal ulcers may result from trauma, decreased tear production (keratoconjunctivitis sicca), aberrant eyelashes (distichiasis and districhiasis), inward rolling of the eyelid (entropion), and inability to blink. Animals with superficial corneal ulcers experience a significant amount of pain. This pain is manifested as excessive tearing, sensitivity to bright light, and squinting (blepharospasm). Corneal ulcers are diagnosed by using fluorescein dye. Fluorescein is a water-soluble dye that will not stain the epithelial layer but stains the underlying layers if the superficial epithelial layer is damaged.

Treatment should be directed first toward correcting the underlying cause. Once this has been accomplished, epithelialization of the ulcerated area is rapid and usually uncomplicated. Broad-spectrum antibiotics are generally used to eliminate infection. It has been shown that ointments may retard healing more than solutions; however, the difference in healing may not be clinically significant. One advantage to solutions is that the dose can be more easily controlled. Systemic medications usually are not necessary with corneal ulcers. Occasionally, a surgical flap over the cornea is necessary until epithelialization is complete.

DERMATOLOGY

Veterinary dermatology is an important part of small animal practice. Veterinary dermatology is a challenging discipline; although there are many causes of skin disease, there are only a limited number of ways in which the skin can react. Consequently, in many cases a specific etiological diagnosis can be difficult to make.

It is beyond the scope of this chapter to consider all of the

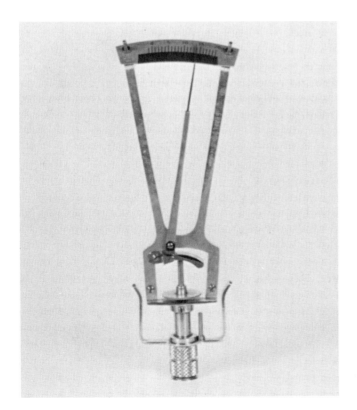

Figure 12-9. Tonometer (Schiøtz Tonometer) used for measurement of intraocular pressure. The tonometer is placed on the cornea to obtain the pressure reading.

common dermatological diseases of dogs and cats. Instead, emphasis is placed on several diagnostic procedures that are commonly performed by veterinary technicians.

Skin Scraping

Skin scraping is one of the most frequently used tests in veterinary dermatology. It should be part of the minimum data base whenever the diagnosis has not been established. The skin scraping is used to identify microscopic ectoparasites such as *Demodex* and *Sarcoptes* as well as dermatophytes. The material and equipment needed to identify ectoparasites include mineral oil, scalpel blade, microscope slide, coverslip, and microscope. The material and equipment used to identify a dermatophyte include saline, scalpel blade, microscope slide, coverslip, potassium hydroxide solution, a heat source (e.g., Bunsen burner), and a microscope.

A representative area should be selected for the skin scraping. In general, an area that has not been disturbed or medicated should be selected. If a dermatophyte is suspected, an area near the margin of the lesion should be selected. If *Demodex* is suspected, a fold of skin should be gently pinched and the skin scraped until there is a slight ooze of blood. When scraping for ectoparasites, a drop of mineral oil should be placed on the scalpel blade so it is possible to transfer the material to a microscope slide. When scraping for dermatophytes, saline or water is used to wet the blade to facilitate the transfer of the specimen to the microscope slide.

Once the accumulated material and mineral oil have been transferred, one or two drops of mineral oil are added, and the mixture is spread evenly with an application stick. A coverslip is added, and the specimen is carefully examined under the microscope. If parasites are not found, demodectic mange is generally eliminated as a diagnostic possibility; however, as many as 8 to 10 sites should be evaluated and found to be negative before eliminating sarcoptic mange as a possibility.

If a dermatophyte is suspected, a potassium hydroxide preparation should be examined. The material is collected, using the technique described, and placed on a microscope slide. Several drops of 10% potassium hydroxide are placed on the sample, a coverslip is added, and the slide is gently heated for 15 to 20 seconds. Alternatively, the preparation can be placed on the microscope stage and heated by the microscope light source for 15 to 20 minutes. Interpretation of the specimens obtained requires patience and experience. Identification of dermatophytosis can be made by finding branching mycelia. The mycelial filaments are uniform in diameter (2 to 6 μm), are divided into compartments, and vary in length and degree of branching. Hair shafts should be carefully examined for spores. The dermatophytes that infect animals generally have ectothrix spores, which form a prominent sheath on the outside of the hair shaft, in addition to growing inside the hair shaft.

If there is any doubt about the interpretation of the potassium hydroxide digestion, a fungal culture should be performed. A culture is considered the most reliable means of identifying dermatophytes.

The equipment needed for culture includes culture media, a sterile scalpel blade, sterile forceps, and alcohol swab. Appropriate culture media include Sabouraud's media and dermatophyte test media (DTM).

Before a specimen is obtained, the area is cleansed with 70% alcohol to reduce bacterial contamination. A small scraping of superficial debris and hair should be obtained, using the sterile scalpel blade and forceps. Alternatively, a small tuft of hair can be plucked from the margin of a lesion, using mosquito hemostats. The hair sample should be deposited partially beneath the surface of the culture medium. The culture medium bottle cap should be left open a fourth-turn to provide aerobic conditions, and the specimen should be incubated at room temperature. Care should be taken not to inoculate the medium with too large a specimen because this may confuse interpretation of the results. A number of commercial media, which contain agents that inhibit the growth of bacteria and indicator dyes that help to differentiate pathogens from saprophytes, are available (e.g., Fungassay, Pitman-Moore).

Another commonly used diagnostic technique in veterinary dermatology is bacterial culture of suspected pyodermal lesions. The technique used to obtain the specimen is extremely important because skin contaminants are usually present. A representative site should be selected, and an unopened lesion should be gently prepared with a surgical scrub. The lesion should be opened with sterile instruments, and a sterile swab should be inserted deep into the cavity or tract. Alternatively, after the area has been scrubbed, a sterile needle is introduced into the unopened lesion, and the purulent material is aspirated into a syringe. Inoculation of the culture medium should be made immediately. Direct smears should also be made immediately and stained with Gram's stain.

CARDIOLOGY

Congestive Heart Failure

Congestive heart failure is a clinical term used to describe the state when the heart is unable to maintain adequate cardiac output. Because of decreased cardiac output, the body's tissues do not receive sufficient blood supply for normal function. The decreased cardiac output and the resultant increase in pressures within the vessels entering the heart stimulate complex compensatory mechanisms that contribute to the clinical signs of congestive heart failure. The term *congestive heart failure* does not indicate a specific etiology.

Tachycardia and cardiomegaly (heart enlargement) are general signs associated with congestive heart failure. However, depending on the principal site of involvement, signs of left-sided or right-sided heart failure will predominate.

Left-sided heart failure results from dysfunction of the left atrioventricular valve (mitral valve), ventricle, or both. Clinical signs associated with left-sided heart failure include cough, exertional dyspnea, orthopnea, and, at times, syncope. Characteristically, early in left-sided heart failure the cough occurs in paroxysms and at night or in the early morning. The cough in left-sided heart failure is usually secondary to the development of pulmonary edema or occurs because the left atrium has enlarged and compressed the left mainstem bronchus. Exertional dyspnea refers to labored breathing associated with increased activity. This may be manifested as decreased exercise tolerance or reluctance to exercise. *Orthopnea* means difficult or labored breathing in the recumbent position. Pulmonary edema refers to the accumulation of abnormal fluid in the interstitial spaces and alveoli of the lungs. It can be detected by auscultating rales (crackles) in the lungs or by observing the characteristic pattern on chest radiographs. Syncope, or fainting, results from decreased cardiac output to the brain.

Right-sided heart failure results from a pathological condition of the right atrioventricular valve (tricuspid valve), right ventricle, or both. Clinical signs associated with right-sided heart failure include hepatic enlargement, ascites, pleural effusion, and subcutaneous edema. Increased pressure in the abdominal veins results in congestion and enlargement of the liver. Increased hydrostatic pressure in capillaries results in leakage of fluid and the subsequent development of ascites, pleural effusion, and subcutaneous edema. Subcutaneous edema is a relatively rare sign in the dog and is seen late in the course of the condition. (Table 12–6 provides a list of signs seen with left- and right-sided heart failure.)

Certain cardiovascular problems result in both left-sided and right-sided heart failure. Obviously, the signs described are not specific for heart disease. Consequently, when evaluating a patient for cough or ascites, the conditions to rule out should include noncardiac problems.

Mitral Insufficiency

Mitral insufficiency resulting from chronic mitral (left atrioventricular) valvular fibrosis is the most frequently diagnosed form of heart disease in the dog. It is followed in prevalence by chronic tricuspid (right atrioventricular) valvular fibrosis, which causes tricuspid insufficiency. *Valvular insufficiency* is a term used to indicate functional incompetence (leakage) of the valve with subsequent regurgitation (backward flow) of blood from the ventricle into the atrium during ventricular systole.

The signs associated with chronic mitral insufficiency are those of left-sided heart failure (e.g., cough, exertional dyspnea, and pulmonary edema). The specific cause of mitral valvular fibrosis is unknown; however, it appears to be associated with aging. Certain breeds appear to be predisposed, the majority of these being small breeds of dogs (e.g., miniature poodles). Mitral insufficiency as a cause of left-sided heart failure is much less common in the cat. The diagnosis of chronic mitral insufficiency is based on the clinical history, auscultation of the heart and lungs, thoracic radiography, and electrocardiography. Although the traditional treatment for this condition has included the use of cardiac glycosides (e.g., digoxin), recent evidence indicates that cardiac contractility is normal to increased in the

majority of these dogs, and therefore digoxin is not indicated until late in the course of the failure state.

Initially, the use of diuretics such as furosemide (Lasix), a sodium-restricted diet, and exercise restriction are the primary mode of therapy. Treatment with vasodilators such as hydralazine (Apresoline), captopril (Capoten), and enalapril (Enacard) are also beneficial. These drugs work by decreasing the resistance against which the heart has to pump. As more long-term data are accumulated, we may find in dogs, as in people, that vasodilators may help to prolong survival of dogs with heart failure if they are begun earlier in the disease state.

Heartworm Disease

Heartworm disease, caused by *Dirofilaria immitis*, is characterized principally by the presence of right-sided heart failure. The adult parasites lodge in the right atrium, right ventricle, right ventricular outflow tract, pulmonary arteries, and venae cavae. The major effect of heartworm disease is to produce pulmonary hypertension (increased blood pressure in pulmonary arteries), which results in right-sided heart failure.

Heartworm disease has a geographical distribution. The highest incidences of infection occur along the southeastern Atlantic and Gulf coasts. Gradually, heartworm disease has spread to most of the eastern and midwestern United States. Small endemic areas have also been reported in the western United States. With the increased travel of dogs from one region to another, heartworm disease is possible anywhere.

Mosquitoes are an intermediate host for the parasite. The disease is spread by mosquitoes ingesting microfilariae (immature parasites, the L_1 larvae) from the blood of an infected dog. The microfilariae undergo maturation within the mosquito to become an infective larva. Infective larvae (L_3 stage) enter the dog through the skin puncture wound produced by the mosquito and migrate to subcutaneous tissue, muscle, or fat. Two more molts occur within the dog's body, and the young adult heartworm arrives in the heart approximately 110 days after infection. The adult female heartworms begin producing circulating microfilariae 6 to 7 months after infection.

The most practical method to detect heartworm disease is to observe the presence of circulating microfilariae in the peripheral blood. The microfilariae of a nonpathogenic filarial worm, *Dipetalonema reconditum*, must be differentiated from those of *Dirofilaria immitis*. The most useful diagnostic characteristics of the microfilariae of *D. reconditum* are the blunt shape of the head and the serpentine progressive movement demonstrated in direct blood smears. There are three basic tests used to detect microfilariae. They include the direct smear, modified Knott test, and filter tests. Each test has its advantages and disadvantages; however, if cost, sensitivity, and ease of species identification are considered, the modified Knott test is preferred. During the past few years, serological testing for heartworm disease has become the preferred method of documenting heartworm infection. There are multiple kits available to detect heartworm antigens in dog serum, and these can be easily performed in practice.

It has been estimated that as many as 25% to 65% of dogs with heartworm disease have no circulating microfilariae. This is referred to as *occult heartworm disease*. If heartworm disease is suspected based on history, physical examination, radiography, and electrocardiography, yet circulating microfilariae are

• Table 12–6 •

CLINICAL SIGNS OF LEFT- AND RIGHT-SIDED HEART FAILURE
CONGESTIVE SIGNS—LEFT 1. Pulmonary congestion and edema resulting in: cough, tachypnea, dyspnea, orthopnea, pulmonary crackles, tiring, hemoptysis, cyanosis 2. Secondary right heart failure 3. Cardiac arrhythmias **CONGESTIVE SIGNS—RIGHT** 1. Systemic venous congestion: High CVP (central venous pressure) Jugular vein distention 2. Liver and spleen enlargement 3. Fluid in chest cavity (pleural effusion) causing: dyspnea, orthopnea and cyanosis 4. Fluid in abdominal cavity (ascites) 5. Subcutaneous edema 6. Fluid in pericardial sac (pericardial effusion)

not present, a serological test for detection of adult heartworm antigens should be performed.

The treatment of heartworm disease can be divided into three phases. The first phase is to kill the adult heartworms (adulticidal therapy) that are present in the heart and blood vessels. The next phase is to eradicate the circulating microfilariae (microfilaricidal therapy). Finally, preventative medication (prophylactic therapy) is administered to those dogs at risk of developing heartworm disease. This would include any dog residing in or traveling to an endemic area.

Adulticide therapy consists of administering thiacetarsamide sodium (Caparsolate, Abbott Laboratories) intravenously. The recommended regimen is to administer the drug twice per day for 2 days. If the injection takes a perivascular route, swelling, inflammation, and tissue necrosis will occur. If it is suspected that extravasation has occurred, the area should be immediately infiltrated with sterile saline and dexamethasone. Thiacetarsamide may produce renal and hepatic toxicity. In addition, an adulticide (Immiticide, Rhone-Merieux) is available for intramuscular administration. It is an arsenical compound given by intramuscular injection into the epaxial muscles in the lumbar region. Two treatments are given 24 hours apart. If needed, a second treatment can be given 4 months later.

The adult heartworms will die slowly over a 2- to 3-week period. Fever, coughing, and, in more severe cases, dyspnea and hemoptysis (coughing up blood) are the signs observed as the worms die and pass to the lungs (pulmonary thromboembolism). Prednisone therapy (1 mg/kg) is the accepted therapy for pulmonary thromboembolism. Aspirin therapy (5 mg/kg once daily) is recommended in dogs with moderate to severe heartworm disease to reduce thromboembolism. It may be started 1 week before treatment and continued 4 to 6 weeks after treatment.

To minimize the development of clinical pulmonary thromboembolism, it is important to restrict exercise for 3 to 4 weeks after adulticide therapy. If the signs associated with pulmonary thromboembolism are severe, hospitalization and administration of bronchodilators, anti-inflammatory drugs, and antibiotics are recommended. DIC may occur in dogs with severe clinical signs. Treatment of advanced DIC is usually unsuccessful.

Microfilaricide therapy is begun 3 weeks after adulticide therapy. Ivermectin (Ivomec), 50 μg/kg orally once, is the current accepted method of treatment for microfilaria, even though it is not FDA approved for this function.

Heartworm disease may be prevented with the use of one of several products. Some of these also have protective activity against some endoparasites. Table 12–7 lists the products currently available for heartworm prevention in the dog.

Cardiomyopathy

Cardiomyopathy is a general term that merely indicates that the basic pathological lesion involves the heart muscle. Cardiomyopathies can be primary or secondary. Primary cardiomyopathies indicate that the myocardial disease is not due to any recurrent or preexisting cardiovascular or systemic disease. Primary cardiomyopathies in cats are further subdivided into hypertrophic, dilated, and restrictive forms. Secondary cardiomyopathies in dogs and cats are less frequent and are due to diseases such as infection, metabolic disorders (e.g., uremia), endocrine problems (e.g., hyperthyroidism), and infiltrative processes (e.g., neoplasia).

• Table 12–7 •

CURRENTLY AVAILABLE HEARTWORM PREVENTATIVES

TRADE NAME	INGREDIENT(S)	COMPANY	ANTI-PARASITIC ACTIVITY
Multiples	Diethylcarbamazine	Multiple	Roundworms Heartworm prevention
Filaribits	Diethylcarbamazine	Pfizer	Roundworms Heartworm prevention
Filaribits-Plus	Diethylcarbamazine Oxibendazole	Pfizer	Hookworms Roundworms Whipworms Heartworm prevention
Heartgard	Ivermectin	Merck-AgVet	Heartworm prevention
Heartgard-30 Plus	Ivermectin Pyrantel pamoate	Merck-AgVet	Heartworm prevention Roundworms Hookworms
Heartgard for cats	Ivermectin	Merck-AgVet	Heartworm prevention Hookworms
Interceptor	Milbemycin oxime	Novartis	Heartworm prevention Hookworms Whipworms Roundworms
Sentinel	Milbemycin oxime Lufenuron	Novartis	Heartworms Fleas Whipworms Roundworms Hookworms

Hypertrophic cardiomyopathy is characterized by increased thickness of the myocardium and a small left ventricular lumen. Clinical signs are seen in middle-aged cats of all breeds. The most prominent sign is the sudden development of respiratory distress secondary to pulmonary edema. Hindlimb paresis (weakness) and severe pain may also be present. These hindlimb signs are due to aortic thromboembolism (blood clots) disrupting the blood supply to the hindlimbs. This problem can usually be diagnosed easily if femoral pulses are found to be poor or absent. Diagnosis of cardiomyopathy is based on history, physical examination, radiography, electrocardiography, and echocardiography. If echocardiography is not available, nonselective angiocardiography may be necessary for diagnosis. The basic initial therapeutic approach may include diuretics (e.g., Lasix, Hoeschst-Roussel Pharmaceuticals), cage rest, oxygen therapy, beta-adrenergic blockers such as propranolol (Inderal, Ayerst Laboratories), and calcium channel blockers such as diltiazem hydrochloride (Cardizem, Marion Merrell Dow). Long-term management consists of diuretics, beta blockers, calcium channel blockers, a sodium-restricted diet (feline H/D, Hill's), aspirin, and restricted activity. Aspirin is used to reduce the likelihood of aortic thromboembolism.

Dilated cardiomyopathy is characterized by extreme ventricular dilation and moderate atrial enlargement. This results in impaired pump function of the ventricle. This type of cardiomyopathy is also known as *congestive cardiomyopathy*. Signs of right-sided heart failure usually predominate. In addition, cats may show a gradual onset of lethargy and anorexia and at times may be presented dehydrated, hypothermic, and in cardiovascular shock. Respiratory distress secondary to pleural effusion and aortic thromboembolism resulting in hindlimb paresis is also occasionally seen. The basic therapeutic approach is to mechanically remove as much fluid as possible from the pleural cavity (thoracocentesis), digitalize the cat (digoxin therapy), and administer diuretics. Aspirin is used as a preventative measure against aortic thromboembolism. Vasodilators, such as nitroglycerin ointment (Nitrol ointment, Kremers-Urban Co.), may have a role in the management of dilated cardiomyopathy.

Some cats with dilated cardiomyopathy have low plasma taurine levels, and cardiac function will increase with oral taurine supplementation of 250 to 500 mg daily. Cardiac function usually improves over a period of months, and if cats are placed on a diet containing ample taurine, cardiac drugs and taurine supplementation may eventually be discontinued. It should be stated that because this association of low taurine levels and cardiomyopathy in the cat has been made, almost all commercial and prescription diets have adequate levels of taurine, so low-taurine dilated cardiomyopathy is much less common than it used to be.

Restrictive cardiomyopathy is the least common form of primary feline cardiomyopathy. A synonym is endomyocardial fibrosis. Respiratory distress is the most common clinical sign. Diagnosis is similar to the other forms of primary cardiomyopathy. Response to therapy is generally poor.

Primary cardiomyopathies in the dog are categorized as dilated (congestive), boxer cardiomyopathy, Doberman pinscher cardiomyopathy, and hypertrophic cardiomyopathy.

Dilated cardiomyopathy is most common in large and giant breed male dogs aged 4 to 6 years; however, English and American cocker spaniels are smaller-breed dogs that may be affected. Presenting signs often include weakness, lethargy, respiratory distress, cough, anorexia, weight loss, and possibly ascites, and syncope. The left ventricle and atrium are dilated with decreased contractility. Diagnosis is confirmed by physical examination, radiography, electrocardiography, and echocardiography. Treatment consists of diuretics, a low sodium diet, arteriolar dilators, and positive inotropes, such as cardiac glycosides. The long-term prognosis is guarded in that most dogs with the dilated form of cardiomyopathy have an average life span of 6 to 8 months after the diagnosis has been made.

TECHNICIAN NOTE

Dilated cardiomyopathy is primarily a disease of large and giant purebred dogs, although medium-sized breeds, such as English and American cocker spaniels, are being diagnosed with increasing frequency with this acquired heart disease.

A specific cardiomyopathy occurs in boxers. These dogs may be asymptomatic or present with syncope and episodic weakness. Arrhythmias are common and may cause sudden death. Diagnosis is confirmed by the same methods as those used in dogs with dilated cardiomyopathy. Treatment with diuretics and antiarrhythmics, such as propranolol, may be useful; however, prognosis is still poor.

Doberman pinschers may present with a primary cardiomyopathy that is similar to congestive or dilated cardiomyopathy. Ventricular contractility is often severely compromised, and atrial arrhythmias are common. These dogs are often in fulminant congestive heart failure and require supportive care with oxygen, diuretics, positive inotropes, and vasodilators. Prognosis is poor.

Hypertrophic cardiomyopathy is the most uncommon primary cardiomyopathy. It is most often seen in German shepherd dogs and other large breeds. Presenting signs are referable to cardiac disease, and sudden death may occur. Treatment with diuretics and propranolol may improve cardiac output and clinical signs.

ENDOCRINOLOGY

Canine hyperadrenocorticism (Cushing's syndrome) is a disorder that results from the excessive production of cortisol by the adrenal cortex. The clinical signs of canine hyperadrenocorticism include polyuria, polydipsia, abdominal distention, polyphagia, muscular weakness, dermatological changes, and reproductive problems (anestrus and testicular atrophy). Cushing's syndrome can result from excessive production of adrenocorticotropic hormone (ACTH) by the pituitary gland (pituitary-dependent hyperadrenocorticism) or from a functional tumor of the adrenal cortex. Pituitary-dependent hyperadrenocorticism is by far the most common, comprising approximately 80% of the cases. Diagnosis is based on measurements of the plasma cortisol levels after stimulation with ACTH or suppression with dexamethasone. Treatment is different for these two conditions. If a functional tumor is present, the recommended treatment is surgical removal. The drug used to treat Cushing's syndrome caused by excessive ACTH production is mitotane (Lysodren, Bristol Laboratories). Side effects associated with the use of mitotane include anorexia, lethargy, vomiting, and depression.

Canine hypoadrenocorticism (Addison's disease) is due to lack of glucocorticoid and/or mineralocorticoid levels and activity. It is generally seen in the middle-aged female and the most common signs are gastrointestinal (vomiting, anorexia), weakness, depression, and collapse. These signs may have a waxing-waning course.

In an acute crisis these patients may present in acute collapse and in hypovolemic shock. The classic laboratory abnormalities are a low serum sodium (Na^+) level, and a high serum potassium (K^+) level, resulting in a low $Na^+:K^+$ ratio (usually less than 25:1). These patients may also be azotemic and have a low urine specific gravity, which could be confused with renal failure.

The most accurate means of diagnosis, is to perform an ACTH stimulation test and show that the patient has a very poor response to this drug, as their cortisol levels will not increase following ACTH administration.

The treatment consists of aggressive fluid therapy, and supplementation with glucocorticoid and mineralocorticoid therapy. Prednisolone sodium succinate and desoxycorticosterone are the glucocorticoid and mineralocorticoid used to treat this disease.

Hypoglycemia

Canine hypoglycemia is a clinical problem associated with a variety of diseases rather than a specific diagnosis itself. The signs associated with hypoglycemia include weakness of the rear legs, generalized weakness, focal or diffuse muscle twitching, incoordination, blindness, generalized seizures, and behavioral changes. These behavioral changes include aggressive behavior, and anxiety as evidenced by incessant running, barking, and loss of bowel and bladder control. These signs tend to be episodic, regardless of the cause of hypoglycemia. Hypoglycemia should be considered a differential diagnosis in any dog that is having seizures or is presented in a coma.

The first step in evaluating a patient with suspected hypoglycemia is to verify or document that hypoglycemia exists. Improper handling of blood samples may result in falsely low blood glucose levels. The blood glucose level can be lowered if the serum is not removed from the clot or if the specimen is stored at room temperature for a prolonged period. It is preferable to remove serum from the clot within 10 to 15 minutes of drawing the blood sample. If this cannot be done, use of sodium fluoride tubes may be helpful.

Once hypoglycemia has been verified, the signalment, history, clinical findings, and further laboratory tests may be needed to reduce the long and rather diverse list of conditions that may cause hypoglycemia. Functional beta-cell tumors (insulinomas of the pancreas), nonpancreatic tumors, hypoglycemia-ketonemia in pregnant bitches, glycogen storage diseases, septic shock, juvenile and neonatal hypoglycemia, canine parvoviral diarrhea, and excessive insulin administration in diabetic patients are all examples of diseases that can cause hypoglycemia.

Hypothyroidism and Hyperthyroidism

Hypothyroidism is one of the most common endocrine disorders in the dog, but it is rare in the cat. Some of the common clinical signs include oily seborrhea, alopecia, thickened skin, weight gain, lethargy, and cold intolerance. There are some breeds with an apparent increased incidence of hypothyroidism, and these are listed in Table 12–8. The thyroid-stimulating hormone (TSH) stimulation test is the most accurate diagnostic test available for assessment of thyroid gland function. This test involves drawing blood before and 6 hours after TSH administration and then measuring the serum T_4 levels on each sample. Most normal animals should increase their baseline T_4 level by 2× and exceed 3 μg/dl at the 6-hour sampling. Treatment of hypothyroidism consists of supplementation with thyroxine (T_4).

Hyperthyroidism is the most common endocrinopathy affecting cats older than 8 years of age, but it is rare in the dog. The most common clinical signs of hyperthyroidism are weight loss despite a good appetite, restlessness, hyperactivity, and diarrhea. In many cases, a thyroid nodule can be palpated in the ventrocervical region of the neck. The diagnosis can usually be confirmed by documenting an elevated serum T_4 level. Treatment may consist of medical therapy with methimazole (Tapazole, Eli Lilly and Co.), surgical removal of the thyroid nodule, and/or radioactive iodine (^{131}I).

Diabetes Mellitus

This endocrinopathy is seen in the older dog and cat, and it is more common in the female dog and the male cat. Common clinical signs include excessive water intake (polydipsia), urination of large volumes of urine (polyuria), weight loss in spite of a good appetite, and rapidly developing lens opacities (cataracts) in the dog. If the dog or cat is ketoacidotic, then weakness, vomiting, depression, and, possibly, coma may develop. The diagnosis of diabetes mellitus is made by documenting hyperglycemia, glucosuria, and, if animal is ketoacidotic, ketonuria or ketonemia.

The technician's role in the treatment of patients with this endocrinopathy is twofold: (1) management of the ill ketoacidotic diabetic in the hospital and (2) education of clients concerning home management and treatment of their pets.

The ketoacidotic diabetic represents a true challenge for the veterinarian and technician alike, and it is important that they work in unison so optimal patient care is achieved. The technician's role involves close monitor of vital signs, ensuring fluids are given at the proper rate, frequent blood glucose determinations, and administering of short-acting (regular/crystalline) insulin. Because the ketoacidotic patient requires such close monitoring, the technician plays a major role in the minute-to-minute and hour-to-hour evaluation of the patient, so minor changes in the patient's condition can be recognized early and the veterinarian be informed. Because of the complexity of the ketoacidotic diabetic, all of these functions should be done under the direct supervision of a veterinarian.

The second aspect of diabetic management involves the instruction of the client concerning home management of the pet. This can be a time-consuming function, and the technician who has a good understanding of diabetes management can be a tremendous asset to the veterinarian. Examples of areas in which the client should be instructed and/or shown include how to (1) mix the insulin, (2) read the syringes, (3) draw up the insulin into the syringe, (4) give the subcutaneous injection, and (5) read urine test strips for urine glucose measurement. In addition, the client needs to be instructed (1) about the type of diet to be fed and how much and when to feed, (2) *not* to give the insulin if the pet does not eat in the morning, and (3) if the pet has a seizure, give the animal Karo syrup orally and call the hospital immediately. All of these items can be compiled into a handout that the technician can develop with the aid of the veterinarian. This handout can then be given to the client, who can refer to it as needed at home.

THERIOGENOLOGY

Postpartum Disorders in the Bitch

The postpartum bitch may be presented to an animal hospital for a variety of serious problems after whelping. These prob-

• Table 12–8 •

BREEDS OF DOGS WITH AN APPARENT INCREASED INCIDENCE OF HYPOTHYROIDISM	
Afghan hound	Golden retriever
Airedale	Great Dane
Beagle	Irish setter
Boxer	Irish wolfhound
Brittany spaniel	Malamute
Chow chow	Miniature schnauzer
Cocker spaniel	Newfoundland
Dachshund	Pomeranian
Doberman pinscher	Poodle
English bulldog	Shetland sheepdog

lems include mastitis, metritis, and eclampsia. *Mastitis* refers to inflammation of one or more mammary glands. In severe cases, affected glands are hot and painful, and the patient is systemically ill. Bitches with septic mastitis are depressed, anorectic, and reluctant to care for the puppies. In less severe cases, the bitch may not be symptomatic; however, the puppies may fail to gain weight or may show signs of septicemia. Systemic antibiotics are used to treat mastitis. Since the affected glands produce abnormal milk, and the antibiotics excreted in the milk may be harmful to the puppies, it is recommended that the puppies be hand-reared.

Severe mastitis may progress to abscess formation or gangrenous mastitis. Surgical drainage and treatment may be required in these cases.

Stasis of milk in the mammary glands can occasionally result in enlarged, painful mammary glands. Galactostasis may be observed during pseudopregnancy or at the time of weaning when the body is attempting to resorb milk. Unlike mastitis, dogs with galactostasis are not systemically ill. Treatment consists of application of cool towels and compresses to decrease inflammation. Care should be taken not to massage the glands because this can stimulate additional milk letdown.

Metritis is a uterine disease of the immediate postpartum period. Signs usually develop within the first week of whelping. Metritis is associated with retained placentas, retained fetuses, and dystocia. Clinical signs suggestive of metritis include fever, depression, and reduced interest in the puppies. A foul-smelling, brown or reddish-brown vaginal discharge may be present; the normal discharge after whelping is nonodorous and greenish. The diagnosis is based on history, clinical findings, and laboratory results. Laboratory tests that are useful include vaginal cytological studies, CBCs, and bacterial cultures.

Initial therapy consists of replacing fluid deficits, treating shock, if present, and initiating antibiotic therapy after cultures have been obtained. Medical drainage of the uterus can be attempted in valuable breeding bitches. In severe cases, ovariohysterectomy may be indicated to save the bitch's life.

Hypocalcemia (eclampsia) usually occurs 2 to 3 weeks postpartum in small bitches with large litters but occasionally can occur before birth. Presenting signs include weakness and trembling and may proceed to tonic convulsions. The temperature is usually elevated during convulsions.

Diagnosis is based on clinical signs in a lactating female. Treatment includes removing the young for 12 to 24 hours, treating the dam with intravenous 10 percent calcium gluconate, and ensuring the dam receives oral calcium lactate or calcium gluconate and vitamin D at home. If the condition recurs, the young should be weaned.

Canine Brucellosis

Canine brucellosis is primarily an infection of the reproductive tract, although other organ systems may be involved. *Brucella canis* has been isolated from dogs with discospondylitis and chronic recurrent fever. Brucellosis is a frequent cause of infertility and other reproductive problems in both males and females.

Definitive diagnosis requires demonstration of the organism by a culture of blood or body fluids. Serological tests can be diagnostic as well. The rapid slide agglutination test is an easy, readily available test; however, false-positive results occur. The rapid slide agglutination can be used as a screen, with positive tests being confirmed using an alternative technique (e.g., agar gel immunodiffusion).

The mode of transmission is venereal. However, infection can also result from the ingestion of infected material, for example, aborted fetuses, placentas, and vaginal discharge. Because of these means of spread, brucellosis can quickly become a kennel-wide problem.

Although a variety of antibiotic combinations have been recommended, therapeutic success cannot be guaranteed. After antibiotic therapy, some dogs will continue to harbor the organism and represent a risk to other dogs. Canine brucellosis is considered a possible zoonotic disease. For these reasons, some experts advocate removal of all infected dogs from the premises. Other experts feel that this position is extreme and instead recommend castration or ovariohysterectomy and antibiotic therapy for infected pet dogs.

Because treatment is not always successful, prevention is emphasized. All dogs should be tested before breeding or before introduction into a kennel.

Pyometritis

Pyometritis is a uterine disease that occurs during the luteal phase of the reproductive cycle. It occurs in both bitches and queens. Pyometritis may be part of a complex that initially starts with cystic changes in the endometrium and endometrial hyperplasia. Prior estrogen therapy may predispose to pyometritis.

Clinical signs are variable. A vaginal discharge may or may not be present, but, if present, the color of the discharge can be green, yellow, or reddish brown. Bitches with pyometritis frequently will be polydipsic and polyuric. Affected animals can be severely depressed and septic or can be clinically normal.

An enlarged uterus on radiographs and leukocytosis with a left shift are considered diagnostic. Fluid therapy to correct fluid and electrolyte deficits followed by ovariohysterectomy is the treatment of choice in nonbreeding animals. In valuable breeding bitches, medical treatment with prostaglandin $F_{2\text{-alpha}}$ has been advocated to preserve the breeding life of the patient. Treatment with prostaglandin $F_{2\text{-alpha}}$ is expensive and potentially dangerous; therefore, it should be strictly reserved for dogs of significant breeding value.

Canine Prostatic Disease

Prostatic disease is occasionally seen in older intact male dogs. Clinical signs include straining to urinate (stranguria), painful urination (dysuria), blood in the urine (hematuria), and/or difficulty in defecation. The conditions that affect the prostate include benign prostatic hypertrophy, bacterial prostatitis, prostatic abscess, prostatic cyst, and prostatic neoplasia.

The following noninvasive techniques are used to evaluate the prostate: rectal palpation, routine radiology, sonography (ultrasound), urethrography, cytological studies, and bacterial cultures of prostatic washes or the prostatic fraction of the ejaculate. Frequently, it is difficult to differentiate neoplasia, infection, and hypertrophy with use of these noninvasive techniques. Consequently, surgical exploration and biopsy may be required to establish a definitive diagnosis.

Treatment varies, depending on the specific process. Dogs with benign prostatic hypertrophy respond to castration. Although estrogen therapy reduces the size of the prostate in benign prostatic hypertrophy, it is not recommended because of possible adverse reactions. Prostatic abscesses and cysts require surgical drainage. Bacterial prostatitis and prostatic abscesses are treated with antibiotics. Prostatic neoplasia is generally highly malignant, and treatment is directed toward palliation rather than cure. Some dogs with prostatic cancer may benefit from castration because the tumors possess testosterone receptors.

GASTROENTEROLOGY

Acute Gastroenteritis

Acute gastroenteritis is one of the more common problems seen in canine practice. Some examples of conditions that may cause this problem include dietary indiscretion, viral gastroenteritis, bacterial gastroenteritis, gastrointestinal foreign bodies, gastrointestinal parasites, intussusception, ingestion of toxins, acute pancreatitis, and hypoadrenocorticism. The clinical history, signalment, and physical examination may suggest the diagnosis. Frequently, response to symptomatic therapy is used to assess whether further diagnostic study is warranted. The intensity and degree of symptomatic and supportive care are determined by the severity of clinical signs.

The fundamental decision of whether to hospitalize the patient is based on a number of factors; they include the hydration status of the dog, severity and frequency of vomiting and diarrhea, presence or absence of blood in the vomitus or stool, and presence of fever or profound lethargy. Non–patient-related factors to be considered include the client's ability to provide adequate care for the patient at home and ability of the client to pay for hospitalized care.

Clinical management of outpatients consists primarily of dietary restriction, administration of locally acting gastrointestinal medications, and use of fluid therapy when indicated. Dietary restriction is the most important aspect of the symptomatic care of acute gastroenteritis. The objective is to rest the gastrointestinal tract. This is accomplished by withholding all food for 12 to 24 hours, depending on the details of the case. If vomiting is severe, water is also withheld. If diarrhea is present and vomiting has not occurred, warm electrolyte-containing solutions can be given by mouth. During this period of symptomatic therapy, it is imperative that the patient be observed closely to prevent ingestion of foreign material and detect any worsening of clinical signs.

After food has been withheld for the prescribed period, small, frequent, bland meals should be offered. These meals should be low in fat, low in fiber, and easily digested and absorbed. These criteria are met by prescription diets, such as Prescription Diet I-D (Hill's), and by homemade diets, such as cottage cheese and boiled rice. These diets should be warmed before feeding. These frequent, small, bland meals should be continued for 2 to 3 days. If the patient is doing well, the regular diet and feeding schedule can be gradually reintroduced over the next 3 to 5 days. If clinical signs recur during this process, the dog should be reevaluated. Further diagnosis, evaluation, and more intensive supportive therapy may be warranted.

Although a vast number of locally acting preparations are available for the treatment of acute gastroenteritis, most have not been proved effective in controlled clinical trials. An over-the-counter preparation containing bismuth subsalicylate (Pepto-Bismol) has been shown to shorten the duration of symptoms in humans with experimental viral enteritis. It is theorized that the beneficial response is not due to the coating action of the product but rather to the salicylate inhibiting prostaglandin synthesis. Prostaglandins play a role in diarrhea by affecting both motility and secretory activity of the gastrointestinal tract. The recommended dose of Pepto-Bismol in the dog is 2.2 ml/kg of body weight three or four times daily. The technician should be aware that Pepto-Bismol may cause the stool to be dark to black, giving the false impression that melena is present when it truly is not.

TECHNICIAN NOTE

Pepto-Bismol causes the stool to be colored black and therefore should not be confused with melena.

In animals that are slightly to mildly dehydrated, some form of fluid therapy is appropriate. Fluids can be administered by mouth if the patient is not vomiting. Commercial water and electrolyte solutions, such as Gatorade, can be used to restore hydration and correct electrolyte imbalances. Alternatively, a homemade solution can be prepared inexpensively. One formula that has been recommended consists of 3.5 g of sodium chloride, 2.5 g of sodium bicarbonate, 1.5 g of potassium chloride, and 20 g of glucose added to 1 liter of water. Approximately 13.6 ml/kg/day of this solution will meet the maintenance requirements of the patient.

If the dog is mildly to moderately dehydrated or is vomiting, subcutaneous fluids are indicated. Lactated Ringer's solution is the fluid of choice. If signs have been prolonged, the lactated Ringer's solution can be supplemented with potassium chloride. Generally, the dose of subcutaneous fluids is 4.5 to 9.0 ml/kg of body weight administered at multiple sites. This can be repeated if necessary.

Client education is an essential part of the symptomatic care for acute gastroenteritis. The client should be informed that a definitive diagnosis has not been established and that merely the symptoms are being treated. If the animal is getting worse or if the signs persist longer than 36 to 48 hours, the animal should be reevaluated. The technician should have a concerned, caring attitude during the outpatient visit so if signs persist, the client will not hesitate to return or call for additional help. In many practices, it is standard procedure to telephone the client to receive follow-up progress reports. This ensures close client contact and thus improves the chances of successful management of the problem.

If initial clinical signs are severe or there is no response to symptomatic therapy, hospitalization is necessary. A major indication for hospitalization is the need for intravenous fluid therapy. Details about intravenous fluid therapy have been discussed earlier.

Dogs with severe acute gastroenteritis may also benefit from the parenteral administration of an antibiotic. Damage to the mucosal barrier of the intestines and altered intestinal motility may result in bacteremia. The parenteral route is preferred in order to provide effective tissue antibiotic levels. This is necessary because of potential decreased intestinal absorption.

Oral administration of antibiotics is not recommended in the vomiting patient. Antibiotics of choice in an adult animal would be a combination of ampicillin and gentamicin. Spectinomycin is a safe alternative for puppies because nephrotoxicity is less than with gentamicin. Specific therapy is indicated if an etiological agent is identified by fecal culture, such as erythromycin for the treatment of *Campylobacter* and chloramphenicol for the treatment of *Salmonella* or *Yersinia*.

The oral administration of aminoglycoside antibiotics (neomycin, gentamicin, kanamycin) is controversial. The proposed justification is that because the aminoglycosides are poorly absorbed from the gut, they will sterilize the gut and prevent absorption of harmful bacteria through the damaged intestinal wall. The counterargument is that this practice may actually do harm. In certain species, the aminoglycosides have been shown to damage the intestinal mucosa. It has been demonstrated that complete sterilization of the gut with any antibiotic or combination of antibiotics is impossible. Instead, oral antibiotics may alter the normal population of bacteria in the intestinal tract so disease-producing organisms may predominate. In certain bacterial gastroenteriditis, antibiotics may prolong the shedding of the infective organism in the feces.

Medications that alter the motility of the gastrointestinal tract may be indicated in cases of severe gastroenteritis. Improved understanding of the pathophysiology of intestinal motility has resulted in the more rational use of medications that are used to symptomatically treat vomiting and diarrhea. Anticholinergics decrease the resistance to intestinal flow and thus are of questionable efficacy in treating diarrhea. Antispasmodics are of minimal benefit as well.

Narcotics and narcotic-like drugs increase the rhythmical segmental contractions of the bowel, slow the passage of ingesta, and thus help to control diarrhea. These drugs should be used cautiously because of potential problems. Generally, they are reserved for more chronic or severe cases that are unresponsive to conservative therapy. A major disadvantage of the narcotic derivatives is that they can cause central nervous system depression. The decreased ingesta flow rate may result in increased absorption of toxins and altered bacterial flora in the gut. These compounds are contraindicated in the presence of intestinal obstruction.

Drugs used for the treatment of acute vomiting can be divided into several categories (see Table 12–9).

Drugs that have been used to decrease gastric acidity include anticholinergics. Anticholinergics probably have no effect on acid secretion. Antacids do not decrease the secretion of acid; however, they neutralize the acid that is produced. Antacids must be given frequently because their duration of action is brief. Paradoxically, if antacids are not given frequently, total daily acid secretion increases. Antacids administered according to a schedule of two or three times per day are probably of no value and may, in fact, be harmful. In most practices, more frequent administration is not practical. Drugs that block H_2 (histamine) receptors inhibit secretion of gastric acid. Cimetidine (Tagamet, SK&F Lab Co.) works by this mechanism. Phenothiazine-derivative tranquilizers—for example, chlorpromazine—work on the vomiting center of the central nervous system. These drugs are effective at controlling vomiting at much lower doses than the usual tranquilizer doses. These agents should be used with caution in dehydrated patients because of their blood pressure–lowering effects. Other antihistamines act by inhibiting a neural center involved in vomiting

called the chemoreceptor trigger zone. Vomiting induced by certain drugs, such as digoxin, is mediated by this center. Vomiting caused by motion sickness or vertigo may also respond to drugs in this group.

When the patient has improved, oral fluids and frequent, small, bland meals can be instituted. After discharge from the hospital, the dog can be treated as already described under outpatient management.

Canine Viral Enteritis

The two most important causes of viral enteritis in the dog are canine coronavirus and canine parvovirus. Other viral agents can occasionally produce gastroenteritis; they include canine distemper and canine rotavirus.

Clinical signs vary from subtle lethargy and anorexia to severe, rapidly fatal hemorrhagic gastroenteritis. Dogs of any age can be affected; however, the more severe cases typically occur between 6 and 20 weeks of age. On physical examination, the pups are usually febrile, depressed, and dehydrated. Vomiting or diarrhea may be observed. The stool may be watery, watery with flecks of blood, or severely hemorrhagic. Occasionally, infected dogs will display abdominal tenderness

• Table 12–9 •

ROSTER OF COMMONLY USED DRUGS FOR THE TREATMENT OF ACUTE GASTROENTERITIS

NARCOTICS
Lomotil (diphenoxalate, atropine)
Donnagel-PG (opium, atropine, hyoscyamine, kaolin, pectin)
Imodium (loperamide)
Diban (opium, atropine)
Parapectolin (paregoric, pectin, kaolin)
TRANQUILIZERS
Thorazine (chlorpromazine)
Darbazine (prochlorperazine, isopropamide)
Tigan (trimethobenzamide)
ANTICHOLINERGICS
Atropine
Scopolamine
Methscopolamine
Robinul-V (glycopyrrolate)
Centrine (aminopentamide hydrogen sulfate)
Diathal (diphemanil methylsulfate, penicillin, dihydrostreptomycin, chlorpheniramine maleate)
Darbazine (prochlorperazine, isopropamide)
Biosol-M (methscopolamine, neomycin)
Amoforal (kanamycin, aminopeptamide hydrogen sulfate, pectin)
Sulkamycin tablets (phthalylsulfacetamide, neomycin, belladonna alkaloids, pectin)
LOCALLY ACTIVE AGENTS
Kaopectate (kaolin, pectin)
Kao-forte (kaolin, pectin)
Pepto-Bismol (bismuth subsalicylate)
SMOOTH MUSCLE RELAXANTS (ANTISPASMODICS)
Oct-Vet (isometheptene)
Novin (dipyrone)
Jenotone (aminopropazine)
Myoquin-65V, Neopavin (ethaverine)
ANTIHISTAMINES
Dramamine (dimenhydrinate)
Bonine (meclizine)
H_2 BLOCKERS
Tagamet (cimetidine)

or pain. The presence of fever is more commonly associated with parvovirus than with coronavirus. A history of vaccination does not rule out viral enteritis because maternal antibodies may have prevented a protective immune response to the vaccination. It should be noted that the gastroenteritis and clinical disease secondary to coronavirus infection is much less severe than that seen with parvovirus infection.

Hemograms are usually normal with coronavirus enteritis but may be abnormal with parvovirus enteritis. Transient leukopenia is present in roughly one third to one half of dogs with parvovirus infections. Severely leukopenic patients may develop secondary infections because of a compromised immune system.

Plain abdominal radiographs do not reveal specific changes. Gastrointestinal contrast study changes may mimic small bowel obstruction. Abnormalities include dilated loops of bowel, tremendously prolonged passage time, and gas-capped fluid lines.

Definitive diagnosis is possible by several techniques. The viruses may be detected in the stool by electron microscopy. An ELISA performed on the feces can detect parvoviral antigen and can be used to demonstrate the virus in the feces during the period of active viral shedding. This period corresponds to the clinical illness. An easy-to-perform in-house test is available to check for parvovirus antigen in the stool (Probe-Canine Parvovirus Antigen test kit, Idexx Labs, Westbrook, ME).

It should be stressed that the treatment of canine viral gastroenteritis is supportive because there are no effective antiviral agents. Treatment includes aggressive intravenous fluid therapy, antibiotics, injectable antiemetics, and keeping the animal clean and comfortable. One other complication seen with parvovirus infection, to which the technician should be alert, is the development of hypoglycemia. If profound weakness and/ or seizures develop, a blood glucose level should be determined.

A myocardial form of canine parvovirus has been described in young pups. This form of the disease is characterized by sudden death in otherwise healthy pups; however, it appears to be becoming less common. This may be due to the fact that most pups have maternal antibodies at the critical period when they are susceptible to the myocardial form.

Both canine parvovirus and coronavirus are highly contagious. The major route of the infection is fecal-oral. Dogs showing clinical signs will shed large numbers of viral particles for 1 to 2 weeks. The canine parvovirus is hardy; therefore, once the environment is contaminated, infective virus will survive for prolonged periods. The virus has been shown to remain infectious in dog feces held at room temperature for longer than 6 months.

Good sanitation will reduce the numbers of infective virus in the hospital environment. Dilute hypochlorite (chlorine bleach and water, diluted to a ratio of 1:32) solutions have significant viricidal properties. Because the virus is ubiquitous, however, the best means of prevention is an appropriate immunization program.

NEPHROLOGY-UROLOGY

Canine Uroliths

A *urolith* is a pathological stone formed from mineral salts found in the urinary tract. Clinical signs depend on location,

number, size, shape, and whether there is concurrent urinary tract infection. Urolith classification is generally based on the predominant mineral component, such as phosphate or urate. In the dog, more than 90% of the uroliths are located in the bladder and urethra and fewer than 10% are located in the kidneys. Although uroliths can occur in any breed, some breeds suspected to be at greater risk include the miniature schnauzer, dalmatian, dachshund, pug, English bulldog, Welsh corgi, basset hound, Pekingese, and Scottish terrier.

If the urolith is located in the bladder, there may be no clinical signs, but more commonly stranguria, increased frequency of urination (pollakiuria), and hematuria will be seen. If the urolith is in the urethra, there may be frequent attempts to urinate and dribbling of urine. If the urethra is completely obstructed by the stone or stones, abdominal distention, pain, anorexia, depression, and vomiting will be observed.

Laboratory findings generally are not specific for uroliths. Radiology, including contrast studies such as cystograms and pneumocystograms, may be necessary to establish the diagnosis. Generally speaking, uroliths are managed surgically. A prescription diet (S/D, Hill's) has been advocated as a means of medically treating phosphate uroliths. The diet is high in sodium and low in protein and phosphorus and has an acidifying effect on urine. Dissolution of the uroliths occurs over a period of weeks. Unfortunately, this medical approach has several important limitations. A prescription S/D diet is effective in the dissolution of only phosphate calculi and is not recommended as a long-term maintenance diet.

The overall recurrence rate for bladder stones is high, approximately 25%. Therefore, efforts to reduce the chance of recurrence are very important. The first step is to analyze the mineral composition of the stone because different stone types are managed differently. It is also important to determine whether infection is present and, if so, which antibiotics are most likely to be effective.

Several preventative measures are appropriate regardless of the stone type. These include elimination of any infection and stimulation of increased urine output. The urine output can be increased by salting the diet and thereby increasing water intake.

Depending on the specific stone type, it may also be desirable to initiate dietary therapy and modify the urine pH. Ammonium chloride is commonly used to acidify the urine, and sodium bicarbonate is used to alkalinize it.

Because the recurrence rate for uroliths is high, client education is extremely important. First, long-term therapeutic compliance will be achieved only if the importance of these measures is stressed to the client. Second, the owner should be aware of signs that indicate recurrence of the problem.

Feline Urological Syndrome

Feline urological syndrome is the term used to describe a condition of unknown etiology in cats characterized by dysuria, hematuria, pollakiuria, urinating in uncommon places, and occasionally urethral obstruction. Urethral obstruction, if it occurs, is potentially fatal because of the associated severe metabolic derangements. The emergency treatment of feline urethral obstruction is covered in Chapter 11.

Because recurrence of the urethral obstruction is frequent, some clinicians prefer to routinely use indwelling urethral catheters for a brief period of time after relief of the obstruction.

The justification for the use of indwelling catheters is to maintain urine flow without the trauma associated with recatheterization and manual compression of the bladder. Indwelling urethral catheters should be used judiciously because of the risk of ascending urinary tract infection and catheter-induced injury to the bladder or urethra. Complications associated with the use of indwelling catheters can be minimized if an appropriate catheter is selected. Commercially manufactured polypropylene catheters (Sovereign tomcat catheters and open-end tomcat catheters, Sherwood Medical Industries) can be either too short or too long. Therefore, care should be taken to select a catheter with an appropriate length. Soft, flexible polyvinyl catheters, such as Sovereign sterile disposable feeding tube and urethral catheter, are preferred because of decreased damage to the urethral and bladder mucosa. To pass these catheters, they are kept frozen until immediately before use. This will make the catheter sufficiently rigid to allow passage in a male cat. The catheter should be well lubricated before passage.

Indwelling urethral catheters are generally secured by suturing the catheter to the prepuce. Adhesive tape is attached longitudinally and transversely to the end of the catheter. If the catheter is wet when the tape is applied, it may not stick. Two simple interrupted sutures on either side of the prepuce penetrate the tape and thus prevent movement of the catheter. If analgesia is required to place the sutures, the prepuce can be numbed by applying an ice cube for 1 or 2 minutes. When the catheter is sutured in place, it should be done in such a way that there is no chance of kinking. An Elizabethan collar can be used to prevent the cat from removing the indwelling catheter.

To prevent ascending urinary tract infection, sterile technique is required when placing and maintaining the indwelling catheter. The collection apparatus should be a closed, sterile system. The entire system—catheter, plastic tubing, and collection bottle—must be sterile initially and must be kept sealed to prevent bacterial contamination. Povidone-iodine ointment should be applied several times a day at the point at which the catheter exits the urethra.

Indwelling urethral catheters should be used for as brief a time as possible. The prophylactic use of antimicrobials does not reduce infection. If infection does develop, it is frequently caused by an organism resistant to the prophylactic antimicrobial.

Because the recurrence rate for feline urological syndrome is high, preventative measures are an important aspect of its medical management. Unfortunately, because the etiology of feline urological syndrome is unknown, preventative measures are largely empirical. The most frequently recommended preventative measures include providing an ample supply of fresh, potable water, cleaning the litter pan frequently, and lightly salting the food to increase water intake and, thus, urine volume. Exclusive feeding of diets that contain 20 mg of magnesium per 100 kcal or less and that maintain a urine pH of 6.4 or less is the most important preventive measure. Certain diets, such as C/D or Feline Maintenance (Hill's), meet this requirement. Although urinary acidification with ammonium chloride has been recommended, it should be emphasized that some diets, such as the ones mentioned above, cause urinary acidification, and additional acidifiers are contraindicated. The basis of acidifying the urine is to increase the solubility of this crystalline material, which is incriminated as the cause of feline urological syndrome.

If ammonium chloride is used with a nonacidifying diet, it should be thoroughly mixed with the food to improve palatability. It should also be administered with every meal. Any change in diet or introduction of a food additive—for example, ammonium chloride or salt—should be done gradually over several days. This will reduce the chances of the cat's rejecting the new or altered food. Enteric-coated ammonium chloride tablets are not effective in the cat.

Chronic Renal Failure

Animals in renal failure should be fed diets containing reduced quantities of high-quality protein and adequate nonprotein calories. This can be accomplished by using prescription diets such as K/D (Hill's). K/D is a moderate protein-restricted diet available for dogs in canned, semimoist, and dry forms. Feline K/D is a canned product suitable for use in uremic cats.

If desired, homemade diets can be used (Lewis et al., 1987). The following is a recipe for a moderately low-protein diet for dogs:

¼ lb. regular ground beef

1 hard-boiled egg, finely chopped

2 cups cooked rice without salt

3 slices white bread, crumbled

1 tsp. calcium carbonate

Balanced vitamin and mineral supplement

The meat should be braised, retaining the fat, and thoroughly mixed with the other ingredients. This recipe will meet the daily requirements of a 13.5-kg dog.

The following is an example of a homemade protein-restricted diet for cats:

¼ lb. liver

2 large eggs, hard boiled

2 cups cooked rice without salt

1 T vegetable oil

1 tsp. calcium carbonate

Balanced vitamin and mineral supplement

Dice and braise the liver, retaining fat. This recipe provides a total of 635 kcal per pound.

Many animals with renal failure are anorectic because of nausea and vomiting. Small, frequent meals are recommended to reduce the nausea. If the animal can tolerate food orally but is not eating, feeding by means of an orogastric tube is recommended. The diets described can be administered through a stomach tube if the ingredients are thoroughly mixed with water in a kitchen blender.

Supportive therapy for chronic renal failure includes the use of phosphorous binders, anabolic steroids, sodium bicarbonate, sodium chloride, calcium, and vitamin D metabolites. The use of these treatments should be based on documented abnormalities because the inappropriate or incorrect use of these agents can do more harm than good.

ORTHOPEDICS
Canine Hip Dysplasia

Hip dysplasia refers to a developmental problem of the canine coxofemoral joint. Subluxation of the femoral head leads to abnormal wear and eventual degenerative joint disease. The acetabulum is more shallow than normal, and the femoral head is flattened.

The etiology of hip dysplasia is multifactorial. Genetics and environmental factors such as nutrition appear to be important. Hip dysplasia is seen in most large breeds and is inherited by a polygenic mode of inheritance. This means that many genes are responsible for its development. It is also quantitative in its expression. In other words, affected dogs can show slight or severe changes. As is characteristic for traits with a polygenic mode of inheritance, hip dysplasia is modified by environmental factors. For example, it has been suggested that dogs fed a high-calorie diet during growth have an increased incidence, whereas dogs fed a low-calorie diet have a decreased incidence.

The Orthopedic Foundation of America in Columbia, MO, is an organization established to evaluate the hip radiographs of potential breeding dogs. Radiologists identify those dogs with radiographically normal hip joints. Unfortunately, because of the factors mentioned, breeding two radiographically normal dogs does not ensure normal progeny. It is better to evaluate entire families (siblings and progeny) when selecting dogs to be included in a breeding program to decrease the incidence of hip dysplasia. It is also important to recognize that good hip joints should not be the sole criterion for selection. Other traits, such as disposition, working ability, and conformation, should also be considered.

The clinical signs of hip dysplasia vary tremendously from occasional slight discomfort to a severe disabling disease. It should be remembered that the clinical signs of hip dysplasia do not always correlate with the severity of hip dysplasia detected radiographically.

Dogs with hip dysplasia will respond differently to varying levels of exercise. Some dogs are most comfortable with minimal activity, yet others do best with a regular regimen of moderate exercise. Swimming is an excellent form of exercise, since muscle tone is increased with the hip joints in a non–weight-bearing position. Any exercise program should be instituted gradually. Forced sudden activity such as ball playing or rough play should be discouraged. Severely affected dogs should be treated symptomatically with analgesics and anti-inflammatory drugs.

Several surgical procedures have been advocated for the treatment of hip dysplasia. They include procedures such as pectineus myotomy, pelvic osteotomy, excision arthroplasty, and total hip prosthesis. A discussion of these surgical procedures is beyond the scope of this chapter.

Intervertebral Disk Disease

Intervertebral disk disease is a relatively common problem affecting the spinal cord of chondrodystrophoid and other breeds. Breeds commonly affected include dachshunds, Pekingese, cocker spaniels, poodles, pugs, and beagles. The chondrodystrophoid breeds tend to develop signs at an earlier age than the nonchondrodystrophoid breeds.

The intervertebral disks are structures located between the vertebrae and function as a shock-absorbing system. The disk itself is composed of two parts—the firm fibrous outer annulus and the softer inner nucleus. In intervertebral disk disease, the annulus undergoes degeneration, and the nuclear material protrudes or is completely extruded. The result is compression of the spinal cord with the subsequent development of neurological signs. These signs vary from simple pain to complete paralysis.

Intervertebral disk disease can be managed either conservatively with cage confinement and anti-inflammatory drugs or more aggressively with neurosurgery. Management decisions are based on the history, neurological signs, and wishes of the owner.

If conservative therapy is elected, the technician plays a vital role. Extreme care should be taken in handling the patient because movement may result in the extrusion of additional disk material and worsening of signs. To reduce handling, these patients should be placed in lower cages whenever possible. Because these patients are frequently in severe pain, gentle, compassionate care is essential. Many cases will benefit from some of the physical therapy techniques described earlier.

Dogs with intervertebral disk disease receiving anti-inflammatory drugs, such as dexamethasone, may develop secondary problems, such as gastrointestinal hemorrhage or acute pancreatitis. Consequently, these patients should be observed closely for fever, anorexia, abdominal pain, hemorrhagic vomiting, and diarrhea.

Recommended Reading

Feldman EC and Nelson RW: Canine and Feline Endocrinology and Reproduction. Philadelphia, WB Saunders, 1987.
Lewis LD, Morris MI, and Hand ___ all Animal Clinical Nutrition III. Topeka, KS, Mark Morris ___
Schultz RD: Theoretical an___ ___ an immunization program for dogs and ___ ___9, 1982.

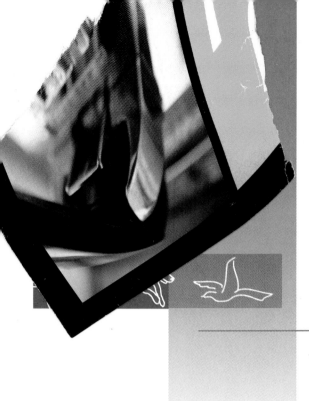

Neonatal Care of Puppy, Kitten, and Foal

Johnny D. Hoskins • Cyprianna E. Swiderski

Caring for the ill puppy, kitten, or foal from birth to young adulthood is often complicated by age-related changes in the body systems. These age-related changes occur because the normal development of specific body systems continues well after birth. Thorough clinical evaluation of the ill puppy, kitten, or foal may include the case history, physical examination, routine laboratory tests, electrocardiography (ECG) (lead II rhythm strip), and, possibly, radiography.

PUPPY AND KITTEN

Physical and Laboratory Examination

The physical examination of a sick puppy or kitten should be conducted in a systematic manner. Additional information on the physical examination is found in Chapter 3. The first skill used in the examination is careful observation of the animal's responses, specifically noting the puppy's or kitten's general condition, mentation, posture, locomotion, and breathing pattern. Next, the body temperature, respiratory and heart rates, capillary refill time, and body weight should be recorded. After completing the observation and vital sign collection phase, the clinician should assess the function of specific body systems (Table 13–1).

Veterinarians often use a commercial laboratory facility for such routine tests as hemograms, serum chemistry profiles, and urine analyses. However, collections from puppies and kittens younger than 6 weeks of age often do not yield adequate samples for testing by these laboratories. As an alternative, the veterinarian can use in-house laboratory tests, including microhematocrit for the packed cell volume (PCV), blood film

examination of erythrocyte and leukocyte morphology, blood glucose and urea nitrogen (BUN) by reagent strip for whole blood, urine evaluation by reagent strip for urinalysis and a urine sediment examination, and total plasma solids and urine specific gravity by refractometer. The results of these few tests may be sufficient to confirm illness or assist in case management of an illness.

ECG can be used to diagnose life-threatening arrhythmias and conduction disturbances in puppies and kittens; however, ECG identification of right- or left-sided chamber enlargement or hypertrophy and alterations in mean electrical axis (MEA) usually is not attempted. The ECGs of young kittens normally have smaller amplitude P waves and QRS complexes than puppies in all leads. Any ECG lead with easily recognizable P waves and QRS complexes can be used to identify arrhythmias.

Real-time, gray-scale ultrasonography is the newest diagnostic tool to be used in puppies and kittens to identify selected abdominal and cardiac diseases. Ultrasonography usually is tolerated better by puppies and kittens and is safer for personnel than routine radiography. For ultrasonography in most puppies and kittens, a 5-MHz ultrasound transducer or, preferably, a 7.5-MHz transducer is required. The higher the transducer frequency, the better is the image resolution but the greater is the ultrasound beam attenuation in soft tissue. Linear array transducers used transrectally for reproductive examination are inadequate for imaging in most puppies and kittens.

Most echocardiography is performed in puppies and kittens that are 6 weeks of age or older. Echocardiography, whether obtained by the M-mode, two-dimensional, contrast, and/or Doppler echocardiographic technology, has facilitated evaluation of puppies and kittens with congenital heart disease

• Table 13–1 •

PHYSICAL EXAMINATION OF PUPPY AND KITTEN

- *Head and Oral Cavity:* Check for malformations of the skull, cleft lip, stenotic nares, or cleft palate. The mucous membranes should be light pink and moist. The teeth, if present, should be examined for early occlusion.
- *Ears:* External ear canals open between 6 and 14 days after birth and should be completely open by 17 days. When ear canals first open, cytological examination shows an abundance of desquamative cells and some oil droplets. A thorough otoscopic examination can be made in kittens older than 4 weeks of age.
- *Eyes and Eyelids:* The eyelids separate into upper and lower eyelids at 5 to 14 days after birth. Menace reflex may not appear until 3 to 4 weeks of life. Reflex lacrimation begins when the eyelids separate, therefore, evaluation of tear production by Schirmer's tear test can be done thereafter. Pupillary light responses are present after the eyelids open but may not be evident until 21 days of age.
- *Nose:* Check appearance and patency of the nostrils and the presence of fluids (mucus, pus, blood, milk, clear discharges)
- *Thorax:* Check the thoracic wall, whether symmetrical or deformed, and auscultate the thorax using a stethoscope with a pediatric chest piece (2-cm bell; 3-cm diaphragm). The heart rate approximates 220 beats/min and the respiratory rate is from 15 to 35 breaths/min during the first 4 weeks of life; they become similar to adults thereafter. The normal heart rhythm of puppies and kittens is a regular sinus rhythm. Heart sounds are localized to the left cardiac apex (left fifth to sixth intercostal space, ventral third of thorax), the left cardiac base (left third to fourth intercostal space above the costochondral junction), or the right cardiac apex (right fourth to fifth intercostal space opposite the mitral valve area). Heart murmurs are the most common type of abnormal sound heard, frequently being a functional murmur and not a murmur associated with congenital heart disease. Absence of lung sounds or audible asymmetry may indicate abnormalities within the thorax and/or lungs.
- *Abdomen:* Unless the liver margins extend beyond the ribs, the liver is not enlarged. The spleen normally is not palpable unless it is enlarged. Both kidneys are palpable in all kittens. The stomach may feel like a large, fluid-filled sac if it is full. The intestines palpate as soft, slightly fluid or gas-filled structures that are freely movable and nonpainful. The urinary bladder can be gently squeezed to determine resistance to urine outflow.
- *Skin and Umbilicus:* The skin should be inspected for wounds, state of hydration, and condition of foot pads. The skin and haircoat should also be examined for evidence of bacterial infection, external parasites, or dermatophytosis. The umbilicus should be carefully inspected for evidence of inflammation and/or infection or abnormalities of the abdominal wall. The umbilical cord normally drops off by 2 to 3 days of age.
- *Limbs, Tail, Anus, and Genitalia:* Check the limbs for deformities or absence of long bones, number and position of toes and pads, position of limbs at rest and during movement, presence of soft tissue (bruises, swelling, wounds), and condition of joints (deformities, range of mobility). The tail is inspected for length, mobility, and deformities. The anus should be evaluated for patency, redness, and signs of diarrhea, and the genitalia should be checked for position and appearance.
- *Nervous System:* Suck reflex is present at birth and disappears by 3 weeks of life. Eliminative behaviors are controlled for first 3 to 4 weeks of life by anogenital reflex.

by improving the diagnostic accuracy and lessening the stress and risk to animals. For echocardiography in puppies and kittens, a 7.5-MHz transducer is preferred. Heart lesions readily identified with M-mode or two-dimensional echocardiography include pericardial effusion, valvular vegetations, chamber size, myocardial hypertrophy, and abnormal cardiac motion. Although specific cardiac lesions cannot always be directly imaged, echocardiography usually demonstrates the secondary effects of a lesion on the heart, such as dilation, hypertrophy, and hyperkinesis.

Contrast echocardiography may be helpful in confirming a right-to-left shunting lesion. Doppler ultrasonography is becoming increasingly available as a noninvasive means of assessing and quantifying the direction and velocity of blood flow within the heart and blood vessels. Doppler imaging of high-velocity, retrograde, or turbulent flow through valves or intracardiac communications provides useful diagnostic and prognostic information in puppies and kittens with congenital heart defects. Interpretation of echocardiography from puppies and kittens requires an awareness of the growth pattern and developmental anatomy of the heart during the first year of life. After birth, there is a decrease in right ventricular mass relative to the left ventricle and to body weight, a decrease that occurs by the third week of life in puppies.

Additional information on ultrasound and radiology can be found in Chapter 9.

A finely tuned technique chart is necessary if good-quality radiographs are to be produced for all body parts of young puppies and kittens. Seldom can a technique chart designed for one x-ray machine be used on another x-ray machine with any

degree of success. Kilovoltage must be greatly reduced for radiography of a young puppy or kitten because of minimal absorption of x-rays by partially mineralized bones and because of the thinness of soft tissue body parts. A general guideline for reducing kilovoltage is to reduce the radiographic exposure to about one half of that used for adult dogs and cats of the same thickness. Extrapolations to thinner dogs and cats can be made based on the fact that each 1 cm of soft tissue is the equivalent of 2 kVp at values equal to or less than 80 kVp. Most radiography of young puppies and kittens will be performed in the 40 to 60 kVp range; therefore, a change of 4 to 6 kVp doubles or halves the film exposure.

TECHNICIAN NOTE

Kilovoltage must be greatly reduced for radiography of a puppy or kitten.

An additional step that can be helpful in producing maximum-quality radiographs in young puppies and kittens is to use a single high-detail intensifying screen within the cassette. The single screen should be adhered to the back inner surface of the cassette. The cassette is then loaded with single-emulsion x-ray film to take advantage of the increased detail that can be produced with the single screen. The screen should be a rare-earth high-detail type. The emulsion side of the x-ray film must be positioned toward the screen.

The development of computer equipment that can average electrical signals by extracting low-amplitude, time-locked potentials from random background electrical activity has provided procedures for non-invasive evaluation of the auditory and visual system. Recording of the brain stem auditory-evoked response (BAER) is the best objective procedure for assessment of hearing in puppies and kittens. The electrical potential from the cochlea, cochlear nerve and brain stem in response to an auditory stimulus is recorded. The BAER approximates functional maturity by 4 to 6 weeks of age. If there is no response at all in puppies or kittens older than 6 weeks of age, the cochlea is not functioning, as may occur with congenital deafness.

The electroretinography (ERG) is the electrical recording of retinal response to light. The ERG approximates functional maturity by 5 to 10 weeks of age. If there is no response at all after 10 weeks of age, the retina is not functioning, as may occur in retinal blindness due to congenital or acquired causes. The visual-evoked response (VER) provides an objective evaluation of the central visual pathways. The VER is the cortical electrical activity that occurs in response to a light stimulus administered to the eye. The VER approximates functional maturity by 6 weeks of age. If there is an altered VER after 10 weeks of age, central visual pathways may not be functioning, as may occur in central blindness due to congenital or acquired causes.

Causes for Neonatal Care

Puppies and kittens commonly present for severe illnesses or rearing as an orphan during the time period between birth and 12 weeks of age. Illnesses may have been acquired in utero, during the birth process (0 to 2 weeks of age) or in the postweaning period of 6 to 12 weeks of age. Illness during the postweaning period is primarily caused by infectious (bacterial, viral, protozoal, and parasitic) diseases and/or malnutrition potentiated by weaning stress, exposure to pathogenic organisms in the immediate environment, and diminished local and/or systemic immunity. In general, most puppy and kitten illnesses will occur because of congenital anomalies, nutritional diseases resulting from improper diets fed to the mother or her young, abnormally low birth weights, traumatic insults during or after the birth process (dystocia, cannibalism, maternal neglect), neonatal isoerythrolysis, infectious diseases, and other miscellaneous factors.

Nutrition of the Orphan Puppy or Kitten. If the mother is healthy and well nourished, the newborn's nutritional needs for the first 3 to 4 weeks of life should be handled completely by her. Indications that the puppy or kitten is not receiving adequate milk are shown by its constant crying, extreme inactivity, and/or failure to attain the weight gains. Puppies should gain 2 to 4 g/day/kg of anticipated adult weight (10% increase in weight per day, doubling birth weight by 10 days); kittens should attain appropriate weight gains of 10 to 15 g/day.

Weaning from mother's milk to other foods should be a gradual process. Kittens should be encouraged to begin eating solid food at 4 weeks of age, puppies at 3 weeks of age. At the beginning of weaning, the kitten or puppy can be offered a mixture of a high-quality food designed for growth and milk or water as a thick gruel (a mixture of 1 part dry food blended with 3 parts water [or milk] or 2 parts canned food blended with 1 part water [or milk]). The puppy or kitten is encouraged to eat gruel by smearing some of the gruel on its lips, being careful not to get any in the nose; or the feeder can touch a finger in the gruel and then into the mouth. Once the puppy or kitten is eating the gruel well, gradually reduce the amount of milk or water in the gruel until the animal is consuming only solid food. Most kittens will wean at 6 to 8 weeks of age, puppies at 5 to 7 weeks of age. Early weaning and separation from littermates before 6 weeks can result in behavioral problems (slowness to learn and more suspicious, cautious, and aggressive actions).

TECHNICIAN NOTE

Caloric needs for most puppies and kittens is 22 to 26 kcal/100 g of body weight.

Because the puppy's or kitten's eating habits are still in the formative stage after weaning, it remains important that easily digested high-quality, high-calorie food be fed daily and fresh water be available. Cow's milk should never be fed to the puppy or kitten in place of plenty of fresh drinking water. Puppies should be fed to attain the average growth rate for that dog breed; overfeeding is not recommended. Kittens should be fed all the food they will consume. Free-choice feeding or feeding at least three times a day is preferred during growth; and any type of supplementation should be avoided.

Commercially prepared milk replacement formulas are preferred for raising motherless puppies or kittens, because they more closely compare to mother's milk. These formulas generally provide 1 to 1.24 Kcal of metabolizable energy per milliliter of formula. Caloric needs for most puppies and kittens is 22 to 26 kcal/100 g of body weight for the first 3 months of age. Therefore, the puppy or kitten should receive daily about 13 ml of formula/100 g of body weight for the first week of life, 17 ml of formula/100 g of body weight for the second week, 20 ml of formula/100 g of body weight for the third week, and 22 ml of formula/100 g of body weight for the fourth week. These amounts of formula are fed in equal portions three or four times daily. Before each feeding, the formula is warmed to about 37.8°C (100°F). For the first feedings, the amount of formula fed should be less than the prescribed amount per feeding. The amount is then gradually increased to the recommended feeding amount by the second or third day and is then increased accordingly as the puppy or kitten gains weight and a favorable response to feeding occurs. When feeding the puppy or kitten formula, always follow the manufacturer's directions on the label for its preparation, and keep all feeding equipment scrupulously clean.

Malnutrition. Malnutrition occurs when basic nutritional requirements for the puppy or kitten are not being met. Malnutrition is especially common during the time when the young depend entirely on the mother. Several factors can contribute to malnutrition in the nursing puppy or kitten. The puppy or kitten may ingest insufficient or inadequate milk because the mother dies; the mother disowns her young; a larger litter is born than can be cared for properly; and partial or complete lactation failure by the mother due to mastitis, metritis, or underdeveloped mammae. In addition, puppies and kittens may be born underdeveloped, be so weak and sick that they cannot suckle, or have a congenital anomaly that precludes adequate milk intake. Failure to provide an adequate growth diet at 3 to 4 weeks of age can also result in malnutrition.

Immediate recognition of a malnourished puppy or kitten is usually based on their smaller, lighter appearance; feeble attempts to feed; and/or inability to attain adequate weight gain for their age. High-pitched, constant crying and inactivity with an accompanying weak sucking reflex are advanced indications that the nursing puppy or kitten is receiving insufficient or inadequate milk. Reduced body tone and muscle strength may be evident on handling. Coexisting congenital anomaly that is not immediately life threatening may be detected on physical examination as well.

TECHNICIAN NOTE

Hypoglycemia and dehydration occur quickly when the puppy or kitten is not adequately fed.

The management of malnutrition in the nursing puppy or kitten generally requires that the proper nourishment be provided. Complications that are frequently encountered during the management of malnutrition are diarrhea, dehydration, hypoglycemia, and hypothermia. If diarrhea occurs during feeding of adequate amounts of commercial milk replacement formula, immediately reduce the amount of solids intake to one half of that offered. This can be done by diluting 1:1 the milk replacement formula with water or preferably with a mixture of equal parts of Ringer's solution and 5% dextrose in water solution. As the condition of feces improves, gradually increase the amount of solids to the recommended level. Hypoglycemia and dehydration occur quickly when the malnourished puppy or kitten is not adequately fed. Milk replacement formula should not be fed to a weak and severely chilled puppy or kitten that possesses a diminished sucking reflex or in which body temperature is below 35°C (95°F). Giving an equal mixture of warm Ringer's solution and 5% dextrose/water solution parenterally or administering orally a warm nutrient-electrolyte solution every 15 to 30 minutes until the puppy or kitten responds can help to alleviate or prevent dehydration and mild hypoglycemia.

Bacterial Infections. When bacterial infections overcome the ability of the puppy's or kitten's immune system to provide adequate protection, life-threatening illnesses such as neonatal sepsis occur. The bacterial invasion of the bloodstream that regularly occurs in puppies and kittens after birth would rarely be of any consequence in healthy adults. However, when overwhelming bacteremia develops in puppies and kittens 4 to 16 weeks of age, the severity of the illness usually influences survival. Factors predisposing puppies and kittens to septicemic conditions include coexistence of inadequate nutrition and thermoregulation, viral infections, parasitism, and developmental and heritable defects of the immune system.

Bloodstream invasion usually occurs by the more common

bacteria, such as *Staphylococcus, Escherichia, Klebsiella, Enterobacter, Streptococcus, Enterococcus, Pseudomonas, Clostridium, Bacteroides, Fusobacterium,* and *Salmonella* spp.; of these, gram-negative bacilli most often occur. Sources from which gram-negative bacilli enter the bloodstream include gastrointestinal tract and peritoneal infection, respiratory tract infection, skin and wound infection, and urinary tract infection.

Signs of Neonatal Illness

The clinical manifestations of neonatal illness do not always allow specific identification of the causative condition. Furthermore, many puppies and kittens have unusual or a wide variety of clinical presentations, which may not be immediately recognized as being associated with a specific illness. Death can occur so suddenly that noticeable signs are virtually absent. More typically, however, puppies and kittens will cry a lot and show signs of restlessness, weakness, hypothermia, diarrhea, altered respiration, hematuria, failure to thrive, and cyanosis, and in advanced stages, they may slough parts of their extremities.

The diagnosis of a neonatal illness is usually based on the case history and physical findings. Ideally, a complete blood count, plasma chemistry profile, urinalysis, urine and/or blood culture, and culture of suspected sources of infection are obtained. When dealing with neonatal sepsis, it is imperative to conduct a thorough search for the primary source of infection and collect appropriate bacterial culture samples before initiating antimicrobial therapy.

The hemograms of septicemic puppies and kittens are usually characterized by a normochromic normocytic anemia. Thrombocytopenia and mild to moderate neutrophilia with a left shift may be present. Another laboratory finding that is consistent with, but by no means specific for, neonatal sepsis is hypoglycemia. The remaining laboratory values from the plasma chemistry profile and urinalysis may reflect a specific organ failure.

Management of Neonatal Illness

Early, prompt care for the ill puppy or kitten is required for satisfactory results. Because many neonatal diseases may cause sudden death, puppies and kittens suspected of having a severe illness should be treated immediately. In most instances, rewarming, fluid replacement, and antimicrobial therapy are started empirically. Severely ill puppies and kittens may also require glucose therapy if hypoglycemia is present (Table 13–2).

TECHNICIAN NOTE

Rewarming, fluid/glucose replacement, and antimicrobial therapy are the hallmarks of management for the ill puppy or kitten.

Meaningful advances in treating bacterial infections have been made in recent years, particularly in the development of antimicrobial agents. Many of these antimicrobial agents have either an increased spectrum of activity or a diminished toxicity

• Table 13–2 •

MANAGEMENT OF SEVERELY ILL PUPPY AND KITTEN

I. External warming procedure
   A. Use circulating hot water blanket and hot water bottle
   B. Take at least 20 to 30 minutes for gradual warming of the patient
   C. Turn the patient every hour
   D. Record rectal temperature every hour (preferred temperature, 100°F)
II. Parenteral fluid therapy
   A. Use multiple electrolyte solution supplemented with 5% dextrose solution
   B. Supplement the fluids with potassium chloride solution if plasma potassium concentration is less than 2.5 mM/liter
   C. Administer warm fluids slowly by intravenous or intraosseous route
III. Glucose replacement therapy
   A. Administer 5% dextrose solution intravenously or intraosseously, to effect
   B. Administer 1 to 2 ml/kg of a 10% dextrose solution to the patient that is profoundly depressed or having seizures
   C. Maintain plasma glucose concentration at 80 to 200 mg/dl for euglycemia
IV. Antimicrobial therapy
   A. Collect bacterial culture samples (whole blood, urine, exudate, feces) before initiation of antimicrobial therapy
      1. For blood culture, collect 1 ml of whole blood aseptically and inoculate blood directly into enriched tryptic or trypticase soy broth, dilute the whole blood 1:5 to 1:10 in enriched broth, and examine broth for bacterial growth 6 to 18 hours later
      2. For urine culture, collect urine by cystocentesis and culture it by standard methods
      3. For exudate and fecal cultures, collect and culture by standard methods
   B. Empirical treatment with antimicrobial agent(s) begins immediately after collection of appropriate bacterial culture samples
   C. Adjust the dosage and dosing interval of antimicrobial agent(s) selected
   D. Administer the antimicrobial agent by intravenous or intraosseous route
V. Provide oxygen and nutritional therapy
   A. Administer oxygen by mask or intranasal catheter to counteract tissue hypoxemia
   B. Encourage food intake once patient is normothermic and adequately hydrated
VI. Monitor the effectiveness of medical management
   A. Observe for improvement in the patient's general demeanor
   B. Regularly assess the cardiopulmonary status (it is extremely easy to overhydrate the severely ill puppy or kitten, and so attentive monitoring of breathing pattern is helpful for early recognition of overhydration)
   C. Weigh the patient three to four times a day to record weight gain
   D. Observe for moistness of mucous membranes and clearness of urine in assessing for adequate hydration (healthy puppies and kittens have clear, colorless urine when normally hydrated—any color to the urine usually indicates dehydration)

relative to previously available antimicrobial agents. However, specific pharmacokinetic data for many of the antimicrobial agents have not been obtained in adults or in puppies and kittens, and therefore the veterinary use of these antimicrobial agents remains somewhat empirical.

Unfortunately, clinical information necessary for appropriate dosing of antimicrobial agents in septicemic puppies and kittens is not always available. Drug distribution, especially in puppies and kittens younger than 5 weeks of age, differs from that of adults because of differences in body composition, such as lower total body fat, higher percentage of total body water, lower concentrations of albumin, and poorly developed blood-brain barrier. Because of these differences, modifications of dosing amounts for adults, as much as 30% to 50% reduction of the adult dose, or changes in dosing frequency may be necessary when antimicrobial agents are administered to septicemic puppies and kittens.

Furthermore, fluid replacement therapy and antimicrobial agents should be administered intravenously or intraosseously in severely ill puppies and kittens because systemic absorption after oral, subcutaneous, or intramuscular administration may not be reliable. Most drugs ingested by the lactating bitch or queen appear in her milk; the amount generally is 1% to 2% of the mother's dose. Therefore, severely ill puppies or kittens should never be treated by treating only the lactating mother. The beta-lactam antimicrobial agents are considered to be the first choice in the treatment of septicemic puppies and kittens. The beta-lactam antimicrobial agents include the penicillins, cephalosporins, and the combination of beta-lactam antimicrobials and beta-lactamase inhibitors.

FOAL

The critically ill foal is perhaps the most intensively managed of all veterinary patients. With the advent of specialized centers for the treatment of foals, great advances have been made in understanding the physiology and disease states of the equine neonate. With these advances, the overall survival rate for foals entering intensive care is improving, and foals of younger gestational age are surviving. The most critical factor influencing a foal's survival is, undoubtedly, diligent nursing care. Successful foal management requires a team approach, and competent veterinary technical support has become the foundation of the team. The skills required of equine neonatal technicians are extensive. This chapter provides only an overview of these skills, and individuals with aspirations in this area should consult other textbooks that focus on equine and human neonatal care. Additional clinical training can be obtained in most university teaching hospitals that have a foal neonatal care unit.

The High-Risk Foal

The term *high-risk foal* refers to the foal that is not necessarily ill but at high risk of becoming ill. Sick foals generally appear normal for the first 24 hours of life and then quickly decompensate. Because survival depends on early recognition of disease, during the period of vague clinical signs, foals at high risk of becoming ill are assumed to be abnormal and are treated accordingly. During the initial examination, physical, historical, and laboratory factors that may classify the foal as high risk are identified.

Assessment of the foal should attempt to identify factors relative to the dam that increase the foal's risk of being diseased. Foals from mares that have had prior foaling difficulties, including abortion, stillbirth, or twinning, are considered to be at high risk. If the mare experienced poor nutrition, vaginal discharge, illness, prolonged transport, or abdominal surgery during gestation, the foal is at high risk of being diseased. Retained, inflamed, or infected fetal membranes; induced or prolonged labor; and dystocia increase the risk of disease in the foal. The mare's udder should be inspected for the presence and quality of colostrum. Good colostrum should be sticky and have a specific gravity of 1.060 on a colostrometer reading. A full, tight udder is presumptive evidence that the foal is not nursing adequately and is not normal.

The classic early signs of disease in the foal are lethargy, depressed suck reflex, depressed appetite, increased recumbency and sleeping, and decreased affinity for the mare. Historical factors relative to the foal that increase its chance of being "high risk" include in utero meconium passage (evidenced by staining of white hair and hooves), the presence of twins, abnormal birth behavior (see physical examination), abnormal physical findings, failure of passive transfer, and prolonged or shortened gestational length.

TECHNICIAN NOTE

Incomplete skeletal ossification is common in immature foals and can result in crushing injury to the carpal and tarsal bones during normal weight bearing. Foals exhibiting signs of immaturity should undergo carpal and tarsal radiography to identify this condition so proper supportive therapy can be instituted.

The equine gestation length may range from 315 to 365 days, with an average of 341 days. Prematurity refers to foals that are born before 320 days of gestational age. Physical signs of prematurity include low birth weight, weakness, delayed standing post partum, soft pliant lips and ears, flexor tendon laxity, prominent forehead, soft silky haircoat, and incomplete ossification of the carpal and tarsal bones. Any of these physical abnormalities will categorize the foal as high risk. The terms *prematurity*, *dysmaturity*, and *immaturity* are often used incorrectly. Dysmature foals are of a gestational age greater than 320 days with physical signs of prematurity. Immaturity is a blanket term encompassing all foals with physical signs of prematurity regardless of gestational age. Because the foal's haircoat matures from the head to the rump, the hindquarters should be closely examined for the presence of silky hair. It is noteworthy that miniature horse foals normally have a prominent forehead. Technicians working with foals should remember that external signs of immaturity correlate with immaturity of other body systems and greater susceptibility to disease and injury. For example, foals with soft silky haircoat are likely to have incomplete skeletal ossification, which can result in crushing injury to the carpal and tarsal bones by simple weight bearing. Individuals involved with foal care should be aware of the fragile nature of the equine neonate and take appropriate precautions.

Physical Examination

Recognizing high-risk foals requires familiarity with normal peripartum history and behavior. After birth, the normal equine neonate will exhibit a suck reflex in 20 minutes, stand within 1 to 2 hours, and nurse within 2 to 3 hours. Foals should urinate within 10 hours of birth and pass meconium, the dark first

feces, by 24 hours of age. The mare should pass her placenta within 4 to 6 hours of delivering the foal.

The physical examination of the foal begins at a distance. The awake foal should be alert and easily aroused by stimuli in its environment. The respiratory rate is 20 to 40 at birth, increasing to 60 to 80 within 1 hour. The respiratory rhythm is regular in the awake state but may be irregular while the foal is sleeping. The degree of inspiratory and expiratory effort should be noted. Foals should develop a strong bond with their mare by 1.5 hours of age. Foals generally sleep by 3 hours after birth and after each feeding. Foals nurse an average of 7 times per day. Head bobbing while searching for the udder is normal. Within 24 hours of birth the normal foal should be strong, alert, and capable of running.

As the examination continues, the foal's body systems should be thoroughly evaluated. Because the foal has its own list of common diseases (Table 13–3), special attention should be directed toward their early identification. The heart rate is 40 to 80 beats per minute within five minutes after birth, increasing to 130 at 6 to 60 minutes and stabilizing at 90 to 100. The heart rate will increase to 130 or higher on exertion (e.g., when standing). Normal rectal temperature ranges from 37.2° to 38.9°C (99° to 102°F). The integument should be inspected for decubital ulcers, urine, and fecal scalding.

Evaluating cardiovascular stability begins by palpating the extremity for temperature and for the quality, regularity, and rate of the arterial pulses. The arterial pulse is easily identified at the facial artery, which courses beneath the ramus of the mandible; the brachial artery, located at the medial aspect of the elbow; and the great metatarsal artery, which is palpable on the lateral aspect of the third metatarsal bone (Fig. 13–1). This latter vessel is ideal for the collection of arterial samples for blood gas analysis. The foal should not have pulse deficits,

• Table 13–3 •

DISEASES OF FOALS	
Infectious	Septicemia/bacteremia, pneumonia, meningitis, omphalophlebitis, nephritis, septic arthritis, osteomyelitis, septic peritonitis
Gastrointestinal	Meconium impaction, gastric and duodenal ulceration, enteritis, peritonitis, intussusception, intraluminal obstruction, volvulus, cleft palate, prognathism, brachygnathism, atresia coli, atresia recti, atresia ani
Respiratory	Respiratory distress complex, pneumonia, meconium aspiration, persistent pulmonary hypertension
Cardiovascular	Ventricular septal defect
Musculoskeletal	Flexural deformities, angular limb deformities, incomplete skeletal ossification, osteochondrosis, physitis, rib fracture
Urogenital	Patent urachus, rupture of the ureter, bladder, urethra or urachus, umbilical hernia, scrotal hernia
Immunological	Failure of passive transfer, combined immunodeficiency
Hematological	Neonatal isoerythrolysis, anemia
Neurological	Neonatal maladjustment syndrome, brain and spinal hemorrhage, epilepsy
Ocular	Corneal ulcer, entropion, ectropion
Miscellaneous	Hypoxemia, hypoglycemia, hypothermia

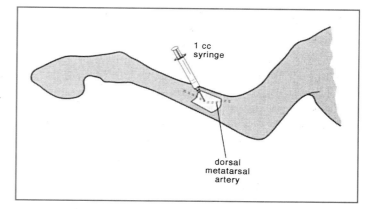

Figure 13-1. Location of dorsal metatarsal artery for collection of arterial blood samples in the foal.

jugular distention, or a jugular pulse. Cardiac auscultation generally reveals a grade II to VI machinery or holosystolic murmur at the left heart base, which abates by 72 hours post partum. Rarely, the murmur may continue for 30 to 60 days. This murmur is suspected to be associated with closing of the ductus arteriosus. Rate and rhythm of the heart should also be assessed. The capillary refill time should be less than 2 seconds. Mucous membranes of the mouth, eyes, nares, vulva, and urethra should be pink and moist. Cyanotic, jaundiced, or injected membranes are abnormal. All membranes should be closely inspected for ulceration or petechiae. It should be noted that membrane color is not an adequate assessment of oxygenation in the foal. Adequate oxygenation can only be assessed by means of arterial blood gas analysis.

A complete auscultation of the lung fields should be performed. The respiratory tract is a major route for exposure to organisms causing septicemia. The boundaries of the equine lung begin at the 17th intercostal space at the level of the tuber coxae and slope in an arc to an area just above the olecranon. Careful auscultation of these areas and the trachea should be performed in a quiet room. As allowed by the foal's temperament and status, a rebreathing bag may help to identify abnormal areas. The benefits of this procedure should be carefully weighed against the potential stress on the foal.

TECHNICIAN NOTE

All high-risk foals should undergo thoracic radiography at admission even if thoracic auscultation is normal.

A foal's lung sounds are normally harsh, making evaluation subjective. An elevated respiratory rate, which exacerbates harsh lung sounds, can occur with many systemic diseases in the absence of lung disease. The slightest wheeze or crackle should be taken seriously. Note that auscultation is extremely insensitive for the detection of lung disease in the foal. The chest should be carefully examined for possible rib fractures. Because pneumonia and other lung diseases can be ruled out only by radiographic examination of the thorax, all high-risk foals should have thoracic radiographs performed on admission.

In examining the gastrointestinal system, the passage of meconium should be ensured because meconium impaction is the primary cause of neonatal colic. Foals should have fecal matter on the thermometer. If none is present, the possibility of a nonpatent gastrointestinal system (atresia ani, atresia coli) in a foal that exhibits abdominal pain or straining to defecate should be considered. Diarrhea is a significant finding because the gastrointestinal system is a second major route for exposure to bacterial organisms causing septicemia. Borborygmi should be detectable by auscultation. Abdominal distention or "pings" noted on auscultation are abnormal findings. The mouth is examined for cleft palate and abnormal dentition. Foals with clefts in the soft palate often require endoscopic examination to identify the abnormality.

The musculoskeletal evaluation focuses predominantly on the joints and growth plates. All joints are placed through their full range of motion to identify contracted tendons. The foal is encouraged to stand and move to identify flexor tendon laxity (walking on heels or fetlocks), lameness, and angular limb deformities. Each joint and physis must be carefully palpated to detect swelling, heat, or pain. Careful palpation of these areas can detect infection before the onset of lameness, improving response to treatment. Any lameness in the foal should be assumed to be infectious until proved otherwise and is an emergency situation. It is a misconception that mares step on their foals.

The urogenital system is another area for intense examination. For many years, the significance of the umbilicus as a major route of infection has been recognized. The umbilical stump, palpable outside the abdomen, consists of remnants of the urachus (which connected to the bladder in utero), one umbilical vein, and two umbilical arteries. Within the abdomen, the umbilical vein courses forward to the liver, and the umbilical arteries travel caudally entering the wall of the bladder. The umbilicus is closely inspected for infection, increased size, and moistness, which suggests patency. Because the predominance of the umbilical structures is within the abdomen, thorough examination requires ultrasonic imaging. The umbilical, inguinal, and scrotal areas are palpated for hernias and distention. Abdominal distention or pitting edema of the perineal or inguinal areas may indicate impatency of the urinary tract. Because of its liquid diet, the normal foal passes dilute urine frequently.

The neurological system of the foal is relatively unique compared with that of the adult horse. When the foal stands for the first time, it assumes a base-wide stance and, as it tries to ambulate, takes exaggerated steps. Exaggerated response to visual, auditory, and tactile stimuli and exaggerated jerky movements are normal. The recumbent foal will normally have hyperreflexive spinal reflexes even as severe as myoclonus (rhythmic muscle contraction) when one is eliciting the patellar reflex. The normal foal also exhibits a crossed extensor reflex (extension of a limb in response to squeezing the opposite limb) for as long as 4 weeks. When restrained, the standing foal initially struggles and then falls limp into the arms of the person restraining it, as if sleeping. Loosening the restraint causes the foal to support its weight again.

During the neurological examination, the eyes must not be neglected. Foals do not have a menace reflex for 2 weeks after birth. When excited, the pupillary light reflex of the foal may be slow. The presence of entropion or ectropion should be noted because such conditions and associated corneal ulceration are common. The eyes are carefully examined for corneal abrasion and ulcers, uveitis, hyphema (blood in the anterior chamber), hypopyon (purulent exudate in the anterior chamber), and congenital cataracts. Detection of hyphema and hypopyon requires diligent examination of the dependent portion of the anterior chamber. The sclera should be checked for hemorrhage and injected blood vessels, which can be the result of trauma during birth or sepsis.

Laboratory Examination

The hematological values and serum chemistry values of the foal differ somewhat from those of the adult horse (Table 13–4). The ranges provided are from the laboratory of the University of Florida College of Veterinary Medicine. Because of inter-laboratory variations in technique and equipment, reference ranges should be established at each laboratory. The packed cell volume (PCV) of the normal foal is greater than that of the adult during the first 24 hours of life and falls into the low normal range of the adult from 2 weeks to 1 year of age. Total red blood cell count (RBC) for the foal remains above that of the adult from birth through 1 year of age. Band neutrophils are uncommon in the normal foal and more than 100 to 150 cells/µl should be considered abnormal. Plasma protein concentrations of the foal are expected to be much lower than those of the adult before absorption of colostral immunoglobulins, but as noted, the normal range of plasma protein concentration in the foal post suckle remains below that of the adult horse. Serum protein concentrations follow a similar trend.

Serum concentrations of alkaline phosphatase (ALP), gamma glutamyl transferase (GGT), sorbitol dehydrogenase (SDH), alanine transaminase (ALT), and glucose in foals are consistently higher than those in adult horses. ALP elevation is attributable to increased bone, intestine, and liver activity. The GGT and SDH activities are attributed to a greater liver activity, perhaps associated with greater liver mass relative to body mass in the foal. ALT changes are of questionable clinical significance because this enzyme is not organ specific in the horse. Foals' higher serum glucose concentrations are attributed to their frequent feeding behavior. Serum creatinine and urea nitrogen may be elevated above levels of normal equine adults during the first 36 to 72 hours of life. The reason for this finding is a subject of debate, but evidence exists to suggest that concentrations of these metabolic by-products increase with placental insufficiency. Creatinine and urea nitrogen values fall below the normal adult values by 1 to 3 days after birth. Urine specific gravity is also low throughout the neonatal period, with values ranging from 1.001 to 1.012. The fall in creatinine and urea nitrogen coupled with urine dilution is associated with the natural diuresis of the foal's total liquid diet.

• Table 13–4 •

SELECTED LABORATORY VALUES OF THE EQUINE NEONATE

AGE	PCV (%)	RBC ($\times 10^6$/µl)	PLASMA PROTEIN (g/dl)	
Presuckle	40–52	9.3–12.9	4.5–5.9	
≤12 hours	37–49	9.0–12.0	5.1–7.6	
1 day	32–46	8.2–11.0	5.2–8.0	
1 day–1 month	28–46	7.2–11.6	5.1–7.9	
Adult	31–47	5.9–9.9	6.2–8.0	
	SERUM PROTEIN (g/dl)	ALP (IU/LITER)	GGT (IU/LITER)	SDH (IU/LITER)
Presuckle				
<12 hours	4.0–7.9	152–2835	13–39	0.2–4.8
1 day	4.3–8.1	861–2671	18–43	0.6–4.6
1 day–1 month	4.4–7.76	137–1462	8–169	0.6–8.4
Adult	5.5–7.9	64–214	5–28	0.5–3.0
	GLUCOSE (mg/dl)	CREATININE (mg/dl)	BUN (mg/dl)	
Presuckle				
<12 hours	108–190	1.7–4.2	12–27	
1 day	121–233	0.4–4.3	9–40	
1 day–1 month	101–221	0.4–2.1	2–29	
Adult	57–96	0.9–2.0	12–24	

Data from Koterba AM, Drummond WH, and Kosch PC: Equine Clinical Neonatology. Philadelphia, Lea & Febiger, 1990; and University of Florida, College of Veterinary Medicine.

Admitting the Sick Foal

The labor involved in admitting, monitoring, and treating a sick foal is intensive. A team approach to the diagnostic workup and management of the foal is integral to success. For this reason, management of the severely compromised neonate has been most successful in a specialized Neonatal Intensive Care Unit.

> **TECHNICIAN NOTE**
>
> Initial management of the foal should identify and treat the three most immediate life-threatening conditions of compromised foals: asphyxia, hypoglycemia, and hypothermia.

Three conditions are immediately life threatening in the compromised foal: asphyxia, hypoglycemia, and hypothermia. Initial management of the foal should address these problems before proceeding to less-threatening problems. Ambulatory foals should be gently restrained during work-up to minimize stress. Recumbent foals should be examined on a well-padded, warm (25°C) surface. As the foal is examined, nasal insufflation of oxygen is warranted if the foal is showing respiratory distress. Although it is ideal to collect blood gas samples before oxygen insufflation and begin intravenous fluid administration after collecting samples for blood culture, the stability of the patient should alter the order of admission protocol as needed.

Once initial parameters are recorded, heat lamps and circulating water blankets are applied if the foal's rectal temperature is less than 37.8°C (100°F). Foals should be warmed slowly to prevent cardiovascular collapse and thermal burns. Heating blankets and heat lamps should not exceed 39.4°C (103°F). Foals are extremely susceptible to burns, and electric dry heat pads are not recommended. Next, a peripheral vein is prepared for venipuncture under sterile conditions. The cephalic vein is ideal, because the jugular vein should be used only for venous catheterization. Blood is collected for aerobic and anaerobic blood culture, CBC, fibrinogen, serum chemistry, electrolyte analysis, and assessment of passive transfer. Once initial blood cultures are collected, a venous catheter is placed if warranted. An arterial blood gas sample is collected. A second set (and possibly a third) of blood cultures is collected in 15 minutes to 1 hour. Appropriate fluid therapy is administered.

> **TECHNICIAN NOTE**
>
> Venous catheters and lines must be placed and maintained under conditions of rigid asepsis.

Venous catheters are a primary iatrogenic portal of infection and *must* be placed and maintained under conditions of *rigid asepsis*. Always clip hair and use sterile solutions to scrub liberally for catheter placement. Wear sterile gloves. Use an extension set on the catheter and wrap the secured catheter with a sterile dressing. The fluid of choice and rate of administration for initial therapy depend on the foal's glucose, electrolyte, and hydration status. As a rule of thumb, 0.45% sodium chloride with 2.5% dextrose solution is a safe initial fluid in the dehydrated foal. The normal maintenance fluid requirement in the equine neonate is 80 to 120 ml/kg/24 hr or 150 to 225 ml/ hr for the average 45-kg foal. Shock fluids can be administered at 20 ml/kg/hr for short periods. Concentrations of dextrose solution from 5% to 10% are warranted in the severely hypoglycemic foal but should be administered with the understanding that hyperglycemia can be detrimental. Bolus dosing of 25% to 50% dextrose solution is not advised.

Once the foal is stabilized, it is weighed, thoracic radiographs are performed, and therapy is determined. Additional diagnostic measures that may be warranted include abdominal ultrasound and radiographs, transtracheal aspirate, arthrocentesis, cerebrospinal fluid collection, urinary catheterization, fecal collection, abdominocentesis, nasogastric intubation, and gastroduodenal endoscopy.

Therapy

Routine Perinatal Therapy

Certain aspects of neonatal care are common to all foals regardless of their risk category. At birth, the umbilicus should be allowed to tear on its own. A dilute (2% to 3.5%) iodine solution should be applied to the umbilical stump. This treatment should be continued four times a day for 1 week, or until umbilical disease abates. Foals from mares that were not vaccinated with tetanus antitoxin in the last 4 to 6 weeks of gestation should receive 1500 IU of tetanus antitoxin intramuscularly. On some farms, an enema is routinely administered after birth. If the foal has not defecated within 24 hours or is straining to defecate, a pediatric Fleet enema or warm, soapy water enema can be administered. This should be done with great care and generous lubrication, as the rectal mucosa of the foal is fragile. Another unfortunately common practice is the routine administration of a single dose of an antibiotic, generally penicillin, after birth. There is no sound rationale for this practice, and it should be strongly discouraged.

Failure of Passive Transfer. Foals are born without appreciable quantities of circulating protective immunoglobulin. The mare's first milk contains colostrum rich in immunoglobulins that the foal must ingest and absorb for adequate immunologic protection. Because the gastrointestinal cells that allow absorption of these immunoglobulins are lost soon after birth, the foal must ingest the colostrum by 6 hours of age. Inadequate absorption of colostrum is termed *failure of passive transfer* and is thought to be associated with increased susceptibility to infection.

Assessing adequate passive transfer is an integral portion of the initial work-up. Although there is some debate over what constitutes adequate passive transfer, most neonatal clinicians agree that high-risk foals should have serum IgG concentrations greater than 800 mg/dl. IgG levels are generally measured 18 to 24 hours after birth to allow time for absorption of ingested colostrum. Several tests that quantify IgG are available, each with its advantage and disadvantage. At this time, the time-honored gold standard is the radial immunodiffusion (RID) test. Although this appears to be the most accurate, the expense, limited availability, and 24-hour testing time preclude its use in routine screening. The concentration immunoassay technology (CITE) test is perhaps the most commonly used screening test because it is quick, accurate, easily performed, and readily available. Of the rapid test methods (zinc sulfate turbidity, latex agglutination, CITE), CITE is the only test that has sensitivity in the 800 mg/dl range.

Ensuring adequate passive transfer is an integral part of treatment for all equine neonates regardless of their disease process. When an immunoglobulin deficit is detected, it can be replaced by one of two methods. The first, oral administration of colostrum from a donor, is ideal but is not generally useful because most foals are too old to absorb colostrum by the time a deficit is detected. Foals should receive 1 to 2 liters of colostrum by 12 to 16 hours of age and have IgG levels measured 16 to 20 hours later. Failure of passive transfer after 24 hours is treated with intravenous administration of plasma from an appropriate donor. Commercial plasma is available and is expensive. Plasma is administered via a sterile intravenous catheter. A general rule of thumb is that 1 liter of plasma raises the IgG level of the 45-kg foal by 200 mg/dl.

Antimicrobials. High-risk foals are likely to suffer from infectious processes. As a matter of course, antimicrobial agents capable of killing both gram-positive and gram-negative bacterial organisms are routinely administered to foals entering intensive care. The antimicrobial agents may be altered as needed based on antimicrobial sensitivities of bacterial organisms isolated from the foal.

Nutrition. Malnutrition decreases growth, immune function, and healing and increases susceptibility to infection. The exact nutritional requirements of the compromised equine neonate are not known. Accepted minimum energy requirements of the normal foal to 30 days of age are in the range of 130 to 150 Kcal/kg/day. Sepsis is known to increase the energy requirements of the human neonate by 100%. The currently accepted minimum energy requirement of the compromised equine neonate is 180 Kcal/kg/day. Achieving this level via the enteral route (using the gastrointestinal tract) is practically impossible, and accordingly many compromised foals require parenteral (intravenous) nutrition to achieve sufficient energy intake. At this time, adequate nutrition is assessed based on weight gain. The healthy 45-kg foal should gain 1.4 to 1.6 kg/day.

Some foals require assistance or encouragement to nurse from their mare. Every effort should be made to feed foals from their mare. Foals that are unable or unwilling to nurse from their mare can be allowed to nurse a bottle or bucket if they maintain a suck reflex. Without a strong suck reflex, the foal will require an indwelling nasogastric tube for feeding. Enteral feeding is ideal because it is physiological, inexpensive, and simple, and it stimulates gastrointestinal maturity. The primary complication associated with enteral feeding is aspiration pneumonia. Before each use of a nasogastric tube, its position within the stomach or distal esophagus must be ensured. Recumbent foals must be placed in sternal recumbency during and for 30 minutes after feeding to prevent regurgitation and aspiration of milk.

Mare's milk is the best source of enteral nutrition for the foal. When available, mare's milk should always be used. To prevent mastitis, the mare's udder and caretaker's hands should always be cleaned before milking and teat dip applied after milking. Several alternatives to mare's milk are available, but all have their drawbacks. Preparations formulated for enteral nutrition of other species are generally not suitable for the foal. Goat's milk is palatable but causes some metabolic abnormalities and should not be utilized alone for extended periods. Goat's milk has a caloric density of 276 Kcal/pint. Milk replacers are readily available and inexpensive but unpalatable and notorious for causing gastrointestinal upsets. Goat's milk can be added to milk replacers to improve palatability. Milk replacers, when fed according to labeled directions, underestimate the caloric requirements of foals by 50% to 70%. Quantities to be fed should be calculated daily based on caloric requirement and foal's body weight. Table 13–5 lists the caloric density of several milk replacers.

When feeding foals, all utensils should be thoroughly cleaned and disinfected before and after use. Once reconstituted, milk should be kept refrigerated. The preparations should be discarded after 2 hours at room temperature. Foals will not nurse from commercial cow nipples but do quite well with a lamb's nipple. Orphan foals should be bucket-fed as soon as possible to limit human imprinting, which can become dangerous as the foal matures. Enteral feeding should be started gradually. Begin at 50 to 100 ml every 30 to 60 minutes. If the foal tolerates these feedings, the volume of milk may be gradually increased, and timing of feedings may be spaced to every 2 hours. Many high-risk foals will not tolerate enteral nutrition, and feeding should be discontinued if regurgitation, abdominal distention, colic, or severe diarrhea occurs. Foals receiving less than 100 Kcal/kg/day should be considered candidates for parenteral nutrition.

Monitoring and Nursing Care

Once the foal has been admitted and initially examined, diligent monitoring is critical. The objective of frequent monitoring is to detect subtle changes in body parameters that signify a worsening or improvement in the foal's status. The primary complications that occur in foals are the development of alternative resistant nosocomial infections, alternate sites of infection (arthritis, osteomyelitis), corneal ulcers, decubital ulcers, and malnutrition. Frequency of monitoring varies with the severity of the patient's illness. Parameters should always be recorded on a flow sheet. Table 13–6 lists parameters that should be monitored and is basically a thorough, foal-oriented, physical examination with the addition of blood pressure, blood gas, and ventilator monitoring as warranted. Pay close attention to the catheter site for evidence of jugular distention, heat, pain, or swelling. Table 13–7 suggests examination parameters that warrant closer attention by the attending clinician.

The hallmarks of nursing care for the foal are cleanliness

• Table 13–5 •

CALORIC DENSITIES OF SELECTED MILK REPLACERS FOR FOALS
Foal Lac: 260 Kcal/pint
Mare's Match: 221 Kcal/pint
Nutri-Foal: 345 Kcal/pint

Foal Lac: Pet Ag Inc., Elgin, IL.
Mare's Match: Land O Lakes, Fort Dodge, IA.
Nutri-Foal: Ross Laboratories, Columbus, OH.

and tender loving care. Working with foals is as much an art as a science. Standing foals are generally restrained against a wall with one hand under the neck, the other under the rump. The recumbent foal can be a challenge to restrain. Techniques are described, but the reality is usually different. Restraint should be safe for the foal, handlers, and associated intravenous lines and equipment.

If more than one foal is being treated, care must be exercised to avoid cross-contamination. All injections are made through skin that is clean after alcohol swabbing of the area has dried. Intramuscular injections are limited to the semimembranosus region and should not be given in the neck or gluteal region. Fluid lines should be changed daily. Once disconnected, fluid lines are contaminated and should be replaced. Multidose vials and catheter caps should be disinfected before needle insertion. Needles and syringes are *not* reused. All intravenous ports should be capped with injection caps. Catheters should be flushed with heparinized saline every 4 hours. The interval for catheter change depends on the type of catheter material and the status of the vein. The commonly used Teflon catheters should be removed and placed in an alternate vein *at least every 72 hours.* Silastic and polyurethane catheters are available and, because of their lower thrombogenicity relative to Teflon, can remain in place for several months if they receive the proper care. These catheters are expensive but quickly become cost-effective over a time course that would require several Teflon catheter changes.

The foal should be kept clean, dry, and warm, and milk

• Table 13–6 •

MONITORING IN THE CRITICALLY ILL FOAL

BODY SYSTEM	PARAMETERS MONITORED DURING PHYSICAL EXAMINATION
Cardiovascular	Pulse: rate, rhythm, and strength
	Heart rate, rhythm, and murmurs
	Mucous membranes: color, CRT, petechiae, injection, and hyperemia
Respiratory	Breathing: rate, effort, and pattern
	Chest excursion
	Lungs: auscultation and percussion
Thermoregulatory	Body temperature: warmth of extremities
Gastrointestinal	Feces: volume and consistency
	Borborygmi: frequency and character
	Abdominal distention, signs of colic and gastric reflux
Urinary	Urination: frequency and volume
	Umbilicus: monitor for patency and signs of infection
Musculoskeletal	Joints: lameness, warmth, and distention
	Tendon and ligament laxity
	Angular limb deformity
Integument	Decubital ulcers; urine and fecal scalding
Ocular	Cornea: abrasions, ulcers, and edema
	Anterior chamber: hypopyon
	Lids: entropion
	Sclera: injection and petechiae
Nervous	Mental status, attitude, and behavior
	Posture and muscle tone
	Gait: limb proprioception
	Cranial nerve and spinal reflexes

CRT, capillary refill time.
From Koterba AM, Drummond WH, and Kosch PC: Equine Clinical Neonatology. Philadelphia, Lea & Febiger, 1990.

• Table 13–7 •

TRENDS OR CHANGES IN CONDITION THAT OFTEN WARRANT INTERVENTION

1. Trends
   a. Increasing or decreasing body temperature
   b. Increasing or increasingly irregular respiratory rate
   c. Increasingly rapid (>120 bpm), slow (<60 bpm), or irregular heart beat
   d. Weakening peripheral pulses
   e. Blood gases
      (1) *Decreasing* Pa_{O_2}: If receiving oxygen therapy, check the flow rate and the pressure gauge for any disconnections or plugs in the tubing. Consider the amount of struggling and the length of time in lateral recumbency. If there are no equipment problems, consider worsening pulmonary function
      (2) *Increasing* Pa_{CO_2}, particularly with increased effort of breathing, suggests that the foal's respiratory system may be failing
      (3) *More negative base excess* implies worsening metabolic acidosis. The cause should be determined
2. Seizure activity
3. Colic
4. Decreased nursing activity
5. Gastric reflux
6. Diarrhea or constipation, excessive straining to defecate
7. Abdominal distention
8. Lack of, or reduced, urination
9. Eye abnormalities, most commonly corneal ulcers
10. Pitting edema, most commonly observed in the subcutaneous tissues of the ventral abdomen and legs, may indicate fluid overload, impaired renal function, infection, or capillary injury

Adapted from Koterba AM, Drummond WH, and Kosch PC: Equine Clinical Neonatology. Philadelphia, Lea & Febiger, 1990.

should be warmed before being fed. All joints should be placed through passive range of motion several times per day. Because of the adverse effects of lateral recumbency on lung pathology and ventilation, foals should be maintained in a semisternal position with their thorax and forelimbs in sternal recumbency and their hips and rear limbs in lateral recumbency. This position can be achieved through the use of wedge-shaped pads or sand bags positioned at the level of the elbows and thorax.

If this position cannot be maintained, the recumbent foal should be turned from side to side every 2 to 4 hours. Foals should be encouraged to stand and ambulate. This effort may range from the handler's suspending the foal and encouraging it to bear weight to him or her taking the foal for casual short walks in the fresh air.

Summary

Working with compromised foals is an exhaustive endeavor. Despite intensive labor, many high-risk foals will still die, usually taking with them a piece of each team member that has worked so hard to save them. Attention to detail must be unrelenting, and with the help of diligent, highly skilled technicians, more will survive.

Recommended Reading

Puppy and Kitten

Boothe DM and Tannert K: Special considerations for drug and fluid therapy in the pediatric patient. Comp Cont Educ Pract Vet 14:313–329, 1992.

Dow SW and Papich MG: Keeping current on developments in antimicrobial therapy. Vet Med 86:600–609, 1991.

Hoskins JD: Veterinary Pediatrics: Dogs and Cats From Birth to Six Months. 2nd ed. Philadelphia, WB Saunders, 1995.

Foal

Clabough DL: Disease of the equine neonate. J Equine Vet Sci 8(1):5–10, 1988.

Drummond WH: Bridging the gap between the human and equine neonate. *In* Rossdale PD (editor): The Application of Intensive Care Therapies and Parenteral Nutrition in Large Animal Medicine. Deerfield, IL, Travenol Labs Inc., 1986, pp 8–9.

Koterba AM, Drummond WH and Kosch PC (editors): Equine Clinical Neonatology. Philadelphia, Lea & Febiger, 1990.

Koterba AM: IV fluid therapy and nutritional support in the sick neonate. Equine Vet Educ 3(1):33–39, 1991.

Madigan JE (editor): Manual of Equine Neonatal Medicine. 2nd ed. Woodland, CA, Live Oak Publishing, 1991.

14 Preventive Health Programs

Johnny D. Hoskins • Tom L. Seahorn • Marjorie S. Gill

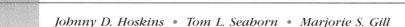

In veterinary practice, preventive health programs are an integral part of providing for the general health needs of dogs, cats, horses, cattle, small ruminants, and swine. Regularly scheduled vaccinations alone do not represent a comprehensive preventive health program. Vaccinations are only one component of a preventive health program that attempts to meet the general health needs of an animal.

The time and effort invested in a preventive health program are rewarding not only to the animal but also to its owner(s) and those persons attending to the health needs of the animal. The veterinary technician can provide direct assistance to the consulting veterinarian by ensuring that the general goals of the preventive health program are met.

PREVENTIVE HEALTH PROGRAM FOR DOGS

For most dogs, a preventive health program usually begins when they are first presented to the veterinary hospital or clinic at 6 weeks of age. A general outline of one preventive health program and its implementation for dogs is presented in Table 14–1.

The Physical Examination

Clinical evaluation of a dog initially focuses on taking a complete case history and performing the physical examination. Basic information about the animal, such as breed, age, and sex, as well as owner concerns or complaints, is essential to the case history. After the case history is obtained, the physical examination should be conducted in a systematic manner. Although the examination may be easier to complete by proceeding from head to tail, it is advisable to examine and record observations according to body systems.

The first skill used in the physical examination is careful observation of the animal's responses to the environment. Specific notes should be made regarding the animal's general condition, mentation, posture, locomotion, and breathing pattern. Next, the body temperature, respiratory and heart rates, capillary refill time, and body weight of the dog are recorded on the health record. The thorax should be thoroughly auscultated and the abdomen palpated for evidence of physical abnormalities. Body weights are recorded for several reasons. First, the weight provides information needed for dispensing medication; and second, it is an immediate indicator of the nutritional status of the animal. The body weight of a growing puppy steadily increasing at each office revisit is an indication that the puppy is receiving adequate nutrition (nutritional information is found in Chapter 26).

TECHNICIAN NOTE

The technician should become skilled in obtaining a history and performing the basic physical examination.

Physical inspection begins by checking the head and oral cavity for evidence of malformation of the skull, cleft lip, stenotic nares, or cleft palate. The mucous membranes should be light pink and moist. The teeth, if present, should be examined for periodontal disease and occlusion problems. Periodontal

• Table 14–1 •

GENERAL OUTLINE OF A PREVENTIVE HEALTH PROGRAM FOR DOGS

I. First office visit for health program—usually at 6 weeks of age
   A. Conduct a general physical examination and record the body weight
   B. Check for external parasites and dermatophytes and initiate appropriate therapy
      1. Fleas, ticks, and ear mites (*Otodectes cyanotis*)
      2. Mange mites, especially *Demodex canis* and *Sarcoptes scabiei*
      3. Dermatophytes, particularly *Microsporum* spp. and *Trichophyton mentagrophytes*
   C. Conduct fecal examination including both direct smear and flotation
   D. Initiate administration of heartworm preventive management
   E. Administer an anthelmintic for hookworms and roundworms and, if tapeworms are present, administer praziquantel or epsiprantel
   F. Vaccinate with DA$_2$PL-PC* and, possibly, with kennel cough vaccine† and canine Lyme borreliosis vaccine
   G. Advise on nutrition and routine grooming
   H. Provide the owner with client education pamphlets on such topics as:
      1. Identification, treatment, and control of fleas, ticks, and ear mites
      2. The benefits of preventive management for canine heartworm disease
      3. Management of normal and abnormal puppy behaviors
      4. Skin, nails, and ear care
      5. "How to" on grooming and nutrition
   I. Fill in the puppy's health record for the owner
II. Second office visit for health program—usually at 9 weeks of age
   A. Conduct a general physical examination and record the body weight
   B. Check for external parasites and dermatophytes and initiate appropriate therapy
      1. Fleas, ticks, and ear mites (*O. cyanotis*)
      2. Mange mites, especially *D. canis* and *S. scabiei*
      3. Dermatophytes, particularly *Microsporum* spp. and *T. mentagrophytes*
   C. Conduct fecal examination including both direct smear and flotation
   D. Adjust the dosage of heartworm preventive according to body weight, especially for diethylcarbamazine (DEC) products
   E. Administer an anthelmintic for hookworms and roundworms and, if tapeworms are present, administer praziquantel or epsiprantel
   F. Vaccinate with DA$_2$PL-PC* and, possibly, with kennel cough vaccine† and canine Lyme borreliosis vaccine
   G. Adjust the nutrition according to health needs and, if needed, change the grooming procedures
   H. Provide the owner with client education pamphlets on such topics as:
      1. Identification, treatment, and control of fleas, ticks, and ear mites
      2. The benefits of preventive management for canine heartworm disease
      3. Dental, skin, nails, and ear care
      4. "How to" on grooming and nutrition
      5. Management of normal and abnormal puppy behaviors
      6. Exercise and its importance
   I. Fill in the puppy's health record for the owner
III. Third office visit for health program—usually at 12 weeks of age
   A. Conduct a general physical examination and record the body weight
   B. Check for external parasites and dermatophytes and initiate appropriate therapy
      1. Fleas, ticks, and ear mites (*O. cyanotis*)
      2. Mange mites, especially *D. canis* and *S. scabiei*
      3. Dermatophytes, particularly *Microsporum* spp. and *T. mentagrophytes*
   C. Conduct fecal examination, including both direct smear and flotation
   D. Adjust the dosage heartworm preventive according to body weight, especially for DEC products
   E. Administer an anthelmintic for hookworms and roundworms and, if tapeworms are present, administer praziquantel or epsiprantel
   F. Vaccinate with DA$_2$PL-PC* and rabies vaccines and, possibly, with kennel cough vaccine† and canine Lyme borreliosis vaccine
   G. Adjust the nutrition according to health needs and, if needed, change the grooming procedures
   H. Provide the owner with client education pamphlets on such topics as:
      1. Identification, treatment, and control of fleas, ticks, and ear mites
      2. Dental, skin, nails, and ear care
      3. "How to" on grooming and nutrition
      4. Management of normal and abnormal puppy behaviors
      5. Recommendations for spaying and castration
      6. Exercise and its importance
   I. Fill in the puppy's health record for the owner
IV. Subsequent visits for health program—usually annual visits‡
   A. Conduct a general physical examination and record the body weight
   B. Check for external parasites and dermatophytes and initiate appropriate therapy
      1. Fleas, ticks, and ear mites (*O. cyanotis*)
      2. Mange mites, especially *D. canis* and *S. scabiei*
      3. Dermatophytes, particularly *Microsporum* spp. and *T. mentagrophytes*
   C. Conduct fecal flotation and a Knott's test or occult heartworm examination, or all tests, for intestinal and heartworm infection screen
   D. Adjust the dosage heartworm preventive according to body weight, especially for DEC products
   E. Administer an anthelmintic according to fecal examination findings
   F. Vaccinate with DA$_2$PL-PC* and rabies and, possibly, with kennel cough vaccine† and canine Lyme borreliosis vaccine
   G. Adjust the nutrition according to health needs and, if needed, change the grooming procedures
   H. Provide the owner with client education pamphlets on such topics as:
      1. Identification, treatment, and control of fleas, ticks, and ear mites
      2. Dental, skin, nails, and ear care
      3. "How to" on grooming and nutrition
      4. Management of normal and abnormal behaviors
      5. Exercise and its importance
   I. Fill in the dog's health record for the owner

*This refers to the use of a vaccine to protect against: D—canine distemper; A$_2$ (canine adenovirus type 2)—infectious canine hepatitis; P—canine parainfluenza; L—leptospirosis; P—canine parvovirus type 2 disease; and C—canine coronavirus disease.
  †This refers to the use of vaccine to protect against canine *Bordetella bronchiseptica*–induced disease. Puppies may be vaccinated with either an intranasal vaccine or a parenteral vaccine.
  ‡A fourth office visit may be desirable at 15 weeks of age for an additional parvovirus-2 vaccine booster in some puppies, especially high-risk breeds such as Doberman Pinscher, Rottweiler, Labrador Retriever, and other presumed high-risk breeds.

disease generally begins in dogs when the first teeth appear in the mouth and continues in variable degrees throughout the animal's life. Frequent dental examinations as part of the preventive health program convey to the owner the need for regularly performed prophylactic dentistry, the importance of providing the right type of food for the control of periodontal disease, and the importance of brushing even a young dog's teeth on a regular basis. Routine dental care and dental surgery are discussed in Chapter 18.

The skin and ears should be inspected for wounds, state of hydration, completeness of hair cover, and condition of foot pads. When necessary, the dermatological examination may also require such diagnostic procedures as exfoliative cytology, bacterial culture and sensitivity testing, skin scrapings, and dermatophyte culture and identification of external parasites (such as ear mites, fleas, ticks, and chiggers). When the observation and basic inspection phase has been completed, the animal is assessed according to specific body systems. Detailed information concerning the history and physical examination may be found in Chapter 3.

Vaccinations

In the general outline of the preventive program, the statement "vaccinate with DA$_2$PL-PC vaccine" refers to the use of a vaccine to protect against the following: D—canine distemper; A$_2$ (canine adenovirus type 2)—infectious canine hepatitis; P—canine parainfluenza; L—leptospirosis; P—canine parvovirus type 2 disease; and C—canine coronavirus disease. A listing of some vaccines currently available is presented in Table 14–2. In addition, a fourth office visit may be desired at 15 weeks of age for an additional canine parvovirus-2 vaccine booster in some puppies, especially the high-risk breeds.

In addition to regularly scheduled DA$_2$PL-PC and rabies vaccinations, other immunizations can be incorporated into the preventive health program, as detailed below.

Infectious Tracheobronchitis Vaccine. Vaccination can be an effective means for preventing or, at least, reducing the incidence of infectious tracheobronchitis (kennel cough) in dogs of all ages. Intranasal vaccination, in particular, provides rapid, long-term protection against *Bordetella bronchiseptica* and parainfluenza virus infection and disease (see Table 14–2). Puppies can be vaccinated intranasally as early as 2 to 4 weeks of age without interference from maternal antibody and it is safe to use in pregnant bitches during all trimesters. One dose is effective for a full year. Adult dogs can receive a one-dose intranasal vaccination at the same time as their puppies or at the time they receive their annual vaccinations. Puppies being prepared for shipment or entering a boarding kennel or veterinary hospital should be vaccinated at least 1 to 2 weeks before admission or shipping. Other infectious tracheobronchitis vaccines available include inactivated *B. bronchiseptica* parenteral vaccine. Parenteral vaccines are administered as two doses 2 to 4 weeks apart. When dogs younger than 4 months of age are being vaccinated, they should be revaccinated after reaching the age of 4 months. Initial vaccination of puppies with parenteral vaccines is recommended at or about 6 to 8 weeks of age.

Canine Lyme Borreliosis Vaccine. Canine *Borrelia burgdorferi* vaccine, available as killed bacteria and recombinant products, provides protection against canine Lyme borreliosis.

According to the manufacturers currently marketing canine *B. burgdorferi* vaccines, puppies 9 to 12 weeks of age or older should receive two doses administered at 2- to 3-week intervals; with annual revaccination a single dose is recommended.

Heartworm Preventive Therapy

Puppies can be started on a heartworm preventive program, using diethylcarbamazine, or ivermectin or milbemycin oxime at 6 to 8 weeks of age. Heartworm preventive products that contain diethylcarbamazine are available for oral administration as a chewable tablet, standard tablet, and syrup from a variety of manufacturers and should be given once a day at a dose rate of 6.6 mg/kg (3 mg/lb) of body weight. Heartworm preventive products that contain ivermectin (Heartgard 30 and Heartgard 30 Plus, MSD AGVET) should be administered orally at the recommended minimum dose level of 6.0 μg/kg of body weight at monthly dosing intervals. A heartworm preventive product that contains milbemycin oxime (Interceptor, Ciba Animal Health) should be administered orally at the recommended minimal dose level of 0.5 mg/kg of body weight at monthly dosing intervals. Heartworm preventive products of any type should be started in heartworm areas 1 month before the beginning of mosquito season and continue until 2 months after the season's end.

Owner Education

Owner education pamphlets on a variety of dog-related topics can be sent home with the owner each time the dog is seen for the preventive health program. Generally, only one or two well-written owner education pamphlets are given to the owner at the end of each office visit.

TECHNICIAN NOTE

The technician should function as a technician-educator as often as possible.

Veterinarians and veterinary technicians are in an excellent position to provide meaningful owner educational services and thus make owners more aware of their dogs and the associated responsibilities of dog ownership. By offering consultative advice and providing owners with educational pamphlets, the veterinary technician not only assists owners who are seeking medical treatment for their dogs but serves a vital role in educating people in the community.

PREVENTIVE HEALTH PROGRAM FOR CATS

For most cats, a preventive health program usually begins when they are first presented to the veterinary hospital or clinic at 8 to 10 weeks of age. A general outline of one preventive health program and its implementation for cats is presented in Table 14–3.

The Physical Examination

Clinical evaluation of a cat initially focuses on taking a complete case history and performing the physical examination. Basic

• Table 14–2 •

CANINE VACCINES*

VACCINE	MANUFACTURER	TYPE	CDV	CAV	CPI	CPV	Lep	Br	Rb	CV	MV	Bo
Adenomune 7	BioCor	A/I	X	X	X	X	X					
Adenomune 5L	BioCor	A/I	X	X	X	X	X					
Adenomune 7L	BioCor	A/I	X	X	X	X	X					
Annumune	Fort Dodge Laboratories	I							X			
Bronchicine	BioCor	I						X				
Bronchi-Shield	Fort Dodge Laboratories	A						X				
CaMune 5	Bayer	A/I	X	X	X	X						
CaMune 7	Bayer	A/I	X	X	X	X	X					
CaMune 7 KP	Bayer	A/I	X	X	X	X	X					
CaMune B	Bayer	I						X				
CaMune C-K	Bayer	I								X		
CaMune DHPL	Bayer	A/I	X	X	X	X	X					
CaMune Parvo	Bayer	A/I				X						
CaMune Parvo-K	Bayer	I				X						
Canine 4	Rhone Merieux	A	X	X	X	X						
Canine 4 + Corona-MLV	Rhone Merieux	A	X	X	X	X				X		
Canine 5	Rhone Merieux	A/I	X	X	X	X	X					
Canine 6	Rhone Merieux	A/I	X	X	X	X	X					
Canine 6 + Corona-MLV	Rhone Merieux	A/I	X	X	X	X	X			X		
Canine 7-Way	DurVet	A/I	X	X	X	X	X					
Canine Corona-MLV	Rhone Merieux	I								X		
Canine Parvo	Rhone Merieux	A				X						
Canine Parvovirus vaccine	DurVet	I				X						
Canine Recombinant Lyme	Rhone Merieux	I										X
CoronaVac	BioCor	I								X		
CoughGuard-B	Pfizer Animal Health	I						X				
CoughGuard-BP	Pfizer Animal Health	A/I			X			X				
CPV/LP	A.M. BioTechniques	A			X	X						
Defensor	Pfizer Animal Health	I							X			X
Duramune Cv-K	Fort Dodge Laboratories	I								X		
Duramune DA$_2$P + Pv	Fort Dodge Laboratories	A/I	X	X	X	X						
Duramune DA$_2$LP + Pv	Fort Dodge Laboratories	A/I	X	X	X	X	X					
Duramune DA$_2$PP + CvK	Fort Dodge Laboratories	A/I	X	X	X	X				X		
Duramune DA$_2$PP + CvK/LCl	Fort Dodge Laboratories	A/I	X	X	X	X	X			X		
Duramune KF-11	Fort Dodge Laboratories	A	X	X	X	X						
Duramune PC	Fort Dodge Laboratories	A/I				X				X		
Dura-Rab 1	ImmunoVet, Vedco	I							X			
Dura-Rab 3	ImmunoVet, Vedco	I							X			
D-Vac-7	Bio-Ceutic Laboratories	A/I	X	X	X	X	X					
Endurall-K	Pfizer Animal Health	I							X			
Endurall-P	Pfizer Animal Health	I							X			
Firstdose CPV	Pfizer Animal Health	A				X						
Firstdose CV	Pfizer Animal Health	I								X		
Firstdose CPV/CV	Pfizer Animal Health	A/I				X				X		
Fromm D	Schering-Plough Animal Health	A	X									
Galaxy Cv	Schering-Plough Animal Health	I								X		
Galaxy D	Schering-Plough Animal Health	A	X									
Galaxy DA$_2$L	Schering-Plough Animal Health	A/I	X	X	X		X					
Galaxy DA$_2$PL	Schering-Plough Animal Health	A/I	X	X	X	X	X					
Galaxy DA$_2$PPv	Schering-Plough Animal Health	A	X	X	X	X						
Galaxy DA$_2$PPvL	Schering-Plough Animal Health	A/I	X	X	X	X	X					

Product	Manufacturer	Type
Galaxy DA₂PPv + Cv	Schering-Plough Animal Health	A/I
Galaxy DA₂PPvL + Cv	Schering-Plough Animal Health	A/I
Galaxy Lyme	Schering-Plough Animal Health	I
Imrab 1	Rhone Merieux	I
Imrab 3	Rhone Merieux	I
Intra-Trac-II	Schering-Plough Animal Health	A
Intra-Trac-II ADT	Schering-Plough Animal Health	A
LymeVax	Fort Dodge Laboratories	I
Naramune-2	Bio-Ceutic Laboratories	A
NasaGuard-B	Pfizer Animal Health	A
Paramune 5	BioCor	A/I
Parvocine	BioCor	I
Parvocine MLV	BioCor	A
Parvoid 2	Schering-Plough Animal Health	A
Performer Borde-Vac	Performer	A/I
PerformerSeven-K	Performer	A/I
PerformerSeven-L	Performer	A/I
Progard-5	Intervet	A
Progard-7	Intervet	A/I
Progard-CPv	Intervet	A
Progard-CvK	Intervet	I
Progard-KC	Intervet	A/I
Progard Puppy-DPv	Intervet	A
Prorab-1	Intervet	I
Quantum vaccine	Schering-Plough Animal Health	A
Quantum 4 vaccine	Schering-Plough Animal Health	A
Quantum 6 vaccine	Schering-Plough Animal Health	A/I
Rabdomun vaccine	Schering-Plough Animal Health	I
Rabdomun 1 vaccine	Schering-Plough Animal Health	I
Rabguard-TC	Pfizer Animal Health	I
Rabvac 1	Schering-Plough Animal Health	I
Rabvac 3	Schering-Plough Animal Health	I
RXV Vac Canine BodyGuard 7	RXV	A/I
Sentrypar	Synbiotics	A
Sentrypar DHP	Synbiotics	A
Sentrypar DHP/L	Synbiotics	A/I
SentryRab-1	Synbiotics	I
Sentryvac-DHP	Synbiotics	A
Sentryvac-DHP/L	Synbiotics	A/I
Solo-Jec-7	Anchor	A/I
Trimune	Fort Dodge Laboratories	I
Tissuvax 6 vaccine	Schering-Plough Animal Health	A/I
UnaMax	A.M. BioTechniques	I
Vanguard 5	Pfizer Animal Health	A
Vanguard 5/CV	Pfizer Animal Health	A/I
Vanguard 5/CV-L	Pfizer Animal Health	A/I
Vanguard 5/L	Pfizer Animal Health	A/I
Vanguard CPV	Pfizer Animal Health	I
Vanguard DA₂MP	Pfizer Animal Health	A
Vanguard DA₂P	Pfizer Animal Health	A
Vanguard DA₂PL	Pfizer Animal Health	A/I
Vanguard 5/B	Pfizer Animal Health	A/I
Vanguard D-M	Pfizer Animal Health	A
Vanguard DMP	Pfizer Animal Health	A

CDV, canine distemper virus; CAV, canine adenovirus (infectious canine hepatitis); CPI, canine parainfluenza virus; CPV, canine parvovirus-2; Lep, leptospirosis (usually *Leptospira canicola* and *Leptospira icterohaemorrhagiae*); Br, *Bordetella bronchiseptica* (kennel cough); Rb, rabies; CV, canine coronavirus; MV, measles virus; Bo, *Borrelia burgdorferi* (Lyme disease); A, attenuated (modified live virus or MLV); I, inactivated (killed); A/I, combination of attenuated and inactivated.

*Compiled with the assistance of *Compendium of Veterinary Products*. Port Huron, MI, North American Compendiums, 1995–1996.

• Table 14–3 •

GENERAL OUTLINE OF A PREVENTIVE HEALTH PROGRAM FOR CATS

I. First office visit for health program (usually at 8–10 weeks of age)
  A. Perform a general physical examination and record the body weight
  B. Check for external parasites and dermatophytes and initiate appropriate therapy for:
    1. Fleas and ear mites (*Otodectes cyanotis*)
    2. Mange mites, especially *Notoedres cati, Demodex* spp., and *Cheyletiella* spp.
    3. Dermatophytes, particularly *Microsporum* spp. and *Trichophyton mentagrophytes*
  C. Perform fecal examination including both direct smear and flotation
  D. Administer an anthelmintic, such as pyrantel pamoate for roundworms and hookworms and praziquantel or epsiprantel for tapeworms (if present)
  E. Vaccinate with FVRC-P,*† *Chlamydia,*‡ feline leukemia virus§ (possibly test for FeLV/FIV before initial FeLV vaccination), and FIP‖ vaccines
  F. Advise on nutrition and routine grooming
  G. Provide the owner with client education pamphlets on such topics as:
    1. Identification, treatment, and control of fleas, ticks, and ear mites
    2. The benefits of vaccination for feline leukemia virus infection
    3. Management of normal and abnormal cat behaviors
    4. Grooming "how to" and nutrition
  H. Fill in the kitten's health record for the owner
II. Second office visit for health program (usually at 12–14 weeks of age)
  A. Perform a general physical examination and record the body weight
  B. Check for external parasites and dermatophytes and initiate appropriate therapy for:
    1. Fleas and ear mites (*O. cyanotis*)
    2. Mange mites, especially *N. cati, Demodex* spp., and *Cheyletiella* spp.
    3. Dermatophytes, particularly *Microsporum* spp. and *T. mentagrophytes*
  C. Perform fecal examination including both direct smear and flotation
  D. Administer an anthelmintic, such as pyrantel pamoate for roundworms and hookworms and praziquantel or epsiprantel for tapeworms (if present)
  E. Vaccinate with FVRC-P,* *Chlamydia,*‡ feline leukemia virus,§ rabies, and FIP‖ vaccines
  F. Adjust the nutrition and grooming procedures
  G. Provide the owner with client education pamphlets on such topics as:
    1. Identification, treatment and control of fleas, ticks, and ear mites
    2. The benefits of vaccination for feline leukemia virus infection
    3. Dental, skin, nail, and ear care
    4. Management of normal and abnormal cat behaviors
    5. Exercise and its importance
    6. Recommendations for spaying, castration, and declawing
  H. Fill in the kitten's health record for the owner
III. Subsequent visits for health program (usually annual visits)
  A. Perform a general physical examination and record the body weight
  B. Check for external parasites and dermatophytes and initiate appropriate therapy for:
    1. Fleas and ear mites (*O. cyanotis*)
    2. Mange mites, especially *N. cati, Demodex* spp., and *Cheyletiella* spp.
    3. Dermatophytes, particularly *Microsporum* spp. and *T. mentagrophytes*
  C. Perform fecal examination (fecal flotation)
  D. Administer an anthelmintic according to fecal examination findings
  E. Vaccinate with FVRC-P,* *Chlamydia,*‡ feline leukemia virus,§ rabies, and FIP‖ vaccines
  F. Adjust the nutrition and grooming procedures
  G. Provide the owner with client education pamphlets on such topics as:
    1. Identification, treatment, and control of fleas, ticks, and ear mites
    2. The benefits of vaccination for feline leukemia virus infection
    3. Dental, skin, nail, and ear care
    4. Management of normal and abnormal cat behaviors
    5. Exercise and its importance
    6. Recommendations for spaying, castration, and declawing
  H. Fill in the cat's health record for the owner

Modified from Hoskins JD: Preventive health program for cats. Vet Technician 9:273, 1988.
*This refers to the use of a vaccine to protect against: FVR—feline viral rhinotracheitis; C—feline calicivirus infection; and P—feline panleukopenia.
†Cats being prepared for shipment or entering a boarding kennel or veterinary hospital or clinic should be vaccinated at least 1 to 2 weeks before admission or shipment.
‡The vaccine currently available apparently produces effective protection only against *Chlamydia psittaci* infections. As with other vaccines for respiratory ailments, complete protection is not afforded; however, clinical signs of conjunctivitis or upper respiratory tract disease, if they do occur, can be restricted to short courses and are mild.
§This refers to the use of a vaccine to protect against feline leukemia virus infection. They are administered subcutaneously in healthy kittens or older cats as two doses, with the second dose given 3 or 4 weeks after the first. Annual revaccination with a single dose is recommended.
‖The Primucell-FIP Vaccine (Pfizer Animal Health) is administered intranasally to healthy cats. Primary vaccination with two doses should be given with the second dose administered 3 to 4 weeks after the first, and single-dose annual revaccination is recommended.

information about the animal, such as breed, age, and sex, as well as owner concerns or complaints, is essential to the case history. After the case history is obtained, the physical examination should be conducted in a systematic manner. Although the examination may be easier to complete by proceeding from head to tail, it is advisable to examine and record observations according to body systems.

The first skill used in the physical examination is careful observation of the animal's responses to the environment. Specific notes should be made regarding the animal's general condition, mentation, posture, locomotion, and breathing pattern. Next, the body temperature, respiratory and heart rates, capillary refill time, and body weight (expressed in pounds, kilograms, or grams) of the cat are recorded on the health record. The thorax should be thoroughly auscultated and the abdomen palpated for evidence of physical abnormalities. Body weights are recorded for several reasons. First, the weight provides information needed for dispensing medication; and second, it is an immediate indicator of the nutritional status of the animal. The body weight of a growing kitten steadily increasing at each office visit is an indication that the kitten is receiving adequate nutrition. Further nutritional information is found in Chapter 26.

Physical inspection begins by checking the head and oral cavity for evidence of malformation of the skull, cleft lip, stenotic nares, or cleft palate. The mucous membranes should be light pink and moist. The teeth, if present, should be examined for periodontal disease and occlusion problems. Periodontal disease generally begins in cats when the first teeth appear in the mouth and continues in variable degrees throughout the animal's life. Frequent dental examinations as part of the preventive health program convey to the owner the need for regularly performed prophylactic dentistry, the importance of providing the right type of food for the control of periodontal disease, and the importance of brushing even a young cat's teeth on a regular basis. Routine dental care and dental surgery are discussed in Chapter 18.

The skin and ears should be inspected for wounds, state of hydration, completeness of hair cover, and condition of foot pads. When necessary, the dermatological examination may also require such diagnostic procedures as exfoliative cytology, bacterial culture and sensitivity testing, skin scrapings, and dermatophyte culture and identification of external parasites (such as ear mites, fleas, ticks, and chiggers). When the observation and basic inspection phase has been completed, the animal is assessed according to specific body systems. Detailed information concerning the history and physical examination may be found in Chapter 3.

Vaccinations

In the general outline of the preventive program, the statement "vaccinate with FVRC-P vaccine" refers to the use of a vaccine to protect against the following: FVR—feline viral rhinotracheitis, C—feline calicivirus infection, and P—feline panleukopenia. A listing of some vaccines currently available is presented in Table 14–4.

Cats being prepared for shipment or entering a boarding kennel or veterinary hospital or clinic should be vaccinated at least 1 to 2 weeks before admission or shipment. In addition to regularly scheduled FVRC-P and rabies vaccinations, other immunizations can be incorporated into the preventive health program, as detailed below.

Feline *Chlamydia* Vaccine. Although feline chlamydiosis is not as prevalent as feline viral rhinotracheitis or feline calicivirus infections, it is evident that in some cat populations chlamydial infection is contributing to persistent conjunctivitis and upper respiratory tract disease. The vaccines currently available apparently produce effective protection only against *Chlamydia psittaci* infections. As with other vaccines for respiratory ailments, complete protection is not afforded; however, clinical signs of conjunctivitis or upper respiratory tract disease, if they do occur, can be restricted to short courses and are mild. Vaccines for feline chlamydiosis can be obtained from several manufacturers in various combinations with the more traditional feline vaccine components (see Table 14–4).

Feline Leukemia Virus (FeLV) Vaccine. Several vaccines are currently available to protect cats of all ages against feline leukemia virus infection (see Table 14–4). The vaccines are administered subcutaneously in healthy kittens or older cats as two doses, with the second dose given 3 or 4 weeks after the first. Annual revaccination with a single dose is recommended. According to the manufacturers, the vaccines cause no interference with simultaneous vaccinations against rabies, panleukopenia, and upper respiratory viruses. The vaccines also do not affect red blood cell or white blood cell counts, weight gain, reproductive capability, or feline leukemia virus testing in kittens vaccinated as young as 6 weeks of age. In viremic cats, vaccines may produce minimal antibody responses and cats remain viremic, but they are not harmed by the vaccination.

Feline Infectious Peritonitis (FIP) Vaccine. A first-generation temperature-sensitive FIP virus (TS-FIPV) vaccine that affords protection against FIP virus challenge is available (Primucell-FIP Vaccine, Pfizer Animal Health). This TS-FIPV vaccine contains attenuated whole coronavirus and is recommended by the manufacturer to be administered intranasally to healthy cats. Primary vaccination with two doses should be given, with the second dose administered 3 to 4 weeks after the first, and annual revaccination with a single dose is recommended. Cats vaccinated twice intranasally with the TS-FIPV vaccine have not developed a febrile response, nor have they had any blood dyscrasia indicative of FIP disease. Likewise, vaccinated pregnant cats, dexamethasone-suppressed cats, feline leukemia virus–infected cats, and feline enteric coronavirus–infected cats have not shown a febrile response or any blood dyscrasia.

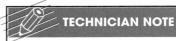

TECHNICIAN NOTE

A new anti-ringworm vaccine available for cats is *Microsporum canis* killed fungal vaccine.

Feline Fungal Vaccine. A *Microsporum canis* killed fungal vaccine that affords protection against ringworm-induced skin lesions is available. The vaccine is used in cats 4 months of age and older as an aid in the prevention and treatment of clinical signs of disease caused by *M. canis*. Vaccination has not been demonstrated to eliminate *M. canis* organisms from infected cats. Primary vaccination with two doses should be given, with the second dose administered 3 to 4 weeks after the first, and revaccination with a single dose every 6 months is recommended.

• Table 14–4 •

FELINE VACCINES*

VACCINE	MANUFACTURER	TYPE	VACCINE COMPONENTS						
			FPV	FVR	FCV	Chl	Rb	FIP	FeLV
Annumune	Fort Dodge Laboratories	I					X		
Dura-Rab 1	ImmunoVet, Vedco	I					X		
Dura-Rab 3	ImmunoVet, Vedco	I					X		
Eclipse 3	Schering-Plough Animal Health	A	X	X	X				
Eclipse 3 KP	Schering-Plough Animal Health	A/I	X	X	X				
Eclipse 3 KP-R	Schering-Plough Animal Health	A/I	X	X	X		X		
Eclipse 4	Schering-Plough Animal Health	A	X	X	X	X			
Eclipse 4 + FeLV	Schering-Plough Animal Health	A/I	X	X	X	X			X
Eclipse 4-R	Schering-Plough Animal Health	A/I	X	X	X	X	X		
Eclipse 4 KP	Schering-Plough Animal Health	A/I	X	X	X	X			
Eclipse 4 KP-R	Schering-Plough Animal Health	A/I	X	X	X	X	X		
Endurall-K	Pfizer Animal Health	I					X		
Endurall-P	Pfizer Animal Health	I					X		
Defensor	Pfizer Animal Health	I					X		
Feline 3	Rhone Merieux	A	X	X	X				
Feline 3 + Imrab 3	Rhone Merieux	A/I	X	X	X		X		
Feline 3 + Leucat	Rhone Merieux	A/I	X	X	X				X
Feline 4	Rhone Merieux	A	X	X	X	X			
Feline 4 Pk	Rhone Merieux	A/I	X	X	X	X			
Feline 4 + Imrab 3	Rhone Merieux	A/I	X	X	X	X	X		
Feline 4 + Leucat	Rhone Merieux	A/I	X	X	X	X			X
Feline 3 vaccine	DurVet	A/I	X	X	X				
Feline 3-C vaccine	DurVet	A	X	X	X	X			
Felin-L	Anchor	A	X						
Felin-RC	Anchor	A	X	X	X				
Felocell CVR	Pfizer Animal Health	A	X	X	X				
Felocell CVR-C	Pfizer Animal Health	A	X	X	X	X			
Felomune CVR	Pfizer Animal Health	A		X	X				
Fel-O-Fax IV	Fort Dodge Laboratories	A/I	X	X	X	X			
Fel-O-Vax Lv-K	Fort Dodge Laboratories	I							X
Fel-O-Vax Lv-K III	Fort Dodge Laboratories	I	X	X	X				X
Fel-O-Vax Lv-K IV	Fort Dodge Laboratories	I	X	X	X	X			X
Fel-O-Vax PCT	Fort Dodge Laboratories	I	X	X	X				
Fel-O-Vax PCT-R	Fort Dodge Laboratories	I	X	X	X		X		
FeTec 3	Bayer	A	X	X	X				
FeTec 3 KP	Bayer	A/I	X	X	X				
FeTec 4	Bayer	A	X	X	X	X			
Fevaxyn 3	Schering-Plough Animal Health	I							X
Fevaxyn 3 + C	Schering-Plough Animal Health	A/I	X	X	X	X			
Fevaxyn FeLV	Schering-Plough Animal Health	I							X
FVR C-P vaccine	Schering-Plough Animal Health	A/I	X	X	X				
FVR C-P-C vaccine	Schering-Plough Animal Health	A/I	X	X	X	X			
FVR C-P (MLV) vaccine	Schering-Plough Animal Health	A	X	X	X				
Genetivac FeLV vaccine	Schering-Plough Animal Health	I							X
Imrab 1	Rhone Merieux	I					X		
Imrab 3	Rhone Merieux	I					X		
Leucat	Rhone Merieux	I							X
Leukocell 2	Pfizer Animal Health	I							X
Panacine RC	Synbiotics	A	X	X	X				
Panacine-5	Synbiotics	A/I	X	X	X	X			X
Panavac RC	Synbiotics	A/I	X	X	X				
Performer-Feline	Performer	A	X	X	X				
Performer-Feline 4	Performer	A	X	X	X	X			
Primucell FIP	Pfizer Animal Health	A						X	
Prorab-1	Intervet	I					X		
Prorab-3F	Intervet	I					X		
Protex-3	Intervet	A	X	X	X				
Psittacoid	Schering-Plough Animal Health	A				X			
Rabdomun vaccine	Schering-Plough Animal Health	I					X		
Rabdomun 1 vaccine	Schering-Plough Animal Health	I					X		
Rabguard-TC	Schering-Plough Animal Health	I					X		
Rabvac 1	Schering-Plough Animal Health	I					X		
Rabvac 3	Schering-Plough Animal Health	I					X		
Respomune-CP	BioCor	A/I	X	X	X				
Rhinolin-CP	Bio-Ceutic Laboratories	A	X	X	X				
Rhinopan 4	BioCor	A	X	X	X	X			
Rhinopan MLV	BioCor	A	X	X	X				
RXV Vac Feline BodyGuard 3	RXV	A/I	X	X	X				
SentryRab-1	Synbiotics	I					X		
Trimune	Fort Dodge Laboratories	I					X		
VacSYN/FeLV	Synbiotics	I							X

FPV, feline parvovirus (feline panleukopenia virus); FVR, feline viral rhinotracheitis; FCV, feline calicivirus; Chl, *Chlamydia psittaci* infection (feline pneumonitis); Rb, rabies; FIP, feline infectious peritonitis; FeLV, feline leukemia virus. A, attenuated (modified live virus or MLV); I, inactivated (killed); A/I, combination of attenuated and inactivated.

*Compiled with the assistance of *Compendium of Veterinary Products.* Port Huron, MI, North American Compendiums, 1995–1996. Inactivated *Microsporum canis* vaccine is available from Fort Dodge Laboratories under the proprietary name Fel-O-Vax MC-K.

Owner Education

Owner education pamphlets on a variety of cat-related topics can be sent home with the owner each time the cat is seen for the preventive health program. Generally, only one or two owner education pamphlets are given to the owner at the end of each office visit.

Veterinarians and veterinary technicians are in an excellent position to provide meaningful owner educational services and thus make owners more aware of their cats and the associated responsibilities of cat ownership. By offering consultative advice and providing owners with educational pamphlets, the veterinary technician not only assists owners who are seeking medical treatment for their cats but serves a vital role in educating people in the community.

PREVENTIVE HEALTH PROGRAM FOR HORSES

A preventive health program for horses should be designed to meet the specific needs of the individual animal or herd. Such programs generally vary from one stable to another and from one veterinary practice to another depending upon expected exposures, management styles, and personal preferences of attending veterinarians and horse owners. An example of one preventive health program for horses is outlined in Table 14–5.

The Physical Examination

New additions to a stable or an established herd should be Coggins test negative for equine infectious anemia (EIA) and quarantined for 1 month before entering the general population. During this time, the first physical examination for the preventive health program can be performed. The physical examination should be completed in a manner that will gain the confidence of the new horse and allow the veterinarian to establish the current health status and soundness of the animal. These observations are then recorded in a permanent medical record at the stable.

In addition to recording the rectal temperature, respiratory rate, and heart rate before and after light exercise, the thorax should be thoroughly auscultated. The horse should be weighed or the body weight estimated with a thoracic tape, both to establish a weight baseline and for future reference in calculating doses. Both eyes should be completely examined for soundness. A dental examination should reveal incisor malocclusion and abnormal wear of the cheek teeth. Similarly, the musculoskeletal system and skin should be examined. Physical examination should be repeated at 2- to 3-month intervals as part of the preventive health program for horses of all ages. Obtaining a history and performing a physical examination are discussed in Chapter 3.

Vaccinations

A variety of vaccines approved for use in healthy horses can be obtained from manufacturers as individual components or in various combinations. A listing of some vaccines currently available is presented in Table 14–6.

Horses that are immunologically naive or have an unknown immunization history should receive an initial immunization followed in 4 weeks by a second immunization.

TECHNICIAN NOTE

Horses that are immunologically naive or have an unknown immunization history should receive an initial immunization followed in 4 weeks by a second immunization.

Further booster vaccinations can be administered as indicated by the risk of exposure and the veterinarian's experience with the vaccine. In rare instances, anaphylactoid reactions associated with the use of any vaccine can occur. This life-threatening crisis must be handled quickly. Accordingly, it is essential that epinephrine be available for the treatment of anaphylactoid reactions. Other complications, such as fever, lameness, and swelling, or abscess formation at the injection site, may also occur with the routine use of these vaccines. The horse owner should always be apprised of these possibilities before any vaccine is administered. Common diseases and vaccines used as an aid in disease prevention are discussed below.

Tetanus Vaccines. Tetanus, or lockjaw, is a disease characterized by muscular rigidity, which may culminate in death from respiratory arrest or convulsions. Tetanus is caused by the toxins produced by the anaerobic bacterium *Clostridium tetani.* Active immunity to tetanus is produced by administration of a tetanus toxoid, which is a purified, inactivated toxin of *C. tetani.*

Tetanus antitoxin is produced by hyperimmunization of donor horses with tetanus toxoid. Administration of antitoxin to unvaccinated horses induces immediate protection, which lasts approximately 2 weeks.

Equine Encephalomyelitis Vaccine. Equine encephalomyelitis is a viral neurological disease of horses caused by eastern, western, and Venezuelan viruses. These viruses are maintained in nature by bird and animal reservoirs and are transmitted to horses by biting insects. Venezuelan equine encephalomyelitis occurs in South and Central America, but has not been diagnosed in the United States for several years. The trivalent vaccine is commonly used for horses in states bordering Mexico to create a buffer zone which may prevent spread of Venezuelan equine encephalomyelitis into the United States. The clinical signs of equine encephalomyelitis may be as subtle as fever and partial anorexia and as severe as marked depression, convulsions, and death. Death rate varies with the type of virus infection, but it may range from 19% to 90%.

The equine encephalomyelitis vaccines currently used for active immunization are inactivated virus vaccines. They should be administered annually before the season of the biting insects. In areas where winter freezes are not common, semiannual vaccinations may be advisable.

Equine Rhinopneumonitis Vaccine. Equine herpesvirus (EHV) has caused sporadic infections and death in horses throughout the world. Four distinct equine herpesviruses have been identified: EHV-1, EHV-2, EHV-3, and EHV-4. EHV-1 and EHV-4 are the cause of rhinopneumonitis. EHV-1 has been exclusively associated with the neurological form of rhinopneumonitis, and it is also responsible for late-gestation abortions, stillbirths, and weak neonatal foals that fail to survive. EHV-4 is

• Table 14–5 •

GENERAL OUTLINE OF A PREVENTIVE HEALTH PROGRAM FOR HORSES

First Quarter: January–March
All Horses
Deworm—minimum of every 8 weeks. Exercise care in choice of anthelmintics for mares in the third trimester. Begin deworming foals at 2 months of age.
Trim feet—every 6 weeks. More frequently in foals requiring limb correction.
Dentistry—check adults twice yearly and float teeth as needed. Remove wolf teeth in 2-year-olds and retained caps in 2-, 3- and 4-year-olds.
    Immunize for respiratory disease: influenza, strangles, and rhinopneumonitis.
Stallions
Perform complete breeding examination. Maintain stallions under lights if being used for early breeding.
Pregnant Mares
Immunize with tetanus toxoid, and open sutured mares 30 days prepartum. Develop a colostrum bank. Ninth-day breeding only for mares with normal foaling history and normal reproductive tract. Wash udders of foaling mares.
Open Mares
Maintain under lights if being used for early breeding. Perform daily teasing. Perform reproductive tract examination during estrus. Mares should not be too fat but in gaining condition during breeding season.
Newborn Foals
Dip navel in disinfectant. Carefully, give a cleansing enema at birth. Administer tetanus prophylaxis if indicated by history.

Second Quarter: April–June
All Horses
Deworm—minimum of every 8 weeks.
Trim feet—every 6 weeks. Don't forget the foals and yearlings.
Dentistry—check teeth and remove or float teeth as needed.
Immunize for equine encephalomyelitis. Administer appropriate vaccine boosters.
Stallions
Maintain an exercise program. Monitor the semen quality.
Broodmares
Palpate at 21, 42, and 60 days after successful breeding.
Foals
Creep-feed the foals and provide free-choice minerals. Immunize at 3 months of age. Group the foals by sex and size when weaned.

Third Quarter: July–September
All Horses
Deworm—minimum of every 8 weeks. Clip and sweep the pastures.
Trim feet—every 6 weeks. Continue corrective trimming on foals.
Dentistry—check teeth and remove or float teeth as needed.
Stallions
Maintain an exercise program.
Broodmares
Administer rhinopneumonitis boosters to pregnant mares according to manufacturer's labeled directions. Administer appropriate vaccine boosters to foals and yearlings. Check condition of mare's udder at weaning and reduce the amount of feed given until milk flow is reduced.
Foals
Administer all appropriate immunizations. Provide free-choice minerals. Maintain a protein supplement in creep feeders.

Fourth Quarter: October–December
All Horses
Deworm—minimum every 8 weeks. Select anthelmintics appropriate for season.
Trim feet—every 6 weeks. Continuous corrective trimming on foals.
Dentistry—check teeth and remove or float teeth as needed.
Stallions
Continue the exercise program. Check immunizations. Perform breeding examination.
Broodmares
Confirm pregnancy. Begin treating the open mares. Check immunizations.

most frequently associated with upper respiratory tract disease in young horses and rarely is a cause of abortion.

Until recently all herpesvirus vaccines were prepared from EHV-1 virus. Vaccination of foals and young horses to prevent EHV-4 infections relied on the induction of cross-reactive antibody to EHV-1. The resulting immunity is short-lived and requires revaccination at 2- to 3-month intervals. Recently new vaccines have been introduced which contain both EHV-4 and EHV-1 and are approved for use in the prevention of respiratory infection.

Pregnant mares should be vaccinated during the fifth, sev-

enth, and ninth months of gestation using an inactivated EHV-1 vaccine. Total protection from abortion cannot be achieved.

Equine Influenza Vaccine. Equine influenza has a worldwide distribution and is frequently seen in mobile populations of horses. Disease outbreaks usually occur in horses 1 to 3 years of age after mixing with infected horses at the racetrack or show ground. Equine influenza may also occur in older horses, but the clinical signs are mild. Infection is characterized by fever, depression, anorexia, muscle soreness, and coughing.

The equine influenza viruses of importance in the United

• Table 14–6 •

EQUINE VACCINES*

| VACCINE | MANUFACTURER | TYPE | VACCINE COMPONENTS | | | | | | | | | | | | | |
			EEE	WEE	VEE	EVA	A1	A2	EHV-1	EHV-4	TT	TAT	RB	ST	ANX	PHF
Anthrax vaccine	Colorado Serum	—													X	
Arvac	Fort Dodge Laboratories	MLV				X										
		I	X	X							X					
		I	X	X	X						X					
Cephalovac VEWT	EquiLabs	I	X	X	X						X					
Encephaloid IM	Franklin	I	X	X												
Encephaloid I.M.	Fort Dodge Laboratories	I	X	X												
Encephalomyelitis vaccine	Colorado Serum	I	X	X												
Encevac with Havlogen	Bayer	I	X	X												
Encevac-T with Havlogen	Bayer	I	X	X							X					
Encevac-T + Havlogen	EquiLabs	I	X	X							X					
Encevac TC-4 with Havlogen	Bayer	I	X	X			X	X			X					
Encevac TC-4 + Havlogen	EquiLabs	I	X	X			X	X			X					
Equibac II	Fort Dodge Laboratories															
Equicine II with Havlogen	Bayer	I					X	X								
Equi-flu	EquiLabs	I					X	X								
Equi-Flu VEWT	EquiLabs	I	X	X	X		X	X			X					
Equiloid	Fort Dodge Laboratories	I	X	X							X					
Equiloid	Franklin	I	X	X							X					
EWT	Schering-Plough	I	X	X							X					
EWTF	Schering-Plough	I	X	X			X	X			X					
Flumune EWT	Pfizer Animal Health	I	X	X			X	X			X					
Fluvac	Fort Dodge Laboratories	I						X								
Fluvac	Franklin	I					X	X								
Fluvac EHV-1	Fort Dodge Laboratories	I					X	X	X							
Fluvac EHV 4/1	Franklin	I					X	X	X	X						
Fluvac EWT	Fort Dodge Laboratories	I	X	X			X	X			X					
Fluvac EWT	Franklin	I	X	X			X	X			X					
Fluvac-T	Fort Dodge Laboratories	I					X	X			X					
		I												X		
Inflogen	Fort Dodge Laboratories	I					X	X								
Inflogen 3	Fort Dodge Laboratories	I					X	X			X					
Mystique	Bayer	I														X
Mystique II	Bayer	I											X			X
PHF-Vax	Schering-Plough	I														X
PHF-VAX + 4	Schering-Plough	I	X	X			X	X			X					X
Pneumabort-K + 1b	Fort Dodge Laboratories	I							X							
Pneunobort-K + 1b	Franklin	I								X	X					
Potomacguard	Fort Dodge	I														X
Potomacguard	Franklin	I														X
Potomacguard EWT	Fort Dodge	I	X	X							X					X
Potomacguard EWT	Franklin	I	X	X							X					X
Potomavac	Rhone Merieux	I														X
Prestige + Havlogen	Bayer	I							X	X						
Prestige + Havlogen	EquiLabs	I							X	X						

Table continued on following page

• Table 14–6 •

			VACCINE COMPONENTS													
VACCINE	**MANUFACTURER**	**TYPE**	**EEE**	**WEE**	**VEE**	**EVA**	**A1**	**A2**	**EHV-1**	**EHV-4**	**TT**	**TAT**	**RB**	**ST**	**ANX**	**PHF**
Prestige II + Havlogen	Bayer	I					X	X	X	X						
Prestige II + Havlogen	EquiLabs	I					X	X	X	X						
Prodigy + Havlogen	Bayer	I							X							
Rabguard-TC	Pfizer Animal Health	I											X			
Rabvac 3	Fort Dodge Laboratories	I											X			
Rhino-Flu T	Fort Dodge Laboratories	MLV, I					X	X	X			X				
Rhinomune	Pfizer Animal Health	MLV							X							
RM Equine Ehrlichia + Imrab	Rhone Merieux	I											X			X
RM Imrab 3	Rhone Merieux	I											X			
RM Imrab Bovine Plus	Rhone Merieux	I											X			
Strepguard with Havlogen	Bayer	I												X		
Strepvax II	EquiLabs	I												X		
Super-Tet with Havlogen	Bayer	I									X					
Tetanus Antitoxin Equine Origin	EquiLabs	Antitoxin										X				
Tetanus toxoid	Fort Dodge Laboratories	I									X					
Tetanus toxoid	Colorado Serum	I									X					
Tetanus toxoid	Franklin	I									X					
Tetanus toxoid—concentrated	Colorado Serum	I									X					
Tetmune EW	Pfizer Animal Health	I	X	X							X					
Tetmune + Duophase	Pfizer Animal Health	I									X					
Tetnogen	Fort Dodge Laboratories	I									X					
Tetnogen-AT	Fort Dodge Laboratories	Antitoxin										X				
Tetanus antitoxin	Sanofi	Antitoxin										X				
Tetanus antitoxin	Fort Dodge Laboratories	Antitoxin										X				
Tetanus antitoxin	Professional Biological	Antitoxin										X				
Tetanus antitoxin	Coopers Animal Health	Antitoxin										X				
Tetanus antitoxin	Colorado Serum	Antitoxin										X				
Thraxol-2	Bayer	—													X	
Triple-E	Fort Dodge Laboratories	I	X	X	X											
Triple E-Ft	Fort Dodge Laboratories	I	X	X	X		X	X			X					
Unitox	EquiLabs										X					
Unitox	EquiLabs	I									X					
Double-EFT	Fort Dodge Laboratories	I	X	X			X	X			X					
Double-ET	Fort Dodge Laboratories	I	X	X							X					
Equi-Flu EWT	Coopers	—	X	X			X	X			X					
Flumune	Pfizer Animal Health	I					X	X								
Rhino-Flu	Pfizer Animal Health	I					X	X	X							
Triple-ET	Fort Dodge Laboratories	I	X	X	X						X					

EEE, eastern equine encephalomyelitis; WEE, western equine encephalomyelitis; VEE, Venezuelan equine encephalomyelitis; EVA, equine viral arteritis; A1, equine influenza myxovirus A-equi 1; A2, equine influenza myxovirus A-equi 2; EHV-1, equine herpesvirus 1; EHV-4, equine herpesvirus 4; TT, tetanus toxoid; TAT, tetanus antitoxin; RB, rabies; ST, strangles; ANX, anthrax; PHF, Potomac horse fever; MLV, modified live virus; I, inactivated.

States are A/1 and A/2. Currently available vaccines contain inactivated virus that includes both A/1 and A/2 strains. The duration of protective immunity from vaccination is short-lived, requiring revaccination every 2 to 3 months.

Strangles Vaccine. Strangles is a respiratory disease caused by infection with the bacterium *Streptococcus equi.* Strangles is a highly contagious disease that is transmitted through direct contact with mucopurulent discharges from infected horses or from contaminated fomites, such as feeding utensils, buckets, or other equipment. Strangles is characterized by sudden onset of fever and upper respiratory catarrh, followed by acute swelling and abscess formation in submaxillary, submandibular, and retropharyngeal lymph nodes.

TECHNICIAN NOTE

Strangles is a highly contagious disease that is transmitted through direct contact with mucopurulent discharges from infected horses or from contaminated fomites.

Several inactivated subunit M protein vaccines and one inactivated whole-cell bacterium are available for intramuscular injection as an adjunct to the prevention of strangles. All of these vaccines may cause postinjection reactions or abscesses at the site of administration.

Equine Viral Arteritis Vaccine. Equine viral arteritis infection may cause subclinical to severe disease and death. The disease is characterized by fever, depression, nasal discharge, lacrimation, coughing, and limb swelling. Several attenuated live virus vaccines have been developed in recent years. Only one serotype of virus appears to be relevant to the protection of horses. The vaccine induces partial to complete protection against the clinical signs of disease, but virus replication will still occur after virus challenge.

Potomac Horse Fever Vaccine. Potomac horse fever (equine monocytic ehrlichiosis) is caused by *Ehrlichia risticii.* It is most prevalent in eastern states, particularly near large waterways, but has been identified in many regions of the United States and in other countries. Although not proven, an insect vector such as the tick is believed to be involved in disease transmission. An approved vaccine is now available for use in the prevention of Potomac horse fever, and its use should be considered in areas where the disease is known to occur.

Anthrax and Rabies Vaccines. Anthrax and rabies vaccines for use in horses are currently available but are not widely used except where a genuine risk is identified.

Dental and Hoof Care

Many of the directional instructions from rider or driver reach the horse through the mouth. If the bit causes pain, the instructions given to the horse may be compromised. Wolf teeth cause extreme pain in some horses, especially with broken snaffle, overdraw checks, and gag bits. The mouth of the young horse

should be examined, and if wolf teeth are present, they should be removed before training begins. Deciduous premolars that are retained and enamel points on cheek teeth may also cause pain in the mouth that interferes with normal feeding and willing response to the bit. In addition, the cheek teeth should also be checked visually or by palpation for evidence of abnormal wear, such as wave mouth, step mouth, or shear mouth. Of course, all dental examinations should include inspection for malocclusion.

The role of the veterinarian and veterinary technician in hoof care is largely advisory and can be given via owner education pamphlets.

TECHNICIAN NOTE

The role of the veterinarian and veterinary technician in hoof care is largely advisory and can be given via owner education pamphlets.

Frequent hoof cleaning helps in the prevention of thrush. Keeping the hooves trimmed short and maintaining the correct hoof-pastern axis also helps to prevent excess stress on tendons and ligaments of the limb. In foals that are born splay-footed or pigeon-toed, frequent hoof trimming can often correct these conformation problems.

Parasites

It is well accepted that the athletic horse cannot perform at its genetic peak potential if handicapped with a heavy parasite load. Likewise, the pet horse may not maintain its well-kept appearance if burdened with external or internal parasites. Therefore, close attention to parasite control is extremely important in a preventive health program. Complete records are essential to ensure that each horse is being adequately treated. Pastured horses should be dewormed every 60 days or more often. Horses that never eat grass may not require deworming as often; in this case, the frequency of deworming should be based on results from fecal flotation examinations. Follow-up fecal flotations on all age groups of horses on a farm will help to determine the efficacy of the anthelmintics used.

Feed additives are available that are lethal to developing house fly and stable fly larvae in treated horse feces (but not effective against existing adult flies). These types of feed additives are to be used with caution, since they are organophosphate larvicides with possible side effects if used concomitantly with other pharmaceutical products. Chapter 6 contains additional information on parasitology.

Nutrition

Horses have evolved as forage eaters and their digestive system is able to handle most forages, such as grass and hay, efficiently. Furthermore, metabolic diseases (such as laminitis and azoturia) are less likely to occur in horses fed diets composed primarily of roughage rather than grain. Therefore, the horse's diet should contain mostly high-quality roughage with just enough grain supplement to maintain body weight. The amount of grain in the diet should increase as the amount of work performed

• Table 14–7 •

GENERAL OUTLINE OF A PREVENTIVE HEALTH PROGRAM FOR BEEF CATTLE

Cow-Calf Herd Recommendation*
At Birth
Ingestion of colostrum within the first few hours after birth is an important factor in baby calf survival. Immunize with oral bovine rotavirus
  and coronavirus enteric disease vaccine if a calf diarrhea problem exists in the herd.
1- to 3-Month-Old Calves
Immunize with a seven-way clostridial diseases product. Deworm with commercial product that is safe for calves.
Preweaning Calves
Deworm with broad-spectrum commercial dewormer and immunize as follows:

IMMUNIZING VACCINE	AGE FOR VACCINE ADMINISTRATION
Brucella abortus, strain 19	5–6 months of age (dependent upon federal and state regulations)
(calfhood vaccination—replacement heifers only)	
Clostridial diseases	5–6 months of age
Clostridium perfringens types C and D, *C. chauvoei*, *C. novyi*, *C.*	
septicum, and *C. sordelli*	
Infectious bovine rhinotracheitis (IBR) and parainfluenza-3 (PI-3)	5–6 months of age, booster at 12–13 months of age
respiratory diseases (inactivated vaccines only)	
Bovine virus diarrhea (BVD) (inactivated vaccines only)	5–6 months of age, booster at 12–13 months of age

Weaning Calves
Deworm with broad-spectrum commercial dewormer and treat for lice and grubs. Castrate the bull calves. Immunize with *Pasteurella*
  (optional) and *Haemophilus* (optional) vaccines.
Prebreeding Replacement Heifers
Deworm with broad-spectrum commercial dewormer and treat for lice. Immunize as follows:

IMMUNIZING VACCINE	TIME OF VACCINE ADMINISTRATION
Infectious bovine rhinotracheitis (IBR) and parainfluenza-3 (PI-3)	10–12 months of age
respiratory diseases	
Clostridial diseases	10–12 months of age
C. perfringens types C and D, *C. novyi*, *C. septicum*, *C. sordelli*,	
and *C. chauvoei*	
Bovine virus diarrhea (BVD)	10–12 months of age
Leptospirosis	10–12 months of age
Campylobacteriosis	10–12 months of age

Prebreeding Cows
Deworm with broad-spectrum dewormer and treat for lice. Immunize for leptospirosis and campylobacteriosis.
Precalving Cows
Immunize as follows:

IMMUNIZING VACCINE	TIME OF VACCINE ADMINISTRATION
Infectious bovine rhinotracheitis (IBR) and parainfluenza-3 (PI-3)	Prior to calving
respiratory diseases (inactivated vaccines only)	
Bovine virus diarrhea (BVD) (inactivated vaccines only)	Prior to calving
Bovine rotavirus and coronavirus enteric diseases	Prior to calving
Escherichia coli enteric disease	Prior to calving
Clostridial diseases	Prior to calving
C. perfringens types C and D, *C. chauvoei*, *C. novyi*, *C. septicum*,	
and *C. sordelli*	

Bulls
Deworm annually with broad-spectrum dewormer and treat for lice and grubs. Immunize as recommended for prebreeding replacement
  heifers annually (see the above section).
Feedlot Recommendations†
On Arrival into the Feedlot
Deworm with a broad-spectrum dewormer and immunize for infectious bovine rhinotracheitis (IBR), parainfluenza-3 (PI-3), bovine virus
  diarrhea (BVD), and clostridial diseases (use seven-way vaccine). Inactivated infectious bovine rhinotracheitis, parainfluenza-3, and bovine
  virus diarrhea vaccines are the safest.
Three–Four Weeks After Arrival into the Feedlot
Implant a commercial implant product. Treat for lice and grubs. Administer booster immunizations if necessary. Abort the heifers if
  necessary. Castrate and dehorn if necessary.

*Other optional vaccines that may be incorporated into the immunization program, depending on individual herd needs and
diseases endemic to the area, include anthrax and anaplasmosis.
  †Other optional vaccines that may be incorporated into the immunization program, depending on individual herd needs
and diseases endemic to the area, include *Haemophilus somnus, Pasteurella* spp., respiratory syncytial virus, leptospirosis,
and anthrax.

increases. A complete vitamin and mineral supplement is usually added to the diet to ensure that the proper balance of vitamins and minerals is received. All guesswork can be removed from ration planning if there is a feed analysis laboratory in proximity. Equine nutrition is discussed in Chapter 26.

Sanitation

Advice on sanitation may be communicated orally to the horse owner or given via owner education pamphlets. The fact that diseases are effectively spread from sick horses to susceptible horses via shared feed and water buckets, bits, twitches, chain shanks, trailers, and clothing is sometimes overlooked. Water and feed buckets should be cleaned and sanitized on a regular basis. Proper manure disposal is also important in preventing the spread of infectious diseases and in controlling flies and internal parasites.

PREVENTIVE HEALTH PROGRAM FOR CATTLE

Preventive health programs for beef and dairy cattle are generally based on recommendations of the consulting veterinarian and the specific needs of the herd and the herdsman. Accordingly, the development of a vaccination program should be based on several factors. First, it is important to have a knowledge of disease conditions present within a given herd and of the disease conditions present in the surrounding area. This should be based on accurate diagnosis or previous diagnoses of diseases in the specific herd and surrounding herds. Second, it is necessary to be familiar with the management procedures present on a farm that allow for a vaccination program designed around the working patterns of the herd; this is especially true for a cow-calf operation. Third, the population variances within a herd should be known. Vaccine choices and the frequency of their use can vary depending on such factors as open versus closed herds, source of new replacement cattle, and feeding practices. General approaches to preventive health programs for beef and dairy cattle are presented in Tables 14–7 and 14–8, respectively.

Vaccinations

Vaccines that may be included in preventive health programs for beef and dairy cattle can be obtained from manufacturers as individual components or in various combinations. A listing of some vaccines currently available is presented in Table 14–9. Diseases for which vaccines are more frequently used in these preventive health programs are detailed below.

Text continued on page 342

• Table 14–8 •

GENERAL OUTLINE OF A PREVENTIVE HEALTH PROGRAM FOR DAIRY CATTLE*

Calves

At Birth
Immunize with bovine rotavirus and coronavirus enteric disease vaccine† and administer orally *Escherichia coli* enteric disease vaccine.
Weaning Age (about 2 months of age) to Breeding Age (about 15 months of age)

Immunizing Vaccine	*Age for Vaccine Administration*
Brucella abortus, strain 19 (calfhood vaccination—replacement heifers only)	4–8 months of age optimal time (dependent upon federal and state regulations)
Clostridial diseases	2–4 months of age
Clostridium perfringens types C and D, *C. chauvoei*, *C. novyi*, *C. septicum*, and *C. sordelli*	
Infectious bovine rhinotracheitis (IBR) and parainfluenza-3 (PI-3) respiratory diseases	4–6 months of age, booster at 12–13 months of age
Bovine virus diarrhea (BVD)	6–8 months of age, booster at 12–13 months of age
Leptospirosis	4–6 months of age, booster in 2 weeks
Campylobacteriosis (if natural breeding)	4–6 months of age, booster at 12–13 months of age

Fresh Cows and Heifers

Immunizing Vaccine	*Time of Vaccine Administration*
Infectious bovine rhinotracheitis (IBR) and parainfluenza-3 (PI-3) respiratory diseases (inactivated vaccines only)	30 days post partum
Bovine virus diarrhea (BVD) (inactivated vaccines only)	30 days post partum
Leptospirosis	30 days post partum
Campylobacteriosis	30 days post partum

Dry Cows and Bred Heifers
The goal of dry cow immunization is to provide for optimal protection for the newborn calf.

Immunizing Vaccine	*Time of Vaccine Administration*
Leptospirosis	At time of dry-off
Bovine rotavirus and coronavirus enteric diseases†	At time of dry-off, booster in 2–3 weeks
Escherichia coli enteric disease†	At time of dry-off, booster in 2–3 weeks
Clostridial diseases	At time of dry-off, booster in 2–3 weeks
C. perfringens types C and D, *C. chauvoei*, *C. novyi*, *C. septicum*, and *C. sordelli*	

*Other vaccines that may be incorporated into the vaccination program, depending on individual herd needs and diseases endemic to the area, include *Haemophilus somnus*, *Pasteurella* spp., *Salmonella* spp., *Clostridium haemolyticum*, anthrax, and anaplasmosis.
†Use if problem of neonatal calf diarrhea exists on the farm.

• Table 14–9 •

CATTLE VACCINES*

VACCINES	MANUFACTURER	TYPE	IBR	PI3	BVD	BRSV	Haemophilus	Pasteurella	Leptospirosis	Clostridium chauvoei	Clostridium septicum	Clostridium novyi	Clostridium sordellii	Clostridium hemolyticum	Clostridium perfringens C and D	Campylobacter	Trichomonas	Escherichia coli	Coronavirus	Rotavirus	Moraxella	Tetanus	Anaplasmosis	Anthrax	Brucella	Rabies	Corynebacterium	Salmonella	Actinomyces	Fusobacterium	Papilloma	Staphylococcus
20/20	Bayer	I																			X											
Absolute	AgriLabs	I						X																								
Alpha-7	Bio-Ceutic	I								X	X	X	X		X																	
Alpha-7	Anchor	I								X	X	X	X		X																	
Anaplaz	Ford Dodge	MLV																					X									
Anthrax spore-vaccine	Colorado Serum	MLV																						X								
Bar Somnus-2P	Anchor	I					X	X																								
Bar Somnus	Anchor	I					X																									
Bar-3/Somnus	Anchor	I	X	X	X		X																									
Bar-4	Anchor	I	X	X	X			X																								
Bar-4/Somnus	Anchor	I	X	X			X	X																								
Bar-Vac 7/Somnus	Anchor	I					X			X	X	X	X		X																	
Bar-Vac-CD/T	Anchor	I													X							X										
BovEye	Pfizer Animal Health	I																				X										
Bovi-K 4	Pfizer Animal Health	MLV/I	X	X	X	X																										
Bovine rhinotracheitis vaccine with Leptospira interrogans serogroup pomona bacterin	Sanofi	MLV/I	X			X			X																							
Bovine rhinotracheitis-parainfluenza-3 vaccine	Colorado Serum	MLV	X	X																												
Bovine rhinotracheitis-virus diarrhea vaccine with Leptospira interrogans serogroup pomona bacterin	Sanofi	MLV/I	X		X				X																							
Bovine Scour Bac oral	Grand	I																	X													
Bovine Pili Shield	Grand	I																	X													
Bovine rhinotracheitis-virus diarrhea-parainfluenza-3 vaccine	Colorado Serum	MLV	X	X	X																											
Bovine 9	Durvet	MLV/I	X	X	X				X							X																
BoviShield IBR	Pfizer Animal Health	MLV	X																													

332

Product	Manufacturer	Type								
BoviShield IBR-BRSV-LP	Pfizer Animal Health	MLV/I	X	X	X			X		
BoviShield IBR-PI3-BRSV	Pfizer Animal Health	MLV	X	X	X			X		
BoviShield 4	Pfizer Animal Health	MLV	X	X	X			X		
BoviShield IBR-BVD-BRSV-LP	Pfizer Animal Health	MLV/I	X	X	X			X		
BoviShield IBR-BVD-LP	Pfizer Animal Health	MLV/I	X	X				X		
BoviShield 4 + L5	Pfizer Animal Health	MLV/I	X	X	X			X		
BoviShield 3	Pfizer Animal Health	MLV	X	X	X					
BoviShield BRSV	Pfizer Animal Health	MLV			X					
BRD-I	Franklin	I		X						
Breed-Back-10	Bio-Ceutic	MLV/I	X	X	X	X		X		X
BreedBack-10	Anchor	MLV/I	X	X	X	X		X		X
BRSV Vac 4	Bayer	MLV	X	X	X					
BRSV Vac 9	Bayer	MLV/I	X	X	X			X		
BRSV Vac	Bayer	MLV		X	X					
BRSV Vac 3	Bayer	MLV	X	X	X					
BRSV-KV	Anchor	I			X					
Brucella abortus vaccine	Colorado Serum	MLV								X
Brucella abortus vaccine	Professional Biological	MLV								X
Brucella abortus vaccine	Coopers	MLV								X
C & D toxoid	AgriLabs	I					X	X		
C & D toxoid	Anchor	I					X	X		
Calf-Guard	Pfizer Animal Health	MLV	X						X X	
Cattlemaster 4	Pfizer Animal Health	MLV/I	X	X	X			X		
Cattlemaster 3	Pfizer Animal Health	MLV/I	X	X	X			X		
CattleMaster BVD-K	Pfizer Animal Health	I		X		X				
CattleMaster 4 + VL5	Pfizer Animal Health	MLV/I	X	X	X		X	X		
CattleMaster 4 + L5	Pfizer Animal Health	MLV/I	X	X	X			X		
Cattle-Vac 9	Durvet	I	X	X	X			X		
Cattle-Vac 4	Durvet	I	X	X	X					
Cattle-Vac 3	Durvet	I	X	X	X					
Cattle-Vac 4-Somnus	Durvet	I	X	X	X					
Cattle-Vac 9-Somnus	Durvet	I	X	X	X	X				
Cattle-Vac 8	Durvet	I	X	X				X		
Clostridium perfringens Types C and D toxoid	Colorado Serum	I						X		
Clostri Shield C	Grand	I				X		X		
Clostri Shield 8	Grand	I			X	X		X		
Clostri Shield 7	Grand	I	X	X	X			X		
Clostridial 7-Way + Somnumune	AgriLabs	I	X	X				X		
Clostridial 8-Way	AgriLabs	I	X	X	X	X		X		
Clostridial 7-Way	AgriLabs	I	X	X	X			X		
Clostridial 4-Way	Lextron	I	X	X						

Table continued on following page

333

• Table 14-9 •

CATTLE VACCINES* (Continued)

VACCINES	MANUFACTURER	TYPE	IBR	PI3	BVD	BRSV	Haemophilus	Pasteurella	Leptospirosis	Clostridium chauvoei	Clostridium septicum	Clostridium novyi	Clostridium sordellii	Clostridium haemolyticum	Clostridium perfringens C and D	Campylobacter	Trichomonas	Escherichia coli	Coronavirus	Rotavirus	Moraxella	Tetanus	Anaplasmosis	Anthrax	Brucella	Rabies	Corynebacterium	Salmonella	Actinomyces	Fusobacterium	Papilloma	Staphylococcus
Clostridial 7-Way	ProLabs	I								X	X	X	X		X																	
Clostridial 7-Way	Lextron	I								X	X	X	X		X																	
Clostridial 7-Way + Somnumune	ProLabs	I					X			X	X	X	X	X	X																	
Clostridial 8-Way	ProLabs	I								X	X	X	X	X	X																	
Clostridium chauvoei-septicum-Pasteurella haemolytica-multocida bacterin	Colorado Serum	I						X		X	X																					
Clostridium chauvoei-septicum-novyi-sordellii bacterin-toxoid	Colorado Serum	I								X	X	X	X																			
Clostridium chauvoei-septicum bacterin	Colorado Serum	I								X	X																					
Clostridium perfringens types C and D-tetanus toxoid	Colorado Serum	I													X							X										
Conquest-1 + 3	Lextron	MLV/I	X	X	X																											
Conquest-4	Lextron	MLV/I	X	X	X	X																										
Conquest-4K	Lextron	I	X	X	X	X																										
Conquest-4K + H.S.	Lextron	I	X	X	X	X	X																									
Conquest-4KW	Lextron	I	X	X	X	X																										
Conquest-8K	Lextron	I	X	X	X	X																										
Conquest-9	Lextron	MLV/I	X	X	X	X			X																							
Conquest-9K	Lextron	I	X	X	X	X			X																							
Cow-Vac 9	Lextron	MLV/I	X	X	X				X							X																
Cow-Vac 9	AgriLabs	MLV/I	X	X	X				X							X																
Defender IBR-BVD-PI3	Premier Farmtech	I	X	X	X																											
Defender IBR-BVD-PI3-L5	Premier Farmtech	I	X	X	X				X																							
Defender 9	Premier Farmtech	I	X	X	X	X			X																							
Defender 9 HS	Premier Farmtech	I	X	X	X	X	X		X																							
Defender IBR-BVD-PI3-BRSV	Premier Farmtech	I	X	X	X	X																										
Defender-4HS	Premier Farmtech	I	X	X	X	X	X																									

Defensor	Pfizer Animal Health	I													X
Discovery BRSV-Kv	Franklin	I				X		X							
Discovery-3 VL5	Franklin	I	X	X	X			X				X			
Discovery-3	Franklin	I	X	X		X									
Discovery-3L5	Franklin	I	X	X	X			X							
Discovery-4	Franklin	I	X	X	X	X									
Discovery-4 + PH	Franklin	I	X	X	X	X	X								
Discovery-4 + Somnus	Franklin	I	X	X	X	X									
Discovery-4L5	Franklin	I	X	X	X	X		X							
Discovery-4L% + PH	Franklin	I	X	X	X	X	X	X							
Discovery-4L5 + Somnus	Franklin	I													
Electroid 7 + H.S. vaccine	Coopers	I							X	X	X	X			
Electroid 7 Vaccine	Coopers	I							X	X	X	X			
Elite 4-HS	Bio-Ceutic	I	X	X	X	X									
Elite 4-HS	Anchor	I	X	X	X	X									
Elite 9-HS	Bio-Ceutic	I	X	X	X	X		X							
Elite 4	Bio-Ceutic	I	X	X	X										
Elite 9	Bio-Ceutic	I	X	X	X			X							
Elite 9-HS	Anchor	I	X	X	X	X									
Elite 4	Anchor	I	X	X	X										
Elite 9	Anchor	I	X	X	X			X							
ENDOVAC-Bovi	Immvac	I												X	
Enviracor	Upjohn	I								X					
Fermicon C-D	Bio-Ceutic	I							X			X			
Fermicon CD/T	Bio-Ceutic	I							X			X			
Fermicon-7/MB	Bio-Ceutic	I							X	X	X	X			
Fermicon-7/Somnugen	Bio-Ceutic	I							X	X	X	X			
Fortress 7	Pfizer Animal Health	I							X	X	X	X			
Fortress CD	Pfizer Animal Health	I							X	X	X	X			
Fortress 8	Pfizer Animal Health	I							X	X	X	X			
Herd-Vac 9	BioCor	MLV/I	X	X		X		X							
Horizon 10	Bayer	MLV/I	X	X	X	X		X							
Horizon 9	Bayer	MLV/I	X	X	X	X		X							
Horizon 4	Bayer	MLV/I	X	X	X	X									
Horizon 7	Bayer	I	X	X											
Horizon 1 + Vac 3	Bayer	MLV/I	X	X	X	X									
IBP-RS	Lextron	MLV	X	X	X										
IBP-RS-L5	Lextron	MLV/I	X	X	X			X							
IBR/Marker-KV	Syntrovet	I	X												
IBR	Sanofi	MLV	X												
IBR/BVD/PI3/L5	Sanofi	MLV/I	X	X	X	X									

Table continued on following page

Table 14-9 • CATTLE VACCINES* (Continued)

VACCINE COMPONENTS

VACCINES	MANUFACTURER	TYPE	IBR	PI3	BVD	BRSV	Haemophilus	Pasteurella	Leptospirosis	Clostridium chauvoei	Clostridium septicum	Clostridium novyi	Clostridium sordellii	Clostridium hemolyticum	Clostridium perfringens C and D	Campylobacter	Trichomonas	Escherichia coli	Coronavirus	Rotavirus	Moraxella	Tetanus	Anaplasmosis	Anthrax	Brucella	Rabies	Corynebacterium	Salmonella	Actinomyces	Fusobacterium	Papilloma	Staphylococcus
IBR-BVD	Sanofi	MLV	X		X																											
IBR-BVD-PI3	BioCor	MLV	X	X	X																											
IBR-BVD-PI3/Bar Somnus-2P	Anchor	MLV/I	X	X	X		X	X																								
IBR-BVD-PI3	AgriLabs	MLV	X	X	X																											
IBR-BVD-PI3	Sanofi	MLV	X	X	X																											
IBR-BVD-PI3/Somnugen-2P	Bio-Ceutic	MLV/I	X	X	X		X	X																								
IBR-BVD-PI3	Durvet	MLV	X	X	X																											
IBR-BVD-PI3-Lepto 5	Durvet	MLV/I	X	X	X				X																							
IBR-BVD-PI3-Lepto 5	BioCor	MLV/I	X	X	X				X																							
IBR-BVD-PI3-Lepto 5 8-Way	AgriLabs	MLV/I	X	X	X				X																							
IBR-BVD-PI3-SomnuMune	AgriLabs	MLV/I	X	X	X		X																									
IBR-BVD-PI3-SomnuTech	BioCor	MLV/I	X	X	X		X																									
IBR-PI3/Bar Somus-2P	Anchor	MLV/I	X	X			X	X																								
IBR-PI3	Sanofi	MLV	X	X																												
IBR-PI3	Lextron	MLV	X	X																												
IBR-PI3-Lepto P	Lextron	MLV/I	X	X					X																							
IL	Lextron	MLV/I	X						X																							
Immu-Coli-B	Sanofi	I																	X														
IP-RS	Lextron	MLV	X	X		X																										
I-Site	AgriLabs	I																				X											
J • Vac J5	Sanofi	I																	X														
Jencine K99 vaccine	Coopers	I																	X														
Lepto 5	Lextron	I							X																								
Lepto Shield 5	Grand	I							X																								
Lepto 5	Durvet	I							X																								
Lepto 5	BioCor	I							X																								
Lepto 5-Way	Sanofi	I							X																								
Lepto 5	AgriLabs	I							X																								

336

Product	Manufacturer	Type
Leptoferm-5	Pfizer Animal Health	I
Leptospira pomona bacterin	Sanofi	I
Leukotox	A.H.A.	I
Lysigin	Bio-Ceutic	I
Nasalgen IP vaccine	Coopers	MLV
Nasal-Ject I.P.	AgriLabs	MLV
OneShot	Pfizer Animal Health	MLV
Pasteurella haemolytica-multocida bacterin	Colorado Serum	I
Piliguard E. coli-1	Schering-Plough	I
Piliguard Pinkeye + 7	Schering-Plough	I
Piliguard Pinkeye-1	Schering-Plough	I
Pilivib Shield	Grand	I
Pneumosyn-H	Franklin	I
Pneumosyn-H + Somnus	Franklin	I
PregGuard	Pfizer Animal Health	MLV/I
Pregsure 9	Pfizer Animal Health	MLV/I
Premier 4	BioCor	I
Premier 9-SomnuTech	BioCor	I
Premier 9	BioCor	I
Premier 8	BioCor	I
Premier 4-SomnuTech	BioCor	I
Presponse	Langford	I
Pre-Vent 6	AgriLabs	I
Pro-Bac 4	A.V.L.	I
Pro-Bac 3	A.V.L.	I
Pro-Bac 3R	A.V.L.	I
Pro-Vac-3/Somnugen	Bio-Ceutic	I
Quadraplex/Somnugen	Bio-Ceutic	I
Rabdomun vaccine	Schering-Plough	I
Rabguard-TC	Pfizer Animal Health	I
Redwol with Spur	Bayer	I
Reprotec-T	Franklin	I
Reprotec-TVL5	Franklin	I
ResProMune 8 IBP-Lepto 5	AgriLabs	I
ResProMune 4 + SomnuMune	AgriLabs	I
ResProMune 10	AgriLabs	I
ResProMune 4 IBP-BRSV	AgriLabs	I
ResProMune 9	AgriLabs	I
Resvac BRSV/Somubac	Pfizer Animal Health	MLV/I
Resvac 2/Somubac	Pfizer Animal Health	MLV/I
Resvac 4/Somubac	Pfizer Animal Health	MLV/I

Table continued on following page

• Table 14-9 •

CATTLE VACCINES* (Continued)

VACCINES	MANUFACTURER	TYPE	IBR	PI3	BVD	BRSV	Haemophilus	Pasteurella	Leptospirosis	Clostridium chauvoei	Clostridium septicum	Clostridium novyi	Clostridium sordellii	Clostridium hemolyticum	Clostridium perfringens C and D	Campylobacter	Trichomonas	Escherichia coli	Coronavirus	Rotavirus	Moraxella	Tetanus	Anaplasmosis	Anthrax	Brucella	Rabies	Corynebacterium	Salmonella	Actinomyces	Fusobacterium	Papilloma	Staphylococcus
Resvac 3/Somubac	Pfizer Animal Health	MLV/I	X	X	X		X																									
RM Imrab Bovine Plus	Rhone Merieux	I																								X						
RM Imrab 3	Rhone Merieux	I																								X						
RS	Lextron	MLV				X																										
RXV 4K-Somnus Vac	RXV	I	X	X	X	X	X																									
RXV Vac SomnuMune	RXV	I	X	X	X	X	X																									
RXV Vac IBR-BVD-PI3	RXV	MLV	X	X	X																											
RXV Vac Cow-Vac 9	RXV	MLV/I	X	X	X				X							X																
RXV 4K Vac	RXV	I	X	X	X	X																										
RXV 4K-L5 Vac	RXV	I	X	X	X	X			X																							
RXV Vac Lepto 5	RXV	I							X																							
RXV Vac Vibrio-Lepto 5	RXV	I							X							X																
RXV 3K-L 5 Vac	RXV	I	X	X	X				X																							
Salmo Shield T	Grand	I																										X				
Salmonella dublin-typhimurium bacterin	Colorado Serum	I																										X				
ScourGuard 3 (K)/C	Pfizer Animal Health	I													X			X	X	X												
ScourGuard 3 (K)	Pfizer Animal Health	I																X	X	X												
Septimune PH/HS	Fort Dodge	I					X	X																								
Septimune PH-K	Fort Dodge	I					X	X																								
Siteguard MLG vaccine	Coopers	I							X																							
Somato-Staph/Lepto-5	Anchor	I							X																							X
Somato-Staph	Anchor	I																														X
Somnu Shield	Grand	I					X																									
Somnu Shield + 7 Way	Grand	I					X			X	X	X	X	X	X																
Somnu Shield XT	Grand	I					X																									
Somnubac	Pfizer Animal Health	I					X																									
SomnuMune	Lextron	I					X																									
SomnuMune	AgriLabs	I					X																									

Product	Manufacturer	Type													
SomnuTech	BioCor	I											X		
StayBred VL5	Pfizer Animal Health	I							X		X		X		
Strategy V4 vaccine	Schering-Plough	I	X	X	X				X						
Strategy V4L5 vaccine	Schering-Plough	I	X	X	X	X			X						
Strategy V4HSL5 vaccine	Schering-Plough	I	X	X	X	X	X		X						
Strategy V4HS vaccine	Schering-Plough	I	X	X	X	X	X								
Syn Shield	Grand	I					X								
Tandem 9 K	Sanofi	I	X	X	X	X			X						
Tandem 4 KL	Sanofi	MLV/I	X	X	X	X									
Tandem 3 KL	Sanofi	MLV/I	X	X	X										
Tandem 2	Sanofi	I	X	X											
Tandem 4KL IBR Plus	Sanofi	MLV/I	X	X	X	X									
Tandem SV+3 IBR Plus	Sanofi	MLV/I	X	X	X	X									
Tandem 3KL IBR Plus	Sanofi	MLV/I	X	X	X										
Tandem 3 K	Sanofi	I	X	X	X										
Tandem 8 K	Sanofi	I	X	X	X	X			X						
Tandem SV+3	Sanofi	MLV/I	X	X	X	X									
Tandem 1	Sanofi	I	X												
Tandem 1 SV	Sanofi	I	X	X	X										
Tandem SV	Sanofi	I	X		X										
Tandem 4 K	Sanofi	I	X	X	X	X									
Tetanus toxoid-concentrated	Colorado Serum	I								X					
Tetanus toxoid	Colorado Serum	I								X					
Tetnogen	Fort Dodge	I								X					
Thraxol-2	Bayer	MLV									X				
Triangle 3	Fort Dodge	I	X	X	X				X						
Triangle 8	Fort Dodge	I	X	X	X	X			X						
Triangle 3 VSL	Fort Dodge	I	X	X	X	X		X	X						
Triangle 9+HS	Fort Dodge	I	X	X	X	X	X		X						
Triangle 4+PH-K	Fort Dodge	I	X	X	X	X	X								
Triangle 4+HS	Fort Dodge	I	X	X	X	X									
Triangle 9+PH-K	Fort Dodge	I	X	X	X	X	X		X						
Triangle 1	Fort Dodge	I		X											
Triangle 4	Fort Dodge	I	X	X	X										
Triangle 9	Fort Dodge	I	X	X	X				X						
TrichGuard V5L	Fort Dodge	I							X				X	X	
TrichGuard	Fort Dodge	I												X	
Trichontrol	Pfizer Animal Health														X	
Trichontrol VL5	Pfizer Animal Health	I							X				X	X	
TriVib 5L	Fort Dodge	I							X					X	
TSV-2	Pfizer Animal Health	MLV	X	X											
Ultrabac 7	Pfizer Animal Health	I					X	X		X					

Table continued on following page

• Table 14-9 •
CATTLE VACCINES* (Continued)

VACCINES	MANUFACTURER	TYPE	IBR	PI3	BVD	BRSV	Haemophilus	Pasteurella	Leptospirosis	Clostridium chauvoei	Clostridium septicum	Clostridium novyi	Clostridium sordellii	Clostridium hemolyticum	Clostridium perfringens C and D	Campylobacter	Trichomonas	Escherichia coli	Coronavirus	Rotavirus	Moraxella	Tetanus	Anaplasmosis	Anthrax	Brucella	Rabies	Corynebacterium	Salmonella	Actinomyces	Fusobacterium	Papilloma	Staphylococcus
Ultrabac 7/Somnubac	Pfizer Animal Health	I					X			X	X	X	X		X																	
Ultrabac CD	Pfizer Animal Health	I										X			X																	
Ultrabac 8	Pfizer Animal Health	I								X	X	X	X	X	X																	
Unitox	EquiLabs	I																				X										
Vib Shield L5	Grand	I							X							X																
Vib Shield Plus	Grand	I														X																
Vib Shield	Grand	I														X																
Vib Shield Plus L5	Grand	I							X							X																
Vibo-5/Somnugen	Bio-Ceutic	I					X		X							X																
Vibo-5	Bio-Ceutic	I							X							X																
Vibralone-H-L5	Bayer	I							X					X		X																
Vibralone-L5	Bayer	I							X							X																
Vibri-Lep-5	Franklin	I							X							X																
Vibrin	Pfizer Animal Health	I														X																

340

Product	Manufacturer	Type									
Vibrio/Leptoferm-5	Pfizer Animal Health	I	X								X
Vibrio-Lepto 5	Durvet	I	X								X
Vibrio-Lepto 5	BioCor	I	X								X
Vibrio-Lepto 5	Lextron	I	X								X
Vibrio-Lepto 5	AgriLabs	I	X								X
Vibrio-Lepto-5/Somnus	Anchor	I	X		X						X
Vibrio-Lepto-5	Anchor	I	X								X
Vira Shield 5 + Somnus	Grand	I	X	X X X	X						
Vira Shield 2	Grand	I		X							
Vira Shield 5	Grand	I	X	X X X	X						
Vira Shield 2 + BRSV	Grand	I		X X	X						
Vira Shield 3	Grand	I	X	X							
Vira Shield 4	Grand	I	X X	X							
Vira Shield 4 + L5	Grand	I	X	X X	X						
Vision 7 Somnus with Spur	Bayer	I			X	X					
Vision 8 with Spur	Bayer	I			X X X	X X	X				
Vision 7 with Spur	Bayer	I			X X X	X	X				
Vision CD • I with Spur	Bayer	I						X	X		
Volar	Bayer	I								X	
Wart Shield	Grand	I									X
Wart vaccine	AgriLabs	I									X
Wart vaccine	Sanofi	I									X
Wart vaccine	Colorado Serum	I									X

IBR, infectious bovine rhinotracheitis; PI3, parainfluenza-3 virus; BVD, bovine virus diarrhea; BRSV, bovine respiratory syncytial virus. I, inactivated (killed); MLV, modified live virus (attenuated); MLV/I, combinations of modified live virus (attenuated) and inactivated.

*Compiled with the assistance of *Compendium of Veterinary Products*, Bayer Commemorative ed., Port Huron, MI, North American Compendiums, 1995.

Campylobacteriosis (Vibriosis) Vaccine. Campylobacteriosis is a venereal disease of cattle caused by the bacterium *Campylobacter fetus* subsp. *veneralis*. Infection of a cow's genital tract often causes early embryonic death resulting in temporary infertility, repeat breeding, delayed conception, and a prolonged calving interval. The *Campylobacter* organism may be transmitted during coitus or by artificial insemination with contaminated semen. Systemic vaccination can cure as well as prevent *Campylobacter* infection. Vaccination of breeding stock is highly recommended.

Trichomoniasis Vaccine. Trichomoniasis, caused by *Trichomonas foetus*, is a venereal protozoal disease of cattle that manifests as infertility, relatively early abortion, or pyometra. It causes virtually no systemic illness, so its presence within a herd may go undetected for long periods of time, resulting in substantial economic losses. The bull serves as an asymptomatic carrier, and the organism may be spread by natural breeding or artificial insemination with contaminated semen. Inactivated protozoal vaccines are now commercially available to aid in prevention of the disease.

Leptospirosis Vaccine. Leptospirosis is a common bacterial disease of cattle that may cause hemolytic anemia, nephritis, decreased milk production, and late-term abortion. Abortion is probably the most economically significant effect of the disease. Regular vaccination of breeding animals for leptospirosis is strongly encouraged. Heifers should be vaccinated two or three times at monthly intervals before breeding and again mid-gestation of the first pregnancy. Because leptospirosis bacterins produce immunity of fairly short duration, annual (prebreeding) or twice-annual (prebreeding and mid-gestation) boosters should be given.

Brucellosis Vaccine. Brucellosis is caused by the organism *Brucella abortus*. Infection in the cow can result in late-term abortion, usually around 5 months or more into gestation, and shedding of the *Brucella* organisms in the milk. In bulls, infection results in orchitis, impaired fertility, and shedding of *Brucella* organisms in the semen. Brucellosis is a serious human health hazard, and known *Brucella*-positive reactors must be culled from the herd and vaccination of replacement heifers performed. *Brucella abortus* strain 19 vaccine is a live bacterial product that confers long-term, cell-mediated protection. Vaccination of females only is accomplished using a strain 19 live culture vaccine. Age of vaccination of heifers is critical and usually determined by federal and state regulations. Vaccination is only undertaken by accredited veterinarians or state or federal animal health representatives. Care must always be exercised when using *B. abortus* vaccine, since accidental injection, ingestion, or exposure through broken skin or mucous membranes can result in human brucellosis (undulant fever).

Anthrax Vaccine. Anthrax is caused by the bacterium *Bacillus anthracis* and is characterized by septicemia and sudden death. Many times, affected animals are simply found dead without any prior signs of illness. Typically, the dead animal exhibits blood oozing from body orifices, failure of blood to clot, and absence of rigor mortis. Differential diagnosis of sudden death in cattle may include anthrax, lightning strike, clostridial diseases, and anaplasmosis. Vaccination for anthrax is recom-

mended 4 weeks prior to anticipated exposure in those areas where the disease has historically been a problem.

Clostridial Vaccines. Clostridial infections are caused by bacteria that live as spores in the soil. These spores may be ingested by cattle as they graze or may enter the body via wound contamination. The more common clostridial infections encountered in cattle are described briefly in the following paragraphs.

Infections with *Clostridium chauvoei* (the causative agent of blackleg), *Clostridium septicum* (the causative agent of malignant edema), and *Clostridium sordellii* primarily affect striated muscles. The spores of these organisms are deposited in muscles by the circulation after ingestion or via wound contamination. When conditions of reduced oxygen tension within these muscles exist (such as trauma during handling, transporting, butting, or riding), the spores vegetate and the resulting organisms multiply. Toxins released by the multiplying organisms rapidly destroy the muscles and cause death through destructive effects on vital organs. Death may occur suddenly, as early as 12 hours after onset of infection.

Infections with *Clostridium novyi* type B and *Clostridium haemolyticum* (also known as *Clostridium novyi* type D) primarily affect the liver. These spores are usually ingested and travel by the circulation to the liver, where they remain latent until some form of liver damage occurs that allows the spores to vegetate and the resulting organisms to multiply. Predisposing conditions that may activate the spores in the liver include liver flukes, migrating parasites, abscesses, bacterial hepatitis, fatty infiltration, and various hepatotoxins. Potent toxins produced by the multiplying bacteria are absorbed systematically and cause death through destructive effects on vital organs and blood vessels. Death may occur suddenly, as early as 24 hours after onset of infection.

Infections with *Clostridium perfringens* types B, C, and D affect primarily the gastrointestinal tract. These organisms are normal inhabitants of the gastrointestinal tract of cattle and tend to proliferate under conditions of reduced oxygen tension created by consumption of large quantities of concentrate feed or when sudden changes in feed occur. With favorable conditions, the organisms multiply rapidly and produce toxins that can cause several intestinal lesions leading to a hemorrhagic, necrotic enteritis and sudden death, particularly in young animals.

TECHNICIAN NOTE

Infections with *Clostridium perfringens* types B, C, and D affect primarily the gastrointestinal tract.

Clostridium tetani is the clostridial organism responsible for tetanus. *Clostridium tetani* is a soil inhabitant that commonly gains entry through contaminated wounds or through uterine infection after calving. Multiplying organisms produce a neurotoxin that affects the central nervous system (CNS). The neurotoxin causes tonoclonic spasms and muscle rigidity that, if untreated, can lead to prostration, convulsions, and death.

Because these clostridial infections commonly occur in

cattle, routine vaccination for clostridial infections is highly recommended.

Anaplasmosis Vaccine. Anaplasmosis in the United States is a common rickettsial disease of cattle and is caused by the intraerythrocytic parasite *Anaplasma marginale*. Affected red blood cells are destroyed by the liver and spleen, resulting in a severe anemia. Clinical signs due to an acute anemia may include pale mucous membranes, weakness, depression or aggressive behavior, and increased heart and respiratory rates. Anaplasmosis often causes sudden death and must be differentiated from anthrax and the clostridial diseases.

An anaplasmosis vaccine is currently available that helps to reduce severe clinical illness and death. One risk in using this vaccine in brood cows is neonatal isoerythrolysis. Neonatal isoerythrolysis is an anemic syndrome initiated by antibodies in the colostrum which, when absorbed, destroy the red blood cells of some newborn calves. When making a decision on whether to vaccinate brood cows for anaplasmosis, the protective benefits of the vaccination should be weighed against potential risks of neonatal isoerythrolysis.

Bovine Respiratory Disease Complex Vaccines. There are several viruses and bacteria that are widespread in the cattle population and are considered to be the major contributors to the bovine respiratory disease complex. Multiple infections may occur with these viruses, and secondary infections with these bacteria often exacerbate the primary diseases produced.

Parainfluenza-3 (PI-3) virus causes a mild respiratory disease that is often associated with shipment of cattle to the feedlot (and, thus, commonly referred to as "shipping fever"). Clinical signs may include fever, serous to mucopurulent nasal discharge, coughing, increased respiratory rate, weakness, depression, and weight loss.

TECHNICIAN NOTE

Parainfluenza-3 virus causes a mild respiratory disease in cattle often associated with shipment to a feedlot and is commonly called "shipping fever."

Infectious bovine rhinotracheitis (IBR) virus causes high fever, nasal discharge, conjunctivitis, increased respiratory rate, coughing, dyspnea, and severe hyperemia of the muzzle (commonly referred to as "red nose").

Bovine virus diarrhea (BVD) virus can cause respiratory disease and is often confused with or obscured by the other viruses of this complex. In addition to the respiratory disease, the virus may also cause a mild transient diarrhea and may be associated with abortions and birth of malformed or weak calves if the primary infection occurs during pregnancy. The chronic form of BVD, known as mucosal disease, often results in ulcerative lesions throughout the alimentary tract, causing persistent diarrhea and usually death. In general, attenuated (modified live virus) vaccines containing infectious bovine rhinotracheitis BVD should *not* be administered intramuscularly to pregnant cows or to calves being nursed by pregnant cows

since abortion may result. Intranasal attenuated infectious bovine rhinotracheitis vaccines *are* safe, however, for pregnant cows or calves being nursed by pregnant cows.

Bovine respiratory syncytial virus (BRSV) has been recognized in recent years as a major viral component of the bovine respiratory disease complex. Infection typically causes anorexia, coughing, increased respiratory rate, serous ocular and nasal discharge, fever, pulmonary edema and emphysema, and subcutaneous edema of the neck and throat. Death may occur rapidly, as early as 48 hours after onset of infection.

The bacteria *Pasteurella multocida* and *Pasteurella haemolytica* are normal inhabitants of the bovine respiratory tract and therefore are common secondary bacterial invaders in cases of primary viral pneumonia in cattle. In addition, these bacteria contribute to a primary fibrinous pneumonia and pleuritis that are readily apparent at necropsy. Clinical signs associated with these *Pasteurella* organisms may include fever, coughing, dyspnea, mucopurulent nasal discharge, depression, anorexia, and, in severe cases, death.

The bacterium *Haemophilus somnus* is another bacterial pathogen that can be a part of the bovine respiratory disease complex. It ranks second to *P. haemolytica* as the most frequent isolate from acute cases of fibrinopurulent pneumonia. *H. somnus* infection often develops as a septicemia, which can progress to fibrinous pleuritis, pericarditis, polyarthritis, or thromboembolic meningoencephalitis (also known as TEME or Sleeper's syndrome).

Many vaccines are currently available for these virus- and bacteria-induced bovine respiratory diseases. The vaccines contain these agents in various combinations and in the attenuated (modified live virus) or inactivated forms. Their routine use will depend on the needs of the herds and herdsman.

Enteric Disease Vaccine. Bovine rotavirus and coronavirus as well as enterotoxigenic bacterial strains of *Escherichia coli* are often isolated from calves with diarrhea. These organisms may occur in combination or with other bacterial, viral, or protozoal pathogens. The combination of enterotoxins produced by *E. coli* and the cytopathogenic effects of rotavirus and coronavirus induces secretion of large amounts of fluid and electrolytes into the lumen of the gut, resulting in diarrhea, dehydration, and, in severe cases, death. Vaccines are currently available for immunization of pregnant heifers or cows before calving. Some of these vaccines are also designed for oral administration to the newborn calf.

Moraxella Vaccine. *Moraxella bovis* is the principal cause of infectious bovine keratoconjunctivitis (IBK). Infection may result in characteristic clinical signs including epiphora, blepharospasm, photophobia, corneal ulcers, corneal edema, and chemosis. Healing may occur at any stage, but occasionally, with or without appropriate treatment, an affected cornea may perforate, resulting in loss of vision. Several inactivated vaccines are now available for protection against infection by *M. bovis*.

External and Internal Parasites

Control of external parasites, especially lice and grubs, may be achieved with repeated applications of approved insecticidal sprays or pour-on products or with the use of ivermectin. Many commercial products are currently available for effective treatment of lice and grubs. Always follow the manufacturer's labeled instructions completely and closely observe the slaughter and milk withdrawal times when using these products. Some products are not recommended for use in Brahmans, Brahman crosses, or exotic cattle breeds.

The most common internal parasites of beef and dairy cattle are the barber's pole worm (*Haemonchus* spp.), the brown stomach worm (*Ostertagia* spp.), the bankrupt worm (*Trichostrongylus* spp.), the hookworm (*Bunostomum* spp.), Cooper's worm (*Cooperia* spp.), the intestinal worm (*Nematodirus* spp.), the nodular worm (*Oesophagostomum* spp.), the lungworm (*Dictyocaulus* spp.), and the liver fluke (*Fasciola* spp.). In general, it is a good idea to deworm calves at least once before weaning and again at weaning. Cows, heifers, and bulls should be dewormed as needed. Many commercial dewormers are currently available. Product choice depends on the parasite(s) diagnosed by fecal examination within a herd and the resistance patterns of those parasites. Cattle raised in locales where liver flukes exist should be treated in the spring or fall or at both times with clorsulon (Curatrem, Merck AGVET; Ivomec-F, Merck AGVET) or albendazole (Valbazen, Pfizer Animal Health). Chapter 6 contains additional information on parasitology and specific drug therapy.

Several commercial implants are currently available for beef cattle that are designed to improve feed efficiency and increase feed savings. Most implants contain anabolic agents, such as estradiol, progesterone, testosterone, zeranol, or combinations of these agents. The type of implant and its scheduled use depend on the sex and age of calves implanted as well as the needs of the herdsman. Ruminant nutrition is discussed in Chapter 27.

Management Recommendations for Dairy Calves

The ultimate goal in raising replacement heifers is to produce a healthy heifer that will calve and enter the milking herd by 24 months of age (see Table 14–8). Probably the single most important factor in successful rearing of baby calves is to see that the calves ingest colostrum soon after birth. If the calf does not nurse on its own shortly after birth, the herdsman should administer at least 2 liters of warm colostrum to the calf within the first hour. During the first 3 days of life, continue to feed colostrum at 10% of the calf's body weight daily, split into two feedings (as an example, a 40-kg calf should receive 2 liters of colostrum twice daily).

After this time, the calf can be switched to whole milk or a good-quality commercial milk replacer administered at 10% of its body weight daily divided into two feedings. For the neonatal calf, it is important to use a milk replacer that contains 20% to 22% crude protein, all of which is milk-derived, and 18% to 20% crude fat. Fresh water should be provided at all times, and grain (18% to 20% protein) and hay should be offered free choice beginning at 7 to 14 days of age.

Calves should be housed in individual huts until weaned. Separating calves helps to control direct transmission of disease, prevents postfeeding sucking among calves, reduces stress of competition, and allows for assessment of individual feed intake and fecal consistency. Most dairy calves should be weaned by 50 to 60 days of age.

PREVENTIVE HEALTH PROGRAM FOR SWINE

An effective and economical preventive health program is an essential part of successful swine production.

TECHNICIAN NOTE

An effective and economical preventive health program is an essential part of successful swine production.

Preventive health programs should be individually designed by the consulting veterinarian and based on the specific needs of the swine herd and the producer. The preventive health programs should include immunization programs for disease prevention, well-proven methods of external and internal parasite control, recommendations for appropriate nutrition, and improvements in general management and sanitation procedures. A general approach to preventive health programs for swine herds and its implementation is presented in Table 14–10.

• Table 14–10 •

GENERAL OUTLINE OF A PREVENTIVE HEALTH PROGRAM FOR SWINE
Prebreeding Recommendations for Boars
Purchase boars 60 days before intended use. Quarantine the new boars for 30 days, then allow fence line contact with gilts and sows for 30 days before breeding. Immunize boars for leptospirosis and erysipelas. Treat for external and internal parasites before breeding.
Prebreeding Recommendations for Sows and Gilts
Immunize for leptospirosis, porcine parvovirus infection,* and pseudorabies* 2–4 weeks before breeding. Flush gilts by increasing feed (energy) intake before breeding to increase ovulations. Treat for external and internal parasites before breeding.
Prefarrowing Recommendations for Sows and Gilts
Limit feed intake to about 4 lb per head per day or feed according to condition to avoid overweight sows or gilts at farrowing. Immunize for colibacillosis,* atrophic rhinitis, erysipelas, transmissible gastroenteritis (TGE), porcine rotavirus infection,* and *Clostridium perfringens* type C* according to the manufacturer's labeled instructions. Treat for external and internal parasites before farrowing with approved products.
Farrowing Recommendations
Gradually increase feed intake so lactating swine are receiving full feed at peak milk production. (Rule of thumb: Feed daily 1 lb of feed for every pig being nursed [e.g., a lactating sow with a litter of 12 pigs should receive at least 12 lb of feed daily].)
General Recommendations for Pigs
At birth
Perform newborn pig procedures (e.g., clip needle teeth, dock tails, castrate, ear-notch, and inject iron dextran).
One Week of Age
Immunize for TGE,* rotavirus,* and for atrophic rhinitis.
Four–Five Weeks of Age
Weaning occurs at this time. Immunize for atrophic rhinitis, erysipelas, and *Actinobacillus* infection.*
Six–Eight Weeks of Age
Treat for external and internal parasites with approved products.
Older Than Eight Weeks of Age
Repeated treatments for external and internal parasites with approved products may need to be done during the growing-finishing period.

*Dependent on problems in the individual swine herd.

Vaccinations

Vaccines that may be incorporated in preventive health programs for swine herds can be obtained from manufacturers as individual components or in various combinations. A listing of some vaccines currently available is presented in Table 14–11. Diseases for which vaccines are commonly used in preventive health programs are described below.

Leptospirosis Vaccine. Leptospirosis is an important bacterial disease that affects domestic animals as well as humans and wildlife. Leptospirosis in swine is characterized by poor production, anemia, kidney disease, and abortions. Abortions are especially common after infection during late pregnancy. Routine vaccination of the breeding swine (such as gilts, sows, and boars) 2 to 4 weeks before breeding has proved to be effective in its prevention. Since immunity is short-lived, semiannual revaccination is generally recommended.

Porcine Parvovirus Vaccine. Porcine parvovirus (PPV) is believed to be the most common cause of infectious reproductive failure in swine. Infection of pregnant sows and gilts can result in stillbirths, mummified fetuses, embryonic death, and infertility (formerly referred to as SMEDI). Prebreeding vaccination is recommended in swine herds experiencing PPV infections.

Transmissible Gastroenteritis Vaccine. Transmissible gastroenteritis (TGE) is a common viral disease of swine. TGE affects swine of all ages but is most devastating to pigs younger than 10 days of age. Clinical signs in very young pigs may include anorexia, vomiting, profuse watery diarrhea, and dehydration, which often progress to death. Older swine can exhibit similar but milder symptoms, and death is rare.

Vaccination of prefarrowing sows and gilts may be necessary for herds in which TGE has been diagnosed as a cause of neonatal diarrhea. In addition, vaccination of pigs within the first week of life may assist in the prevention of postweaning scours.

Porcine Rotavirus Vaccine. Porcine rotavirus infection causes a gastroenteritis that may be characterized by vomiting, watery diarrhea, dehydration, and death in young pigs. It is generally difficult to differentiate porcine rotavirus infection from TGE. Porcine rotavirus infection commonly occurs in both nursing and weaned pigs, and many swine herds have serological evidence of its presence. Vaccination of prefarrowing sows and gilts, nursing pigs, and pigs 7 to 10 days before weaning is recommended for the prevention of post-weaning scours in herds where porcine rotavirus infection has been diagnosed as a cause of enteric disease in young pigs.

***Clostridium perfringens* Type C Vaccine.** The bacterium *C. perfringens* type C can cause enteric disease in young pigs. In peracute infection, there is a rapid onset of bloody diarrhea and death within the first 2 days of life. Acutely infected young pigs usually develop a red-brown liquid feces and die within 2 days after onset of enteric disease. The subacute infection may result in persistent diarrhea, emaciation, and death after 5 to 7 days of age. In chronic infections, a gray mucoid diarrhea occurs that lasts for about 7 days. Some of these patients will die, while others survive and typically become chronic poor doers.

Vaccination of prefarrowing sows and gilts effectively assists in the control of *C. perfringens* type C infections in nursing pigs.

Neonatal Porcine Colibacillosis Vaccine. Neonatal porcine colibacillosis is caused by bacterial enterotoxigenic strains of *Escherichia coli*. The results are diarrhea, dehydration, and, in severe cases, death. Vaccination of healthy, pregnant sows and gilts provides good protection against neonatal colibacillosis in their nursing pigs.

***Bordetella, Pasteurella, Actinobacillus,* and *Mycoplasma* Vaccines.** *Bordetella bronchiseptica* is considered to be the major cause of atrophic rhinitis in swine. In young pigs, atrophic rhinitis is characterized by acute rhinitis that results in destruction of the nasal turbinates. Destruction of the turbinates leads to impaired filtering of air in the nasal passages, decreased rate of weight gain, and increased incidence of respiratory infections, including pneumonia. Vaccination of pregnant swine and nursing pigs can often reduce the incidence of clinical atrophic rhinitis. *Pasteurella multocida* is a common bacterial pathogen of the respiratory tract of swine. In combined infections, *P. multocida* and *B. bronchiseptica* can cause a more severe form of atrophic rhinitis than in cases where either agent occurs alone. Several inactivated vaccines containing *P. multocida* are currently available.

Actinobacillus pleuropneumoniae, the most common causative respiratory agent of swine, causes a severe and often fatal disease affecting swine of all ages. Manifestations of the disease are fibrinopurulent bronchopneumonia and fibrinous pleuritis. Acute *Actinobacillus* infections can cause death within 12 hours after the onset of clinical signs (such as coughing, cyanosis, and blood-tinged nasal discharge). However, some individuals may die suddenly without development of clinical signs. Chronic infections are usually subclinical and are characterized by decreased performance and an extended finishing period.

Mycoplasma hyopneumoniae is the most common cause of chronic pneumonia in swine. The disease is not usually evident until pigs are 3 to 6 months old. It is characterized by a chronic, nonproductive cough, often induced by exercise. The greatest economic loss from the disease is decreased growth rate; for every 10% of lung affected by pneumonia, average daily gain is reduced by 5.3%. Morbidity is variable and mortality is low in uncomplicated cases. Secondary bacterial infections may exacerbate clinical signs.

Porcine Reproductive and Respiratory Syndrome Vaccine. Porcine reproductive and respiratory syndrome (PRRS) is also known as swine infertility and respiratory syndrome (SIRS), mystery swine disease, and blue ear disease. It is a recently recognized viral disease of swine which causes respiratory problems in all ages of pigs as well as reproductive problems in breeding swine. Clinical signs include transient, mild anorexia; lethargy; and fever in grower-finisher pigs and breeding animals. Cyanosis of the ears (blue ear disease), vulva, tail, abdomen, or snout is occasionally reported. Viral infection of breeding gilts or sows may result in premature farrowings with small, weak, or stillborn piglets and an increased incidence of fetal mummies. Respiratory distress, ("thumping") and open-mouth breathing in suckling and weanling pigs may occur. The virus tends to increase the incidence of secondary respiratory infections in young pigs. Chronic infection in nursery and grower-

Text continued on page 351

• Table 14–11 •

			\vbox{\hbox{SWINE VACCINES*}}	

VACCINES	MANUFACTURER	TYPE	Bordetella	Pasteurella	Haemophilus/Actinobacillus	Mycoplasma	Erysipelas	Clostridium	Escherichia coli	Rotavirus	TGE	Leptospirosis	Parvovirus	Pseudorabies	Salmonella	Streptococcus	EMC	Anthrax	Influenza	PRRS	Tetanus
Anthrax spore vaccine	Colorado Serum	MLV																X			
AR-M-Pac	Schering-Plough	I	X	X		X															
AR-P+D	Schering-Plough	I	X	X																	
AR-Pac-P	Schering-Plough	I	X	X																	
AR-Pac-P+D	Schering-Plough	I	X	X																	
AR-Pac-P+ER	Schering-Plough	I	X	X			X														
AR-Pac-PD+ER	Schering-Plough	I	X	X			X														
AR-Parapac	Schering-Plough	I	X	X	X		X														
Atrobac 3	Pfizer Animal Health	I	X	X			X														
Borde Shield 4	Grand	I	X	X			X														
Borde-Cell	AgriLabs	I	X																		
Bordegen P/D vaccine	Schering-Plough	I	X	X																	
Bordetella bronchiseptica intranasal vaccine	MVP	MLV	X																		
Borditech P.E.	BioCor	I	X	X			X														
BratiVac	Pfizer Animal Health	I										X									
BratiVac-6	Pfizer Animal Health	I										X									
Breed Sow 6	AgriLabs	I										X	X								
Breed Sow 7	AgriLabs	I					X					X	X								
C & D toxoid	Anchor	I						X													
C & D toxoid	AgriLabs	I						X													
Clostri Shield C	Grand	I						X													
Clostridium perfringens type C and D toxoid	Colorado Serum	I						X													
Clostridium Bac with Imugen II	Oxford	I						X													
Clostridium perfringens types C and D tetanus toxoid	Colorado Serum	I						X													X
Colimix	Central Biologics	I							X												
Colipig	Sanofi	I							X												
Durvac RP1+D	Durvet	I	X	X																	
Durvac RPE+D	Durvet	I	X	X			X														
Durvac APB	Durvet	I			X																
Durvac HP-APB+ER	Durvet	I			X		X														
Durvac AR-PP	Durvet	I	X	X	X		X														
Durvac TGE-Rota-C	Durvet	MLV/I							X	X	X	X									
Durvac P-Strep	Durvet	I			X											X					
Durvac RP2+D	Durvet	I	X	X			X		X												
Durvac Myco	Durvet	I				X															
Durvac Parvo-Lepto 5	Durvet	I										X	X								
Durvac *S. suis*	Durvet	I														X					
Durvac *Salmonella*	Durvet	I													X						
E-Bac	Oxford	I					X														
EMC Vac	Oxford	I															X				

• Table 14–11 •

SWINE VACCINES* (Continued)																					
											VACCINE COMPONENTS										
VACCINES	MANUFACTURER	TYPE	*Bordetella*	*Pasteurella*	*Haemophilus/Actinobacillus*	*Mycoplasma*	*Erysipelas*	*Clostridium*	*Escherichia coli*	*Rotavirus*	TGE	*Leptospirosis*	*Parvovirus*	*Pseudorabies*	*Salmonella*	*Streptococcus*	EMC	*Anthrax*	*Influenza*	PRRS	*Tetanus*
Emulsibac* H.P.	MVP	I			X																	
Emulsibac-SS	MVP	I														X						
ENDOVAC-Porci	Immvac	I													X							
Equisimilis Shield	Grand	I														X						
ER Bac	Pfizer Animal Health	I					X															
ER Bac/Leptoferm	Pfizer Animal Health	I					X					X										
Ery Shield	Grand	I					X															
Erycell	Grand	MLV					X															
Ery-Mune C	Anchor	I					X															
Erysipelas	AgriLabs	I					X															
Erysipelas	Lextron	I					X															
Erysipelas	Durvet	I					X															
Erysipelas	BioCor	I					X															
Erysipelothrix rhusiopathiae bacterin	Colorado Serum	I					X															
Erysipelothrix rhusiopathiae bacterin	Sanofi	I					X															
Erysipelothrix rhusiopathiae–Haemophilus parasuis bacterin	Nobl	I			X		X															
EVA	Pfizer Animal Health	MLV					X															
FarrowSure PRV	Pfizer Animal Health	MLV/I					X					X	X	X								
FarrowSure B	Pfizer Animal Health	I					X					X	X									
FarrowSure B-PRV	Pfizer Animal Health	MLV/I					X					X	X	X								
FarrowSure	Pfizer Animal Health	I					X					X	X									
Feeder Pig Bac 5	Oxford	I			X		X									X						
Feeder Pig Bac 4	Oxford	I			X		X															
Fermicon C-D	Bio-Ceutic	I						X														
Genesis B-P + D	AgriLabs	I	X	X																		
Haemo Shield P	Grand	I		X	X																	
IntestiMune 4	Lextron	MLV/I						X	X	X	X											
IntestiMune TGE Rota	Lextron	MLV								X	X											
IntestiMune EC	Lextron	I						X	X													
Lepto Shield 5	Grand	I										X										
Lepto 5	AgriLabs	I										X										
Lepto 5	Lextron	I										X										
Lepto 5	Durvet	I										X										
Lepto 5	BioCor	I										X										
Leptoferm-5	Pfizer Animal Health	I										X										
Lepto-Parvo	Nobl	I										X	X									
Leptospira pomona bacterin	Sanofi	I										X										
LitterGuard LT	Pfizer Animal Health	I							X													
LitterGuard LT-C	Pfizer Animal Health	I						X	X													
LitterGuard	Pfizer Animal Health	I							X													

Table continued on following page

• Table 14–11 •

SWINE VACCINES* (Continued)

VACCINES	MANUFACTURER	TYPE	Bordetella	Pasteurella	Haemophilus/Actinobacillus	Mycoplasma	Erysipelas	Clostridium	Escherichia coli	Rotavirus	TGE	Leptospirosis	Parvovirus	Pseudorabies	Salmonella	Streptococcus	EMC	Anthrax	Influenza	PRRS	Tetanus
Maxi/Guard Nasal Vac	Addison	MLV	X																		
MaxiVac-Flu	Syntro Vet	I																	X		
MaxiVac-M	Syntro Vet	I				X															
M-Pac	Schering-Plough	I				X															
Myco Silencer	Oxford	I				X															
Mycoplasma hypopneumoniae bacterin	Nobl	I				X															
Nitro-Sal	Arko	MLV													X						
Optivac-GI	Nobl	MLV											X								
Oravac-Ery	Nobl	MLV					X														
Para Shield	Grand	I				X															
Parapleuro Shield P	Grand	I		X	X																
Parapleuro Shield P + BE	Grand	I	X	X	X		X														
Parvo Shield	Grand	I											X								
Parvo Shield L5	Grand	I										X	X								
Parvi Shield L5E	Grand	I					X					X	X								
Parvo-Lepto Vac	Oxford	I										X	X								
Parvoplex-6 Way	Lextron	I										X	X								
Parvotech Lepto 5	BioCor	I										X	X								
Parvo-Vac/Leptoferm-5	Pfizer Animal Health	I										X	X								
Pilimune	Oxford	I							X												
Pleuro Ban Plus	A.A.H.	I			X																
Pleuro Ban-E	A.A.H.	I			X		X														
PleuroGuard 4	Pfizer Animal Health	I	X	X	X		X														
Pleuromune with Imugen II	Oxford	I			X	X															
Pleuromune-S with Imugen II	Oxford	I			X											X					
Pneu Pac-ER	Schering-Plough	I				X	X														
Pneu Pac	Schering-Plough	I				X															
Pneumosuis III	Pfizer Animal Health	I				X															
Porcimune B vaccine	Schering-Plough	I	X						X												
Porcimune vaccine	Schering-Plough	I							X												
Porcine Pili Shield	Grand	I							X												
Postwean Scour Bac	Grand	I							X												
ProSystem 4*3	Ambico	I						X	X												
ProSystem 3	Ambico	I							X												
ProSystem B*P*M	Ambico	I	X	X		X															
ProSystem 1	Ambico	MLV									X										
ProSystem 2C	Ambico	MLV								X											
ProSystem 2*1	Ambico	MLV								X	X										
ProSystem 2	Ambico	MLV								X											
ProSystem A	Ambico	I			X																
ProSystem 2*1*4*3/B*P*E	Ambico	MLV/I	X	X			X	X	X	X	X										
ProSystem B*P	Ambico	I	X	X																	
ProSystem 2*1*3	Ambico	MLV/I							X	X	X										

• Table 14–11 •

SWINE VACCINES* (Continued)

VACCINES	MANUFACTURER	TYPE	Bordetella	Pasteurella	Haemophilus/Actinobacillus	Mycoplasma	Erysipelas	Clostridium	Escherichia coli	Rotavirus	TGE	Leptospirosis	Parvovirus	Pseudorabies	Salmonella	Streptococcus	EMC	Anthrax	Influenza	PRRS	Tetanus
ProSystem B*P*E/4*3	Ambico	I	X	X			X	X	X												
ProSystem 2*3	Ambico	MLV/I							X	X											
ProSystem 2*4*3	Ambico	MLV/I						X	X	X											
ProSystem B*P*E	Ambico	I	X	X			X														
ProSystem 2*1*4*3	Ambico	MLV/I						X	X	X	X										
PRV/Marker	SyntroVet	MLV												X							
PRV/Marker-KV	SyntroVet	I												X							
PRV/Marker Gold-XL	SyntroVet	MLV												X							
PRV/Marker-KV	SyntroVet	I												X							
PRV/Marker Gold	SyntroVet	MLV												X							
PRV/Marker Gold	Schering-Plough	MLV												X							
PRV/Marker Gold-MaxiVac Flu	Syntro Vet	MLV/I												X					X		
PR-Vac Plus	Pfizer Animal Health	MLV												X							
PR-Vac-Killed	Pfizer Animal Health	I												X							
PR-Vac	Pfizer Animal Health	MLV												X							
RespiSure	Pfizer Animal Health	I				X															
Respogen	Oxford	I				X															
RespPRRS	Nobl	I																		X	
Rhi-Co-Pig D	Sanofi	I	X	X					X												
Rhinicell	Grand	MLV	X																		
Rhinicell + E	Grand	MLV	X				X														
Rhinipig-D	Sanofi	I	X	X																	
RhiniTech-P.E.	Lextron	I	X	X			X														
RhiniTech-P.E.	AgriLabs	I	X	X			X														
Rhinobac 3	Pfizer Animal Health	I	X	X			X														
Rhinogen CTSE	Oxford	I	X	X			X									X					
Rhinogen CT 5000	Oxford	I	X	X																	
Rhinogen PE	Oxford	I	X	X			X														
Rhinogen CTE 5000	Oxford	I	X	X			X														
Rhusigen Vaccine	Schering-Plough	I					X														
RM Porcine Myco Hyo	Rhone Merieux	I				X															
Rotamune with Imugen II	Oxford	I								X											
Rota-Vac TGE	Pfizer Animal Health	MLV								X	X										
RXV Vac Parvomune Lepto 5	RXV	I										X	X								
RXV Vac Erysipelas	RXV	I					X														
RXV Vac RhiniTech-P.E.	RXV	I	X	X			X														
RXV Vac Lepto 5	RXV	I										X									
RXV Vac Streptomune	RXV	I														X					
Salmo Shield C	Grand	I																			
Salmo Shield 2	Grand	I													X						
Salmo-Bac	AgriLabs	I													X						
Salmonella Bac with Imugen II	Oxford	I													X						
Salmonella bacterin	Pfizer Animal Health	I													X						

Table continued on following page

• Table 14–11 •

SWINE VACCINES* (Continued)																					
													VACCINE COMPONENTS								
VACCINES	MANUFACTURER	TYPE	Bordetella	Pasteurella	Haemophilus/Actinobacillus	Mycoplasma	Erysipelas	Clostridium	Escherichia coli	Rotavirus	TGE	Leptospirosis	Parvovirus	Pseudorabies	Salmonella	Streptococcus	EMC	Anthrax	Influenza	PRRS	Tetanus
SC-54	Nobl	MLV													X						
Score	Oxford	I	X	X			X														
Scourmune	Schering-Plough	I							X												
Scourmune-C	Schering-Plough	I						X	X												
Scourmune-CR	Schering-Plough	I						X	X	X											
Scourmune-CRT	Schering-Plough	MLV/I						X	X	X	X										
ScourShield	Pfizer Animal Health	MLV/I						X	X	X	X										
Sow Bac-E	Oxford	I	X	X			X		X												
Strep Shield	Grand	I														X					
Strep Bac with Imugen II	Oxford	I														X					
Suis-Bac	AgriLabs	I														X					
Suvaxyn HerdFend Thrix	Fort Dodge Laboratories	I					X														
Suvaxyn MaternaFend 7	Fort Dodge Laboratories	I	X	X			X		X												
Suvaxyn GestaFend 5+B	Fort Dodge Laboratories	I										X									
Suvaxyn RespiFend APP	Fort Dodge Laboratories	I			X																
Suvaxyn GestaFend 1	Fort Dodge Laboratories	I											X								
Suvaxyn GestaFend 5	Fort Dodge Laboratories	I										X									
Suvaxyn MaternaFend 4	Fort Dodge Laboratories	I							X												
Suvaxyn GestaFend 7+B	Fort Dodge Laboratories	I					X					X	X								
Suvaxyn RespiFend MH	Fort Dodge Laboratories	I				X															
Suvaxyn GestaFend 7	Fort Dodge Laboratories	I					X					X	X								
Suvaxyn RespiFend 3DT	Fort Dodge Laboratories	I	X	X			X														
Suvaxyn RespiFend 2DT	Fort Dodge Laboratories	I	X	X																	
Suvaxyn HerdFend PrV gpl-	Fort Dodge Laboratories	I												X							
Suvaxyn GestaFend 6	Fort Dodge Laboratories	I										X	X								
Suvaxyn GestaFend 8+B	Fort Dodge Laboratories	MLV/I					X					X	X	X							
Swine Master H/P	AgriLabs	I				X															
Swine Master A.P.E.	AgriLabs	I				X	X														
Swine Tech/PR-CP-EC	Premier Farmtech	I						X	X	X											
Swine Master 8	AgriLabs	MLV/I	X	X			X	X	X	X	X										
Swine Tech/BB-ER-PM-PS	Premier Farmtech	I	X	X	X		X														
Swine Tech MM-ER-PM	Premier Farmtech	I	X	X			X														
Swine Master B-P-E+D/C-E	AgriLabs	I	X	X			X	X	X												
Swine Tech/CP-EC	Premier Farmtech	I						X	X												
Swine Tech/AP-PS+ER	Premier Farmtech	I			X		X														
Swine Tech/PS	Premier Farmtech	I			X																
Swine Master F.P.	AgriLabs	I	X	X	X		X														
Swine Master B-P-E+D	AgriLabs	I	X	X			X														
Swine Tech/BB-PM+D	Premier Farmtech	I	X	X																	
Swine Tech/AP	Premier Farmtech	I			X																
Swine Tech/AP-ER	Premier Farmtech	I			X		X														
Swine Master H.P.+P.	AgriLabs	I		X	X																
Swine Master B-P+D/M	AgriLabs	I	X	X		X															

• Table 14–11 •

SWINE VACCINES* (Continued)

VACCINES	MANUFACTURER	TYPE	Bordetella	Pasteurella	Haemophilus/Actinobacillus	Mycoplasma	Erysipelas	Clostridium	Escherichia coli	Rotavirus	TGE	Leptospirosis	Parvovirus	Pseudorabies	Salmonella	Streptococcus	EMC	Anthrax	Influenza	PRRS	Tetanus
Swine Tech/Strep S	Premier Farmtech	I														X					
Swine Master-R.T.C.E.	AgriLabs	MLV/I						X	X	X	X										
Swine Master-T	AgriLabs	MLV									X										
Swine Master-R.T.	AgriLabs	MLV								X	X										
Swine Tech/BB-ER-PM-EC	Premier Farmtech	I	X	X			X		X												
Swine Master-R.	AgriLabs	MLV									X										
Swine Tech/PR-TGE-CP-EC	Premier Farmtech	MLV/I						X	X	X	X										
Swine Tech/*Salmonella* C + T	Premier Farmtech	I													X						
Swine Tech BB-ER-PM + D	Premier Farmtech	I	X	X			X														
Tetanus toxoid	Fort Dodge Laboratories	I																			X
Tetanus toxoid	Colorado Serum	I																			X
Tetanus toxoid–concentrated	Colorado Serum	I																			X
Tetanus toxoid	Franklin	I																			X
Tetnogen	Fort Dodge Laboratories	I																			X
TGE Shield	Grand	I																			
TGE vaccine	Pfizer Animal Health	MLV									X										
TGE Cell	Grand	MLV									X										
TG-Emune Rota with Imugen II	Oxford	MLV								X	X										
TG-Emune with Imugen II	Oxford	I									X										
TGE-Vac C	Bayer	MLV						X			X										
Thraxol-2	Bayer	MLV																X			
Tolvid II	Oxford	MLV												X							
Toxivac EC	Nobl	I	X	X			X	X	X												
Toxivac AD	Nobl	I	X	X																	
Toxivac AD + E	Nobl	I	X	X			X														
Toxivac + Parasuis	Nobl	I	X	X	X		X														
Turbinator BPAD	Lextron	I	X	X																	
Turbinator 3 + D	Lextron	I	X	X			X														
Unitox	EquiLabs	I																			X
WeanVac 3	Pfizer Animal Health	I	X		X		X														

*Compiled with the assistance of *Compendium of Veterinary Products*. Bayer Commemorative ed., Port Huron, MI, North American Compendiums, 1995.

†TGE, transmissable gastroenteritis; EMC, encephalomyocarditis virus; PRRS, porcine reproductive and respiratory syndrome; ‡I, inactivated (killed); MLV, modified live virus (attenuated); MLV/I, combination of modified live virus (attenuated) and inactivated.

finisher pigs may result in decreased growth rate and feed efficiency and increased morbidity and mortality due to secondary infections. A vaccine for PRRS has recently been approved.

Erysipelas Vaccine. Erysipelas is caused by the bacterium *Erysipelothrix rhusiopathiae*, and can occur as acute septicemia, skin discoloration (commonly known as "diamond skin

disease"), chronic arthritis, and vegetative endocarditis. Erysipelas is extremely common among swine herds, and therefore routine vaccination of gilts and sows before farrowing and of pigs at weaning is highly recommended.

Pseudorabies Vaccine. Pseudorabies is a viral disease of swine that is characterized by fever, vomiting, encephalitis, and sudden death in nursing pigs, and abortion, stillbirths, or mummies in pregnant swine. Vaccines are currently available, but their use is limited by state regulations.

Streptococcus Vaccine. *Streptococcus suis* is a primary cause of meningitis and septicemia in postweaning pigs. It has also been associated with pneumonia and arthritis in pigs, and abortion and infertility in sows and gilts. Peracute cases may die suddenly, while less severe cases exhibit CNS signs often followed by death. *Streptococcus suis* can pose a significant human health hazard. Available vaccines may help to reduce the losses caused by *S. suis*.

Encephalomyocarditis Vaccine. Encephalomyocarditis (EMC) virus primarily infects the heart and brain of swine. Mortality can be up to 100% among pigs less than 1 week old. Although mortality from EMC declines as pigs mature, older pigs do become clinically ill. Not all weaned pigs with EMC infections show clinical illness and a normal-appearing pig may die suddenly, especially if excited or forced to exercise. A very small lesion in the cardiac conduction system can result in death. There is a vaccine available which markedly reduces gross and microscopic lesions caused by EMC virus in weaned pigs. Vaccination is recommended in herds experiencing problems with EMC virus.

External and Internal Parasites

Control of external parasites, especially lice (*Haemophilus suis*) and mange mites (*Sarcoptes scabiei* var. *suis*), may be done with repeated applications of approved insecticidal sprays or pour-on products or with the use of ivermectin. Treatment of external parasites should be done at the same time as treatment for internal parasites; however, always read the manufacturer's labeled instructions, since some types of sprays and pour-on products cannot be used concomitantly with dewormers or may not be used safely in pregnant or young nursing swine.

The most common internal parasites of swine are the roundworm (*Ascaris suum*), the whipworm (*Trichuris suis*), the threadworm (*Strongyloides* spp.), the nodular worm (*Oesophagostomum* spp.), the lungworm (*Metastrongylus* spp.), the red stomach worm (*Hyostrongylus rubidus*), and the kidney worm (*Stephanurus dentatus*). Many commercial dewormers are currently available. Product choice should depend on the parasites diagnosed by fecal examinations within a herd, convenience of administration, and cost-effectiveness. In general, it is a good idea to deworm adults before breeding, sows and gilts before farrowing, and pigs once or twice after weaning and once during the growing-finishing period. Chapter 6 contains additional information on parasitology and specific drug therapy.

PREVENTIVE HEALTH PROGRAM FOR SMALL RUMINANTS

In North America, sheep and goats are managed under a wide variety of conditions, including extensive range operations, semiconfinement, total confinement, and hobby farm systems, and as backyard pets. Meat-producing goats have gained popularity in recent years. One primary task of the small ruminant veterinarian and veterinary technician is to educate the producer about the value of careful observation, animal identification, and record-keeping for improvement of herd and flock health and productivity. With adequate information, the veterinarian and veterinary technician can then make sound recommendations concerning nutrition, vaccination, parasite control, and management geared to the needs of a particular herd or flock.

Vaccinations

The number of vaccines licensed for use in small ruminants is limited. The veterinarian's first choice should be a licensed vaccine used in accordance with label instructions; however, products licensed for use in other species (particularly in cattle) frequently are considered to be effective in sheep and goats. Use of vaccines depends upon the disease incidence within a given herd or flock, but vaccination for enterotoxemia and tetanus should be included in every herd and flock health program (Table 14–12).

Enterotoxemia Vaccine. Toxins produced by *Clostridium perfringens* types C and D may cause enterotoxemia in young sheep and goats. The organism is present in the gastrointestinal tract of healthy animals but may overgrow and produce potent toxins in the presence of rich ingesta and bowel stasis. Enterotoxemia is most likely to occur in young animals nursing from dams that are heavy milk producers or in animals receiving heavy grain rations as in feedlot situations. It is for this reason that the disease is called "overeating" disease. Enterotoxemia is easily prevented by vaccination of the dams before lambing and kidding and vaccination of lambs and kids several times at 2- to 4-week intervals beginning at 6 to 8 weeks of age. Vaccination for enterotoxemia is effective and should be a part of all herd health programs.

Tetanus Vaccine. Tetanus is caused by a toxin produced by the anaerobic organism *Clostridium tetani*, a bacterium that may be carried into wounds or surgery sites. Clinical signs may include muscular stiffness ("sawhorse" stance), difficulty in swallowing ("lockjaw"), prolapse of the third eyelids, labored breathing, and exaggerated response to external stimuli. Since small ruminants are particularly susceptible to infection, vaccination for tetanus at the time of vaccination for enterotoxemia is vital (combination products are available). In addition, booster vaccination is recommended any time an animal is wounded or has undergone any surgical procedure (such as dehorning, castration, or tail docking).

Contagious Ecthyma Vaccine. Contagious ecthyma (soremouth, orf) is a viral infection of goats. Kids are primarily affected but may spread the disease to the udder of the doe. Clinical signs include papules, vesicles, pustules, and scabs on the lips, muzzle, eyelids, oral cavity, udder, teats, and feet. Affected kids usually exhibit a decrease in feed consumption, and some kids become depressed, anorectic, and febrile. Contagious ecthyma is transmissible to humans, and so it is advisable to wear gloves when handling infected animals. Effective live virus vaccines are available but are not recommended for closed herds that are not experiencing contagious ecthyma. Proper precautions, such as wearing gloves during vaccine administration and disposal of contagious ecthyma vaccine containers, are necessary to prevent risks to human health.

Foot Rot Vaccine. *Bacteroides nodosus* is the primary causative agent of foot rot in sheep. It is a highly contagious disease

• Table 14–12 •

VACCINES	MANUFACTURER	TYPE	Anthrax	Clostridium chauvoei	Clostridium septicum	Clostridium novyi	Clostridium sordellii	Clostridium haemolyticum	Clostridium perfringens C and D	Escherichia coli	Pasteurella	Tetanus	Bacteroides nodosus	Fusobacterium	Bluetongue	Campylobacter	Chlamydia	Ecthyma	Epididymitis	Rabies	Corynebacterium	Salmonella
Anthrax spore vaccine	Colorado Serum	MLV	X																			
	Anchor	I																				
Bar-Vac-CD/T	Anchor	I							X			X										
Bluetongue Vaccine	Colorado Serum	MLV													X							
C & D toxoid	Anchor	I							X													
C & D toxoid	AgriLabs	I							X													
Campylobacter fetus bacterin	Colorado Serum	I														X						
Campylobacter fetus-Chlamydia psittaci-Escherichia coli bacterin	Grand	I								X						X	X					
Case-Bac	Colorado Serum	I																			X	
Caseous D-T	Colorado Serum	I							X			X									X	
Chlamydia psittaci bacterin	Colorado Serum	I															X					
Clostri Shield C	Grand	I							X													
Clostri Shield 8	Grand	I		X	X	X	X	X	X													
Clostri Shield 7	Grand	I		X	X	X	X		X													
Clostridial 7-Way	AgriLabs	I		X	X	X	X		X													
Clostridial 8-Way	AgriLabs	I		X	X	X	X	X	X													
Clostridial 4-Way	Lextron	I		X	X	X	X															
Clostridial 7-Way	Lextron	I		X	X	X	X		X													
Clostridial 7-Way	ProLabs	I		X	X	X	X		X													
Clostridial 8-Way	ProLabs	I		X	X	X	X	X	X													
Clostridium perfringens types C and D toxoid	Colorado Serum	I							X													
Clostridium perfringens types C and D–tetanus toxoid	Colorado Serum	I							X		X											
Clostridium chauvoei-septicum-novyi-sordellii bacterin toxoid	Colorado Serum	I		X	X	X	X															
Clostridium chauvoei-septicum–Pasteurella haemolytica-multocida bacterin	Colorado Serum	I		X	X						X											
Clostridium chauvoei-septicum bacterin	Colorado Serum	I		X	X																	
Covexin 8 vaccine	Coopers	I		X	X	X	X	X	X			X										
Defensor	Pfizer Animal Health	I																		X		
Electroid 7 vaccine	Coopers	I		X	X	X	X		X													
Enzabort Eae-Vibrio	Colorado Serum	I														X	X					
Fermicon C-D	Bio-Ceutic	I							X													
Fermicon CD/T	Bio-Ceutic	I							X			X										
Footvax vaccine	Coopers	I											X									
Ovine ecthyma vaccine	Colorado Serum	MLV																X				

Table continued on following page

• Table 14–12 •

OVINE VACCINES* (Continued)

VACCINES	MANUFACTURER	TYPE	Anthrax	Clostridium chauvoei	Clostridium septicum	Clostridium novyi	Clostridium sordellii	Clostridium haemolyticum	Clostridium perfringens C and D	Escherichia coli	Pasteurella	Tetanus	Bacteroides nodosus	Fusobacterium	Bluetongue	Campylobacter	Chlamydia	Ecthyma	Epididymitis	Rabies	Corynebacterium	Salmonella
Ovine Pili Shield	Grand	I								X												
Ovine ecthyma vaccine	Bayer	I																X				
Pasteurella haemolytica-multocida bacterin	Colorado Serum									X												
Prorab-1	Intervet	I																		X		
Rabdomun vaccine	Schering-Plough	I																		X		
Rabguard-TC	Pfizer Animal Health	I																		X		
Ram epididymitis bacterin	Colorado Serum	I																	X			
Redwol + Spur	Bayer	I							X													
RM Imrab 3	Rhone Merieux	I																				
RM Imrab Bovine Plus	Rhone Merieux	I																		X		
Siteguard MLG vaccine	Coopers	I		X	X	X	X	X	X													
Super-Tet + Havlogen	Bayer	I																				
Tetanus toxoid–concentrated	Colorado Serum											X										
Tetanus toxoid	Fort Dodge	I										X										
Tetanus toxoid	Franklin	I										X										
Tetanus toxoid	Colorado Serum	I										X										
Tenogen	Fort Dodge	I										X										
Tetnogen-AT	Fort Dodge	I																				
Thraxol-2	Bayer	MLV	X																			
Ultrabac CD	Pfizer Animal Health	I							X													
Ultrabac 7	Pfizer Animal Health	I		X	X	X	X		X													
Ultrabac 8	Pfizer Animal Health	I		X	X	X	X	X	X													
Unitox	EquiLabs	I							X													
Vision CD + Spur	Bayer	I							X													
Vision 7 + Spur	Bayer	I		X	X	X	X		X													
Vision 8 + Spur	Bayer	I		X	X	X	X	X	X													
Volar	Bayer	I												X								

I, inactivated (killed); MLV, modified live virus (attenuated).
*Compiled with the assistance of *Compendium of Veterinary Products*. Bayer Commemorative ed., Port Huron, MI, North American Compendiums, 1995.

and is probably the most common disease of sheep in the United States, causing more economic loss than any other disease. Lameness in one or more feet is the most obvious clinical sign. The development of foot rot is facilitated by wet environmental conditions. A vaccine is available which, when combined with regular foot trimming and foot baths, significantly reduces the incidence of disease within a flock.

Bluetongue Vaccine. Bluetongue is a viral disease of ruminants; however, clinical disease is largely restricted to sheep. Clinical signs may include oral ulcers; edema of the face, lips,

muzzle, and ears; excessive salivation; cyanosis of the tongue (thus the name); and lameness caused by coronitis. Teratogenic effects include abortions, stillbirths, and weak, live "dummy lambs." An attenuated live virus vaccine is available for prebreeding vaccination of healthy sheep and goats; vaccination of pregnant females may produce teratogenic effects.

Campylobacteriosis (Vibriosis) Vaccine. Campylobacteriosis is caused by *Campylobacter fetus* subsp. *fetus* and *Campylobacter jejuni*. The principal clinical sign with this disease is abortion, which usually occurs in the last 6 weeks of pregnancy.

Losses from abortion may be substantial in individual flocks. Vaccines for *Campylobacter* alone, or in combination with *Chlamydia*, are now available for prevention of abortion in sheep.

Chlamydia Vaccine. *Chlamydia psittaci*, the cause of enzootic abortion of ewes (EAE), is a major cause of abortion in sheep and goats. Abortions or stillbirths with placentitis usually occur in the fourth or fifth month of gestation; other animals in the flock or herd may concurrently show signs of arthritis or pneumonia. Vaccines for *Chlamydia* alone, or in combination with *Campylobacter*, are now available for prevention of abortion in sheep.

Foot Care. Foot rot is one of the most common diseases of sheep and goats.

TECHNICIAN NOTE

Foot rot is one of the most common diseases of sheep and goats.

It is highly contagious, and infection can result in lameness in a significant number of animals within a herd or flock. Frequent foot trimming combined with foot baths, foot soaks, or vaccination, or a combination of these, is important in the control of the disease. Repeated foot soaking alone is an economical, practical, and effective treatment for foot rot in large commercial operations where hoof trimming is impractical. Products typically used for foot baths or foot soaks include zinc sulfate, copper sulfate, and formalin. There is some evidence of genetic susceptibility to development of foot rot in sheep; therefore, culling of animals with recurring infections may be helpful.

Nutrition. Sheep and goats should be fed a good-quality commercial feed labeled for that particular species. Feeding horse or cattle feeds to small ruminants may result in copper toxicity since the copper levels in those feeds are much higher than normally tolerated by sheep and goats. Feed commercial feeds according to the manufacturer's recommendations and based on the needs and use of the animal. Good-quality roughage may be fed free choice. Since castrated lambs and kids (wethers) are predisposed to the development of urinary calculi, it is advisable to feed a diet of good-quality roughage or pasture and no grain. If grain must be fed, it would be advisable to supplement their feed with salt and a urinary acidifier such as ammonium chloride (see Chapter 27).

External and Internal Parasites. There are few effective anthelmintics labeled for use in small ruminants. Most small ruminant veterinarians utilize cattle dewormers for the treatment of external and internal parasites in sheep and goats. Products commonly used include ivermectin, fenbendazole, albendazole, and levamisole. Caution should be exercised when using these products in lactating does and animals intended for slaughter. Recommendations for extra label use of these products and suggested milk and slaughter withdrawal times may be obtained from the Food Animal Residue Avoidance Data Bank.

Frequency of deworming varies according to several factors, including concentration of animals in a given area and environ-mental conditions. Severe gastrointestinal parasitism can be life-threatening, especially in subtropical climates, where it may be necessary to deworm small ruminants as often as every 4 weeks during the hot, humid summer months. Routine fecal examinations, either individual or composite samples, may be useful to determine the frequency of deworming and the effectiveness of various anthelmintics. See Chapter 6 for more information.

Recommended Reading

Dogs and Cats

Hoskins JD: Feline infectious peritonitis: A current update. Vet Technician 12:193–201, 1991.

Hoskins JD: Tick-borne zoonoses: Lyme disease, ehrlichiosis, and Rocky Mountain spotted fever. Semin Vet Med Surg (Small Anim) 6(3):236–243, 1991.

Hoskins JD: The puppy's first veterinary examination: Physical examination and preventive health program. Vet Technician 12:521–528, 1991.

Hoskins JD: Veterinary Pediatrics: Dogs and Cats from Birth to Six Months, 2nd edition. Philadelphia, WB Saunders, 1995.

Horses

George LW: Diseases of the nervous system. *In* Smith BP (editor): Large Animal Internal Medicine. St Louis, Mosby–Year Book, 1990, pp 917, 1023.

Martens JG, and Martens RJ: Equine herpesvirus type 1: Its classifications, pathogenesis, and prevention. Vet Med 86:936, 1991.

Messer NT, IV: The use of biologics in the prevention of infectious diseases. *In* Smith BP (editor): Large Animal Internal Medicine. St Louis, Mosby–Year Book, 1990, p 1478.

Wilson JH, and Erickson DM: Neurological syndrome of rhinopneumonitis. Proceedings of the American College of Veterinarians Internal Medicine Forum, New Orleans, May 30–June 2, 1991, p 419.

Cattle

Aldridge B, Garry F and Adams R: Role of colostral transfer in neonatal calf management: Failure of acquisition of passive immunity. Compendium Continuing Educ Pract Vet 14:265–270, 1992.

Baker JC and Velicer LF: Bovine respiratory syncytial virus vaccination: current status and future vaccine development. Compendium Continuing Educ Pract Vet 13:1323–1335, 1991.

Heinrichs AJ: Milk replacers for dairy calves—Part I. Compendium Continuing Educ Pract Vet 16:1605–1619, 1994.

Larson BL: Immunization to decrease pregnancy wastage in beef cattle. Part II. Available vaccines. Compendium Continuing Educ Pract Vet 18:571–580, 1996.

Smith BP: Large Animal Internal Medicine. St Louis, Mosby–Year Book, 1996.

Spire MF: Immunization of the beef breeding herd. Compendium Continuing Educ Pract Vet 10:1111–1118, 1988.

Swine

Christianson WT and Joo HS: Porcine reproductive and respiratory syndrome: A review. Swine Health Production 2(2):10–28, 1994.

Cowart RP. An outline of swine diseases, 1st ed. Ames, Iowa State University Press, 1995.

Fedorka-Cray PJ, Hoffman L, Cray WC, et al: *Actinobacillus* (*Haemophilus*) *pleuropneumoniae*. Part I. History, epidemiology, serotyping, and treatment. Compendium Continuing Educ Pract Vet 15:1447–1455, 1993.

Primm ND, Friendship RM, and Hall WF: Deworming strategies for swine. Part II. Anthelmintics and their use in the control of endoparasites. Compendium Continuing Educ Pract Vet 12:889–896, 1990.

Small Ruminants

Council report. Vaccination guidelines for small ruminants (sheep, goats, llamas, domestic deer, and wapiti). J Am Vet Med Assoc 205:1539–1544, 1994.

Robinson A, and Wolf C: American Association of Small Ruminant Practitioners survey of biologic usage. Symposium on Health and Disease of Small Ruminants, 1991, pp 197–214.

Zajac AM and Moore GA: Treatment and control of gastrointestinal nematodes in sheep. Compendium Continuing Educ Pract Vet 15:999–1011, 1993.

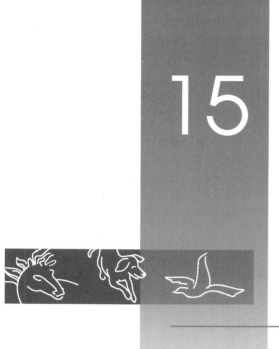

15 Veterinary Anesthesia

Janyce L. Cornick-Seahorn

INTRODUCTION

Anesthesia is a necessary part of veterinary medicine for restraint, elimination of pain sensation during surgical and medical procedures, control of seizure activity, and humane euthanasia. Anesthesia is an area in which veterinary technicians can contribute significantly to their employers and their patients.

Anesthesia is defined as total loss of sensation in a body part (local anesthesia) or in the entire body (general anesthesia), which results from administration of a drug (or drugs) that depresses the activity of part or all of the nervous system. The safe and effective use of anesthetic agents requires a general understanding of their pharmacological actions and the refinement of several technical and interpretive skills for a variety of animal species. Anesthesia requires thorough preanesthetic evaluation of every patient and formulation of an anesthetic plan based on the patient, the surgical or medical procedure to be performed, drug availability, and the experience of the anesthetist. Careful patient monitoring is essential throughout the anesthetic period.

Five topics are discussed in this chapter, including (1) anesthetic pharmacology, (2) anesthetic equipment, (3) anesthetic monitoring and ventilatory support, (4) anesthetic management of selected domestic species, and (5) anesthetic emergencies.

PHARMACOLOGY OF ANESTHETIC AGENTS

Preanesthetic agents are an important part of safe patient management. Drugs most commonly used as preanesthetic agents in veterinary medicine include anticholinergic agents, tranquilizers, sedatives, opioids, and combinations of an opioid with a tranquilizer or sedative (neuroleptanalgesic combinations). These agents are used in the practice of anesthesia to (1) aid in animal restraint; (2) allay apprehension and minimize pain; (3) decrease the quantity of potentially more severe cardiopulmonary depressant drugs used to produce sedation, analgesia, or general anesthesia; (4) produce a safe, smooth, and uncomplicated induction, maintenance, and recovery from general anesthesia; (5) minimize the adverse and potentially toxic effects of concurrently administered drugs used for general anesthesia; and (6) minimize autonomic reflex activity.

 TECHNICIAN NOTE

Preanesthetic agents facilitate animal restraint, reduce patient anxiety, and smooth both induction and recovery.

Anticholinergic Agents

These agents are used to prevent bradycardia associated with increased vagal tone and to prevent excessive upper airway and salivary secretions. Atropine and glycopyrrolate are the two most commonly used drugs. Although atropine is more economical to use, glycopyrrolate offers some advantages, including a longer duration of action, less tendency to promote cardiac arrhythmias, and perhaps less suppression of intestinal motility (Short, 1987). Glycopyrrolate appears to increase heart rate less than does atropine; this may be beneficial in animals with heart disease in which the increase in myocardial oxygen consumption associated with a profound increase in heart rate could be detrimental. Glycopyrrolate, unlike atropine, does not cross the placental barrier, thus having no effect on the fetus during cesarean section.

Although many veterinarians use anticholinergic agents as a routine part of a preanesthetic regimen, their use has become more selective and is based on the needs of the individual patient, the anticipated response to the anesthetic agents, and the tendency to develop bradycardia or excessive salivation. Procedures that may increase vagal tone include traction on abdominal organs and procedures involving the neck, throat, and eye. Anesthetic agents that promote bradycardia include opioids, alpha₂ agonists, barbiturates, and gas anesthetics. Dissociative agents, such as ketamine, may cause excessive salivation, which may be minimized by using an anticholinergic agent.

The use of anticholinergic agents is controversial in large animal species. They are never used routinely in horses because of the potential to cause ileus and colic. Nor are they recommended for use in ruminants because the secretions become more viscid and difficult to clear from the respiratory tract. Anticholinergic agents may be used in swine in conjunction with drugs known to promote bradycardia or excessive salivation. Anticholinergic agents should be used in horses and ruminants only when life-threatening bradycardia develops. (See Table 15–5 for normal ranges for heart rate.)

Tranquilizers and Sedatives

These agents are used to depress the central nervous system (CNS), to aid in restraint, and to reduce anxiety and struggling. This action helps to minimize stress during both induction and recovery and to reduce the requirements for the more potent agents used for induction and maintenance of anesthesia.

Tranquilizers used in veterinary medicine include phenothiazines such as acepromazine (PromAce, Fort Dodge), benzodiazepines such as diazepam, midazolam, and zolazepam (Telazol, AH Robins). Acepromazine calms animals and decreases motor activity; however, animals may be readily aroused by external stimuli, especially animals that are highly excitable or apprehensive. Acepromazine itself does not provide analgesia but may enhance the analgesic effects of concurrently used drugs. Acepromazine has a long duration of action and is dependent on metabolism by the liver; thus acepromazine should be avoided in patients with liver disease and in geriatric and pediatric patients. Other side effects and contraindications are listed in Table 15–1.

Benzodiazepine tranquilizers, including diazepam and midazolam, produce minimal tranquilization and may even increase excitability in dogs, cats, and horses. Benzodiazepines are rarely used alone but are useful for potentiating the effect of concurrently used premedications (such as opioids), for providing muscle relaxation in association with the dissociative drugs (such as ketamine), and for reducing the requirements for induction agents (such as barbiturates). Because of minimal cardiopulmonary effects, they are useful in geriatric and pediatric animals and animals with heart disease. Benzodiazepines have anticonvulsant activity and are useful in patients with a history of seizures or any neurological disorder. Diazepam is usually used intravenously because its carrier, propylene glycol, causes pain when given intramuscularly. Midazolam is water soluble and may be used intramuscularly or intravenously.

Xylazine, detomidine (Dormosedan) and medetomidine (Domitor) are alpha₂ agonists that provide excellent sedation, muscle relaxation, and analgesia. Because of the profound cardiovascular effects (see Table 15–1), including bradycardia, conduction disturbances, and myocardial depression, alpha₂ agonists should be used only in healthy dogs and cats. Concurrent use of anticholinergic agents will help prevent bradycardia; however, this practice is controversial. Thermoregulation is impaired for several hours following xylazine administration, so extremes in environmental temperature must be avoided. Xylazine and detomidine are commonly used in horses. Xylazine is used in ruminants; large and small ruminants are sensitive to xylazine and low doses must be used (Table 15–2). Reversal agents, including yohimbine (Yobine), tolazoline (Tolazine) and atipamezole (Antisedan) are available for veterinary use.

Opioids

Opioids are commonly used in veterinary medicine to produce analgesia and sedation. In horses and cats, they should be used in conjunction with a tranquilizer or sedative because excitement is likely when pure opioids, such as morphine or oxymorphone, are used. Opioids promote bradycardia, which is responsive to anticholinergic agents, but depression of cardiac contractility is minimal. Opioids produce respiratory depression; thus, apnea and hypoventilation during general anesthesia are more likely to occur when opioids are used. Ventilatory support may be required to alleviate this effect, especially in animals with underlying respiratory abnormalities (such as pneumonia or diaphragmatic hernia).

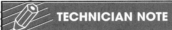

TECHNICIAN NOTE

An induction protocol should facilitate a smooth transition from consciousness to unconsciousness and provide adequate relaxation and immobilization for atraumatic endotracheal intubation.

Thermoregulation is impaired by opioids, which may delay the return of normothermia following anesthesia. External stimuli should be minimized prior to general anesthesia in animals that have received pure opioids because they are hyperresponsive, especially to noise. An advantage of opioids is the availability of opioid antagonists (such as naloxone) to reverse their effects (see Table 15–2).

Neuroleptanalgesia is defined as a state of profound CNS depression and analgesia produced by the combination of a tranquilizer or sedative with an opioid agent (see Tables 15–2 and 15–9). Animals may become unconscious but remain responsive to external stimuli. These drug combinations provide more profound analgesia and calming than is the case when either agent is used alone and may provide adequate analgesia and restraint for procedures such as radiography, wound debridement, suturing of skin lacerations, and ear treatment. When a neuroleptanalgesic combination is used for premedication, dosage requirements of the agents used for induction and maintenance are greatly reduced.

• Table 15–1 •

EFFECTS OF ANESTHETIC DRUGS USED FOR PREMEDICATION AND INDUCTION

DRUG	CARDIOVASCULAR	PULMONARY	ADVERSE EFFECTS	CONTRAINDICATIONS
Premedications				
Acepromazine	Hypotension Antiarrhythmic effect	Minimal	Penile paralysis (stallions) Lowers seizure threshold Promotes hypothermia	Liver disease History of seizures Dehydration Hypovolemia Shock Heart disease Geriatric patients Pediatric patients
Diazepam	Minimal	Minimal	Hypotension if injected too rapidly Burns when given IM	Should not use alone because excitement is possible
Xylazine/detomidine/ medetomidine	Bradycardia Conduction disturbances Hypotension Arrhythmias with halothane anesthesia in dogs and cats	Respiratory depression	Impaired thermoregulation Hyperglycemia Profound muscle relaxation may exacerbate upper respiratory abnormalities	Heart disease Geriatric patients Pediatric patients Ruminants require *low* doses
Opioids	Minimal Bradycardia that is responsive to anticholinergic administration	Respiratory depression	Impaired thermoregulation (panting in dogs) Hyperresponsive to external stimuli Excitement in cats and horses (pure agonists)	Use with tranquilizer or sedative in horses and cats
Induction Agents				
Barbiturates	Myocardial depression Arrhythmias Hypotension	Respiratory depression (apnea)	Excessive salivation Laryngospasm Tissue necrosis with perivascular injection	Heart disease Liver disease Geriatric patients (low doses) Pediatric patients (low doses) Sighthounds (methohexital only) Obese animals (dose on lean weight)
Ketamine/tiletamine	Increase in heart rate and blood pressure Some direct myocardial depression	Minimal Apneustic breathing May cause apnea when given IV	Profuse salivation Muscle rigidity when used alone Convulsions with high doses Poor visceral analgesia	Never use alone except in cats Must have good sedation prior to administration in horses (IV only) Animals with seizure history
Propofol	Myocardial depression Hypotension	Apnea	None	None
Guaifenesin	Minimal	Minimal	Tissue necrosis with perivascular injection	

IM, intramuscular; IV, intravenous.

• Table 15–2 •

DOSAGES* (mg/kg) OF COMMONLY USED ANESTHETIC AGENTS FOR PREMEDICATION AND CHEMICAL RESTRAINT

AGENT	DOG	CAT	HORSE	COW	GOAT/ SHEEP	PIG
Anticholinergics						
Atropine	0.02–0.04	0.02–0.04	—	0.04 (max. 20 mg)	0.04	0.04
Glycopyrrolate	0.011	0.011	—	—	—	0.003
Tranquilizers						
Acepromazine	0.055–0.22	0.11–0.22	0.022–0.088	0.044–0.088	0.044–0.088	0.1–0.22
Diazepam	0.22	0.22	0.022–0.088	0.022–0.088	0.022–0.088	0.22–0.44
Midazolam	0.22	0.22	—	—	—	—
Sedatives						
Xylazine	0.44–1.1	0.44–1.1	0.44–1.1	0.022–0.11	0.022–0.066	1.1–2.2
Detomidine	—	—	0.01–0.02	—	—	—
Medetomidine	.01–.04	.01–.04	—	—	—	—
Opioids						
Oxymorphone	0.01–0.05	0.055–0.011†	0.011–0.044†	—	—	—
Butorphanol	0.11–0.44	0.22–0.44	0.011–0.044	0.011–0.022	0.022–0.044	0.22–0.33
Morphine	0.44–1.1	0.11–0.22†	0.044–0.11†	—	—	0.44–0.88
Meperidine	0.44–1.1	0.22–0.44†	0.22–0.66†	—	—	0.44–1.1
Pentazocine	0.22–0.44	0.11	0.44–0.88	—	—	—
Buprenorphine	0.01–0.04	0.01–0.03	0.01–0.02	—	—	—
Neuroleptanalgesic Combinations						
Droperidol-fentanyl (Innovar)	1 ml/15–30 kg	—	—	—	—	1 ml/23 kg
Acepromazine	0.1–0.22	0.1–0.22	—	—	—	—
Oxymorphone	0.11–0.22	0.055–0.11	—	—	—	—
Acepromazine	0.22	0.22	0.044	—	—	—
Butorphanol	0.22	0.22–0.44	0.022	—	—	—
Xylazine	0.22	0.22	0.66	0.022	0.022	—
Butorphanol	0.11–0.22	0.22–0.44	0.022–0.044	0.022–0.055	0.022	—
Reversal Agents						
Yohimbine‡ (alpha₂ antagonist)	0.11	0.11	0.11	0.11	0.11	0.11
Tolazoline (alpha₂ antagonist)	2.0–5.0	2.0	4.0	1.1	2.0	—
Atipamezole (alpha₂ antagonist)	0.2–0.35	0.2	—	—	—	—
Naloxone (opioid antagonist)	0.0066	0.0066	0.0055–0.022	—	—	0.0066

*Most agents may be used intravenously (IV) or intramuscularly (IM). As a general rule, use higher dose range IM and lower dose range IV.

†Use these opioids in these species *only* in conjunction with a tranquilizer or sedative.

‡Administer yohimbine "to effect" in large animal species. Calculate recommended dose and give in 1/4 increments until reversal of sedation is observed. Adapted from Muir WW: Handbook of Veterinary Anesthesia. St Louis, Mosby–Year Book, 1989, pp. 20–21.

Dissociative Agents

Dissociative agents are usually used as part of an induction or maintenance protocol, but they may be used alone in cats as a premedication to produce immobilization for intravenous catheter placement and short noninvasive procedures and to facilitate induction of general anesthesia. They are discussed in more detail in the following paragraphs.

Induction and Maintenance

Induction agents are incorporated into an anesthetic plan to facilitate smooth and rapid transition from consciousness to unconsciousness for maintenance of general anesthesia. Agents most commonly used include the ultrashort-acting barbiturates, guaifenesin, dissociative agent combinations, propofol and gas anesthetics via mask delivery. *Agents for maintenance* of anesthesia are most commonly the gas anesthetic agents. Effective anesthetic maintenance for short periods of anesthesia may be achieved using various combinations of those drugs used for induction.

Ultrashort-Acting Barbiturates

This group of drugs includes thiopental (thiobarbiturate) and methohexital (oxybarbiturate). They may be used without preanesthetic medication to produce rapid loss of consciousness; however, because of some undesirable cardiopulmonary effects (see Table 15–1), it is safer to use premedications to facilitate intravenous injection and to reduce the dosage required to achieve unconsciousness. The degree of respiratory depression associated with barbiturate administration is related to dosage and rate of administration. One should be prepared to intubate and provide ventilatory support if transient apnea occurs.

Detrimental cardiopulmonary effects are more likely to occur when large doses are administered rapidly and when higher concentrations are used. Although solutions up to 10% in strength are used in large animals, it is preferable to use a solution no stronger than 5% in small animals and safest to use a 2.0% or 2.5% solution. More dilute solutions will reduce the likelihood of adverse effects and cause less tissue necrosis with accidental perivascular injection. Should perivascular administration occur, 2% lidocaine diluted 1:9 with sterile saline should be infiltrated into the injection site. Barbiturates are metabolized by the liver and should be avoided in animals with liver disease. Recovery from thiopental anesthesia is due to redistribution to muscle. Repeated bolus doses to maintain anesthesia are not recommended because this practice will contribute to a rough and prolonged recovery.

Sighthounds (greyhounds, Irish wolfhounds, whippets) are unable to metabolize thiobarbiturates effectively, resulting in a prolonged recovery. An alternative induction method for sighthounds is with methohexital (6 to 11 mg/kg), which acts in much the same way as the thiobarbiturates but is effectively metabolized. Excitement during recovery may be more pronounced with methohexital administration, especially following short procedures, so preanesthetic tranquilization is recommended.

Propofol

Propofol (Rapinovet) is a nonbarbiturate, intravenously administered anesthetic agent which produces a rapid loss of consciousness for induction of anesthesia. The drug is noncumula-tive, being rapidly metabolized (even in the presence of liver dysfunction). Thus, propofol provides a smooth and rapid recovery and may be used for maintenance of anesthesia by infusion (0.4 mg/kg/minute) or repeated bolus, as well as for induction. The major side effects are transient apnea and cardiovascular depression. Both effects may be minimized by using adequate premedication to facilitate minimal dosage requirements and by titrating slowly to effect. Propofol is significantly more expensive than thiopental (13 times more expensive per 10 kg body weight). The propofol formulation is a milky-white emulsion containing soybean oil, egg lecithin, and glycerol. These carrier agents support bacterial growth; therefore, once opened (20-ml vials), the remainder should be placed in a sealed sterile vial and refrigerated, then discarded after 24 hours. This further raises the cost of the product.

Dissociative Agent Combinations

Dissociative agents produce immobilization and superficial analgesia. Swallowing and ocular reflexes remain intact, and muscle tone is increased. These agents may be administered intramuscularly or intravenously; however, intramuscular administration requires higher doses and results in a prolonged recovery. The intramuscular route is most commonly used in cats, dogs, small ruminants, and swine and is *never* used in horses.

TECHNICIAN NOTE

Dissociative agents increase respiratory secretions and salivation and some animals may require administration of an anticholinergic agent to ensure a patent airway.

Concurrent administration of an anticholinergic agent may be needed in some species (cats, dogs, swine) owing to excessive salivation. Although some direct depression of heart function occurs, an increase in sympathetic tone compensates for this effect by increasing heart rate and arterial blood pressure. This effect on heart rate and blood pressure offers an advantage over the thiobarbiturates for use in debilitated and septic patients or patients with heart disease. Since elimination of ketamine depends on both liver metabolism and renal excretion, high dosages should be avoided in animals with liver or kidney disease.

Ketamine offers an alternative method of induction for sighthounds and is most commonly used in combination with diazepam for this purpose. *Telazol* (AH Robins) is a commercial drug combination containing equal parts of zolazepam (benzodiazepine) and tiletamine (dissociative) that may be used for both induction and maintenance of anesthesia. Although approved only for intramuscular use, intravenous administration of very low doses provides an effective method for induction and for short-term anesthesia (Table 15–3).

Guaifenesin

Guaifenesin is an intravenously administered central-acting muscle relaxant that potentiates the effects of concurrently used

• Table 15–3 •

AGENT	DOG	CAT	HORSE	COW	SHEEP/ GOAT	PIG
DRUGS (mg/kg)* COMMONLY USED FOR INDUCTION OR FOR SHORT-DURATION ANESTHESIA						
Thiopental	8.8–13	8.8–13	6.6–11	4.4–11	4.4–11	8.8–13
Propofol	2–6	2–6	—	—	—	—
Guaifenesin	44–88	—	66–132	66–132	66–132	44–88
Ketamine	—	2.2–18	—	—	2.2–6.6	2.2–6.6
Telazol	2.2–11†	2.2–11†	—	4.4–11	2.2–11	4.4–11†
Guaifenesin-thiopental	33–88	—	44–88	44–88	—	33–88
	2.2–6.6	—	2.2–6.6	2.2–6.6	—	2.2–6.6
Guaifenesin-ketamine	33–88	—	44–88	44–88	44–88	—
	1.1	—	1.1–1.5	0.6–1.1	0.6–1.1	—
Acepromazine-ketamine	0.11	0.22†	—	—	—	0.44†
	11.0	4.4–11†	—	—	—	2.2–6.6†
Xylazine-ketamine	0.66–1.1†	0.66–1.1†	1.1	0.044–0.088†	0.044†	2.2–4.4†
	2.2–11†	4.4–22†	2.2	2.2–6.6†	2.2–6.6	2.2–11†
Diazepam-ketamine	0.25	0.25	—	—	0.25–0.55	0.22–0.44
	5.0	5.0	—	—	4.4	4.4
Xylazine-telazol	0.44†	0.66†	1.1	0.022–0.11†	0.044–0.088†	0.66–1.1†
	6.6†	2.2–6.6†	1.1–2.2	2.2–6.6†	2.2–6.6†	4.4–6.6†
Xylazine-guaifenesin-ketamine	(See tables giving specific species protocol.)					

*Dosage is for intravenous use unless otherwise designated.
†Indicates protocols that may be used intramuscularly in some species.
Adapted from Muir WW: Handbook of Veterinary Anesthesia. St Louis, Mosby–Year Book, 1989, p. 76.

preanesthetic and anesthetic agents, allowing for lower dosages of these agents to be used. Guaifenesin is used in large animals as part of an induction protocol and may also be incorporated into the anesthetic plan for maintenance of anesthesia with injectable agents. Cardiopulmonary effects are minimal, and there is a wide margin of safety. Excessive dosages may result in paradoxical muscle rigidity of the forelimbs and neck and an apneustic breathing pattern, which is more likely to occur in young animals. Administration is best performed through an indwelling venous catheter because large volumes must be administered to achieve the desired effect and perivascular injection is caustic to tissues.

Epidural Analgesia

Epidural analgesia provides a method of complete anesthesia (local anesthetics such as lidocaine and bupivacaine) or supplemental analgesia both intra- and postoperatively (opioids). (See Chapter 20 on pain management) The site of injection is at the lumbosacral intervertebral space which allows entry of a needle into the epidural space (Heath et al., 1989; Klide and Soma, 1968).

Local anesthetics provide total analgesia and muscle relaxation to the caudal portion of the body which will facilitate surgery of the hindlimbs, perineal region, and abdomen. The cranial extent of the analgesia varies from patient to patient and supplemental anesthesia may become necessary for some animals. This technique is good for cesarean section, because of minimal fetal effects, and for high-risk patients. Side effects may include hypotension due to vasodilation (which may be minimized by fluid loading prior to administration) and, in rare cases, respiratory arrest if excessive cranial migration occurs.

Animals receiving local anesthetics epidurally should never be placed in a head-down position. Dosage is approximately *1 ml per 4.5 kg for both 2.0% lidocaine and 0.5% bupivacaine* with a duration of action of 1½ to 2 hours and 4 to 6 hours,

respectively. Dosage should be reduced by 50% if cerebrospinal fluid is observed in the hub of the needle, and by 10% to 20% in obese and pregnant animals. Contraindications include patients with sepsis, clotting abnormalities, or infected skin.

Inhalation Anesthetics

Inhalation agents used in veterinary medicine include isoflurane, halothane, and methoxyflurane. Another inhalant agent, sevoflurane, which acts similarly to isoflurane, has recently been introduced for veterinary use. These agents produce general anesthesia, which includes unconsciousness, muscle relaxation, and analgesia, and are suitable for use in all species. Advantages include more rapid control of changes in depth of anesthesia and a more rapid recovery. However, these agents produce profound effects on cardiopulmonary function and patients must be closely monitored throughout the anesthetic period. The use of gas anesthetics requires more complex and expensive equipment than that used with injectable techniques, and an understanding of this equipment is necessary to use the agents safely and effectively.

TECHNICIAN NOTE

Mask induction should be reserved for high-risk patients that are adequately sedated. This technique greatly increases waste gas contamination of the work environment.

Some properties of the gases (Table 15–4) must be reviewed to appreciate the anesthetic vaporizers used to deliver the gases and the speed at which the agents exert their anesthetic effect. *Vapor pressure* of a gas determines the maximum

• Table 15–4 •

CHARACTERISTICS OF COMMONLY USED INHALATION AGENTS IN VETERINARY MEDICINE

AGENT	VAPOR PRESSURE (mm Hg)	SOLUBILITY COEFFICIENT	MAC VALUES				INDUCTION		MAINTENANCE	
			Dog	Cat	Horse	Pig	SA	LA	SA	LA
Isoflurane	240	1.4	1.5%	1.6%	1.3%	1.47%	2%–4%	4%–5%	1%–3%	2%–3%
Halothane	244	2.4	0.87%	1.19%	0.9%	1.25%	2%–4%	3%–5%	0.5%–1.5%	1%–2%
Methoxyflurane	23	13.0	0.23%	0.16%	0.3%	*	2%–3%	†	0.2%–1%	†
Sevoflurane	157	0.68	2.38%	2.58%	2.31%	—	—	—	—	—

MAC, maximum allowable concentration; SA, small animal; LA, large animal.
*Value not available.
†Methoxyflurane is not used routinely in large animals.

concentration that may be achieved in the carrier gas (oxygen) at any given temperature. For example, methoxyflurane, with a low vapor pressure (23 mm Hg), may only reach a maximum concentration of 3.5% at room temperature, whereas halothane and isoflurane, both with vapor pressures of approximately 240 mm Hg, may reach a maximum concentration of 32% at room temperature. This means that a precision vaporizer (see discussion of equipment), which delivers a precise concentration of anesthetic gas according to settings on the vaporizer, is required to avoid potentially lethal concentrations of isoflurane and halothane. On the other hand, methoxyflurane may be used with a nonprecision vaporizer for which exact concentration settings are absent, since it is impossible to achieve the same excessive concentrations possible with the other two agents.

Solubility determines the speed of induction and recovery of the anesthetic gas and is most frequently defined as its distribution between blood and gas phases. Methoxyflurane with a very high solubility is dissolved to a high degree in the blood. This delays the development of a tension (partial pressure) of anesthetic gas in the blood, which is essential for the gas to pass into the brain and render the patient unconscious. This high solubility of methoxyflurane is manifested clinically as a very slow induction of and recovery from general anesthesia, making it undesirable for use as an induction agent. Halothane is much less soluble than methoxyflurane, and isoflurane is the least soluble of the three. Both halothane and isoflurane may be used effectively to achieve induction of anesthesia via mask delivery, and the recoveries are much more rapid. Seroflurane is the least soluble gas agent and produces a more rapid induction and recovery than isoflurane.

Minimum alveolar concentration (MAC) is a measure of anesthetic potency by which the gas anesthetic agents may be compared and is used as a guide to deliver adequate but not excessive concentrations for surgical procedures. MAC is defined as the minimum concentration of anesthetic in the alveoli at 1 atm that prevents a response in 50% of patients exposed to a painful stimulus. The MAC values have been determined for the commonly used gas anesthetics for many animal species (see Table 15–4). For most surgical procedures in most species, 1.5 to 2.0 times MAC is adequate to maintain a surgical plane of anesthesia. Factors that may decrease the MAC requirement include age (older patients require less), hypothermia, administration of other depressant drugs (such as opioids, tranquilizers), anemia, and diseases such as septicemia.

The anesthetic gases cause a dose-dependent depression of heart function, with isoflurane having the least effect on the heart at clinically used concentrations. All three gases cause respiratory depression, and ventilation should be assisted (see Ventilatory Support) to minimize the development of hypercapnia and atelectasis. Halothane has the additional undesirable characteristic of sensitizing the heart to catecholamines, which can result in the development of arrhythmias. Methoxyflurane is less likely to induce arrhythmias, and isoflurane does not have this effect. Isoflurane, although more expensive than halothane, is the safest and most versatile anesthetic gas because it may be used in young, old, debilitated, and diseased patients with the fewest detrimental effects.

ANESTHETIC EQUIPMENT

Anesthetic equipment should be organized in a specific location in the hospital, usually the surgery preparation area. This area should be quiet and away from the mainstream hospital traffic. Once the technician knows what anesthetic drugs and equipment the veterinarian wants to have available, adequate supplies should be stocked and maintained.

Basic equipment and supplies that should be available to provide anesthesia include needles and syringes, intravenous catheters, tape for securing catheters, heparinized saline (2 units of heparin per milliliter of 0.9% saline), endotracheal tubes in a variety of sizes, laryngoscope, lubricant for the endotracheal tubes, ophthalmic lubricant, an oxygen source and method of delivery, an apparatus for manual ventilation (i.e., Ambu bag [see Fig. 15–19] or anesthesia machine), and a selection of anesthetic agents. If gas anesthesia is used in the practice, an anesthesia machine, breathing systems, and a selection of rebreathing bags and face masks should be available. An emergency drug box (discussed under Anesthetic Emergencies) should also be accessible in this area.

Catheters

Intravenous administration equipment and catheters are covered in Chapter 10. As a general rule of anesthesia, dependable venous access, as with an intravenous catheter taped or glued securely in place, should be available in all anesthetized patients. An intravenous catheter provides a route of administration for polyionic fluids to maintain homeostasis; for additional drugs to maintain anesthesia, which is especially important when injectable techniques are used; and for emergency drug administration if cardiopulmonary arrest occurs.

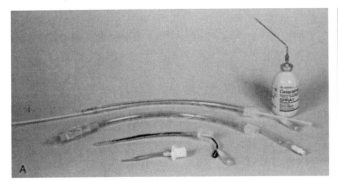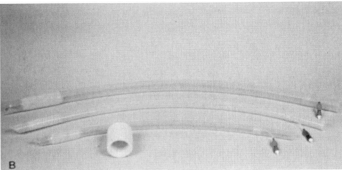

Figure 15-1. A, Representative sizes of cuffed endotracheal tubes appropriate for use in small animals, small ruminants, and swine. The top tube and the third tube from the top contain two types of stylets in place as they might be used clinically to facilitate intubation. A noncuffed Cole tube is also shown (bottom). Right, Topical anesthetic spray (Cetacaine, Cetylite Industries Inc., Pennsauken, NJ) for desensitizing the larynx before intubation. B, Cuffed tubes (Biovona, Gary, IN) that are used for horses and cattle. An oral speculum, which is placed between the equine incisors to facilitate intubation, is also shown.

Endotracheal Tubes

The endotracheal tube provides the connecting link between the patient's airway and the anesthetic equipment. Although it is not essential to place an endotracheal tube when injectable anesthesia is used, tubes must be available in rare instances when respiratory arrest dictates the need for artificial ventilation and delivery of oxygen or when the risk of regurgitation and aspiration is increased (as in patients who have not adequately fasted, who have a history of vomiting, or who are pregnant). Some veterinarians prefer to place an endotracheal tube routinely during injectable anesthesia as a precautionary measure. Cuffed tubes (Fig. 15–1) are most commonly used and provide for an effective seal within the airway to prevent aspiration and to facilitate effective ventilatory support. Cuffed tubes are available in a wide variety of sizes according to internal diameter (ID) in millimeters, with sizes 2.5 to 14 mm ID appropriate for dogs, cats, swine, and small ruminants and sizes 16 to 30 mm ID for large ruminants and horses. Noncuffed (Cole) tubes (see Fig. 15–1) are used in very small patients (such as newborn kittens and puppies, ferrets, birds) because they preserve a larger airway diameter.

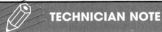

> **TECHNICIAN NOTE**
>
> All anesthetized animals should be intubated to ensure and protect the airway. Intubation, while not essential for short procedures which utilize injectable agents, should be performed on those animals at increased risk of regurgitation (not fasted, history of vomiting, pregnant).

Laryngoscopes

Laryngoscopes facilitate intubation in many species and are especially beneficial in small ruminants, swine, and cats. These instruments consist of a battery-containing handle with a detachable blade. Blades come in a variety of shapes and sizes.

Two styles commonly used in veterinary anesthesia are shown in Figure 15–2.

Anesthetic Machines

The primary purposes of an inhalation anesthetic machine and breathing system are to deliver oxygen, to deliver a controlled amount of an inhalation anesthetic agent, and to provide a method of assisting ventilation. The variability of anesthetic machines, which are offered in a wide variety of types and sizes by numerous manufacturers, presents a challenge to the veterinary anesthetist; however, all machines have the same basic components (Fig. 15–3) (Dorsch and Dorsch, 1984a; Hartsfield, 1987).

The four basic components of an anesthetic machine are a *compressed gas source* (oxygen and sometimes nitrous oxide); the *pressure regulator,* which reduces and controls the pressure of gas leaving the compressed gas source to a lower pressure that will not damage the flowmeter; the *flowmeter,* which precisely controls the flow of gas entering the patient's breathing system; and the *vaporizer,* which facilitates delivery of a controlled concentration of an inhalation anesthetic agent into the patient's breathing system.

Another feature is the pressure gauge, which reflects the amount of gas remaining in the compressed gas tank (see Fig. 15–3). Specifically, a full oxygen tank maintains a pressure of approximately 2200 psi, and that pressure decreases proportionately as the tank empties. An oxygen flush valve, which is included on most anesthetic machines, delivers oxygen directly and rapidly (35 to 75 liters/minute) to the common gas outlet of the machine, thus bypassing the vaporizer and quickly filling the breathing system with pure oxygen (see Figs. 15–3 and 15–6).

Older machines may flush through the vaporizer (see Fig. 15–4), which presents an inherent danger if the flush valve is engaged while the vaporizer is turned on. The flush valve may be used to quickly decrease the inhalation anesthetic concentration present in the breathed gases for a rapid decrease in anesthetic depth or rapid recovery from anesthesia. Use of the flush valve should be avoided as a method of filling the rebreathing bag unless a change in depth of anesthesia is desired.

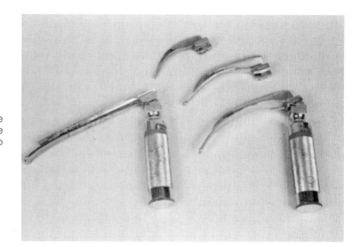

Figure 15-2. Laryngoscopes used in veterinary medicine. The three blades on the right are different-sized McIntosh blades. The blade on the left is a Miller blade, which is long enough to facilitate intubation of small ruminants and swine.

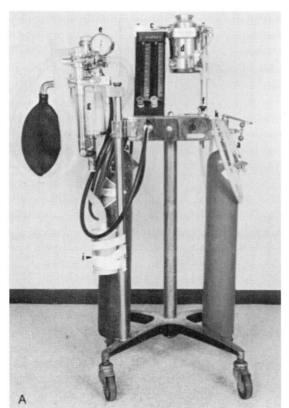

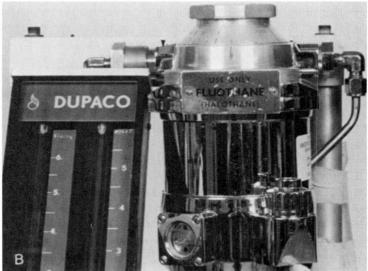

Figure 15-3. A, A basic veterinary anesthetic machine with a circle breathing system for use in animals of 7 to 135 kg. Components include compressed gas sources for both oxygen and nitrous oxide (a), built-in pressure regulator (b), flowmeters (c), and a precision vaporizer (d) located out of the system. Also included are a pressure manometer (e), oxygen flush valve (f), soda lime canister (g), and common gas outlet (h), which delivers oxygen and anesthetic gas to the breathing system. A waste gas-capturing device (i), located below the breathing system, is connected by corrugated tubing to the ``pop-off'' valve (j). The hoses that attach at the back of the machine (k) allow connection to a central hospital gas pipeline system. B, A Fluothane Tec (Fluotec 3, Matrix Medical Inc, Orchard Park, NY) vaporizer showing calibration of output in volumes percent. The vaporizer is set at 0.5%. Button at the left of the vaporizer (arrow) is a locking mechanism that must be depressed to activate the control dial.

Vaporizers convert a volatile liquid inhalation anesthetic into a vapor for delivery into the patient's breathing system. Classification of vaporizers is a complex task, and more detailed descriptions are available (Hartsfield, 1987; Dorsch and Dorsch, 1984d; Bednarski, 1991). Most newer vaporizers (precision) provide precisely determined vapor concentrations according to the settings on the vaporizer, regardless of temperature and incoming gas flow rate (see Fig. 15–3). Nonprecision vaporizers are low-efficiency vaporizers that volatilize the anesthetic agent without producing a precisely known vapor concentration, and their output varies with temperature, gas flow rate through the vaporizer, and the patient's ventilation (Fig. 15–4). A more specific set of criteria exists for classification of vaporizers, and this includes a method of regulating output concentration, a method of vaporization, location of the vaporizer in relation to the breathing system, a method of temperature compensation, and agent specificity (Hartsfield, 1987; Dorsch and Dorsch, 1984d; Bednarski, 1991).

Location of the vaporizer may be out of the breathing system (out-of-the-system) or in the breathing system (in-the-system) as illustrated in Figure 15–5. There is an inherent danger in the use of an in-the-system (nonprecision) vaporizer. While an out-of-system vaporizer can never deliver a concentra-

tion higher than what is set on the vaporizer dial (because fresh gas flow passes through the vaporizer one time only), an in-the-system vaporizer receives, in addition to fresh gas flow, a gas mixture containing anesthetic gas not taken up by the patient; therefore, vapor concentration in the breathed gas may increase over time. This increase is exacerbated by low fresh gas flows, which allow exhaled gases already containing anesthetic vapor to recirculate more times, and by ventilation, with greater ventilation resulting in increased vaporization. The latter effect theoretically provides a built-in safety factor *if* the animal is breathing spontaneously, because as anesthetic depth increases, ventilation becomes depressed, allowing anesthetic concentration in the breathed gases to decrease. Controlled ventilation is not safe to use with an in-the-system vaporizer.

Breathing Systems

The most commonly used breathing system is the circle rebreathing system, meaning that the patient rebreathes the gas mixture within the circle (Figs. 15–3 through 15–6). Three sizes are available, including pediatric (<7 kg), standard adult circle (7 to 135 kg) (see Fig. 15–3), and large animal (>135 kg) (see Fig. 15–6). These systems vary in internal volume owing to differences in diameter of the connecting Y-piece, breathing tubes, breathing tube connectors, one-way valves, and the size of the rebreathing bags used (Hartsfield, 1987).

Gases move in one direction owing to the presence of one-way valves, and carbon dioxide produced by the animal is neutralized by soda lime or barium hydroxide lime contained in the absorbent canister (see Figs. 15–3 and 15–6). Most absorbent granules contain an indicator dye, which becomes visible owing to a color change as the granules become exhausted. Although no set guidelines exist for when to change the absorbent granules, a general rule is that a strong color indicates the point of clinical exhaustion and should be changed when the color shift is present in two thirds of the absorbent (Dorsch and Dorsch, 1984b).

Rebreathing bag selection may be made by multiplying the patient's tidal volume (10 ml/kg) times six. Rebreathing bags available for animals less than 135 kg include 1-, 2-, 3-, 5- and 6-liter sizes, and for animals greater than 135 kg, they include 15-, 20- and 30-liter sizes.

Fresh gas flow rates vary with personal preference. A setting that just meets the patient's metabolic oxygen needs (small animal = 8 to 10 ml/kg/minute; large animal = 2 to 3 ml/kg/minute) is termed a "closed" circle system, in which the overflow or 'pop-off' valve is closed and flow rates are adjusted to maintain a constant volume in the rebreathing bag. Although this system is more economical, retains more heat and humidity, and causes less environmental pollution, hypoxia may develop if the patient is not closely monitored. The system must be flushed two to four times during the first 15 minutes of anesthesia, and every 30 minutes thereafter, to prevent nitrogen (which is exhaled by the patient) from building up within the system. In a "semiclosed" circle system, defined by fresh gas flows of three times the patient's metabolic oxygen needs (small animal = 30 ml/kg/minute; large animal = 6 ml/kg/minute), the pop-off valve is open. Although these flow rates are less economical and result in more pollution, they ensure greater patient safety. Regardless of the flow rate used for maintenance, flow rates for mask induction and for a short period following intubation and connection to the breathing system (2 to 5 minutes) should

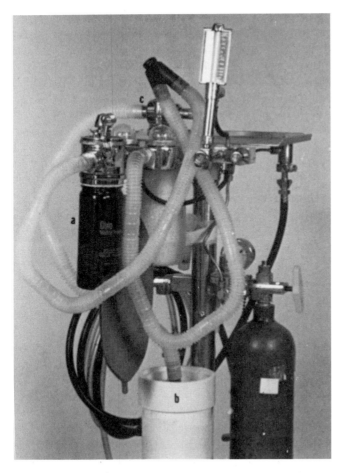

Figure 15–4. A basic veterinary anesthetic machine with a circle breathing system. The nonprecision vaporizer (a) is located within the breathing system for delivery of methoxyflurane. The mouthed scavenger system (b) is connected to the pop-off valve (c).

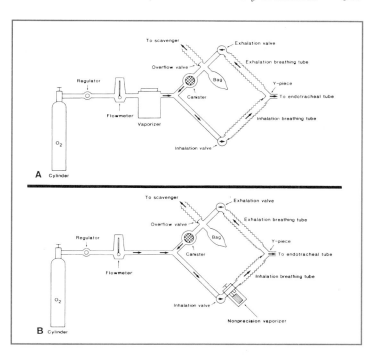

Figure 15–5. A, Diagram of the relationship of an out-of-the-system precision vaporizer to the various components of an anesthetic machine and a circle breathing system. B, Diagram of the relationship of an in-the-system nonprecision vaporizer to the various components of an anesthetic machine and a circle breathing system. (From Harstfield SM: Machines and breathing systems for administration of inhalation anesthetics. *In* Short CE (ed): Principles and Practice of Veterinary Anesthesia. Baltimore, The Williams & Wilkins Co., 1987, p. 403. © 1987, The Williams & Wilkins Company, Baltimore.)

be increased (except for in-the-system vaporizers) to facilitate delivery of anesthetic gas to the patient and to aid in denitrogenation of the patient. A rate of two to three times the calculated maintenance flow rate will be adequate.

Non-rebreathing systems are also used in veterinary medicine for patients weighing less than 7 kg. Non-rebreathing (NRB) systems are simple to use and inexpensive, do not require carbon dioxide absorbent, and impart minimal resistance to breathing. Disadvantages include decreased economy and increased pollution due to the high flow rates required to remove carbon dioxide and a greater loss of heat and humidity.

Flow rates vary according to the particular system used but are approximately 100 to 300 ml/kg/minute with a minimum flow of 500 ml/minute. A commonly used NRB system in veterinary medicine is the Bain coaxial system (Fig. 15–7).

In veterinary hospitals in which inhalation anesthetics are used, it is important to minimize environmental exposure of attending personnel to waste gases (also see Chapter 36). Reduction of environmental pollution is facilitated by scavenging the waste gas exiting through the pop-off valve, checking equipment frequently for leaks (see under Preparation of Equipment and Supplies) and practicing techniques that minimize

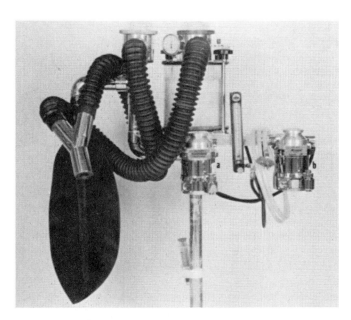

Figure 15–6. Large animal anesthetic machine with circle breathing system. This machine is equipped with both a halothane (a) and an isoflurane (b) precision vaporizer, which may be used interchangeably.

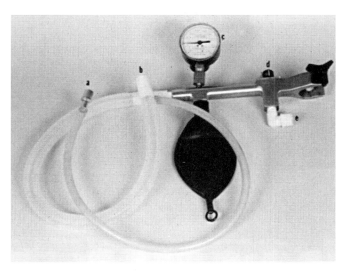

Figure 15–7. Bain circuit non-rebreathing system attaches to (a) the common gas outlet of the anesthetic machine. (b) Patient connection end. The system is also equipped with a pressure manometer (c); a ``pop-off'' valve (d), which remains open except during assisted ventilation; and an interface for connection to a waste gas scavenging system (e).

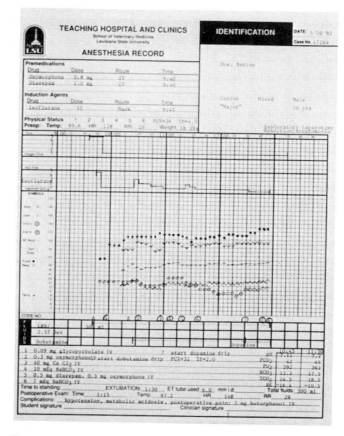

environmental pollution (Dorsch and Dorsch, 1984c; Paddleford, 1987; Muir et al., 1989). Although a cause-and-effect relationship has not been clearly demonstrated, studies of operating room personnel suggest that exposure to trace anesthetic gases may be a contributing factor in spontaneous abortion, congenital abnormalities, cancer, hepatic disease, renal disease, and neurological disease (Dorsch and Dorsch, 1984c; Paddleford, 1987). Scavenging systems must include the gas-capturing device, the interface, and the disposal system, and detailed descriptions are available (Dorsch and Dorsch, 1984a and c; Paddleford, 1987). Considerations that help to minimize waste gas exposure include the following:

1. Fill vaporizers at the end of the workday when fewer people are present, taking care to avoid spillage.
2. Use low-flow techniques when possible.
3. Have patients recover in well-ventilated areas and leave the patient attached to the breathing system as long as possible so that expired gases can be scavenged.
4. Do not turn on the vaporizer until the patient is connected to the machine.
5. When disconnecting the patient from the machine, turn off the vaporizer and occlude the Y-piece until the patient is reconnected.
6. Use mask or chamber inductions only when considered necessary for the safety of the patient or for unrestrainable patients.

Figure 15–8. A sample anesthetic record that allows for sequential recording of heart rate, respiratory rate, and arterial blood pressures. Also included is a summary of the preanesthetic findings and the dose, route, and time of administration of drugs used.

MONITORING

Intraoperative monitoring is essential to successful anesthesia because chemical restraint and general anesthesia impose a great stress on homeostasis in both normal and debilitated patients. Since irreversible brain and cellular changes occur in 3 to 5 minutes following the cessation of blood flow that occurs with cardiac arrest, vital signs should be assessed and recorded every 5 minutes. Life-threatening changes must be detected early so that action can be taken to avoid permanent damage to the patient.

The anesthetic record is a concise method for recording time of administration and doses (in milligrams) of anesthetic agents used and physiological data measured throughout the anesthetic period. The record serves as a legal document, prompts the anesthetist to evaluate and record the patient's vital signs at regular intervals, permits recognition of trends in one or more of the recorded values that might signal an impending problem, and provides information for any subsequent anesthetic procedures in the same patient (Fig. 15–8).

Monitoring includes both physical and technical methods. Physical methods parallel those skills involved in performing a physical examination plus assessment of muscle tone and eye reflexes. Technological methods use sophisticated equipment

to quantify various aspects of homeostasis. Monitoring should focus on the cardiovascular and pulmonary systems, the CNS, and body temperature because these are most affected by anesthetic drugs and surgical procedures. The preanesthetic physical status of the patient (see Preanesthetic Evaluation), the anesthetic protocol used, the procedure to be performed, and the anticipated duration of anesthesia help to determine the sophistication of the monitoring techniques used.

Cardiovascular system monitoring involves integrated assessment of heart rate and rhythm, pulse quality, capillary refill time (CRT), and mucous membrane color. Heart rate and rhythm may be assessed by external auscultation or with an esophageal stethoscope in small animals (Fig. 15–9). During the surgical procedure, direct auscultation may be difficult, especially in large animals, and palpation of a peripheral pulse

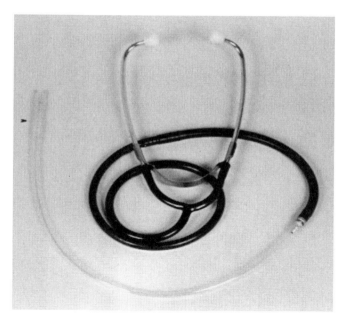

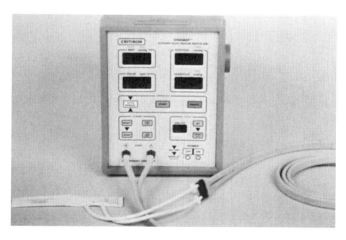

Figure 15-10. Oscillometric peripheral pulse monitor for indirect monitoring of systolic, diastolic, and mean arterial blood pressures. This monitor also records pulse rate (Dinamap, Critikon, Tampa, FL).

Figure 15-9. Esophageal stethoscope (arrow) allows auscultation of heart sounds during the anesthetic monitoring period. The device may be coupled to a stethoscope or an amplifier for transmission of audible heart sounds.

is more reliable. Peripheral pulses used to assess rate and quality include the femoral, dorsal metatarsal, digital, and lingual arteries in dogs; the femoral artery in cats and swine; the facial, transverse facial, and lateral metatarsal arteries in horses; and the auricular, digital, coccygeal, and dorsal metatarsal arteries in ruminants. A continuous electrocardiogram (ECG) determines whether cardiac rate and rhythm are normal and aids in early detection of arrhythmias. Lead II is used in small animals, and a base-apex lead placement, recorded in lead II, is useful in large animals. Lead placement for a base-apex ECG (right arm over heart; left arm over jugular furrow; left leg over point of shoulder) will yield a large positive R wave. It is important to remember that a normal ECG only indicates normal electrical activity and yields no information regarding heart contractility or tissue perfusion.

Adequate perfusion is assessed by subjective evaluation of mucous membrane color, CRT (normal <2 seconds), and pulse quality.

Pulse oximetry is a noninvasive method of monitoring pulse rate and the amount of oxygen carried by hemoglobin in the arterial blood (Jones, 1996). Most pulse oximeters provide a digital display of pulse rate and the percent oxygen saturation of hemoglobin (Sao_2). The Sao_2 should be maintained above 95% in animals breathing 100% oxygen and above 90% in animals breathing room air. Values below 90% signal an arterial oxygen partial pressure (Pao_2) of less than 60 mm Hg, which defines hypoxemia.

Several sources of error can limit the usefulness of pulse oximetry, including hypotension, tachycardia, hypothermia, movement, and poor probe positioning. These potential sources of error should be considered when interpreting the values, and other methods should be used in overall patient assessment. As a general rule, the closer the oximeter pulse rate is to the actual heart rate, the more accurate the Sao_2 value. Sites for probe placement in animals include the tongue (not for adult horses

and cattle), lip fold, toe web, ear, skin folds, vulva, and nasal septum. A reflectance probe is also available, which may be used in the rectum or esophagus.

Arterial blood pressure may be measured by either direct or indirect methods. Indirect methods, which include the oscillometric pulse monitor (Fig. 15–10) and the ultrasonic Doppler apparatus (Fig. 15–11), require placement of an inflatable cuff on a peripheral artery. These methods are easy to use but are less accurate than direct methods and are not applicable to all species or breeds because of variations in limb shape and size.

For direct pressure monitoring, a catheter is placed in a peripheral artery and connected via heparinized saline-filled tubing to a pressure transducer (Fig. 15–12) or aneroid manometer (Fig. 15–13). Direct methods require more technical skill and knowledge of the equipment. The aneroid manometer is relatively inexpensive and gives a continuous value for mean arterial pressure, whereas a pressure transducer records mean, systolic, and diastolic arterial pressures but requires expensive

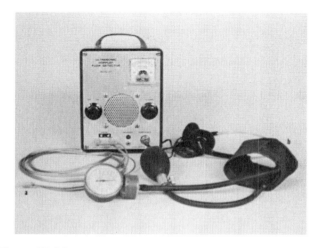

Figure 15-11. Ultrasonic Doppler apparatus for indirect monitoring of systolic arterial blood pressure. An electronic activated crystal (a), positioned distal to an occlusive cuff (b), senses blood flow in a peripheral artery, which is audibly broadcast.

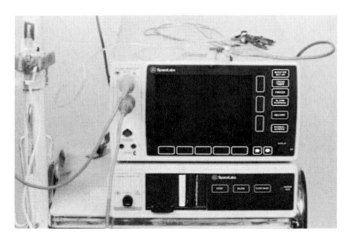

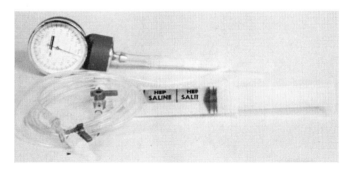

Figure 15-13. An aneroid manometer provides direct measurement of mean arterial blood pressure. The device is attached (arrow) to a catheter placed in a peripheral artery, and the air-water interface within the connecting tubing should be placed at the level of the patient's heart.

Figure 15-12. A computed electrocardiograph monitor for recording a continuous electrocardiogram. The monitor is also equipped with a pressure transducer (a), which may be connected (b) to a catheter placed in a peripheral artery for direct measurement of systolic, diastolic, and mean arterial blood pressures. This monitor will also continuously record body temperature (c; probe not shown) (Spacelabs Inc, Redmond, WA).

equipment. Blood pressure monitoring aids in the assessment of depth of anesthesia and adequacy of tissue perfusion; a minimum of 60 mm Hg mean arterial pressure should be maintained in all patients to ensure adequate perfusion to vital organs (brain, heart, lungs, kidneys) (Haskins, 1987). Normal values for arterial blood pressure are listed in Table 15–5.

The *pulmonary system* is monitored by assessing breathing rate and rhythm. Although these assessments yield minimal information regarding adequacy of ventilation, sudden changes in the ventilatory pattern may signal an impending problem.

For example, the onset of apnea during anesthesia may indicate excessive anesthetic depth. An increase in rate following initiation of surgery may indicate that the anesthesia is too light.

Respiratory monitors, which sound an audible beep with each expiration, provide a method for monitoring breathing rate. The monitor is placed on the endotracheal tube and is especially useful in small patients and birds whose respirations may be difficult to assess by either chest wall excursions or movement of the rebreathing bag.

Most anesthetic agents are potent respiratory depressants, and apnea following anesthetic induction is not uncommon. Ventilation should be supported at this time (two to four breaths per minute) to ensure adequate delivery of oxygen and anesthetic gas until spontaneous ventilation returns (see Ventilatory Support).

The degree of collapse of the rebreathing bag provides a

• Table 15–5 •

REFERENCE INTERVALS FOR COMMONLY MEASURED CARDIOVASCULAR AND RESPIRATORY TESTS, BODY TEMPERATURE, AND LABORATORY VALUES IN COMMON DOMESTIC SPECIES						
COMPONENT	**DOG**	**CAT**	**HORSE**	**COW**	**GOAT/SHEEP**	**PIG**
Heart rate	70–180	145–200	30–45	60–80	60–90	60–90
Respiratory rate	10–40	20–40	8–20	20–40	15–40	10–40
Temperature (°F)	101–104	101–104	99.5–101.5	100.5–102.5	101–104	101–103
Packed cell volume	35–54	27–46	25–45	23–43	30–50	30–48
Total protein	5.7–7.8	6.3–8.3	6.0–8.5	6.7–8.6	6.3–7.1	6.0–7.5
Systolic arterial pressure* (mm Hg)	110–160	(Arterial blood pressure values tend to decrease during general anesthesia, especially with inhalation anesthetics and especially in debilitated patients. The exception is in cattle, which tend to show an increase in blood pressure during general anesthesia. As a general rule, mean arterial blood pressure should be maintained above 60–70 mm Hg during general anesthesia in all species.)				
Diastolic arterial pressure* (mm Hg)	70–90					
Mean arterial pressure* (mm Hg)	80–110					
Arterial pH*	7.35–7.45					
$Paco_2$* (mm Hg)	35–45					
Pao_2* (mm Hg)	80–110	(As high as 500 when patient is breathing 100% oxygen)				
HCO_3^-* (mEq/liter)	17–30	(Mean = 24: higher values refer to horses and ruminants; lower values refer to dogs and cats)				
Co_2, total (mEq/liter)	18–31					
Base excess* (mEq/liter)	⁻4–⁺4					

$Paco_2$, partial pressure of arterial carbon dioxide; Pao_2, partial pressure of arterial oxygen; HCO_3^-, bicarbonate.
*Values are similar for all species; differences are explained in the table.

crude estimation of tidal volume. Arterial carbon dioxide ($Paco_2$) and oxygen (Pao_2) partial pressures provide the most accurate method of determining adequacy of ventilation; however, equipment for measuring blood gases is expensive and available only in large veterinary hospitals.

Capnometry provides a noninvasive method for monitoring breathing rate and adequacy of ventilation (Jones, 1996). The capnometer measures the partial pressure of carbon dioxide in expired gases and quantitates the end-tidal (end of expiration) carbon dioxide partial pressure (ET-Pco_2). The ET-Pco_2 is a close estimate of $Paco_2$ and should be maintained between 35 and 45 mm Hg. An increase indicates hypoventilation and the need for ventilatory assistance (see Ventilatory Support). The capnometer attaches to the patient's endotracheal tube and also provides a digital respiratory rate and an audible beep with each expiration.

Central nervous system evaluation yields information regarding depth of anesthesia and includes assessment of the position of the eye in the orbit and depression of eye reflexes (Table 15–6). Loss of the anal reflex is a crude indicator of excessive anesthetic depth. Degree of muscle relaxation (such as jaw tone) and absence of voluntary movement also aid in the evaluation of anesthetic depth. Muscle relaxation may be an unreliable indicator in animals given ketamine. Indicators of light anesthesia may include shivering and tensing of the neck and shoulder muscles.

TECHNICIAN NOTE

Since anesthetized patients hypoventilate during anesthesia, ventilation should be assisted to combat the development of hypercapnia and atelectasis.

VENTILATORY SUPPORT

General anesthesia depresses respiration; therefore, ventilatory support is often necessary during general anesthesia. Special consideration must be given to high-risk patients, such as animals with pulmonary and pleural cavity disease, abdominal distention, diaphragmatic hernia and obesity, and in animals

• Table 15–6 •

EYE SIGNS* DURING MAINTENANCE OF ANESTHESIA

| | PLANE OF ANESTHESIA | | |
SIGN	Too Light	Adequate	Too Deep
Corneal reflex	Brisk	Present	Absent
Palpebral reflex	Brisk	Slowed	Absent
Lateral nystagmus	Present	Absent or occasional	Absent
Unstimulated blinking	Present	Absent	Absent
Eyeball position	Centered	Rotated anteromedially	Centered
Tearing	Present	Absent or reduced	Absent

*Not useful after administration of dissociative anesthetics.
From Hubbell JAE: Monitoring. *In* Muir WW and Hubbell JAE (editors): Equine Anesthesia Monitoring and Emergency Therapy. St Louis, Mosby–Year Book, 1991, p. 155.

undergoing open chest procedures. Although ventilatory assistance is not vital to the survival of most patients undergoing general anesthesia, ventilation should be assisted to aid in the maintenance of normal ventilation ($Paco_2 = 35$ to 45 mm Hg) and to minimize atelectasis, which occurs over time.

Assisted ventilation involves closing the pop-off valve and compressing the rebreathing bag. Many anesthesia machines are equipped with a pressure manometer, which measures the pressure inside the breathing system (see Figs. 15–3 and 15–6). A peak inspiratory pressure of 15 to 25 cm H_2O (small animals) and 25 to 30 cm H_2O (large animals) is sufficient to deliver an adequate tidal volume to the patient. Higher pressures may be needed in animals with open thoracic cavities or with primary lung disease. Ventilation should be assisted once or twice per minute, and the animal should be "sighed" once every 5 to 10 minutes. The latter involves slightly higher peak inspiratory pressures to specifically combat atelectasis.

Most veterinary hospitals are not equipped with mechanical ventilators; however, several types of ventilators are available and will enhance the quality of anesthesia (Fig. 15–14) (Muir et al., 1989; Shawley, 1987). More detailed descriptions of mechanical ventilators and their use are available in the literature (see Muir et al., 1989; Shawley, 1987).

ANESTHETIC MANAGEMENT

Several principles apply to the perianesthetic management of veterinary patients regardless of species. These are outlined and specific differences between species are noted in Table 15–7.

Preanesthetic Evaluation

The patient's history should be reviewed and a thorough physical examination performed, giving special attention to the cardiovascular and pulmonary system, prior to anesthesia (see Table 15–5). Minimal laboratory data consist of packed cell volume (PCV) and total protein concentration (see Table 15–5) in healthy animals. For high-risk patients, such as geriatric animals and animals with systemic diseases, a CBC, serum chemistry panel, electrolyte concentrations, and urinalysis should also be performed. An ECG should be recorded in traumatized and geriatric patients and in patients with evidence of cardiac arrhythmias or murmurs. Thoracic radiographs are indicated in patients with evidence of cardiac or pulmonary disease and those with a history of trauma. Abnormalities detected on physical examination and laboratory evaluation (such as anemia, respiratory distress, dehydration and electrolyte imbalance) should be corrected whenever possible prior to anesthetic induction.

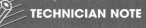

TECHNICIAN NOTE

Animals must be fasted prior to induction of general anesthesia to prevent regurgitation. Nonfasted animals should only be anesthetized in an emergency situation.

On the basis of the foregoing information, the animal's physical status should be established (Table 15–8). The physical

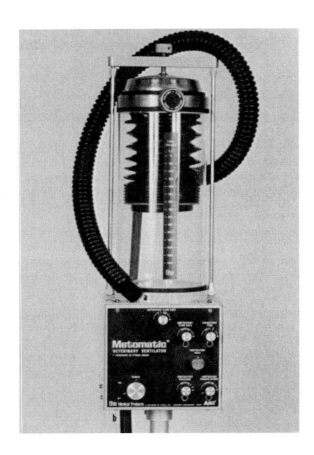

Figure 15-14. Metomatic veterinary ventilator for small animals. Tidal volume settings facilitate use in patients up to approximately 80 kg. The ventilator hose (a) is connected to the breathing system where the rebreathing bag is placed and the breathing system "pop-off" valve is closed. The waste gas scavenging system is then connected to the ventilator pop-off device (b) (Ohio Medical Products, Madison, WI).

• Table 15-7 •

	FASTING* (HOURS)		INTUBATION				
SPECIES	Food	Water	Technique	Desensitize Larynx	Laryngoscope Required	REGURGITATION POSSIBLE†	COMMENTS
Dog	12	12	Visualization	No	No‡	Yes	—
Cat	12	12	Visualization	Yes	No‡	Yes	May need stylet
Horse	8-12	2	Blind	No	No	No	Oral or nasal
Cattle	36-48	12-24	Digital	No	No	Yes	Use guide tube
Sheep, goat, calves	18-24	2	Visualization	Yes	Yes‡	Yes	Use guide tube
Swine	8-12	2-4	Visualization	Yes	Yes	Yes	Use guide tube

*Does not apply to neonates less than 1 month of age.

†The incidence of regurgitation increases when animals are not adequately fasted, in animals with a history of vomiting, and in pregnant animals. Regurgitation may occur in horses presented for colic which have gastric distention.

‡A laryngoscope may be needed to visualize the larynx in some brachycephalics and in dogs with pigmented mucosa. Although a laryngoscope is not essential for intubating cats, it may be necessary in some patients. Intubation may be performed blindly in small ruminants, but it is much more difficult and there is an increased risk of esophageal intubation, which may predispose to regurgitation and aspiration.

• Table 15–8 •

PHYSICAL STATUS CLASSIFICATIONS AS DEFINED BY THE AMERICAN SOCIETY OF ANESTHESIOLOGISTS		
CLASSIFICATION	**DEFINITION**	**EXAMPLE**
I	Normal animal admitted for elective surgery	Elective castration
II	Animal with slight to moderate systemic disturbance	Obesity, dehydration
III	Animal with major systemic disturbance which limits activity but is not incapacitating	Heart disease, anemia, severe fracture
IV	Animal with very severe systemic disturbance that could lead to death if surgical or medical intervention is not applied	Frequent arrhythmias, ruptured bladder, internal hemorrhage, severe pneumothorax
V	Animal in a moribund state that will probably die despite surgical or medical intervention	Prolonged gastric dilation/volvulus, severe trauma with shock

status indicates the risk for development of anesthetic complications in the individual patient and aids in the selection of an anesthetic protocol. The animal should be *fasted* prior to anesthesia; the duration varies among species (see Table 15–7). Neonates, birds, and patients under 2 kg should not be fasted because of limited glycogen stores and high metabolic rates.

Preparation of Equipment and Supplies

Selection of an anesthetic protocol is based on several factors, including the animal's temperament and physical status, the procedure to be performed, the available anesthetics, the familiarity of personnel with the drugs available, and the amount of assistance. Suggested protocols utilizing both inhalation and injectable techniques for the common domestic species are listed in Tables 15–9 to 15–13.

TECHNICIAN NOTE

Preparation of equipment and drugs is essential for successful anesthesia.

An anesthetic preparation checklist should be devised to optimize organization so that anesthetic induction and maintenance will be smooth and uncomplicated. Preparations may be completed after the animal has been premedicated and should include the following:

I. Organize necessary supplies for intravenous catheterization, including appropriate catheters, tape, heparinized saline, and antiseptics for sterile preparation of the skin site.
II. Organize equipment for endotracheal intubation, including appropriately sized tubes that have been checked for cuff leaks, laryngoscope, stylet and topical anesthetic spray if needed for the particular species, an oral speculum for

• Table 15–9 •

SUGGESTED PROTOCOLS FOR CHEMICAL RESTRAINT AND GENERAL ANESTHESIA IN DOGS	
NEUROLEPTANALGESIC COMBINATIONS FOR CHEMICAL RESTRAINT	
1. Acepromazine	0.22 mg/kg IV (maximum: 4 mg)
Oxymorphone	0.22 mg/kg IV (maximum: 4 mg)
2. Acepromazine	0.22 mg/kg IV (maximum: 4 mg)
Butorphanol	0.22–0.44 mg/kg IV
3. Atropine	0.044 mg/kg SC
Xylazine	0.22 mg/kg IV followed by:
Butorphanol	0.11–0.22 mg/kg IV
For animals in which acepromazine and xylazine should be avoided:	
4. Diazepam	0.22 mg/kg IV
Oxymorphone	0.22 mg/kg IV (maximum: 4 mg)
5. Diazepam†	0.22 mg/kg IV
Butorphanol	0.22–0.44 mg/kg IV
PROTOCOL FOR PHYSICAL STATUS I AND II ANIMALS	
Premedication	Acepromazine: 0.11 mg/kg IM (maximum: 2 mg)
	OR
	Acepromazine: 0.11 mg/kg IM (maximum: 2 mg) plus
	Butorphanol: 0.22–0.44 mg/kg IM
Induction	Thiopental
Maintenance	Halothane, isoflurane, or methoxyflurane
PROTOCOL FOR PHYSICAL STATUS ≥III ANIMALS	
Premedication	Neuroleptanalgesic combinations number 4 or 5 listed above. Alternate administration of ¼ calculated dose of each drug beginning with opioid until total dose has been administered or until desired degree of sedation is achieved.
Induction	Mask with isoflurane
	OR
	Ketamine: 2.2–4.4 mg/kg IV "to effect"
	OR
	Propofol: 2–4 mg/kg IV "to effect"
Maintenance	Isoflurane (if available). Halothane may be used but delivered concentrations should be minimized.
INJECTABLE PROTOCOLS FOR SHORT-DURATION ANESTHESIA*	
1. Atropine	0.044 mg/kg SC
Xylazine	0.66–1.1 mg/kg IV or IM
Ketamine	6.0–12.0 mg/kg IV or IM
2. Diazepam	0.25 mg/kg Mix and inject IV.
Ketamine	5.0 mg/kg Provides 10–15 minutes of anesthesia.
3. Atropine	0.044 mg/kg SC
Xylazine	0.44–0.88 mg/kg IV or IM
Telazol	4.4–11.0 mg/kg IV or IM

IV, intravenous; SC, subcutaneous; IM, intramuscular.
*Protocols 1 and 3 may be used IV or IM. Use higher dose range when administering IM. The IM route will be slower in onset of effect and will give a longer duration of anesthesia and a longer recovery.
†Midazolam may be used in place of diazepam at the same dose and may be administered IM, SC, or IV.

cattle, gauze or tape to secure the tube in place, sterile lubricant to facilitate passage of the tube into the trachea, and a syringe to inflate the endotracheal tube cuff.

III. Prepare the anesthesia machine and select a breathing system according to the animal's size (see selection criteria under Anesthesia Equipment):

A. Fill vaporizer and check the oxygen supply.

B. Evaluate soda lime absorbent and refill if material is exhausted.

C. Turn on flowmeter to check for free movement of indicator.

D. Close pop-off valve and pressurize the breathing system to 40 cm H_2O (on the pressure manometer) using the oxygen flush valve. This may be accomplished by placing your thumb over the patient connection. The system should maintain pressure if no leaks are present.

E. Connect the breathing system to the waste gas scavenging system.

IV. Calculate the oxygen flow rate according to patient size and breathing system used.

V. Organize fluids for administration and calculate the appropriate administration rate (see below).

• Table 15–10 •

SUGGESTED PROTOCOLS FOR CHEMICAL RESTRAINT AND GENERAL ANESTHESIA IN CATS

PROTOCOL FOR PHYSICAL STATUS I AND II ANIMALS

Premedication	Acepromazine: 0.06 mg/kg	
	Ketamine: 15 mg/kg	Mix and give IM
	OR	
	Butorphanol: 0.44 mg/kg SC	
Induction	Mask with halothane or isoflurane.	
	OR	
	Ketamine: 2.2–4.4 mg/kg IV "to effect"	
	OR	
	Thiopental: 4.0–8.0 mg/kg IV	
Maintenance	Halothane or isoflurane	

PROTOCOL FOR PHYSICAL STATUS ≥III ANIMALS

Premedication (if needed)	Butorphanol: 0.44 mg/kg SC	
Induction	Mask with isoflurane	
	OR	
	Diazepam: 0.25 mg/kg	Mix and give IV "to effect."
	Ketamine: 5.0 mg/kg	
	OR	
	Propofol	
		2–4 mg/kg IV "to effect."
Maintenance	Isoflurane (if available). Halothane may be used, but delivered concentrations should be minimized.	

INJECTABLE PROTOCOLS

1. Butorphanol	0.44 mg/kg	
Telazol	6–11 mg/kg	Mix and give IM.
2. Butorphanol	0.44 mg/kg	
Xylazine	0.44 mg/kg	
Ketamine	15–22 mg/kg	Mix and give IM.
3. Diazepam and ketamine may be used as above to provide 10–15 minutes of anesthesia.		
4. Acepromazine	0.1 mg/kg	
Butorphanol	0.44 mg/kg	
Ketamine	15–22 mg/kg	Mix and give IM.

IM, intramuscular; IV, intravenous

• Table 15–11 •

SUGGESTED PROTOCOLS FOR CHEMICAL RESTRAINT AND GENERAL ANESTHESIA IN HORSES

STANDING CHEMICAL RESTRAINT

1. Xylazine	0.44–0.66 mg/kg IV	(Give xylazine first.)
Butorphanol	0.022–0.044 mg/kg IV	
2. Detomidine	0.022 mg/kg IV	
3. Acepromazine	0.022–0.044 mg^g IV	(Give acepromazine
Xylazine	0.44 mg/kg IV	20 minutes prior to
Butorphanol	0.022 mg/kg IV	administration of other agents.)

PROTOCOLS FOR INDUCTION OF ANESTHESIA PRIOR TO MAINTENANCE WITH AN INHALATION AGENT

1. *Premedication*	Xylazine: 1.1 mg/kg IV	(Give xylazine and wait 3–5 minutes
Induction	Ketamine: 2.2 mg/kg IV	before administering ketamine.)
2. *Premedication*	Xylazine: 0.44 mg/kg IV	
	OR	
	Acepromazine: 0.044 mg/kg IV	
Induction	5% guaifensin IV "to effect"	
	Thiopental bolus: 4.4–6.6 mg/kg IV	
3. *Premedication*	Xylazine: 0.22–0.44 mg/kg IV	(This protocol works well in old,
Induction	5% guaifenesin "to effect"	debilitated, and colic patients.)
	Ketamine: 1.5–1.8 mg/kg IV	

INJECTABLE PROTOCOLS FOR INDUCTION AND MAINTENANCE OF GENERAL ANESTHESIA

Xylazine and ketamine as listed above provides 8–12 minutes of anesthesia. Duration of anesthesia may be extended by:

1. Administering butorphanol (0.022 mg/kg IV) or diazepam (0.055 mg/kg IV) prior to ketamine administration.

OR

2. Simultaneous administration of 50% of the original dose of xylazine and ketamine at 15–20 minute intervals. Do not repeat more than two times.

OR

3. Administering a combination of 1 liter of 5% guaifenesin containing 1 mg/ml of ketamine and 0.5 mg/ml of xylazine. The combination is administered at a constant drip (approximately 2.2 ml/kg/hour) until the procedure ends.

IV, intravenous.

VI. Calculate dosage for induction drugs. Withdraw drugs from bottles into labeled syringes.

Endotracheal Intubation

Endotracheal intubation techniques in a variety of species are described in Table 15–7. Several principles should be remembered when performing intubation in any species:

1. Inject air into cuff before use to check the cuff's ability to hold volume.

2. Always have two or three tube sizes readily available for each patient in case the first selection is too small or too large.

3. For cats, dogs, small ruminants, and swine, positioning the animal in sternal recumbency so that the head and neck are in a straight line offers the best visualization of the larynx for successful intubation. Some anesthetists prefer dorsal recumbency to perform intubation in swine. Horses and adult cattle

• Table 15–12 •

SUGGESTED PROTOCOLS FOR CHEMICAL RESTRAINT AND GENERAL ANESTHESIA IN RUMINANTS

CATTLE

Premedication Xylazine: 0.022–0.066 mg/kg IM (may not be required depending on animal's temperament and available restraint)

Induction 1 liter of 5% guaifenesin plus 2–3 mg/ml of thiopental (give until animal assumes recumbency and can be intubated)

OR

1 liter of 5% guaifensin plus 1.0–2.0 mg/ml of ketamine given "to effect"

Maintenance Halothane or isoflurane

INJECTABLE PROTOCOLS FOR INDUCTION AND MAINTENANCE OF ANESTHESIA

1. 1 liter 5% guaifenesin plus 2 mg/ml thiopental may be used for induction and maintenance: 1 liter will provide induction and 30–45 minutes of anesthesia for a 500-kg animal. If a second bottle is required, only 1 mg/ml of thiopental should be added to the guaifenesin.

2. 1 liter 5% guaifenesin plus 1 mg/ml of ketamine plus 0–50 mg of xylazine (total). Omit xylazine if the animal was premedicated with xylazine. This combination may be used for induction (2.2–4.4 ml/kg) and maintenance (2.2 ml/kg/hour), and 1 bottle may last 30–90 minutes depending on the animal's size and type of procedure.

SHEEP AND GOATS

Premedication Acepromazine: 0.055–0.11 mg/kg IV or IM

Diazepam: 0.22–0.55 mg/kg IV (usually not required because animals are easy to restrain)

Induction Thiopental: 11 mg/kg IV (Give "to effect" to facilitate intubation.)

OR

Diazepam (0.25–0.5 mg/kg) plus ketamine (4.4 mg/kg): Mix and give IV "to effect" to facilitate intubation. (This combination is good for debilitated, old, or diseased animals.)

Maintenance Halothane or isoflurane

INJECTABLE PROTOCOLS FOR INDUCTION AND MAINTENANCE OF ANESTHESIA

1. Xylazine: 0.11 mg/kg IM followed in 15 minutes by ketamine: 11.0 mg/kg IV (This combination provides 30–45 minutes of anesthesia. The recovery is prolonged but may be shortened by reversing the xylazine.)

2. Diazepam and ketamine as described above under induction provides 5–10 minutes of anesthesia.

3. Telazol: 2.2–6.6 mg/kg IV or IM provides 20–30 minutes of anesthesia.

IM, intramuscular; IV, intravenous.

are usually intubated while positioned in lateral recumbency with the head, neck, and back placed in a straight line to facilitate introduction of the tube into the larynx (Figs. 15–15 and 15–16). Horses may also be intubated via the ventral meatus of the nasal cavity (a smaller tube must be used) with the head positioned as described above, and this position may be indicated for procedures involving the oral cavity. This method is especially applicable to foals and may be performed in the awake foal with minimal sedation to facilitate a rapid method of induction with inhalation anesthetics (Fig. 15–17).

4. A stylet with an atraumatic tip may be necessary in some situations. A rigid stylet will provide support for very flimsy tubes and will facilitate proper placement. In species such as small ruminants, swine, and sometimes cats, an atraumatic stylet such as a dog urinary catheter will facilitate introduction of the tube into the larynx. These species have a sensitive larynx, which is prone to laryngospasm. Visualization is poor in small ruminants and swine owing to their narrow oral cavity, and use of both a laryngoscope and a stylet is especially beneficial. In adult cattle, one can introduce a nasogastric tube into the trachea by digitally palpating the laryngeal opening. The endotracheal tube is then guided over the smaller and longer nasogastric tube and into the trachea. *The use of a wire or any sharp instrument as a stylet is not advised; severe and even fatal tracheal trauma could result!*

5. The conservative use of a topical anesthetic agent in the laryngeal area (see Fig. 15–1), specifically in cats, swine, and small ruminants, will facilitate intubation with minimal trauma.

6. Adequate anesthesia and muscle relaxation are important for successful intubation. This will avoid unnecessary laryngeal trauma and excessive autonomic nervous system stimulation, which may give rise to cardiac arrhythmias.

7. The endotracheal tube should be long enough to reach midway between the larynx and carina so that accidental dislodgment does not occur. It should not be too long because this can increase the risk of endobronchial intubation, and an excessive tube length that extends beyond the oral cavity constitutes dead space, which can contribute to hypercapnia.

8. Proper tube placement may be assessed by (a) visualization of the tube passing between the arytenoid cartilages (not applicable in horses and cattle), (b) condensation of respiratory gases on the inside of the tube with expiration, (c) only one tubular structure (trachea) palpable in the neck region, (d) auscultation of lung sounds during assisted ventilation, and (e) absence of vocalization.

9. The cuff should be inflated just enough to form an effective seal within the trachea. This can be assessed by closing the pop-off valve, assisting ventilation, and listening for air escaping around the cuff or checking for the smell of anesthetic gas.

10. Secure the tube to the patient by tying gauze tightly around the tube and then securing it around the head (cats, brachycephalic breeds) or to the upper or lower jaw. This is usually not necessary in horses and adult cattle.

Fluid Administration During Anesthesia

Fluid administration is important to the maintenance of homeostasis during anesthesia and provides venous access for the delivery of agents used intraoperatively for supportive therapy (such as antibiotics, inotropic agents), for maintenance of anesthesia (injectable anesthetic agents), and for cardiopulmonary resuscitation. Imbalances may occur owing to blood loss, drying of exposed tissues, removal of effusions, and the hypotensive

• Table 15–13 •

SUGGESTED PROTOCOLS FOR CHEMICAL RESTRAINT AND GENERAL ANESTHESIA IN SWINE		
Premedication	Atropine: 0.044 mg/kg IM Xylazine: 1.1–2.2 mg/kg IM Ketamine: 2.2–4.4 mg/kg IM OR	Can mix and give as one injection.
	Atropine: 0.044 mg/kg IM Xylazine: 1.1 mg/kg IM Telazol: 6.0 mg/kg IM (decrease to 2.0–3.0 mg/kg for swine >50 kg)	Can mix and give as one injection.
Induction	Mask with halothane or isoflurane to facilitate intubation or maintain on mask.	
Maintenance	Halothane or isoflurane	
Injectable Protocols for Maintenance of Anesthesia		
Premedication	See above protocols. These combinations will facilitate catheter placement in an ear vein.	
Induction	1 liter of 5% guaifenesin plus 1 mg/ml xylazine and 1 mg/ml ketamine.	
Maintenance	Drip at an approximate rate of 2.2 ml/kg/hour.	

effects of anesthetic agents. The following guidelines will keep fluid therapy during anesthesia simple and effective:

I. Fluids most commonly used are polyionic isotonic crystalloid solutions, such as lactated Ringer's solution (LRS). For neonates (< 1 month of age), very small patients, and birds, use 5% dextrose or supplement LRS with 5 or 10 ml of 50% dextrose per 100 ml of LRS for a dextrose concentration of 2.5% or 5.0%, respectively.

II. For healthy animals during routine procedures the following fluid rates are suggested: *small animals, 10 to 20 ml/kg/hour; large animals, 5 to 10 ml/kg/hour. Exceptions to the foregoing fluid rates include:*

A. Increasing the administration rate in animals with preexisting dehydration, excessive intraoperative blood loss, or hypotension, and during cardiopulmonary resuscitation.

B. Decreasing the administration rate in animals that have significant cardiac or renal disease or are hypoproteinemic. These situations make the animals more prone to the development of pulmonary edema because they are unable to handle the additional fluid load.

III. Blood lost during surgery should be replaced at a volume of three times the approximate loss in addition to the

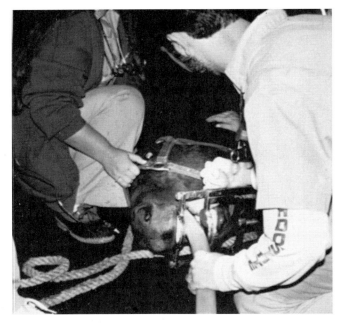

Figure 15–15. Positioning a horse to facilitate endotracheal intubation using the blind technique. An oral speculum is positioned between the incisor teeth to hold the mouth open, and the tongue is pulled out of the mouth.

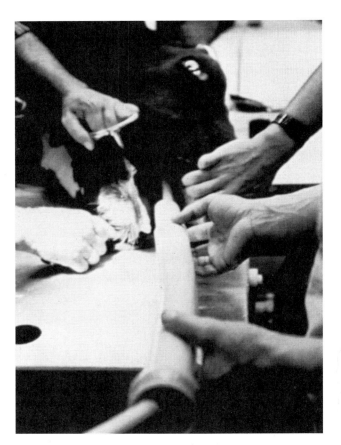

Figure 15–16. Endotracheal intubation of adult cattle requires placement of an oral speculum, digital palpation of the larynx, and introduction of a nasogastric tube into the trachea to guide the endotracheal tube into the trachea.

basic fluid rate during anesthesia. Ideally, when blood loss is significant, the PCV and total protein should be monitored to avoid excessive dilution. An acute fall in PCV below 20% should be treated with packed red cells or whole blood. Total protein should not fall below 3.5 g/dl because of the increased risk of developing pulmonary edema.

Induction and Maintenance

Guidelines for induction and maintenance are as follows:

1. Turn on oxygen flow a few minutes prior to connection of the patient to the breathing system to fill the system with oxygen.
2. Connect the endotracheal tube to the breathing system and turn on the vaporizer to the appropriate induction setting (see Table 15–4).
3. Assess pulse rate and quality.
4. Assess respiration. If the animal is apneic or the rate is slow, assist ventilation.
5. Apply ophthalmic ointment.
6. Reduce vaporizer settings to the appropriate maintenance concentration as indicated by the patient's anesthetic depth.
7. Begin intravenous fluid administration.
8. Begin monitoring and instrumentation with available monitoring equipment.
9. Record all pertinent information in the anesthetic record and begin recording vital signs every 5 minutes (see Fig. 15–8).
10. When using injectable techniques in horses and adult cattle, procedures should be limited to 1 hour. For procedures lasting longer than 1 hour, an oxygen source should be available to insufflate oxygen (10 to 15 liters/minute) into the nares to prevent the development of hypoxia due to hypoventilation and atelectasis. The anesthetic period should also be limited to 1 hour in small animals when injectable protocols are used. For longer procedures, oxygen should be administered through an endotracheal tube or, preferably, inhalation anesthesia should be used.

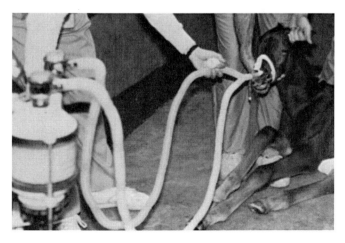

Figure 15-17. Newborn foal with an endotracheal tube introduced through the ventral meatus of the nasal cavity into the trachea for induction of anesthesia with isoflurane.

Padding and Positioning of the Patient

Proper padding and positioning depend on the procedure to be performed and the particular species.

1. Dogs, cats, neonates of all species, and all other small species should be placed on a covered heating pad or circulating water blanket when available to minimize hypothermia. *Never* place the animal directly on a heating pad or water blanket.
2. When securing limbs to the surgery table, do not apply ties too tightly and do not apply excessive traction to the forelimbs. Both actions may result in neurological damage and the latter may impede ventilatory effort.
3. Ensure that the head and neck are positioned to avoid kinking of the endotracheal tube or disconnection from the breathing system.
4. Assure that appropriate expansion of the thorax is not compromised.
5. For horses and adult cattle, adequate padding, such as a thick foam pad, water-filled pad, or air dunnage bag, is essential to prevent the development of postoperative myositis and neuropathy. For procedures in the field, a grassy area offers the best padding. The down eye should be protected and the head padded if possible.
6. For horses and cattle in lateral recumbency, the upper fore- and hindlimbs should be supported so that they are parallel to the table surface. The down forelimb should be pulled forward to avoid entrapment of the brachial plexus between the rib cage and humerus.
7. Always remove the halter from horses during general anesthesia to avoid damage to cranial nerves by the metal connectors.
8. Ruminants should be placed in right lateral recumbency *when possible* so that the rumen is on the up side. During lateral recumbency, the neck should be elevated with a soft pad so that the head angles downward to promote flow of saliva and regurgitation (if it occurs) out of the oral cavity.
9. Because of the high incidence of regurgitation in mature ruminants, an endotracheal tube should be placed and the cuff inflated (even if injectable anesthetics are used) before positioning the animal (especially in dorsal recumbency).

TECHNICIAN NOTE

Hypothermia is a significant problem during general anesthesia, especially in small animals, and can be life-threatening. Precautions to minimize heat loss should always be part of anesthetic management.

Recovery

Guidelines for recovery from anesthesia vary according to species.

Dogs and Cats

1. Flush the breathing system with pure oxygen and continue oxygen delivery for 5 to 10 minutes.

2. Deflate the cuff (*if* the animal is not at risk for regurgitation) and extubate only *after* swallowing is observed. Suction the oral cavity prior to extubation if excessive secretions have collected. Maintain the tube in place as long as possible in brachycephalic breeds, which are prone by conformation to upper airway obstruction following anesthesia.
3. Position the animal in sternal recumbency with the head extended if possible. This is especially important in brachycephalic breeds.
4. Most animals are hypothermic following general anesthesia, and an external heat source will hasten recovery and return to normothermia. Hot-water bottles, heating pads, or a circulating water blanket may be used, but *never* place it directly on the patient's skin.
5. Changing the animal's position and rubbing the body will hasten recovery.
6. Use analgesics (such as opioids) postoperatively if the procedure was invasive (such as orthopedic surgery, thoracotomy, abdominal surgery).
7. Some patients may need continued intravenous fluid therapy (e.g., patients with renal disease, dehydration) and the suggested maintenance rate is 60 ml/kg/24 hours.
8. Check the animal frequently until it can maintain sternal recumbency and stand unassisted.

Horses

1. When inhalation anesthesia is used, the horse should be placed in a padded dark room and allowed to recover unassisted. Extubate with the cuff deflated when swallowing is observed. A safer method to ensure a patent airway throughout recovery is to extubate when anesthesia is discontinued and place a smaller noncuffed tube into the trachea via the nasal passage and secure it to the muzzle with tape. This tube may be left in place until the horse is standing.
2. If available, insufflate oxygen (10 to 15 liters/minute) via the recovery tube or nasal cavity for 15 to 30 minutes following the end of anesthesia.
3. For recoveries in the field, the halter should be replaced so that the animal can be assisted during recovery. The eye should be covered to minimize external stimulation.
4. Some horses have a rough recovery regardless of the technique used. Administration of a sedative such as xylazine or a tranquilizer such as acepromazine or diazepam in low doses will quiet the animal until it is ready to rise unassisted.

Ruminants

1. If inhalation anesthesia is used, 100% oxygen should be administered for 5 to 10 minutes after anesthetic delivery is discontinued.
2. Ruminants should be positioned in sternal recumbency as soon as possible to promote eructation and minimize the chance of regurgitation.
3. Extubation should be performed with the cuff *inflated* only after swallowing is observed.

4. A stomach tube should be passed to decompress the rumen if bloat has developed intraoperatively.
5. Ruminants generally recover smoothly from general anesthesia and minimal assistance is required.

Swine

1. Continue oxygen for 5 to 10 minutes after anesthetic delivery has been discontinued when inhalation techniques have been used.
2. Extubate with the cuff deflated (unless there is evidence of regurgitation) when swallowing is observed.
3. Position the animal in sternal recumbency as soon as possible and allow the animal to recover in a cool and quiet environment.

POSTOPERATIVE ANALGESIA

Any procedure considered to be painful to humans should be considered painful to animals and if there is any doubt whether or not an animal is in pain, it should be treated (Tranquilli et al., 1989). In large animals, nonsteroidal anti-inflammatory agents, such as phenylbutazone or flunixin meglumine, are most commonly used. In small animals, systemic administration of opioids, such as oxymorphone, butorphanol, morphine, or buprenorphine, is excellent for postoperative pain management (see Table 15–2 for dosages). Buprenorphine offers the advantage of prolonged duration of effect (8 to 12 hours). While butorphanol and buprenorphine are useful in cats, the pure opioid agonists (oxymorphone and morphine) may elicit an excitatory response and should be used in conjunction with a tranquilizer.

An alternative to systemic opioid administration is epidural administration, offering the advantages of longer duration of action and elimination of side effects such as respiratory depression and bradycardia. Epidural morphine *(0.1 mg/kg) diluted in saline (1 ml/5 kg not to exceed 6 ml) or a local anesthetic* provides a duration of action of 10 to 24 hours. Butorphanol *(0.2 mg/kg)*, oxymorphone *(0.1 mg/kg)*, and buprenorphine *(0.003 to 0.005 mg/kg)* may also be used epidurally, but have a shorter duration than morphine (Carroll, 1996). Systemic and epidural opioids are also useful for pain management in small ruminants and swine (epidural dosages as listed above). Additional information concerning pain management may be found in Chapter 20.

ANESTHETIC EMERGENCIES

Anesthesia causes a stress to homeostasis, including respiratory and cardiac depression, which may increase the risk of cardiopulmonary arrest, especially in high-risk patients. Cardiopulmonary arrest is the sudden cessation of ventilation and effective circulation that requires rapid emergency intervention (cardiopulmonary resuscitation) to prevent death. Physical status categorization alerts the anesthetist to the likelihood that complications that may lead to arrest could occur in a particular patient and stresses the importance of careful monitoring throughout the anesthetic period. Complications may occur at any time during the anesthetic period, including induction, maintenance, and recovery.

Cardiopulmonary resuscitation (CPR) is subdivided into

• Table 15–14 •

READINESS CHECKLIST FOR CARDIOPULMONARY RESUSCITATION
• Well-lighted area with adequate workspace
• Clippers
• Emergency drugs (see Table 15-15)
• Endotracheal tubes
• Tracheostomy tubes
• Face masks
• Method for artificial ventilation (anesthesia machine or Ambu bag)
• Oxygen source
• Gauze for securing endotracheal tube
• Needles and syringes
• Laryngoscope
• Aspiration device
• Intravenous catheters
• Electrocardiograph machine
• Defibrillator

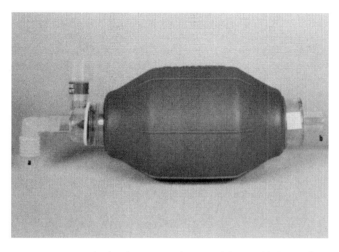

Figure 15–19. Ambu bag may be used to ventilate patients during cardiopulmonary arrest. The bag is attached to the endotracheal tube (a) and squeezed to deliver a breath. Some Ambu bags are equipped with tubing for connection to an oxygen source (b).

four phases, including readiness and prevention, recognition and basic cardiac life support, advanced cardiac life support, and postresuscitative care.

Readiness and Prevention

Hospital personnel should be prepared to handle cardiopulmonary arrest by identifying an area in the hospital that is well-lighted and stocked with emergency equipment and drugs (Table 15–14; Figs. 15–18 and 15–19). Staff member involved in resuscitation should have an assigned role, which should be practiced periodically in mock drills to improve response time and the quality of treatment.

Prevention, as it applies to anesthetic-related cardiopulmonary arrest, involves recognition of high-risk patients and the application of appropriate and effective monitoring of all anesthetized patients. Clinical signs that may indicate an impending arrest include cyanosis; changes in respiration, such as apnea, tachypnea, dyspnea, or a marked abdominal effort associated with breathing; and changes associated with the cardiovascular system, such as bradycardia, tachycardia, weak, irregular or

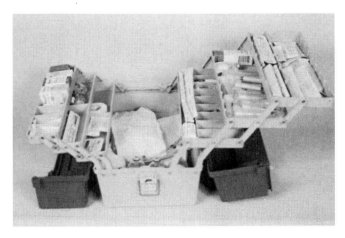

Figure 15–18. Example of a utility box used to organize emergency equipment and drugs for anesthetic emergencies.

absent pulse, pale mucous membranes, and increased CRT. Hypothermia may increase the risk of arrest by contributing to the development of bradycardia and excessive anesthetic depth. A body temperature less than 30°C (86°F) predisposes to life-threatening ventricular arrhythmias. Recognition and correction of some potentially life-threatening problems are listed in Table 15–15.

Recognition and Basic Life Support

Early recognition of cardiopulmonary arrest, if prevention was ineffective, is critical to successful resuscitation and is optimized by effective patient monitoring. The initial actions to be taken in the arrest of an anesthetized patient are to discontinue delivery of the anesthetic agent, flush the breathing system with pure oxygen, and increase the fluid administration rate. Reversal of anesthetic agents, such as opioids or xylazine, may also be indicated in the anesthetized patient with cardiac arrest. The basic life support techniques should be initiated concurrently and include the following:

1. *Airway.* If the animal is not already intubated (as with injectable techniques), an endotracheal tube is placed. If the animal is already intubated, the tube should be checked for proper placement and patency. If an endotracheal tube cannot be placed or is not patent owing to an obstruction, a tracheostomy should be performed or the tube changed, respectively.
2. *Breathing.* Breathe for the patient using the anesthesia machine or an Ambu bag (see Fig. 15–19), preferably with 100% oxygen, at a rate of 20 breaths per minute performed simultaneously with every third to sixth chest compression, depending on the compression rate.
3. *Circulation.* If a pulse or heartbeat cannot be detected, external cardiac compressions should be initiated, the goal being to maintain adequate blood flow to the brain and heart until normal heart rhythm can be restored. In most animals, compressions are performed

• Table 15–15 •

DIFFERENTIAL DIAGNOSIS AND TREATMENT OF COMPLICATIONS THAT MAY OCCUR DURING ANESTHESIA

ABNORMALITY	POTENTIAL CAUSES	TREATMENT
Bradycardia	Excessive anesthetic depth Drugs: opioids, xylazine, gas anesthetics Hyperkalemia Vagal reflex (intubation, oculocardiac reflex) Visceral manipulation Hypothermia Terminal stages or hypoxia Exogenous and endogenous toxemias	Correct underlying cause if possible Administer anticholinergic agent Administer sympathomimetic agent Dopamine: 2–20 µg/kg/minute* Dobutamine: 2–20 µg/kg/minute* Ephedrine: 0.05–0.5 mg/kg bolus* Isoproterenol: 5–10 µg/kg/minute*
Tachycardia	Drugs: ketamine, thiobarbiturates, anticholinergics, sympathomimetics Hypokalemia Hyperthermia Inadequate anesthetic depth Hypercapnia, hypoxemia Anemia, hypovolemia Hyperthyroidism, pheochromocytoma Anaphylaxis	Correct underlying cause if possible

Atrial and ventricular premature contractions	Light anesthesia
	Deep anesthesia
	Hypoxia, hypercapnia
	Hypovolemia
	Exogenous catecholamine therapy
	Digitalis toxicity
	Hypokalemia
	Hyperkalemia
	Hypercalcemia
	Certain anesthetics (xylazine, halothane, thiobarbiturates)
	Endocarditis or myocarditis
	Severe hypothermia
	End-stage visceral organ failure
	Intracranial disorders
		Correct underlying cause if possible
		Evaluate anesthetic depth
		Check anesthetic machine and oxygen flow
		Assist ventilation
		If arrhythmia persists and meets one or more of the following criteria:
		  (1) >20 per minute
		  (2) Increasing in frequency
		  (3) Multifocal
		  (4) Occurring in runs
		  (5) Causing significant effect on pulse
		Treat arrhythmia as follows:
		  (1) Turn off anesthetic gas
		  (2) Increase fluid administration rate
		  (3) Administer lidocaine IV (maximum: 4 doses)
		    Dog: 2.2 mg/kg
		    Cat, horse: 0.5 mg/kg

Hypotension	Hypovolemia (i.e., blood loss)
	Sepsis
	Shock
	Drugs (thiobarbiturates, inhalant)
		Increase fluid administration rate
		Decrease aesthetic concentration
		Administer sympathomimetic agents
		  Dopamine: 2–20 µg/kg/minute*
		  Dobutamine: 2–20 µg/kg/minute*
		  Ephedrine: 0.055–0.55 mg/kg bolus (small animals)*
		    0.022 mg/kg bolus (horse)*

Tachypnea	Pain Hypoxia Hypercapnia Hyperthermia Acidosis Drugs (i.e., doxapram)	Correct underlying cause if possible
Apnea	Hypothermia Hyperventilation with 100% O_2 Drug effects (thiopental, ketamine) Deep anesthesia Aminoglycoside administration	Correct underlying cause if possible Assist ventilation until spontaneous ventilation returns

IV, intravenous.
*These drugs may cause cardiac arrhythmias. Monitor electrocardiogram during administration.

• Table 15–16 •

EMERGENCY DRUG DOSAGES AND DEFIBRILLATION SETTINGS USED FOR CARDIOPULMONARY RESUSCITATION				
DRUG	**CONCENTRATION**	**DOSAGE**	**INDICATION**	**COMMENTS**
Epinephrine	1 mg/ml	0.02–0.2 mg/kg (SA) 0.0011–0.0055 mg/kg (LA)	Initiate heartbeat Increase heart rate Increase contractility Improve blood flow during CPR	Dose may be repeated every 5 minutes
Atropine	0.5 mg/ml	0.044 mg/kg (SA) 0.011 mg/kg (LA)	Increase heart rate Treat ventricular asystole	
Lidocaine	20 mg/ml	2.2 mg/kg (dogs) 0.5 mg/kg (cats) 0.5 mg/kg (LA)	Treat ventricular arrhythmias	
Prednisolone sodium succinate (Solu-Delta-Cortef)	10 mg/ml 50 mg/ml	22 mg/kg (SA) 2.2 mg/kg (LA)	Shock and ischemia Stabilize cellular membranes Prevent cerebral edema	
OR Dexamethasone sodium phosphate	4 mg/ml	2.2–4.4 mg/kg		
Sodium bicarbonate	1 mEq/ml	0.5–1.0 mEq/kg per 5 minutes of arrest	Treat metabolic acidosis	Use after 10 minutes of arrest or with preexisting acidosis only
Calcium chloride	100 mg/ml	10 mg/kg (SA) 2.2 mg/kg (LA)	Prevent arrhythmias associated with hyperkalemia Treat hypocalcemia	Has been incriminated in reperfusion injury
Hypertonic saline	70 mg/ml	4 ml/kg	Treat hypovolemic shock Restore vascular volume	Must be used with isotonic fluids
Furosemide	50 mg/ml	1.1 mg/kg	Treat pulmonary and cerebral edema	Monitor hydration status
Mannitol	200 mg/ml	0.55–1.1 mg/kg	Treat cerebral edema Protect brain against reperfusion injury	Monitor hydration status
Doxapram	20 mg/ml	1.1–4.4 mg/kg (SA) 0.22 mg/kg (LA)	Initiate breathing	Better to treat underlying problem
Direct current defibrillation	Body wt. External Internal	<8 kg / 2 w-s/kg 0.5–2.0 w-s/kg 8–40 kg / 2–5 w-s/kg >40 kg / 5–10 w-s/kg	Treatment of ventricular fibrillation	

SA, small animal; LA, large animal; CPR, cardiopulmonary resuscitation; w-s, watt-second (joules), which defines units of energy output produced by an electrical defibrillator.

at the level of the costochondral junction between the fourth and eighth ribs at a rate of 80 to 120 per minute, with the animal in lateral recumbency. In barrel-chested dogs, such as the brachycephalic breeds, compressions may be more effective placed in a ventrodorsal direction with the animal stabilized in dorsal recumbency. Abdominal wrapping or interposed rhythmic abdominal compressions may help to improve forward blood flow by increasing the intrathoracic pressure generated.

Advanced Life Support

These techniques include diagnosis of the type of arrest, the use of emergency drugs, defibrillation and internal cardiac massage.

1. *Drugs.* Venous access is critical in the successful treatment of cardiac arrest. Although a central venous catheter (placed via the jugular vein) offers the most effective route for drug administration, such catheters

are not placed routinely, and placement following arrest is difficult and time-consuming. Drugs may be given by a peripheral venous catheter, if effective blood flow has been established by compression techniques, and a fluid bolus should follow administration of every drug used. The tracheal route via the endotracheal tube is effective for epinephrine, atropine, and lidocaine administration. Dosages should be twice those given intravenously, the dose should be diluted in 3 to 10 ml of saline, and several rapidly applied ventilations should follow administration to ensure distribution to the pulmonary vasculature. The intraosseous route (via the tibial tuberosity, greater tubercle of the humerus, trochanteric fossa of the femur, wing of the ilium) may also be used for fluid and drug administration if venous access cannot be achieved. Table 15–16 lists some of the commonly used emergency drugs, indications for their use, and dosages.

2. *Electrocardiogram.* An ECG should be recorded as

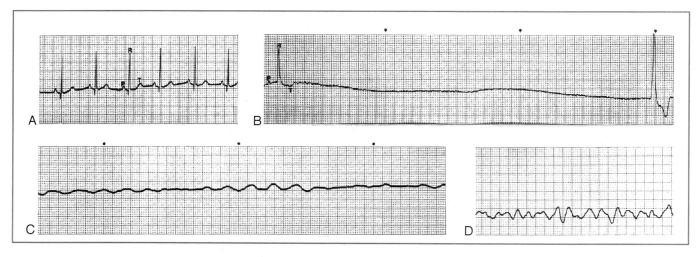

Figure 15–20.   Representative electrocardiogram tracings of the different types of cardiac arrest. A, Electromechanical dissociation presents as a normal tracing, but no palpable pulse is associated with the electrical activity. B, Ventricular asystole presents as a flat tracing. Fine (C), and coarse (D), ventricular fibrillation present as wavy lines. It is important to distinguish between fine and coarse ventricular fibrillation because the latter is easier to convert to normal rhythm with defibrillation techniques. (From Tiley LP: Essentials of Canine and Feline Electrocardiography. 3rd ed. Philadelphia, Lea & Febiger, 1992.)

soon as possible during the course of resuscitation to identify the type of arrest so that specific therapy for conversion to normal rhythm can be applied. The three types of cardiac arrest include ventricular asystole, ventricular fibrillation, and electromechanical dissociation. Figure 15–20 illustrates the three types of arrest, and Table 15–17 lists the specific treatment steps for each type of arrest.

3. *Fluid therapy.* Cardiac arrest is a rapidly vasodilating disease process, and fluid therapy, most often with an isotonic polyionic solution such as LRS, is essential. Never use dextrose-containing fluids during resuscitative efforts because dextrose may exacerbate brain damage. It is recommended that fluids be given

rapidly as calculated boluses so that overhydration, which may predispose to pulmonary and cerebral edema, is avoided. For cats, boluses of 20 ml/kg are recommended, and for dogs and most other species, boluses of 40 ml/kg are recommended. These boluses may be repeated as needed throughout resuscitation to maintain an effective circulating volume. Three percent to 7% hypertonic saline (4 ml/kg) has been shown to be beneficial in resuscitation efforts, in conjunction with isotonic fluid administration, to rapidly restore vascular volume and reduce the risk of development of pulmonary and cerebral edema.

4. *Internal cardiac massage.* If external techniques and drug administration have not established effective

• Table 15–17 •

CLASSIFICATIONS OF CARDIAC ARREST AND SUGGESTED TREATMENT PROTOCOL		
ARRHYTHMIA	**TREATMENT**	**DOSAGE**
Ventricular asystole	Epineprhine	0.02–0.2 mg/kg IV or IT*
	Atropine	0.044 mg/kg IV or IT
	Prednisolone sodium succinate (Solu-Delta-Cortef)	22 mg/kg IV
	Sodium bicarbonate (if >10–15 minutes)	1.0 mEq/kg IV
Ventricular fibrillation	Precordial thump	(if defibrillator not available)
	Epinephrine	0.2 mg/kg IV or IT
	Defibrillate	(see Table 15–15)
	Defibrillate	(double original dose)
	Lidocaine	2.2 mg/kg IV or IT (cats: 0.5 mg/kg)
	Sodium bicarbonate (if >10–15 minutes)	1.0 mEq/kg IV
Electromechanical dissociation	Epinephrine	0.2 mg/kg IV or IT
	Prednisolone sodium succinate (Solu-Delta-Cortef)	22 mg/kg IV
	OR	
	Dexamethasone sodium phosphate	2.2 mg/kg IV
	Sodium bicarbonate	1.0 mEq/kg IV

*IT, intratracheal administration: double the recommended intravenous dose.

circulation in 5 minutes or if the heart has not resumed normal rhythm in 10 minutes, a thoracotomy and internal massage should be performed at the left fourth or fifth intercostal space. This procedure should be performed immediately in very large or barrel-chested animals or in animals with fractured ribs or pneumothorax.

Postresuscitative Care

Patients may suffer arrest again following successful resuscitative efforts. Careful monitoring of the ECG, pulse quality, respiratory pattern, body temperature, and CNS (pupillary responses, mentation, seizure activity) is essential for several hours after the primary event. Neurological damage may become evident 24 to 48 hours after the arrest, so serial neurological examinations should be performed. Oxygen therapy should be administered for a period of time, depending on the condition of the patient.

Cardiopulmonary arrest in the anesthetized patient may be successfully treated only if the anesthetist recognizes the arrest early through careful monitoring and acts rapidly and correctly to reestablish normal cardiac rhythm before permanent organ damage occurs.

References

Bednarski RM: Anesthetic equipment. *In* Muir WW, Hubbell JAE (editors): Equine Anesthesia: Monitoring and Emergency Therapy. St Louis, Mosby–Year Book, 1991, pp. 325–351.

Carroll GL: How to manage perioperative pain. Vet Med 91:353–357, 1996.

Dorsch JA and Dorsch SE: The anesthesia machine. *In* Tracy TM (editor): Understanding Anesthesia Equipment, 2nd ed. Baltimore, Williams & Wilkins, 1984a, pp. 38–76.

Dorsch JA and Dorsch SE: The breathing system. IV. *In* Tracy TM (editor): Understanding Anesthesia Equipment, 2nd ed. Baltimore, Williams & Wilkins, 1984b, pp. 210–246.

Dorsch JA and Dorsch SE: Controlling trace gas levels. *In* Tracy TM (editor): Understanding Anesthesia Equipment, 2nd ed. Baltimore, Williams & Wilkins, 1984c, pp. 247–288.

Dorsch JA and Dorsch SE: Vaporizers. *In* Tracy TM (editor): Understanding Anesthesia Equipment, 2nd ed. Baltimore, Williams & Wilkins, 1984d, pp. 77–135.

Hartsfield SM: Machines and breathing systems for administration of inhalation anesthetics. *In* Short CE (editor): Principles and Practice of Veterinary Anesthesia. Baltimore, Williams & Wilkins, 1987, pp. 395–418.

Haskins SC: Monitoring the anesthetized patient. *In* Short CE (editor): Principles and Practice of Veterinary Anesthesia. Baltimore, Williams & Wilkins, 1987, pp. 455–477.

Heath RB, Broadstone RV, Wright M, et al.: Using bupivacaine hydrochloride for lumbosacral epidural analgesia. Compendium Continuing Educ Pract Vet 11:50–55, 1989.

Jones JL: Noninvasive monitoring techniques in anesthetized animals. Vet Med 91:326–336, 1996.

Klide AM and Soma LR: Epidural analgesia in the dog and cat. J Am Vet Med Assoc 153:165–173, 1968.

Muir WW, Hubbell JAE, and Skarda RT: Handbook of Veterinary Anesthesia. St Louis, Mosby–Year Book, 1989.

Paddleford RR: Anesthetic waste gases and your health. *In* Short CE (editor): Principles and Practice of Veterinary Anesthesia. Baltimore, Williams & Wilkins, 1987, pp. 607–620.

Shawley RV: Controlled ventilation and pulmonary function. *In* Short CE (editor): Principles and Practice of Veterinary Anesthesia. Baltimore, Williams & Wilkins, 1987, pp. 419–425.

Short CE: Anticholinergics *In* Short CE (editor): Principles and Practice of Veterinary Anesthesia. Baltimore, Williams & Wilkins, 1987, pp. 8–15.

Tranquilli WJ, Fikes LL, and Raffe MR: Selecting the right analgesics: Indications and dosage requirements. Vet Med 84:692–697, 1989.

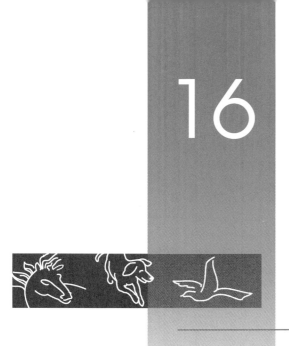

16 Surgical Instruments and Aseptic Technique

Randall Fitch • Jacqueline R. Davidson • Daniel J. Burba

INTRODUCTION

Surgery has a code of conduct which must be followed for the handling and processing of surgical instruments, and for the preparation of the patient and surgical team. A team approach provides the best possible patient care. All members of the surgical team must work cohesively and be completely familiar with instrumentation and aseptic technique. The technician is an invaluable part of the surgical team and can greatly enhance the quality and efficiency of the surgical procedure.

The veterinary technician is required to assist the veterinarian with many surgical procedures performed in large and small animal practices. The technician may need to provide nonsterile support by preparing the patient for surgery, acting as a circulating nurse in the operating room, and taking responsibility for the care, cleaning, packing, and sterilization of the instruments. In addition, the technician is often responsible for ordering surgical instruments and implants; therefore familiarity with this equipment is essential. The technician may also need to provide sterile support as a surgical scrub nurse or surgical assistant, so the principles of aseptic technique should be as second nature. As a surgical assistant the technician can be of great value by anticipating instruments which the surgeon will need and by aiding in tissue retraction and hemostasis. The technician's nonsterile or sterile participation is vitally important to the surgical team. These roles can be quite challenging and competent technicians achieve their own expertise in these areas.

INSTRUMENTATION

Thousands of different surgical instruments are available and new instruments are continually being designed to increase the efficiency and ease of performing procedures. Each instrument is designed for a specific purpose such as cutting, holding, clamping, or retracting. The surgical technician must know the purpose of each instrument in order to anticipate when it will be used and to understand how to handle and care for it.

TECHNICIAN NOTE

Each instrument is designed for a specific purpose such as cutting, holding, clamping or retracting.

General Surgery Instruments

Scalpel

The scalpel is the best instrument for incising tissues with minimal trauma. Generally, scalpel handles with interchangeable, disposable blades are used (Fig. 16–1). The *no. 3 Bard-Parker handle* uses detachable blades nos. 10, 11, 12, and 15 and is the most applicable for small animal surgery. The *no. 4 Bard-Parker handle* is larger and uses detachable blades nos. 20, 21, and 22. This handle is most commonly used for large animal surgery.

Electrosurgery

Electroscalpels are sometimes used to cut tissue. They cut by passing a high-frequency alternating electrical current through a small point of contact with the tissue (Fig. 16–2). Proper

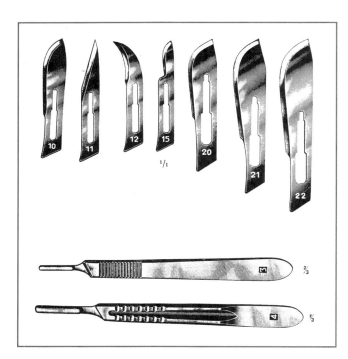

Figure 16-1. Scalpel handles and attachable surgical blades. Surgical blades Nos. 10, 11, 12, and 15 are interchangeable and mount onto the No. 3 Bard-Parker scalpel handle. Surgical blades Nos. 20–22 are interchangeable and mount onto the No. 4 Bard-Parker scalpel handle. The No. 3 scalpel handle and No. 10 blade are commonly used in small animal surgery. The No. 4 handle and No. 20 blade are commonly used in large animal surgery.

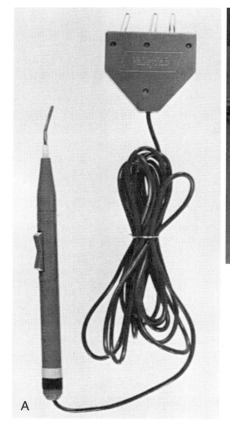

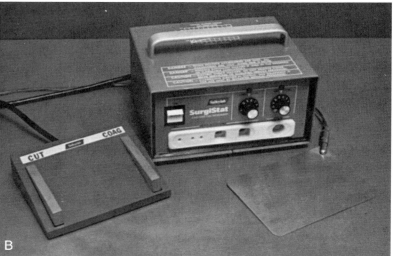

Figure 16-2. Electrosurgery equipment. A, Electrosurgery handpiece with a cutting/coagulation hand control. B, Electrosurgical foot switch, power source, and ground plate. The handpiece is kept sterile. The animal must be well grounded with good contact against the ground plate for the electrosurgery unit to function correctly. This unit provides two different modes of current (for coagulation and cutting).

grounding through a metal plate placed under the patient is essential to ensure good cutting performance and to avoid possible electrical burns. In addition to cutting tissue, electrocautery can provide rapid coagulation. Cutting or coagulation can be performed through the same handpiece and is controlled by a switch on the sterile handpiece or by a foot switch. Electrosurgery may provide many advantages over the steel scalpel including reduced surgery time, less blood loss, better visibility, and reduced need for ligatures. However, improper use will lead to greater tissue damage, delayed wound healing, greater scar width, and possibly skin burns. The technician is often responsible for ensuring that the patient is properly grounded and that the power level is adjusted according to the surgeon's needs.

Scissors

Scissors are used for sharp and blunt tissue dissection, and for cutting sutures and bandage materials. Dissecting scissors are made for accurate cutting and dissection of tissue. Many types of operating scissors are available. *Operating scissors* may vary by the type of blades (straight or curved), the type of points (blunt-blunt, blunt-sharp, or sharp-sharp), and the cutting edge of the blades (plain or serrated) (Fig. 16–3C). *Mayo dissecting scissors* (Fig. 16–3D) are heavy, straight, or curved scissors commonly used for cutting tough tissues such as heavy connective tissue. *Metzenbaum dissecting scissors* (Fig. 16–3E) are fine, curved scissors used for more delicate tissues such as fat and thin muscle. Metzenbaum scissors are the instrument of choice for soft tissue dissection with minimal surgical trauma. Special scissors are designed for cutting sutures. Stitch scissors or *Littauer suture removal scissors* (see Fig. 16–5A) should be used to cut all sutures except wire sutures. Dissecting scissors, such as Metzenbaum scissors, should not be used for cutting sutures because this dulls their edges and causes the blades to separate and lose their effectiveness. However, an older pair of operating scissors may be designated as suture scissors. *Wire suture-cutting scissors* are designed to cut wire, but they may also be

used to cut suture material (see Fig. 16–5B). *Lister bandage scissors* are available for cutting bandage material (see Fig. 16–5C). To prolong the life of a scissors, it should be used only for its intended purpose.

TECHNICIAN NOTE

Scissors are specifically designed for many purposes including sharp and blunt dissection of many different tissues, and for cutting sutures and bandage materials.

Needle Holders

Needle holders are specifically designed for holding curved suture needles during suturing and for performing instrument suture ties. *Mayo-Hegar* and *Olsen-Hegar* needle holders are two commonly used needle holders (Fig. 16–3A and B). The Olsen-Hegar needle holder has a built-in scissors. Suture material can be placed and cut with the same instrument; therefore, a separate suture scissors is not required. This may have an advantage for the veterinary surgeon who is performing surgery alone. The major disadvantage of this needle holder is that the suture may be cut accidentally. This can result in delay or complications, especially when a continuous suture pattern is used.

Needle holders consist of a set of jaws, a hinge or box lock, and handles with a ratcheted locking device (Fig. 16–4). The size and design of these components vary greatly depending on their intended use. The jaws commonly have tungsten carbide inserts which provide excellent grip. The tungsten carbide insert is hard, resistant to wear, and can be replaced when worn, thereby prolonging the life of the instrument. Worn inserts can result in improper closure of the jaws or sharp edges that inadvertently cut suture. Needle holders are available in different sizes, depending on the needle sizes they are designed

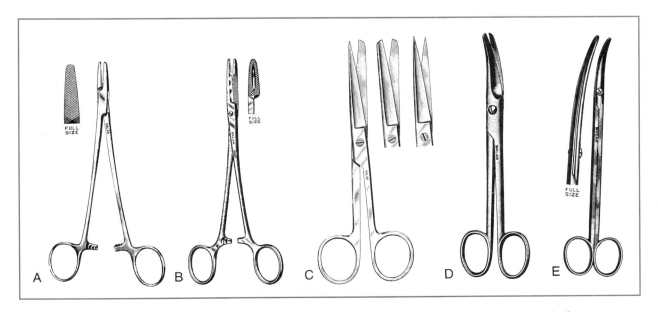
Figure 16-3. Needle holders. A, Mayo-Hegar. B, Olsen-Hegar (cutting scissors incorporated). Operating scissors. C, Operating scissors: sharp-blunt, blunt-blunt, and sharp-sharp. D, Mayo dissecting scissors. E, Metzenbaum dissecting scissors.

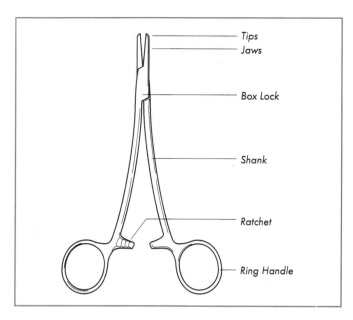

Figure 16-4 labels (top to bottom):
Tips
Jaws
Box Lock
Shank
Ratchet
Ring Handle

Figure 16-4. Basic components of a surgical instrument (Mayo-Hegar needle holder).

to hold. Improper use of needle holders (such as using a needle holder that is too small for the size of the needle or using the needle holder to bend or twist wire) may not only damage the jaws but may also spring the box lock and ratchet.

TECHNICIAN NOTE

Needle holders are designed for handling the suture needle and performing instrument suture ties.

Thumb Forceps

Thumb forceps are special tissue forceps designed to hold and easily release tissue with a simple finger motion (similar to tweezers). They have a spring action and the jaws are opposed by compressing the two metal handles together. Several different jaw surfaces are available and are designed for use with various tissues (Fig. 16–5D–G). *Brown-Adson thumb forceps* have multiple intermeshing teeth with a broad tip, providing good tissue and needle handling. They are commonly used during suturing and wound closure. *Rat-tooth thumb forceps* have large interdigitating teeth and are primarily used for skin or fascia. *Adson thumb forceps* have delicate intermeshing teeth ("rat-toothed") that provide a good, atraumatic grasp of delicate tissues. They are commonly used during dissection. *Cooley* and *DeBakey thumb forceps* have long, narrow jaws with multiple delicate sets of teeth which are especially good for vascular surgery. *Russian thumb forceps* have a broad curved surface good for needle handling, but are traumatic when used to hold tissues (Fig. 16–6A). *Dressing thumb forceps* do not have teeth and are used for applying and removing dressings (Fig. 16–6B). They are not designed to grasp tissue and are undesirable for this use because the surgeon must squeeze hard and crush the

tissue in order to grasp it. Thumb forceps are available in a variety of sizes depending on the intended surgery. For example, thoracic forceps have very long handles to enable the surgeon to reach tissues deep within the chest, but these same forceps would be too cumbersome and awkward to use on the skin.

TECHNICIAN NOTE

Thumb forceps are commonly used in the surgeon's nondominant hand to hold tissues throughout surgery during incision, dissection, and suturing.

Tissue Forceps

Tissue forceps are locking self-retaining instruments which clamp on to tissues. They have different teeth patterns which allow them to grip various types of tissues without slipping. *Allis tissue forceps* are sturdy and provide a secure grasp of tissue but they also crush it (see Fig. 16–8C). Therefore, they are very traumatic and should only be used on tissue that is being removed. *Babcock forceps* are shaped similarly to the Allis forceps, but are designed for gentle tissue handling by means of a smooth grasping surface and less tip compression (see Fig. 16–8D). The Doyen intestinal tissue forceps, as an example, is a less traumatic, more delicate instrument used to occlude and hold intestine. The disadvantage of less traumatic tissue forceps is that they are less secure on the tissues.

TECHNICIAN NOTE

Tissue forceps are used to clamp and hold tissues with a self-locking mechanism.

Towel clamps are forceps used to attach towels and drapes to each other and to the patient. These forceps have pointed tips that curve and join like ice tongs. *Backhaus towel clamps* and *Roeder towel clamps* are two common designs (see Fig. 16–8E and F). The Roeder towel clamp has a metal bead or ball stop attached to the jaws which prevents deep tissue penetration and prevents the towel from slipping toward the box lock of the forceps.

Hemostatic Forceps

Hemostatic forceps are tissue forceps used to clamp blood vessels or tissue to stop bleeding. These are all crushing instruments and are used primarily to stop bleeding by collapsing the lumen of the vessel. These forceps come in several lengths and may be straight or curved. Most hemostatic forceps have transverse grooves on the inside surface of the jaws to better grasp the tissue. *Halsted mosquito hemostats* are small and delicate, designed for occluding small vessels (Fig. 16–6C). When using hemostatic forceps, the tips of the forceps should be used to grasp only as much tissue as necessary. *Crile forceps* and *Kelly forceps* (Fig. 16–7A and B) are larger, sturdier hemostatic forceps and are used on larger vessels. They differ in that the jaws of the Crile forceps are transversely grooved for the

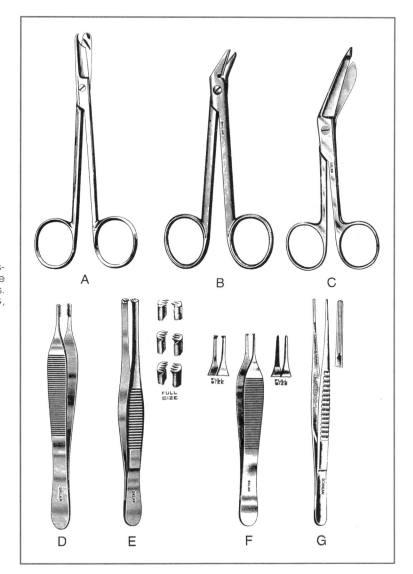

Figure 16-5. Scissors. A, Littauer suture-removal scissors. B, Wire suture-cutting scissors. C, Lister bandage scissors. Thumb Forceps. D, Brown-Adson thumb forceps. E, Rat tooth thumb forceps. F, Adson thumb forceps. G, DeBakey vascular thumb forceps.

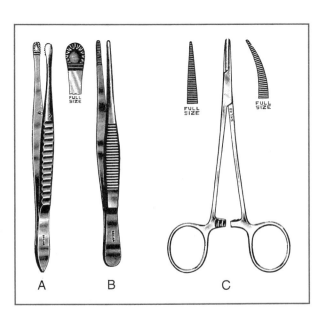

Figure 16-6. Thumb forceps. A, Russian thumb forceps. B, Dressing thumb forceps. Hemostatic forceps. C, Halsted mosquito hemostatic forceps.

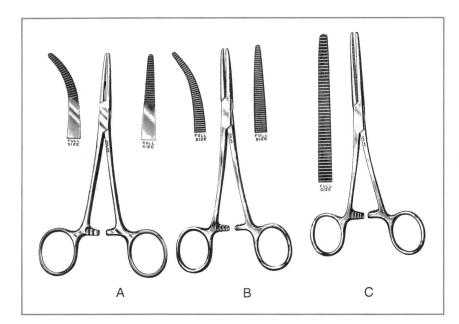

Figure 16–7. Hemostatic forceps. A, Kelly forceps. B, Crile forceps. C, Rochester-Pean forceps.

entire length whereas only the distal halves of the Kelly forceps are grooved. *Rochester-Pean forceps* are large, transversely grooved forceps that are useful for the control of large tissue bundles and vessels (Fig. 16–7C). *Rochester-Ochsner forceps* are similar to the Rochester-Pean forceps but have interdigitary teeth at the tips (Fig. 16–8A). This modification helps prevent tissue from slipping from the forceps. Rochester-Oschner forceps are used most commonly in orthopedic or large-animal surgery. *Rochester-Carmalt forceps* are large crushing forceps with longitudinal grooves to prevent tissue slippage and the cross-grooves at the tip help to provide more traction (Fig. 16–8B). These forceps are used for clamping across tissue that contains vessels. The Rochester-Carmalt forceps are commonly used prior to ligation for crushing the ovarian pedicle of vessels or the body of the uterus during an ovariohysterectomy (spay) operation. When clamping across vessels and tissue stumps for ligation, the forceps should be applied with the concave surface facing upward to facilitate tying the ligature.

TECHNICIAN NOTE

Hemostatic forceps are used to clamp, crush, and hold blood vessels with a self-locking mechanism.

Retractors

Tissue retraction is required to provide good visibility of the surgical site. Retractors may be hand-held or self-retaining. A surgical assistant is needed to maintain the position and tissue tension of a hand-held retractor. Hand-held retractors provide specific, firm tissue retraction while avoiding extra hands in the surgical wound which can interfere with the surgeon's instruments or view. The *Army-Navy retractor* and the *Senn retractor* are double-ended hand-held retractors commonly used to retract skin, fat, or muscle (Fig. 16–9A and C). The Army-Navy retractor is smooth-bladed, while the Senn has one smooth blade and one blade with three finger-like, sharp, or blunt prongs (see Fig. 12–9C). The *malleable retractor* is made of thin metal which is easily bent to the desired curvature (Fig. 12–9B). It can be used to retract muscle and is also commonly used to retract abdominal organs. The *Snook ovariohysterectomy hook* is a specialized type of hand-held retractor used to retrieve the horn of the uterus from the abdomen to perform an ovariohysterectomy (Fig. 16–9D). The *Hohmann retractor* consists of a single blade and a handle that are used to lever tissues out of the way for better visibility. These are used almost exclusively in orthopedic surgery and can provide superior visibility in certain situations such as joint surgeries.

TECHNICIAN NOTE

Retractors rather than hands are used to retract tissues and provide good visibility of the surgical site.

Self-retaining retractors maintain the tips in the desired position by some type of locking mechanism on the retractor handle. The advantage of the self-retaining retractors is that they maintain tissue distraction so the surgeon and the assistant have their hands free for other tasks. The *Balfour retractor* is used to retract the abdominal wall to provide increased exposure of the abdominal cavity (Fig. 16–10A). The two wire-like blades are used to distract the abdominal incision and the solid spoon-like blade is hooked onto the sternum to distract cranially. The *Finochietto rib spreader* is used to distract the ribs to provide an unobstructed view of the surgical field within the thoracic cavity (Fig. 16–10B). The ratcheted part of the retractors is positioned at the dorsal aspect of the thoracic incision so that it does not interfere with the surgeon. *Gelpi retractors* (Fig. 16–11A) and *Weitlaner retractors* (Fig. 16–11B) are self-retaining retractors commonly used for muscle retraction, especially in orthopedic and neurological surgery.

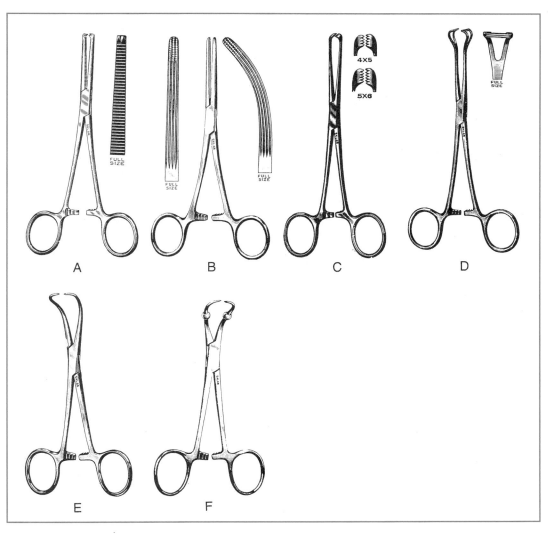

Figure 16–8. Hemostatic forceps. A, Rochester-Ochsner forceps. B, Rochester-Carmalt forceps. Tissue forceps. C, Allis tissue forceps. D, Babcock tissue forceps. Towel clamps. E, Backhaus towel clamp. F, Roeder towel clamp.

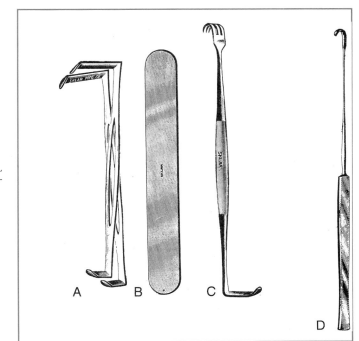

Figure 16–9. Hand-held retractors. A, Army-Navy retractor. B, Malleable retractor. C, Senn retractor. D, Snook ovariohysterectomy hook (spay hook).

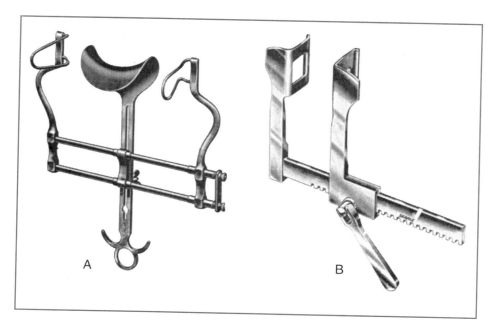

Figure 16–10. Self-retaining retractors (general surgery). A, Balfour abdominal retractor. B, Finochietto rib retractor.

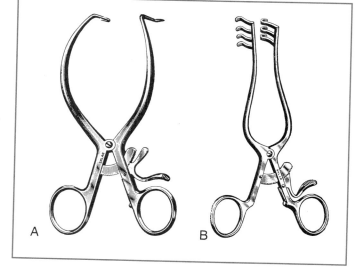

Figure 16–11. Self-retaining retractors (orthopedic and neurologic). A, Gelpi retractor. B, Weitlaner retractor.

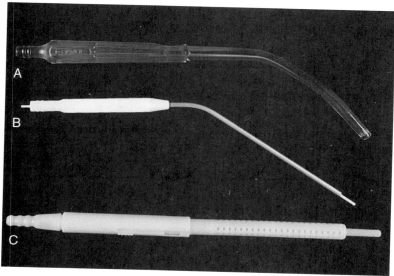

Figure 16–12. Suction tips. A, Yankauer. B, Frazier. C, Poole.

• Table 16–1 •

STAPLING EQUIPMENT			
NAME	**FUNCTION**	**TYPES OF SURGERY**	**COMMENTS**
TA	Thoracoabdominal	Commonly used for lung resection	Places double or triple row of staples
GIA	Gastrointestinal anastomosis	Gastrointestinal resection and anastomosis	Places four rows of staples and cuts between the middle two rows
EEA	End-to-end anastomosis	Gastrointestinal anastomosis	Staples two intestinal segments together in a circular manner with a functional lumen
Skin and fascial stapler		Closes skin and fascial planes	Places single staple; much faster than suturing
LDS	Ligate-and-divide stapler	Vascular stapler—ligates and divides blood vessels	Places two staples on a vessel and cuts between them

Suction Tips

Several different suction tips are commonly used (Fig. 16–12). The *Poole tip* is used primarily in the abdominal or thoracic cavities because it has an outer sleeve with small holes to prevent tissue from becoming entrapped in the tip (especially the omentum in abdominal surgeries). The *Frazier tip* is most commonly used in orthopedic and neurological surgery. The *Yankauer tip* is a general-purpose suction tip. The suction tip is inserted into a sterile suction tube which is attached at the other end to a suction canister outside of the sterile field.

Stapling Equipment

Several different surgical stapling devices are available for an array of purposes. There are many advantages to using stapling devices in both large and small animal surgery. Stapling devices provide a easier, faster, competent alternative to hand suturing techniques. Some stapling devices both cut and staple. The staplers are named by an abbreviation of their designed function (Table 16–1). A number is used after the name which indicates the length of the row of staples (e.g., a TA 30 places thoracoabdominally (TA) two rows of staples 30 mm long; Fig. 16–13).

Michel Skin Clips

Drape material is often attached to the incised skin edge during surgical procedures to minimize contamination of the surgical field by the surrounding skin. The use of Michel skin clips is one method of attaching the drape to the wound edges (Fig. 16–14). One end of the Michel clip-applying-and-removing forceps grips the edges of the clip. When the handles are squeezed the clip bends to pinch the edges of the drape and the skin together. The other end of the forceps has jaws to remove the clip by clamping onto it. The curvature of the clip is reversed to disengage it from the incision edge. There are alternatives to Michel clips, including the use of suture, "scalp clips," towel clamps, and adhesive drapes.

Ophthalmic Instruments

Ophthalmic surgery requires the use of delicate instruments, which may be easily damaged if improperly handled. Basic ophthalmic instruments include specialized scalpels, scissors, thumb forceps, needle holders, and retractors (Fig. 16–15).

Orthopedic Instruments
Rongeurs

Rongeurs have sharp cupped tips which are used to cut small pieces of dense tissue such as bone, cartilage, or fibrous tissue.

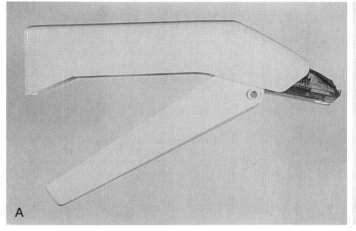

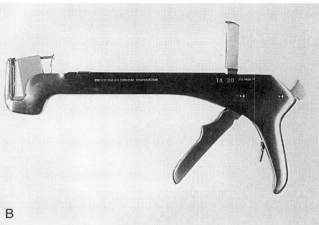

Figure 16–13. Surgical stapling equipment. A, Surgical skin stapler applies a single staple with each squeeze of the trigger (staple guns commonly hold 25 to 35 staples). B, Thoracoabdominal stapler (TA 30) applies two rows of staples simultaneously to provide a tight instantaneous closure.

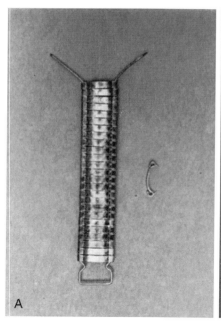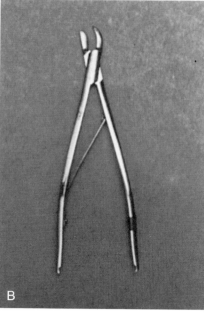

Figure 16-14. A, Michel skin clips. B, Michel clip forceps. Michel skin clips are used in surgical draping to secure the drape to the skin incision.

Rongeurs have a single-action or double-action mechanism (Fig. 16–16). Double-action rongeurs have a smoother cutting action and are mechanically stronger than the single-action forceps, but they are also bulkier. Therefore, the double-action rongeurs are preferred for removing larger and denser tissue. Single-action rongeurs are more commonly used in confined areas, as in removing bone to perform spinal surgery. Bone-cutting forceps are similar to rongeurs but have paired chisel-like tips. They are used for cutting bone and should not be mistaken for wire cutters.

Bone-Holding Forceps

Bone-holding forceps are heavily constructed forceps designed to hold bone and bone fragments to reduce the fracture and maintain alignment while orthopedic implants (screws, pins, wires, or plates) are applied (Fig. 16–17). Most bone-holding forceps are self-retaining. The *Kern bone-holding forceps* has a racheted handle which allows it to be clamped securely on the bone, while the *self-retaining bone-holding forceps*, also known

as "speed locks," has a nut which tightens against one handle to squeeze the handles together.

Curettes

Curettes are used to scrape away hard tissue for uses such as removal of necrotic bone or unhealthy cartilage. One of their most common uses is to remove cancellous bone from the medullary cavity inside bones (tibia, humerus, ilium) for use as a bone graft. Cancellous bone grafts are used commonly in fracture repair. Curettes are designed with a small cup-like structure at one or both ends of a handle (similar to an ice cream scoop). The cup has a sharp cutting edge and is available in various sizes (Fig. 16–18A).

Periosteal Elevators

Periosteal elevators are instruments that are commonly used to pry and undermine periosteum and other soft tissues from the surface of bone. They have a blade-like structure at one or both

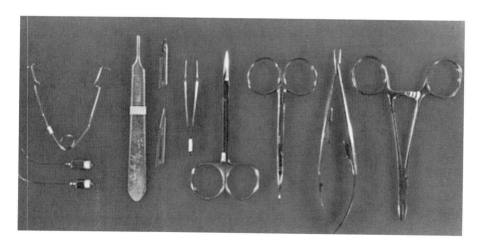

Figure 16-15. Common ophthalmic instruments. From left to right: lid speculum (above) and lacrimal cannulas (below), No. 3 scalpel handle and No. 15 and No. 11 surgical blades, thumb forceps, iris scissors, tenotomy scissors, Castroviejo needle holder, and Collier needle holder.

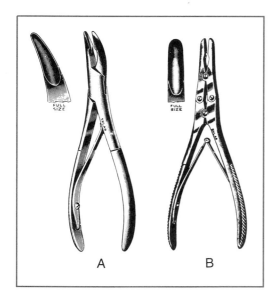

Figure 16-16. Rongeurs. A, Single-action rongeur. B, Double-action rongeur. The rongeurs are forceps that have cupped jaws for cutting away bone. They are commonly used in orthopedic and neurologic surgery, especially for hemilaminectomy procedures.

ends of a handle. The blades have sharp or blunt edges and are available in various sizes (Fig. 16–18B).

Osteotomes and Chisels

Osteotomes and chisels are used with a steel or plastic mallet to cut or shape bone and cartilage. The difference between the osteotome and chisel is the shape of the cutting edge. The cutting edge of the osteotome is tapered on both sides while the chisel is tapered only on one side (Fig. 16–18C). Osteotomes and chisels are used by pounding on the flared end of the handle with a mallet.

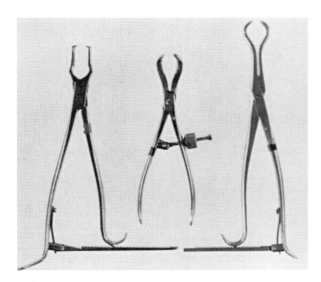

Figure 16-17. Bone-holding forceps. Kern forceps (left), speed lock forceps (center), and Richard's forceps (right). Bone-holding forceps are commonly used in open reduction of fractures.

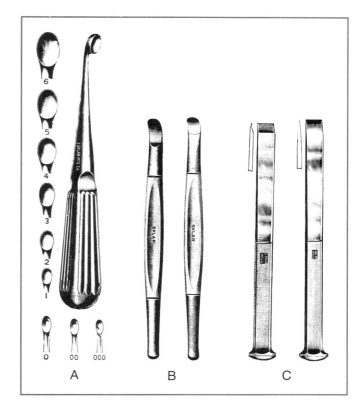

Figure 16-18. A, Curettes are commonly used for obtaining cancellous bone graft. B, Periosteal elevators are commonly used in surgical approaches to bone. C, Chisel (left) and osteotome (right) are used to cut bone in procedures such as femoral head and neck osteotomies.

Gigli Wire

Gigli wire is used to cut bone by placing the wire around the bone and drawing it back and forth in a sawing fashion. T-shaped handles hook onto the wire to give the surgeon a firm grasp of the wire.

Trephines

Trephines are T-shaped tubular instruments with a cylindrical cutting blade (Fig. 16–19). Trephines are usually used to remove a core of bone for biopsy.

Power Equipment

Some power equipment is commonly used in orthopedic and neurological surgery. Although some drills are electric (Fig. 16–20C) or battery-powered, many orthopedic drills and saws are powered by nitrogen gas which is supplied via a sterile hose (Fig. 16–20A and B). A Hall air drill is a specialized high-speed burr which is used to grind away bone for certain neurological and orthopedic procedures (Fig. 16–21).

Orthopedic Implants

Bone Pins

Bone pins vary in diameter, length, and type of points. *Steinmann pins* are smooth, round pins made of stainless steel and are commonly used in veterinary medicine. They range in

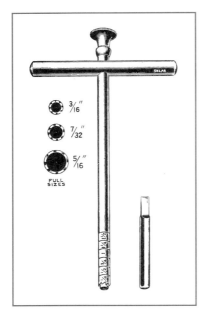

Figure 16–19. Trephine is most commonly used to obtain a bone biopsy.

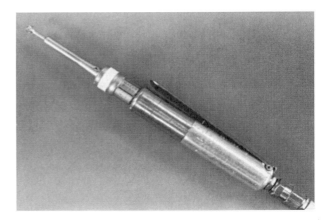

Figure 16–21. Hall air drill. The rotating mechanical burr tip is used to remove bone and is commonly used in neurologic surgeries such as laminectomies and cervical vertebral decompression surgeries (ventral slot decompression).

Steinmann pins but smaller and can be used to pin small bone fragments. The available sizes are 0.035-inch, 0.045-inch and 0.062-inch diameter.

Interlocking Nails

Interlocking nails are similar to intramedullary pins but have preplaced holes through the pin which allow screw placement. Interlocking nails have more rigid fixation than intramedullary pins. Equipment is similar to that required for pins, but specialized equipment is needed for screw placement.

diameter from one-sixteenth to one-fourth inch. Three different types of pin points are available, including chisel, trocar, or threaded trocar (Fig. 16–22). A Jacobs pin chuck is required to insert the pin into the bone, and a pin cutter is necessary to cut it to the proper length (Fig. 16–23). Steinmann pins are often placed in the medullary cavity (intramedullary) of long bones for fracture fixation. Kirschner wires (K-wires) are similar to

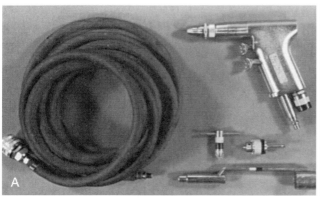

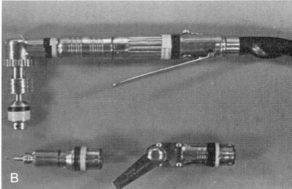

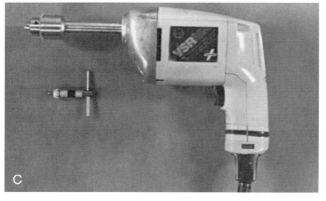

Figure 16–20. Orthopedic drills. A, ASIF drill is an air-powered drill that requires a connection to a pressurized nitrogen tank. B, OEC drill is an air-powered drill with two additional connection options: a mechanical burr and an oscillating saw. C, Variable-speed electric drill is not a surgical-grade drill, but it is commonly used because it is inexpensive. Electric drills may require a sterile shroud to maintain sterility. Cordless drills are more convenient and sterility is more easily managed.

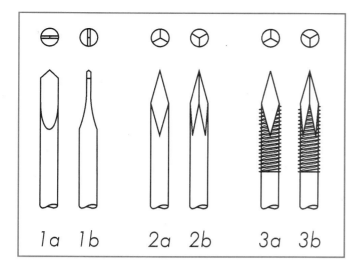

Figure 16–22. Steinmann intramedullary pin points: 1a and 1b, Chisel tip is a sliding tip used to slide in the medullary cavity along the inner cortical surface. 2a and 2b, Trocar tip is a cutting tip. 3a and 3b, Threaded trocar tip can be used for better anchorage in bone.

Orthopedic Wire

Orthopedic wire is a monofilament, stainless steel wire which is supplied on spools. The common sizes used in small animal surgery are 22 gauge, 20 gauge, and 18 gauge (Table 16–2). It is most commonly applied in a cerclage fashion by encircling

• Table 16–2 •

COMMONLY USED ORTHOPEDIC WIRE SIZES

| | SIZE | |
GAUGE	Inches	Millimeters
22	0.025	0.64
20	0.032	0.81
18	0.040	1.02

the bone or bone fragments and twisting the ends in a "twist-tie" manner. Orthopedic wire is often used for fracture repair in combination with pins or bone plates.

External Fixators

External fixation is a means of stabilizing fractures using pins placed through the skin and bone. The pins are held rigid by a connecting bar which is attached to the pins several centimeters from the skin (Fig. 16–24). The whole apparatus is removed

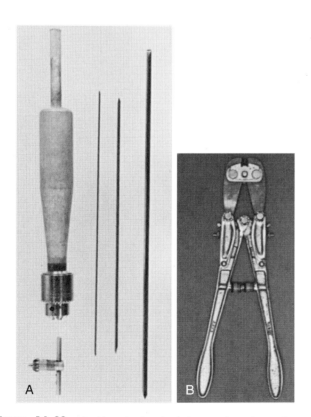

Figure 16–23. A, Hand chuck, key, and various sizes of Steinmann pins. The hand chuck is used to insert pins into bone. B, Pin cutter.

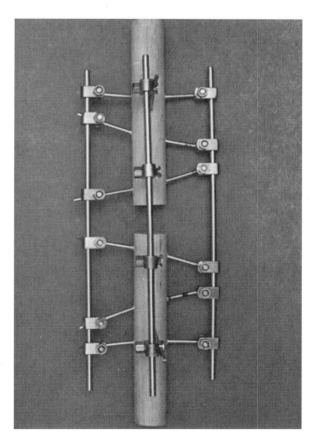

Figure 16–24. External fixation. An external fixator placed on a wooden dowel fracture model. External fixators come in many configurations, but the basic components consist of the transcortical pins, fixator clamps, and connecting bar. The pins are placed through the skin and bone (represented by the wooden dowel), whereas the clamps and connecting bar are attached on the outside of the limb approximately 1 inch away from the skin. Methyl methacrylate (bone cement) is commonly used in place of the clamps and connecting bar. The entire device is removed after healing.

following fracture healing (generally 8 to 16 weeks). The Kirschner-Ehmer (K-E) apparatus uses special clamps to attach the connecting bar to the pins and is commonly used. Acrylic (methyl methacrylate) can be used as a substitute for the metal connecting bars. Dental acrylics and hoof wall repair acrylics are commonly used because they are less expensive than surgical grades of acrylic. The acrylic connecting bar is more versatile and lighter than the metal K-E apparatus.

Bone Screws

The two basic screw types are cortical and cancellous screws. Cortical screws are fully threaded screws that are designed to be placed in dense (cortical) bone. Cancellous screws are either partially threaded or fully threaded and are made with wider and deeper threads than cortical screws in order to engage a larger surface area in the softer cancellous bone (Fig. 16–25).

A variety of sizes (length and diameter) of bone screws exist. Commonly used screws in small animal surgery are 2.7- and 3.5-mm-diameter cortical screws and 4.0-mm-diameter cancellous screws. All of these screws are driven by the same screwdriver with a hexagonal head. Smaller screws include 1.5- and 2.0-mm-diameter screws which require smaller corresponding equipment including a small cruciate-head screwdriver. Larger screws such as 4.5-, 5.5-, and 6.5-mm-diameter screws are commonly used in large animal surgery. These also require larger equipment and a large hexagonal screwdriver. The screws are designed to work in concert with a bone plate of a specific size. A depth gauge is used during surgery to determine the appropriate screw length.

The majority of bone screws used in veterinary surgery are designed to be placed in pretapped, drilled holes. This means the threads are cut in the drilled hole with a bone tap (an instrument with sharp threads) before the screw is placed. However, pretapping is not absolutely required, especially when using cancellous screws.

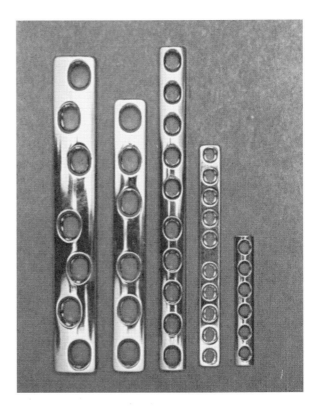

Figure 16–26. Orthopedic bone plates. Various sizes, lengths, and shapes of bone plates are available. Bone plates are named by their type, size of screw used, and number of holes. For example, the plate on the left is a seven-hole, broad 3.5-mm dynamic compression plate.

Bone Plates

Bone plates are available in various types, sizes, and lengths (Fig. 16–26). Bone plates are named by the number of screw holes and by the screw diameter size that best fits the plate. For example, 3.5-mm screws are used to secure a 3.5-mm plate. Instrumentation required to apply a bone plate is highly

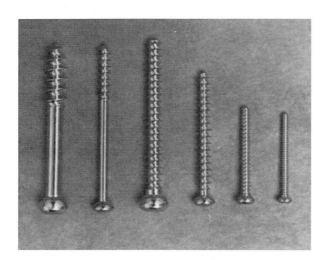

Figure 16–25. Orthopedic screws. Various sizes and lengths of partially threaded cancellous screws (left) and fully threaded cortical screws (right). Cortical screws are fully threaded and have proportionately smaller threads than the larger threaded cancellous screws. Screw sizes are listed by their outside thread diameter.

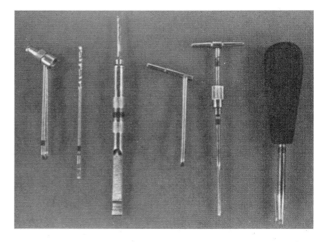

Figure 16–27. Bone plating equipment. From left to right: drill guide, drill bit, depth gauge, tap sleeve (to prevent soft tissues from being caught on the bone tap), bone tap, and screwdriver.

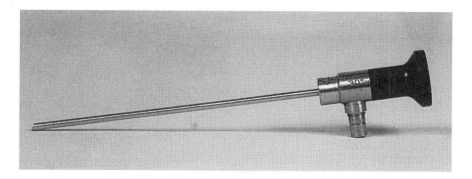

Figure 16-28. A 4-mm (outer diameter) arthroscope.

specialized and includes drills, drill bits, drill guides, depth gauges, bone taps, tap sleeves, screws, plate benders, and screwdrivers (Fig. 16–27). Bone plates are placed on the surface of bones; therefore special equipment is required to bend the plate to the contour of the bone. The plate is secured to bone with screws. More equipment is required to implant a bone plate than other types of orthopedic fixation, but plate fixation is much more stable in most cases.

Arthroscopic Instruments and Equipment

Introduction

The arthroscope is used as a diagnostic and surgical tool in veterinary surgery. It is used mostly to examine various joints of the horse including the scapulohumeral, humeroradial, carpal, fetlock, distal interphalangeal, coxofemoral (foals only), stifle, and tarsocrural. Arthroscopy is utilized primarily to remove osteochondral chip fragments, which occur in racehorses, and osteochondrotic lesions on the articular surface in joints of young horses. The arthroscope has been used to visualize intra-articular fractures for lag screw fixation such as third carpal bone slab fractures in horses. The arthroscope has also been used to perform tenoscopy of the digital flexor tendon sheath and sinuscopy of the paranasal sinuses through trephined holes in the facial bones overlying the sinuses of horses. Most of the equipment used in veterinary arthroscopy has been adapted from human arthroscopy. New technology is constantly being developed which will no doubt influence the veterinary field. This section is intended to allow the veterinary technician to become more familiar with the instruments and techniques of equine arthroscopy.

Arthroscope

There is a selection of different arthroscopes that have been developed with various diameters and viewing angles. Richard Wolf Medical Instruments (Rosemont, Ill.), for example, has developed a 5-mm-OD (outer diameter) arthroscope with either a 10-, 25-, or 70-degree lens angle; a 4-mm-OD with a 10-, 25-, 70-, or 110-degree lens angle; a 2.7-mm-OD with a 5-, 25-, or 70-degree lens angle; and a 1.9-mm-OD with a 5- or 25-degree lens angle. A 4-mm-OD 25- or 30-degree angled lens scope is generally what most equine surgeons use (Fig. 16–28).

Ancillary Arthroscopic Equipment

Along with the arthroscope come various instruments used to introduce the scope into the joint and attachments for television viewing and fluid hookup. Stab incisions are made in the skin,

over the joint space, through which the arthroscope and hand instruments will be inserted once the animal is positioned for surgery, and the site is surgically prepared (Fig. 16–29).

Sharp Trocar, Sleeve

A pointed instrument called a sharp trocar is inserted inside a hollow, cannula-type instrument called the sleeve (Fig. 16–30). The trocar and sleeve unit are used to penetrate the fibrous portion of the joint capsule through a stab incision (Fig. 16–30).

Blunt Obturator

Once the sharp trocar has penetrated the fibrous joint capsule, the sharp trocar is replaced with a conical (blunt) obturator (Fig. 16–31), which is used to penetrate the synovial membrane of the joint capsule and advance the sleeve into the joint space with less risk of damaging the articular cartilage (Fig. 16–32). At this point the obturator is withdrawn from the sleeve. The joint space is distended with a sterile balanced electrolyte solution (fluids) prior to placement of the sleeve in the joint, so a rush of fluids through the barrel of the sleeve will occur as the obturator is being removed. The obturator is replaced with the arthroscope (Fig. 16–33), which is designed to lock onto the sleeve once it is slid into position in the sleeve (Fig. 16–34).

Light Cable, Light Projector, and Television Camera

Once the arthroscope is positioned in the joint a fiberoptic light cable (Fig. 16–35) is attached directly to the optical light port

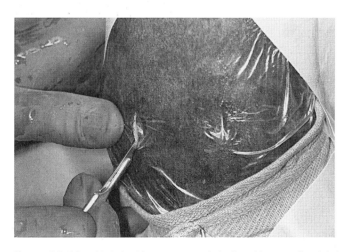

Figure 16-29. Stab incisions are made in the skin over the joint space of a horse, through which the arthroscope and hand insruments will be inserted.

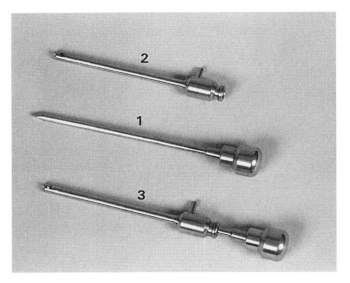

Figure 16–30. The sharp trocar (1) fits inside the arthroscope sleeve (2). The unit (3) is used to penetrate the fibrous joint capsule through a stab incision in the skin.

on the arthroscope (Fig. 16–36). A high-intensity light generated from a specially designed light projector is fed through the fiberoptic cable and through the arthroscope to illuminate the joint space (Fig. 16–37). A television camera (Fig. 16–38) then is attached to the eyepiece of the scope, (Fig. 16–39). Most arthroscopes today are coupled to a television camera, which allows the surgeon and surgical team to view the joint on a television monitor (Fig. 16–40). A television monitor has the advantage of a larger image. This greatly improves the visualization of the intra-articular space compared with direct viewing through the eyepiece of the arthroscope. This method also provides better aseptic technique, because the surgeon's face is not near the surgical field and an assistant can operate the camera-scope unit, allowing the surgeon more freedom. A monitor also allows several people to observe the procedure simultaneously and a videotape record can be made for future replay.

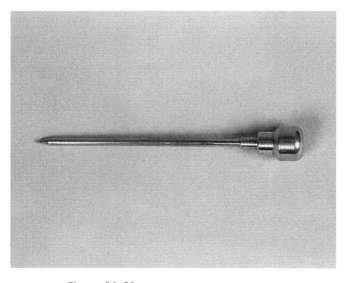

Figure 16–31. Conical (blunt) obturator.

Fluid Delivery Systems

Fluids, usually a balanced electrolyte solution, are infused into the joint under pressure to maintain distention of the joint capsule which is essential for visualization of the intra-articular space. Gas insufflation, using carbon dioxide or nitrous oxide, has also been used as a method of distending the joint. However, a special system with a pressure-regulated device is required. One disadvantage of gas is that it does not allow for lavage of the joint space if osteochondral chip fragments become dettached in the joint. The fluids are infused into the joint space through the sleeve, around the arthroscope. The sleeve has at least one stopcock which is used as an ingress port to connect a sterile fluid line (Fig. 16–41).

Pressurized Bag System

There are various systems available to deliver fluid to the joint. One system is a pressurized bag design. A pneumatic pressure "cuff" is slipped around a bag containing sterile fluids. The cuff is inflated with air which squeezes the fluid bag, thus pressurizing the fluids (Fig. 16–42). The amount of pressure is regulated by the amount of cuff inflation.

Motorized Pump System

Another type of system uses a motorized pump to regulate the fluid rate through the fluid lines connected to the arthroscope. One example of this type of system uses sterile silicone tubing which is threaded around the rollers of an infusion pump (Masterflex, Cole-Parmer, Chicago) (Fig. 16–43). The speed of the rollers is regulated by the surgeon or assistant using sterile handles that are attached to the pump switches (Fig. 16–43).

Automated pressure-sensitive pump systems are also available, which incorporate a pressure feedback control through a separate fluid line connected to an egress cannula placed into the joint through a remote site. This allows the pump to maintain a preset pressure in the joint without the need of the surgeon having to adjust the fluid pressure.

Hand Instruments for Arthroscopic Surgery

There are numerous hand instruments of various types that are available or that have been adapted for arthroscopy. The hand instruments are used to remove or retrieve osteochondral chip fragments, debride articular cartilage or subchondral bone, or probe cartilage or cartilage lesions. The instruments are inserted into the joint through a separate stab incision and the arthroscopic operation is performed via a technique called triangulation (Fig. 16–44). Only the most commonly used instruments are discussed here.

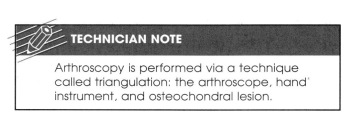

TECHNICIAN NOTE

Arthroscopy is performed via a technique called triangulation: the arthroscope, hand instrument, and osteochondral lesion.

Blunt Probe

This instrument is used to probe a site in the joint to determine such aspects as cartilage integrity or the extent of a cartilage lesion (Fig. 16–45).

Text continued on page 405

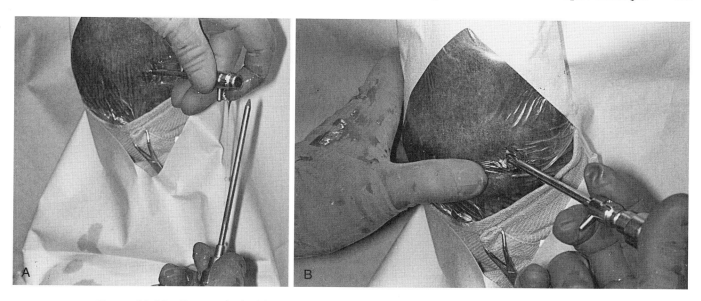

Figure 16-32. The conical obturator replaces the sharp trocar in the sleeve and is used to penetrate the synovial membrane portion of the joint capsule (A), and advance the sleeve further into the joint (B).

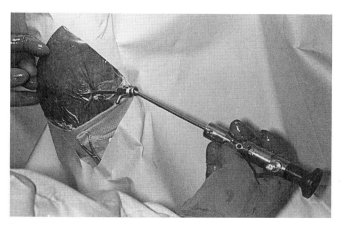

Figure 16-33. Once the sleeve is in position in the joint, the obturator is removed and the arthroscope is placed into the sleeve.

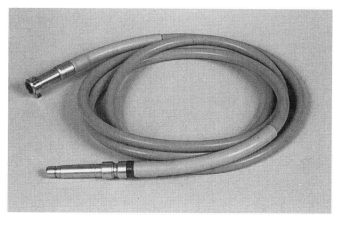

Figure 16-35. Fiberoptic light cable.

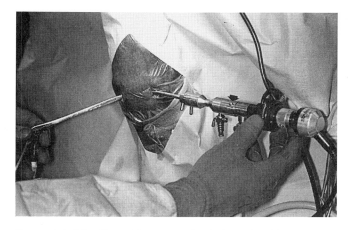

Figure 16-34. The arthroscope is designed to lock (arrow) onto the sleeve to prevent dislodgement during surgery.

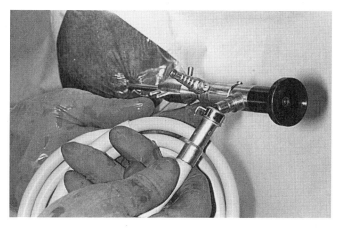

Figure 16-36. The fiberoptic light cable attaches to the light port of the arthroscope.

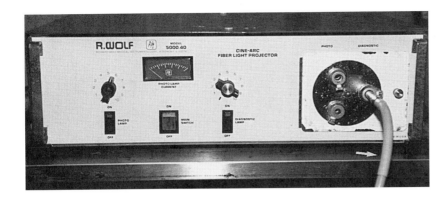

Figure 16-37. Light projector is designed to project light through a fiberoptic light cable (arrow) of the arthroscope.

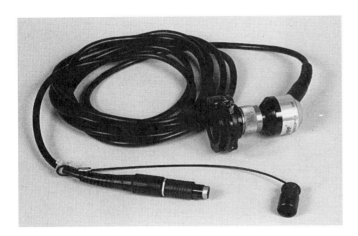

Figure 16-38. Television camera is designed for arthroscopic surgery.

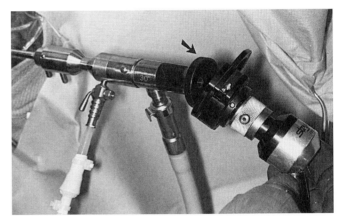

Figure 16-39. The television camera couples to the eyepiece (arrow) of the arthroscope.

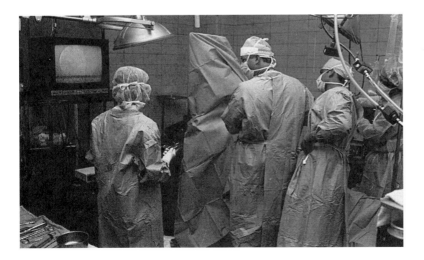

Figure 16-40. Most arthroscopic procedures are viewed on a television monitor.

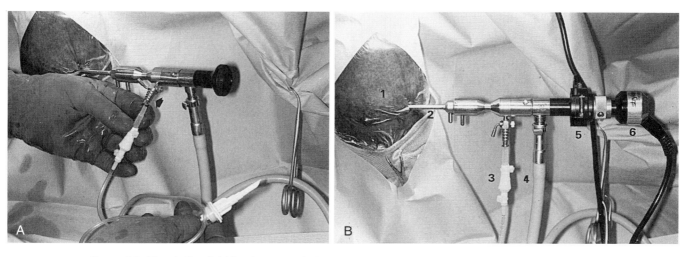

Figure 16-41. A, The fluid line is connected to the stopcock of the arthroscope (arrow). B, Carpus of a horse (1), sleeve (2), fluid line (3), light cable (4), arthroscope (5), and camera (6).

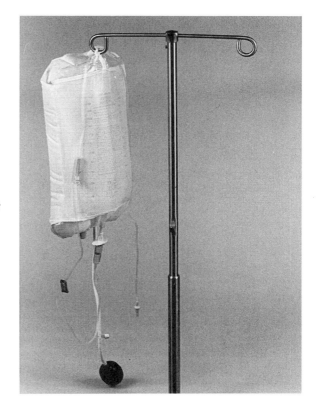

Figure 16-42. Pressurized bag of fluids can be used to distend a joint during arthroscopy.

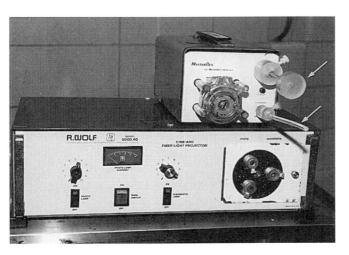

Figure 16-43. Infusion pump used to infuse sterile fluids into a joint during arthroscopy. Sterile handles (arrows) are connected to the switches to allow an assistant to regulate the speed and amount of fluids going into the joint.

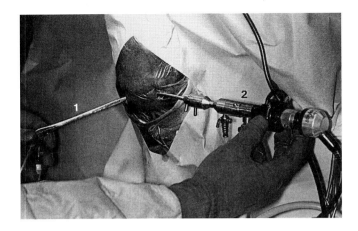

Figure 16–44. Arthroscopy is performed via triangulation of the hand instrument (1) and arthroscope (2) with the intra-articular lesion.

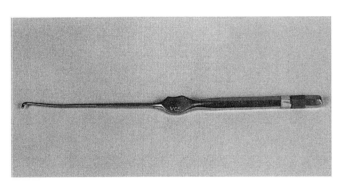

Figure 16–45. Blunt arthroscopy probe.

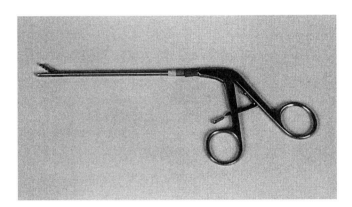

Figure 16–47. Forceps used in arthroscopy.

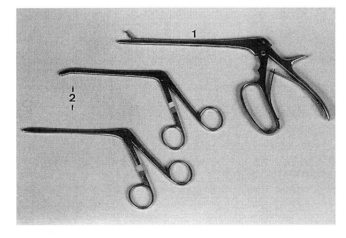

Figure 16–46. Rongeurs used in arthroscopy: Ferris Smith (1) and Love and Gruenwald (2).

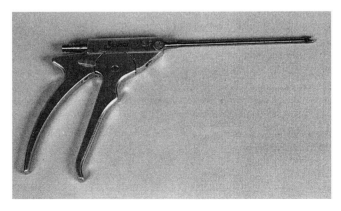

Figure 16–48. The Dyonics DynoVac suction forceps.

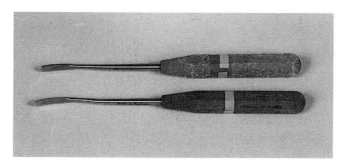

Figure 16–49. Elevator and osteotome used in arthroscopy.

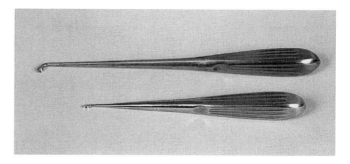

Figure 16–50. Small cupped bone curettes used in arthroscopy.

Rongeurs and Grasping Forceps

Various types and sizes of rongeurs have been adapted for use in arthroscopy. These instruments have a beveled edge along the cupped jaws to cut the attachments of an osteochondral chip fragment as it is being removed (Fig. 16–46). Forceps are used primarily to retrieve loosely attached fragments (Fig. 16–47). There are specially designed forceps that have a suction attachment to the hollow shaft of the instrument which allows evacuation of small fragments through the shaft as the surgeon grasps the fragments with the jaws of the instrument (Fig. 16–48).

Elevators and Osteotomes

These instruments have small beveled heads that are designed to cut or break down the attachments of an osteochondral chip fragment and elevate it from the parent subchondral bone bed (Fig. 16–49).

Curettes

These instruments are inserted into the joint to debride a defect left in the articular cartilage or subchondral bone after removal of an osteochondral chip fragment or osteochondrotic lesion (Fig. 16–50).

Motorized Burrs

These burrs are often referred to as a motorized arthroplasty system. The system consists of a small rounded burr attached to a power-driven shaft. The burr and shaft are enclosed in a sleeve, with a portion of the burr protected to prevent inadver-

tent damage to surrounding articular cartilage (Fig. 16–51). This instrument is also used to debride a defect left in the articular cartilage or subchondral bone after removal of an osteochondral chip fragment or osteochondrotic lesion. The speed of rotation of the burr can be adjusted, and is usually operated at several thousand revolutions per minute. Most systems operate with an on/off foot pedal switch for the surgeon.

Instrument Packs

Most veterinary hospitals and clinics organize their surgical instruments into several different instrument packs based on the type of surgical procedure. Surgical pack organization is dependent on the type of practice and surgeries performed, but some examples are as follows: general packs for soft tissue surgeries, bone packs for orthopedic surgeries, emergency packs for emergency and minor procedures, and neurological packs for spinal surgeries (Tables 16–3 and 16–4). The use of a pack system helps to organize the instruments, to have the most commonly used instruments readily available, and to eliminate unnecessary resterilization of infrequently used instruments. For example, all commonly used instruments for spinal surgery are organized in one pack so that it is opened, used, cleaned, sterilized, and repacked only when necessary. Infrequently used instruments are typically wrapped individually. Large and bulky instruments are also packed separately.

Within each pack there should be a system for packing instruments so that they are placed in the same position on the

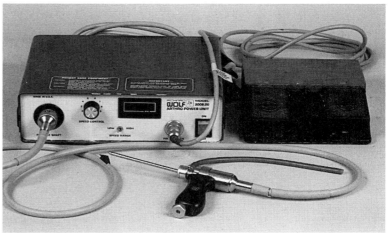

Figure 16–51. Motorized arthroplasty system with burr attachment (arrow).

• Table 16–3 •

SMALL ANIMAL INSTRUMENT PACKS		
SOFT TISSUE/GENERAL PACK	**EMERGENCY PACK**	**ORTHOPEDIC PACK**
No. 3 scalpel handle	No. 3 scalpel handle	Army-Navy retractors
Brown-Adson thumb forceps	Brown-Adson thumb forceps	Senn retractors
Adson thumb forceps	Needle holder, Olsen-Hegar	Rongeurs
Needle holder, Mayo-Hegar	Mayo scissors, curved	Large Kern bone-holding forceps
Mayo scissors	Mosquito hemostats (3 curved, 3 straight)	Small Kern bone-holding forceps
Metzenbaum scissors	Crile or Kelly forceps (1 curved, 1 straight)	Bone curette
Wire suture scissors	Allis forceps	Periosteal elevator
Mosquito hemostats (4 curved, 4 straight)	Towel clamps (4)	Steinmann pins (5/64, 3/32, 7/64, 1/8,
Crile forceps (1 curved, 1 straight)	Towels (4)	9/64, 5/32, 3/16, 1/4)
Carmalt forceps (2 curved)	Sponges	Kirschner wire (0.035, 0.045, 0.062)
Allis forceps (2)	Sterilization indicator	Jacobs chuck and key
Ovariohysterectomy hook (Snook hook)		Roll 18-gauge stainless steel wire
Towel clamps (8)		Roll 20-gauge stainless steel wire
Towels (6)		Roll 22-gauge stainless steel wire
Stainless steel bowl		Metal ruler
Sponges		Michel clips and applicator
Lap sponges (2)		Sterilization indicator
Sterilization indicator		

tray each time (Fig. 16–52). This makes it easier to inventory the instruments and facilitates finding the instruments quickly during a procedure.

Instrument Care

Almost all surgical instruments are made of stainless steel which is rust-resistant and retains a keen edge. The two common instrument finishes are polished or satin. The polished finish tends to reflect light and can hinder the vision of the surgeon, but it resists spotting and discoloration. The satin or dull finish was developed to eliminate glare and lessen the surgeon's eye strain, but is less resistant to spotting and discoloration.

Good-quality instruments are expensive but will last for years if treated properly. All instruments should be handled gently and delicate instruments should be separated from the general instruments before cleaning. Multiple-component instruments should be disassembled prior to cleaning. Power equipment should be cleaned separately to ensure that water does not get inside the components.

Immediately after their use, instruments should be rinsed with cold water to prevent blood and organic debris from drying in the serrations, hinges, box locks, or ratchets. Each instrument is scrubbed with a soft brush in warm water with a neutral pH instrument detergent. Abrasive cleaning agents should never be used on surgical instruments. Saline solutions are corrosive to stainless steel, so instruments should be rinsed with deionized or distilled water. Some hospitals have ultrasonic (high-frequency sound) cleaners (Fig. 16–53) which clean the instruments in areas that the brush cannot reach. The ultrasonic cleaner is used following manual cleaning. Instruments should be thoroughly dried before autoclaving to prevent rust spots.

Ideally, instruments with a working action, such as a hinge or box lock, should be treated with an instrument lubricant or instrument "milk" after each cleaning. Only water-soluble lubricants are recommended for instrument lubrication. These lubricants are nonoily and nonsticky and do not interfere with steam sterilization. Lubricants usually contain a rust-inhibiting agent that is useful in preventing electrolysis on points and

edges. Ultrasonic cleaners effectively remove all lubricant from the instruments so lubrication should be done after ultrasonic cleaning. Working components of power equipment should also be lubricated to maximize efficiency and to prolong the working lifetime of the equipment. Before instruments are repacked for sterilization they should be thoroughly inspected for cleanliness, stiff or "frozen" hinges, improper jaw alignment, and worn or broken parts.

Drapes and Gowns

Either paper or cloth surgical drapes and gowns may be used. Paper drapes and gowns are designed to be disposable and the

• Table 16–4 •

LARGE ANIMAL STANDARD AND EMERGENCY PACKS	
STANDARD PACK	**EMERGENCY PACK**
No. 3 scalpel handle	No. 3 scalpel handle
No. 4 scalpel handle	No. 4 scalpel handle
Rat-tooth thumb forceps (3)	Rat-tooth thumb forceps
Adson thumb forceps (3)	Brown-Adson thumb forceps
Needle holders (2)	Needle holder
Mayo scissors (1 curved, 1 straight)	Mayo scissors (1 curved, 1 straight)
Operating scissors (sharp-sharp)	Mosquito hemostats (2 curved, 2 straight)
Metzenbaum scissors (1 curved, 1 straight)	Allis tissue forceps (2)
Bandage scissors	Towel clamps (4)
Mosquito hemostats (4 straight, 4 curved)	Towel
Kelly or Crile forceps (2 straight, 2 curved)	Sponges
Ochsner forceps, 15-cm (1 curved, 1 straight)	Sterilization indicator
Allis tissue forceps (2)	
Towel clamps (16)	
Towels (4)	
Saline bowl	
Sponges	
Sterilization indicator	

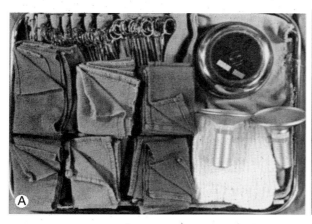
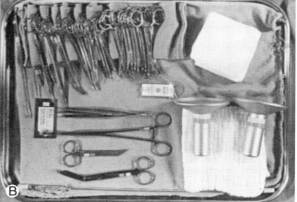

Figure 16-52. A, Properly organized instrument set (gauze sponges are underneath saline bowl). B, Towels and saline bowl have been removed.

manufacturer recommends they be used only once. However, if the paper item has not been soiled, it may be repacked, resterilized, and used again.

Cloth drapes and gowns are designed for repeated use, but they require washing after each use. Immediately soaking the cloth in cold water will prevent blood and other fluids from setting. All cloth drapes and gowns should be washed in a mild detergent and thoroughly dried prior to sterilization.

✎ TECHNICIAN NOTE

Accordion folding of drape allows easy unfolding and placement on the patient.

Gown packs are prepared so that the gown can be unfolded and put on without contaminating it. The gowns must always be folded in the same manner (Fig. 16–54).

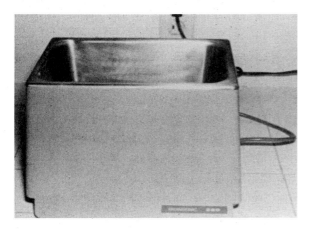

Figure 16-53. Ultrasonic cleaner. The ultrasonic cleaner is used to remove tightly bound soil on instruments that is not completely removed by other cleaning processes. The instruments are placed in water inside the tub shown and should be rinsed after ultrasonic cleansing.

Drape packs must also be specially prepared to prevent contamination as they are unfolded and applied to the patient.

"Accordion folding" allows easy unfolding and placement of the drape (Fig. 16–55). Many specifically designed drapes are also available, including adhesive drapes, transparent drapes, fenestrated drapes, stockinettes, and compressive wraps. When the drapes and gowns have been properly folded, they are usually double-wrapped in paper or cloth (Fig. 16–56).

ASEPTIC TECHNIQUE

Asepsis is defined as freedom from infection. Aseptic technique includes all steps taken to prevent contamination of the surgical site by infectious agents. A thorough understanding of aseptic technique is required to properly sterilize the surgical equipment and clean the operating room. Certain principles of aseptic technique must also be followed when scrubbing the surgical site and placing sterile drapes on the patient. The technician may need to act as a circulating nurse by getting the patient in the operating room and opening sterile equipment for the surgeon. Additionally, the technician may be called upon to "scrub in" as a scrub nurse or surgical assistant to organize and pass instruments to the surgeon or to assist with the surgical procedure. A working knowledge of aseptic technique is necessary to perform these tasks correctly and also to monitor for inadvertent "breaks" in sterile technique.

Microorganisms must be introduced into the surgical site for infection to develop. The source of microorganisms includes exogenous and endogenous routes. Exogenous sources of contamination include the air, the surgical instruments and supplies, the patient's skin, and the surgical team. Endogenous contamination arises from within the patient and may reach the wound through the blood stream. Examples of endogenous sources are bacteria from gingivitis or dermatitis.

During every surgery, some bacterial contamination occurs at the surgical site. Whether the contamination progresses to an infection depends on many factors, including the general health of the patient, the degree of tissue damage in the wound, the virulence of the infectious agent, and the number of infectious agents. The factor over which the surgical team has the most control is the number of infectious agents that are introduced into the wound by an exogenous route. Strict adherence to the

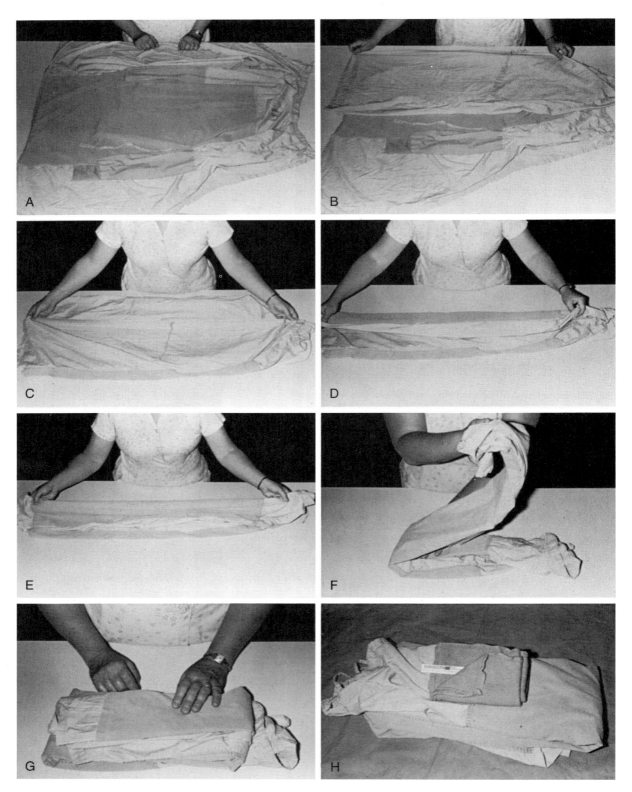

Figure 16-54. Method of folding a surgical gown. A, The gown is spread on a countertop with the outside of the gown facing up. B, The near edge of the gown is folded to the center. C, Next, the far edge of the gown is folded toward the center to meet the near edge. D, The gown is folded in half. E, The gown is folded in half again. F and G, The gown is folded lengthwise in accordian fashion into thirds. H, A hand towel and sterilization indicator are placed on top, and the gown is ready for wrapping.

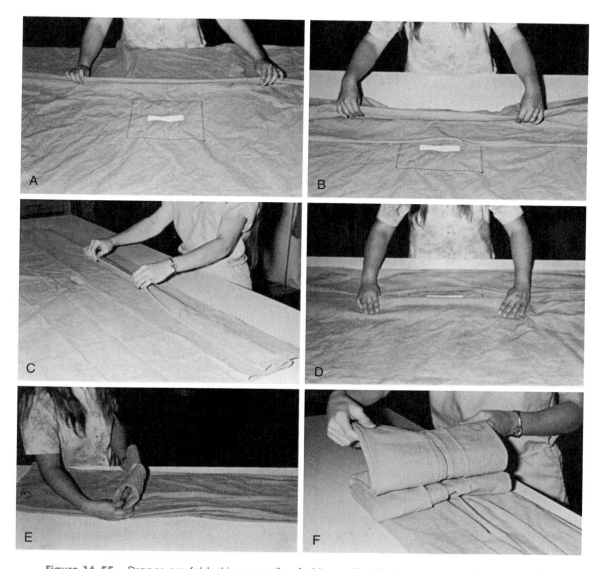

Figure 16-55. Drapes are folded in accordion fashion so that they are easily unfolded onto the patient. A–C, One side of the drape is folded to the center in accordian fashion. Each fold is approximately 15 cm wide. D, The opposite side is folded in a similar manner. E and F, Lengthwise, the drape is again folded to the center of the fenestration in accordian fashion. These folds are also approximately 15 cm in width.

Illustration continued on following page

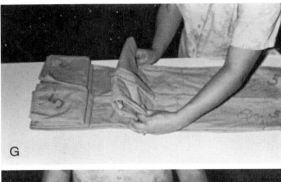

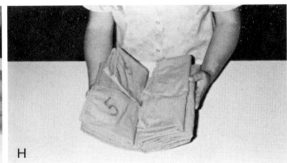

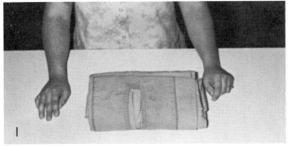

Figure 16-55 *Continued* G, The opposite side is folded in the same manner. H, The two sides are folded together, and the drape is ready for wrapping (I).

principles of aseptic technique will minimize exogenous wound contamination and prevent many infections from developing.

All procedures do not require the same degree of vigilance regarding aseptic technique. For example, the debridement of a cutaneous abscess is considered to be a contaminated or dirty surgery so aseptic technique would not be strictly followed. The wound would be scrubbed but surgical instruments may be disinfected (cold sterilization) rather than sterilized (steam autoclave or gas sterilization) and the surgeon may wear sterile gloves but forgo complete sterile surgical attire. It may actually be preferable for the patient to remain outside the operating room since excessive contamination could result. In contrast, total hip replacement surgery involves the implantation of synthetic material and infection can be devastating to the success of the surgery. In such a case, the surgical team adheres strictly to aseptic protocol. The surgeon will determine the degree to which the principles of asepsis are to be followed in each case.

Sterilization. *Sterilization* is the complete destruction of living organisms. The purpose of sterilization is to destroy all pathogenic organisms and spores that may be present on instruments and materials. *Disinfection* implies destruction of the vegetative forms of bacteria but not the spores. Both sterilization and disinfection are used to prepare medical and surgical materials. The process used depends on the nature of the material and its intended use. Methods of sterilization and disinfection can be classified as either physical or chemical.

Physical Methods of Sterilization

The three general types of physical methods used for sterilization include filtration, radiation, and heat. Filtration and radiation are primarily used during the production and packaging of certain surgical products.

Filtration

Filtration is the separation of particulate material from liquids or gases. Pharmaceuticals are commonly sterilized by filtration.

Radiation

Certain materials that cannot be sterilized by heat or chemicals are sterilized by radiation. Sterilization is achieved by radiant energy which destroys microorganisms without a significant elevation of temperature. Gloves and some suture materials are sterilized by radiation during the manufacturing process.

Thermal Energy

The most common method used for sterilization is heat. The mechanism by which heat destroys microorganisms is not completely understood, but it is believed that death is the result of protein denaturation. This is probably a gradual process and may be reversible during the early stages of sterilization. The thermal susceptibility of microorganisms is influenced by several factors, including inherent resistance, individual variation, and age (young bacteria are more susceptible). There is no one temperature at which all microorganisms are killed instantly. The death of bacteria and spores is a function of temperature and duration of heat.

The two basic types of heat sterilization are moist heat and dry heat. Dry heat is used to sterilize materials that cannot tolerate moist heat but can withstand exposure to high temperatures. Oils, powders, and petroleum products are most effectively sterilized by dry heat. In addition, needles and sharp instruments are not corroded or rusted by dry heat. Dry heat is more difficult to control than moist heat and the sterilization time is longer. Additionally, the high temperatures required are destructive to rubber goods and fabrics and may destroy the temper of metal instruments.

Both dry and moist heat destroy bacteria through protein denaturation; however, dry heat kills by protein oxidation whereas moist heat kills by coagulation of critical cellular proteins. Moisture facilitates the coagulation of proteins; thus moist heat kills bacteria and spores at lower temperatures and shorter exposures than dry heat.

Moist heat sterilization is accomplished by either boiling water or steam under pressure. Boiling water at ambient pres-

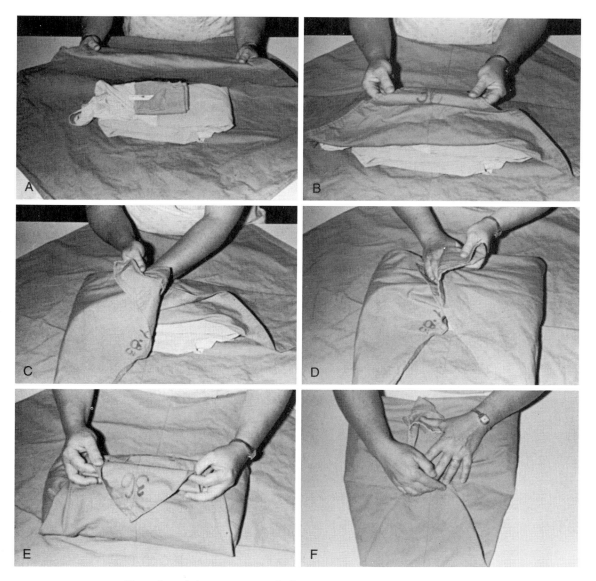

Figure 16–56. Wrapping of drape or gown. A, The gown, along with a hand towel and sterilization indicator, is placed diagonally onto the nonfenestrated drapes. B–E, The corners are folded over the gown. F, Three corners of the second drape are folded in a similar manner.

Illustration continued on following page

sures is not a reliable means of sterilization because of its relatively low temperature. The bactericidal effect of boiling water can be enhanced by alkalinization with sodium hydroxide (0.1 g/dl) or sodium carbonate (2 g/dl). The addition of these agents reduces instrument corrosion, but they can not be used with glassware or rubber goods. Boiling water is considered to be a disinfecting agent, but is rarely used.

The most common method of sterilization is saturated steam under pressure. Increased pressure causes steam to achieve a higher temperature. Materials to be sterilized in this manner must be penetrable by steam and not damaged by either heat or moisture. Sterilizers that employ steam under pressure are called *autoclaves* (Fig. 16–57).

Autoclave Sterilization

Autoclave sterilization is technique-sensitive. An autoclave load is not sterile unless the steam has penetrated the packs com-

pletely so that all materials have been exposed to steam at the proper temperature and for the proper duration. Adequate steam penetration requires that the packs be properly prepared and loaded into the autoclave. Operating instructions accompanying the autoclave should be followed completely.

Proper pack preparation begins by checking that all materials are thoroughly clean and free from grease, oil, or protein materials. Materials need to be packed as loosely as is practical to ensure good steam penetration. It is recommended that packs be no larger than 30 cm × 30 cm × 50 cm and weigh no more than 5.4 kg, but it depends on the type of material being autoclaved. In many practices, the pack size is limited by the size of the autoclave.

Packs must be properly wrapped with steam-permeable wrappers. Double-thickness muslin (thread count of 140 threads per 6.45 cm²) is a good wrapping material and will protect the surgical supplies following sterilization. Paper

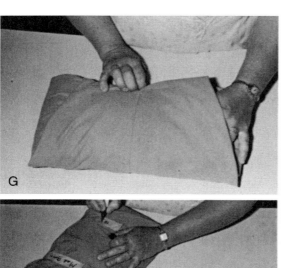

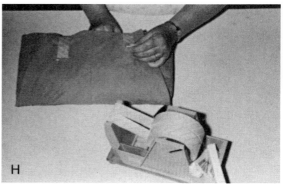

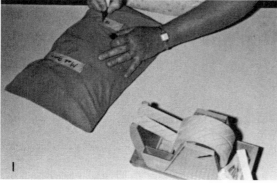

Figure 16-56 *Continued* G, The remaining corner is folded under and then folded over the top. H, The pack is secured with autoclave tape and is labeled with contents, date, and initials of the individual preparing the pack (I).

(crepe) can be used as a wrapping material, but waxed paper is unsuitable. Each pack must be labeled identifying the pack contents, the person who prepared it, and the date it was sterilized.

The autoclave should be loaded with a space of 2.5 to 7.5 cm around each pack. Packs should be arranged so that steam can readily flow from top to bottom in the autoclave. For example, a large pack should not be placed on top of several small ones because it will impede the flow of steam down through the spaces between the smaller packs. Alternatively, packs may be positioned vertically (on edge) to facilitate steam flow.

A number of minimum time-temperature standards have

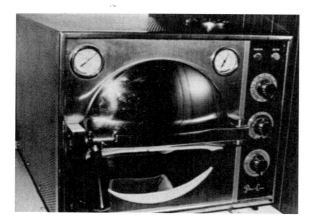

Figure 16-57. Autoclave. The autoclave uses saturated steam under pressure to achieve high temperatures capable of sterilizing instruments. Particular care must be taken to correctly load the autoclave.

been established for routine sterilization of surgical packs. Exposure to saturated steam at 121°C (250°F) for 13 minutes is considered to be a safe minimum standard. In general, 5 to 10 minutes at this temperature will destroy most resistant microbes, and an additional 3 to 8 minutes provides a margin of safety. Timing of the exposure begins when the temperature in the exhaust line reaches the desired level, at which point the entire contents of the sterilizing chamber are completely exposed to steam. The time required for the sterilizing temperature to be reached is referred to as the heat-up time and is extremely short (about 1 minute) in prevacuum and pulsing-type sterilizers. Large linen packs require both a longer heat-up time and a longer exposure time. General guidelines for their saturation are 30 to 45 minutes at 121°C (250°F) in gravity displacement sterilizers and 4 minutes at 131°C (270°F) in prevacuum sterilizers.

Emergency sterilization of instruments, also called "flash" sterilization, is usually performed in prevacuum sterilizers. The recommended exposure time is 3 minutes at 131°C (270°F). The unwrapped instruments are placed in a perforated metal tray for sterilization and then carried to the operating room using detachable handles.

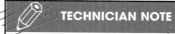
TECHNICIAN NOTE

The safe minimal standard for autoclave sterilization is 121°C (250°F) for 13 minutes.

At the end of the sterilizing cycle, the autoclave door is unlocked and "cracked." If the autoclave door is opened wide, the cool air from outside will condense the steam in the materials, causing them to become soggy. After about 10 minutes, the

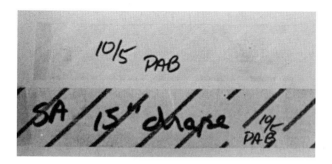

Figure 16-58. Autoclave tape before (above) and after (below) sterilization. Notice the appearance of the black line stripes.

moisture remaining in the materials has vaporized and escaped through the cracked door, and the materials should be thoroughly dry.

Paper-wrapped products should not remain in the autoclave longer than 15 to 20 minutes after cracking the door. If left too long, the heat will dry the paper, making it brittle and likely to crack and split when handled.

Sterilization Quality Control

The only practical and reliable assurance that sterilization has been achieved is through proper technique and the use of dependable sterilization indicators. An indicator should be placed in the central, least accessible portion of each pack. After the pack is opened, the indicator is checked before using the materials.

There are four types of sterilization indicators used in autoclaves: (1) autoclave tape, (2) fusible melting pellet glass type, (3) culture tests, and (4) chemical sterilization indicators. These indicators are meant to be used in combination because no one test alone can provide quality assurance of sterility.

Autoclave tape is useful for identifying packs and articles that have been exposed to steam, but it does not ensure that the proper requirements of time, temperature, and steam have been met (Fig. 16–58). The fusible melting pellet glass type indicates that a temperature of approximately 118°C (244°F) was reached, but there is no assurance of proper length of time or of a saturated steam atmosphere. Culture test indicators consist of test strips that contain a controlled-count spore population of some particular strain of bacterium. This biological challenge test is very helpful since it is the only test that proves sterility was achieved and microorganisms were killed. The

disadvantage of this test is that the results are not immediately available and it does not assess steam penetration. Chemical sterilization indicators are available in many types (Fig. 16–59) and they undergo color changes when subjected to saturated steam for adequate periods of time. Most practices will use a combination of autoclave tape and a centrally placed chemical sterilization indicator to assure sterility of the surgical pack.

> ### ✎ TECHNICIAN NOTE
>
> The four types of sterilization indicators are (1) autoclave tape, (2) melting glass pellets, (3) culture tests, and (4) chemical sterilization indicators.

In the newer *prevacuum* sterilizers, an air removal test can be run daily to ensure that air is sufficiently removed from the autoclave. In *gravity displacement* sterilizers, temperature graphs can be kept as a record of autoclave performance. Therefore, quality assurance occurs at two levels, one to ensure that the pack runs through a sterilization cycle and another to ensure that the autoclave system is working properly. Quality control is essential to any surgical practice, because failure of proper sterilization can have far-reaching consequences.

Care and Handling of Sterile Packs

Sterile packs should be stored in a dust-free, dry, and well-ventilated area away from contaminated equipment. Storage in closed cabinets is preferable to open shelving. Safe pack storage times are listed in Table 16–5. If a pack is dropped, the tape sealing the pack is broken, or the pack wrap becomes wet, punctured, or torn, the pack should be considered contaminated. If there is any doubt as to the sterility of an item, consider it unsterile.

> ### ✎ TECHNICIAN NOTE
>
> Ethylene oxide is the most commonly used type of chemical sterilization.

Chemical Methods of Sterilization

Chemical sterilization is performed with certain liquids or gases. Liquid chemicals can be used for instrument sterilization. The

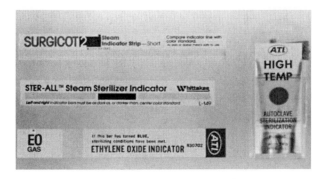

Figure 16-59. Various sterilization indicator strips.

• Table 16–5 •

SAFE STORAGE TIMES FOR STERILE PACKS		
WRAPPER	**CLOSED CABINET**	**OPEN CABINET**
Single-wrapped muslin	1 week	2 days
Double-wrapped muslin	7 weeks	3 weeks
Single-wrapped crepe paper	At least 8 weeks	3 weeks

most common agent used for liquid sterilization is glutaraldehyde. Gas sterilization is used for items which cannot tolerate the high temperatures or steam associated with autoclaving (some power equipment or plastic products). The most common agent used for gas sterilization is ethylene oxide.

Ethylene Oxide

Ethylene oxide is a colorless gas at room temperature. It is flammable, explosive, toxic, irritating to skin and mucous membranes, and therefore a potential health hazard. Ethylene oxide penetrates paper and plastic film packaging. The item to be gas-sterilized is wrapped in plastic packaging and heat-sealed prior to sterilization. Plastic film packaging materials that are suitable for ethylene oxide sterilization include polyethylene, polypropylene, and polyvinyl chloride.

Ethylene oxide destroys metabolic pathways within the cells by alkylation and it is capable of killing all microorganisms. Effective sterilization with ethylene oxide is dependent on the concentration of gas, exposure time, temperature, and relative humidity. The activity of ethylene oxide is enhanced by increasing the temperature or the gas concentration. Ethylene oxide sterilizers usually operate at temperatures between 21° and 60°C (70° and 140°F). The activity of ethylene oxide approximately doubles with each 10°C increase in temperature. Doubling the ethylene oxide concentration decreases the sterilization time by approximately one half. Moisture is necessary for the lethal action of ethylene oxide and optimal relative humidity for sterilization with ethylene oxide is 40%. Exposure time varies from 48 minutes to several hours, but 12 hours of exposure is commonly used when sterilizing at room temperature.

All materials sterilized with ethylene oxide should be quarantined in a well-ventilated area for a minimum of 24 hours following sterilization. Color-coded chemical sterilization indicators are commonly placed within the packs when using ethylene oxide sterilization (Fig. 16–59). Biological indicators are available for ethylene oxide sterilization and are the only truly reliable test for sterility. Since results are unavailable for several days, biological indicators are most commonly used to evaluate the sterilization system and not individual packs.

Gas plasma sterilization is quickly replacing ethylene oxide because it is safer for the environment and personnel. Many human hospitals and university veterinary hospitals have converted to this system. In ethylene oxide systems, the chlorofluorocarbon component (CFC-12) of a 12/88 ethylene oxide system was banned by the Food and Drug Administration (FDA) as of January 1, 1996 and is no longer manufactured. Therefore, many hospitals had to recalibrate their ethylene oxide system or convert to a gas plasma system.

Chemical Disinfection

A *disinfectant* is an agent that destroys disease-producing microorganisms or inactivates viruses. In general, disinfectants are chemical agents that are applied to inanimate objects to destroy the vegetative form of bacteria but not necessarily the spore forms. Disinfectants that are capable of destroying vegetative bacteria, plus spores, tubercle bacilli, and viruses, may be used as chemical sterilizers.

Disinfection time is the time required for a particular agent to produce its maximum effect. It is influenced by many factors, including the nature of the material being disinfected, the degree of soil and microbial contamination, and the concentration and germicidal potency of the disinfectant.

Antisepsis is the prevention of infection by destruction or inhibition of the infectious agents, generally bacteria. Antiseptics are used on skin and living tissue and antisepsis is accomplished by topical treatment with antiseptic agents such as an iodine or chlorhexidine scrub. A glossary of key terms used in describing aseptic technique may be found in Table 16–6.

Antiseptic and Disinfectant Compounds

Iodine

Iodine compounds are effective antimicrobial agents, but have limited activity against bacterial spores. Iodine solutions are used for surgical preparation, topical wound therapy, and joint and body cavity lavage (Table 16–7). Iodine compounds are available as aqueous solutions, tinctures, and iodophors. *Aqueous solutions* contain higher levels of free iodine than iodophors and therefore have greater bactericidal activity. However, aqueous solutions are also cytotoxic and cannot be used in living tissue unless they are greatly diluted. Aqueous iodine also stains materials and is corrosive to instruments.

Tincture of iodine is a solution of 2% iodine in 50% ethyl alcohol and is intended for use on intact skin. It is not commonly used in veterinary practice.

Iodophors contain iodine complexed with surfactants or polymers, so free iodine is released slowly. The adverse properties of staining and irritation are reduced and delivery of iodine to the tissues is enhanced. *Povidone-iodine* is the most commonly used iodophor and is available as scrubs or solutions. Dilution of stock solutions (common dilutions include 1:10, 1:50, and 1:100) increases the bactericidal activity and decreases

• Table 16–6 •

GLOSSARY OF KEY TERMS	
Antiseptic	An agent capable of preventing infection by inhibiting the growth of infectious agents. This term is generally applied to living tissues.
Autoclave	Sterilizers that use saturated steam under pressure to achieve high temperatures for sterilization. Minimal exposure to saturated steam is 13 minutes at 121°C (250°F).
Disinfectant	An agent that destroys of inhibits microorganisms. Typically refers to inanimate objects.
Ethylene oxide	A gas chemical sterilization agent used to sterilize objects that cannot withstand heat.
Flash sterilization	Emergency sterilization in which the object (instrument) is placed unwrapped in an autoclave and taken directly to the surgery following sterilization. Recommended exposure is 3 minutes at 131°C (270°F).
Sterilization	The destruction of all microorganisms. This term is generally applied to inanimate objects.

• Table 16–7 •

COMMON ANTISEPTIC AND DISINFECTANT AGENTS

AGENT	EXAMPLES	COMMON USES	SPECTRUM OF ACTIVITY	RESIDUAL ACTIVITY
Povidone-iodine detergent	Betadine scrub (Purdue-Frederick) (brown sudsy solution)	Preoperative scrubs	Bacteria, viruses, fungi, protozoa, yeast	4–6 hours, but inactivated by organic debris and alcohol
Povidone-iodine solution	Betadine solution (Purdue-Frederick) (brown solution)	Preoperative antiseptic application; wound lavage when diluted 1:100	Bacteria, viruses, fungi, protozoa, yeast	4–6 hours, but inactivated by organic debris and alcohol
Chlorhexidine detergent	Nolvasan scrub (Fort Dodge Laboratories) (blue solution); Hibiclens scrub (Stuart Pharmaceuticals) (pink solution)	Preoperative scrubs	Bacteria, viruses, fungi, yeast	2 days; not inhibited by organic matter or alcohol; less skin irritation
Chlorhexidine solution	Nolvasan solution (Fort Dodge Laboratories) (nonsudsy blue solution)	Preoperative antiseptic application; wound lavage when diluted 1:40	Bacteria, viruses, fungi, yeast	2 days; bactericidal, but not cytotoxic in open wounds at diluted concentrations
Alcohol: isopropyl and ethanol	Many manufacturers	Surgical preparations; disinfection antisepsis; do not use in open wounds	Bacteria, some fungi	None
Phenols Hexchlorophene	pHisoHex scrub (Sanofi; Winthrop) (white)	Preoperative hand scrub	Bacteria (more effective against gram-positive than gram-negative species)	Up to 2 days
Glutaraldehyde		Cold sterilization; not intended for living tissues	Bacteria, viruses, fungi, yeast, spores	None; causes skin irritation

the cytotoxicity. The residual bacterial activity of povidone-iodine is 4 to 6 hours, but this is greatly diminished in the presence of organic matter.

Povidone-iodine is one of the most common surgical scrubs used in veterinary hospitals. Although it is a relatively safe skin preparation there are several concerns regarding its use. Alcohol, lavage solutions, or organic debris such as blood will destroy the residual bactericidal activity. Povidone-iodine can cause skin irritation or acute contact dermatitis in up to 50% of canine patients and it may be a problem for some hospital staff. Rarely, individuals who have repeated contact with iodine scrub solutions may develop systemic iodine toxicity, resulting in metabolic acidosis and thyroid dysfunction.

> **TECHNICIAN NOTE**
>
> The two most commonly used antiseptic agents are povidone-iodine and chlorhexidine.

Chlorhexidine

Chlorhexidine is an antiseptic agent that is available in aqueous, tincture, and detergent formulations. It is an effective antimicrobial agent with activity against bacteria, molds, yeasts, and viruses. Chlorhexidine has a rapid onset and a long residual activity which is not affected by alcohol, lavage solutions, or organic debris. It has become a popular surgical scrub because of its effectiveness and because it is nonirritating to the skin. In several human studies chlorhexidine has been found to be superior to povidone-iodine as a surgical hand scrub. The effectiveness of povidone-iodine and chlorhexidine is similar when they are used as surgical scrubs for canine surgery.

As a lavage solution for open wounds, chlorhexidine must be diluted 1:40 with sterile water or saline to produce a 0.05% solution. At this concentration, chlorhexidine has significant antibacterial activity with no cytotoxicity and is superior to povidone-iodine, saline, and other antiseptics. Higher concentrations can cause inflammation and cytotoxicity, so they are not recommended in open wounds. When chlorhexidine is mixed with electrolyte solutions (such as lactated Ringer's solution), it will precipitate, but this does not affect antimicrobial activity and the solution can still be used for wound lavage.

> **TECHNICIAN NOTE**
>
> Chlorhexidine is an effective antimicrobial agent with rapid onset and long residual activity.

Alcohols

Widely used as disinfectant and antiseptic agents, alcohols are organic solvents that evaporate rapidly, leaving no residue. Alcohols are bactericidal, but ineffective against spores and fungi. They have no residual effects and are inhibited by organic debris. Ethyl and isopropyl alcohols are more effective than methyl alcohol as disinfecting agents. Alcohols should

never be used in open wounds because they are both painful and cytotoxic.

Phenols

Phenols (carbolic acid) have been used historically as both antiseptics and disinfectants, but phenols have been routinely replaced by newer, safer, and more effective agents. Hexachlorophene, a skin preparation, was one of the most popular phenols but it has been replaced by povidone-iodine and chlorhexidine.

Quaternary Ammonium

Quaternary ammonium compounds are synthetic cationic detergents which act on cell membranes and are effective against bacteria, but not spores or some viruses. Very bland and nontoxic, these agents are quite popular. Benzalkonium chloride is the most commonly used quaternary ammonium compound and is used as a disinfectant.

Chloride

Chloride compounds were among the first agents to be used as medical disinfectants and found popularity for wound treatment in World War I as Dakin's solution. Antimicrobial chlorine compounds, specifically the hypochlorites, have broad bactericidal and virucidal activity, but can be cytotoxic when improperly used on living tissues. Presently, sodium hypochlorite (bleach) is commonly used as a disinfectant in many hospitals.

Aldehyde

Formaldehyde and glutaraldehyde are the most commonly used aldehydes in veterinary medicine. They are both toxic and irritating which restricts them from use on living tissues. They are very effective antimicrobial agents, but may require several hours of exposure time. Formaldehyde is commonly used in the preservation of tissue specimens. Glutaraldehyde is commonly used for chemical sterilization in cold trays and for endoscopy equipment.

Cold Sterilization

Cold sterilization refers to soaking instruments in disinfecting solutions such as chlorhexidine or glutaraldehyde. Metal trays used to soak instruments in disinfectant are called "cold trays" (Fig. 16–60). Since sterility cannot be guaranteed, cold-sterilized instruments should be used only for minor procedures (superficial lacerations, dental procedures) or for equipment that cannot tolerate other forms of sterilization such as endoscopic equipment. Exposure times should exceed 3 hours and the equipment must be rinsed thoroughly before use.

> **TECHNICIAN NOTE**
>
> The arthroscope, fiberoptic light cable, and camera should never be steam-sterilized.

Sterilization of Arthroscopic Equipment

Most of the hand instruments and ancillary equipment can be steam-sterilized. They can also be gas-sterilized with ethylene oxide or cold-sterilized using a glutaraldehyde-based solution

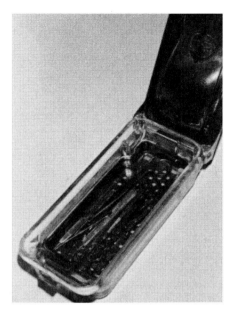

Figure 16-60. Cold pack sterilization tray. Instruments are kept submerged in a disinfectant solution and retrieved by lifting the rack. Instruments are only used for minor procedures because instrument sterility is not guaranteed.

(Cidexplus, Johnson & Johnson Medical Inc, Arlington, Tex.) (Fig. 16–61). Cold sterilization affords the ability to use the equipment more than once in a single day, unlike steam and gas sterilization in most situations. The arthroscope, light cable, and camera can be gas- or cold-sterilized, but *not* steam-sterilized.

With cold sterilization, the instruments are soaked for a minimum of 20 minutes in the Cidexplus just prior to surgery. The electrical plug of the camera cable and light source end of the light cable are not submerged in the cold sterilization solution, which would damage them. These ends are draped out over the top of the container with the Cidexplus (Fig. 16–62). The surgeon or assistant double-gloves and removes the instruments from the solution. The instruments are then placed in a

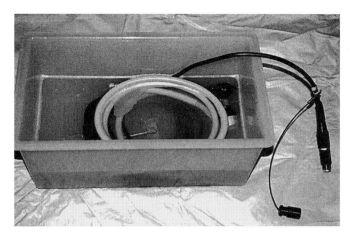

Figure 16-62. The electrical plug of the camera cable is draped over the top of the cold sterilization container to prevent it from being submerged, which could damage it.

sterile autoclave tray containing sterile water (Fig. 16–63). Once the instruments have been submerged in the water, each piece is gently agitated, individually removed from the tray, rinsed with sterile water by a scrub nurse or other assistant, and transferred to the instrument table. The surgeon or assistant removes his or her outer gloves and dries the instruments. It is important that the Cidexplus be thoroughly rinsed from the instruments. Glutaraldehyde can cause a chemical synovitis and is injurious to chondrocytes. A double rinse further reduces the amount of glutaraldehyde residue remaining on the instruments.

 TECHNICIAN NOTE

Glutaraldehyde causes a chemical synovitis and is injurious to chondrocytes.

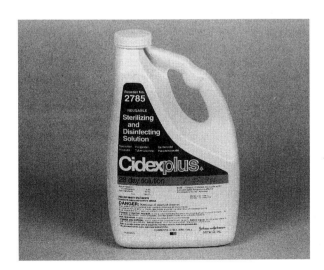

Figure 16-61. Cold sterilization solution (Cidexplus, Johnson & Johnson Medical Inc.).

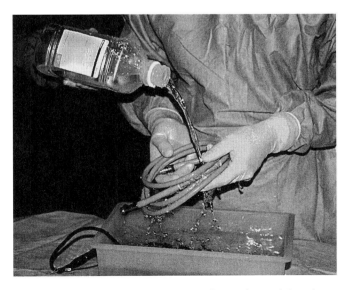

Figure 16-63. Once the arthroscopic equipment has been cold soaked, it is rinsed and transferred aseptically to a sterile tray that contains sterile water.

Operating Room Preparation

Operating room cleanliness is essential to proper aseptic technique. A routine daily and weekly cleaning schedule should be established to keep the operating room clean and dust-free. The surgery table should be cleaned and disinfected, and soiled areas of the floor should be cleaned and disinfected by damp mopping after each surgery throughout the day. It is preferable to perform thorough daily cleaning at the end of the day because cleaning creates airborne dust which takes several hours to settle. (The operating room is never dry-mopped or dusted because this produces excessive airborne dust.) Buckets should be emptied and cleaned. The operating table and all equipment should be cleaned and damp-dusted with a disinfectant solution. The casters on equipment should be cleaned, and the floor should be mopped.

Once a week, the operating room should undergo a thorough cleaning in which movable equipment is removed and cleaned with a disinfectant solution. Permanent structures such as walls, windows, window sills, light fixtures, and the surgical table should also be wiped clean. Radiators or air vents should be cleaned and cabinets should be emptied, washed, and restocked. The operating room floor should be scrubbed and disinfected. Disinfectant can be applied with a mop, although this may actually spread dirt and microorganisms throughout the room. To avoid this, the mop head should be laundered daily and not stored in used disinfectant solution. The wet-vacuum method in which the clean floor is flooded with disinfectant solution and then vacuumed is superior to mopping. All cleaning equipment used in the operating room should be kept separate from all other cleaning equipment.

Operating room design is important for ease of cleaning. The operating room should be simple and uncluttered. Commonly used equipment and materials should be readily available, but excess stock should not be stored in the operating room. When additional equipment is needed it is brought to the operating room by the circulating nurse.

Daily cleaning of the surgical preparation room is also important. The surgical preparation room is subject to continual contamination and must be kept tidy and clean. Sinks and plumbing fixtures should be scrubbed. Buckets and vacuum canisters are emptied and cleaned. Furniture and cabinets should be damp-dusted and the floor scrubbed. If there are holding cages in the preparation room, they should be cleaned and disinfected. All surgical preparation solutions and supplies should be replenished.

Patient Preparation

Surgical Clip

The surgical preparation can begin the day before surgery. The animal should be bathed (small animal) and a rough clipping performed at the surgical site. In the rough clipping, the hair is shaved in the same direction as the hair growth.

On the day of surgery, the surgical site is prepared after the animal is anesthetized. In the final surgical clip, the hair is shaved against the direction of hair growth to achieve the closest shave possible (using a no. 40 clipper blade for small animals and no. 10 for large animals). A wide region of skin is shaved around the proposed surgical incision. A general rule is to shave at least 4 inches in every direction from the proposed incision. Long hair that originates outside this area, but falls into the field, should also be clipped. If an open wound is present, it should be packed with a sterile, water-soluble lubricant prior to shaving. The lubricant traps hair and debris, which can be flushed away before skin preparation. Areas with obvious signs of infection should be clipped last so that the clippers will not spread infected fluids and debris toward the intended incision site. Once the surgical clip is completed a vacuum cleaner may be used to eliminate loose hairs on the skin. The surgical clip and scrub should be thorough but gentle. Unnecessary roughness will result in inflamed or traumatized skin which can cause greater postoperative complications.

Surgical Scrub

Initial skin preparation is done in the preparation room. The skin is initially washed to remove gross contamination. The surgical scrub is usually performed by alternating between an antiseptic scrub (such as povidone-iodine or chlorhexidine scrub) and alcohol. (Remember not to use alcohols or detergents in open wounds, eyes, or mucous membranes.) The surgical site is scrubbed a minimum of three separate times or until the sponges do not pick up dirt. It is extremely important to begin the scrub over the proposed incision site, and to scrub outward in a circular pattern, never going back toward the center with the same gauze sponge (Fig. 16–64). An antiseptic solution may be applied to the surgical site via a spray bottle or sterile sponge after the final surgical scrub. The animal is moved to the operating table and positioned. If contamination occurs the area is rescrubbed. Many veterinarians prefer to routinely have the surgical site rescrubbed after the animal is positioned on the operating table.

> **TECHNICIAN NOTE**
>
> It is generally recommended that the surgical site be scrubbed and rinsed three times. An antiseptic solution is often applied to the skin following the scrubs.

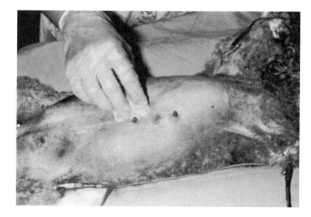

Figure 16–64. The surgical preparation should begin at the proposed incision site and should progress outward, never returning to the proposed incision line with the same gauze sponge. Examination gloves worn during the preparation decrease contamination from human hands.

There are many common modifications to the surgical preparation technique. For example, in preparation for feline orchiectomy (castration) the scrotal hair is plucked rather than clipped. Feline onychectomy (declawing) and tail docking and dewclaw removal of neonatal puppies are commonly performed without clipping the hair. The surgical site is soaked or gently scrubbed with detergent and swabbed with alcohol or antiseptic solution. Bovine and porcine castrations are performed without clipping the hair and an alcohol or antiseptic wash is usually used. Equine castrations may be prepared with three thorough washes using chlorhexidine or povidone-iodine solution diluted in water.

Patient Positioning

The veterinarian should be consulted as to how the animal will be positioned during surgery. The majority of surgical procedures are performed using a few basic positions. The position of the animal is described by the region of the body that is contacting the table. For example, right lateral recumbency means the animal is lying on its right side, dorsal recumbency means the animal is on its back, and sternal recumbency means the animal is on its belly. Patient positioning can be facilitated by the use of adjustable surgical tables, portable tabletop V troughs, sandbags, or vacuum-activated "beanbags."

In orthopedic surgery the affected leg is often suspended from an overhead support or IV (intravenous) stand during skin preparation and initial surgical draping. The advantage of "hanging the leg" is that it allows aseptic preparation of the entire circumference of the limb, so the surgeon can manipulate it during surgery. It is often necessary for the surgeon to manipulate the limb to properly position it and provide the best exposure of the surgical site. To hang the leg, the distal limb is wrapped (using gauze or an examination glove covered with tape) to cover any unclipped areas, and strips of tape ("stirrups") are extended from the end of the foot. The leg is suspended by these stirrups (Fig. 16–65). The entire limb circumference is clipped and scrubbed from the highest point (distal limb) to the level of the inguinal or axillary region. The skin preparation is usually extended to the dorsal and ventral midlines to allow adequate room for sterile towels to be draped on the body. The surgeon covers and holds the foot with a sterile wrap while the circulating nurse cuts the stirrups. The surgeon then completes the draping process. A cotton stockinette or adhesive drape is often used to cover the entire leg and further isolate the incision site from the surrounding skin. The stockinette-covered limb is passed through a hole in a sterile drape. Once the skin incision has been made, stockinette or drape is sutured or clipped to the skin edges.

TECHNICIAN NOTE

The dorsal recumbent position is commonly used for abdominal surgical procedures.

Surgical Team Preparation

Attire

Surgical attire, the surgical scrub suit, and proper gowning and gloving procedures are important aspects of aseptic technique.

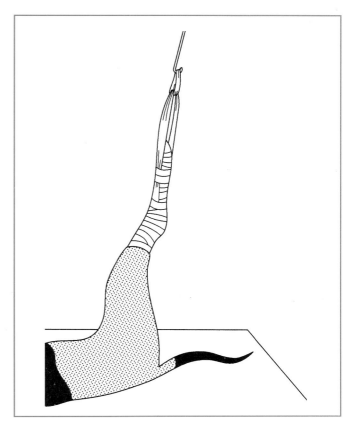

Figure 16–65. Hanging leg surgical preparation. This is commonly used for orthopedic surgeries of legs including the shoulder and hip. The operated limb is suspended by tape stirrups that cover all distal leg hair. The surgical scrubs are started at the highest aspect of the clipped leg and worked downward with gravity in a circular fashion. At surgery, the taped foot is wrapped in a sterile towel, and the stirrups are cut.

Street clothing, especially shoes, are a major source of contamination and should not be worn into the operating room. Shoes worn in the operating room should not be worn as street shoes, or shoe covers should be worn. Cotton scrub suits should be worn during surgery. The shirt should be tucked into the pants to reduce the amount of skin debris dispersed into the room. When preparing an animal for surgery, surgical scrubs should be protected by a smock or laboratory coat.

Surgical caps and masks are essential. The surgical cap is designed to cover the hair and prevent airborne contamination. Several types of surgical head covers are available to accommodate long hair or to cover beards (Fig. 16–66). The mask is worn to filter air exhaled from the nose and mouth. Masks are effective filters for relatively short periods only and should be changed between operations.

Hand Scrub

The purpose of scrubbing the hands and arms is to remove dirt and decrease the concentration of bacterial flora. The surgical cap and mask must be donned, and all jewelry removed from hands and arms before beginning the sterile hand scrub. Once the scrubbing has begun, the hands and arms should not touch unsterile objects. If this occurs, the scrub is started over.

The hands and arms are lathered for about 1 minute without a brush and then rinsed in running water. While scrubbing,

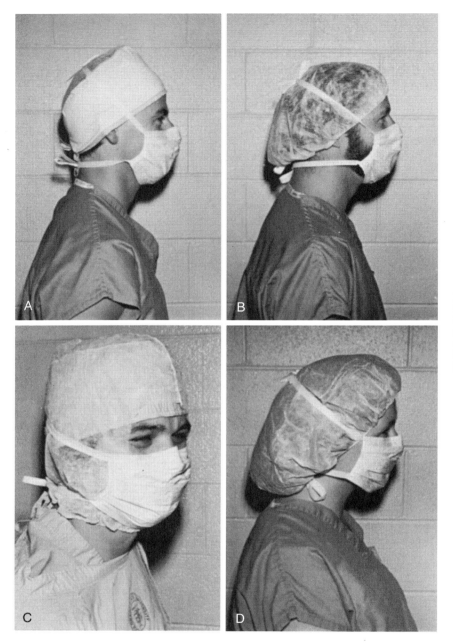

Figure 16-66. Surgical caps and masks. A, Cap and mask suitable for short-haired individual. B, Inappropriate coverage of sideburns and beard by a cap and mask. C, Hoods available for individuals with long hair, sideburns, or beard. D, Bouffant-type head cover for long hair.

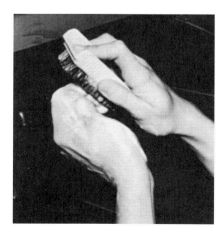

Figure 16-67. Surgical hand scrub. Each surface of every finger should be thoroughly scrubbed, with special attention paid to the fingernails.

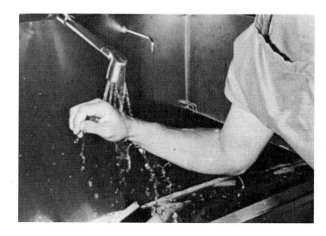

Figure 16-68. The hands, forearms, and brush are thoroughly rinsed between scrubs. Keep hands above elbows.

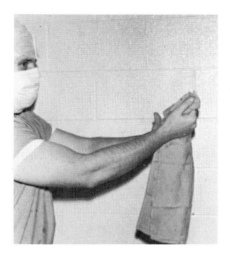

Figure 16–69. One hand and arm are dried at a time, using a double-thickness (folded longitudinally) towel. The hand is dried first and then the arm, using half the towel. The other hand and arm are dried in a similar manner, using the other half of the towel. The towel should be held so that it does not brush against the body.

the hands are always held above the level of the elbows so the water drains off the elbows. Soap is applied to a sterile brush and a systematic scrub is begun. Scrub all four sides of each finger, with special attention to the fingernails (Fig. 16–67). The back, both sides, and the palm of the hand are scrubbed. Next, the wrist and forearm are scrubbed, working toward the elbow. After both hands and arms have been scrubbed, they are rinsed in running water (Fig. 16–68). The entire scrub process is then repeated.

The two basic types of surgical scrubs are anatomical and timed. The anatomical scrub is performed by counting the number of brush strokes used on each skin surface. Ten brush strokes are made on each surface of the hands and arms before rinsing. This is performed four times. The more commonly used timed scrub is performed by repeated scrubs over a set period of time. The initial scrub of the day should last about 10 minutes. For subsequent scrubs between surgeries, 5 minutes is adequate unless gross contamination has occurred.

> **TECHNICIAN NOTE**
>
> The surgical hand scrub requires that all surfaces of the fingers, hand, and forearm be scrubbed. Skin-soap contact time should last 10 minutes.

Gowning and Gloving

The hands and arms are thoroughly dried (Fig. 16–69) before gowning and gloving. The sterile gown is picked up and held by inside shoulder seams, allowing it to unfold. Sometimes it is necessary to gently shake the gown to completely unfold it. Hands should be approximately at chest level, and the gown should be held out away from the body. The sleeve openings are located, and the arms are slid into the sleeves (Fig. 16–70). The gown is secured at the neck and waist by a nonsterile assistant.

The two methods of gloving are *closed gloving* and *open gloving.* The risk of contamination is minimized with closed gloving (Fig. 16–71) since the outside of the gloves never contact skin. There is a much higher risk of contamination during open gloving (Fig. 16–72) and it is generally reserved for minor procedures when a gown is not worn. If it is necessary to replace gloves during surgery, it is preferable to have a nonsterile assistant remove the old gloves and simultaneously pull the

Figure 16–70. A, The gown is picked up at the shoulder seams, with only the inside of the gown touched. The gown is unfolded and held away from the body at shoulder height. B, The arms are slid into the sleeves.

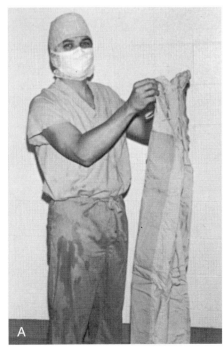

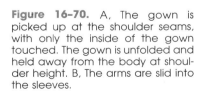

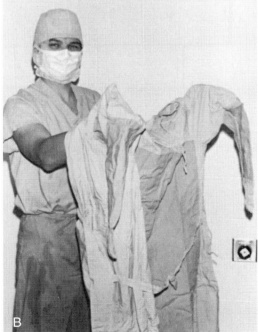

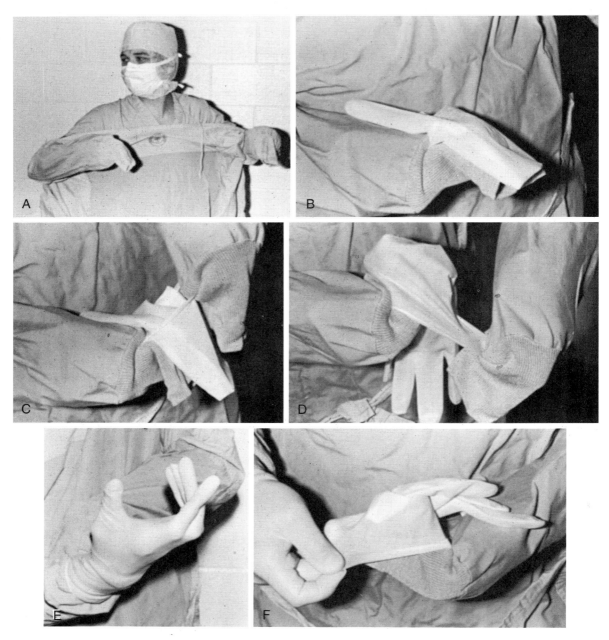

Figure 16–71. Closed gloving. A, When performing closed gloving, the hands are kept inside the sleeves while gloving takes place. B, The palm side of the glove is grasped at the cuff through the sleeve. C, The opposite side of the cuff is grasped in the other hand and D, pulled over the top side of the hand. E, The hand is slid completely into the glove. F, The opposite hand is gloved in a similar fashion. At no time should skin be visible while performing closed gloving.

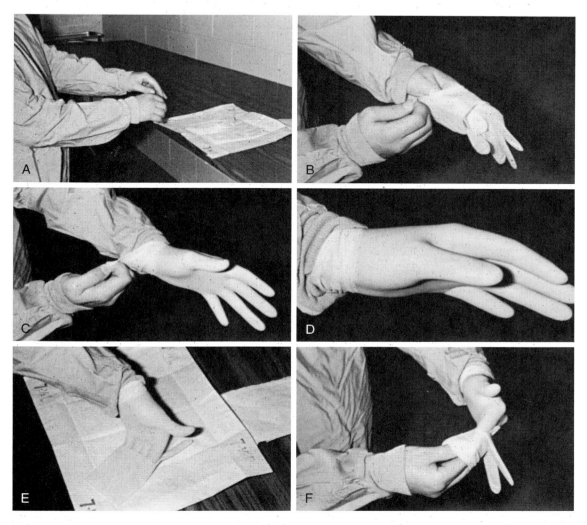

Figure 16-72. Open gloving. A, When performing open gloving, the hands are extended out of the sleeves while gowning. B, The palm side of the left glove is grasped at the fold by the right hand and is pulled onto the left hand. C and D, The left glove is pulled to the level of the sleeve and released. E, The gloved fingers of the left hand are then slid into the fold of the right glove. F, The fingers of the right hand are slid into the glove.

Illustration continued on following page

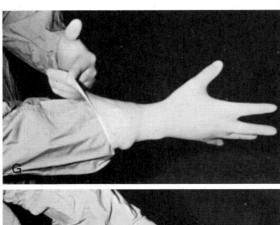

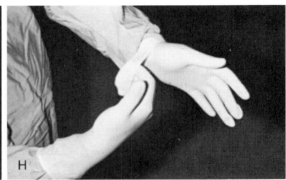

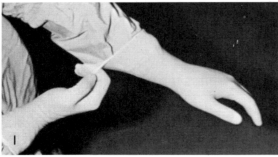

Figure 16-72 *Continued* G, Using the left hand, the glove is pulled up over the gown sleeve. H and I, The fingertips of the right hand are slid under the cuff of the left hand, and the glove is pulled over the sleeve. You will notice that ungloved fingers contact only the inside of the glove.

gown sleeve so the hands remain inside the sleeves. If the old gloves are removed in this manner, new gloves can be put on by the closed gloving method. If a surgical assistant is not available during a sterile procedure, the surgeon will have to use the open gloving technique when glove contamination occurs.

The Sterile Field

It is important for the entire surgical team to be aware of the sterile field, even if they are not "scrubbed in." Sterile personnel should only touch sterile items or areas. To maintain sterility of an item while removing it from its wrap, it should be grasped by a gloved hand or sterile instrument and lifted up and out. The edges of a sterile container are considered to be contaminated so items should not be dragged over the edge of the

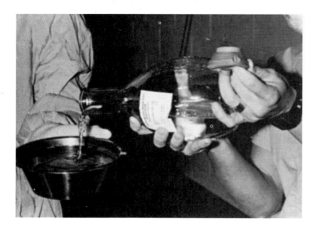

Figure 16-73. When pouring sterile fluids, one should hold the fluid container far enough away so that it does not come in contact with the sterile bowl yet it should be held close enough so that fluids do not splash.

container. The gown is considered to be sterile on the front of the sleeves and from the waist to shoulder level in front only. The back of a gowned person is considered to be nonsterile and should not be turned toward the sterile field. Draped tables are considered to be sterile only at table level, so if a sterile item extends below the table it is considered to be contaminated and should no longer be touched by sterile personnel.

TECHNICIAN NOTE

The two methods of gloving are *closed gloving* and *open gloving.*

Nonsterile personnel should only touch nonsterile items or areas and should not lean over a sterile field. Only the outside of sterile wraps should be touched by ungloved hands, and they should always be opened away from the body. When fluids are poured into a sterile bowl, the fluid container should not touch the bowl, nor should the fluids be poured from such a height that they splash (Fig. 16–73).

Recommended Reading

Berg RJ: Sterilization. *In* Slatter DH (editor): Textbook of Small Animal Surgery. Philadelphia, WB Saunders, 1993, pp 124–129.
Fries CL: Assessment and preparation of the surgical patient. *In* Slatter DH (editor): Textbook of Small Animal Surgery. Philadelphia, WB Saunders, 1993, pp 137–147.
Hurov L: Handbook of Veterinary Surgical Instruments and Glossary of Surgical Terms. Philadelphia, WB Saunders, 1978.
Knecht CD, Allen AR, Williams DJ, et al: Fundamental Techniques in Veterinary Surgery, 3rd ed. Philadelphia, WB Saunders, 1987, pp 2–25.
Knecht CD, Allen AR, Williams DJ, et al: Fundamental Techniques in Veterinary Surgery, 3rd ed. Philadelphia, WB Saunders, 1987, pp 73–103.

Lemarie RJ and Hosgood G: Antiseptics and disinfectants in small animal practice. Compendium Continuing Educ Pract Vet 17:1339–1352, 1996.

McIlwraith CW: Diagnostic and Surgical Arthroscopy in the Horse, 2nd ed. Philadelphia, Lea & Febiger, 1990, pp 5–20.

Nieves MA, Merkley DF, and Wagner SD: Surgical instruments. *In* Slatter DH (editor): Textbook of Small Animal Surgery. Philadelphia, WB Saunders, 1993, pp 154–168.

Pavletic MM: Surgical stapling. Vet Clin North Am 24:225–429, 1994.

Sumner-Smith G: Surgical nursing and anesthesiology. *In* Catcott EJ (editor): Animal Health Technology, 2nd ed. Santa Barbara, CA, American Veterinary Publications, 1977, pp 183–199.

Tracy DL and Warren RG: Small Animal Surgical Nursing. St Louis, Mosby–Year Book, 1983, pp 1–73.

Tracy DL and Warren RG: Small Animal Surgical Nursing. St Louis, Mosby–Year Book, 1983, pp 74–172.

Tracy DL and Warren RG: Instrumentation. Small Animal Surgical Nursing. St Louis, Mosby–Year Book, pp 173–244.

Wagner SD: Preparation of the surgical team. *In* Slatter DH (editor): Textbook of Small Animal Surgery, 2nd ed. Philadelphia, WB Saunders, 1993, pp 130–137.

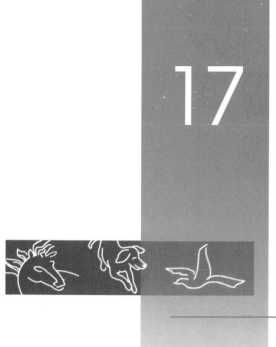

17

Surgical Assistance and Suture Material

Erick L. Egger

ROLE OF THE VETERINARY TECHNICIAN IN SURGICAL ASSISTANCE

The purpose of surgery in veterinary medicine is primarily that of service. In cases of clinical disease or injury, surgery is used to relieve suffering and improve the quality of life for the animal patient and consequently the owner. Veterinary surgery is also performed to maintain or increase the economical value of animals that are used for food, breeding, show, or competitive purposes. The veterinary technician's role is to assist in providing this specialized service to the animal and owner. The technician accomplishes this by both helping the surgeon and protecting the patient. Surgical assistance includes improving the surgeon's visualization by providing retraction and hemostasis in the surgical field, being familiar with the objectives of the technique, and manipulating the instrumentation and tissues into position for completion of the surgical task. The second charge of the technician is to protect the patient from hazards of surgery, such as infection, by maintaining an aseptic surgical field and expediting surgical completion by anticipating needs for proper instrument and suture readiness. Since the surgeon is often concentrating on the surgical procedure, the technician must also be constantly aware of the patient's anesthetic and cardiovascular status while assisting.

PROPER TISSUE HANDLING TECHNIQUES

Each of the various body tissue systems has specific attributes that require consideration when being surgically approached. If the technician understands the general surgical principles of each system, the appropriate actions and measures to be taken in each specific case will be apparent.

Skin

The preparation of the patient's skin for surgery has been described in Chapter 16. One must remember that preparation results in an *aseptic* but not *sterile* skin. This means that the

---

 TECHNICIAN NOTE

Surgical preparation of the skin results in an aseptic, not sterile, skin.

---

number of bacteria have been reduced below the number required to overwhelm the body's defense mechanism. However, with a depressed immune system or prolonged surgery, these resident bacteria can start to multiply and result in infection. Therefore, the surgeon and assistant should avoid unnecessary direct handling of the skin with the gloves or instruments that will be used in the deeper incision. These items could then carry organisms into the deeper tissues. For lengthy or complicated procedures, a sterile plastic drape (Barrier, Johnson & Johnson) that directly adheres to the skin surface may be used (Fig. 17–1). A spray adhesive may be applied to the skin to augment the plastic's ability to remain in place throughout the surgery. The incision is made directly through the plastic drape. Alternatively, sterile towels or drapes may be applied to the margins of the skin incision to protect the deeper incision (Fig. 17–2). These towels may be attached with additional towel clamps spaced every 5 to 10 cm along the incision (Fig. 17–3) or by suturing the rolled edge of the towel or drape to the subcutaneous tissue with a simple continuous pattern of a

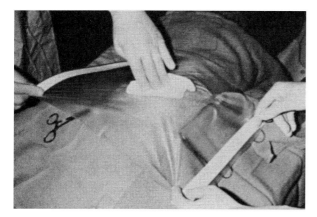

Figure 17-1. Application of a sterile plastic drape that adheres directly to the skin and minimizes potential contamination.

strong, inexpensive suture material. For orthopedic surgery, the limb is often enclosed in a sterile stockinette to allow movement and manipulation and to limit exposed skin. The edges of the incised stockinette are, likewise, often attached to the surgical incision. This can be accomplished by suturing as previously described or by the use of Michel clips (Fig. 17–4). The cut edge of the stockinette should be rolled under so that cut

TECHNICIAN NOTE

The skin incision should be performed with a sharp scalpel blade.

fragments of the stockinette material will not fall into the incision. The rolled-under stockinette is usually pulled over the skin edge and attached to the subcutaneous tissue to com-

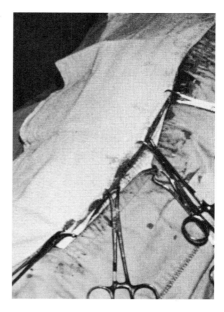

Figure 17-3. Use of towel clamps to attach towels to the incision margins.

pletely cover the cut skin edge. This will also control much of the minor hemorrhage that occurs following skin incision.

The skin incision itself should be performed with a sharp scalpel blade. A scissors will crush and shear skin as it cuts. Skin is generally sensitive to this form of injury and will commonly react with severe swelling and scar formation. Since the skin is relatively thick and elastic, it will also tend to force or "spring" the blades of the scissors apart, damaging the instrument. A sharp incision with a scalpel blade results in the most rapid healing and the least amount of scar formation. Skin incision with an electroscalpel somewhat delays healing and generally results in a larger scar. The principles and use of the electroscalpel are discussed later under Electrosurgery.

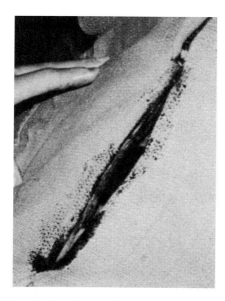

Figure 17-2. Application of sterile towels to skin margins to protect the deeper incision.

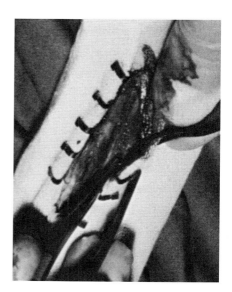

Figure 17-4. Use of Michel clips to attach the edge of the stockinette to the skin incision margins.

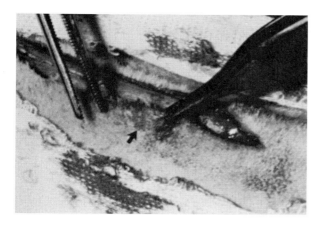

Figure 17-5. Smooth-jawed instruments hold tissue by pressure and can damage it by crushing (arrow).

Any instrument used to hold or manipulate skin should grip the tissue with teeth or hooks. Instruments that have smooth tips hold the tissue by pressure, which tends to crush skin and damage it in much the same way as scissors do (Fig. 17–5).

Hollow Organ Surgery

Surgery of the hollow organs (i.e., stomach, intestines, bladder, esophagus) requires both complete control of luminal contents to avoid contamination and careful handling to avoid damage to these delicate tissues. Whenever possible, the surgical site is isolated from the body cavity with saline-moistened laparotomy sponges. Specific intestinal forceps (Doyen) have been developed and can be used to prevent luminal content leakage when performing enterotomies or intestinal resections (Fig. 17–6). However, even these specialized clamps can damage tissues if tightened excessively or left in place too long (Fig. 17–7). Consequently, many surgeons prefer the assistant to occlude the intestinal lumen by using moistened gloved fingers (Fig. 17–8). Large, hollow organs such as the stomach or urinary bladder often cannot be exteriorized. Consequently, the incision

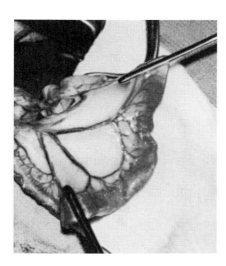

Figure 17-6. Use of Doyen intestinal forceps to prevent luminal content leakage during an enterotomy or a resection.

is made into the most elevated portion of the viscus to avoid leakage into the body cavity. This is usually accomplished by placing *stay sutures* at four points around the incision. Stay sutures are simple loops of suture that pass through the outer layers of the viscus and are held together at their ends with a clamp (Fig. 17–9). The surgical assistant supplies traction to the clamps to keep the incision in the desired location and elevated to avoid content leakage. (Fig. 17–10).

Musculoskeletal Surgery

Surgery of the musculoskeletal system often requires surgical assistance. Although muscle itself is highly vascular and has great healing ability, bone has a limited blood supply and heals slowly. Consequently, as the assistant retracts and manipulates fractures, all efforts should be made to preserve soft tissue attachment to bone. The assistant must also be cognizant of adjacent structures and protect them from damage by bony fragments or the surgeon. The most significant endangered structures are nerves. Specifically, the radial, ulnar, and ischiatic nerves course very closely to commonly occurring fractures and their surgical exposures. The surgical assistant must be familiar with the anatomical location of these structures.

Retraction Techniques

Retraction of tissues is often used to increase visibility and ease of manipulation in the incision. This can be accomplished with hand-held retractors by which the assistant provides traction in one direction with one retractor and countertraction in the opposite direction with a second retractor (Fig. 17–11). Retractors are available with various tips and blades to be used on different tissues. Care should be taken that retractors do not slide around or pull out of the incision, as this causes significant tissue trauma. Consequently, sharp-tipped retractors that maintain a grip on the tissue (without crushing) are often preferable to blunt-tipped retractors, particularly for muscle and skin retraction. Self-retaining retractors are also often used to free the assistant for other duties (Fig. 17–12). Excessive retraction for prolonged periods must be avoided with self-retaining instruments.

TECHNICIAN NOTE

The surgical assistant must be familiar with vital structures to avoid injury during retraction of tissues during surgery.

Manual traction on adjacent tissues is often used to increase visibility or expose organs. Deep structures of the right half of the canine or feline abdominal cavity may be visualized by retracting the proximal duodenum, which holds the abdominal viscera behind the mesentery, to the left, thus exposing the right kidney and ureter (Fig. 17–13). The left half of the abdominal cavity may likewise be visualized by retracting the abdominal viscera to the right, behind the mesocolon of the descending colon (Fig. 17–14). The pancreas is best exposed by traction on the adjacent duodenum. As when using fingers for occluding

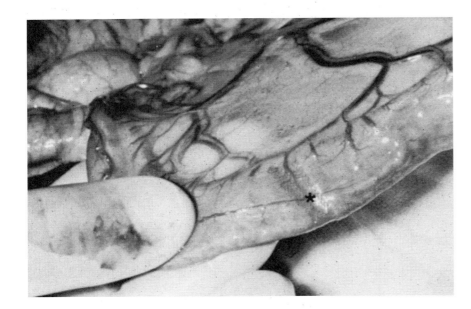

Figure 17-7. Area of intestinal damage (asterisk) from excessive tightening of a Doyen intestinal clamp.

Figure 17-8. Use of moistened gloved fingers to occlude the intestinal lumen.

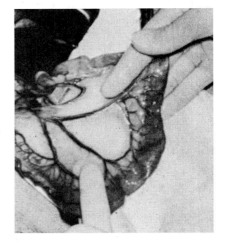

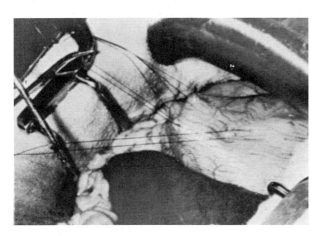

Figure 17-9. Stay sutures are passed through the outer layers of hollow organs. Both ends are held with a clamp.

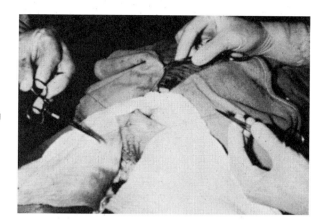

Figure 17-10. The assistant elevates the area of incision by applying traction to the stay sutures.

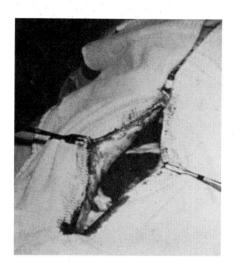

Figure 17-11. Exposure in the incision can be increased with hand retractors by the application of traction in one direction and countertraction in the opposite direction.

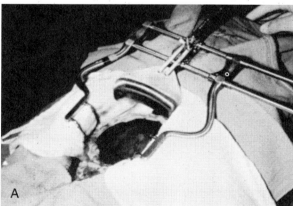

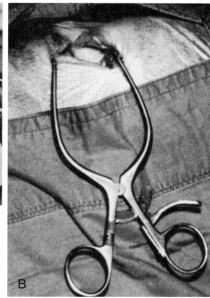

Figure 17-12. A, Use of a blunt-tipped self-retaining retractor (Balfour) in an abdominal incision during an exploratory laparotomy. B, Use of a sharp-tipped self-retaining retractor (Gelpi) between muscles during an arthrotomy.

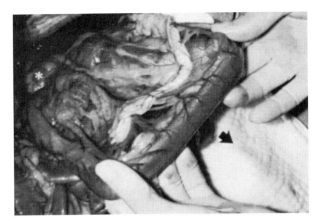

Figure 17-13. Retraction of the proximal duodenum to the left (arrow) exposes the right kidney (asterisk).

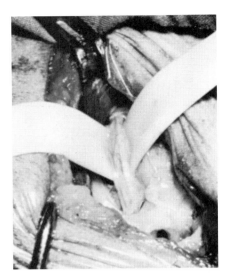

Figure 17-15. A Penrose drain is passed behind a nerve and used as a retractor.

the intestinal lumen, gloves should be moistened and excessive pressure should be avoided.

Nerves or large blood vessels are often retracted to improve visualization or to avoid potential damage. Careful blunt dissection is used to free the nerve or vessel from surrounding tissue. A broad, flat band, such as a Penrose drain or moistened umbilical tape, is passed around the structure (Fig. 17–15), and the ends are clamped together much like a stay suture. The assistant can gently retract the nerve or vessel to one side, carefully avoiding entanglement with other instruments or equipment (Fig. 17–16).

HEMOSTASIS

The surgical assistant is often responsible for maintaining hemostasis during surgery. Hemostasis is needed both to limit the volume of blood loss and to obtain optimal visibility in the incision. Hemostasis can be obtained by a variety of methods with which the surgical assistant should be familiar.

Sponge Hemostasis

Gauze sponge is often used to remove existing hemorrhage from incised tissues. Since any dry material is damaging to body

tissues, many assistants slightly moisten sponges with saline before using them in the incision. The sponge should be applied with a blotting type of motion. A wiping motion will irritate tissue and will often renew bleeding by pulling the forming blood clots out of incised capillaries. Sustained pressure through gauze sponges can be used to control bleeding from small vessels. The pressure apparently stops hemorrhage by collapsing the vessels until clotting can occur. With persistent hemorrhage, pressure may need to be sustained for up to 5 minutes to allow adequate coagulation.

Sponge Complications

Gauze sponges are extremely irritating and will cause severe tissue reaction, adhesions, and drainage if they are left in a closed incision. The abdominal and thoracic cavities are particularly hazardous locations for sponges to become lost. Consequently, many surgical assistants count sponges in such areas to make sure all sponges have been removed. Before surgery

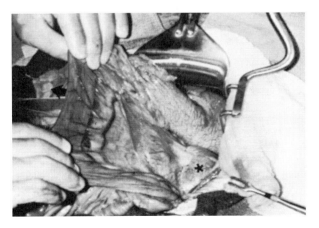

Figure 17-14. Retraction of the descending colon to the right (arrow) exposes the left kidney (asterisk).

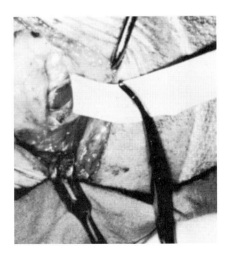

Figure 17-16. The ends of the drain are clamped together, and the nerve is pulled to one side to avoid damage.

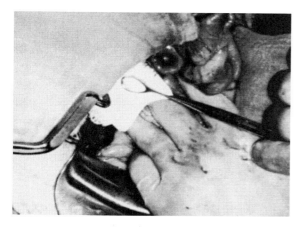

Figure 17-17. Gauze sponge held in a sponge forceps.

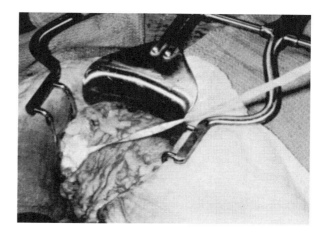

Figure 17-19. The tail is left extending out of the incision, allowing easy retrieval.

begins, sterile sponges are counted out in piles on the Mayo stand. Usually, two or three piles of ten sponges are used to start. The total number is recorded, and all other sponges (such as those used for skin preparation) are removed from the area. If additional sponges are required during surgery, they are supplied in packs of ten, and their number is added to the total. The used sponges are saved in a separate pile and are counted at the termination of the procedure before the incision is closed. The number of used sponges plus the remaining clean sponges must equal the total amount to account for all sponges.

TECHNICIAN NOTE

The surgical assistant should always count sponges in and out of the large body cavities (thorax or abdomen).

For use in particularly deep incisions, sponges may be held in a sponge forceps (Fig. 17–17) or tied with a long piece of umbilical tape (Fig. 17–18). The end of the tape (called the tail) is left extending out of the incision as the sponge is used (Fig. 17–19). The sponge can then be easily removed by pulling the tail.

Hemostatic Forceps

Hemorrhage from larger vessels can be occluded by clamping with a hemostatic forceps. The clamp should be applied perpendicular to the tissue surface and the bleeding vessel, with a minimal amount of adjacent tissue being grasped in the tips of the clamp (Fig. 17–20). Some surgeons twist off small vessels after clamping, but many surgeons have found this technique to be unreliable for hemostasis.

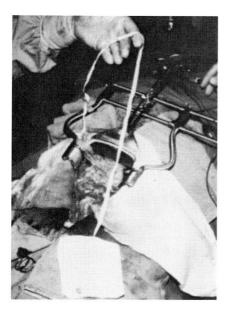

Figure 17-18. Gauze sponge tied to a long piece of umbilical tape.

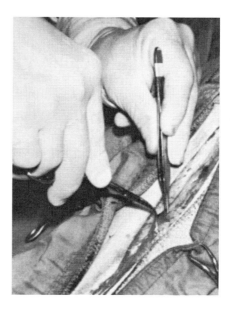

Figure 17-20. A hemostatic forceps is perpendicularly applied to the bleeding vessel with an minimal amount of adjacent tissue included.

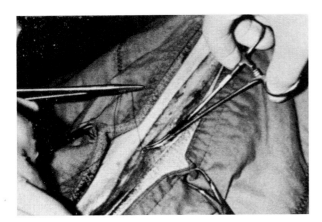

Figure 17-21. Lowering the handles of the hemostatic forceps raises the tips, forcing the ligation loop to form around the vessel.

Figure 17-22. The tips of the scissors are used to cut off excess suture.

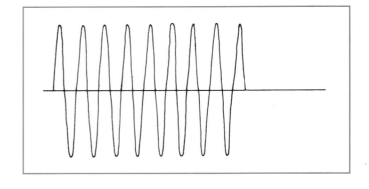

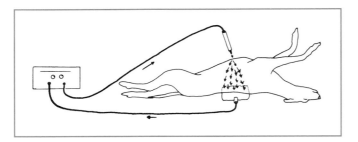

Figure 17-23. Diagram of electrical current passing from the handpiece, dispersing in the body, and returning to the generator via the ground plate.

Figure 17-24. Diagram of the undamped sine wave current, which ``cuts'' tissues.

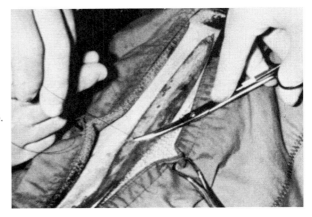

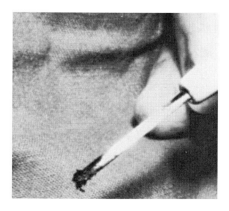

Figure 17-25. Build-up of protein on the handpiece tip, which prevents passage of current.

Suture Ligation

A bleeding vessel that has been clamped can be ligated to achieve permanent hemostasis. After the suture material is passed around the vessel, the assistant lowers the handles of the clamp, which raises the tips (Fig. 17–21). This causes the ligation loop to form around the vessel and not the instrument. As the first throw of the knot is pulled tight, the assistant releases the clamp. This allows the vessel to totally collapse, thus occluding the lumen. However the assistant should return the vessel to its origin before releasing the clamp so the knot is not snapped off the cut end of the vessel. After the surgeon finishes the knot, the assistant cuts off excessive suture, using the tips of the scissors (Fig. 17–22). Care must be taken not to pull the ligature off the end of the vessel. Only enough material to secure the knot should be left. Arteries are commonly ligated twice, particularly if more than 2 mm in diameter.

Electrosurgery

Electrosurgery offers a means of stopping hemorrhage after a vessel has been cut with electrocoagulation or preventing hemorrhage by incising with an electroscalpel. Either coagulation or incision can be obtained by passing an electrical current from a unipolar handpiece to a small contact area on the patient. The current then spreads out through the body and returns to the current generator via a ground plate (Fig. 17–23).

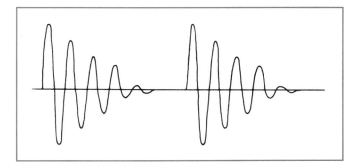

Figure 17-26. Diagram of the damped sine wave current, which causes coagulation.

Electroscalpel

Electrocutting occurs when the current generated is an undamped sine wave (Fig. 17–24). It causes microcoagulation of the tissue proteins at a small point of contact. A slow, steady motion of the handpiece is used to create an incision. As the protein coagulation occurs, carbon tends to build up on the active tip of the handpiece (Fig. 17–25). This carbon tends to insulate the current and should be periodically removed by the assistant who scrapes it with a hard metallic edge such as a scalpel handle.

Electrocoagulation

Electrocoagulation uses a damped electrical wave (Fig. 17–26) to produce protein coagulation of the blood elements within the blood vessel wall. Electrocoagulation should be used only on vessels smaller than 1.5 mm. Larger vessels should be ligated. The current can be applied through a hemostatic forceps clamped on the vessel (Fig. 17–27). Current can be directly applied to the vessel from the handpiece tip only if all blood and fluid, which would dissipate the current, have been blotted away. Most modern electrosurgical generators allow the blending of cutting and coagulation currents to achieve a truly bloodless incision (Fig. 17–28).

Bipolar Electrocautery

Bipolar electrocautery utilizes a thumb forceps–like handpiece (Fig. 17–29). The vessel to be cauterized is grasped between the blades of the forceps, and the coagulating current runs from one blade to the other, not through the body (Fig. 17–30). This form of electrocoagulation is particularly useful in neurosurgery in which unipolar currents can stimulate unwanted muscle contractions and injure the central nervous system.

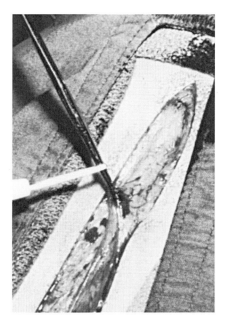

Figure 17-27. Application of current to a bleeding vessel by touching the handpiece to the hemostatic forceps.

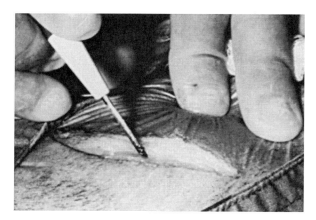

Figure 17–28. A bloodless incision can be obtained by blending cutting and coagulating currents.

Safety with Electrosurgery

Since electrosurgery will result in spark formation, it should *not* be used when explosive anesthetics, such as ether and cyclopropane, are present. Likewise, some antiseptic preparation materials (alcohol-based) and adhesive agents are volatile and should be avoided or allowed to dry thoroughly before using electrosurgery. The patient must have good electrical contact, using a conductive gel or fluid to a large area of ground plate to avoid a burn at the point of current grounding (Fig. 17–31). An electrical shock to hands holding the clamp or electrosurgical handpiece is usually caused by a hole in the glove. Regloving should alleviate the problem. Continued shocking reflects poor grounding or an equipment malfunction that should be checked by a qualified service representative.

TECHNICIAN NOTE

Electrosurgery should not be used in the presence of explosive anesthetics (ether) or alcohol-based antiseptic materials.

Tissue healing following the use of the electroscalpel has been shown to be significantly delayed. Likewise, the incidence of incisional infection is somewhat increased. Therefore, techniques of asepsis and atraumatic tissue handling must be strictly adhered to when using electrosurgery.

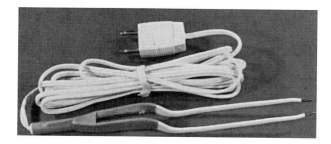

Figure 17–29. The thumb forceps-like handpiece used for bipolar cautery.

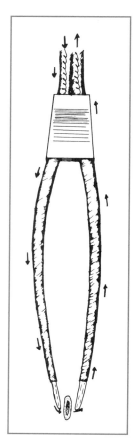

Figure 17–30. Diagram of the bipolar coagulation current as it passes from one tip of the handpiece to the other.

Biological Coagulants

Biological agents, such as gelatin sponge (Gelfoam, Upjohn) or cellulose gauze (Surgicel, Johnson & Johnson) (Fig. 17–32), can be used to achieve hemostasis on tissues that tend to continually ooze or to pack small bleeding cavities (Fig. 17–33). These agents promote coagulation and provide a lattice for the forming clot to adhere to. They are normally absorbed in 2 to 6

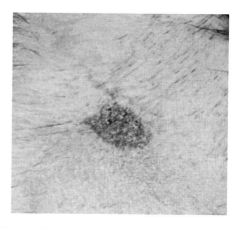

Figure 17–31. Cautery burn caused by inadequate conductive contact to the grounding plate.

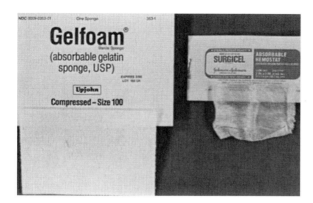

Figure 17–32. Biological hemostatic agents such as gelatin foam or cellulose sponge promote coagulation and clot adherence.

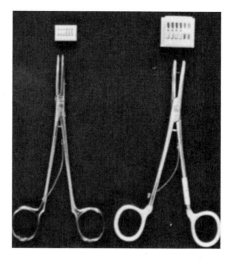

Figure 17–34. Metallic hemostatic clips are available in several sizes.

weeks, depending on the area of implantation and the specific material.

Chemical Cauterization

Chemical cauterization by agents such as phenol and silver nitrate will achieve hemostasis by denaturing the proteins of the tissues they contact, thus sealing small blood vessels. However, these agents are difficult to apply without contacting and damaging adjacent soft tissues. This usually precludes their use in general surgery.

Metal Clips

Metal clips made of noncorrosive materials (Surgiclip, Versaclip) and the specialized forceps to apply them are available in a variety of sizes and designs (Fig. 17–34). They are very effective and rapid in application. Their use in veterinary surgery is becoming more widespread as their expense relative to convenience decreases. Vascular stapling devices that automatically occlude both sides of a vessel with small metallic staples, as well as divide it, are available (LDS, U.S. Surgical Corp.) and are commonly used in human surgery. While the staple cartridges are expensive, the supplying company will often lease the application device.

INCISION IRRIGATION AND SUCTION

Incision irrigation and suction (lavage) serve four main purposes. The first is to physically dilute and remove bacteria carried into the incision from the skin or the air or from spillage from incising a contaminated or infected structure, such as the intestine. The body has a tremendous ability to resist infection from low numbers of bacteria. Consequently, lavaging the site after the initial skin incision, and periodically throughout the procedure to decrease bacterial numbers, will dramatically reduce the incidence of infection. Second, irrigation and suction are used to remove hemorrhage, increasing visibility at the surgical site. This makes both hemostasis and surgical manipulations easier to accomplish. Third, lavage keeps the tissues moist, particularly during longer procedures. If the tissues desiccate (dry out), cell damage and death occur. This decreases the rate of healing and increases the incidence of infection by devitalizing the natural cellular defense mechanisms. There is an old surgical saying that "moist tissues are happy tissues." Finally, lavage is used to dilute and remove irritating and degenerative material, such as urine, bile, or bony fragments. Although these materials will not cause infection, they can cause undesirable biological reactions and should be removed.

Lavage Fluid

Many different fluids are used for lavage, but they all have common characteristics. The fluid should be a physiologically neutral, isotonic solution (i.e., buffered normal saline or lactated Ringer's solution), meaning it has the same pH (acidity) and osmolality (mineral concentration) as serum. Excessively acid or basic fluids can promote bacterial growth and cause cell damage. Hypotonic (less concentrated) solutions, such as distilled water, will be imbibed by the tissues, resulting in significant edema. Hypertonic (more concentrated) solutions will pull water out of tissues and result in dehydration. This reaction is occasionally used to reduce preexisting edema.

Antiseptic and antibiotic agents are commonly added to the irrigation solution. Povidone-iodine (Betadine, Purdue-Frederick) is used to make a 10% solution with saline. The addition of 10 ml of chlorhexidine hydrochloride (Nolvasan solution,

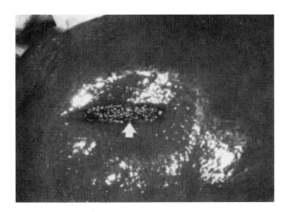

Figure 17–33. Cellulose sponge packed into a bleeding crevice (arrow) in a liver.

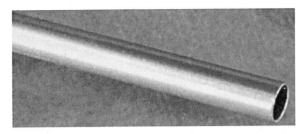

Figure 17–35. The single-orifice suction tip is used for precise control.

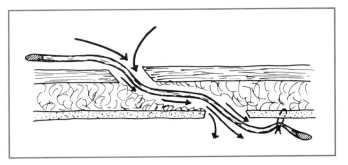

Figure 17–37. Diagram of discharge escaping around the outside of a Penrose drain.

Fort Dodge Laboratories) per 1 ml of saline also makes a useful lavage solution. Care should be taken not to use scrub materials for antiseptic solutions, since they contain detergents that are highly irritating to tissues. Aminoglycoside antibiotics (e.g., gentamicin) should not be used in lavage of the abdominal and thoracic cavities, since they may be rapidly absorbed and may cause a neuromuscular respiratory paralysis. Antibiotic solutions in general should not be used with cancellous bone grafts, since the antibiotic will diminish the graft's biological activity.

> ✎ **TECHNICIAN NOTE**
>
> Scrub solutions should not be used for antiseptic irrigation solutions because they contain detergents that are irritating to delicate tissues.

Lavage Technique

Irrigation solutions can be applied with a bulb syringe or a large syringe to obtain a hydraulic cleansing effect. They should

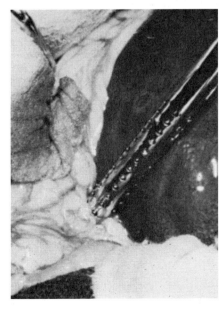

Figure 17-36. The multiple fenestrated suction tip is used to remove large volumes of fluids and avoid omental occlusion.

be warmed to body temperature to avoid causing hypothermia. This is particularly important in very small or debilitated patients. Cloth drapes should not become excessively damp during surgery, since this will allow capillary movement of bacteria from the underlying nonsterile area. Alternatively, waterproof draping materials such as baby crib sheets, may be used.

Suction of the surgical incision requires a suction tip, tubing, and a suction bottle. The suction tip may have a single orifice or multiple fenestrations. The single-orifice tip is most useful in orthopedic surgery, neurosurgery, and general surgery, in which the exposure is limited and relatively small amounts of liquid must be removed from very precise areas (Fig. 17–35). The multiple fenestrated tips are used in thoracic and abdominal procedures in which large volumes of fluid are removed (Fig. 17–36). Fenestrated tips also reduce the incidence of plugging with movable soft tissue, such as omentum and mesentery. The surgical assistant controls the strength of suction by occluding the vent hole in the handle of the suction tip. If the tip becomes plugged, it can be cleared by passing a stylet made of slightly smaller stainless steel wire. Periodic suction of clean irrigation solution during the surgical procedure will reduce the incidence of suction tube plugging and make cleaning of the tube much easier.

SURGICAL DRAINS

Postoperative drainage of the surgical area may be indicated for several different reasons. Any incision that is thought to be infected should be allowed to discharge. This can be accomplished by leaving the wound open or by inserting a drain. A drain is also indicated when soft tissues cannot be opposed to obliterate dead space. Serum tends to accumulate in such spaces and seromas can develop if a drainage route is not established. Finally, drainage may be indicated as a method of removing lavage solution that remains after surgery. This occurs most commonly with abdominal procedures in large animals.

Two types of drains are commonly used in veterinary surgery. *Penrose drains* are thin-walled, collapsible, latex rubber tubes. Discharge escapes by moving along the *outside* of the drain (Fig. 17–37). Therefore, the holes in the tissues through which the drain runs must be kept spread open and clean for the drain to work properly. Cleanliness is particularly important, since the hole and drain can act as an avenue for retrograde infections. *Suction drains* are thick-walled tubes of rubber or Silastic. Suction is applied to the outside end of the drain and discharges are pulled through the lumen of the tube. Multiple openings are created in the wall of the tube on the

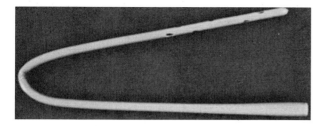

Figure 17–38. Multiple openings on the implanted end of a suction drain.

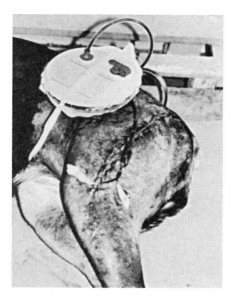

Figure 17–40. A commercially available spring-activated constant-suction device.

implanted end (Fig. 17–38). This decreases the problem of soft tissues obstructing the drainage. A fenestrated Penrose drain can be placed over the end to further maintain flow, particularly in the abdominal cavity in which the omentum tends to isolate the drain (Fig. 17–39). Suction must be maintained for this type of drain to work. Spring-activated devices are commercially available (HemoVac) (Fig. 17–40). A homemade device can be made from a large injection syringe and a hypodermic needle (Fig. 17–41).

 TECHNICIAN NOTE

Surgical drains are used to provide an open site of discharge in infected tissues, evacuate dead space, and remove lavage solutions.

SURGICAL THEATER CONDUCT

The principles of aseptic technique and proper preparation are discussed in Chapter 16. The surgical assistant should review these concepts and be constantly cognizant of them during surgery. The assistant must monitor not only his own activity but also the surgeon's and that of anyone else in the surgical theater. Ignoring a break in aseptic technique, regardless of the origin, results in contamination and leads to infection. This may destroy an otherwise perfectly performed surgical procedure unless the break is recognized and proper steps are taken to rectify it. Unnecessary traffic and visitors in the surgery suite should be avoided, not only during the procedure but at all times, to help control dust and aerial contamination of the facility.

Nonpertinent conversation should be kept to a minimum during surgery, since it detracts from concentration, and speech quickly moistens the material of the mask, reducing its filtering ability.

Some surgeons prefer hand signals to speech for requesting instruments. This further reduces necessary talking and increases efficiency. The assistant should discuss any such arrangements with the surgeon and be familiar with signals before surgery begins. To be truly efficient and effective as a surgical assistant, the veterinary technician must be familiar with the procedure being performed. This allows readiness of proper instruments and supplies and minimizes the time spent explaining positioning and retraction. This may require maintenance of a card file detailing necessary equipment and a brief review of the operative technique for each procedure (Fig. 17–42).

The surgical assistant is responsible for organizing the instrument set and passing instruments to the surgeon. Although no specific organizational scheme is universally used because of the variation in instruments and specialty equipment, the surgical assistant should be consistent in the general arrangement of the instrument stand. This will save time and effort for the assistant and speed up the procedure. In general, the most-

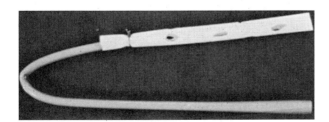

Figure 17–39. Placing a fenestrated Penrose drain over the end of a suction drain decreases occlusion from the omentum.

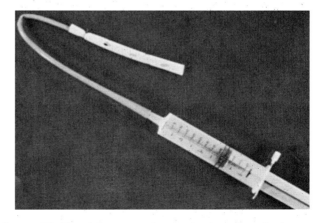

Figure 17–41. A homemade constant-suction device constructed from a large syringe and hypodermic needle.

SURGEON: Dr. McCurnin	**PROCEDURE:** Anterior Cruciate Repair
GLOVE SIZE: 7½	**POSITION OF PATIENT:** VD, leg hung
SKIN PREP: Standard	**DRAPES:** 25 cm fenestrated drape 17.5 cm × 15 cm back table drape
SUTURES AND NEEDLES	**INSTRUMENTS AND EQUIPMENT**

TIES:
 	
PERITONEUM:
 	
FASCIA:
 	
SUB-CU: 2-0 chromic gut, cutting
 	
SKIN: 2-0 nylon, cutting
 	
RETENTION:
 	
OTHER: joint capsule: 0 Prolene, Taper
 	
DRESSINGS:
	BASIC:
	      Standard set
	      Bone set
	      Suction hose
	      Large Frazier tip
	      Cautery
	      Stockinette
	
	EXTRA INSTRUMENTS:
	      Stryker saw
	      *Chronic: Round file
	                  Small rongeur

Figure 17–42. A technique card that is used to detail the necessary equipment for each surgical procedure.

used instruments are placed in the front of the tray, and specialty instruments are placed toward the back (Fig. 17–43). A specific region should be reserved for the saline bowl, suture, and sponges. The saline bowl should be placed either inside a sterile tray or on waterproof drapings to prevent wicking from underlying nonsterile surfaces (Fig. 17–44). Technicians should follow the progress of the procedure closely to anticipate the surgeon's needs. When passing instruments, the assistant should firmly "snap" the handle or handles into the open hand of the surgeon (Fig. 17–45). This keeps the instrument firmly under control and in position for use. When the surgeon has finished with an instrument, it should be quickly wiped clean of blood and tissue and returned to its position on the instrument stand. Prolonged soaking of instruments in water (particularly saline) should be avoided since this ultimately causes corrosive damage to sharp cutting edges and hinges.

SUTURE MATERIAL

Suture is any material that holds tissues together until they heal. The use of suture has been documented since the first century A.D. However, it was not until the advent of sterilization and aseptic technique that suture became commonly used. During the late 1800s and early 1900s, suture materials were derived mainly from natural sources. Synthetic suture materials first became available in the 1930s and are still being developed.

Some uses of suture include the following:

1. Apposing the edges of an incision or wound
2. Obliterating open space in which serum would tend to accumulate
3. Tightening and stabilizing joints that have sustained ligament injury or have luxated

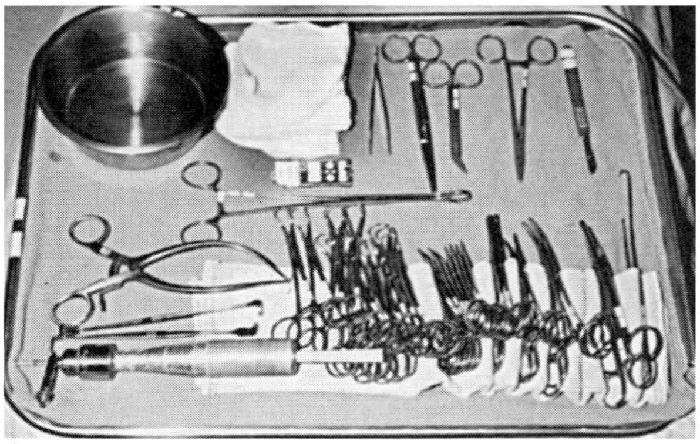

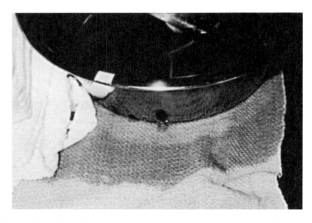

Figure 17–43. Example of a typical instrument arrangement on the Mayo stand.

Figure 17–44. The saline bowl is placed inside a sterile tray to avoid wick contamination after spillage.

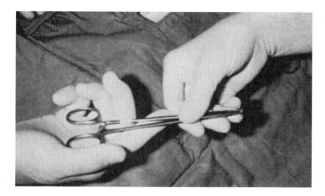

Figure 17–45. Instruments are passed, ready for use, into the open hand of the surgeon.

4. Strengthening or replacing weakened tissues, as in hernias
5. Ligating blood vessels or tissues that will be removed

Qualities of the Ideal Suture Material

The ideal suture material would have the following qualities:

1. Able to be used for any procedure with the same characteristics in all tissues
2. Easily handled and tied by the surgeon
3. Cause minimal tissue reaction and not support, spread, or sequester bacterial growth
4. High tensile strength in a small diameter, yet not cut through tissues
5. Knot securely with a minimum number of throws and small knot size
6. Easy and economical to produce and sterilize
7. Not induce allergic, electrolytic, or neoplastic changes
8. Hold tissues until healing occurs, then resorb with minimum tissue reaction

Obviously, no such suture material exists or probably ever will since several of these attributes are contradictory. Consequently, we must be aware of the advantages and disadvantages of all available sutures and choose the one most appropriate for the use at hand. The technician will need to become familiar with all sutures used by the surgeon.

Suture Nomenclature

Suture material can be classified by a number of characteristics. *Absorbable suture* is broken down and resorbed by the body, resulting in a loss of tensile strength within 60 days. Consequently, it should be used in tissues that heal rapidly to adequate strength. *Nonabsorbable suture* does not significantly weaken with time. It is used in areas that heal slowly and are subject to disruptive stresses. *Multifilament* or *braided suture* material is made up of a number of very small elements that are braided or twisted together to form the desired diameter (Fig. 17–46). Multifilament suture tends to be relatively strong, handles well, and has good knot-holding abilities. However, many braided sutures induce significant tissue reaction and can harbor bacteria, leading to intractable suture tract infections if they become contaminated. Moreover, most braided suture will

exhibit capillary or "wicking" characteristics in which fluids travel along the length of the suture between the filaments. Therefore, multifilament suture should not be used in hollow organs or in the skin when part of the suture is exposed to a contaminated environment and the wicking fluid can carry bacteria into the body. *Monofilament suture* (Fig. 17–47) avoids the capillary problem and has a low coefficient of surface friction, making it easy to generally pull through tissues. However, the low surface friction results in poor knot security, necessitating many throws on each knot. Some monofilament suture also has a tendency to return to its original shape (called memory), resulting in poor handling characteristics (Fig. 17–48).

TECHNICIAN NOTE

Suture material can be classified as absorbable or nonabsorbable, monofilament or multifilament.

Absorbable Suture Material

Surgical gut is collagenous protein obtained from the submucosal layer of sheep small intestine. It was originally known as kit gut (meaning fiddle string, as the material was used for stringed instruments). Over the years, the term "kit" was mistakenly changed to "cat," resulting in the common misnomer "catgut." When implanted in tissues, surgical gut incites an inflammatory reaction that ultimately resorbs the suture by phagocytosis. The severity of reaction, and consequently the rate at which the gut loses strength, can be decreased by tanning the material with chromic salts. Surgical gut has been classified into four groups: *plain, mild, medium* and *extra chromic* treated with resorption times of 10, 20, 30, and 40 days, respectively. Since surgical gut is broken down by phagocytosis, implantation in inflamed, highly vascular, or biologically active tissue will result in a faster rate of resorption. Because medium chromic gut is relatively inexpensive and has predictable handling and knotting charac-

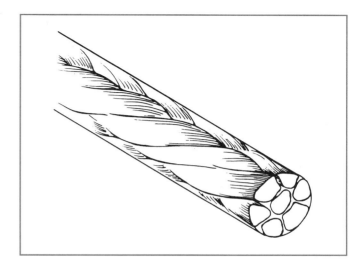

Figure 17–46. Constructed multifilament suture. (From Alexander EL: Alexander's Care of the Patient in Surgery. 8th ed. St. Louis, The CV Mosby Co., 1987.)

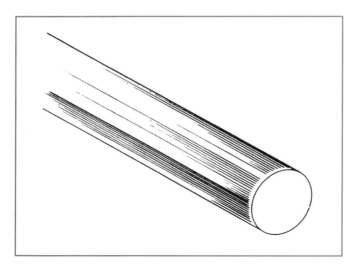

Figure 17-47. Monofilament suture. (From Alexander EL: Alexander's Care of the Patient in Surgery. 8th ed. St. Louis, The CV Mosby Co., 1987.)

teristics, it is still one of the most popular absorbable sutures for ligations in veterinary practice. However, its variability in rate of tensile strength loss, particularly in response to an inflammatory environment, should be considered and has led most surgeons away from its use for closure of support layers.

Other absorbable suture materials, such as collagen, kangaroo tendon, and fascia lata, have been developed but have shown few distinct advantages over surgical gut.

Synthetic Absorbable Suture Material

Synthetic absorbable sutures have been developed to avoid the variation of resorptive rates in inflammatory environments. Polyglycolic acid (Dexon, Davis-Geck) is a synthetic polyester polymerized from hydroxyacetic acid. It is produced in fine filaments that are braided into sutures of various sizes. Consequently, it has excellent handling and knot-holding characteristics. Dexon is broken down in the body by enzymatic hydrolysis, which does *not* induce a significant inflammatory reaction. Furthermore, the rate of absorption is not affected by placement in an inflamed or infected environment. Dexon loses about 33%

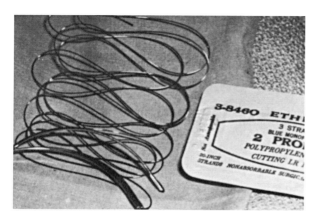

Figure 17-48. Memory is the tendency of suture to return to its package shape.

of its tensile strength in 7 days and 80% of this strength within 2 weeks. Some studies have shown that Dexon absorbs more rapidly in the presence of urine. Overall, it has a superior initial strength, but it loses its strength more rapidly than surgical gut.

Polyglactin 910 (Vicryl, Ethicon) is a copolymer of lactic and glycolic acids. Its production and resorption processes are similar to those of Dexon. Vicryl also has a high initial strength that declines rapidly when implanted. Likewise, it has good handling qualities and knot security.

Poliglecaprone (Monocryl, Ethicon), polydioxanone (PDS, Ethicon) and polyglyconate (Maxon, Davis-Geck) are newer synthetic polyester materials that are pliable enough to be produced and used in monofilament form. Consequently, they have significantly less tissue drag in placement. However, they do possess some memory characteristics and must have multiple throws to knot securely. The process of resorption is similar to that of the other synthetic absorbables. Monocryl absorbs at a rate similar to medium chromic gut. Its predictability may lead to its replacing gut for many applications in the future. PDS and Maxon are significantly stronger, retaining 74% strength at 2 weeks, 58% strength at 4 weeks, and 41% of their original strength at 6 weeks after implantation. Consequently, they are particularly useful in slow-healing tissues. The major disadvantage of these sutures is their expense, which is approximately twice that of surgical gut and one and one-half times that of Vicryl or Dexon in comparable sizes.

 TECHNICIAN NOTE

Absorbable sutures retain their tensile strength in tissues for several weeks, while nonabsorbable sutures last 60 days or more.

Nonabsorbable Suture Material

Nonabsorbable suture retains its tensile strength for more than 60 days. It can be natural fiber, metallic, or synthetic and will be described according to origin.

Silk is one of the first and still most commonly used nonabsorbable materials. It is obtained from the cocoon of the silkworm and is braided or twisted into multifilament strands. It has excellent handling and knotting qualities. However, it can induce a severe soft tissue reaction, allow capillary migration of contamination (wicking), and serve as a nidus for infection. Despite its nonabsorbable classification, the inflammatory reaction usually results in complete loss of tensile strength within 6 months.

Cotton and linen are natural fibers that are also used to make suture. They both increase slightly in strength when wet but otherwise behave very much like silk. They have seen limited use in veterinary surgery.

Metallic sutures have been used since the 14th century, when the biologically nonreactive nature of gold was first described. Stainless steel is the major metallic suture in use today. It is biologically inert and will not support bacterial growth. Also, steel retains its high tensile strength when implanted. Consequently, it is particularly useful in infected wounds or tissues that are expected to be stressed while healing slowly. Stainless steel suture is available in monofilament and multifilament forms. The major disadvantage of steel is its poor handling quality and its tendency to kink. Silver, aluminum, and tantalum sutures have some limited use in human surgery.

Synthetic Nonabsorbable Suture Material

Polyamide (nylon) is a polymerized plastic that is available as suture in both monofilament and braided forms. It does not cause tissue reaction when implanted, but it gradually loses its tensile strength over several years. It is somewhat stiff, slippery, and has significant memory, making handling and knot security exacting.

Polypropylene (Prolene, Ethicon) is a synthetic plastic that is similar to nylon. However, polypropylene does not weaken with time, making it useful when permanent suture support is needed.

Polybutester (Novafil, Davis-Geck) is a similar synthetic suture that is much more elastic. This means it can stretch and return to its original length without breaking. This makes it useful for repairing ligaments and other structures that must stretch under weighted motion.

Polyester fibers (Mersiline, Ethicon; Dacron, Davis-Geck) are braided to form a strong noncapillary suture. Handling quality is good, but five or six throws are required for good knot security. It also has significant tissue drag and induces just slightly less tissue reaction than silk. Some manufacturers coat the polyester fibers with Teflon (Tevdek and Polydek, Deknatel) or silicone (Ticron, Davis-Geck) to reduce drag and reaction. However, chronic infection and draining fistulas remain a common complication of polyester use.

Polymerized caprolactum (Vetafil, B. Braun Melsungen AG) is made of synthetic fibers coated with a smooth plastic-like material. It has high tensile strength and does not induce a significant tissue reaction. However, it will act as a nidus for continued infection if contaminated. Chemical sterilization is not adequate, and the material must be heat-sterilized before it is buried in tissue. Consequently, it is used most commonly for skin closure.

Suture Size and Strength

TECHNICIAN NOTE

Oversized sutures do not strengthen a wound and may lead to overtightening and strangulation of tissues.

The size or diameter of suture has been classified by the U.S. Pharmacopeia. Table 17–1 lists the established limits of surgical gut from 7–0 to no. 3. Other suture materials use the same sizing limits and have extended down to an 11–0 nylon for microvascular anastomosis and up to no. 7 stainless steel for orthopedic use. The appropriate-sized suture for each procedure needs to be no stronger than the tissue on which it is used. Oversized sutures do not strengthen a wound and may lead to overtightening and strangulation of tissues. In addition to suture tensile strength, knot security should be considered when selecting suture size. Since the knot is the strength-limiting area of most suture, and the relative knot security decreases as suture size increases; smaller suture offers a me-

• Table 17–1 •

LIMITS ON SUTURE DIAMETER				
	MILLIMETERS		**LIMITS ON KNOT-PULL TENSILE STRENGTH**	
SIZE	**Minimum**	**Maximum**	**kg**	**lb**
7-0	0.025	0.064	0.06	0.125
6-0	0.064	0.113	0.16	0.35
5-0	0.113	0.179	0.32	0.7
4-0	0.179	0.241	0.68	1.5
3-0	0.241	0.318	1.13	2.5
2-0	0.318	0.406	1.18	4.0
1-0	0.406	0.495	2.50	5.5
1	0.495	0.584	3.40	7.5
2	0.584	0.673	4.80	9.0
3	0.673	0.762	5.22	11.5

From United States Pharmacopeia, 16th ed. Rockville, Md, US Pharmacopeial Convention, 1960.

chanical advantage. This is particularly true of the synthetic monofilament sutures, which have a low coefficient of friction (slippery). Besides untying, knotting decreases a suture's strength by converting the longitudinal tensile force into a shearing force that collects at the base of the knot, at which point strands cross and angle. The process of tying the knot also weakens suture by abrading its surface as strands cross. This is particularly true of surgical gut sutures and braided sutures. Excessive suture material should be cut off, leaving the ends just long enough to secure the knot on buried sutures. Of course, this length varies with surface friction and knot security. In general, multifilament and metallic sutures can be cut off quite close to the knot (about 2 mm). Monofilament sutures with memory and polyesters need to have 3 to 4 mm left to prevent knot untying. Skin sutures usually have about 0.5- to 1.0-cm tails to aid in easy removal (Fig. 17–49).

Suture Reaction

As previously noted, some suture material induces more tissue reaction than others. In descending order of reactiveness, surgi-

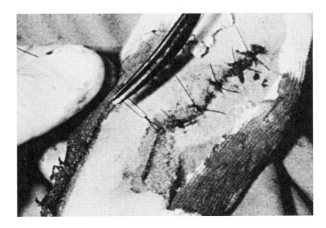

Figure 17–49. Skin sutures are cut off, leaving 5-mm to 1-cm tails to allow easy removal.

cal gut is most reactive, followed by multifilament natural fiber, synthetic multifilament suture, synthetic monofilament suture, and finally metallic suture. Recognizing a suture's reactivity becomes particularly important when suture reaction might affect function of the tissue as in neurosurgery or cardiovascular surgery.

Tissue reaction also impedes healing of normal tissue. The presence of infection or contamination has a much greater effect on the more reactive sutures. For example, the inflammatory process associated with infection will often phagocytose surgical gut at an increased rate, leading to resorption before healing and wound dehiscence. Likewise, the presence of silk has been shown to increase the incidence of infection 10,000-fold in contaminated incisions. Finally, nonabsorbable suture, such as silk or polyester, may cause ulceration of the gastrointestinal tract or serve as the nidus for stone formation in the urinary bladder or gallbladder if it penetrates the lumen of those hollow organs.

Preparation of Suture Material

A number of methods are used by suture producers to sterilize various suture materials. Many prepackaged sutures are sterilized by gamma irradiation. Ethylene oxide is used on those products that will not tolerate irradiation. Steam sterilization (autoclaving) can be used on some materials, with variable damaging effects. The following describes the effects of autoclaving.

I. Severe damage, destroys tensile strength
   A. Surgical gut
   B. Polyglycolic acid (PDS)
   C. Polyglactin (Vicryl)
II. Mild damage, reduces tensile strength
   A. Silk
   B. Linen
   C. Cotton
III. Tolerates at least three autoclavings without loss of tensile strength
   A. Polyester
   B. Nylon
   C. Polypropylene
   D. Metallics

Sutures that can be steam-sterilized are often bought in bulk and are sterilized in the practice. When preparing such suture, an appropriate number of strand lengths (usually 30 to 60 cm) should be cut and coiled or loosely wound around a

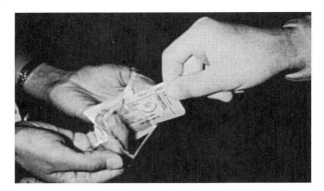

Figure 17–51. Peeling back the outer covering of a prepackaged suture material.

card or sponge (Fig. 17–50). This will avoid repeated autoclaving, which will damage even the most steam-tolerant material.

Prepackaged suture material is opened (by a nonsterile assistant) onto the instrument tray by peeling back the outer packaging (Fig. 17–51). The surgical assistant opens the inner pack by tearing off one end and grasping the suture end or swaged needle with needle holders as directed on the package (Fig. 17–52). Before use, the suture should be stretched slightly to overcome memory, but not snapped as this commonly leads to contamination of the suture end. Any excessive preserving fluid should be wiped off. The tissue drag of many sutures (particularly the synthetic multifilaments) can be reduced by moistening with sterile saline. However, this will reduce the tensile strength of silk, and surgical gut will imbibe water to swell and soften. Multifilament suture strands tend to accumulate blood as they pass through tissue and should be wiped off with a moistened sponge between use.

Suture Needles

Suture needles vary considerably in shape, point design, method of attachment to the suture (eye), and size. The size

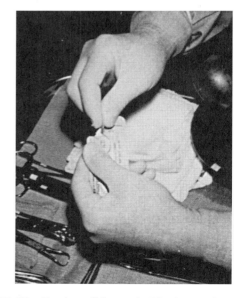

Figure 17–52. Tearing off the end of the inner suture package.

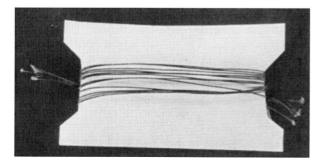

Figure 17–50. Precut strands of suture loosely wrapped around a card.

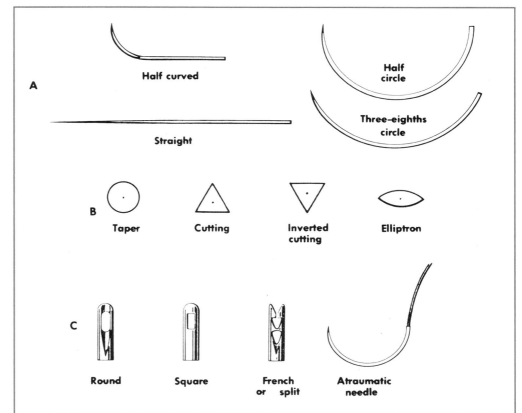

Figure 17-53. A, The size and shape of the needle are chosen according to the thickness of the tissue. B, The needle point design is determined according to the toughness of the tissue on which it is used. C, The needle is attached to the suture either by threading through an eye or being swaged. (Courtesy of Sherwood Davis & Geck, Milford, NJ.)

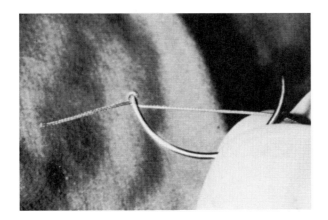

Figure 17-54. Double threading should be avoided because it results in a large bulk of suture that causes severe tissue drag.

Figure 17-55. Threading of a French eye needle by passing the suture through the complete eye and pulling it down through the spring eye.

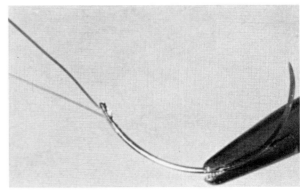

and shape of the needle are determined by the thickness of tissue being sutured and the depth of the incision (Fig. 17–53A).

TECHNICIAN NOTE

Cutting-edged needles should not be used when an air- or watertight suture line is required (lung, urinary bladder, intestine, and so forth).

The point design varies with the toughness of tissue being sutured (Fig. 17–53B). Skin, eye tissues, and some facial tissues are sutured with a *cutting-edged needle. Reverse-cutting needles* (K needles) are preferred by some surgeons for their increased needle shank strength. Cutting-edged needles actually incise a slightly larger hole than the size of the needle shank. Although this makes passage of the needle and suture easier, a true incision that can leak is created. Therefore, cutting-edged needles should not be used when an air- or watertight suture line is required. *Taper needles* do not actually cut tissue, but spread it open around the needle and following suture. This spreading effect avoids hemorrhage and results in a sealed suture line. Taper needles and reverse-cutting needles are used in suturing most hollow organs.

The needle can be attached to the suture by three different methods (Fig. 17–53C). Single-eyed needles have one hole in the head of the needle. The eye should be single-threaded, since double threading leaves a large bulk of suture around the shank (Fig. 17–54), which will cause excessive tissue drag and damage as the needle is passed. A curved needle is threaded from within the curve so that the short end of the suture falls away from the outside curve. About 10 cm of suture should be pulled through the eye. These steps will help to prevent the suture from pulling out of the eye during suturing. Spring- or French-eyed needles have a complete eye and an incomplete "spring" eye. Suture is threaded through the complete eye and is then forced back through the spring eye, which grips the suture end (Fig. 17–55). Eyeless or swaged needles are attached directly to the end of the suture by the factory. The surgeon draws a single strand through the tissue and uses a new sharp needle with every strand. Therefore, swaged needles are the most atraumatic and are becoming the most popular surgical needle.

Recommended Reading

Evans HE and Christenson GC: Miller's Anatomy of the Dog, 3rd ed. Philadelphia, WB Saunders, 1993.

Slatter D: Textbook of Small Animal Surgery, 2nd ed. Philadelphia, WB Saunders, 1993, pp 168–191, 204–211.

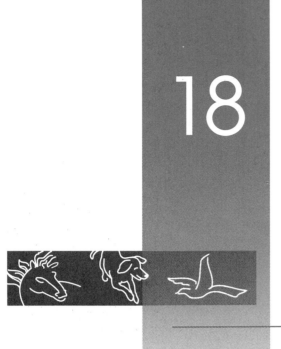

18 | Small Animal Surgical Nursing and Dentistry

Ashley B. Oakes • Matt G. Oakes

GENERAL PRINCIPLES OF SURGICAL NURSING

The role of the veterinary technician in veterinary surgery can best be discussed by dividing the duties into preoperative, operative, and postoperative considerations. Before surgical intervention, the patient must be properly evaluated, prepared, and monitored. The veterinary technician is responsible for the adequate restraint of the patient prior to anesthetic induction (see Chapter 1), the knowledge of proper anesthetic techniques and monitoring (see Chapter 15) and an understanding of surgical instrumentation and aseptic technique (see Chapter 16) and positioning requirements. These techniques are discussed in detail in this text and should be reviewed before operative assistance techniques.

Many operative procedures require the assistance of a veterinary technician. A working knowledge of common surgical procedures will help to make the veterinary technician proficient at surgical assistance. Procedures that often require such assistance include orthopedic surgery (retraction, reduction, traction, countertraction), open chest procedures (artificial ventilation, retraction), and complicated abdominal procedures (diaphragmatic hernia repair, renal surgery, tumor resection). An understanding of aseptic technique, a familiarity with surgical instrumentation, and a working knowledge of the specific surgical procedure are prerequisites for proper intraoperative assistance. Surgical assistance is discussed in Chapter 18.

Small animal surgical nursing includes many aspects of the primary care of the veterinary surgical patient. This chapter deals primarily with the postoperative care and evaluation of patients by the veterinary technician. In addition, the more commonly performed small animal surgical and dental procedures are discussed, with emphasis on the role of the veterinary technician.

Patient Monitoring

Postoperative care can be divided into immediate and delayed categories. The veterinary technician should continue patient monitoring in the immediate postsurgical period in a fashion similar to preoperative and intraoperative monitoring (e.g., respiratory rate, heart rate, reflex changes). The postoperative phase is a critical transition period and must be monitored continuously until the patient is safely extubated, normothermic, and in sternal recumbency.

As the patient becomes more conscious and aware of its surroundings, evaluation of discomfort at the surgical site should be made.

TECHNICIAN NOTE

If the patient is having an unusually "stormy" recovery that can be related to surgical pain, the veterinarian should be alerted, and a proper analgesic should be prescribed. When in doubt, it should be assumed that the patient is having some degree of postoperative pain.

In the daily evaluation of any postsurgical patient, the technician should be aware of several important indicators. First, the patient should be evaluated for its general appearance, attitude, and appetite. A general examination should include temperature, pulse, and respiration. Abnormalities in these can often be the first changes to occur in significant postoperative complications. Second, a visual and palpable inspection of the surgical wound should be made. Common abnormalities in the early postoperative period (1 to 3 days) include redness, swelling, drainage, excessive licking, and dehiscence (wound breakdown).

Incision Evaluation

An incision should be evaluated with respect to the type of surgical procedure performed on the patient. Elective operations, such as ovariohysterectomy and castration, can be expected to produce mild redness and swelling with no drainage from the incision site. However, if the wound was contaminated (e.g., laceration, perianal wound) or if the surgical exposure was extensive, the incision can be expected to be somewhat swollen, reddened, and warm to the touch and have mild to moderate drainage in the first 24 to 48 hours postoperatively. Swelling secondary to surgical trauma can be expected to resolve in several days. However, *seromas* (serum pockets) and *hematomas* (pockets of hemorrhage) may persist and should be treated early. They are recognized by localized areas of fluctuant fluid-filled swellings and are treated by drainage, warm compresses, and bandaging. If the swelling occurs 4 to 6 days postoperatively, is warm to the touch, and is associated with an elevated body temperature, the possibility of an abscess or cellulitis (infection along tissue planes) must be considered. These conditions must be treated by drainage, warm compresses, and systemic antibiotics.

Wound dehiscence is defined as the separation of all layers of an incision or wound. Early recognition is imperative in any wound but especially in abdominal and thoracic incisions.

TECHNICIAN NOTE

Dehiscence of an abdominal wound may result in evisceration of the abdominal organs, with subsequent contamination and infection. Dehiscence of a thoracic wound will result in a severe open *pneumothorax* (air within the chest causing collapse of the lungs), a problem that may result in sudden death.

Critical evaluation of surgical wounds is of paramount importance for the ultimate welfare of the patient.

During the first 12 to 24 hours after surgery, it will become apparent which patients will aggressively lick at their suture line. It is important to recognize these patients early to prevent subsequent wound dehiscence and infection.

Patient Restraint

There are several methods that can be used effectively to prevent postoperative self-trauma. They are divided into two groups: (1) chemical restraint agents and (2) mechanical restraint devices.

The most commonly used chemical restraint agents are tranquilizers and noxious-tasting agents. Tranquilizers must be used with some caution, since they are often insufficient when used alone and may have undesirable side effects. In combination with other devices (e.g., Elizabethan collar, side bar), however, they can be useful. Acepromazine (Ayerst) is the most commonly used tranquilizer in veterinary medicine.

Noxious-tasting agents must also be used with discretion. Some commonly used substances include Variton (Schering), bitter apple, obtundia, Tabasco, Stoma-Nil (Dow Hickam), and various thumb-sucking preparations. The agent is placed directly on the skin, or it can be impregnated into bandage material. The agent should not be placed directly on the incision because it could be irritating. Alternating various substances helps to prevent the patient from becoming accustomed to the taste of one. The combined use of mechanical restraint devices and chemical restraint agents has been helpful in controlling intractable patients.

Mechanical restraint devices include the Elizabethan collar, the body brace, the side bar, hobbles, and various bandages. The assembly, materials necessary, specific indications, contraindications, and complications have been adequately described elsewhere (Seim et al., 1990) and are beyond the scope of this chapter. A properly selected, constructed, and applied device will be well tolerated by the patient and effective for its desired purpose.

Suture Removal

Suture removal is commonly performed by the technician. Most sutures are removed 10 to 14 days postsurgically. Incision healing should be evaluated prior to suture removal. Suture scissors allow removal with minimal discomfort to the patient (Fig. 18–1).

COMMON SURGICAL PROCEDURES

The veterinary technician must have a working knowledge of common surgical procedures in order to properly prepare the patient preoperatively, act as an efficient surgical assistant, and

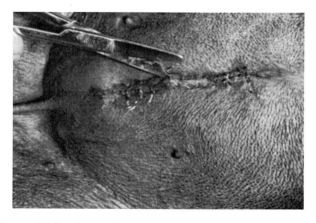

Figure 18-1. Proper instrumentation and technique for removal of sutures.

manage the immediate and long-term postoperative care. The remainder of this chapter reviews the most commonly performed small animal surgical procedures in a veterinary practice. A brief description of the procedure, with emphasis on the role of the veterinary technician, will be given.

Elective Surgery Versus Nonelective Surgery

It is ideal to perform surgery on a healthy patient, thus allowing the surgeon to choose the best time to operate. This is known as an *elective* surgical procedure. Occasionally, a patient will be admitted to the hospital requiring immediate surgery. The patient is often compromised. This is not the ideal time to perform the operation, but it must be done as a lifesaving measure. This is known as *nonelective* or emergency surgery.

Tail Docking on Puppies

Definition. Tail docking refers to partial amputation of the tail. Tails are docked to conform with standards set for certain breeds. The American Kennel Club has a recommended tail length for each breed. This standard should be followed carefully unless the owner or breeder specifies otherwise. Tail docking should be performed at an early age (3 to 5 days). This allows the procedure to be performed without general anesthesia.

Technique. The pup should be cradled in the palms of both hands, with the hindlegs held between the index and middle fingers and the tail directed toward the surgeon (Fig. 18–2). The surgical site is prepared in the usual manner. The desired length of remaining tail is marked, and the skin of the tail is retracted craniad. The tail is amputated with a pair of scissors, bleeding is controlled with electrocautery or pressure, and the skin is released, allowing it to retract over exposed bone. One simple interrupted absorbable suture is placed to appose the skin edges.

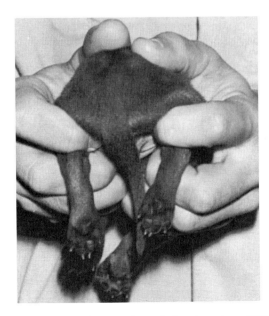

Figure 18–2. Patient properly restrained and positioned for tail-docking procedure.

Aftercare. The pups should be returned to the mother. The procedure is relatively atraumatic to the pups, and they will begin to nurse minutes after surgery. The suture remains until it is absorbed or licked out by the mother.

Dewclaw Removal on Puppies

Definition. The claws located on the medial aspect of the fore- and hindlegs are known as dewclaws. Dewclaws are commonly removed from the fore- and hindfeet of purebred dogs for show purposes, and from hunting dogs because they may be torn as the dog runs over densely shrubbed terrain. It should be remembered that in certain breeds (e.g., Great Pyrenees, Newfoundland) the presence of dewclaws is necessary for proper show quality. Dewclaws should be removed at an early age (3 to 5 days). It is generally performed at the same time as tail docking.

Technique. The surgical site is prepared in the usual manner. The pup is cradled in the palm of one hand, and the extremity is extended with the other hand. Scissors are used to clip the dewclaws off. Hemorrhage is controlled with electrocautery or pressure. The skin edges may be left unsutured or apposed with one absorbable suture.

Aftercare. The pups are returned to the mother immediately.

Tail Docking and Dewclaw Removal in the Adult

Tail docking and dewclaw removal should ideally be done within the first week of life. In some instances, adult dogs are presented for one or both procedures.

Technique for Dewclaw Removal. The patient must be placed under general anesthesia. The surgical site is clipped and prepared in the usual manner, and an elliptical incision is made at the base of the dewclaw. The dewclaw is dissected and is transected at the carpometacarpal joint in the front paw or the tarsometatarsal joint in the hindpaw. Hemorrhage is controlled with electrocautery and pressure. The skin edges are apposed with a subcuticular suture pattern. A foot bandage is used to prevent swelling and self-trauma. An Elizabethan collar should be used if needed.

Technique for Tail Amputation. The tail should be clipped and hung from an intravenous stand, the skin should be prepared in the usual manner, and the end of the tail should be covered with a sterile stockinette. A tourniquet is placed at the base of the tail, and the tail is amputated at the desired location by skin incision and transection of the coccygeal vertebra at the appropriate site. Blood vessels are identified and ligated. The skin edges are sutured over the remaining vertebrae, and the tourniquet is removed. The tail can be bandaged or left unbandaged. In any case, an Elizabethan collar should be placed on the patient postoperatively. The patient should be examined frequently during the first 6 to 8 hours to be certain that the tail cannot be traumatized.

Feline Onychectomy

Definition. Onychectomy (declawing) involves removal of the claw and its associated third phalanx. The third phalanx must be removed to ensure adequate excision of germinal epithelium. If this is not accomplished, regrowth of the claw may occur.

Indications. Onychectomy is an elective procedure to prevent furniture mutilation by the cat. Most veterinarians recommend declawing the front feet only. This does not significantly impair the cat's ability to climb trees or defend itself from intruders. Onychectomy is often performed at the same time as castration or ovariohysterectomy, but young cats (8 to 16 weeks) tend to have less hemorrhage and postoperative pain.

Technique. The feet are surgically scrubbed but need not be clipped unless the patient is a long-haired breed. A tourniquet is placed above the elbow. A Rescoe nail trimmer is positioned snugly onto the dorsal surface of the toe between the second phalanx and third phalanx. During positioning of the nail trimmer, the claw should be pulled cranially. As little skin as possible should be excised. The cutting edge of the Rescoe nail trimmer is positioned at the cranial edge of the foot pad. As the cutting edge is advanced, the pad is moved caudally while rotating the nail dorsally and caudally. The third phalanx is then excised by the Rescoe nail trimmer (Fig. 18–3). Care is taken to avoid cutting the foot pad or leaving any portion of the third phalanx. Each nail is amputated in a similar fashion.

The paws are bandaged snugly with strips of tape and a gauze sponge. The sponge is placed over the excised digits. Strips of tape are placed longitudinally along the leg and distally around the paw (Fig. 18–4). Tape is then placed circumferentially around the paw up to the elbow. Care is taken to lay tape on the leg and not to pull too tightly. Tube gauze (Fig. 18–5) can also be used, but its expense precludes its use in most practices. The tourniquets are removed as soon as bandaging

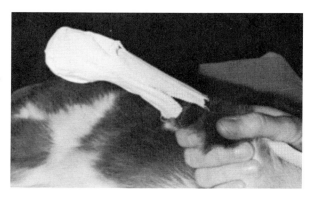

Figure 18-4. Tape and gauze used to bandage paws after onychectomy.

is complete. The bandages should not be left on longer than 24 hours.

✎ **TECHNICIAN NOTE**

The bandage from an onychectomy should be removed within 24 hours.

The patient generally remains in the hospital until the bandages are removed. Most cats allow removal of the bandages by carefully cutting the bandage apart longitudinally and gently peeling it off the leg. If the patient is intractable, the bandage may be cut and the cat returned to its cage. The patient will then remove the bandage on its own. In severely intractable patients, a light dose of intravenous ketamine may be necessary to remove the bandages safely. Patients are generally kept for observation 12 hours after bandage removal. If no signs of hemorrhage occur, the patient can be discharged.

When patients are discharged, it is important to inform owners that the litter must be changed to shredded paper for the first 5 to 7 days at home. This prevents contamination of the paw with litter and subsequent infection.

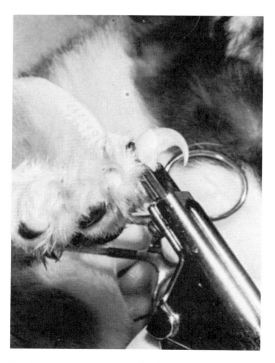

Figure 18-3. Proper placement of claw and third phalanx in the cutting edge of the Rescoe nail trimmer for an onychectomy.

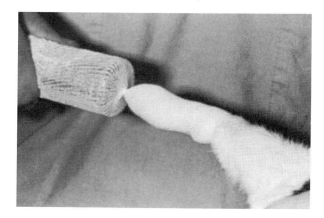

Figure 18-5. Tube gauze used to bandage paws after onychectomy.

Complications. Onychectomy complications can be divided into those that occur in the early postoperative period and those that occur in the late postoperative period. Early complications include loose bandages and postoperative bleeding. Onychectomy patients should be checked frequently for evidence of loose, bloody bandages or complete bandage removal and severe hemorrhage. In the event of hemorrhage, the paws should be rebandaged snugly. Late complications include regrowth of the claws, chronic lameness, or both. Claw regrowth requires reoperation and removal of remaining germinal epithelium. Chronic lameness without evidence of regrowth may be seen with incomplete removal of the phalanx or cut foot pads. For this reason, it is essential that the pads be preserved during the operative procedure.

Variations of the above-described technique have been used to successfully declaw the cat. Included are blade excision of the third phalanx, suturing the defect after claw excision, and the use of cyanoacrylic tissue adhesive to close the wound. The most acceptable technique is that with which the veterinarian is most familiar.

Celiotomy

Definition. *Celiotomy* (laparotomy) is a surgical incision into the abdominal cavity. There are several locations in which the incision can be made: ventral midline, paramedian, paracostal, parapreputial, and flank (Fig. 18–6). The most commonly used incision site is ventral midline.

Indications. A celiotomy incision can be performed in an elective procedure or in a nonelective procedure. Some of the common elective procedures include ovariohysterectomy, cystotomy, cesarean section, intestinal surgery, gastric surgery, and retained abdominal testicles. Some common nonelective procedures include gastric dilation and volvulus (bloated-twisted stomach), intussusception, gastrointestinal foreign bodies, ruptured spleen, penetrating foreign bodies (e.g., knife wound, arrow wound, bullet wound), severe abdominal bleeding, and diaphragmatic hernia. In some instances, the patient is presented for an unknown abdominal problem. These patients may need elective or nonelective celiotomy, referred to as an *exploratory celiotomy*. Exploratory celiotomy is often performed for abdominal masses of unknown origin and is used as a diagnostic tool.

Technique. The patient is placed in dorsal recumbency. Larger dogs should be placed in a vee trough to support their shoulders. Smaller dogs and cats can be placed on moldable beanbags or sandbags. All patients should be placed on a circulating water heater, but this is especially important for smaller dogs and all cats. The abdomen is widely clipped from 2 cm craniad to the xiphoid cartilage to 2 cm caudad to the pubis. The skin is aseptically prepared in the usual fashion (see Chapter 16).

The various incisions (paramedian, paracostal, and so on) are all slight variations of the ventral midline incision (see Fig. 18–6). For this reason, emphasis will be given to the ventral midline incision.

The line of the incision is from the xiphoid process to the pubis. The length used varies with the type of procedure (see specific procedures). The incision is made with a scalpel blade or electrocautery in the cutting mode. The incision is carried through the subcutaneous tissue to the level of the linea alba, which is elevated with forceps to pull it away from the underlying abdominal viscera. This will prevent the inadvertent puncture of abdominal organs when entering the peritoneal cavity. A scalpel blade is used to nick through the linea alba into the peritoneal cavity. The incision is extended the desired length with scissors. Moistened laparotomy pads (sponges) are used to protect the incision edges. A Balfour self-retaining abdominal retractor can be introduced, if necessary, into the incision to facilitate visualization of abdominal structures (exploratory celiotomy). It is important to remember that minimal manipulation of abdominal viscera is the rule. Whenever retraction or manipulation of structures is necessary, atraumatic technique is mandatory. Retract viscera with moistened laparotomy pads, manipulate viscera with moistened gloves, blot any excess hemorrhage with moistened sponges (do not wipe surfaces with sponges), and when using suction be careful not to suck the walls of visceral structures against the suction orifice.

TECHNICIAN NOTE

A thorough inspection of the abdomen should be made prior to closure to avoid leaving instruments or sponges in the abdominal cavity. A preoperative and postoperative sponge count is recommended.

The postoperative sponge count should be made prior to closing the abdomen.

The abdomen is sutured closed in three layers. The linea alba is the layer of strength and must be securely closed. The subcutaneous tissues are then sutured to decrease the amount of dead space. This helps reduce the frequency of postoperative hematoma or seroma formation. The skin is then sutured to complete the celiotomy closure. (For additional information about sutures, see Chapter 17.)

Postoperative Considerations. During the first 24 hours, the skin incision should be examined carefully for evidence of self-trauma. If problems arise, an Elizabethan collar should be

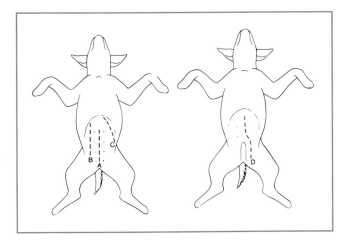

Figure 18–6. Locations for celiotomy incisions. A, Ventral midline. B, Paramedian. C, Paracostal. D, Parapreputial.

considered. If there is evidence of dehiscence, the veterinary technician should notify the veterinarian immediately. Emergency closure may be necessary.

Ovariohysterectomy in the Dog and Cat

Definition. An ovariohysterectomy involves the surgical removal of the uterus and ovaries. The uterus is removed with the ovaries to prevent subsequent development of uterine disease. If any ovarian tissue is inadvertently missed, the animal will continue to have heat cycles.

Indications. In the normal female, the principal objective is prevention of estrus and the accompanying problems associated with bloody discharge, attraction of male dogs or cats, accidental matings, pregnancy, and unwanted puppies or kittens.

Other indications for ovariohysterectomy include endocrine imbalances, infections, injuries, cysts, tumors, and congenital abnormalities. Endocrine disturbances are associated with varied clinical manifestations, such as sterility, skin lesions, mammary tumors, pseudocyesis (false pregnancy), and nymphomania. Among the uterine diseases that may require ovariohysterectomy are metritis, pyometra, endometrial hyperplasia, neoplasia, injury, neglected dystocia, and congenital abnormalities.

Although the operation can be done at almost any age and at any phase of the reproductive cycle, it is best performed either before puberty or during anestrus. About 6 months of age is generally considered best. At this age, the animal can be anesthetized with relative safety.

> **TECHNICIAN NOTE**
>
> The incidence of mammary neoplasia can be greatly reduced in the dog by spaying before the first heat.

The female cat may be spayed any time after 5 months of age.

The surgery is most hazardous during estrus and pregnancy and in old, obese females. The blood supply to the reproductive tract and the risk of intraoperative hemorrhage are increased during estrus and pregnancy. The most favorable time to spay a mature bitch is 3 to 4 months after estrus. Female cats may be spayed during heat with minimal increased risk. After whelping, the operation should be done as soon as the puppies or kittens have been weaned and lactation has ceased, about 6 to 8 weeks following parturition. Gestation does not alter the usual 6- to 8-month estrus cycle.

Technique. The patient is clipped and aseptically prepared for a routine ventral midline celiotomy. The skin incision is made from the umbilicus caudally 3 to 6 cm in a dog and from 2 cm caudad to the umbilicus caudally 3 to 4 cm in length in a cat. When the abdominal cavity is entered, the uterine horns are located and exteriorized from the abdomen. The ovarian arteries (pedicles) are ligated with the appropriate-sized absorbable suture material. The uterine body is then exteriorized and li-

gated. The abdominal cavity is carefully examined for hemorrhage. The celiotomy incision is closed in a routine fashion.

Complications. The most common postoperative complication of ovariohysterectomy is abdominal hemorrhage. The patient should be carefully monitored during the first 3 to 6 hours postoperatively. Temperature, pulse, respiration, and character of mucous membranes should be examined periodically.

When monitoring the patient's body temperature, it should be appreciated that all postoperative patients experience hypothermia. It is considered a good sign if periodic readings show a trend toward an increasing body temperature. If the temperature remains low or continues to fall, it may be an indication of potential problems. Attempts should be made to maintain the patient at normal body temperature during recovery.

The pulse should be evaluated with respect to rate and character. If it becomes rapid and weak, it may be a sign of hemorrhage, developing shock, or both. Frequent evaluation to determine the trend of the pulse rate and its character is necessary to properly evaluate the patient.

Respiratory rate may help to determine the patient's postoperative condition. If the patient is experiencing significant blood loss, the respiratory rate may increase significantly.

The mucous membranes should be examined frequently. They should be evaluated with respect to color and capillary refill time. Normal mucous membranes should be pink and have a capillary refill time of less than 2 seconds.

> **TECHNICIAN NOTE**
>
> If the mucous membranes become pale, and the refill time is greater than 2 seconds, the patient may be experiencing significant blood loss.

One abnormal sign at one given time is not enough to diagnose a significant problem. All indicators (temperature, pulse, respiration, and mucous membranes) should be evaluated serially to determine a trend in the patient's condition. It is this trend that will determine the severity of the postoperative problem and dictate the appropriate treatment. A detailed description of shock is given in Chapter 11.

In severely hemorrhaging patients, the veterinary technician may observe weakness, abdominal enlargement, bleeding from the incision, or a combination of these. They generally occur late and denote a prolonged episode of hemorrhage.

When the patient is suspected of having significant internal bleeding, a packed cell volume (PCV), a total protein determination, and paracentesis (abdominal tap) should be performed to confirm the diagnosis. Reoperation in the severely bleeding patient may be necessary to save the life.

Body weight gain may occur as a late sequela to ovariohysterectomy in the bitch. The reasons for this excessive weight gain are poorly understood but may be partially due to ovarian endocrine deficiency. In most instances, obesity can be controlled by proper diet and exercise.

Canine Castration

Definition. Canine castration involves the removal of both testicles.

Indications. There are numerous indications for canine castration, the most common being an elective procedure in the young male dog to help prevent roaming, aggressiveness, unwanted breeding, or a combination of these. The optimal age for elective castration is 6 to 9 months. Several medical problems may also be treated by castration, including prostate disorders, anal and perianal tumors, perineal hernias, and testicular tumors. Preanesthetic evaluation should include palpation of both testicles to detect retained testicles prior to surgery.

Technique. The abdomen is clipped from the tip of the prepuce to the margin of abdominal skin and scrotal skin (Fig. 18–7). The clipped area should extend widely into the inguinal region. Ideally, the scrotum itself should not be clipped. The scrotum has very delicate, thin skin that is easily subject to clipper burn and laceration. If, however, there are long scrotal hairs protruding into the surgical field, they can and should be clipped. Care should be taken, however, not to touch the clippers to the scrotal skin.

The animal is secured in dorsal recumbency, and a standard surgical preparation of the prescrotal skin (craniad to the scrotum) is performed. Again, when scrubbing the scrotal skin, care should be taken not to be as aggressive as on the abdominal skin.

A midline incision is made in the prescrotal skin. With gentle pressure, one of the testicles is pushed craniad into the incision. The testicle is then exteriorized through the incision by carefully incising over the common tunic (tissue that encases the testicle). The major vessels are then easily identified and ligated with two absorbable sutures. The remaining scrotal ligament is gently dissected from the testicle. The opposite testicle is handled in a similar fashion. The incision is closed with a continuous subcuticular suture pattern.

Complications. Several postoperative complications can occur. The veterinary technician is most commonly the first person to observe early postoperative complications.

If the presurgical preparation is not done carefully so as to preclude scrotal dermatitis (clipper burn, excessive scrubbing), the patient will lick aggressively at the scrotum and the incision. This often results in severe inflammation and swelling of the scrotal and prescrotal skin. If not detected early, the results can be suture removal and wound dehiscence. The best treatment for this complication is prevention. If scrotal dermatitis does

occur, the patient should be immediately placed in an Elizabethan collar. The scrotum and incision are then treated with an anti-inflammatory and antimicrobial ointment combination.

TECHNICIAN NOTE

The most common complications associated with canine castration are secondary to self-trauma.

Another less common complication is hemorrhage. When the testicles are removed from the scrotal sac, a significant amount of free space remains in the scrotum. If there is any hemorrhage, either from the subcutaneous tissue or common tunic, the space will fill with a considerable amount of blood before there is enough pressure to create hemostasis, resulting in a large hematoma within the scrotum. If detected early, before the scrotum is full, cold compresses can be applied with slight pressure to the scrotal area to encourage hemostasis. If the scrotum is full, its surgical removal may be necessary.

Feline Castration

Definition. Feline castration involves the removal of both testicles.

Indications. The major indications for feline castration are to prevent fighting, roaming, and urine spraying, and to decrease urine odor. Castration in the cat may provide a rapid response (2 to 4 weeks) to these objectionable characteristics. Preanesthetic evaluation should include palpation of both testicles to confirm the sex of the cat and to detect retained testicles prior to surgery.

Technique. There are several acceptable techniques for feline castration. The patient is generally placed in dorsal recumbency with the legs tied craniad (Fig. 18–8). The scrotal hairs are gently plucked from the scrotum with the thumb and finger. This is easily accomplished by grasping the base of the scrotum by the thumb and index finger of one hand, and gently pushing the testicles into the scrotum. With the other hand, the thumb and finger are used to gently strip the hair from the scrotal skin. Unlike the dog, the cat is not susceptible to severe scrotal dermatitis. The scrotum is then scrubbed and draped in an aseptic manner.

An incision is made directly through the scrotum. The testicle is protruded through the incision by gentle pressure with the thumb and index finger. The testicle and its spermatic cord (vessels) are exteriorized and then may be ligated with suture, ligated with metal clips, or tied in a knot on itself, or the vessels can be separated from the vas deferens and tied in a square knot. The scrotum is left unsutured.

Complications. Scrotal swelling and bleeding are the two most common complications of feline castration. Scrotal swelling is due primarily to traumatic surgical preparation and hair plucking. An Elizabethan collar may be necessary to control licking. Hemorrhage from a scrotal vessel may be detected

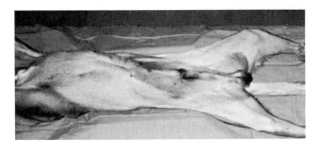

Figure 18-7. Proper positioning and preparation for canine castration.

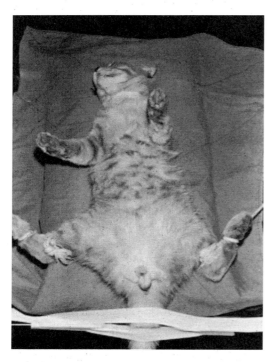

Figure 18-8. Proper positioning and preparation for feline castration.

immediately postoperatively. Cold compresses on the scrotum for 5 to 7 minutes will help to encourage hemostasis.

When the patient is sent home, the owner should be informed to change the litter from gravel type to shredded newspaper for the first 5 to 7 days. This will prevent pieces of litter from contaminating the surgical site.

Cesarean Section

Definition. *Dystocia* (Greek: *dys*, difficult + *tokos*, birth) literally translated means difficult birth. Cesarean section derived its name from Caesar, allegedly the first to be born by such a technique. The procedure involves making an incision into the abdominal cavity and then into the uterus to deliver the newborn.

Indications. Cesarean section is indicated when a bitch or queen cannot deliver the pups or kits through the birth canal by normal uterine contractions, because of either maternal or fetal abnormalities. Some of the common causes of dystocia are seen in Figure 18–9. Normal stages of parturition are discussed in Chapter 13.

Preoperative Considerations. The aim of treatment should be the successful delivery of live and undamaged pups or kits without harm to the dam. Before medical therapy can be instituted, a diagnosis of the cause of dystocia must be made. Medical therapy may do more harm than good when used in the wrong type of dystocia. An example would be giving a drug (oxytocin) that would increase uterine muscular contraction in a bitch that has a malpositioned pup. When proper diagnosis of the type of dystocia is made, and medical therapy is either contraindicated or not effective, the dam should be prepared for surgery.

The anesthetic regimen is of prime importance when considering cesarean section. In order to get strong, healthy pups or kits, the agents used should have minimal effects on the newborn. A detailed discussion of anesthetic regimens for the dystocia patient is given in Chapter 15.

Technique. The patient is clipped *prior to* anesthesia. After anesthetic induction and maintenance, the patient is placed in dorsal recumbency. It is important to remember that the increased weight of the pups or kits on the diaphragm may compromise the normal breathing capacity of the dam.

TECHNICIAN NOTE

It is important to do as much preoperative preparation in lateral recumbency as possible, and then place the patient in dorsal recumbency just prior to the surgical preparation.

A ventral midline celiotomy is performed (see Fig. 18–6A). The uterus is exteriorized and isolated with surgical towels. Uterine isolation helps prevent the uterine contents from entering the abdominal cavity. An incision is made into the dorsal aspect of the uterine body. Care is taken not to cut the fetus. The fetus and fetal membranes are advanced through the uterine incision by applying gentle pressure to the uterine wall. Upon presentation, the fetal membranes are removed, the umbilicus is clamped or ligated, and the newborn is handed to the assistant. Each successive newborn is handled in a similar fashion until all pups or kits are delivered. The uterine incision is closed in two layers. The celiotomy incision is closed in a routine fashion. The skin can be closed with stainless steel sutures in an interrupted pattern or with a synthetic nonabsorbable suture in a *continuous* pattern. This will discourage the pups or kits from removing the sutures when they are nursing.

Immediate Care of the Newborn. The assistant should be ready to grasp the pup or kit from the surgeon and immediately place it in a dry towel. The assistant can then massage the animal gently to stimulate respiration, dry any secretions around the mouth and nose, and dry the remainder of the body to decrease the chance of hypothermia. The mouth should be inspected for evidence of mucus that may be plugging the airway. At the same time, a quick examination for the presence of cleft palate is made. If the mouth and nostrils are clogged with mucus, the pup or kit should be cradled in the palm of the right hand with the left hand stabilizing the animal; it is then swung smartly downward in an arc, which removes any fluid by centrifugal force (Fig. 18–10). Weak newborns or those with faint respirations may be stimulated by injecting doxapram (a respiratory stimulant) in the umbilical vein or under the tongue, using a 25-gauge needle and a tuberculin syringe. A thorough examination for congenital defects is made, and the pup or kit is placed in an incubator or warm, padded area.

The animals can be safely returned to the dam as soon as she has recovered from anesthesia. Care should be taken not to return them so early that the dam may unknowingly harm them by stepping or lying on them. The dam should be re-

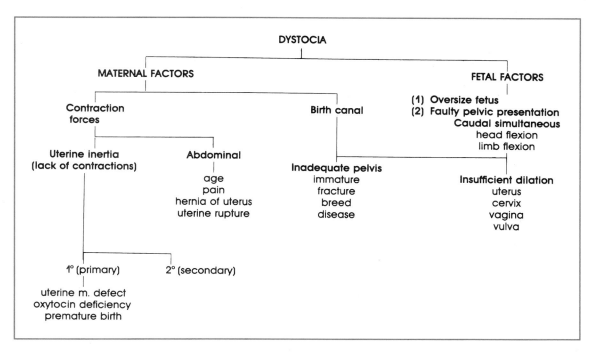

Figure 18-9. Common causes of dystocia.

turned to her home environment as soon as possible so that she can begin caring for her newborn pups or kits.

Cystotomy

Definition. Cystotomy involves incising through the urinary bladder wall to expose the lumen (inside of the bladder).

Indications. The most common indication for cystotomy in small animals is cystic calculi (bladder stones). A cystotomy is also indicated when tumors, mucosal outpouchings, congenital defects, or traumatic rupture occurs.

Technique. The abdomen is widely clipped from the xiphoid to the pubis. In male dogs, care is taken to clip the hair from the prepuce. The preputial orifice and penis are then gently flushed with a 1% povidone-iodine (Betadine) solution. A stiff polyethylene male urinary catheter is aseptically passed from the tip of the penis into the urinary bladder. This will allow flushing of any urethral calculi back into the bladder for easy removal. Although it is more common for urinary stones to lodge in the urethra of the male, a urethral catheter should also be passed in the female, as urethral calculi have been reported.

The animal is placed in dorsal recumbency and prepared for surgery with a standard skin preparation. In male patients, the abdominal skin incision will curve laterally to avoid the prepuce (see Fig. 18–6D). Care should be taken to thoroughly prepare this area aseptically.

In the female, a standard caudal midline celiotomy is performed (see Fig. 18–6A). In the male, a caudal midline skin incision is made from the umbilicus to the sheath of the penis and is then extended lateral to the sheath. Major vessels lateral to the prepuce are encountered—the caudal superficial epigastric artery and vein—which are ligated and transected. The sheath is retracted laterally, and a ventral midline celiotomy is

performed. The bladder is exteriorized and packed off with laparotomy pads to preclude urine spillage into the celiotomy incision. An incision is made on the ventral aspect of the bladder, in a relatively avascular area, between preplaced stay sutures. A urine culture is immediately taken, the cystic calculi are removed and submitted for stone analysis, and the entire

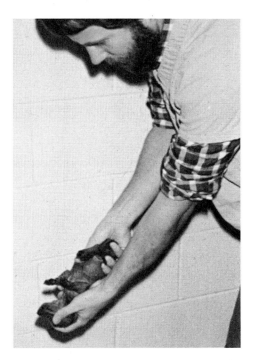

Figure 18-10. Removal of mucus and fluid from nostrils and mouth of the newborn pup can be accomplished safely by cradling the pup in the hand and swinging it smartly downward in an arc.

tract (bladder to urethra) is flushed with sterile physiological saline solution until all calculi have been removed. The bladder wall is inspected for abnormalities and is then closed with a simple interrupted or inverting suture pattern. The laparotomy pads are removed, the abdomen is lavaged with sterile physiological saline solution, and the incision is closed in a routine fashion.

Postoperative Considerations. The immediate postoperative care of the cystotomy patient includes monitoring the patient's urination. During the first 48 to 72 hours postoperatively, a mild hematuria (bloody urine) with or without blood clots can be expected. Owners should be informed of this if the patient is released during this time.

> ✏️ **TECHNICIAN NOTE**
>
> During the first 48 to 72 hours following a cystotomy, a mild hematuria with or without blood clots can be expected.

Following surgical removal of cystic calculi, the major treatment regimen begins—calculi prophylaxis. The stone must be analyzed, the culture and sensitivity must be evaluated, and the client must be informed about recurrence of cystic calculi. Some stones have a specific treatment and dietary regimen that must be strictly adhered to to prevent the reformation of calculi. The prompt treatment of urinary tract infections with the appropriate antibiotics is also very important in preventing stone formation.

Prescription Diet (S/D Hills) has been developed as a nutritional aid for the dissolution of struvite uroliths. This diet increases the solubility of struvite crystals by maintaining an acid urine.

Feline Perineal Urethrostomy

Definition. Perineal urethrostomy is performed in male cats with recurrent urethral obstruction to provide a larger-diameter opening in the penis that will allow passage of urine crystals and mucus.

Indications. The most common indication for a perineal urethrostomy is multiple episodes of feline urological syndrome. Other less common indications include rupture of the penile urethra secondary to traumatic catheterization, or rupture secondary to blunt trauma (e.g., hit by car, abdominal kick).

Preoperative Considerations. A cat with feline urological syndrome can present for examination with an array of clinical findings. The presentation is often dependent upon the duration and completeness of the urinary obstruction. If the patient is brought for examination early, there is little chance that other organ systems are affected. If the patient is presented 12 to 24 hours after a complete obstruction, severe electrolyte abnormalities, cardiac arrhythmias, kidney dysfunction, and shock can be present. These patients must have the obstruction removed and become stabilized, and normal renal function must be restored prior to surgery. This is a *true* emergency situation.

Technique. The hair on the perineum and external genitalia is clipped. The patient is placed in a perineal position (ventral recumbency with the perineum elevated approximately 30 degrees). The tail is extended directly over the dorsal midline and immobilized with tape. A purse-string suture is placed in the anus to eliminate fecal contamination of the surgical field. Standard skin preparation is performed (Fig. 18–11).

If the cat is intact, he is first castrated (see Feline Castration). An elliptical skin incision around the scrotum and prepuce is made. The urethra is dissected free from its pelvic attachments. A catheter is placed in the urethra, and a longitudinal incision is made through the penile urethra extending craniad to the level of the pelvic urethra. The diameter of the pelvic urethra is approximately two times that of the penile urethra. This allows normal urination in the face of crystalluria (sand-like material in the urine) and mucous plugs. The urethral mucosa is sutured to the skin. This results in a new, permanent opening that will easily accommodate the excess mucus and crystals.

Postoperative Considerations. The purse-string suture is removed. Immediate postoperative care includes placement of an Elizabethan collar and examination of the surgical site for evidence of hemorrhage. The Elizabethan collar is essential to keep the patient from licking the sutures. Occasionally, especially in intact male cats, postoperative hemorrhage may be a problem. In such instances, cold compresses can be gently applied to the surgical site to control hemorrhage. Rarely is the bleeding severe enough to require additional surgery or transfusion.

During the first 2 to 3 days postoperatively, the bladder should be gently expressed to determine that a normal flow of urine exists. Postoperative catheters are *discouraged* because of the increased incidence of strictures. The perineal urethrostomy site should be manipulated as little as possible. Ointments and warm cleansings are also discouraged. This may delay healing or aggravate hemorrhage. When the patient is dismissed from the hospital, the use of shredded paper in the litter box is recommended for the first 7 to 10 days at home.

The most common late postoperative complication is stricture. This is generally manifested by chronic stranguria (straining to urinate). Stricture requires reoperation.

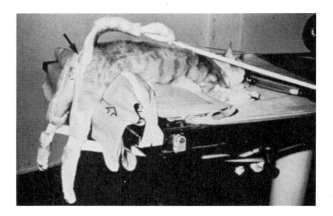

Figure 18-11. The perineal position can be used in the dog or cat. Open arrow, padding in front of the legs. This cat is positioned for a perineal urethrostomy. Arrow, pursestring suture in the anus.

Hernias

The strict definition of *hernia* is protrusion of an organ from its normal cavity (generally abdominal cavity) through a congenital or acquired defect in the wall of that cavity. The most common hernias in the dog and cat are umbilical hernias, inguinal hernias, and diaphragmatic hernias.

Umbilical Hernia

Definition. An umbilical hernia is one in which bowel or, more commonly, omentum protrudes through a defect in the abdominal wall under the skin at the umbilicus. This hernia is most commonly congenital, and it is recognized on physical examination by the presence of a swelling at the umbilicus. Very small hernias in young dogs (2 to 4 months of age) are often self-limiting. Larger hernias in older dogs (6 to 9 months of age) generally require surgical repair. The most common complication of larger umbilical hernias is strangulation of the intestine. Some of the smaller umbilical hernias are repaired during ovariohysterectomy.

Technique. The abdomen is widely clipped from xiphoid to pubis. The patient is placed in dorsal recumbency, and a standard skin preparation is performed. An elliptical skin incision is made around the hernia. The skin is dissected away from the hernial sac, the contents are exposed, and are either replaced into the abdominal cavity (intestine) or excised (falciform or omental fat). The edges of the hernial ring are trimmed to ensure healing of the defect. The abdomen is closed in a routine fashion as for the celiotomy incision.

Postoperative Considerations. Postoperative care is similar to that given for any celiotomy incision.

Inguinal Hernia

Definition. An inguinal hernia is one in which intestine, uterus, broad ligament, or other abdominal organ protrudes through the inguinal canal. This is more common in the bitch than in the male dog. An inguinal hernia is diagnosed on physical examination by the presence of a soft, doughy, non-painful mass in the inguinal region. It does not spontaneously regress and should be surgically repaired when diagnosed, because the abdominal contents may become entrapped within the hernial sac.

Technique. The abdomen is widely clipped from the umbilicus to and including the inguinal area. The patient is placed in dorsal recumbency, and a standard skin preparation is performed. A midline incision is made in the caudal abdominal region just across from the inguinal hernia. The inguinal ring is exposed with its hernial sac and external pudendal vessels. The hernial sac is emptied of its contents and is excised and sutured along with the margin of the inguinal ring. Care is taken during closure to avoid the external pudendal vessels that exit from the caudal medial aspect of the ring. The skin incision is then closed as for a celiotomy closure.

Postoperative Considerations. The incision is monitored as for any abdominal incision.

Diaphragmatic Hernia

Definition. A diaphragmatic hernia exists when abdominal organs protrude through an opening in the diaphragm into the thoracic cavity. Diaphragmatic hernias may be congenital or traumatic. Any patient with a history of trauma or suspected trauma should be examined for a diaphragmatic hernia. Diaphragmatic hernias may be life-threatening. They may be insidious and difficult to identify. Signs may be masked by other problems.

An animal with a massive hernia will have a diminished intrathoracic space as a result of migration of abdominal contents into the thoracic cavity, resulting in a reduction of lung volume. Presumptive diagnosis is based on a thorough physical examination. The classic signs of diaphragmatic hernia are a "tucked-up" abdomen, intestinal sounds in the chest, muffled heart and lung sounds, and dyspnea. The diagnosis is confirmed by chest radiograph.

Once the diagnosis of diaphragmatic hernia has been made, the patient should be stabilized prior to anesthesia. This includes *minimal* stress, oxygen cage confinement to allow maximal oxygenation of available lung capacity, and constant monitoring for respiratory insufficiency or arrest. Rarely is diaphragmatic hernia repair an emergency. Only in cases of massive hernia or severe gas distention of a herniated viscus (stomach, intestine) is immediate operation necessary.

TECHNICIAN NOTE

Diaphragmatic hernia patients should have oxygen cage confinement to allow maximal oxygenation, minimal stress, and constant monitoring for respiratory insufficiency prior to surgery.

Technique. The most critical time for the diaphragmatic hernia patient is at anesthetic induction. It is very important to be thoroughly familiar with induction procedures as well as resuscitative techniques in the event of respiratory or cardiac arrest (see Chapter 13).

The skin is widely clipped from just ahead of the xiphoid process to the pubis. The patient is placed in dorsal recumbency on an incline, with the head slightly higher than the hindquarters. This will allow any easily movable viscera to "slide" from the thorax back into the abdominal cavity, allowing an increase in lung capacity and easier breathing.

A ventral midline celiotomy from xiphoid to umbilicus is performed. The edges of the incision are protected with laparotomy pads, and a Balfour self-retaining abdominal retractor is placed to enhance visualization. The diaphragmatic defect is inspected, and any herniated viscera are gently reduced into the abdominal cavity. A thorough inspection of abdominal and thoracic viscera is made to rule out organ rupture or vascular compromise.

Diaphragmatic hernia repair requires working in a deep cavity. Gentle retraction of viscera to expose the defect is necessary throughout the procedure to preclude damage to abdominal organs. The diaphragmatic defect is sutured with a nonabsorbable suture material in a simple continuous suture pattern. This will effect an airtight and watertight seal. The completed suture line is inspected for leaks by filling the abdominal cavity with warm, sterile physiological saline solution. The lungs are then inflated, and the incision is inspected for bubbles. Air is evacuated from the chest by thoracocentesis through the diaphragm. The celiotomy is closed in a routine fashion.

Postoperative Considerations. The patient should be monitored carefully for signs of respiratory distress. If dyspnea occurs, the chest should be evacuated with a hypodermic needle, three-way stopcock, and a large syringe. A rapid return to normal negative thoracic pressure and normal lung capacity should occur.

In some patients, an indwelling chest tube is placed for the first 1 to 2 days postoperatively. In these cases, periodic aspiration using positional changes (right lateral recumbency, left lateral recumbency, standing on hindlegs, standing on front legs) will afford maximal removal of air and fluid. During the drain management period, it is of utmost importance to keep the patient from chewing a hole in the drain or removing it from the chest cavity. Removal can result in acute death. It is also imperative to keep all connections on the chest drain airtight. Leaks will result in a pneumothorax, respiratory difficulty, and possibly death. Proper management of a chest drain requires full-time patient monitoring.

A chart quantitating the amount of air and fluid removed during a given period of time (12 to 24 hours) will help to determine when the drain should be removed. Generally, the drain can safely be removed as the amount of air and fluid decreases toward zero.

Mammary Neoplasia

General Considerations. Mammary cancer is the most frequently occurring neoplasm in the female dog, and mammary gland neoplasms are the third most frequently found tumors in the female cat.

In dogs there is a significantly higher incidence of mammary gland tumors in nonspayed females or females that are spayed at an age older than 2½ years. Spaying prior to the first estrus cycle provides a definite protective factor.

In the initial stages, the tumor will usually appear as a hard lump in any of the glands of the mammary chain. Long-standing or fast-growing tumors may present a sizeable mass with ulceration and drainage. Early diagnosis and therapy will give the best possible prognosis for mammary gland cancer.

Before surgery can be considered, an examination for possible metastasis (spread) of the tumor is done. Malignant tumors will generally metastasize to the lymph nodes and lungs. Biopsy of regional lymph nodes and chest radiographs may detect metastases. About 50% of mammary tumors in the dog are malignant, and about 80% to 90% of mammary tumors in cats are malignant.

Surgery is currently considered the most effective therapy. Early surgery can cure up to 50% of canine mammary gland cancer. The primary objective of surgical treatment is complete removal of the tumor tissue.

Technique. The skin is clipped widely to include all affected mammary glands. The patient is placed in dorsal recumbency, and a standard skin preparation is performed. An elliptical incision is made, attempting to include a 1-cm margin around the tumor. The skin, mammary gland, and tumor are gently undermined and removed. The skin incision is often gaping after tumor excision, requiring a meticulous subcutaneous closure. Subcutaneous tissues are closed with a simple interrupted pattern using absorbable suture material. The skin is closed in a routine fashion. The excised mammary masses are placed in formalin and sent to a laboratory for histopathological evaluation.

Postoperative Considerations. Major complications that can occur postoperatively are generally related to the tension placed on the skin to adequately close the wound. Dehiscence is not common, but the incision should be examined daily for evidence of separation. Bruising along the incision edges is common and is no cause for alarm. Immediate postoperative hemorrhage can occur. In the event of oozing blood, an abdominal bandage should be applied with gentle pressure. This will help ensure hemostasis and is also comfortable for the patient. The incisions are often very long and must be kept clean and dry at all times. Dogs that prefer to lie on the incision should be well padded or bandaged. If the patient irritates the incision by licking, an Elizabethan collar should be applied until suture removal.

NEUROLOGICAL PATIENT CARE

General Considerations. The most common neurological disorder in the dog is spontaneous intervertebral disk disease. Disks are normally found between vertebral bodies in the spine and act as shock absorbers during spinal movements. With time, the disks can undergo degeneration and calcification. When this occurs, the normal shock absorber–like effect is impaired, and extrusion (rupture) of the disk material into the spinal canal can occur. This puts pressure on the spinal cord and can cause an array of neurological deficits or pain.

One neurosurgical procedure occasionally performed in small animal practice is *intervertebral disk fenestration*. In this procedure, each disk that is calcified or that may become calcified is removed (scraped) from the intervertebral space. This procedure is performed to *prevent* rupture of the disk material into the spinal canal. Dogs may develop spontaneous intervertebral disk extrusions in the cervical spine (neck) or the thoracolumbar spine (lower back). If the disk has already ruptured, a "decompressive" procedure must be performed. The most common decompressive procedures are the ventral slot (for cervical disk rupture) and hemilaminectomy or dorsal laminectomy (for thoracolumbar disk rupture). The most commonly affected breed is the dachshund, but the beagle, Pekingese, poodle, and terrier breeds are also frequently presented with disk herniation.

The pre- and postoperative care of neurological patients is dependent on their neurological status. Patients that have the ability to walk (ambulatory status) on presentation can be managed much like any other animal in the hospital, except that they must be handled with care so as not to exacerbate their cervical or thoracolumbar disk herniation. Patients that have motor weakness (inability to walk normally) or paralysis (inability to walk) on presentation demand frequent attention and careful pre- and postoperative care.

Surgical Technique. When a patient with a herniated cervical or thoracolumbar disk is anesthetized, the normal protective

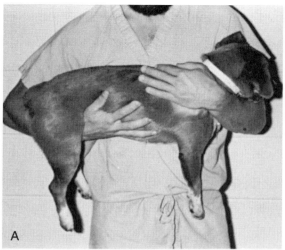
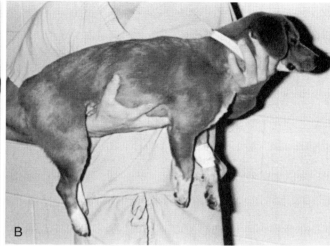
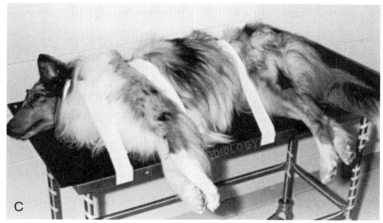

Figure 18-12. Proper technique for transporting an anesthetized patient with a spinal problem. A, Thoracolumbar support. B, Cervical support. C, Patient secured to rigid platform.

abilities of muscle support and conscious perception of pain are removed. It then becomes the responsibility of the veterinary technician, anesthesiologist, and surgeon to protect the patient from further neurological deficits by handling the spine with extreme care. It is important to keep the neck and back as straight as possible when moving the patient from one location to another. This needed support can be achieved in various ways. The patient can be taped to a rigid, flat surface or can be cradled in the arm, being careful to completely support the affected area (Fig. 18–12). The means of transportation may often be dictated by the size of the patient, but, generally speaking, a rigid, flat surface is the preferred method.

Patients undergoing cervical disk surgery are placed in dorsal recumbency with the head and neck in slight extension (Fig. 18–13). The ventral aspect of the neck is widely clipped from the manubrium sterni to the cranial aspect of the larynx. A standard skin preparation is performed. A ventral midline incision is made through the skin and muscles to expose the intervertebral spaces. A dental tartar scraper, curved needle, fenestration hook, or curette can be used to remove the disk material from the interspace. The fenestration technique is carried out from the C2 to C3 disk space to the C6 to C7 disk space. If decompression is needed, an oblong slot is made through the vertebral bodies into the spinal canal using a pneumatic or electric-powered burr. The disk material is then carefully removed from the spinal canal. The surgical wound is closed in layers with a continuous suture pattern using an absorbable suture. The skin is closed in a routine fashion.

Patients undergoing thoracolumbar disk surgery are placed in ventral recumbency (Fig. 18–14). The back is widely clipped from the midthoracic region to the pelvis. A standard skin preparation is performed. A skin incision is made from T11 to L6. Careful dissection between epaxial muscles (muscles of the back) allows palpation and limited visualization of the disk spaces. Each space between T10 and L5 is curetted with a technique similar to that described for cervical disk fenestration.

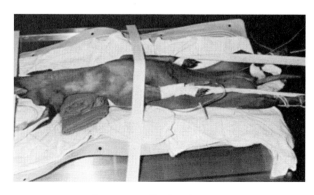

Figure 18-13. Proper positioning for cervical disk surgery.

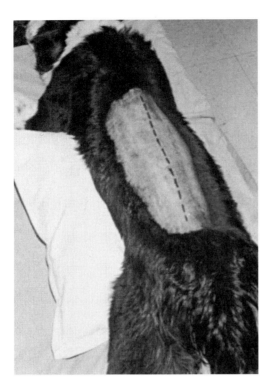

Figure 18-14. Proper positioning for thoracolumbar disk surgery.

If decompression is needed, a portion of the bony lamina covering the spinal cord is removed with a pneumatic or electric-powered burr or bone rongeurs. The ruptured disk material is then carefully removed from the spinal canal. The muscles, subcutaneous tissue, and skin are closed in a routine fashion.

Postoperative Considerations. Postoperative management for the nonambulatory patient is demanding. These patients are subject to decubital ulcers (bed sores or pressure sores), urinary bladder infections, joint stiffness, muscle atrophy (muscle wasting), pneumonia, and gastrointestinal ulceration. Preventing these conditions from occurring is the main objective of proper postoperative management and should include the following:

1. Passive range-of-motion exercises and whirlpool baths to encourage joint motion and muscular activity
2. Urinary bladder expression four to five times a day to keep the urinary bladder empty, thus lowering the incidence of infections secondary to large residual volumes
3. Turning the patient frequently to reduce the incidence of pneumonia
4. Keeping the patient well padded to prevent the formation of decubital sores
5. Using an elevated, perforated, rubber-coated rack to keep the patient from urinating and defecating on itself (Fig. 18–15)
6. Observation of the stool for evidence of fresh blood (bright red on feces) or digested blood (dark, tarry feces), which may be an indicator of colonic or gastric ulceration, respectively; this may be observed following cortisone therapy

7. Observation for vomiting, especially if the vomitus contains coffee ground–like material, indicative of gastric bleeding

As can be seen from the list, the veterinary technician and veterinarian must work diligently and continually to properly manage the nonambulatory neurological patient back to health.

ORTHOPEDIC SURGERY

Long Bone Fractures

Preoperative Considerations. When a patient is presented at the veterinary hospital with a fracture, several steps must be taken to ready the patient for a permanent repair. First, the patient must be stabilized with respect to all other body systems (treated for shock, chest injuries, abdominal injuries). Second, any open wounds associated with the fracture should be managed, and, third, the fracture must be immobilized by means of a bandage, cast, or sling. Once these three things have been achieved, fracture repair can be safely considered. Most long bone fractures are not life-threatening and do not require emergency surgery.

TECHNICIAN NOTE

Most long bone fractures are not life-threatening and do not require emergency surgery.

Operative Considerations. An extensive clip is required on all limb preparations. The surgeon and assistant will manipulate the limb during reduction and repair. For this reason, the limb is clipped from the level of the metacarpus or metatarsus to the scapula or pelvis, respectively, including the medial and lateral aspects of the extremity. This may vary slightly, depending on the particular bone that is fractured, but the general rule should be a wide and thorough clip. The remaining hair at the tip of the paw is covered with a rubber glove and is taped to the clipped skin (Fig. 18–16).

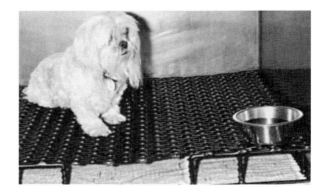

Figure 18-15. Spinal trauma patient on an elevated rack. The rack protects the patient from being soiled with urine and feces and helps prevent decubital sores.

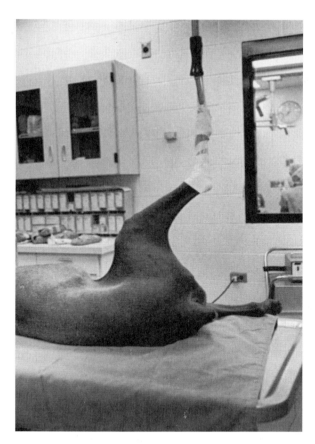

Figure 18–16. Properly prepared extremity must include a thorough clip of the medial and lateral aspects, and proper covering of the paw.

Positioning. Patient positioning depends on the specific bone that is fractured. Generally, the following positions are recommended for each fracture:

1. Femur: lateral recumbency, affected side up
2. Tibia-fibula: lateral recumbency, affected leg down
3. Humerus: lateral recumbency, affected leg up
4. Radius-ulna: dorsal recumbency, affected leg craniad
5. Pelvis: lateral recumbency, affected leg up

With so much skin exposed, skin preparation is time-consuming, but it must be meticulous. The surgeon eventually covers the extremity with a sterile stockinette, but this should not preclude an adequate skin preparation.

Surgical Assistance. Orthopedic procedures are often very difficult and time-consuming, and may demand the help of an assistant. Often, the veterinary technician is called upon to participate as a surgical assistant and, therefore, should have a general understanding of orthopedic tissue handling.

Several basic maneuvers commonly needed by the surgeon are often performed by the veterinary technician. They include retraction, muscle fatigue, alignment and reduction, and suction of the field. Proper techniques for each are discussed separately.

Retraction. Care should be taken to preserve the soft tissues in the operative field. It will be necessary to have functional muscle groups remaining when the bone is repaired. Retraction should be firm but not so traumatic as to bruise or tear the muscle.

Muscle Fatigue. Large-breed dogs, or fractures that are 3 to 5 days old may be difficult to reduce because of heavy muscle mass or severe muscle contraction, respectively. In such cases, constant steady traction on the muscle groups will cause them to fatigue and relax, thus facilitating reduction.

Alignment and Reduction. In order to repair fractured bones, the ends must be reduced and aligned. It is often necessary for an assistant to hold reduction during the fixation of the fracture. For rapid bone healing to occur, the fractured bone must be held in rigid fixation. Pins, wires, screws, and plates of stainless steel may be used to achieve the necessary fixation.

Suction. Whenever a fracture occurs, bleeding into the fracture site can be massive. Some continuous oozing occurs during fixation. A clean surgical field is of the utmost importance in facilitating early and accurate reduction and fixation.

Postoperative Considerations. Some postoperative orthopedic patients may require external coaptation. The patients should be managed as described in Chapter 17. Other patients may require range-of-motion exercises, but the majority require limited activity. It is important to realize the relatively unsure gait of a three-legged dog or cat, and, when exercising it, one must be certain to avoid slippery surfaces (vinyl or wet floors). Cement, grass, gravel, or dirt provides a much more sure-footed environment. Physical therapy should become part of most fracture patients' rehabilitation therapy. Flexing and extending the affected limb along with muscle massage will improve blood flow and muscle tone as well as reduce muscle contraction (Fig. 18–17). Therapy should be done for a period of 5 minutes each time, repeated two to three times per day. A demonstration by the technician of the proper technique will aid the client in understanding the therapy.

Joints

Preoperative Considerations. The majority of orthopedic procedures involving the joints are elective and rarely need emergency care. The preoperative management includes limiting the patient's activity. External coaptation is rarely necessary. The indications for joint surgery involve dislocations, ligament ruptures, infections, fractures involving the joint surfaces, joint capsule biopsy, and osteochondrosis (lytic lesions of the articular cartilage).

Operative Considerations. An extensive clip, as for fractures, should also be done for joint surgery. Positions will vary depending upon the joint involved. Generally, the following positions are recommended for each joint:

1. Hip: lateral recumbency, affected leg up
2. Stifle: lateral recumbency, affected leg up, or dorsal recumbency (can be used for unilateral or bilateral stifle surgery—surgeon's preference)
3. Shoulder: lateral recumbency, affected leg up
4. Tarsus: lateral recumbency, affected leg up
5. Elbow: lateral recumbency, affected leg up
6. Carpus: lateral recumbency, affected leg up

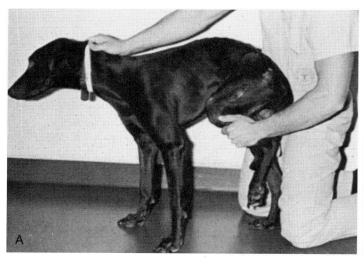
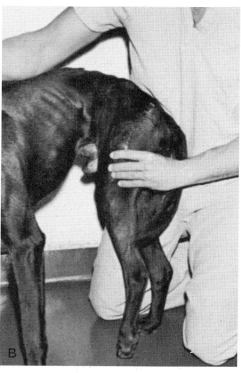

Figure 18-17. Proper technique for (A) passive range-of-motion exercises and (B) muscle massage.

Intraoperative assistance in joint surgery is similar to that necessary in fracture repair. Some special precautions should be taken while joints are exposed.

Retraction. Care should be taken *not* to place retractors in direct contact with the articular cartilage. Cartilage has a relatively poor response to trauma. When exposure of the joint is necessary, sharp retraction of the joint capsule will decrease trauma.

TECHNICIAN NOTE

Care should be taken *not* to place retractors in direct contact with the articular cartilage. Cartilage has a relatively poor response to trauma.

Flush. The cartilage should be frequently flushed with saline to keep it from drying out during the procedure. This is true of all tissues, but especially the articular cartilage because of its poor regenerative ability.

Postoperative Considerations. Postoperative care of patients undergoing joint surgery can be variable, depending on the surgical procedure, the joint involved, and the surgeon's preference. Generally, the joint is immobilized for 1 to 2 weeks, is gradually exercised with passive range-of-motion exercises for 7 to 10 days, then is gradually (1 to 2 weeks) worked back to normal activity.

CLIENT EDUCATION

When a patient is discharged from the professional care available in a veterinary hospital, it becomes the responsibility of the hospital staff to instruct the client to provide the same type of care at home. This requires that time be spent with the client and the pet to educate the client on appropriate treatment techniques. There are several methods of client education in surgical cases, the degree of difficulty of which is often associated with the type of surgical procedure performed (e.g., ovariohysterectomy versus disk fenestration).

Whenever a patient is sent home with a sutured skin incision, the client must be instructed to observe the incision daily for evidence of swelling, redness or drainage and to feel the incision for heat. The client should also watch the animal for aggressive licking, removal of skin sutures, or both.

If a patient is sent home with a bandage, a written discharge form should be given to the client describing in detail the proper management necessary to prevent complications.

In orthopedic cases, as well as in many elective soft tissue surgery cases, the owner should be instructed specifically on what kind of limited activity should be enforced. If passive range-of-motion exercises are expected, the client should be given both oral and written instruction in providing the correct care. A demonstration by the technician of the correct method of therapy is helpful.

In many instances, such as complicated orthopedic and neurological discharges, a handout explaining in detail the care necessary is very informative and gives a handy reference for the client to refer to if a problem arises.

The use of visual aids, such as a skeleton or overlay books that illustrate anatomy, can be effective in helping the client understand the scope of the problem. Clients are generally willing and capable of handling the postoperative patient, and with a little help from the veterinary hospital staff, a predictably successful end result can be expected to occur.

VETERINARY DENTISTRY

Veterinary dentistry has been practiced for decades. It has only been over the past 15 years, however, that the significance of dental problems in companion animals has been acknowledged and treated by methods other than tooth extraction. With the resources available to perform endodontic, periodontic, orthodontic, and restorative procedures, extraction may not be the only option for a diseased tooth. An understanding of the different types of dental problems and how they should be treated is important so that the client can be informed of the treatment options available.

This section provides a detailed discussion of periodontal disease and its prevention. Also included is an overview of the specialty branches of veterinary dentistry. Since veterinary technicians often perform dental scaling and polishing procedures, it is important that they have detailed knowledge of the necessary equipment and its proper use and care. Suggested readings can be found at the end of this chapter for more detailed discussions of each specialty area.

Periodontics and Periodontal Disease

Periodontics is the branch of dentistry concerned with the study and treatment of the periodontium. The periodontium is composed of the supporting structures of the tooth. These supporting structures are the *gingiva*, periodontal ligament, alveolar and supporting bone (tooth socket), and the cementum of the tooth root (Fig. 18–18). Healthy *gingiva* has a sharp, tapered edge (margin) that lies closely against the crown of the tooth (Fig. 18–19). The free gingiva forms a moat around the tooth called the gingival sulcus. The epithelial attachment of the gingiva to the cementum of the tooth root forms the bottom extent of the gingival sulcus. The depth of this sulcus ranges from 1 to 3 mm in a healthy mouth of a dog and is up to 1 mm deep in the cat.

Periodontitis means inflammation of the structures around the tooth (Greek *peri*, around + *odous*, tooth + *itis*, inflammation). It is the most common disease of animals and humans and is caused by plaque. Approximately 80% of dogs and 70% of cats have some form of periodontal disease by age 3.

Plaque is a white slippery film that collects around the gingival sulcus of the tooth. Plaque is composed of bacteria, food debris, exfoliated cells, and salivary glycoproteins. Over time, plaque will mineralize on the teeth to form dental calculus, a brown or yellow deposit (Fig. 18–20). As the plaque collects around the tooth, it damages the gingival tissues by releasing bacterial endotoxins. The animal's immune system further damages these tissues through the release of harmful by-products from white blood cells as they attempt to destroy the bacteria. In the early stages, the *gingiva* becomes inflamed and bleeds easily. This stage is called gingivitis (Fig. 18–20). As the disease progresses and destruction of the periodontium begins to occur (such as loss of alveolar bone, periodontal ligament, and gingiva), this stage of disease is termed *periodontitis* (Fig. 18–21).

> ### ✏ TECHNICIAN NOTE
>
> The key to prevention of periodontal disease is to minimize plaque accumulation by means of proper diet, routine professional dental scaling and polishing, and daily teeth brushing or mouth rinsing.

Periodontal disease is difficult to control once it has developed. For this reason, great emphasis must be placed on its prevention. Although many diseases can contribute to the se-

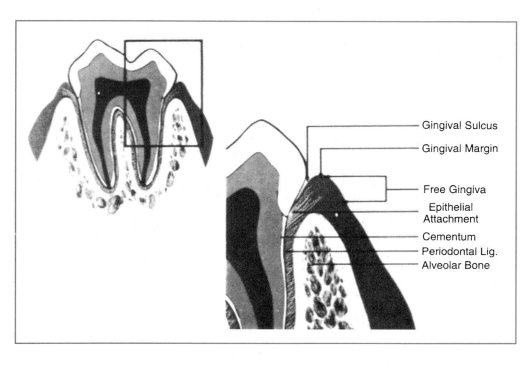

Figure 18-18. Structures collectively referred to as the periodontium. The tooth is suspended in the socket by the periodontal ligament. (From Bojrab MJ and Tholen M: Small Animal Oral Medicine and Surgery. Philadelphia, Lea & Febiger, 1990.)

Gingival Sulcus
Gingival Margin
Free Gingiva
Epithelial Attachment
Cementum
Periodontal Lig.
Alveolar Bone

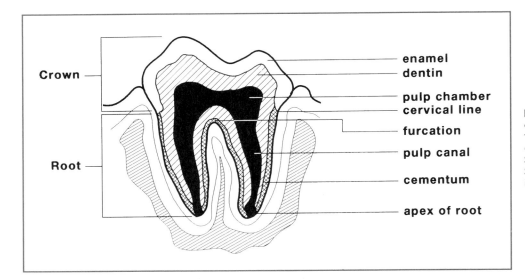

Figure 18-19. Typical external and internal gross anatomy of a tooth. The model is a premolar. (From Bojrab MJ and Tholen M: Small Animal Oral Medicine and Surgery. Philadelphia, Lea & Febiger, 1990.)

verity of periodontal disease, there is only one primary cause: plaque.

When periodontitis is already present, destruction of the periodontal tissues has begun and will continue if not treated. Once the periodontal ligaments are destroyed, they are extremely difficult to replace. As the tooth begins to lose its periodontal tissue, it becomes more susceptible to plaque accumulation in the deep periodontal pockets that form around the tooth root(s). When the tooth loses a significant portion of its periodontium, it becomes mobile (loose) and will eventually fall out. This is nature's way of clearing the infection from the body. The infection, however, is usually present for months to years before the tooth is eventually lost. During this time, the bacteria can gain entrance to the animal's blood stream and become systemic, spreading to numerous organs such as the liver, kidney, heart, and lungs.

For patients with periodontal disease, the treatment goal is to remove the plaque and calculus from the teeth and to minimize plaque reattachment. Treatments to minimize plaque accumulation include those listed for prevention of periodontal disease, as well as periodontal surgery when deep periodontal pockets have formed around tooth roots.

Root planing and subgingival curettage are important procedures in periodontal treatment. *Root planing* is the removal of calculus and necrotic cementum from the diseased tooth roots (Fig. 18–22). The root surface must be thoroughly cleaned before healing can occur. Curettes are used to clean the root

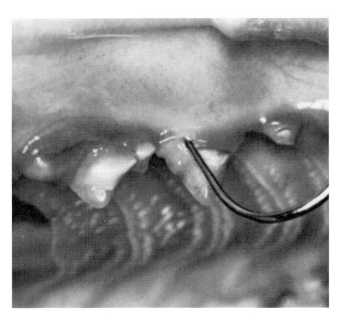

Figure 18-20. The calculus and plaque deposits on these teeth have caused the gingivae to become inflamed (gingivitis). A dental explorer is used to detect subgingival (under the gingiva) calculus or dental abnormalities.

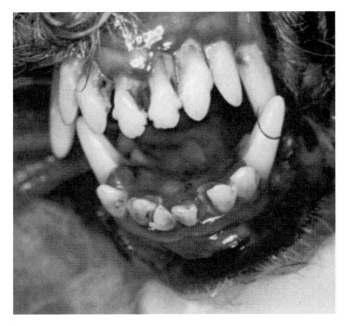

Figure 18-21. Periodontal disease has destroyed a significant portion of the alveolar bone and periodontal ligament of these incisor teeth. The gingivae have receded from the crowns of these teeth, and the tooth roots are now exposed.

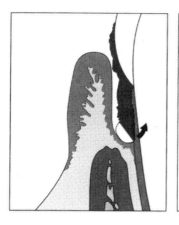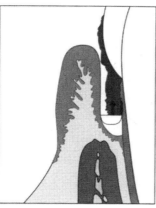

Figure 18-22. Root planing. Left, the curette is inserted into the pocket with its curved edge against the epithelium. It is turned to engage the cutting back in the necrotic cementum and debris. Right, the curette is withdrawn, removing the subgingival debris and necrotic cementum and scraping the pocket epithelium. (From Emily P and Penman S: Handbook of Small Animal Dentistry, 2nd Edition, Pergamon Press Ltd, Oxford, England, 1994.)

surface using multiple overlapping strokes in vertical, horizontal, and oblique directions until the root surface is as smooth as glass. Pressure created with each stroke ranges from firm to light as the tooth root is cleaned. Care must be taken not to gouge the root surface. The gingiva covering these roots must be cleaned of foreign debris and granulation tissue. This procedure is called *subgingival curettage* and curettes are used for this procedure as well. The blade of the curette is directed toward the pocket lining and digital pressure is placed on the gingival tissue to support it while the tissue is debrided.

Subgingival curettage and root planing can be done without incising and elevating the gingival tissue as long as there is sufficient access to the roots and gingival epithelium to thoroughly debride the area. This process is called closed root planing. If the gingiva impedes proper cleaning of the tooth roots, the gingiva should be incised and reflected to allow visualization and instrumentation of the roots for proper debridement. This technique is termed *open root planing*. The gingival tissue is sutured in proper position once the procedure is complete. In some cases the gingival flap is repositioned apically (moved toward the root tip) to reduce the depth of the periodontal pocket.

A grading system is helpful to categorize periodontal disease and determine appropriate treatment. Grade I periodontal disease is a reversible gingivitis and requires routine dental cleaning. Grade II periodontal disease is an early form of periodontitis. There is some attachment loss (approximately 1 to 2 mm) and root planing or subgingival curettage may be required. Grade III periodontal disease is considered a moderate degree of periodontitis; attachment loss is in the range of 3 to 6 mm and root planing, subgingival curettage, and periodontal surgery are often required. These teeth have a fair to guarded prognosis. Grade IV periodontal disease is severe periodontitis; attachment loss is greater than 6 mm and the tooth has a poor prognosis. Many of these teeth are extracted. Efforts to save these teeth require root planing, subgingival curettage, periodontal surgery and possibly periodontal splinting. (The attachment losses mentioned above apply to dogs, not cats.)

Loose teeth can be stabilized by splinting them to adjacent teeth to prevent their loss while the periodontium is healing. A thorough dental cleaning with radiographs, root planing, and subgingival curettage must be performed prior to splinting the loose teeth. Splinting is performed only if the pet owner is willing to provide dental home care and have the teeth professionally cleaned as needed. If the splints and teeth are not properly cleaned by the owner, the splints will retain foreign debris and worsen the condition. Pets with advanced periodontal disease may require professional dental cleaning every 3 to 4 months.

Proper Diet

TECHNICIAN NOTE

Dry pet food is the diet of choice for minimizing the rate of plaque accumulation on the dentition. Hill's t/d is a prescription diet specifically developed to remove dental calculus.

The semimoist and canned pet foods are tacky and tend to stick to the teeth. This accelerates plaque accumulation.

Tartar control pet products have recently entered the marketplace. The active ingredients are sodium hexametaphosphate (HMP) and sodium tripolyphosphate. The tartar control products work by sequestering the calcium in plaque fluids to reduce calculus formation. Research studies on dogs and cats have shown that these products can reduce calculus up to 46% in dogs and 30% in cats.

Hill's Pet Nutrition has produced a dog food called t/d which is nutritionally balanced and designed to help minimize calculus build-up. The t/d biscuit fibers are longer than traditional fibers and are primarily oriented in one direction to keep the biscuit from crumbling readily when the dog bites into it. This design allows the biscuit to mechanically scrape the sides of the teeth clean as the teeth penetrate the biscuit. In order for this product to be effective, the pet should not eat any other brand of pet food or be fed table scraps.

Proper chew toys should be encouraged. Rawhide bones and chews are excellent for exercising the teeth and periodontium to help maintain a healthy mouth. Some pets have a desire to chew on hard objects such as rocks. Hard objects can damage the teeth and should be removed from the pet's environment when possible.

Dental Scaling and Polishing

Prior to beginning the dental cleaning procedure, the dental treatment area should be prepared. The proper instruments should be out for easy access, and they should be clean and sharp. The patient should be examined by the veterinarian prior to anesthesia for evidence of bacterial infection of the periodontium. When oral infection is present, preoperative antibiotics should be given to help prevent the systemic spread of oral bacteria to internal organs. Patients with periodontitis should begin antibiotic treatment at least 3 days prior to the dental cleaning procedure.

The patient is anesthetized and a cuffed endotracheal tube is used to prevent water and foreign debris from entering the trachea. Care should be taken not to overinflate the endotracheal tube cuff, which could damage the trachea. In 1994 the American Veterinary Medical Association Professional Liability Insurance Trust received 18 claims on pets (all cats) diagnosed with subcutaneous emphysema following an anesthetic procedure. All cases were intubated and 16 were under anesthesia for dentistries. The cause of the subcutaneous emphysema was not confirmed in every case but tracheal tears were found in some of the cases. To avoid injury to the trachea, disconnect the animals from the anesthesia circuit when repositioning them, minimize movement of the endotracheal tube, and inflate the cuff just enough to stop the leak of anesthetic gases.

> **TECHNICIAN NOTE**
>
> To avoid injury to the trachea, disconnect the patient from the anesthesia circuit when repositioning is needed, minimize movement of the endotracheal tube, and inflate the cuff just enough to stop the leak of anesthetic gases.

The patient's head should be placed on a slight incline (nose downward) if possible. This can be done by tilting a surgery table, or placing a rolled towel under the animal's neck to ensure that the pharynx is higher than the nose (Fig. 18–23). This allows water and debris to run out of the mouth while mechanical scalers are being used.

Once the anesthetized patient is prepared, the technician should don the proper attire and begin the dental cleaning. Proper attire consists of a mask, gloves, eye protection (glasses or a shield), cap, and laboratory coat. It is important to wear these protective coverings because large numbers of bacteria are aerosolized during the mechanical scaling procedure, and these could be inhaled or could saturate clothing, leading to contamination of other areas in the hospital.

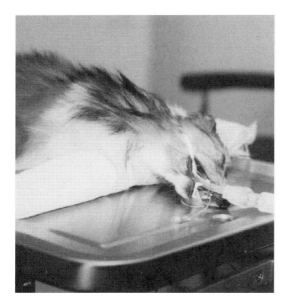

Figure 18–23. Proper patient positioning for dental scaling and polishing. Note that the head is placed in a downward position.

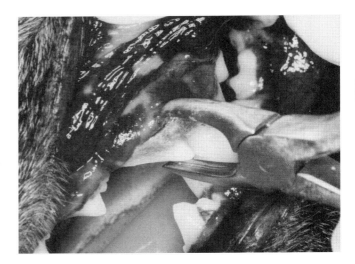

Figure 18–24. Large pieces of calculus can be quickly removed with forceps. Care should be taken not to place excessive pressure on the tooth, especially cusp tips, to avoid fracturing the tooth.

The dental cleaning begins with a thorough examination of the oral cavity. Clinical findings should be recorded at either the beginning or the end of the procedure. Important findings to include are areas of ulceration, missing teeth, loose teeth, periodontal pockets, receded gingiva, degree of periodontal disease, fractured teeth, and so forth.

Large pieces of calculus can often be easily removed with calculus-removing forceps (Fig. 18–24). If the patient has minimal amounts of calculus present, the calculus can be removed with hand scaling instruments alone. Electric and air-driven mechanical scalers can be used on patients with significant amounts of calculus present (most patients!) because they remove calculus rapidly (Fig. 18–25). Since the mechanical vibrations of the tips of these scalers dislodge the calculus, minimal pressure is used when operating these instruments. Most of these instruments generate heat owing to the rapid vibrations, so it is imperative to use irrigation to cool the working tips of these instruments so that the pulp tissue does not receive thermal damage (Fig. 18–25).

> **TECHNICIAN NOTE**
>
> When using mechanical scalers, the instrument must be kept moving on the tooth surface and should not be on the tooth for more than 10 to 15 seconds to avoid heat buildup.

If the scaling of a tooth is not completed in 10 to 15 seconds, the adjacent tooth can be scaled while the first tooth cools. Once cool, the first tooth can be scaled again.

Most dental cleaning procedures require the use of mechanical and hand scalers. Hand scalers can be used to reach those areas that are inaccessible to the mechanical scaler.

There are a large number of different types of dental scalers and curettes on the market. It is important to understand the different components of these instruments so they can be used

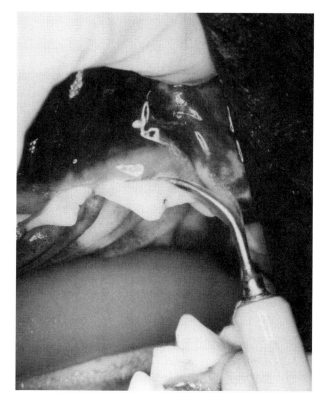

Figure 18-25. An ultrasonic scaler is used to clean the tooth of calculus and plaque deposits. The water helps cool the instrument tip and flush debris off the tooth and gingiva.

for working in the anterior segment of the mouth and in deep periodontal pockets. An angled shank improves instrumentation in the distal segment of the mouth where space is minimal.

The working end does the work of the instrument and has several components: the blade or cutting edge, back, face, heel, and the toe or tip. The blade is the portion which cleans the tooth and gingival pocket epithelium. The face of the working end is the flat surface which creates one of the edges of each blade. The back is the rounded bottom of the working end. These instruments can be purchased as single- or double-ended depending on whether they have a working end at one or both ends of the handle. Double-ended scalers are designed so that one end adapts to the anterior surface of the tooth and the other end adapts to the distal surface. The term *scaler* includes supragingival (above the gingival margin) and subgingival (below the gingival margin) scalers. All curettes can be used subgingivally because they have a round toe and back to help prevent damage to the gingival tissue (Fig. 18-27). They may be used supragingivally as well. Supragingival scalers are not to be used subgingivally because they have a pointed tip which could damage the gingival sulcus (Fig. 18-26B). Supragingival scalers are often referred to as "scalers" and subgingival scalers as "curettes." Curettes and scalers should be held in a modified pen grasp (Fig. 18-28). The thumb and index finger hold the handle close to the shank. The middle finger is placed just in front of the index finger to further support the instrument. The ring finger is placed on a stable surface (as the tooth or gingiva) to act as a fulcrum and support the hand. The strokes of the scaler should be made through the wrist and not the fingers to avoid operator hand fatigue.

To remove subgingival calculus from the gingival sulcus, the curette is placed to the bottom of the gingival sulcus with its curved smooth back toward the gingival epithelium. Once it is seated at the bottom of the sulcus, the cutting edge is turned to engage the calculus on the tooth root. The curette is then pulled toward the crown to dislodge the calculus and remove it from the sulcus, as illustrated for root planing (see Fig. 18-22). This pull stroke is repeated until all the calculus has been removed from the tooth. Proper instrument positioning takes practice and concentration. It is important to master this tech-

properly and aid your decision on which instruments to purchase. Scalers and curettes are designed with three main components: the handle, shank, and working end (Fig. 18-26). The handles can be purchased in slim to wide diameters and be hollow or solid, based on personal preference. The shank attaches the handle to the working end and allows adaptation of the working end to the tooth surfaces. The shank is the most variable part of the curette. A relatively straight shank is good

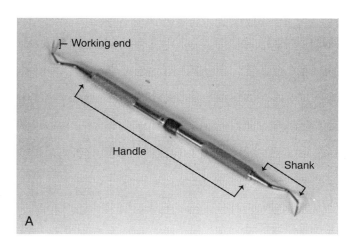

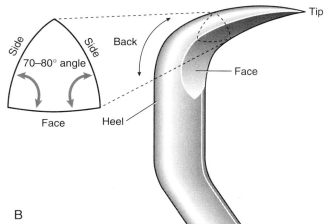

Figure 18-26. A, Supragingival scalers are used to scale the crowns of the teeth. A jacquette scaler is shown here. B, Drawing of the working end. The face of the instrument joins the sides to create a blade edge of 70 to 80 degrees.

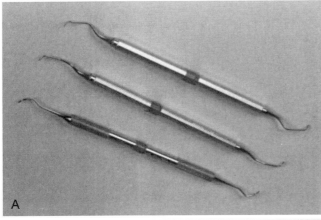

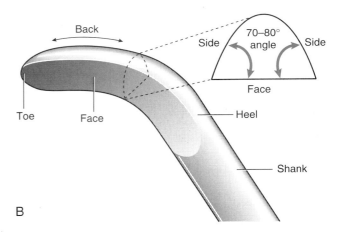

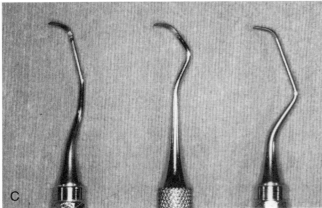

Figure 18-27. Curettes can be used subgingivally (below the gingival margin) to scale tooth roots and debride the gingival sulcus. Note the rounded toe and curvature of the instrument. Curettes are available with different angles to the shank to improve access to the tooth roots. A, Double-ended curettes. B, Drawing of the working end. C, Shank and working end of curettes.

nique to ensure that the gingival tissue is not damaged by the instruments and the subgingival calculus is completely removed.

After the teeth have been properly scaled, they must be polished. This step is performed to smooth the microscopic pits and scratches on the tooth surface created by the scaling procedure. If this step is skipped, the plaque will rapidly return because of increased surface area created by the scratches. Polishing is achieved using a slow-speed handpiece with a prophy cup attached and filled with prophy paste. Enough pressure should be applied to just flare the edge of the prophy cup. Flaring the edge will allow it to be gently inserted into the gingival sulcus to polish subgingivally (Fig. 18–29).

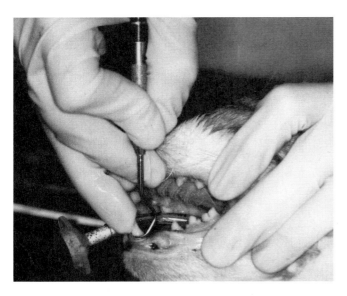

Figure 18-28. The scaler is held in a modified pen grasp.

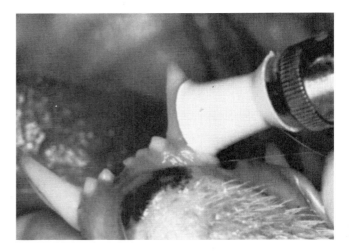

Figure 18-29. Polishing the teeth after scaling is extremely important to prevent rapid plaque accumulation after the teeth have been cleaned. The flared edge of the prophy cup can be placed into the gingival sulcus to polish subgingival enamel.

All surfaces of the tooth crown should be polished. The rotational speed should be kept slow (4000 rpm or less) and the polisher should be constantly moved on the tooth surface to prevent thermal damage to the tooth and gingiva. The tooth should not be polished for more than 5 seconds or thermal damage could result. If the polishing is not completed in 5 seconds, another tooth should be polished, and the unfinished tooth can be polished once it has been given time to cool.

> **TECHNICIAN NOTE**
>
> All surfaces of the tooth crown should be polished. The rotational speed should be kept slow and the polisher should be constantly moved on the tooth surface to prevent thermal damage to the tooth and gingiva.

Ample prophy paste should be kept in the prophy cup to help prevent excessive heat generation and to smooth the tooth surface. Several polishing pastes are available. For routine dental cleanings, the fluoride-containing pastes are preferred. Fluoride strengthens enamel, decreases tooth sensitivity, has antimicrobial properties, and decreases the rate of plaque reattachment. The zirconium silicate pastes (sodium or potassium aluminum silicates) are very effective polishing pastes and will not abrade the tooth enamel.

The oral cavity is rinsed of prophy paste and calculus after all surfaces of the teeth have been polished. The gingival sulcus must be irrigated to remove debris and bacteria. Irrigating systems or syringes can be purchased or a blunt 18-gauge needle on a syringe can be used. A dilute 0.1% chlorhexidine solution is an excellent irrigation agent, but other solutions can be used such as physiological saline, 3% hydrogen peroxide, or zinc ascorbate.

The teeth are checked for any abnormalities and remaining plaque after they have been scaled and polished. Plaque disclosing solutions, such as Reveal (Henry Schein Inc.), are available to enhance visualization of areas of plaque retention. Drying the teeth with air will further enhance visualization of any remaining plaque and calculus.

A dental explorer is used to check for subgingival pathologic changes such as root caries or erosion, calculus, and tooth root furcation exposure. Explorers come in a variety of shapes to aid exploration of the periodontal pockets in the different areas of the mouth (Figs. 18–20 and 18–30). Commonly used explorers are the shepherd's hook for dogs and the no. 6 for cats. The tip of the explorer has a sharp delicate point that gives good tactile sensation to the operator's hand when exploring the subgingival area.

A periodontal probe (see Fig. 18–30A) must be used to check the level of epithelial attachment in the gingival sulcus of each tooth. The probe is placed parallel to the long axis of the tooth root and multiple sites along each tooth should be checked (Fig. 18–31). The clinical probing depth of any periodontal pocket should be recorded on the pet's dental chart, and is a measurement taken from the gingival margin to the epithelial attachment level (base of the pocket).

Periodontal probes come in a wide variety of calibrations, which are either color-coded or notched and measure pocket depths up to 10, 11, or 12 mm. The probes are either round or flat. It is useful to have a variety of probes but the most popular probe is a color-coded probe that measures 3-, 6-, 9-, and 12-mm increments. Factors which affect the probing depth of a periodontal pocket are epithelial attachment level, alveolar bone loss, gingival margin swelling (reversible), and gingival recession. Gingival recession should be measured with the periodontal probe from the level of the cementoenamel junction (CEJ) of the tooth to the gingival margin and recorded on the dental record. This value plus the clinical probing depth will equal the amount of attachment loss for that particular tooth (attachment loss = clinical probing depth + gingival recession). Any problems noted during the dental cleaning should be brought to the attention of the veterinarian and dental radiographs should be taken if indicated.

All tooth extractions should be performed by the veterinarian. Multirooted teeth may require sectioning before extraction. Gingival tissue may need to be reflected and buccal cortical bone removed in order to extract teeth with large roots and a healthy periodontium. Complications associated with extractions include hemorrhage, damage to surrounding soft tissue or the orbital cavity from sharp elevators, and fracture of the alveolar bone, mandible, or maxilla, especially when the animal has significant bone loss from chronic periodontitis.

Proper elevation of the root prior to removal with forceps helps to prevent fracture of the tooth root. If the root does fracture, the retained root tip should be removed to prevent infection of the alveolar socket. After scaling, polishing, and sulcus irrigation have been performed and all problems have been addressed, the animal can be allowed to recover from anesthesia.

Dental Home Care

The final stage of the dental cleaning is client education on dental home care treatment along with the dispensing of dental home care products. There are many products available to encourage good compliance and meet individual needs.

When the owner comes to pick up the pet, he or she should be taken into an examination room, where the technician can demonstrate the proper brushing technique on a dental model. The owner should be instructed to start slowly with the pet and to use ample praise. The owner should then be asked to repeat the brushing procedure on a dental model to ensure correct technique. The pet can then be brought in to the owner. The owner should be shown how to properly grasp the muzzle so that the pet is not injured when brushing the teeth. Daily dental home care is the best way to prevent the accumulation of plaque. For owners with busy schedules, however, an alternate-day or twice-weekly home care session will still provide benefits to the pet.

> **TECHNICIAN NOTE**
>
> The key to success with dental home care is finding a product that works well for the owner and is acceptable to the pet. With patience, praise, and guidance, the owner should be able to find a dental home care treatment that will work for his or her pet.

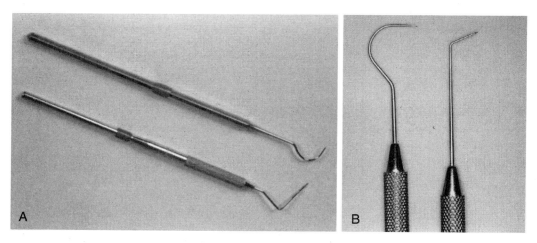

Figure 18-30. A, Dental explorer (top) and periodontal probe (bottom). The periodontal probe is marked in millimeter increments to measure periodontal pocket depth. The dental explorer has a fine tip and is used to detect subgingival calculus and tooth abnormalities. B, Shepherd's hook explorer (left) and No. 6 explorer (right).

The owner should be informed of any dental problems the pet may have as well as the date on which the pet's next dental cleaning will be due. As a general rule, pets with healthy mouths or mild to moderate gingivitis will benefit from annual dental cleanings. Those with early periodontitis will probably require a dental cleaning every 6 to 8 months, and those with moderate to severe periodontitis may require a dental cleaning every 3 to 4 months.

The key to success with dental home care is finding a product that works well for the owner and is acceptable to the pet. There are many different types of toothbrushes available.

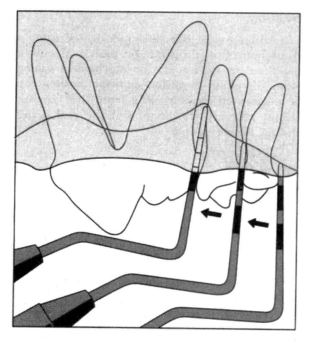

Figure 18-31. Multiple sites on a tooth should be probed to detect any deep pockets present. (From Emily P and Penman S: Handbook of Small Animal Dentistry, 2nd Edition, Pergamon Press Ltd, Oxford, England, 1994.)

Dog and cat toothbrushes can be purchased, or the owner can buy a child's soft-bristled toothbrush. Some pets will not tolerate a toothbrush and may respond better if the owner uses a sponge-type swab or a gauze pad wrapped around the owner's finger. If this is unacceptable to the pet, or if the owner risks being bitten, a mouth rinse or spray can be used.

Pet toothpaste formulas are well tolerated by most pets because they like the malt, poultry, or beef flavoring that has been added. Human toothpaste should not be used on pets. The flavors of the veterinary chlorhexidine and zinc ascorbate oral rinses and spray products are not as well liked by pets. However, they are excellent for keeping oral bacterial levels under control and for healing damaged gingival tissue. They can be applied more quickly than pastes and are easier to use on animals that will not tolerate much handling.

A new product is a bioadhesive pellet (Stomadhex, Immunovet, Tampa, Fl.) that releases chlorhexidine diacetate and niacinamide into the oral cavity as it is slowly dissolved. The tablet is placed on the labial mucosa once daily for the desired length of treatment. This may be beneficial for pets that do not tolerate toothbrushing well or that are too tender to be brushed after periodontal therapy. With patience, praise, and guidance, the owner should be able to find a dental home care treatment that will work for his or her pet.

Sharpening Dental Scalers

Dental scalers must be kept sharp to work properly. Dull instruments burnish calculus into the tooth rather than remove it, and can cause operator hand fatigue. There are several different methods to sharpen scalers. A helpful instructional textbook is *Smarten Up, Sharpen Up* by Hu-Friedy, which is available through most dental supply companies. An oiled sharpening stone should be used to sharpen dental scalers. The finer grades of sharpening stones (e.g., the Arkansas stone) maintain a smoother cutting edge, remove less metal, and as long as instruments are sharpened frequently the sharp edge is rapidly restored. A thin layer of oil should be placed on the surface of the stone before sharpening. The instruments should be cleaned before sharpening and sharpening should be performed in a well-lighted area.

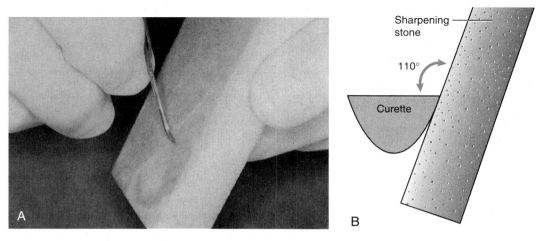

Figure 18-32. A, The sharpening stone should be kept at an angle of 100 to 110 degrees to the scaler face to maintain the proper shape of the instrument. B, Curette face in cross section to sharpening stone showing the 100- to 110-degree angle.

A simple sharpening method is the moving flat stone, stationary instrument technique. The flat stone is held at an angle of 100 to 110 degrees to the face of the curette or sickle scaler (Fig. 18–32). This angle will maintain the 70- to 80-degree bevel of the cutting edge (Figs. 18–26B and 18–27C). Begin sharpening with short up and down strokes starting at the heel of the instrument and working toward the toe or tip of the instrument. Your dominant hand should hold the stone and the other hand should hold the instrument with the face up and parallel to the floor. The instrument hand should be braced on a stable surface such as a counter or tabletop. Sharpening always finishes on a down stroke and greater pressure is placed on the down strokes than on the up strokes. Once the stone reaches the tip of the scaler the stone is removed on completion of the down stroke. The rounded toe must be maintained on curettes to avoid soft tissue trauma. As the stone approaches the toe, the sharpening is continued, maintaining the same angle around the toe to finish on the down stroke.

The instruments should be checked for sharpness on an acrylic stick. A sharp instrument easily engages the acrylic and shaves thin strips off with little effort. The sharpening procedure is repeated until the instrument is properly sharpened. The wire edges are then removed from the face of the instrument by rolling a round stone over the face a few times (Fig. 18–33). Finally, the instrument is cleaned of oil and metal debris and sterilized.

Instruments need to be sharpened based on use. If a scaler is used very little it may be able to go through three or four procedures without dulling. If a dental case requires extensive hand scaling the scaler may require sharpening after that case. A good rule of thumb is to check your scalers frequently with an acrylic stick to identify the dull instruments.

Dental Radiography

Dental radiography is an important tool in the diagnostic and prognostic evaluation of oral disorders in veterinary medicine. As advances have been made in veterinary dentistry, there has been a demand for high-quality dental radiographs to evaluate teeth and oral structures more accurately. The use of dental radiograph machines and intraoral dental film in veterinary medicine has increased dramatically during this time.

Traditionally, radiographs of the teeth, mandible, and max-illa were taken to evaluate disorders such as oral masses, fractured jaws and teeth, and facial pain and swelling. Many veterinarians are now using this diagnostic aid to assess problems such as discolored teeth, feline odontoclastic resorptive lesions, and periodontal disease and to aid in the treatment of endodontically compromised teeth, dental restorations, and difficult extractions.

Dental radiographs can be taken with the film placed in the mouth (intraoral technique) or outside the mouth (extraoral technique). Intraoral dental film is a nonscreened flexible film (Fig. 18–34). Regular screened or nonscreened x-ray film can be used for extraoral radiographic views (Chapter 9) and a limited number of intraoral views. Nonscreened x-ray films provide greater detail than the screened films but require increased exposure times.

There are several advantages of the intraoral radiographic technique over the extraoral technique. Perhaps the greatest advantage of the intraoral technique is the ability to minimize the superimposition of teeth and surrounding structures on the area of study. Intraoral dental film can be purchased in sizes

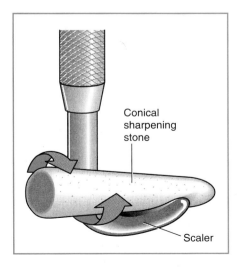

Figure 18-33. The conical sharpening stone is rolled across the face of the scaler to remove wire edges.

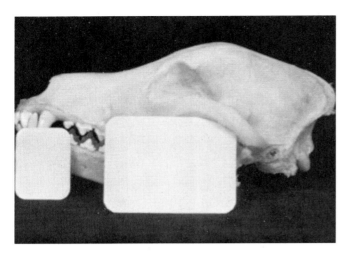

Figure 18-34. Intraoral dental film. Size 2 (left) and size 4 (right) intraoral films are shown.

small enough to fit in the mouth next to the tooth or teeth to be studied. The closer the x-ray film is to the subject of interest (the tooth), the better the detail. The aiming cylinder of the dental radiograph machine can be moved and angled to radiograph the tooth of interest and be placed close enough to the tooth to eliminate the opposite dental arcade.

When using the extraoral technique, there is usually some degree of superimpositioning of teeth from the other arcades that are in the path of the primary beam. The teeth in the opposite arch may obstruct the view of the teeth of interest, and dental abnormalities could be missed.

The film focal distance (FFD) for the dental radiograph machine is 16 inches or less, in contrast to the standard radiograph machines for which an FFD of 36 to 40 inches is commonly used. The shorter FFD of the dental radiograph machine allows closer placement of the anode to the tooth, eliminating the opposite dental arcade or surrounding soft tissue or bone from the path of the primary beam. The shorter FFD also minimizes harmful scatter radiation, as does the small cone

size and lead lining, which many of the dental radiograph cones contain.

The extraoral views require the patient to be placed in many different positions so that the skull is angled in order for the primary beam to avoid the surrounding oral structures. This proper positioning takes time and skill. Intraoral dental film can be placed in the mouth, and the tube head of the x-ray machine can be moved instead of the patient. The patient is placed in dorsal recumbency to radiograph the mandible and in ventral recumbency to radiograph the maxilla. A complete evaluation of all four oral quadrants requires at least six views.

Intraoral dental film can be processed by hand or "piggybacked" to a regular film with electrical tape and automatically processed. Extraoral nonscreened x-ray film may not be compatible with the automatic processor's developer and might require hand developing. The extraoral nonscreened x-ray film is considerably more expensive than the smaller intraoral dental film. If rapid developer and fixative are used, intraoral dental film can be hand-developed in approximately 2 minutes, which is helpful in minimizing anesthesia time.

To use the intraoral radiographic technique, one must master the bisecting angle technique. This method minimizes distortion of teeth caused by the angle of the primary beam to the object (tooth) and the inability to place the film parallel to the maxillary teeth and the mandibular canines and incisors. The reader is referred to the suggested reading section for a detailed discussion and illustration of this technique. By directing the primary x-ray beam perpendicular to a line that bisects the angle created by the plane of the tooth and the intraoral film, an image with minimal distortion can be made on the x-ray film, preventing foreshortening or elongation of tooth roots (Fig. 18–35).

Endodontics

Endodontics deals with the study and treatment of the inside of the tooth (pulp) and periapical tissues. The periapical tissue is located around the tip (apex) of the tooth root. The tooth pulp consists of nerves, blood vessels, lymphatics, and connective tissue. The pulp tissue is found in the pulp chamber (crown) and pulp canal (root) of the tooth and enters the tooth through

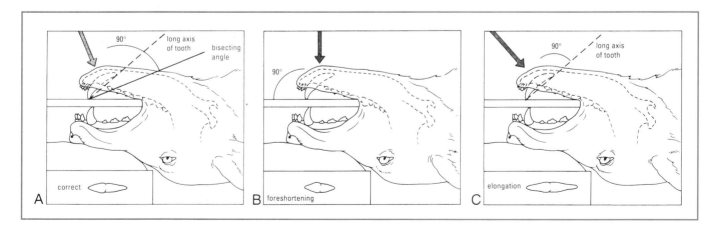

Figure 18-35. A, Bisection angle technique produces an accurate image of the tooth. B, Direction of the x-ray beam at right angles to the film shortens the tooth's image. C, Direction of the x-ray beam at right angles to the long axis of the tooth elongates the tooth's image. (From Emily P and Penman S: Handbook of Small Animal Dentistry, 2nd Edition, Pergamon Press Ltd, Oxford, England, 1994.)

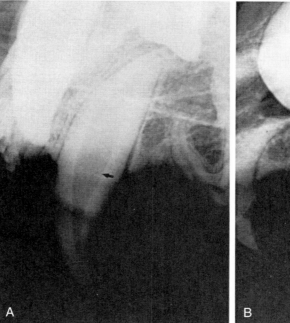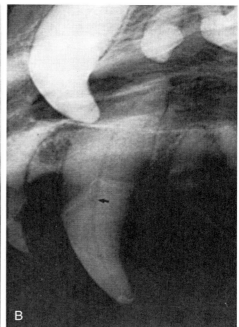

Figure 18-36. A, Large pulp chamber and canal in a young cougar's canine tooth (arrow). B, As the animal ages, dentin is deposited, and the pulp chamber and canal narrow (arrow).

numerous small openings in the apex of the tooth root called the apical delta.

The dental pulp is important to the development of the tooth in a young animal. It supplies the nutrients needed by the odontoblasts to deposit dentin. This makes the tooth walls thicker, so the tooth is stronger. Once the dog or cat is past 10 to 18 months of age, the majority of the dentin has been deposited, the tooth walls are fairly thick, and the root apex should be closed. As the animal continues to age, the pulp chamber and canal will become smaller because the odontoblasts will continue to deposit dentin (Fig. 18–36).

Treatment of teeth with endodontic disease depends on the age of the animal, duration of endodontic disease, and anatomy of the tooth. Conventional root canal therapy is usually performed on dogs and cats 12 months of age and older. Treatment involves removing the dead or dying pulp tissue from the tooth with small files or reamers, disinfecting the root canal, and filling the canal (obturation) with an appropriate material to seal the apex from the periapical tissues. Radiographs are necessary to ensure that a proper apical seal has been achieved.

Among the most common causes of endodontic disease in dogs and cats are pulp exposure from fracture of a tooth and attrition (wear) of the tooth. Many dogs will cause severe attrition of their teeth by chewing on hard objects such as rocks or fences. The teeth most commonly fractured are the canines and the maxillary fourth premolar (carnassial) teeth (Fig. 18–37). Attrition usually occurs on the incisors and canines but can be seen on the premolars and molars as well. If the attrition occurs slowly, the odontoblasts will deposit tertiary dentin over the pulp tissue to prevent pulp exposure as enamel and dentin are lost. The pulp tissue may be visualized through the tertiary dentin as a brown or red dot (Fig. 18–38). A dental explorer should be run over the tooth surface to make sure the pulp tissue is not exposed. When the pulp tissue is exposed, the tip of the dental explorer will drop down into the pulp chamber as it crosses the surface of the tooth.

In fresh fractures the tooth may bleed from the center. If the tooth is treated within the first 48 hours, a vital pulpotomy procedure can usually be performed. This involves removing the coronal pulp tissue (the pulp tissue in the tooth root remains), covering the pulp tissue with calcium hydroxide, and sealing the coronal exposure site with appropriate dental restorative materials.

All teeth with exposed pulp tissue should be treated either by endodontic treatment (root canal, pulp capping, pulpotomy) or by extraction. If left untreated, infection from the exposure site will spread to the periapical tissues, and a periapical abscess may develop. This condition is seen fairly frequently in dogs with maxillary carnassial tooth abscesses. The owner will notice swelling or a draining tract just below the dog's eye and treatment is usually sought (Fig. 18–39). Surprisingly, only about

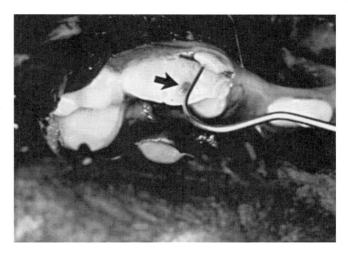

Figure 18-37. Slab fractures of the maxillary fourth premolar teeth are a common problem in dogs. This fracture extends subgingivally, and the pulp tissue has been exposed (arrow).

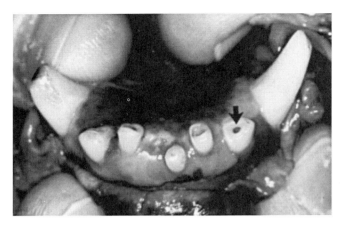

Figure 18–38. Severe attrition of the incisor and canine teeth. The brown or red dots (arrow) in the center of these teeth are the pulp tissues below the less-opaque tertiary dentin.

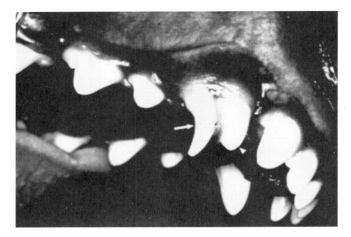

Figure 18–40. A retained deciduous maxillary canine tooth (arrow) has displaced the permanent canine tooth mesially (toward the nose) (arrowhead). The abnormal tooth alignment can lead to periodontal disease and interference with other teeth or oral soft tissues.

20% of periapical abscesses will form a fistula to the skin, which means that unless the teeth of these pets are being examined for endodontic disease, many abscesses go untreated. These abscesses can be very painful and are a source of infection, which can spread to other teeth and the blood stream.

Other signs of endodontic disease include discolored teeth and painful teeth. Diagnosing a painful tooth in an animal can be difficult, but when there is a question, a dental radiograph can be taken to assess the periapical area for signs of disease.

Orthodontics

Orthodontics is concerned with the correction and prevention of irregularities and malocclusion of the teeth. The primary reason for performing orthodontic correction of malaligned teeth in veterinary medicine is to alleviate a painful malocclusion or a malocclusion that will lead to endodontic or periodontal disease. When genetic malocclusions are suspected, the owner should be counseled on the problem in order to prevent breeding of these animals and the propagation of inferior genes.

Interceptive orthodontics involves the extraction of retained deciduous teeth, which will usually cause displacement of the permanent dentition (Fig. 18–40). This treatment can be

extremely beneficial, and many abnormally erupting permanent teeth will correct spontaneously after extraction of the retained deciduous teeth. The most important factor determining success with this treatment is early detection of the problem. Many companion animals have completed their vaccination series by the time they reach this mixed dentition stage and will not be seen again until 6 months of age if the owner has elected to neuter the pet. To prevent this condition from going undetected, the owner should be instructed to monitor the dentition closely to ensure that the deciduous tooth is shed prior to the emergence of the permanent tooth. Dental models can be used to show the owner the difference between deciduous teeth and permanent teeth. Dental recheck examinations can be scheduled so that a dental problem does not go undetected.

Some of the most common dental malocclusions seen are lingually displaced mandibular canine teeth (Fig. 18–41), mesially displaced maxillary canine teeth (Fig. 18–42), and even or level bites. These malocclusions can be corrected by orthodon-

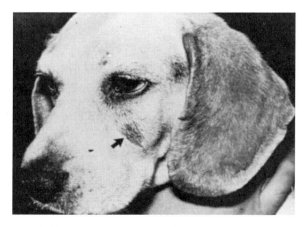

Figure 18–39. Patient with a maxillary tooth abscess. Arrow, draining tract fistula.

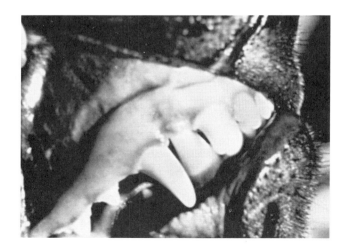

Figure 18–41. Lingually displaced mandibular canine tooth. The mandibular canine is displaced toward the tongue and is striking the gingival tissue.

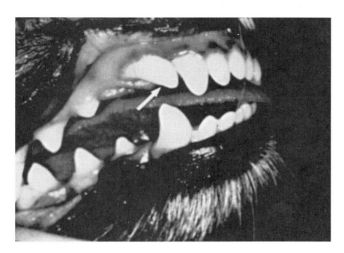

Figure 18–42. Mesially displaced maxillary canine tooth. The maxillary canine tooth is displaced mesially (arrow) and is striking the mandibular canine tooth when the mouth is closed.

tics in most cases, but the owner must be willing to invest the time to clean the oral appliance and return for rechecks as needed. Orthodontic treatment generally costs more than tooth extraction and involves more anesthetic procedures, but it is less invasive than extraction. Orthodontics can be an important treatment option when considering alternatives to extraction of large teeth such as the canines or multiple teeth, such as the six incisors in a dog with an even bite. Many of the cases that present with the malocclusions listed above can be corrected rapidly with orthodontic treatment.

Odontoplasty or pulp capping is another option for ani-

mals with malocclusions, particularly severe malocclusions. These procedures entail shortening the tooth to remove the interference it is causing with another tooth or surrounding soft tissue. This method is less invasive than extraction, removes the animal's source of discomfort, and achieves results more quickly than does orthodontics. However, it does permanently alter the appearance of the tooth (Fig. 18–43).

Restorative Dentistry

The goal of restorative dentistry is to restore a tooth, as closely as possible, to its natural structure and function. No restorative material is as strong as the original tooth structure, so an attempt is always made to preserve as much of the original tooth as possible. Indications for restorative dentistry include teeth with dental caries (cavities), fractured teeth, and endodontically treated teeth.

Dental caries rarely occurs in the dog and cat. When present, the carious tooth structure must be completely removed and the defect restored. If left untreated, the caries will dissolve the enamel and dentin and gain access to the pulp tissue. The tooth will eventually be destroyed.

A common problem of feline dentition is the development of idiopathic feline odontoclastic resorptive lesions (Fig. 18–44). It is estimated that 20% of cats are affected by this problem. The lesions are usually found at the neck of the tooth (the junction of the enamel of the crown and the cementum of the tooth root), which is often hidden by the free gingival tissue. Cats must be examined closely for these lesions. Often the gingival tissue over these lesions is inflamed. A dental explorer must be used to check for irregularities below the gingivae. Early detection and restoration of these lesions may prevent the continued resorption of the tooth. Many of these teeth are

Figure 18–43. The mandibular canine tooth (arrow) has been shortened to prevent it from impinging on the palate. The maxillary canine tooth (arrowhead) is displaced mesially, preventing the mandibular canine tooth from returning to its normal position.

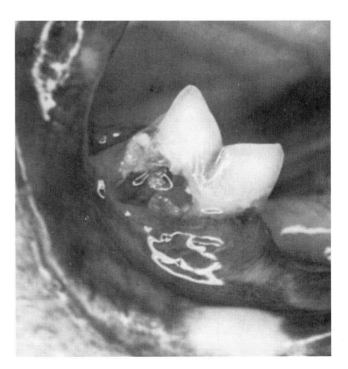

Figure 18–44. Feline odontoclastic resorptive lesion. The large erosion on this tooth involves the distal root and cervical portion of the tooth crown. A dental radiograph is necessary to evaluate the tooth roots.

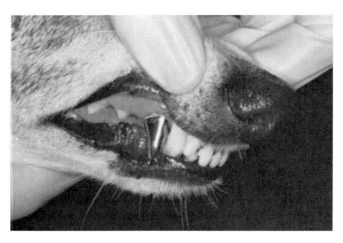

Figure 18–45. A non–precious metal crown has been cemented to the maxillary canine tooth after the tooth was traumatically fractured and received endodontic treatment.

identified in the advanced stages of the disease with pulp exposure and root resorption. When the resorption has progressed this far, the tooth cannot be saved and should be extracted. Dental radiographs of these teeth are necessary to evaluate the severity of resorption.

Fractured teeth are frequently restored to return function and maintain periodontal health. The tooth has a natural design to allow self-cleaning and deflection of food away from the gingival sulcus. When the teeth lose this proper contour they can become predisposed to periodontal disease. Fractured teeth can be restored with restorative materials alone or in combination with retention pins or posts or both. Pins and posts do not add strength to the restoration but aid in retaining the restoration.

Another option available for restoring a tooth with loss of coronal structure is to cover the crown of the tooth with a prosthetic crown. The silver-colored metal crowns, which are made of nonprecious metals, are the most common type used because of their greater strength and lower cost when compared with gold or porcelain crowns. The teeth most commonly crowned in dogs are the canines and maxillary fourth premolars (Fig. 18–45). In the cat, the canine is the most commonly crowned tooth.

Veterinary dentistry is a specialty field in veterinary medicine. Advanced procedures require a strong background knowledge of the materials used, the anatomy and physiology of the teeth and periodontium, and the principles applied to each procedure. It is important for the general practitioner and veterinary technician to be able to identify dental abnormalities and to be able to recommend treatment alternatives to the owner. The pet can then be referred for advanced dental procedures if the owner wishes to pursue treatment.

Recommended Reading

Bojrab MJ, and Tholen M: Small Animal Oral Medicine and Surgery. Philadelphia, Lea & Febiger, 1990.
Holmstrom SE, Frost P, and Gammon RL: Veterinary Dental Techniques. Philadelphia, WB Saunders, 1992.
Seim HB III, Creed JF, and Smith KW: Restraint techniques for prevention of self-trauma. *In* Bojrab MJ (editor): Current Techniques in Small Animal Surgery, 3rd ed. Philadelphia, Lea & Febiger, 1990.

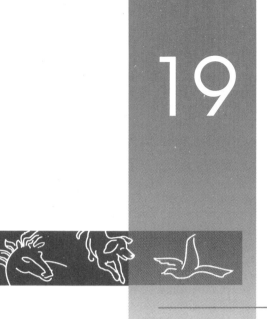

19 Wound Management and Bandaging

Giselle Hosgood • *Daniel J. Burba*

The veterinary technician can play an important role in assisting the veterinary surgeon in the management of wounds. The nature of the wound often dictates the method of wound management. To understand the methods of wound management, a knowledge of the physiology of wound healing and the factors that alter wound healing is required. The methods of wound management, the role of bandaging in wound management, and the different types of bandages are then more clearly understood.

WOUND HEALING

A wound is created when an insult, either purposeful, such as surgery, or incidental, such as trauma, disrupts the normal integrity of the tissue. Wound healing is a complex biological event that is well characterized at the microscopic level but its regulation at the molecular level is only just beginning to be understood. The process of wound healing begins immediately after the insult and is described in four physical phases: the inflammatory, debridement, repair, and maturation phases (Fig. 19–1 and Table 19–1). Wound healing is a dynamic process, and more than one phase of wound healing is usually occurring at any time.

Peptide growth factors appear to play a key role in initiating and sustaining the phases of wound healing (Table 19–2). The platelet appears to initiate the wound healing process through the release of growth factors; the process is then amplified or sustained by wound macrophages, endothelial cells, and fibroblasts. The *inflammatory phase* begins immediately after injury. Hemorrhage fills the wound and cleans the wound surface. The blood vessels constrict immediately to slow hemorrhage, but vasoconstriction lasts only 5 to 10 minutes. The blood vessels then dilate and leak fluid containing clotting elements into the wound. This fluid, combined with blood, causes a blood clot to form. The blood clot stabilizes the wound edges and fibrin within the clot provides the limited wound strength of this phase. In a sutured wound, the sutures will also provide wound strength at this time. The blood clot will dry and form a scab, which protects the wound, prevents further hemorrhage, and allows healing to progress under its surface. The scab does not provide any wound strength. The blood vessels also leak white blood cells into the wound. This marks the beginning of the debridement phase.

The *debridement phase* begins approximately 6 hours after injury, when white blood cells, namely neutrophils and monocytes, appear in the wound. These cells remove necrotic tissue, bacteria, and foreign material from the wound. The white blood cells, in combination with the fluid that has leaked into the wound, form the exudate commonly associated with wounds.

TECHNICIAN NOTE

There is minimal wound strength during the first 3 to 5 days of wound healing, known as the lag phase.

The *repair phase* begins after the blood clot has formed and necrotic tissue and foreign material have been removed from the wound. The repair phase, which is usually active by 3 to 5 days after injury, is associated with invasion of fibroblasts into the wound. The fibroblasts produce collagen that will

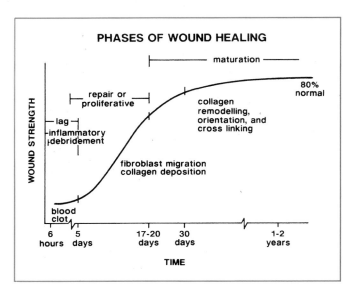

PHASES OF WOUND HEALING

Figure 19-1. Schematic representation of the phases of wound healing and associated changes in wound strength.

mature into fibrous or scar tissue. The repair phase is characterized by a significant increase in wound strength. In contrast, the first 3 to 5 days after injury are associated with a minimal increase in wound strength. Consequently, the first 3 to 5 days are also known as the "lag phase" of wound healing.

• Table 19–1 •

CHARACTERISTICS OF THE MICROSCOPIC PHASES OF WOUND HEALING	
PHASE	**CHARACTERISTICS**
Inflammatory	Begins immediately after injury; characterized by formation of blood clot; platelets stimulate other stages by release of growth factors
Debridement	Part of inflammatory phase; characterized by influx of white blood cells (macrophages, monocytes) into wound; occurs approximately 6 hours after injury; wound healing is sustained by release of growth factors from multiple cell types
Repair (fibroblastic)	Begins 3–5 days after wounding; characterized by invasion of fibroblasts and development of granulation tissue; wound strength increases exponentially
Maturation	Characterized by remodeling of the collagen of the scar and slow gain in wound strength; begins approximately 3 weeks after injury and may take weeks to years to complete

Capillaries appear in the wound at the same time fibroblasts appear. The combination of new capillaries, fibroblasts, and fibrous tissue forms the characteristic red, fleshy granulation tissue that fills the wound, often lying underneath the scab.

TECHNICIAN NOTE

Healthy granulation tissue is red and very vascular, and important in wound healing.

Granulation tissue characteristically appears in the wound after 3 to 5 days. Poor granulation tissue is white and has a high fibrous tissue content with fewer capillaries. Granulation tissue is important in wound healing as it fills the tissue defect, protects the wound, provides a barrier to infection, provides a surface for new epithelial cells to form across, and provides a source of special fibroblasts called *myofibroblasts*, which are responsible for wound contraction.

TECHNICIAN NOTE

Myofibroblasts within the granulation tissue are responsible for wound contraction.

The formation of new epithelium on the wound surface (epithelialization) occurs during the repair phase and begins once an adequate granulation tissue bed has formed. New epithelium is usually visible on a wound in 4 to 5 days. In an incised wound that is sutured, in which the skin edges are close, epithelialization can occur almost immediately (as early as 24 to 48 hours after injury), as there is no defect that needs to be filled with granulation tissue. The normal epithelial cells at the edge of the wound divide and produce new cells that migrate across the granulation tissue. Some hair follicles and sweat glands may also regenerate, depending on the extent of damage. The new epithelium is only one cell layer thick initially and is fragile, but it gradually thickens over time as more cell layers form.

TECHNICIAN NOTE

Visible wound contraction occurs 5 to 9 days after injury.

Wound contraction helps to reduce the size of the wound but occurs totally independent of epithelialization. No new skin is formed during contraction. Wound contraction is a result of contraction of the myofibroblasts in the granulation tissue, which pulls the full-thickness skin edges inward. If the skin around the wound is tight and under tension, wound contraction will be limited. Visible wound contraction usually occurs 5 to 9 days after injury.

The *maturation phase* is the final phase of wound healing,

• Table 19-2 •

CHARACTERISTICS OF SELECTED GROWTH FACTORS AND THEIR ROLE IN WOUND HEALING		
GROWTH FACTOR	**SOURCES**	**EFFECT ON WOUND HEALING**
Platelet-derived growth factor (PDGF)	Platelets, macrophages, fibroblasts, endothelial cells	Stimulates replication of fibroblasts and vascular smooth muscle
Transforming growth factor-β (TGF-β)	Macrophages, lymphocytes, fibroblasts, bone cells, keratinocytes, platelets	Inhibits replication of most cells (keratinocytes, endothelial cells, lymphocytes, and macrophages); may inhibit or stimulate fibroblasts; may have a modulating effect on wound healing
Transforming growth factor-α (TGF-α)	Macrophages, eosinophils, keratinocytes	Stimulates replication of epithelial cells, fibroblast and endothelial cells; more potent effect on endothelial cells than epidermal growth factor
Epidermal growth factor (EGF)	Almost all body fluids, platelets	Stimulates replication of epithelial cells, fibroblasts, and endothelial cells
Insulin-like growth factor (IGF)	Most tissues, fibroblasts, macrophages	Stimulates replication of fibroblasts, endothelial cells, bone cells, neural tissues, and hemopoietic cells
Fibroblast growth factor (FGF)	Fibroblasts, bone cells, smooth muscle cells, endothelial cells, astrocytes	Stimulates replication of neural tissue, bone cells, muscle cells, and fibroblasts

during which the wound strength increases to its maximum level because of changes in the scar. Remodeling of the collagen fibers in the fibrous tissue, with alteration of their orientation and increased cross-linking, improves wound strength. The number of capillaries in the fibrous tissue gradually decreases, causing the scar to become paler. The maturation phase begins once collagen has been adequately deposited in the wound and may continue for several years. The wound never regains the strength of normal tissue.

TECHNICIAN NOTE

The wound never regains the strength of normal tissue.

Factors Affecting Wound Healing

Many factors affect wound healing, including host factors affecting the health of the animal, the characteristics of the wound, and external factors directly affecting the wound.

Host Factors

Old animals tend to heal slowly, probably because they are often debilitated and have other ongoing health problems. Animals that are malnourished or have a disease causing low serum protein concentrations below 2/g/dl (such as liver disease with poor protein production; kidney disease with excessive loss of protein) will have delayed wound healing and decreased wound strength. In addition, the lag phase of wound healing will be prolonged in these animals.

Wound healing is delayed by certain diseases, such as hyperadrenocorticism or Cushing's disease, in which there is an excess of circulating corticosteroids. Corticosteroids delay all phases of wound healing.

Animals with diabetes mellitus have delayed wound healing and a predisposition to wound infection. Animals with liver disease may have clotting factor deficits in addition to low serum protein concentrations.

TECHNICIAN NOTE

Corticosteroids delay all phases of wound healing.

Wound Characteristics

Foreign material in the wound, such as sutures, surgical implants, drains, or extraneous material, can cause an intense inflammatory reaction that interferes with normal wound healing. Soil particles can contain specific infection-enhancing factors.

TECHNICIAN NOTE

Presence of foreign material within a wound delays wound healing.

Compared with a sharp surgical incision, the use of an electroscalpel or electrocoagulation during surgery causes more necrosis at the wound margin, increases the chance of wound infection, and results in a slower gain in early wound strength.

TECHNICIAN NOTE

Electrosurgery delays the gain of wound strength.

Contaminated tissue becomes infected if the bacteria multiply to a critical number of 10^5 organisms per gram of tissue and then invade the tissue. Whether this occurs depends on the degree of tissue trauma, the amount of foreign material present, the delay between injury and treatment, and the effectiveness of host defenses. Infection stops the repair phase.

Bacterial toxins and associated inflammation directly damage the cells. The wound exudate produced during inflammation can accumulate and separate the tissue, leading to wound infection and delayed wound healing.

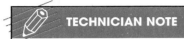

> **TECHNICIAN NOTE**
>
> Infection stops wound repair.

The blood supply to the wound is obviously important for wound healing and is responsible for delivering oxygen and metabolic substrates to the cells. Damage to the blood supply during surgical treatment should be avoided. Tight bandages that compromise the wound's blood supply should not be used. Movement in a healing wound is also detrimental, as it disturbs the fine cellular structures of the healing tissue. Movement across a wound should be limited. It may be necessary to apply a bandage to the affected limb to reduce movement.

> **TECHNICIAN NOTE**
>
> 10^5 microorganisms/g tissue is the critical number for wound infection.

External Factors

Certain drugs and radiation therapy delay wound healing. Corticosteroids depress all phases of wound healing and increase the chance of wound infection. Anti-inflammatory drugs (aspirin, phenylbutazone, ibuprofen) have little effect on wound strength but will suppress early inflammation. Prolonged aspirin therapy may delay blood clotting. Chemotherapeutic drugs can have an adverse affect on wound healing, depending on their mechanism of action and the time of administration in relation to the time of injury. Radiation can have a profound adverse affect on wound healing, depending on dose and time of exposure in relation to time of injury.

WOUND CARE

Immediate Wound Care

The wound should be covered with a clean, dry bandage as soon as possible after injury to prevent further contamination and reduce hemorrhage. The bandage should remain in place until definitive treatment is initiated. Antibiotic ointments or powders act only as foreign bodies and delay wound healing and thus should not be applied.

Once the animal is stabilized and other, life-threatening injuries have been treated, the wound can be prepared for treatment. The bandage is removed, and the wound is packed with sterile gauze or filled with sterile water-soluble lubricant (K-Y jelly, Johnson & Johnson) or temporarily closed with su-

tures, towel clamps or Michel clips. This allows skin around the wound to be clipped and prepared for aseptic surgery without the introduction of hair into the wound.

> **TECHNICIAN NOTE**
>
> Prepare a wound as for aseptic surgery.

Hair from the edges of the wound can be removed by means of scissors dipped in mineral oil to prevent hair from falling into the wound. Once the skin is prepared, the K-Y jelly can be flushed out or the sponges removed from the wound.

Wound Lavage

Wound lavage is necessary to remove debris and loose particles and tissue from the wound. It also reduces the number of bacteria in the wound. If infection is suspected, a piece of tissue should be sampled for bacterial culture before lavage. Large volumes of warm, sterile, normal saline are preferred for lavage.

> **TECHNICIAN NOTE**
>
> Wound lavage with warm, sterile, normal saline is preferred.

Antibiotics should not be added to the fluid. Soaps, detergents, and antiseptic solutions should not be used, as they damage the tissue. The mechanical action of the lavage is the most important factor for successful lavage. Moderate pressure (7 psi) can be generated with a 35-ml syringe and 19-gauge needle; this method is more effective than pouring fluid over a wound. The syringe can be connected to a bag of fluid with a three-way stopcock to facilitate refilling of the syringe (Fig. 19–2). A pulsating, high-pressure (70 psi) stream can be generated by means of a Water Pik (Teledyne), which is even more effective in reducing bacterial population and removing necrotic tissue and foreign material from heavily contaminated wounds.

Wound Debridement

Wound debridement is necessary to remove all contaminated, devitalized or necrotic tissue, and foreign material from the wound (Table 19–3). This can be performed surgically by excising the affected tissue in layers, beginning at the surface and progressing to the wound depths. Alternatively, the entire wound can be excised *en bloc* if there is sufficient healthy tissue surrounding the wound and vital structures can be preserved. Enzymatic debridement with a commercial solution containing trypsin (Granulex, Beecham) can be used for wounds that are not suitable for surgical debridement. Enzymatic debridement is slower and may damage normal tissue.

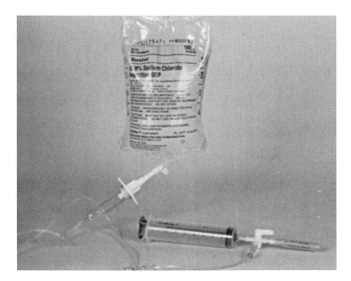

Figure 19-2. Connection of a 35-cc syringe and 19-gauge needle to a three-way stopcock and bag of sterile normal saline solution to facilitate copious lavage of a wound.

Wound Closure

Selection of one of the four methods of wound closure depends on the nature of the wound Table 19–4. *Primary wound closure* results in healing by first intention. First intention healing, known as appositional healing, is achieved by the suturing or grafting of a wound soon after injury. Primary wound closure is indicated in fresh, clean, sharply incised wounds with minimal trauma and minimal contamination that are seen within hours of injury. Wounds treated within 6 to 8 hours of injury are treated within the "golden period," that is, bacteria contaminating the wound have not multiplied to the critical number of 10^5 organisms per gram of tissue and the tissue has not become

• Table 19–3 •

METHODS AND INDICATIONS OF WOUND DEBRIDEMENT	
METHOD	**INDICATIONS**
Layered debridement	Conservative debridement beginning at superficial layers of wound and progressing to depths; indicated for large wounds with substantial tissue trauma
En bloc	Complete excision of wound; indicated for small wounds in areas with loose skin that can be closed
Enzymatic	Use of trypsin products that dissolve necrotic tissue; very slow method of debridement; indicated in minimally contaminated or traumatized wounds or as an adjunct to surgical debridement

• Table 19–4 •

METHODS OF WOUND CLOSURE	
METHOD	**COMMENTS**
Primary closure	First intention healing; closure of a wound with sutures; indicated for fresh clean wounds with minimal contamination or trauma
Delayed primary closure	Closure of a wound before 3–5 days after injury; i.e., before development of granulation tissue; indicated for moderately contaminated or traumatized wounds
Secondary closure	Closure of a wound after 3–4 days; i.e., after granulation tissue has developed in the wound; indicated in severely contaminated or traumatized wounds that require considerable debridement and prolonged wound management; takes advantage of the positive effects of granulation tissue
Second intention healing (contraction and epithelialization)	Wound allowed to heal without surgical closure; relies on contraction and epithelialization; may not be possible or desirable in all wounds

infected. Wounds treated after the golden period should not be closed, since infection is likely.

Delayed primary closure is primary closure of a wound 1 to 3 days after injury, before granulation tissue has appeared in the wound. It is indicated for mildly contaminated, minimally traumatized wounds that require some cleansing and debridement, or for relatively clean wounds seen 6 to 8 hours after injury. This method allows any local contamination or infection to be controlled before closure.

Healing by contraction and epithelialization is defined as second intention healing and is indicated for dirty, contaminated, traumatized wounds when cleansing and debridement are necessary and when closure may be difficult. Adequate, loose skin surrounding the wound is necessary to allow contraction. Closure by second intention may not always be desirable because the new epithelium is fragile and easily abraded. In addition, contraction may impede normal function, depending on the location of the wound.

Secondary closure results in third intention healing. The wound is sutured at least 3 to 5 days after injury. Granulation tissue will be present in the wound by the time of closure. The granulation tissue helps to control infection in the wound and fills in the tissue defect. Secondary closure is indicated when (1) the wound is severely contaminated or traumatized, (2) epithelialization and contraction will not completely close the wound, or (3) second intention healing is undesirable.

The decision whether to treat a wound primarily or to have it remain open initially and follow up with delayed closure, second intention healing, or secondary closure depends on the (1) time lapse since injury; wounds greater than 6 to 8 hours old should be kept open initially; (2) degree of contamination;

• Table 19–5 •

FACTORS IMPORTANT IN WOUND MANAGEMENT DECISION-MAKING
FACTORS FOR CONSIDERATION
Time since injury
Degree of wound contamination
Degree of tissue trauma
Thoroughness of initial debridement
Blood supply of wound
Animal's physical status
Wound tension and possibility of closure
Location of wound

wounds obviously contaminated should be kept open initially and thoroughly cleansed; (3) amount of tissue damage; wounds with substantial tissue damage have reduced host defenses, are more likely to become infected, and consequently should remain open initially; (4) thoroughness of debridement; if the initial debridement was conservative, the wound should remain open until definitive debridement is performed; (5) blood supply to the wound; a wound with questionable blood supply should remain open until the extent of nonviable tissue is determined; (6) the animal's health; if the animal is unable to endure prolonged surgical debridement, the wound should be kept open and possibly undergo enzymatic debridement until the animal can withstand surgery; (7) closure without tension or dead space; if excessive tension or dead space is present, the wound should be allowed to remain open because dead space allows accumulation of fluid, separation of tissues, and formation of seromas, which may predispose to infection and delay wound healing; and (8) location of the wound; certain locations may not be amenable to closure (such as a large wound on a limb) (Table 19–5).

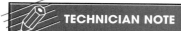

TECHNICIAN NOTE

Nonadherent bandages are indicated in granulating wounds.

WOUND BANDAGING

Bandaging promotes wound healing by protecting the wound from additional trauma and contamination, by preventing wound desiccation, by preventing hematoma and seroma formation through compression and obliterating dead space, and by immobilizing the wound to prevent cellular and capillary disruption. Bandaging minimizes postoperative edema around incisions and minimizes exuberant granulation tissue formation in open wounds on the lower limb region (below the carpus or tarsus) of horses. In addition, the bandage can absorb wound exudate and debride the wound of foreign material and loose tissue that adheres to the bandage as it is removed. Covering a wound with a bandage promotes an acid environment at the wound surface by preventing carbon dioxide loss and ab-

sorbing ammonia produced by bacteria. An acid environment increases oxygen dissociation from hemoglobin and subsequently increases oxygen availability in the wound. The bandage also keeps the wound warm. Higher temperatures improve wound healing and facilitate oxygen dissociation. (Table 19–6)

A bandage usually consists of three layers: the primary or contact layer, the secondary or padded conforming layer, and the tertiary or holding and protective layer. The primary bandage layer contacts the wound surface (if present) and may be adherent or nonadherent and occlusive or semiocclusive. Adherent bandages are indicated if some debridement is still necessary. Wounds discharging large amounts of exudate or containing embedded debris are often covered with an adherent, absorbent type of dressing such as a small stack of gauze pads, disposable baby diaper, cotton (such as combine), and the like, in what is called a *dry-dry bandage*, to absorb exudate and allow debris to adhere. The same absorbent material soaked with saline creates a *wet-dry bandage* to "rehydrate" and loosen dried or thick exudate and debris from a wound, facilitating its removal. Nonadherent bandages are required when healthy granulation fills the wound, to avoid disruption of this tissue during removal of the contact layer. Semiocclusive, nonadherent bandages are preferred, as they allow air to penetrate to the wound surface and exudate to escape from the wound surface. Occlusive bandages should not be used if wound exudate is present, as they keep the exudate at the wound surface, and this causes maceration of the wound and adjacent healthy tissue.

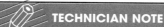

TECHNICIAN NOTE

Wet-dry bandages facilitate removal of debris and viscous exudate from a wound.

The secondary layer is an absorbent, padded, conforming layer of cast padding or roll cotton. The tertiary layer is the holding and protective layer, which uses some form of gauze and elastic or adhesive tape to hold the bandage in place.

Specific bandages and their indications for use in small animal practice are described below. The standard procedure for application of any bandage requires (1) application of anchoring tape strips (stirrups) to the distal portion of the limb; (2) application of a primary bandage layer over the wound, if present; (3) application of the padded secondary layer over the

• Table 19–6 •

BENEFICIAL EFFECTS OF BANDAGING A WOUND
Protects from further contamination
Prevents wound desiccation
Prevents hematoma and seroma formation
Immobilizes the wound and prevents cellular disruption
Minimizes surrounding edema
Absorbs wound exudate and debris
Promotes retention of carbon dioxide and creation of an acid environment, which facilitates oxygen dissociation
Keeps wound warm, which facilitates healing

stirrups; (4) application of the gauze tertiary layer; (5) application of the splint; (6) reflection and twisting of the stirrups to adhere to the gauze layer; and (7) application of the protective tertiary layer of tape, (Table 19–7). The middle two toes should always be exposed to allow assessment of color, warmth, and swelling. A stockinette can be applied under the secondary layer to help prevent the bandage from slipping. Other modifications are acceptable.

> **✎ TECHNICIAN NOTE**
>
> The middle two toes should always be exposed to allow assessment of color, warmth, and swelling.

WOUND BANDAGING IN SMALL ANIMALS

Casts

Fiberglass cast materials are currently used almost routinely because of their light weight, extreme rigidity, rapid setting time, and ventilation and waterproof properties. Casts are indicated for stabilization of certain fractures distal to the elbow or stifle, and for immobilization of limbs to protect ligament or tendon repairs. The cast material is applied instead of a tertiary layer; however, minimal padding is suggested to avoid cast loosening and movement and excessive compression (Fig. 19–3). It is advisable to monitor animals with casts at least weekly.

Bandages and Splints

The *Robert Jones bandage* is most commonly used for temporary immobilization of fractures distal to the elbow or stifle

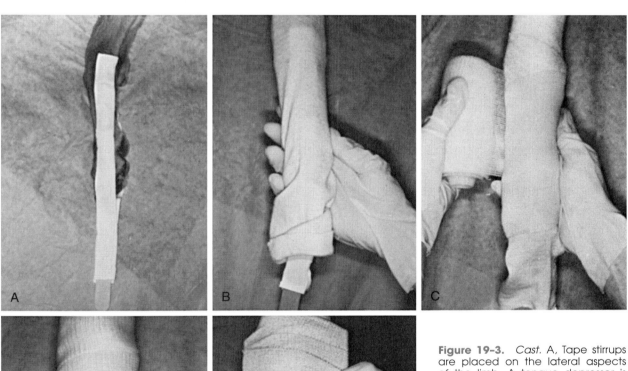

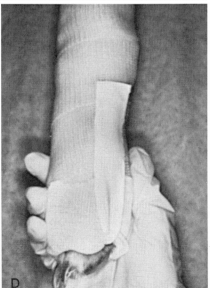

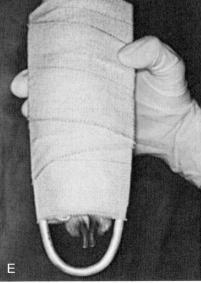

Figure 19–3. *Cast.* A, Tape stirrups are placed on the lateral aspects of the limb. A tongue depressor is placed between them to prevent adherence of the stirrups to each another. B, A stockinette is applied over the limb. A lightly padded, secondary layer is then applied firmly around the leg. C, The fiberglass casting material is applied firmly but not tightly to the leg, with care taken to avoid compression of the cast material with the fingers. D, The stockinette ends are reflected over the cast, and the tape stirrups are reflected onto the cast. Protective tape is applied over the ends of the cast. E, A walking bar can be applied to the cast at this point. The two middle toes are exposed.

• Table 19–7 •

STEPS IN BANDAGE PLACEMENT*

Apply anchoring tapes (stirrups)
Apply primary (contact) layer on wound
Apply secondary (padded) layer
Apply tertiary (conforming) gauze layer
Apply splint
Reflect, twist, and adhere stirrups to gauze
Apply tertiary (protective) tape

*Some steps may not be indicated.

before surgery. It is a large bulky bandage that provides rigid stabilization owing to the extreme compression of the thick cotton secondary layer (Fig. 19–4). The Robert Jones bandage is not appropriate for fractures of the femur or humerus.

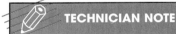

TECHNICIAN NOTE

Casts must be monitored weekly.

The *modified Robert Jones bandage* or simple padded bandage is a less bulky bandage and is used to reduce postoperative swelling of limbs (Fig. 19–5). It provides little or no splinting of the limbs. Less padding is used in the secondary layer, and cast padding is used instead of roll cotton.

TECHNICIAN NOTE

The Robert Jones bandage is not appropriate for fractures of the femur or humerus.

A *chest* or *abdominal bandage* is applied in the standard three layers. These bandages should be applied firmly but without constricting the chest or abdomen (Fig. 19–6). If an abdominal bandage is used to control abdominal bleeding, the layers are applied more firmly. A rolled towel can be used to reinforce the bandage along the midline and is applied before application of the protective tape. The effectiveness of a compression bandage lasts for only 1 to 2 hours, and it should not remain in place longer than 4 hours.

Distal limb splints can be made with tongue depressors for very small animals, or with aluminum splints, cast material, or

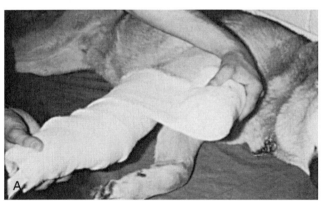

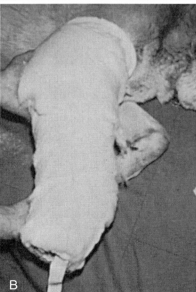

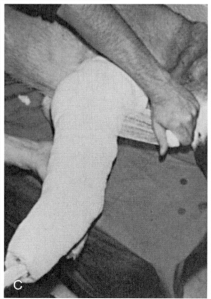

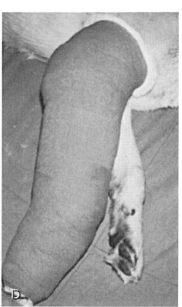

Figure 19-4. *Robert-Jones.* A, Tape stirrups are applied, and the limb is wrapped in a secondary layer of roll cotton. B, The roll cotton is compressed tightly with a gauze tertiary layer. C, Protective tape is then firmly applied. (Courtesy of Dr. John Berg.)

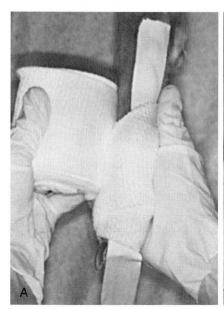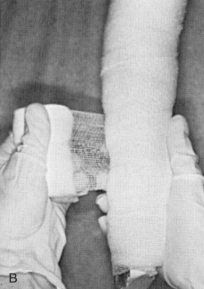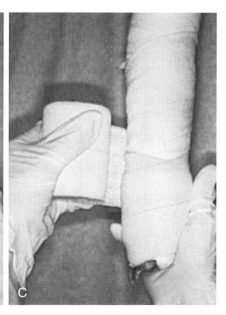

Figure 19-5. *Modified Robert-Jones or simple padded bandage.* A, Tape stirrups and a padded secondary layer are applied to the limb. B, This is followed by a gauze tertiary layer. C, The stirrups are reflected to adhere to the gauze, and the bandage is covered by protective tape.

thermoplastics (Fig. 19–7). They are indicated for temporary immobilization or definitive stabilization of certain fractures of the distal radius and ulna, carpus, tarsus, metacarpals and metatarsals, and phalanges. They can also be used to support a traumatized distal limb. The limb should be well padded to avoid pressure points. The splint should always be placed on the caudal aspect of the limb.

TECHNICIAN NOTE

The splint is always placed on the caudal (plantar) aspect of the limb.

Slings

The *Ehmer sling* is used specifically to immobilize the hindlimb after reduction of craniodorsal coxofemoral luxation, and to prevent weight-bearing after surgery on the pelvis. Correct application results in internal rotation and adduction of the coxofemoral joint (Fig. 19–8). Minimal padding is suggested, and the sling is usually applied with adhesive tape alone to prevent slippage.

TECHNICIAN NOTE

The 90-90 flexion sling is critical in preventing quadriceps contracture after distal femoral fracture repair in young animals.

The *90-90 flexion sling* is applied with the stifle and hock placed in 90-degree flexion, and no attempt is made to adduct

and internally rotate the coxofemoral joint (Fig. 19–9). The 90-90 flexion sling is used to prevent stifle joint stiffness and hyperextension caused by quadriceps muscle contracture after distal femoral fracture repair in young animals. It can also be used as a non–weight-bearing sling to protect other surgical procedures of the hindlimb.

The *Velpeau sling* holds the flexed forelimb against the chest and prevents movement in all joints (Fig. 19–10). It is used as a non–weight-bearing sling for the forelimb. The Velpeau sling is indicated after reduction of scapulohumeral joint luxation or to immobilize scapula fractures.

The *carpal flexion sling* is a non–weight-bearing forelimb sling (Fig. 19–11). The degree of carpal flexion can be reduced by partially cutting the crisscross of tape formed at the caudal aspect of the carpus.

Hobbles can be applied to the hindlimbs to prevent excessive abduction of the limbs. They are specifically indicated after reduction of ventral coxofemoral luxation and to prevent excessive tension in the inguinal region. They can be used to prevent excessive activity after pelvic fracture repair or for nonsurgical, conservative management of pelvic fractures (Fig. 19–12).

Aftercare of Casts, Bandages, Splints, and Slings

Close monitoring of animals with casts, bandages, splints, or slings is extremely important and should be performed daily in the inpatient and at least weekly in the outpatient. Client education for the outpatient is essential. The toes should be monitored daily for warmth, color, and swelling. Abnormal findings are indicative of a tight cast. Monitoring the bandage for a foul odor that would indicate tissue damage is necessary. Observing for areas of chafing from the cast is important. The animal should be restrained from chewing at the bandage (e.g., by

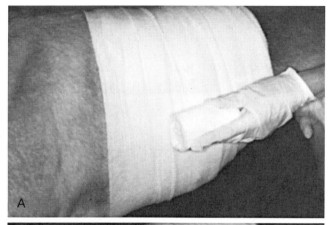

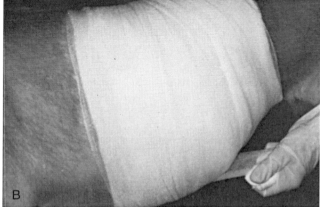

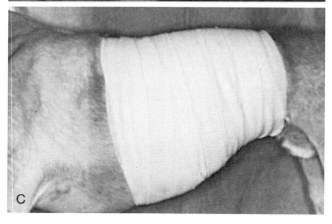

Figure 19-6. *Abdominal or chest bandage.* A, After a primary layer is placed on the wound, the padded secondary layer is applied. B, This is followed by a gauze tertiary layer. C, Protective tape is then applied.

means of an Elizabethan collar), and exercise restriction to short-leash walks is indicated. While the animal is outside, the bandage should be protected from dirt and moisture by application of a plastic bag or other waterproof material. The plastic covering should not remain on for more than 30 minutes,

as it prevents the bandage from breathing, and the underlying tissue can become moist and macerated.

WOUND MANAGEMENT OF HORSES

Wound Care

Basic wound management is no different in large animals than in small companion animals. However, the size and nature of the animal as well as location of the injury may dictate the way a wound is approached. Thus some additional points will be briefly discussed.

When preparing a wound on a horse, K-Y jelly (Johnson & Johnson) or saline-soaked gauze can be used to fill the depths

---

TECHNICIAN NOTE

Close monitoring of animals with bandages, casts, splints, or slings is imperitive to avoid serious complication.

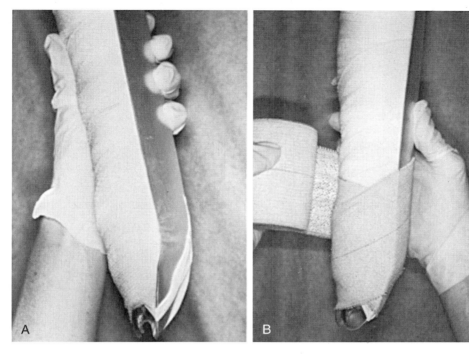

Figure 19–7. *Splint.* A, After application of a modified Robert-Jones or simple padded bandage (see Fig. 19–5), the splint is applied to the caudal aspect of the limb, and the stirrups are reflected onto the splint. B, Protective tape is then applied to hold the splint in place.

of the wound. Electric clippers are usually used to clip the hair from around the edges of the wound. However, if clippers are not available, the wound edges can be lathered with antiseptic scrub (Betadine Scrub, Triad Medical Products), and a straight-edge razor or no. 22 scalpel blade (Bard-Parker, Becton Dickinson AcuteCare) can be used to shave the hair (Fig. 19–13).

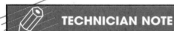

TECHNICIAN NOTE

It is important to clip or shave the hair from around a wound.

Various methods can be used to lavage a wound, as described earlier in this chapter. Another available method of wound lavage is the Pulsavac Wound Debridement System (Zimmer, Snyder Laboratories) (Fig. 19–14), which is effective in removing debris from wounds. It is equipped with a hand-held spray nozzle that has a trigger to regulate fluid flow. The system can be attached to a vacuum to create suction, which facilitates removal of the lavage solution and debris when the coned head, at the end of the spray nozzle, is placed directly over the wound.

In most cases, local anesthesia with tranquilization or general anesthesia is needed before a wound can be properly treated. If tranquilization is used, local or regional anesthesia is necessary to debride and close the wound. Local infiltration is performed by injecting a local anesthetic, mepivacaine (Carbocaine-V 2%, Winthrop Veterinary, Sterling Animal Health Products) or lidocaine (AmVet Pharmaceuticals), approximately 1 cm from the wound edge, subcutaneously around the entire

wound. A 22-gauge hypodermic needle is used in most situations and is reinserted repeatedly through the skin, each time at the end of the bleb formed by the preceding injection of local anesthetic (Fig. 19–15). In this way, the patient will not react to the succeeding injections. If the wound is located on the distal limb, a ring block or nerve block (such as a palmar nerve block) can be utilized to anesthetize the limb distal to the block.

The same considerations for wound closure in small companion animals apply to large animals as well. It is important to remember that open wounds on the distal aspect of the limb (below the carpus or tarsus) of the horse are notorious for developing exuberant granulation tissue. Exuberant granulation tissue, commonly referred to as "proud flesh," can form rapidly in horses. Various measures must be undertaken to keep exuberant granulation tissue in check, or it can become excessive (Fig. 19–16). Methods of controlling granulation tissue include immobilizing the limb (as with a cast), wound bandaging, surgical excision, caustic agents such as equal parts of copper sulfate and boric acid powder, cryotherapy, electrocautery, or topical corticosteroids. Regardless of the decision to allow a wound on the limb of large animals to heal by first or second intention, a bandage should be placed on the limb.

TECHNICIAN NOTE

Open wounds on the distal aspect of a horse's limb most often develop exuberant granulation tissue (``proud flesh''), which can impede healing.

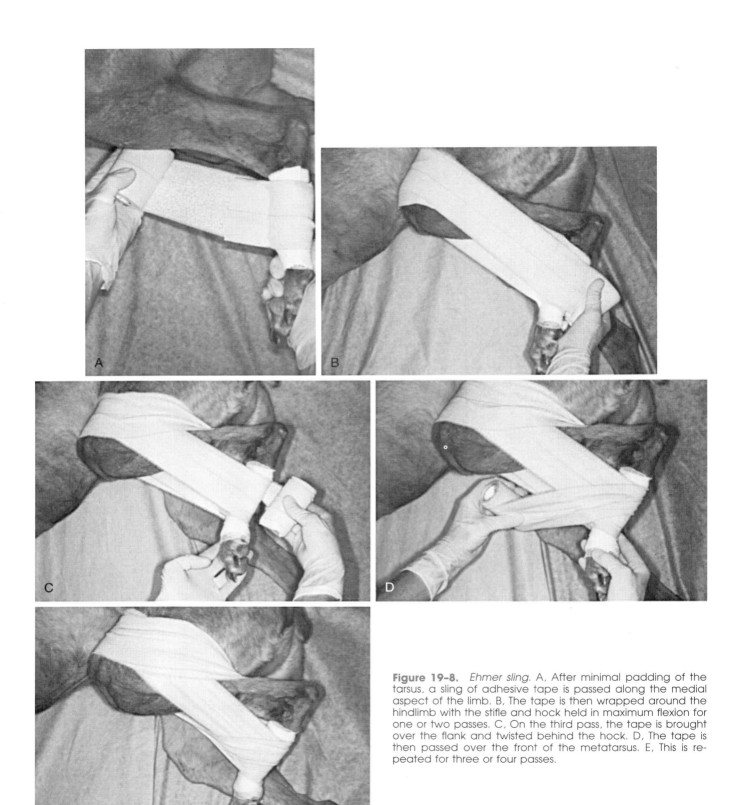

Figure 19-8. *Ehmer sling.* A, After minimal padding of the tarsus, a sling of adhesive tape is passed along the medial aspect of the limb. B, The tape is then wrapped around the hindlimb with the stifle and hock held in maximum flexion for one or two passes. C, On the third pass, the tape is brought over the flank and twisted behind the hock. D, The tape is then passed over the front of the metatarsus. E, This is repeated for three or four passes.

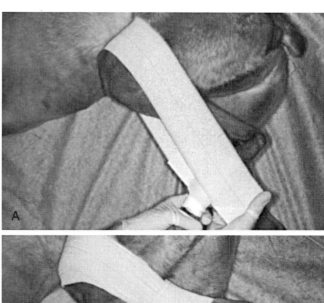

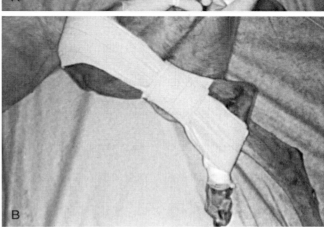

Figure 19-9. *90–90-degree flexion sling.* After minimal padding of the tarsus, a sling of adhesive tape is passed along the medial aspect of the limb (see Fig. 19–8A). A, The tape is then wrapped around the hindlimb with the stifle and hock held in 90-degree flexion. B, A second layer of tape is passed horizontally around the tibia to hold the previous layer in place.

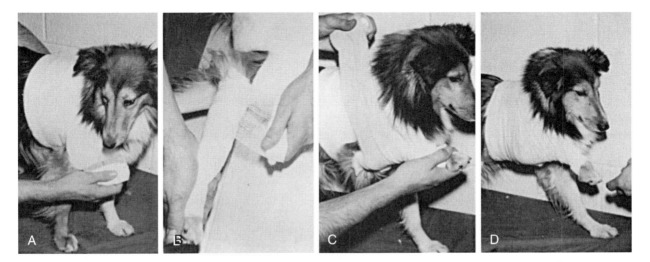

Figure 19-10. *Velpeau sling.* A, The chest wall and shoulder are covered with a lightly padded secondary layer and a gauze tertiary layer. B, The forelimb is bandaged similarly. C and D, The forelimb is flexed against the chest wall, with care taken to avoid extreme flexion of the elbow, and covered by a sling of protective tape. The foot is exposed. (Courtesy of Dr. John Berg.)

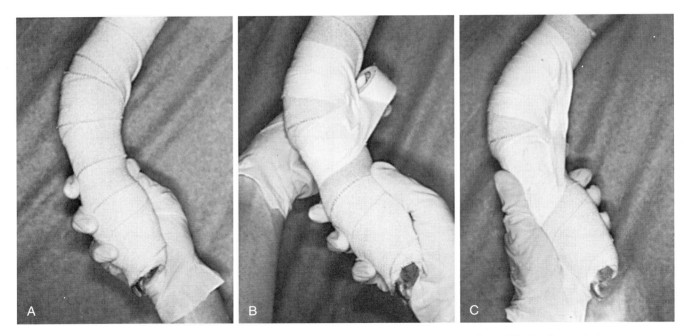

Figure 19-11. *Carpal flexion sling.* A, With the carpus in flexion, a minimally padded soft padded bandage is applied. B, Tape is then applied in a figure-of-eight fashion around the carpus to support the carpus. C, The tape begins in the middle of the carpus and extends distally and proximally, forming a web of tape behind the carpus.

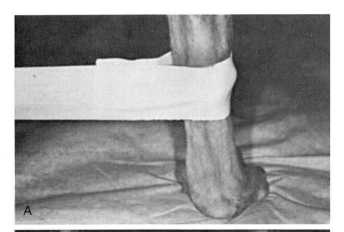

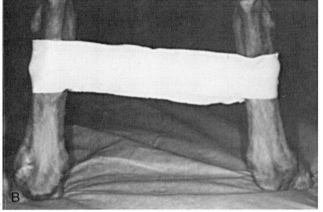

Figure 19-12. *Hobbles.* A, Adhesive tape wide enough to cover half of the metatarsal region is placed loosely around the metatarsal region. B, The tape is then adhered together between the legs and placed around the opposite metatarsus. The hindlimbs are positioned apart at a distance equal to the width of the pelvis.

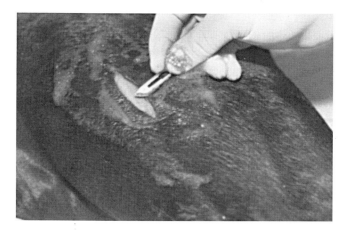

Figure 19-13. Once the hair has been lathered with antiseptic (Betadine) scrub, a No. 22 scalpel blade can be used to shave away the hair from the wound edge.

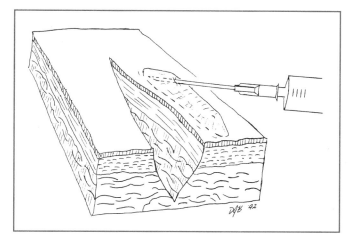

Figure 19-15. Proper technique of infiltration of a wound edge with a local anesthetic. The needle should enter through the skin at the point of the last injection.

BANDAGING AND CAST APPLICATION TECHNIQUES FOR HORSES

Introduction

Bandages and casts serve many purposes and can be named for the location and purpose they cover and serve respectively. Various materials are available for use in a bandage or cast, but the important aspect is their proper application and function. Development of good bandaging and cast application skills is important to ensure proper function of the bandage or cast. The application and purpose of the different types used on horses will be discussed.

Bandages

Lower Limb Wound Bandage

A *lower limb wound bandage* covers a wound on a limb distal to the carpus or tarsus. When the wound is traumatic, after it

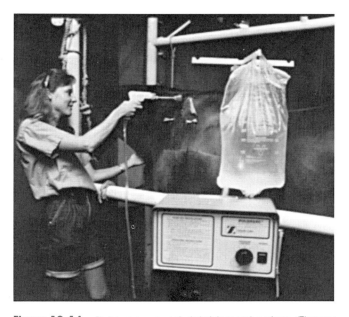

Figure 19-14. Pulsavac wound debridement system (Zimmer, Snyder Laboratories) is used to apply a high-pressure (70 psi) stream of lavage solution to a wound, which removes loose debris from the wound. (Courtesy of Dr. Michael A. Collier.)

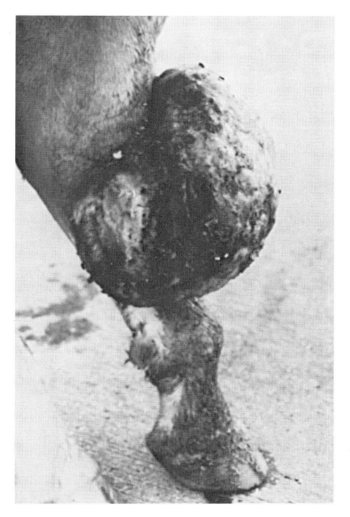

Figure 19-16. Excessive exuberant granulation tissue on the dorsal aspect of the proximal metatarsus of a horse. (Courtesy of Dr. R. Stuart Shoemaker.)

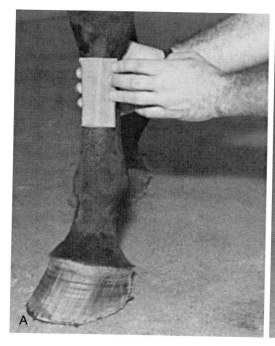
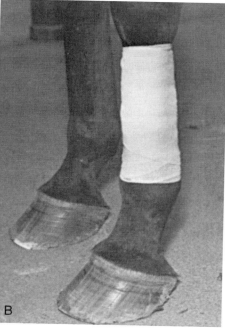

Figure 19-17. Application of wound dressing on the distal region of the limb of a horse. A, Nonadherent dressing is applied directly over the wound. B, Conforming gauze (Kling) is used to maintain a nonadherent dressing over the wound.

has been cleaned and debrided, a topical medication is usually applied if it is left unsutured. Topical preparations usually are not applied to a surgical incision. A nonadhering dressing (Telfa pad, Kendall; Adaptic, Johnson & Johnson) is then placed directly over the wound. The wound dressing is secured to the limb with rolled conforming gauze (Kling, Johnson & Johnson). The conforming gauze is wrapped around the limb with *light* pressure, overlapping, and without wrinkles to avoid pressure lines, which may cause skin sloughing if applied too tightly. It is wrapped proximal and distal to the wound approximately 2 to 4 cm (Fig. 19–17).

TECHNICIAN NOTE

The "barber pole" method of applying white tape to secure a bandage prevents a tourniquet effect from developing.

The padded layer is applied next. Combine cotton sheets cut from a roll, rolled cotton, layered cotton sheet, quilted leg wraps, or a military field bandage can be used (Fig. 19–18). If cotton sheets are available, five are used, folded in half and neatly rolled. The fifth sheet is folded in the opposite direction to the other sheets to conceal the edges. The padded layer is secured to the limb with a roll of conforming gauze (brown gauze, J. R. Raynor; Kling, Johnson & Johnson). Pressure is applied when wrapping to compress and conform the padding to the limb. The outer shell of the bandage is finished using elastic wrap (Vetrap, Animal Care Products/3M; Ace bandage, Johnson & Johnson), adhesive elastic tape (Elastikon, Johnson & Johnson), or a flannel track wrap. The end of the Ace or track wrap is secured with white tape cut into strips or placed around the bandage in a "barber pole" fashion (Fig. 19–19). The barber pole method prevents a tourniquet effect from

developing around the leg. Elastikon (Johnson & Johnson) is placed around the top and bottom of the bandage, with half of the tape sticking to the wrap and half to the skin, to prevent slippage and debris (such as bedding shavings) from getting down inside the bandage.

Lower Limb Support Bandage

This type of bandage is used to provide support of the soft tissues (such as ligaments and tendons) of the limb contralateral to the injured leg, which is bearing excessive weight because of decreased weight-bearing on the injured limb. The bandage also minimizes static limb edema in a confined, inactive horse. A support bandage is placed on the lower limb, just like the

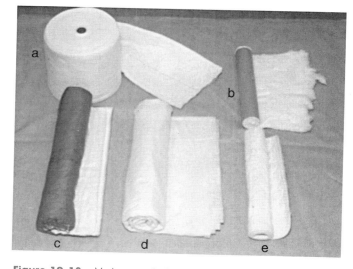

Figure 19-18. Various materials can be used for the padded layer in a leg bandage for large animals. a, Cotton combine. b, Rolled cotton. c, Military field bandage. d, Cotton sheets. e, Quilted leg wraps.

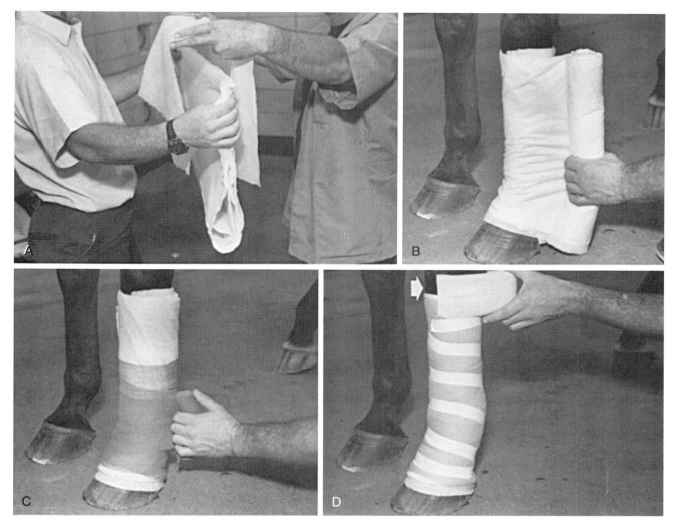

Figure 19-19.   Application of padded layer of a wound bandage. A, The wrap used is constructed by taking five cotton sheets and folding them in half, with the fifth sheet folded opposite the other sheets to conceal the edges. This is then rolled. B, Cotton wrap is applied snugly around the limb. C, Conforming gauze is used to secure the padded layer to the limb. D, An elastic wrap is used to form the outer shell of the bandage. White tape is applied in a "barber pole" fashion to secure the wrap. Wide adhesive tape is used to provide a seal between the skin and bandage (arrow).

wound bandage described above except that the underlying wound dressing and inner conforming gauze layer are not utilized. It is also unnecessary to place wide adhesive elastic tape (Elastikon) around the top and bottom.

Carpal Bandage

This type of wound bandage is used primarily as a counter-pressure bandage after an arthrotomy or arthroscopic surgery. However, it can be used to cover wounds of the carpus. Precautions must be considered to prevent ischemic necrosis of the skin over the accessory carpal bone. One method of protection is the use of a doughnut pad, made from a 2.5-cm-thick piece of orthopedic felt (12 cm × 18 cm). An elliptical hole (2.5 cm × 5 cm) is cut out of the center of the pad, and then the hole is positioned over the accessory carpal bone and secured to the limb with a piece of tape lightly applied around the limb. A nonadherent dressing is placed over the wound or operative site, and the carpus is wrapped with conforming gauze. A

figure-of-eight pattern can be used for wrapping. Because this is a high-motion region, an adhesive elastic tape is then used to form the outer shell of the bandage. The adhesive elastic tape is secured directly onto the skin, at the top and bottom of the wrap, to prevent slippage. A vertical cut is made in the bandage over the accessory carpal bandage to relieve the pressure on this area (Fig. 19–20). A support bandage can be placed on the lower part of the limb as an additional measure to prevent slippage.

> **TECHNICIAN NOTE**
>
> Steps must be taken to reduce pressure over the accessory carpal bone when bandaging the carpus of a horse.

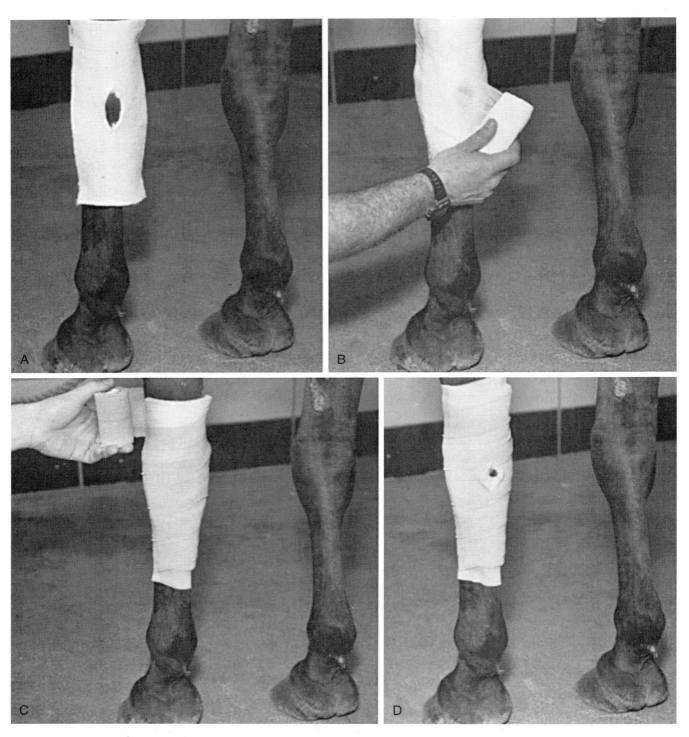

Figure 19-20. Equine carpal bandage. A, A ``doughnut'' pad made from orthopedic felt is placed over the accessory carpal bone. B, Nonadherent dressing is placed over the surgical site, and the carpus is wrapped with conforming gauze in a figure-of-eight fashion. C, Wide adhesive tape is used to cover and secure the bandage to the limb. D, A vertical cut is made in the bandage over the accessory carpal bandage to relieve pressure from the area.

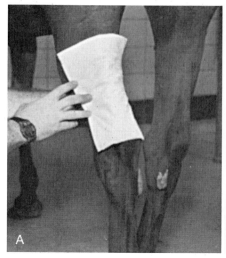
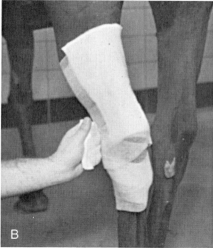
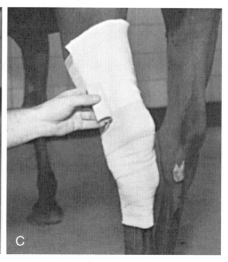

Figure 19-21. Equine hock bandage. A, Padding is placed over the gastrocnemius tendon and point of hock to prevent pressure necrosis when the tarsus is bandaged. B, Nonadherent dressing is applied over the surgical site, and the tarsus is wrapped with conforming gauze. C, Wide adhesive tape is used to cover and secure the bandage to the limb. No pressure is applied as the point of the hock is being covered.

Hock (Tarsal) Bandage

This bandage is used for the same purpose as the carpal bandage, but it is generally more difficult to apply. The bandage may be resented by some horses, who may try to dislodge it by kicking repeatedly with the affected limb. Several different methods may be used to apply a hock bandage. One method is to use a piece of padding (such as cotton combine), which can be placed over the gastrocnemius tendon and point of the hock to prevent pressure necrosis, before securing the nonadhering wound dressing. *Very* light pressure is applied as the conforming gauze is placed over the point of the hock. A layer of padding can be placed around the hock and secured with conforming gauze. The bandage material and application used for the outer shell are the same as for the carpal bandage (Fig. 19–21). No pressure is applied as the point of the hock is covered. A support bandage can be placed on the lower part of the limb as an additional measure to prevent slippage.

TECHNICIAN NOTE

Steps must be taken to reduce pressure over the gastrocnemius tendon when bandaging a horse's hock.

Forelimb Full-Length (Stack) Bandage

This type of bandage is used to cover a wound of the upper limb, to provide support of the limb, or to provide padding under a full limb splint. A support bandage is first placed on the lower part of the limb. Then a wound or support bandage, depending on the circumstances, is "stacked" or placed directly above (proximal) the lower bandage to cover the upper part of the limb (Fig. 19–22). A doughnut pad can used under the bandage, and a vertical cut can be made in the bandage, over the accessory carpal bone, to prevent pressure necrosis of the skin over the prominence.

Robert Jones Bandage

This is a thick, bulky, full-length bandage designed to provide immobilization of a limb. It is used as a temporary measure of immobilization and support in emergency situations, such as long bone fractures, in which the animal is going to be transported for surgical repair. Unfortunately, it is often not effective enough in immobilizing the limb. The bandage is devised by applying multiple layers (four to six of rolled cotton or cotton sheets to the full length of the limb, in a stack bandage configuration, with elastic wrap (Vetrap, Animal Care Products/3M; Ace

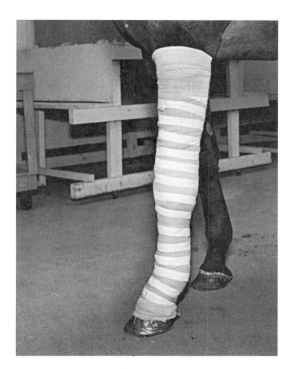

Figure 19-22. Forelimb full-length (stack) bandage.

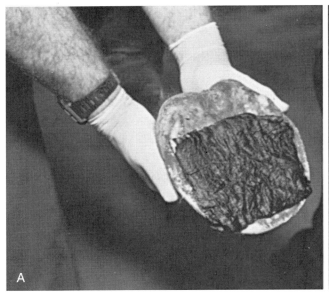

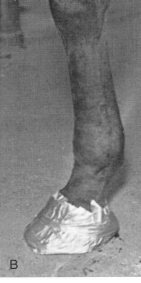

Figure 19–23. Technique for applying an equine foot bandage. A, Cotton soaked in medication is placed on the bottom of the sole. B, The foot is then wrapped with an adhesive tape (duct tape).

bandages, Johnson & Johnson) applied between layers of cotton. This increases the rigidity of the bandage. In large animals, a piece of rigid material (such as a metal bar or a wooden slat) must be incorporated into the bandage for the entire length of the limb, on two sides, to help achieve a rigid, immobilizing bandage.

 TECHNICIAN NOTE

Two pieces of rigid material, positioned 90 degrees to each other, and that run the length of the entire limb, should be incorporated into a Robert Jones bandage when applied on a large animal.

Foot Bandage

This bandage is used to retain a dressing on the hoof, primarily the sole, in the treatment of a subsolar abscess or puncture. When adequate drainage has been established in the sole, the area being treated is flushed with a mixture of equal parts of hydrogen peroxide and strong iodine (5% to 7%). The sole is then covered with cotton that has been soaked in iodine. The entire foot is then wrapped with adhesive tape (Duct tape, 3M; Elastikon, Johnson & Johnson). The tape can be carried above the coronary band, but excessive pressure is avoided around this area (Fig. 19–23). A useful addition to this type of bandage is a protective boot (Medi-Boot, Tex-Sol Plastics) placed over the bandage or a hard plastic sole pad placed underneath the tape to provide additional protection (Fig. 19–24).

Head Bandage

This type of bandage is used to cover wounds of the face, sinuses, mandible, or eye. A piece of orthopedic stockinette (10 or 15 cm) is pulled over the horse's head and positioned just behind the commissures of the mouth back to the throat latch. Holes are then cut in the stockinette over the eyes and the ears.

The ends of the stockinette are usually taped to the skin with elastic adhesive tape (Elastikon, Johnson & Johnson) (Fig. 19–25).

Abdominal Bandage

This bandage is used by some equine surgeons to provide additional support and to reduce or prevent ventral edema formation following abdominal surgery. A layered cotton pad constructed from cotton sheets, cotton combine, or a military

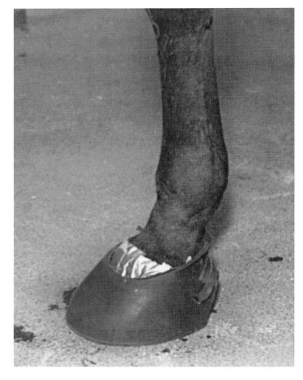

Figure 19–24. A boot can be placed over the foot wrap to provide additional protection.

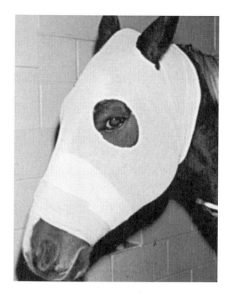

Figure 19-25. Head bandage made from orthopedic stockinette. (Courtesy of C. Wayne McIlwraith.)

field bandage is placed over the ventral incision. Elastic adhesive tape (Elastikon, Johnson & Johnson) is then used to snugly encircle the entire abdomen and retain the pad in position along the entire length of the incision (Fig. 19–26).

Splints

A splint is an addition of a rigid material to a limb bandage to reinforce immobilization of a particular part of a limb. Various materials can be used as the reinforcement, including wooden slats, metal bars, low-temperature thermoplastic, and casting material. However, the most common material used is polyvinyl chloride (PVC) pipe, because of its light weight and strength (Fig. 19–27). The pipe used is 10 cm in diameter and is split in half. It can be bent by heating with a cutting torch to conform to the fetlock angulation. The length and width of the splint varies with the size of the leg and the area being splinted. Depending on the amount of immobilization, splints can be placed the full length of the forelimb or from just below the carpus or tarsus all the way to the ground surface. In most situations, they are placed on the flexor surface of the limb.

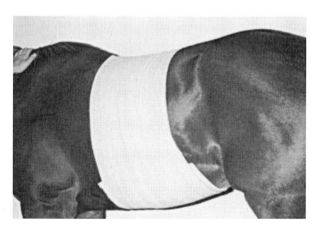

Figure 19-26. Abdominal bandage. (Courtesy of C. Wayne McIlwraith.)

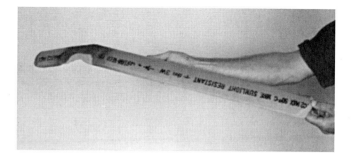

Figure 19-27. PVC piping is commonly used to make limb splits for large animals.

Splints are used in situations such as extensor or flexor tendon lacerations, flexure deformities in foals, or as needed limb support (as in radial nerve paresis).

A thick bandage is first placed on the limb. It should be long enough to cover the limb above as well as below the ends of the splint. This will prevent pressure sores from developing. Once the bandage is in place, the splint is secured to the limb with adhesive tape (Fig. 19–28). Splints should be reset frequently (at least twice a day) in foals.

✎ TECHNICIAN NOTE

It is important that a bandage cover the limb well above and below the ends of a splint to prevent pressure sores.

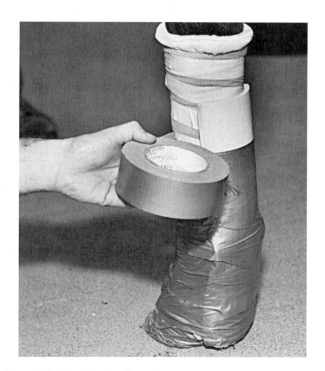

Figure 19-28. Application of a lower limb splint. A thick bandage is placed on the limb. The splint (PVC pipe) is positioned along the flexor surface and secured to the bandage with duct tape.

Casts

A cast is the most frequently used external coaptation to manage various orthopedic injuries or problems when maximum support and immobilization are required. Casts are commonly used for lower limb problems; however, full-limb application is sometimes indicated in large animals. Indications for use of a cast include lower limb fractures, as an adjunct to internal fixation, tendon lacerations, support of the lower limb during recovery from orthopedic surgery, heel bulb lacerations, and luxations of the tarsus, fetlock, or pastern.

For optimal effectiveness in immobilization, a cast must immobilize the joint proximal and distal to the injury. Full-limb casts must extend up to the elbow or stifle as far as possible. The most frequently used material today is fiberglass. Fiberglass (such as Delta-Lite, Johnson & Johnson) is appealing because it is lightweight, strong, and relatively easy to apply. However, some veterinarians prefer to use a layer of the traditional plaster of Paris initially under the fiberglass. Plaster conforms well to the contour of the limb, reducing the risk of pressure sores.

✎ **TECHNICIAN NOTE**

In order to effectively immobilize a fracture, a cast must immobilize the joint proximal and distal to the injury.

Before cast application is begun, several things must be considered. It is important that a limb cast be applied properly or serious problems such as pressure necrosis can occur. Because of its importance, application of a limb cast is described here in detail.

Before the procedure is begun, all the materials needed should be collected: orthopedic stockinette (3-inch), orthopedic felt, towel clamps, white tape (1-inch), wire (approximately 30 cm), ⅛-inch drill bit and hand drill, broom handle, hoof-trimming equipment, bandage scissors, and cast material (Fig. 19–29). It is important that the cast be applied properly, especially if it is to remain on the limb for a prolonged period (4 to 6 weeks).

✎ **TECHNICIAN NOTE**

It is best to apply a cast with the horse under general anesthesia.

Generally, it is best to apply the cast with the horse under general anesthesia. The horse is positioned in lateral recumbency so that the limb to which the cast will be applied is uppermost. Debris is cleaned from the sole, the horseshoe removed, and the hoof trimmed. The limb is placed in an extended position perpendicular to the body. Effective support of the leg to maintain the limb in alignment is essential. Traction using wire looped through holes drilled in the hoof can be helpful. Two holes are drilled in the hoof wall 5 cm apart near the toe, in the same direction as that in which a horseshoe nail is driven. The ends of the wire are twisted together to form a

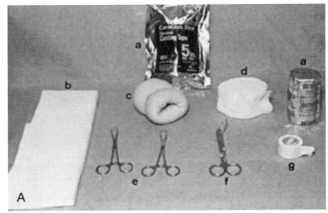

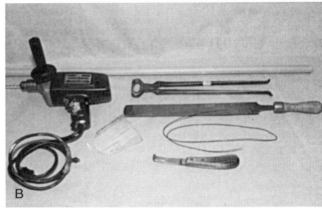

Figure 19-29. Materials needed to apply a limb cast on a large animal. A, Cast material (a), orthopedic felt (b), orthopedic stockinette (3-inch) (c), cast padding (d), towel clamps (e), bandage scissors (f), and white tape (1-inch) (g). B, Wire (approximately 30 cm), 1/8-inch drill bit and hand drill, wooden wedge block, broom handle, and hoof-trimming equipment.

loop through which a broom handle is placed to apply traction (Fig. 19–30).

The frog can be packed with povidone-iodine (Betadine Solution, Purdue Frederick), especially if thrush is present. If a wound is present, a three-layer bandage consisting of a nonadhering dressing, conforming gauze, and adhering elastic tape is used to cover it. The skin must be clean and dry. It can be powdered with talcum or boric acid to help keep the area dry under the cast. The limb is then covered with a double layer of stockinette. The length of the region to receive the cast is measured, and approximately 20 cm is added to this to determine the length of stockinette needed. One end is rolled outward and the other is rolled inward until they meet at the midpoint of the stockinette (Fig. 19–31).

✎ **TECHNICIAN NOTE**

Towel clamps are used to secure the orthopedic stockinette to the medial and lateral aspect of the limb, above the area to which the cast will be applied.

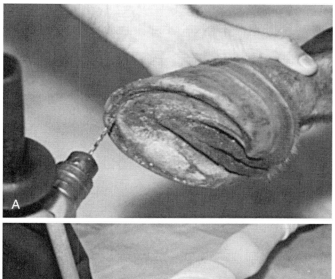

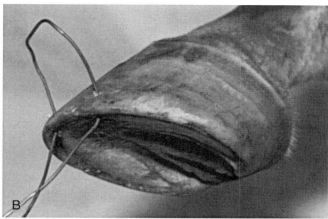

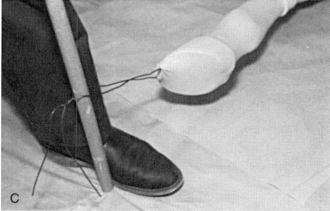

Figure 19-30. Traction can be applied to a limb before cast application by drilling two holes in the toe of the hoof (A) and threading a loop of wire through the holes (B), with a broomstick placed in the loop to apply traction (C).

The traction wire is threaded through the opening in the stockinette. The broom handle is placed through the wire loop and traction is applied. The outward roll is first unrolled up the leg. A twist is placed in the stockinette just beneath the toe, and the inward roll is unrolled up the leg (Fig. 19–32). Any wrinkles are smoothed out, and towel clamps are used to secure the stockinette to the medial and lateral aspect of the limb, above the area to which the cast will be applied.

A strip of orthopedic felt (5 to 7 cm wide) is placed around the leg at the most proximal limit of the cast. This is held in place with 1-inch white tape (Fig. 19–33). Additional padding on the leg should be avoided because this can become compressed, thus allowing the leg to move within the cast and cause sores. When a full-limb cast is used, a doughnut pad cut from orthopedic felt is placed over the accessory carpal bone of the forelimb. A thin strip of orthopedic felt is placed over the gastrocnemius tendon and the point of the hock of the hindlimb to prevent the development of pressure sores. A roll of support foam (Custom Support Foam, 3M) can be applied

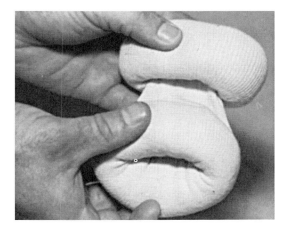

Figure 19-31. Orthopedic stockinette used under a cast is prerolled. One end is rolled outward and the other is rolled inward until they meet at the midpoint of the stockinette.

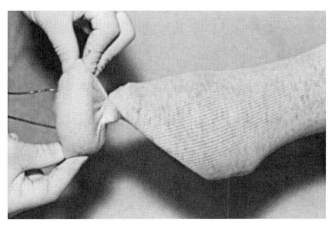

Figure 19-32. A twist is placed in the stockinette just beneath the toe, and the inward roll is unrolled up the leg.

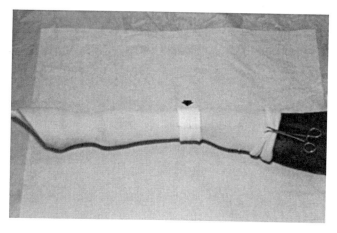

Figure 19-33. Before cast material application, the orthopedic stockinette is secured with towel clamps to the medial and lateral aspect of the limb, above the area to receive the cast. A strip of orthopedic felt (5 to 7 cm wide) (arrow) is placed around the leg at the most proximal limit of cast. This is held in place with 1-inch white tape.

next. Although not necessary, it is applied over the stockinette and was developed to provide padding under a cast to reduce the development of sores (Fig. 19–34).

Two layers of 3-inch plaster material are first carefully and snugly applied to the limb. To prevent pressure sores, it is important that these layers be applied without wrinkles. Appli-

cation of the cast material is usually started at either the proximal or the distal aspect of the limb. We prefer to start distally (Fig. 19–35). A roll of plaster is started at the level of the fetlock and worked distally, then proximally. Approximately 1 cm of the orthopedic felt is left exposed above the top of the cast to prevent formation of a sore.

> **TECHNICIAN NOTE**
>
> Excessive padding under a cast should be avoided.

Next the fiberglass cast material is applied. Usually it is easier to begin with 3-inch material because it conforms to the limb better. The cast material is overlapped by one third to one half. As the fiberglass casting material is worked toward the foot, the traction wires are cut, and an assistant holds the leg out at the upper limb region or by resting it on the palms of the hands placed under the metacarpus or metatarsus region. It is imperative to prevent finger imprints in the cast because they could cause a pressure sore to develop (Fig. 19–36).

> **TECHNICIAN NOTE**
>
> It is very important that the initial layer of casting material be applied to the limb without wrinkles or finger imprints, which may create sores.

More pressure is applied to the succeeding layers of fiberglass. This will allow them to laminate better. Generally, two layers of 3-inch fiberglass cast material are applied, followed by two or three layers of 4- or 5-inch fiberglass. At the time the last roll of cast material is applied, the stockinette is unclamped and the excess is cut off, leaving approximately 4 cm. This 4-cm excess is turned down over the top of the cast and incorporated in the last layer.

A wooden wedge block or a 3-inch roll of wet plaster cast

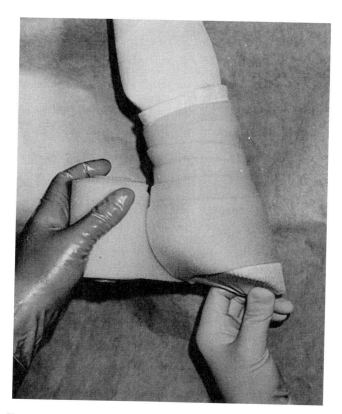

Figure 19-34. A roll of support foam (Custom Support Foam, 3M) can be applied over the stockinette to provide padding under the cast to reduce formation of cast sores.

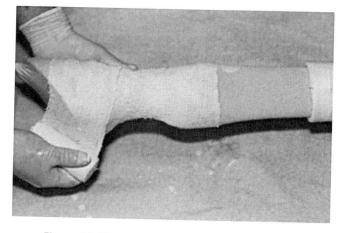

Figure 19-35. Application of the plaster of Paris.

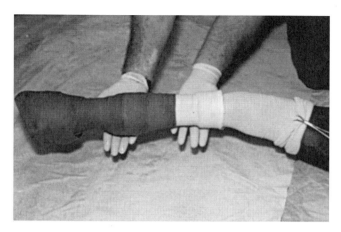

Figure 19-36. As the fiberglass cast material is being applied, an assistant holds the leg out at the upper limb region by resting it on the palms of the hands under the metacarpus/metatarsus region. This method prevents finger impression from being made in the uncured cast material.

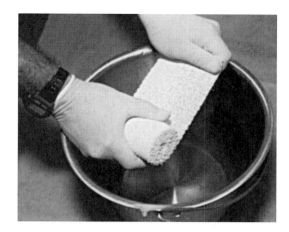

Figure 19-38. The end of the plaster cast material is held away from the roll while it is being moistened.

material is placed underneath the heel and also incorporated with the last layer (Fig. 19–37). A heel wedge allows the horse to walk more easily while wearing a cast because it decreases the breakover force, reduces pressure on the dorsal proximal limits of the cast at the metacarpus or metatarsus, and allows more even axial weight-bearing down through the cast.

It is best to wear gloves, especially when applying the fiberglass. To save time in identifying the end on a wetted plaster roll, unroll 2 to 3 inches of the plaster material and hold onto it while wetting the roll in a bucket of warm water (Fig. 19–38). The excess water is removed by shaking and squeezing the roll. Do not squeeze excessively or excessive plaster will be lost. Fiberglass material is held in a bucket of clean water until thoroughly wet, and the excess water is shaken out.

When application of the cast is completed, the outer layer is smoothed by running your hand cream–covered gloved hands up and down the cast. Hand cream provides a slick surface, which allows a smooth finish to be placed on the final layer. The hand cream should only be used following the completion of the cast, since it may interfere with curing and bonding of the deeper layers. The bottom of the cast is pro-

tected from wear by capping it with hard acrylic (Technovit, Jorgensen Laboratories) (Fig. 19–39). An elastic adhesive tape is placed around the top of the cast and attached to the skin or a piece of stockinette is pulled over the top and taped to the cast and the limb above the cast to prevent debris (wood shavings) from getting down inside the cast (Fig. 19–40).

Stall confinement is mandatory after cast application. The patient must be monitored daily. Indications for cast change or removal include breakage, increased lameness, swelling, or exudates coming out of the top of the cast. Horses vary in their reaction and tolerance to a cast. If there is any doubt, a cast should be removed and the limb evaluated.

TECHNICIAN NOTE

The large animal patient must be confined to a stall and monitored daily after cast application.

Foot Cast

This type of cast affords the ability to immobilize lacerations of the coronary band and heel bulb (Fig. 19–41) without the

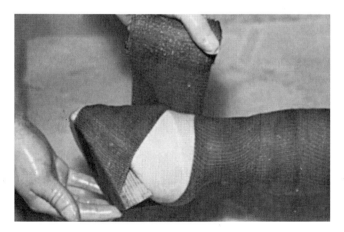

Figure 19-37. A wooden wedge block is placed underneath the heel and incorporated with the last layer of cast material.

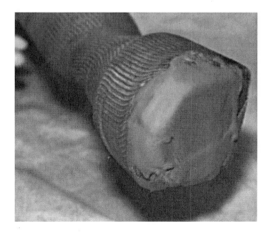

Figure 19-39. The bottom of the cast is protected from wear by capping it with hard acrylic (Technovit).

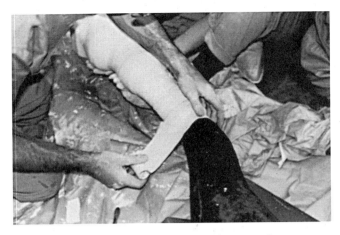

Figure 19-40. Elastic adhesive tape is placed on top of the cast to form a seal between the skin and cast that prevents debris from getting down inside the cast.

expense and involvement of a half-limb cast. The cast reduces motion and gaping of the wound and physically impedes the formation of exuberant granulation tissue in open wounds. The combination of suturing and casting provides the best cosmetic and functional end result, no matter how old the laceration. If exuberant granulation tissue is present, it is surgically excised before application of the cast.

A foot cast is applied in the same manner as a half-limb cast, but with a few alterations. Antimicrobial ointment and wound dressing are applied over the wound (Fig. 19–42). The foot is held in a near-normal standing position during application of the casting material. A heel block is not used. The top of the cast should stop just distal to the fetlock joint. It is important that none of the casting material impinge upon the joint; otherwise a sore will develop due to the motion of the joint (Fig. 19–43). The cast is left in place for 14 to 21 days, depending on the amount of tension required to close the wound and the amount of tissue deficit that was left to heal by

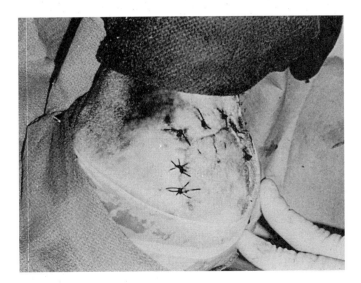

Figure 19-41. A heel bulb laceration on a horse that has been sutured.

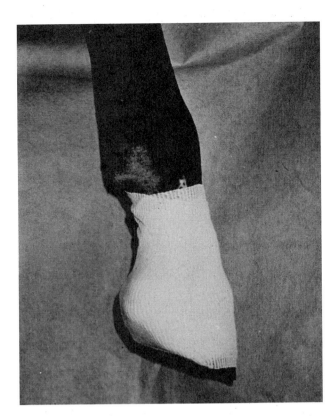

Figure 19-42. Wound dressing is applied over a heel bulb or coronary band laceration before casting.

second intention (Fig. 19–44). The cast is left on longer with greater suture tension and tissue deficit.

Tube Casts

In most cases, a cast completely encloses the foot. However, casts are modified for other purposes as well. *Tube* or *sleeve casts* are a special type of cast used in foals for the treatment of angular limb deformities associated with defective ossification in the carpus or tarsus (Fig. 19–45). By not incorporating the foot, these casts allow continued use of flexor tendons and prevent laxity that may develop with full-limb casts in foals.

To apply the cast, the foal is anesthetized or heavily sedated and placed in lateral recumbency. A double layer of stockinette (2-inch diameter) is placed over the entire limb. A strip (3 to 5 cm wide) of orthopedic felt is placed around the limb a few centimeters distal to the olecranon and at the level of the fetlock. The limb is positioned as straight as possible, and a layer of plaster of Paris followed by two or three layers of fiberglass (3-inch) is applied to the limb to the level of the orthopedic felt pads. The ends of the stockinette are folded over and incorporated into the last layer of cast.

Cast Removal

Removal of a cast is best performed with the animal standing. During cast removal there is a risk of reinjury to the limb in the animal trying to recover from anesthesia. However, general anesthesia is used if the cast is being changed. The cast is split on the medial and lateral surface, and the cut is continued under the foot with a Stryker saw (Fig. 19–46). With this ap-

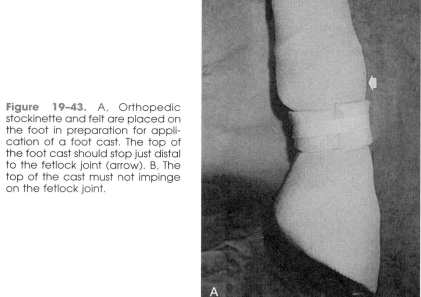

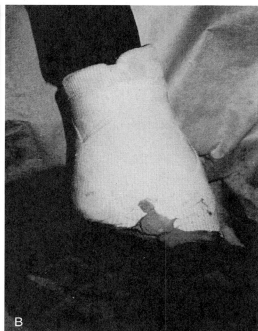

Figure 19-43. A, Orthopedic stockinette and felt are placed on the foot in preparation for application of a foot cast. The top of the foot cast should stop just distal to the fetlock joint (arrow). B, The top of the cast must not impinge on the fetlock joint.

Figure 19-44. A foot cast, applied to manage coronary band and heel bulb lacerations, is left in place for 14 to 21 days.

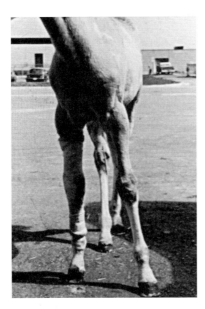

Figure 19-45. Tube cast on a foal with defective ossification of the carpal bones. (Courtesy of C. Wayne McIlwraith.)

proach, injury to the flexor and extensor tendons can be avoided. When cutting over bony prominences, one should be careful to avoid lacerating the skin. Once the cast is completely cut, the two halves are separated with cast spreaders. A support wrap is then placed on the limb.

> **TECHNICIAN NOTE**
>
> A cast is split on the medial and lateral surfaces to avoid injury to the flexor and extensor tendons.

BANDAGING AND CAST APPLICATION TECHNIQUES FOR CATTLE

Limb Bandaging and Cast Application

The principles applied to these procedures are the same in cattle as in horses, but there are specific techniques related to cattle. Cattle often are not as cooperative as horses, and more restraint is required.

With cattle, a cast can be applied directly over the dewclaws without causing major problems. Sores from motion of the cast can occur in this area because of the inability to closely fit the cast. This can be remedied by placing a pad of orthopedic felt, with holes cut out for the dewclaws, between the dewclaws (Fig. 19–47).

Application of a Claw Block

A wooden block is applied to an unaffected claw for various reasons: to alleviate weight-bearing on adjacent claw if it is fractured or injured, or to protect an operated area by raising it higher off the ground after amputation of an adjacent claw. The block is usually made from a piece of wood 5 cm thick and cut

to the shape of the sole surface of the claw. Grooves are cut in the ground surface for traction (Fig. 19–48).

The claw is first trimmed and debris is removed by means of an electric sander or rasp. This is an important step for effective bonding of the acrylic to the claw. The block is then bonded to the horny surface of the claw with acrylic cement, such as Technovit (Jorgensen Laboratories) (Fig. 19–49).

Modified Thomas Splint

Despite advances in external and internal skeletal fixation, modified Thomas splints are still often used in cattle and small ruminants as a means of external skeletal fixation. The modified Thomas splint is often used in combination with internal fixation or a cast. The indications for its use include fractures of the tibia or radius, or ligamentous injuries of the stifle. Pressure sores in the inguinal or axillary region are a problem when a Thomas splint is used, despite padding of the metal ring.

Application of a modified Thomas splint in large ruminants does require special equipment, such as a conduit bender, to bend the round rod iron used to construct the splint. The design of the splint varies somewhat among clinicians, but the purpose is the same.

The animal is first placed in lateral recumbency with the affected leg uppermost. A template to fit the individual animal,

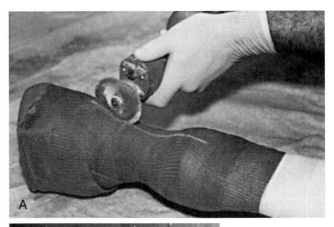

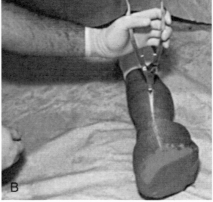

Figure 19-46. Removal of a limb cast from a horse. A, With a Stryker saw, the cast is split on the medial and lateral surface, and the cut is continued under the foot. B, Once the cast is completely cut, the two halves are separated with cast spreaders.

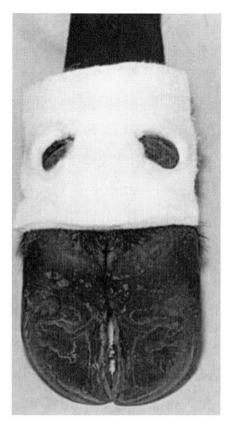

Figure 19-47. A piece of orthopedic felt, with holes cut out, can be placed between the dew claws to reduce pressure sores and motion under a cast.

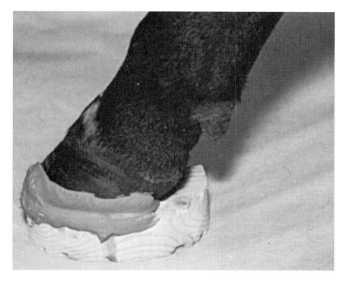

Figure 19-49. A wooden block is cemented to the unaffected claw with acrylic.

devised from a nasogastric tube or other similar flexible tubing, is used to construct the ring that will encircle the proximal part of the leg (Fig. 19–50). The ring should be large enough not to impinge on any bony prominences. The rod iron is bent in a ring the same size as the template. The variation in design occurs with the extensions that come off the ring to support the animal's limb.

One design has the extensions coming off cranially and caudally to the leg. The extensions of the splint must be shaped to conform to the angles of the hock and stifle. These extensions are also bent away (lateral) from the flat plane of the ring to allow the ventral part of the ring to fit into the axillary or inguinal region. Another design has the extensions coming off

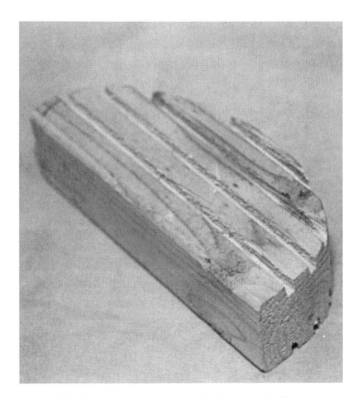

Figure 19-48. A claw block made from wood. Grooves are cut in the block to improve traction and bonding.

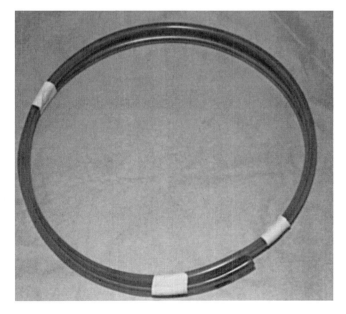

Figure 19-50. A nasogastric tube can be used as a template to construct the ring of a modified Thomas splint that will encircle the proximal portion of the leg.

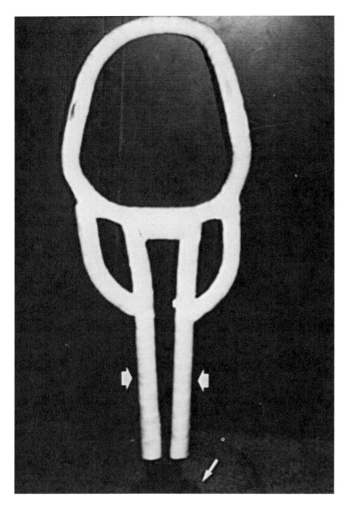

Figure 19-51. A modified Thomas splint. Extensions of the splint (large arrows) come off the ventral aspect of the ring and are positioned medial to the leg. A plate with threaded rods is constructed to fit under the animal's foot (small arrow). (Courtesy of Dr. Dwight F. Wolfe.)

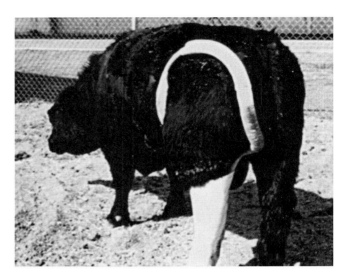

Figure 19-52. The limb and modified Thomas splint are covered with layers of cast material and thereby incorporated to stabilize the limb. (Courtesy of Dr. Dwight F. Wolfe.)

the ventral aspect of the ring (Fig. 19–51). The ring is then bent so that the extensions are positioned medial to the limb, and to fit the contour of the upper limb (Fig. 19–52).

A foot plate is constructed with two threaded rods attached to the extensions of the splint (Fig. 19–51). A piece of rod iron can be used instead and bent in a U shape and positioned under the foot and connected to the ends of the extensions of the splint. Some splints are devised with extensions that are threaded so that the length of the splint can be adjusted. The ring is lightly padded with cotton. Holes are drilled into the toes of the hoof wall and wired to the bottom of the splint. A slight amount of traction should be applied to the limb as the splint is applied. Traction should be minimal within the splint, so as not to create excessive pressure in the axillary or inguinal regions, which could interfere with venous drainage or distract the fracture fragments.

Once the splint is in position, the limb and splint are then covered with layers of cast material, and thereby incorporated together (Fig. 19–52). Cast material should first be placed around the carpus or tarsus to give these areas initial support from bowing medially. The cast material should be applied as proximal as possible.

Recommended Reading

Small Animal

Fowler D: Principles of wound healing. *In* Harari J (editor): Surgical Complications and Wound Healing in the Small Animal Practice. Philadelphia, WB Saunders, 1993, pp 1–32.

Knecht CD, Allen AR, Williams DJ, et al: Fundamental Techniques in Veterinary Surgery, 2nd ed. Philadelphia, WB Saunders, 1981.

Mason LK: Treatment of contaminated wounds. *In* Harari J (editor): Surgical Complications and Wound Healing in the Small Animal Practice. Philadelphia, WB Saunders, 1993, pp 33–62.

Lozier SM: Topical wound management. *In* Harari J (editor): Surgical Complications and Wound Healing in the Small Animal Practice. Philadelphia, WB Saunders, 1993, pp 63–88.

Swaim SF and Henderson RA: Small Animal Wound Management. Philadelphia, Lea & Febiger, 1990.

Large Animal

Adams SB, and Fessler JF: Treatment of radial-ulnar and tibial fractures in cattle, using a modified Thomas splint-cast combination. J Am Vet Assoc 183:430–433, 1983.

Arighi M: Drains, dressings, and external coaptation devices. *In* Auer JA (editor): Equine Surgery. Philadelphia, WB Saunders, 1992, pp 159–176.

Fiberglass Casting Techniques. Product information pamphlet. NJ, Pitman-Moore, 1984.

Lindsay WA: Wound treatment in horses: Healing by third intention. Vet Med 83:506–514, 1988.

Peyton LC: Wound healing in the horse. Part II. Approach to the treatment of traumatic wounds. Compendium 9:191–202, 1987.

Stashak TS: Bandaging and casting techniques. *In* Stashak TS (editor): Equine Wound Management. Philadelphia, Lea & Febiger, 1991, pp 258–272.

Turner AS: Large animal orthopedics. *In* Jennings PB (editor): The Practice of Large Animal Surgery. Philadelphia, WB Saunders, 1984, pp 768–780.

20 Pain Management

Jill E. Sackman

The veterinarian and veterinary technician together have an obligation to recognize and alleviate animal pain. This task is difficult, for only human patients can point to their specific source of discomfort and describe it. We must assume that veterinary patients experience pain under any circumstance in which humans would feel pain. There are, in fact, many similarities between animals and humans in the anatomical and chemical pathways of pain perception. Differences that do exist are generally attributed to alternative pathways for pain and not the absence of them. For many years there has been an erroneous but well-meaning belief that pain in animals is beneficial—that it provides a constant reminder to the patient to avoid movement that might cause further injury. This line of thought is illogical in that uncontrolled pain may lead to prolonged hospitalization, poor wound healing, and an increased rate of complications and mortality in both animals and humans. Recently it has become widely acknowledged that the recognition and alleviation of pain in animals is the essence of good patient care.

ORGANIZATION OF PAIN-CONDUCTING SYSTEMS

Peripheral Nervous System

The transmission of a painful sensation involves stimulation of receptors and peripheral nerves in the traumatized tissue with subsequent conduction through the spinal cord to multiple areas in the brain. When a painful stimulus occurs, a chain of events that lead to the sensation of pain is initiated. The degree of tissue sensitivity to pain is directly related to the density of pain receptors present. Pain receptors respond to traumatic stimuli by converting the chemical, mechanical, or thermal insult into nerve impulses. These impulses are conducted from the peripheral tissue to the spinal cord and brain. Tissues containing a high density of pain receptors include skin, periosteum, joint capsule, muscle, tendon, and arterial wall (Guyton and Hall, 1996). The tissue of the brain is one of the most important pain-free regions in the body.

> **TECHNICIAN NOTE**
>
> Tissues containing a high density of pain receptors include skin, periosteum, joint capsule, muscle, tendon, and arterial wall.

Peripheral nerves that transmit the sensation of pain to the central nervous system vary in size and in the speed with which they conduct sensation (Fig. 20–1). Nerve fibers with a myelin sheath *(A delta fibers)* are larger and conduct pain much more rapidly than the smaller unmyelinated ones *(C fibers)*. Evidence indicates that A delta and C nerve fibers are capable of producing two distinct sensations of pain. Most painful events initially produce a sharp prickling pain followed by a dull burning sensation. The fast-conducting A delta fibers appear to be responsible for the rapid initial sharp sensation (Guyton and Hall, 1996). The subsequent burning or throbbing pain involves conduction by the slower C fibers.

Some of the most intensely painful sensations result from chemical injury such as that associated with inflammation. Chemical substances such as prostaglandins, histamine, and

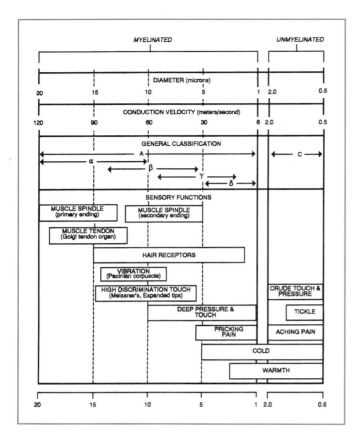

Figure 20-1. Physiological classifications and functions of peripheral sensory nerve fibers.

proteolytic enzymes are made by the body during inflammation. These substances are so potent that they not only stimulate pain receptors but can actually damage them. One of the most important classes of chemical mediators of pain formed during inflammation are the metabolic products of arachidonic acid. This group of metabolites includes the prostaglandins and leukotrienes. Prostaglandin production from arachidonic acid is blocked by nonsteroidal anti-inflammatory drugs (NSAIDs), of which aspirin is an example.

TECHNICIAN NOTE

Some of the most intensely painful sensations result from chemical injury such as that associated with inflammation.

Tissue Damage as a Cause of Pain

Tissue ischemia can be an important source of pain. When blood flow to a tissue is blocked, the tissues become painful within a short period of time. The greater the rate of the tissue's metabolism, the more rapidly the pain appears. The cause of pain during ischemia is probably due to build-up of lactic acid during anaerobic tissue metabolism. It is also possible that the release of chemical substances, such as histamine and prostaglandins, that occurs with cell damage may also be involved during ischemia.

Muscle spasm is a frequently documented cause of pain. Spasm-associated pain may result from the direct stimulation of mechanical pain receptors during the spasm or from chemical receptors as a result of muscle ischemia. Muscle spasm is known to cause a decrease in blood flow as well as an increase in the rate of muscle metabolism, both of which increase the risk of ischemia. Additional instances in which mechanical receptors might be stimulated to transmit pain include a crushing injury or a sharp blow.

Thermal receptors are stimulated by extremes of temperature as occurs with burns or frostbite. Often clinical pain results from the stimulation to some degree of all the receptor subtypes and not simply a single one.

Central Nervous System

The pathways for pain transmission in the central nervous system (CNS) are considerably more complex than those in the periphery. Nerve fibers transmitting pain impulses from the peripheral nerves enter the spinal cord through the dorsal nerve roots. Once the fibers have entered the spinal cord, they may associate with several types of neural hormones (such as substance P, somatostatin, cholecystokinin), which play a role in suppressing or augmenting the transmission and subsequent sensation of pain.

Once the impulse reaches the spinal cord, nerve fibers segregate into neural tracts, which carry specifically grouped fiber types (Fig. 20–2). The spinothalamic tract is important in the transmission of pain impulses through the spinal cord and to the brain. The nerve fibers or axons, which travel in the *spinothalamic tract*, terminate in several areas of the thalamic area of the brain and brain stem. The fibers terminating in the thalamus are involved in the perception and conscious discriminatory aspects of pain, including location, nature, and intensity. Pain fibers also reach the *reticular activating system* (RAS) in the brain and cause the animal to become stimulated and alert to the sensation. The stimulation of the RAS is also responsible for the sleeplessness and restlessness associated with painful episodes (Guyton and Hall, 1996).

Endogenous Opioids

The intensity of pain can be modified substantially in the body by the release of opiate-like (opioid) compounds that are naturally present in the central nervous system. Specific areas in the brain and spinal cord are capable of producing natural opioid compounds which, when they bind at opiate receptors, cause the relief of pain (analgesia). Natural opioid compounds have generated considerable interest in recent years. Since their discovery in the 1970s, more than 20 different naturally occurring opioids have been found, including beta-endorphin, beta-lipotrophin, gamma-endorphin, dynorphin, leu-enkephalin, and met-enkephalin. Evidence indicates that both stress and trauma can stimulate the CNS to release the endogenous opioid compounds, thus stimulating the body's own analgesic system.

Pain Localization

The localization of pain to a particular area of the body is the responsibility of the CNS. Pain can be poorly localized because sensory nerve fibers may be present in low densities in the peripheral tissue or because pain pathways frequently branch and converge, making it difficult for the brain to localize the sensation. For example, the pain resulting from gastroesopha-

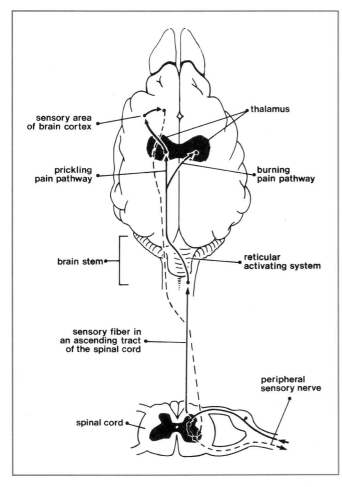

Figure 20-2. Transmission and segregation of nerve fibers carrying pain impulses within the central nervous system.

geal acid reflux in humans is felt as a diffuse burning sensation only vaguely localized to the sternum. A dull, poorly defined burning sensation is felt instead of well-localized pain, partly because of the poor sensory innervation that internal organs (viscera) have. Pain inflicted to tissues with a high density of pain receptors, such as the skin, is generally much more precisely localized than the pain associated with internal organs.

In clinical practice, pain associated with the viscera of the thorax and abdomen is often used to help diagnose disease. The sensation of pain experienced from visceral tissues is different from surface or somatic (such as skin) pain. Somatic pain from the skin is highly localized because of the large number of pain receptors present in this area. Visceral tissues, such as the bladder or intestinal tract, by contrast, are poorly innervated. Because of poor visceral innervation, abdominal and thoracic pain often occur only following extensive, diffuse irritation. Common causes of visceral pain include leakage of damaging substances (such as bile, gastric acid) from the gastrointestinal tract leading to peritonitis or overdistention of the intestinal tract, which might occur with an obstruction or gastric torsion.

RECOGNIZING PAIN IN ANIMALS
Problems with Evaluation

Recognizing pain and anxiety in animals is critical prior to appropriate analgesic selection and pain relief. An animal con-

fronted with a painful situation may exhibit specific behavior patterns, often secondary to stimulation of the autonomic nervous system. The typical nervous system response to pain and stress forms the basis of the classic fight-or-flight reaction. Autonomic nervous system stimulation results in the release of epinephrine and norepinephrine (catecholamines) from the adrenal glands, resulting in elevated heart rate, blood pressure, and respiratory rate, and pupillary dilation (mydriasis). The fight-or-flight response, however, is not unique to painful situations; it may occur in purely stressful situations, such as the anxiety of being in the veterinarian's office. Because of its nonspecific nature, it is not possible to use autonomic stimulation as the sole criterion for pain evaluation. In addition to catecholamines, cortisol is released following pain and anxiety. Cortisol, like catecholamines, is released nonspecifically in response to stressful situations. Other nonspecific physiological signs that animals may exhibit with pain and anxiety include neutrophilia and lymphocytosis (secondary to elevated epinephrine); hyperglycemia (especially in cats); and polycythemia (secondary to splenic contraction).

TECHNICIAN NOTE

Recognizing pain and anxiety in animals is critical prior to appropriate analgesic selection and pain relief.

Signs of Pain and Distress: Animal Variability

Common physiological responses to pain include increased heart rate and blood pressure, pupillary dilation, increased respiratory rate, and arousal (Table 20–1). It is essential for the veterinary staff to be aware of normal physiological values, typical physical appearance, and behavior patterns for each species and breed seen in the practice. Behavioral responses to pain and anxiety vary not only by species involved but also between breeds and even among individuals. As an example, the behavioral response that a stoic hound might exhibit to

• Table 20–1 •

COMMON CLINICAL SIGNS OF PAIN OR DISTRESS	
SYSTEM	**SIGNS**
Cardiovascular	Elevated heart rate and blood pressure, decreased peripheral circulation, prolonged capillary refill, cool extremities (ears, paws)
Respiratory	Rapid, shallow breaths; panting
Digestive	Weight loss, poor growth (young), vomiting, inappetence, constipation, diarrhea, salivation
Musculoskeletal	Unsteady gait, lameness, weakness, tremors, shivering
Urinary	Reluctance to urinate, loss of house training
Laboratory findings	Neutrophilia, lymphocytosis, hyperglycemia, polycythemia, elevated cortisol, elevated catecholamines

postoperative pain will be considerably different from that of the nervous toy breeds. The veterinary staff is more likely to become aware of the pain and anxiety experienced by the toy breed than those experienced by the less vocal hound. Furthermore, behavioral responses to pain may vary between individuals or even families within a breed, making generalizations about signs of discomfort extremely difficult.

Clinical Evaluation of Pain

In many cases, an animal initially reacts to a painful situation by retreating in an attempt to remove itself from the source of discomfort. If this reaction fails to bring relief, the animal may rely upon other behavioral responses such as vocalization, increased attempts to escape, pacing, guarding, sleeplessness, and aggression (Table 20–2). Animals that are experiencing acute postoperative or traumatic pain may also respond by biting, licking, or scratching at the source of discomfort. Chronic, low-grade pain in animals is often associated with prolonged hospitalization, radiation, and chemotherapy; severe osteoarthritis may be manifested by failure to groom, lack of interest in surroundings, reluctance to move, anorexia, weight loss, constipation, and dysuria. Animals experiencing chronic pain may be withdrawn and quiet, unlike the seemingly "energized" state observed in animals experiencing acute pain. It is important to remember that not all signs of pain may be present at one time, and no single sign is a reliable indicator of the level of pain experienced.

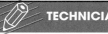

TECHNICIAN NOTE

Animals that are experiencing acute postoperative or traumatic pain may respond by biting, licking, or scratching at the site of discomfort.

CONTROL OF PAIN IN ANIMALS

Patient evaluation to identify the clinical signs of pain and distress is an area in which veterinary technicians can contribute

significantly. The veterinary technician is often the one involved most closely with the minute-by-minute treatment and monitoring of postoperative surgical and intensive care patients. The observant technician can contribute a great deal to pain relief by being observant and learning to recognize the clinical signs of discomfort in his or her patients. By recognizing that a patient is in pain, the technician can promptly alert the attending clinician and help in the formulation of an appropriate analgesic plan.

There are two main types of analgesics that are often considered in the control of pain in companion animals: non-narcotic anti-inflammatory drugs (mild analgesics) and narcotics (strong analgesics). The clinical indications for the use of each of these families of drugs are often very different. Likewise, their mechanism of action and adverse effects also differ significantly.

In the first section we examine the indications and adverse effects of the narcotic (opioid) analgesics, which are the most commonly used analgesics in the postoperative patient. The anti-inflammatory analgesics, covered later, are predominantly employed for mild to moderate chronic pain associated with the musculoskeletal system. Finally we consider the use of tranquilizers along with analgesic drugs to treat the anxiety often associated with pain and distress in companion animals.

Environment and Nursing Care

Environmental factors often affect the emotional component of pain perception in both humans and animals. It is important to provide as clean and comfortable a recovery and intensive care environment as possible. Keep the surroundings as familiar as possible to the animal, including providing toys or blankets from home or visits by owners in chronically hospitalized patients. When possible, animals will often recover better at home from noncritical illnesses if owners are able to provide good nursing care. Recovery areas should be quiet and located away from busy areas with loud animal and human noise. Imagine the distress a cat feels postoperatively listening to a howling dog in a cage below it. Remember that anxiety has the ability to amplify an animal's pain and discomfort. Try to provide as stress-free an environment as possible (Fig. 20–3).

During patient recovery, interaction with humans may also help to relieve stress and anxiety. Talking to an animal, stroking,

• Table 20–2 •

POSTOPERATIVE PAIN EVALUATION			
TYPE OF SURGERY	**SIGNS OF PAIN**	**SUSPECTED PAIN LEVEL**	**DURATION**
Head, ear, oral, dental	Rubbing; shaking; salivating; reluctance to eat, swallow, or drink; irritability; vocalizing	Moderate to high	Intermittent
Ophthalmologic	Rubbing, vocalizing, reluctance to move	High	Intermittent to continual
Orthopedic	Guarding, aggression, abnormal gait, self-mutilation, reluctance to move, dysuria, constipation	Moderate	Intermittent
Abdominal	Guarding, splinting, abnormal posture, vomiting, inappetence	Mild to moderate	Intermittent
Cardiovascular/thoracic	Changes in respiratory rate and pattern, reluctance to move, vocalizing	Moderate to high	Continual
Perirectal	Licking, biting, scooting, self-mutilation, constipation	Moderate	Intermittent

From Johnson JM: The veterinarian's responsibility: Assessing and managing acute pain in dogs and cats. Part I. Compendium Continuing Educ Pract Vet 13:804–807, 1991; Wright EM, Marcella KL, Woodson JF: Animal pain: Evaluation and control. Lab Anim 14:20–36, 1985; and author's clinical experience.

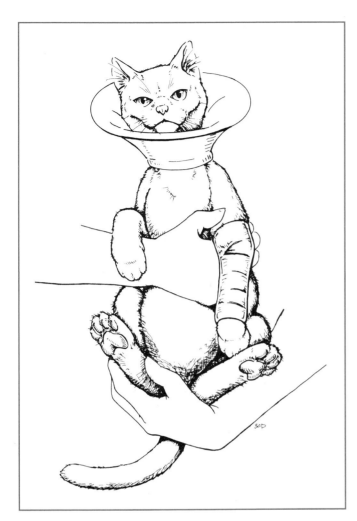

Figure 20–3. Good nursing care is critical to the management of patients experiencing pain and distress.

and petting can help to reduce restlessness, rapid breathing, increased heart rate, and other signs of discomfort. Also remember that an animal's pain may be greatly exacerbated by frequent moving, monitoring, or administration of medications. Prepare a dry, comfortable area for the patient and schedule treatments and monitoring so that the animal is moved and disturbed a minimal amount. Finally, be aware that some patients will experience a great deal of anxiety over not being able to go outdoors to urinate or defecate. For dogs that are able to walk, provide them an opportunity to get outside at least twice daily.

ANALGESIC DRUGS: THE NARCOTICS

Narcotic drugs (opioids) are the oldest and most extensively studied analgesic drugs available. When morphine is administered to humans, it is said to either diminish the intensity of pain or eliminate it altogether. Narcotics control pain but preserve many of the other senses (such as touch, vibration, vision, and hearing). The analgesic effect of narcotics is due to their interaction at specific opioid receptors located within the CNS. Opioid receptors are present in both the brain and the spinal

cord, making the alteration of pain sensation possible at multiple areas (Branson et al., 1995).

Five categories of receptors for opioid drugs have been described to date. Each receptor subtype produces a slightly different response following binding of an opioid drug (Table 20–3). For example, the mu receptor subtype will cause respiratory depression, sedation, euphoria, and addiction when a drug stimulates it. Another receptor subtype, the kappa receptor, produces analgesia and sedation without the drug addiction response.

Opioids referred to as *pure agonists* are substances that exert their effects by only stimulating opioid receptors. An example of a pure agonist is *morphine*. The subclass of drugs known as the opioid *antagonists* bind at opioid receptors, but block or fail to elicit a response. The antagonists bind the opioid receptors and displace agonists such as morphine. The antagonists are often referred to as "narcotic reversal" agents because of their ability to reverse the effects of the opioid agonists by displacing them at the receptor level. The classic opioid antagonist is *naloxone*.

The final category of opioid drugs is the *mixed agonist/antagonist*. These substances have been synthesized to act like agonists at some of the opioid receptors and antagonists at others. A good example of this class of drug is *butorphanol*. Butorphanol acts like naloxone at the mu receptor, but binds like an agonist at the kappa receptor. This mixed effect allows butorphanol to be a good analgesic without having the addictive properties of morphine.

In general, the narcotic drugs produce minimal cardiovascular effects and are safe in patients with cardiac disease. They are known to produce bradycardia and can produce hypotension if they stimulate the release of histamine (morphine and meperidine). Their effects on the respiratory system include respiratory depression (decreased rate and tidal volume) and a decreased sensitivity of the respiratory center to increasing levels of carbon dioxide. Narcotics can also cause salivation, nausea, vomiting, and nonpropulsive intestinal motility (segmental contractions). Along with their analgesic effects, these drugs will produce sedation and in some animals dysphoria (hallucinations) (Short, 1987).

The narcotic drugs are extensively metabolized by the liver and excreted in the urine. Animals with liver disease or neonates with poorly developed hepatic metabolism require reduced dosages of narcotics to avoid prolonged drug effects.

Morphine

Morphine is considered to be the prototypic narcotic analgesic (Fig. 20–4). Two advantages of morphine are analgesia and sedation. The effects of morphine are reversed with narcotic antagonists, such as naloxone. Adverse effects of morphine administration include depression of the respiratory and central nervous systems. Morphine is also known to stimulate the chemoreceptor trigger zone (CTZ) in the brain stem and cause vomiting (Branson et al., 1995).

 TECHNICIAN NOTE

Morphine is considered to be the prototypic narcotic analgesic.

• Table 20–3 •

DRUG	RECEPTOR ACTIVITY		
	Mu	**Kappa**	**Sigma**
Agonist opioids: fentanyl, morphine, meperidine, oxymorphone	Agonist	Agonist	Agonist
Butorphanol	Weak antagonist	Agonist	Antagonist
Pentazocine	Weak antagonist	Agonist	Antagonist
Buprenorphine	Weak agonist	Antagonist	Antagonist
Nalorphine	Weak agonist	Antagonist	Antagonist
Naloxone	Antagonist	Antagonist	Antagonist

Depression of the respiratory and central nervous systems may limit the use of morphine in many clinical situations, such as shock, severe head injury, and any disease in which respiratory function is compromised (such as pneumonia, pneumothorax). The use of morphine is not recommended during intraocular ophthalmic surgery because of its ability to increase pressure within the eye. As with most of the narcotics, morphine is metabolized by the liver and excreted through the kidneys. Care should be taken when administering morphine to animals with renal or hepatic compromise, since drug elimination may be prolonged. At higher doses, morphine can be excitatory for cats, cattle, swine, and horses. Morphine given in lower doses or combined with a tranquilizer appears to reduce the undesirable effects in cats.

Meperidine

Meperidine (Demerol, Winthrop Pharmaceuticals) is a synthetic opioid agonist with approximately one fifth of the analgesic effect of morphine. Meperidine is painful if given intramuscularly (IM), and if injected rapidly intravenously (IV), it can cause severe hypotension. Because of its mild sedative effects, meperidine is frequently used as a preoperative sedative. Owing to meperidine's rapid metabolism and weak analgesia, it is relatively ineffective for postoperative pain control.

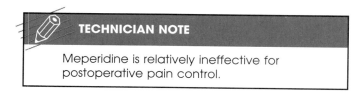

TECHNICIAN NOTE

Meperidine is relatively ineffective for postoperative pain control.

Fentanyl

Fentanyl (Sublimaze, Janssen) is a synthetic opioid with approximately 100 times the potency of morphine and 500 times the potency of meperidine. Fentanyl acts rapidly after IV or IM injection. Profound analgesia and respiratory depression develop within 6 to 8 minutes after injection. Auditory sensitization and elevation of the thermoregulatory center leading to panting also frequently occur. Since bradycardia is commonly produced, concurrent use of atropine or glycopyrrolate is recommended. Extreme caution should be used if fentanyl is administered concurrently with barbiturates (such as thiamylal or thiopental) because bradycardia, hypotension, and respiratory depression can be difficult to reverse (Branson et al., 1995).

Fentanyl has a short duration of action, with peak effects lasting for only 30 to 45 minutes. Like morphine and meperidine, the effects of fentanyl can be reversed with narcotic antagonists such as naloxone. Although fentanyl is an excellent analgesic, its use in veterinary medicine has largely been abandoned (with the exception of administration by continuous IV infusion) because of its short half-life. Fentanyl is most commonly available as a neuroleptanalgesic (narcotic and tranquilizer mix), for which purpose it is combined with the tranquilizer droperidol (Innovar, Pitman-Moore) (Fig. 20–5).

Several new synthetic compounds related to fentanyl have recently been developed, but because of their short half-life, use of these drugs in veterinary medicine will probably be limited. One such drug is afentanyl which has an ultra-short duration of action. Because of rapid body clearance, afentanyl allows for excellent control of blood concentrations during IV infusion. Sufentanil, also related to fentanyl, has a half-life intermediate between afentanyl and fentanyl. Sufentanil appears to have fewer adverse side effects than do the others, perhaps because of its high opioid receptor specificity (Short, 1987).

Oxymorphone

Oxymorphone (P/M Oxymorphone HCl, Pitman-Moore) is a semisynthetic narcotic analgesic that is approximately 10 times as potent an analgesic as morphine. It has a duration of action from 4 to 6 hours. Adverse effects are similar to those of

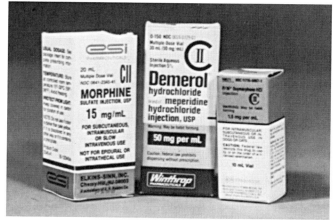

Figure 20–4. Narcotic agonists commonly used for pain control in small animal practice.

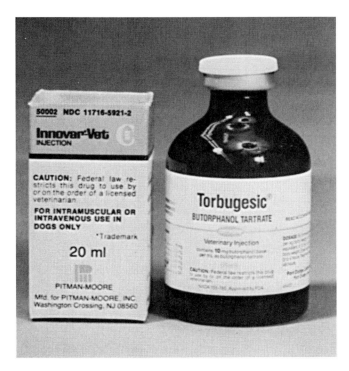

Figure 20–5. Butorphanol is a popular nonschedule, mixed agonist/antagonist analgesic. Fentanyl is combined with droperidol in the neuroleptanalgesic Innovar.

morphine; however, it appears to cause less respiratory depression and gastrointestinal stimulation. Oxymorphone can cause significant auditory sensitization. Bradycardia is frequently observed if an anticholinergic (such as atropine or glycopyrrolate) is not administered concurrently. Elevation of the thermoregulatory center may lead to panting, as seen with other opioids. Oxymorphone is considered an excellent analgesic for moderate to intense pain because of its potency and duration of action.

TECHNICIAN NOTE

Oxymorphone is considered an excellent analgesic for moderate to intense pain because of its potency and duration of action.

Epidural Use of Opioids

Because of significant success with the epidural use of opioid compounds in humans, much attention has recently focused on their use in companion animals (Popilskis et al., 1991; McMurphy, 1993). Instead of being given systemically, epidural opioids are administered through spinal needles or catheters (Fig. 20–6) on top of the outer meningeal covering of the spinal cord (dura mater). Because of the high density of opioid receptors in the spinal cord, epidural administration of opioids offers the advantage of prolonged analgesia (up to five times longer than IM administration) without prolonged sedation and respiratory depression.

Opiates deposited epidurally enter the spinal cord by three pathways: (1) diffusion across the meninges, (2) along nerve

roots, and (3) by uptake into the spinal arteries and epidural veins. The onset of action of epidural opioids varies markedly among drugs depending upon their molecular weight, ionization, and lipid solubility. Lipid-soluble drugs such as fentanyl have rapid onset of action and very short duration, whereas water-soluble morphine has a delayed onset and long duration.

For postoperative epidural analgesia in veterinary patients, morphine is used most commonly. Subarachnoid or epidural administration of preservative-free morphine (Duramorph PF, Elkins-Sinn, Cherry Hill, N.J.; Astromorpho/PF, Astra Pharmaceutical Products, Westborough, Mass.) has been shown to be safe and efficacious. Epidural morphine is an excellent technique for providing postoperative analgesia after pelvic or hind-limb surgery. Administered at the lumbosacral space, it has been used after thoracic surgery, but depends upon cephalad migration of the drug within the cerebrospinal fluid (CSF). The dose of epidural morphine commonly used in dogs and cats is 0.05 to 0.1 mg/kg of preservative-free drug. Epidural morphine should be administered 30 to 60 minutes prior to recovery from anesthesia. Duration of analgesia is from 6 to 24 hours.

Mixed Action Agonist/Antagonist Narcotic Analgesics

Butorphanol

Butorphanol (Torbugesic, Fort Dodge) belongs to a group of synthetic analgesics with combined agonist and antagonist

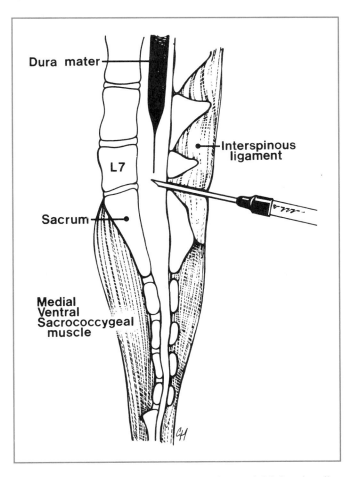

Figure 20–6. Epidural administration of an opioid drug has the advantage of providing analgesia for longer durations than systemic opioid use.

properties. Butorphanol is considered to be a weak antagonist at the mu receptor but a strong agonist at the kappa receptor. Butorphanol is three to five times more potent an analgesic than morphine. The antagonist activity of butorphanol is nearly 50 times less than that of naloxone. The respiratory depression produced by butorphanol is similar to that of morphine; however, butorphanol reaches a "ceiling" effect beyond which higher doses fail to increase the depression. The ceiling on respiratory depression makes butorphanol a somewhat safer drug than morphine. Butorphanol is also a well-recognized antitussive and has also been used as an antiemetic in cancer patients. Similar to other narcotics, butorphanol is metabolized by the liver and has a plasma half-life of 3 to 4 hours in dogs.

In animal studies, butorphanol seems to be less addictive than other narcotics; therefore, it remains a Food and Drug Administration (FDA) nonschedule drug (no records of inventory and use need be kept, as is the rule for other narcotics).

Recent studies in the dog indicate that butorphanol will provide visceral analgesia (such as gastrointestinal) if given subcutaneously, but only for 23 to 53 minutes. In the cat, butorphanol provides somatic (such as skin) analgesia for up to 118 minutes, but only at doses of 0.8 mg/kg. Visceral analgesia in the cat can be achieved for as long as 360 minutes if 0.1 mg/kg is administered IV. Butorphanol appears to have a relatively short duration of action and is a better analgesic for visceral pain than for somatic pain. Clinically, butorphanol appears to act as a good analgesic for mild to moderate pain in the dog and cat. Because of its short analgesic half-life, butorphanol has to be administered frequently.

Much interest has focused recently on the use of butorphanol for its partial narcotic reversal (antagonist) abilities. Because butorphanol blocks agonist effects at the mu receptor, much of the respiratory depression and sedation associated with the pure agonists can be reversed, yet analgesia will be maintained owing to continued kappa receptor agonist activity. Recent work has indicated that analgesic doses of butorphanol can reverse oxymorphone sedation equally as well as low doses of naloxone.

Buprenorphine

Buprenorphine (Buprenex, Norwich Eaton) is a mixed agonist/antagonist that has become popular in Europe as an analgesic and sedative drug. This drug differs from butorphanol in that its association and dissociation with the opioid receptors occur slowly. Because of its slow receptor association, it may take up to 30 minutes after IV injection for buprenorphine to take effect. Buprenorphine has a longer duration of action than butorphanol because of its tight binding to, and slow dissociation from, opioid receptors. Because it binds tightly to the opioid receptor, its effects can be difficult to reverse with naloxone. An important adverse effect following injection of buprenorphine is its delayed respiratory depression. It has been recommended that animals given buprenorphine be observed closely for at least 2 hours following administration.

Pentazocine

Pentazocine (Talwin-V, Upjohn) is also a member of the narcotic agonist/antagonist family. The drug became popular in the 1960s because its potential for abuse was lower than that of many of the other narcotics available. Unlike the FDA sched-

ule II drugs, pentazocine is a schedule IV drug, requiring only a current drug inventory list.

The major effects of the drug are similar to those of the other narcotics. Cardiovascular and respiratory depression are minimal. Unfortunately, pentazocine has a short analgesic half-life (15 minutes), appears to be a poor analgesic in the dog and cat, and is relatively ineffective for most types of postoperative pain.

Narcotic Antagonists

Relatively minor structural changes to opioids can convert a drug with primary agonist activity to one with antagonist action. Narcotic antagonists allow for the quick reversal of a narcotic overdose and its associated respiratory depression, sedation, and analgesia.

Naloxone

Naloxone (P/M Naloxone HCl, Pitman-Moore) (Fig. 20–7) is a pure antagonist with 50 times the reversal potential of butorphanol. Naloxone is regarded as a pure competitive antagonist at all the opioid receptors and is not regulated by the Controlled Substances Act. Small doses of naloxone (0.4 to 0.8 mg), if administered IM or IV, rapidly reverse the effects of morphine-like opioids.

In patients with respiratory depression, an increase in respiratory rate occurs within 1 to 2 minutes following naloxone

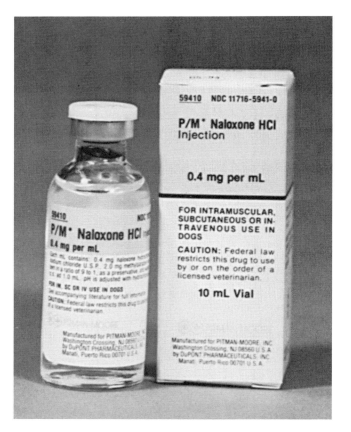

Figure 20–7. Naloxone is a pure opioid antagonist capable of reversing both the analgesic and untoward effects of opioid drugs.

administration. The sedative, cardiovascular, and analgesic effects of the opioids are also rapidly reversed. Antagonist effects will last for 1 to 4 hours, depending on the initial dose given. When naloxone is being used to reverse a pure agonist, readministration may be necessary, since many of the narcotics will last longer than naloxone. At low doses, naloxone has a high binding affinity for the mu receptor, which is responsible for respiratory depression and sedation; much higher doses are needed to antagonize the kappa receptor.

> **TECHNICIAN NOTE**
>
> Naloxone rapidly reverses the effects of morphine-like opioids and is not regulated by the Controlled Substances Act.

Nalorphine

Nalorphine (Nalline, MSD-Agvet) is a morphine derivative that is classified as a partial agonist, but it reverses the effects of many of the opioids. Nalorphine is a schedule III drug, which means that it is less addictive than a schedule II drug such as morphine. In the presence of narcotic agonists, nalorphine acts as a partial antagonist. Like butorphanol, nalorphine may be used alone for sedation and analgesia. The drug has the advantage of having less CNS and respiratory depression than the pure agonists.

MANAGEMENT OF CONTROLLED SUBSTANCES

Controlled substances, as defined by the Controlled Substance Act of 1970, include opioids (narcotics), barbiturates, hallucinogens (ketamine), amphetamines, and other addictive or habituating drugs. This act regulates the manufacturing, distribution, and dispensing of controlled substances. The licensed veterinarian wishing to prescribe or maintain controlled drugs must register with the Federal Drug Enforcement Agency (DEA).

Controlled substances must be kept in a locked cabinet or safe with attachment to a concrete floor. Strict inventory, including patient/client name and volume dispensed, is required by law (Branson et al., 1995).

Controlled drugs are listed in five different schedules (C-I, C-II, C-III, C-IV, C-V). *Schedule I* drugs have a high abuse potential and are not currently accepted in the United States for treatment. Examples include heroin, lysergic acid diethylamide (LSD), mescaline, and marijuana. *Schedule II* drugs have a high abuse potential and can produce severe psychic and physical dependence in humans. Examples include morphine, meperidine, oxymorphone, and pentobarbital. *Schedule III* drugs have less abuse potential than those in schedules I and II. Abuse of these drugs leads to moderate or low physical dependence. Examples include preparations with low levels of morphine as well as nalorphine, ketamine, and barbiturates. *Schedule IV* drugs are considered to have a low abuse potential and include phenobarbital and diazepam (Valium). Additional information on controlled substances may be found in Chapter 25.

NONSTEROIDAL ANTI-INFLAMMATORY DRUGS (NSAIDs)

Inflammation

Non-narcotic analgesics include the large family of drugs frequently referred to as nonsteroidal anti-inflammatory drugs or NSAIDs. NSAIDs exert their analgesic effects in the peripheral tissues primarily by blocking the production of prostaglandins. Prostaglandins are normally produced in tissues during the process of inflammation.

Inflammation may be considered as a series of events (Fig. 20–8) that are mediated by substances such as vasoactive amines (histamine, serotonin), leukocyte products (lymphokines, oxygen radicals, interleukins), and substances that are formed from the metabolism of arachidonic acid (prostaglandins and leukotrienes). Arachidonic acid, a phospholipid, is present in cell membranes, and when released, it can be metabolized to form prostaglandins and leukotrienes (Fig. 20–9).

> **TECHNICIAN NOTE**
>
> Non-narcotic analgesics include the large family of drugs frequently referred to as nonsteroidal anti-inflammatory drugs or NSAIDs.

Inflammation begins with local tissue injury. Vasoactive substances released from both blood cells (leukocytes and platelets) and cells in the peripheral tissue results in the production of pain, heat, and swelling. Fluid exudation from capillaries can cause swelling and pain secondary to the pressure exerted on local nerve endings. Along with the vascular changes, neutrophils and monocyte-macrophages migrate to the injured tissue to ingest and destroy foreign material. During this process,

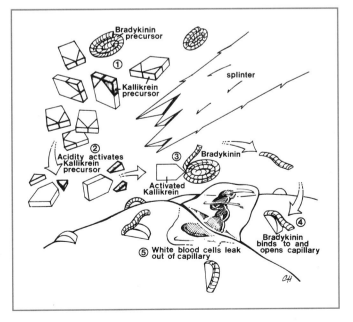

Figure 20–8. The inflammatory process involves the generation of many substances responsible for causing pain and swelling.

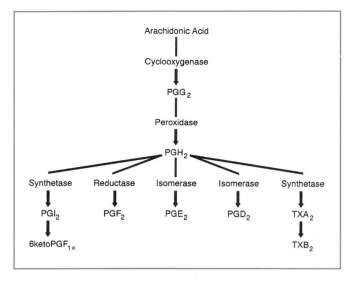

Figure 20-9. Many different prostaglandins (PG) are generated enzymatically after the release of arachidonic acid from cell membranes.

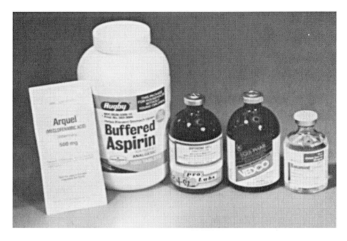

Figure 20-10. Nonsteroidal anti-inflammatory drugs commonly used in treating musculoskeletal pain in veterinary practice.

toxic oxygen radicals and enzymes are released into the local tissues, further exacerbating the inflammatory process (Insel, 1996).

NSAIDs control pain by inhibiting *cyclooxygenase*, a major enzyme in the arachidonic acid pathway leading to the production of prostaglandins. Cyclooxygenase also converts arachidonic acid to thromboxane (causes platelet aggregation) and prostacyclin (inhibits platelet aggregation). An important point to remember is that by blocking cyclooxygenase, NSAIDs inhibit the production of the prostaglandins involved in inflammation as well as those involved in regulating such important functions as blood flow and gastric secretion.

Salicylate Analgesics

Salicylate analgesics were first introduced into clinical medicine in the late nineteenth century. Salicylates commonly used in veterinary practice include aspirin (Fig. 20–10) and bismuth subsalicylate (Pepto-Bismol, Procter & Gamble). Salicylates are effective in relieving pain associated with peripheral inflammation, such as muscle and joint disease, but have virtually no effect on deep or visceral pain. Salicylates have antipyretic effects because of their ability to reduce the prostaglandin-induced fever response. Aspirin, like other NSAIDs, inhibits the generation of thromboxane and thus decreases platelet aggregation.

Salicylates are readily absorbed through the gastrointestinal tract and quickly enter synovial fluid, peritoneal fluid, milk, saliva, and placental membranes. These drugs are metabolized in the liver by the enzyme glucuronyl transferase. Once processed in the liver, metabolic by-products are excreted through the kidney. The drug half-life of salicylates is higher in cats than in dogs because the cat has considerably lower levels of hepatic glucuronyl transferase, and subsequently a decreased ability to metabolize the drug (Boothe, 1995).

Clinical use of aspirin has centered around the management of inflammatory (such as rheumatoid arthritis) and degenerative joint diseases (Fig. 20–11). Aspirin may be used in the

cat as long as it is administered no more often than every 36 to 48 hours.

Clinical signs of toxicity associated with salicylates, as well as other more potent NSAIDs, include nausea and bloody vomitus (hematemesis) associated with gastric ulceration (Fig. 20–

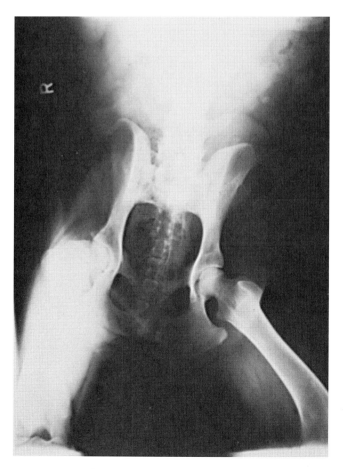

Figure 20-11. Severe right coxofemoral osteoarthrosis amenable to treatment with nonsteroidal anti-inflammatory drugs.

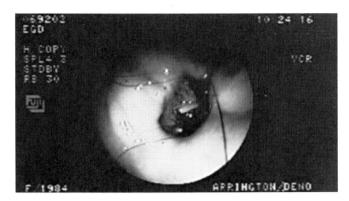

Figure 20-12. Endoscopic view of deep gastric ulcer secondary to chronic nonsteroidal anti-inflammatory drug use in a dog.

12), renal disease, and bleeding tendencies secondary to platelet aggregation inhibition. Gastrointestinal ulceration is the most commonly encountered adverse reaction secondary to NSAID use in the dog. Ulceration occurs secondary to direct irritation of the drug on the gastric mucosa and, importantly, secondary to prostaglandin inhibition. Prostaglandins produced by the gastric mucosa are normally involved in increasing gastric mucus and bicarbonate production, thus helping to coat the stomach lining, neutralize acid produced, and protect the mucosa from irritation. Prostaglandins are also involved in decreasing the volume and acidity of gastric secretion. By inhibiting prostaglandin production, NSAIDs contribute to decreased gastrointestinal protective mechanisms and predispose an individual to ulcer formation.

Propionic Acid Derivatives

Naproxen

There are a considerable number of propionic acid derivatives on the market, most of which act by inhibiting cyclooxygenase. Naproxen (Naprosyn, Syntex), an NSAID, has effective anti-inflammatory, analgesic, and antipyretic properties and is an effective cyclooxygenase inhibitor. Naproxen has approximately 20 times the potency of the related drug ibuprofen. In humans, naproxen has been used successfully to treat degenerative joint disease as well as post-traumatic soft tissue injury (Boothe, 1995).

The toxicity of naproxen is similar to that of other nonsteroidal drugs. Gastrointestinal ulceration leading to perforation and peritonitis has been reported. Because naproxen has a long duration of action in the dog, it can be administered once daily. Because of convenient single daily dosing, naproxen has gained some popularity in treating pain related to orthopedic conditions. The use of naproxen should be limited to dogs in which salicylates do not control pain. If clinical signs of gastric upset occur, administration should be discontinued immediately.

Ibuprofen

Ibuprofen was the first phenylpropionate to be marketed in the United States and has been used successfully to treat rheumatoid and osteoarthritis in humans. In humans, ibuprofen is considered to have less of an analgesic effect than aspirin; however, it is preferred in many cases because it appears to be associated with a lower incidence of gastric bleeding.

The most common form of ibuprofen is available without prescription as 200-mg tablets under a wide variety of proprietary names (Advil, Whitehall; Medipren, McNeil; Midol, Upjohn; Motrin IB, Upjohn; Nuprin, Bristol-Myers).

Studies on ibuprofen use in the dog indicate that gastric irritation and repeated vomiting began after 2 to 4 days of administration and continued days after the drug was discontinued. These studies indicate that dogs are more sensitive than humans to ibuprofen's gastric irritating effects. Ibuprofen offers no advantage over other NSAIDs, and because of significant gastrointestinal irritation, its use in the dog is not recommended.

TECHNICIAN NOTE

Ibuprofen offers no advantage over other NSAIDs, and because of significant gastrointestinal irritation, its use in the dog is not recommended.

Ketoprofen

Ketoprofen (Ketofen, Fort Dodge) is a propionic acid NSAID approved for use in humans and horses. It is a strong cyclooxygenase inhibitor and is subsequently a powerful analgesic and anti-inflammatory drug.

In a multicenter clinical trial, ketoprofen used IV at 2 mg/kg exhibited a potent analgesic effect in the management of pain in horses with colic (Longo et al., 1992). An excellent response was obtained in 89.5% of the horses, without any local or general side effects noted.

Fenamic Acids

Meclofenamic Acid

Meclofenamic acid (Arquel, Fort Dodge) inhibits cyclooxygenase and may also block cell surface receptors for prostaglandins. The drug has gained popularity for treating musculoskeletal pain that is refractory to aspirin. Toxic side effects have been observed in dogs and include diarrhea, vomiting, and gastrointestinal ulceration.

Meclofenamic acid is frequently used in dogs when aspirin therapy has failed to relieve pain associated with chronic degenerative joint diseases such as elbow and hip dysplasia.

Flunixin Meglumine

Flunixin meglumine (Banamine, Schering-Plough) is an NSAID with both analgesic and antipyretic activity. Like other NSAIDs, flunixin inhibits the enzyme cyclooxygenase, blocking the production of prostaglandins. Flunixin is considered to be one of the most potent cyclooxygenase enzyme inhibitors available. The analgesic potency of flunixin is greater than that of phenylbutazone, meperidine (narcotic), or codeine (narcotic).

Flunixin is recommended for relief of persistent, severe inflammation and pain associated with degenerative joint disease that is unresponsive to milder NSAIDs such as aspirin. Because flunixin is a potent inhibitor of prostaglandin synthesis, it also frequently causes severe gastrointestinal ulceration and bleeding. Its use in the dog should not exceed 1 mg/kg once daily for 3 days. Flunixin meglumine is particularly useful for visceral analgesia in horses. Toxicity in horses is rare; it appears to have a wider margin of safety than phenylbutazone.

Pyrazolone Derivatives

Phenylbutazone

Phenylbutazone (Butazolidin, Coopers) has analgesic, anti-inflammatory and antipyretic properties similar to those common to the salicylate analgesics. As a member of the pyrazolone family, it has been associated with significant toxic effects in humans and, less commonly, in animals. Phenylbutazone in humans is known to cause fatal blood disorders (agranulocytosis). Prolonged use in the dog has also led to similar blood diseases.

Clinically, phenylbutazone has been used in the dog for treatment of painful arthritis and skeletal muscle disease and is considered to inhibit cyclooxygenase activity more effectively than aspirin, but less effectively than meclofenamic acid and naproxen. Phenylbutazone is known to cause gastrointestinal ulceration, renal and hepatic disease, and, rarely, bone marrow suppression with prolonged use. Phenylbutazone is commonly used in horses for the control of musculoskeletal and visceral pain. The drug has a narrow margin of safety, and when compared to flunixin meglumine and ketoprofen, was found to cause a higher incidence of gastrointestinal ulceration (Boothe, 1995).

Dipyrone

Dipyrone (Dipyrone Injectable, Butler) is chemically related to phenylbutazone and shares with it similar analgesic, antipyretic, and anti-inflammatory properties. Like phenylbutazone, dipyrone may cause bone marrow suppression (agranulocytosis) if used for prolonged periods (Boothe, 1995). Dipyrone has also been reported to prolong bleeding through the suppression of prothrombin formation. Recommendations for the use of dipyrone are similar to those for phenylbutazone.

Oxicam Derivatives

Piroxicam

Piroxicam (Feldene, Pfizer) is a potent NSAID that has gained tremendous popularity in human medicine for treating bone and joint diseases. One advantage of piroxicam is its long half-life, which allows single daily dosing. Piroxicam has been used to treat musculoskeletal pain in dogs refractory to the less potent NSAIDs. Although little information exists about piroxicam use in dogs, toxicity appears to be similar to that of other NSAIDs. Nausea, vomiting, and gastric ulceration are common with prolonged piroxicam use.

PSYCHOTROPIC AGENTS

Tranquilizers

Animals experiencing pain and anxiety occasionally benefit from the effects of tranquilizers used in conjunction with analgesic drugs (Fig. 20–13). Tranquilizers provide sedation, some muscle relaxation, and antianxiety effects. It is important to remember that tranquilizers provide minimal analgesia, and that it is inappropriate to use these drugs alone for postoperative pain control. The phenothiazines (such as acetylpromazine,

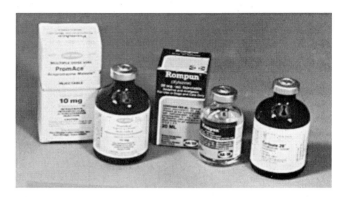

Figure 20-13. Tranquilizers, alpha-2 agonists, and steroids may have a role in the management of pain and distress in small animal patients.

chlorpromazine, promazine) are used extensively for their sedative effects. Other useful tranquilizers include the benzodiazepine diazepam (Valium, Roche) and butyrophenones (droperidol and lenperone). The use of tranquilizers after surgery should be limited to providing sedation and relaxation to animals with pain-related distress and apprehension. Combining narcotics with low doses of tranquilizers often provides the most effective control of pain after surgery in anxious patients.

Alpha₂-Adrenergic Agonists

Xylazine

Xylazine (Rompun, Haver/Diamond Scientific) (Fig. 20–13) binds at alpha₂ receptors in the CNS, causing its sedative and analgesic effects. Many of the side effects of xylazine are secondary to its binding at peripheral alpha₂ receptors. Peripheral alpha₂-receptor stimulation causes vasoconstriction with an increase in arterial blood pressure. This increase in blood pressure is often followed by hypotension and arrhythmias (second-degree heart block). Xylazine can also cause smooth muscle relaxation and vomiting. One significant advantage of xylazine is that its effects may be reversed with the antagonists yohimbine, atipamezole, or idazoxan (Short, 1987).

Xylazine hydrochloride is a potent visceral analgesic in the horse, but is less effective for peripheral pain. In the dog and cat, xylazine provides 15 to 30 minutes of analgesia and is not generally considered to be very potent. Because of its short duration of analgesia and significant cardiovascular effects, xylazine is primarily used as an adjunct to other drugs to provide sedation in the dog and cat. Concurrent administration of atropine is recommended to counteract xylazine's cardiovascular side effects.

Detomidine

Detomidine (Dormosedan, Orion) is a sedative-analgesic originally developed for horses and cattle. Detomidine is more potent than xylazine and has a greater central alpha₂-adrenoreceptor specificity.

Detomidine has similar cardiovascular effects as xylazine when administered at 10 to 60 μg/kg IV. Sedation and analgesia are of a longer duration than xylazine. Administration of detomidine with opioids eliminates the excitation seen in horses given opioids alone (Gross and Booth, 1995). The combination of

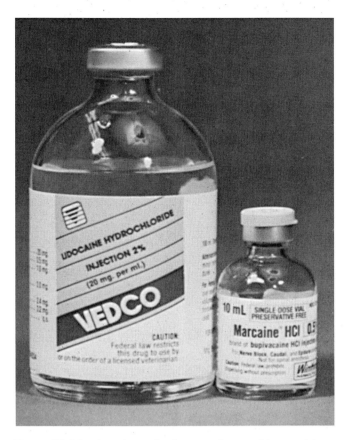

Figure 20-14. Local anesthetics may be used to provide regional analgesia.

detomidine and butorphanol gives effective sedation and analgesia with little cardiovascular effects; detomidine (10 to 15 μg/kg IV) precedes butorphanol (20 to 30 μg/kg IV).

Corticosteroids

Corticosteroids work to suppress the tissue inflammatory response to chemical, thermal, traumatic, and anaphylactic injury. The anti-inflammatory response of corticosteroids results from their ability to inhibit fibroblastic and leukocytic activity and stabilize lysosomal (proteolytic enzyme–containing organelles) membranes in leukocytes and damaged tissues. Corticosteroids also suppress plasma exudation from capillaries and subsequent edema formation. Fibroblastic activity and collagen production are impaired, leading to decreased scarring and slower wound healing.

Corticosteroids principally act by dampening the fire of inflammation and not by eliminating the cause of it. Significant impairment of wound healing and masking of the underlying disease can occur with prolonged high doses of corticosteroids.

Useful corticosteroids for treatment of inflammation include the short-acting cortisone, hydrocortisone, prednisone, and prednisolone. The anti-inflammatory effects of prednisolone and prednisone are approximately five times greater than those of cortisone. Corticosteroids are frequently used as short-term (3 to 5 days) anti-inflammatory drugs in the treatment of acute exacerbations of chronic musculoskeletal pain (such as osteoarthritis of the elbow or hip).

Selective Nerve Blocks

The use of local anesthetics to selectively block peripheral nerves following surgery allows for the relief of pain without the significant side effects associated with other systemic analgesics such as the opioids. Selective blocking of intercostal nerves prior to chest wall closure after thoracic surgery has been shown to provide analgesia equal to that of systemic morphine (Thompson and Johnson, 1991). The technique involves injecting 0.5% bupivacaine (Marcaine, Winthrop Pharmaceuticals) (Fig. 20–14) of intercostal nerves as they pass behind the head of the ribs (Fig. 20–15) for two to three rib spaces in front of and behind the thoracotomy incision. A maximum total dose of 4 to 5 mg/kg in dogs and 2 to 3 mg/kg in cats should be used. Complete blocking of the intercostal nerves with bupivacaine will provide analgesia for 4 to 5 hours. Selective intercostal nerve blocks have a distinct advantage in not producing the respiratory depression associated with narcotic use.

Recently, analgesia in dogs for thoracotomy-associated pain has been achieved by instilling 1.5 mg/kg of 0.5% bupivacaine through chest tubes placed during surgery (Thompson and Johnson, 1991). The analgesia provided is considered to be equal to either systemic morphine or intercostal nerve block. The technique involves instilling the appropriate dose of bupivacaine through the chest tube followed by flushing the tube with 5 ml sterile physiological saline. The dog is then rolled on its back, slightly tilted to the incision side for 10 to 15 minutes. This technique allows the local anesthetic to block the nerve roots at the site of the incision.

Local nerve blocks are also used for injection of transected nerves following thoracic or pelvic limb amputation (Fig. 20–16). Significant postoperative pain is often associated with cut nerve fibers following limb amputation. Analgesia may be provided by injecting 0.5% bupivacaine (0.5 ml per nerve, not to exceed 4 to 5 mg/kg in the dog) into the nerve stump prior to wound closure.

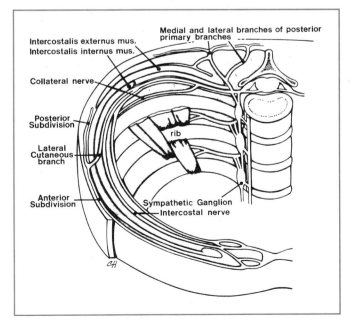

Figure 20-15. Intercostal nerve blocks may be used to provide regional analgesia after thoracic surgery.

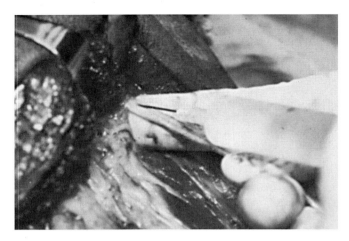

Figure 20-16. Bupivacaine injected into the severed sciatic nerve stump after rear limb amputation helps to provide regional analgesia.

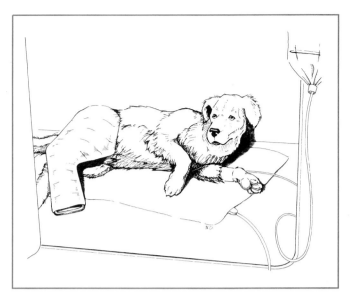

Figure 20-17. Avoid excessive movement in patients recovering from painful surgeries.

TREATMENT OF PAIN IN DOGS AND CATS

The first step in the management of pain in animals is recognizing the behavioral and physiological signs associated with significant discomfort. Recognize that abnormal respiration, rapid heart rate, aggression, changes in appetite, and grooming behavior can all be associated with pain. It is critical to remember that no single sign is definitive in determining whether an animal is experiencing discomfort. It is helpful to remember, when clinical signs are confusing, that if the patient experienced a procedure that would be painful to you, it is likely that it was painful to the animal.

Good nursing care is critical in the management of pain. Providing clean, dry, comfortable bedding in an area free from noise and confusion goes a long way in relieving the distress and anxiety associated with pain. Many patients will benefit

• Table 20–4 •

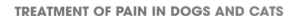

DRUG	**POTENCY***	**DOSE**	**ANALGESIC DURATION**	**COMMENTS**
Morphine	1	0.25–5.0 mg/kg IM, SQ	4 hours	Causes respiratory depression and vomiting; elevates intracranial and intraocular pressure; metabolized by liver
Meperidine	0.2	2–10 mg/kg IM, SQ	2 hours	Causes hypotension with IV injection; painful on injection; metabolized by liver
Oxymorphone	10	0.005–0.2 mg/kg IM, SQ, IV; do not exceed 60 mg total dose	6 hours	Causes respiratory depression, auditory hypersensitivity, and altered thermoregulation; metabolized by liver
		Epidural: 0.1 mg/kg	10 hours	
Butorphanol	5	0.4–0.6 mg/kg IM, SQ, IV	4 hours	Agonist/antagonist; antitussive, antiemetic; ceiling on respiratory depression
Buprenorphine	25–50	0.006–0.01 mg/kg IM, SQ, IV	6–8 hours	Agonist/antagonist; prolonged (≥30 minutes) time from administration to onset of action; long duration; difficult to reverse with naloxone
Pentazocine	0.3	2–3 mg/kg IM	2 hours	Agonist/antagonist; poor analgesic
Fentanyl	100	0.04–0.08 mg/kg IM, SQ, IV	2 hours	Causes respiratory depression, auditory sensitization, decreased cardiac output, bradycardia; metabolized by liver
Nalorphine	0.8	11–22 mg/kg IM, SQ, IV	2–3 hours	Agonist/antagonist
Naloxone		0.04 mg/kg IM, SQ, IV; may be repeated as necessary	2 hours	Pure opiate antagonist; GABA-receptor antagonist

IM, intramuscularly; SQ, subcutaneously; IV, intravenously; GABA, gamma aminobutyric acid.
*Morphine is used as a standard of potency.

• Table 20–5 •

			ANALGESIC	
DRUG	**POTENCY***	**DOSE**	**DURATION**	**COMMENTS**
Morphine	1	0.1 mg/kg IM, SQ	4 hours	Overdose causes excitation; causes respiratory depression, emesis; elevates intraocular pressure; metabolized by liver
Meperidine	0.3	2–10 mg/kg IM	2 hours	Hypotension with IV injection; painful on injection; metabolized by liver
Oxymorphone	10	0.1 mg/kg IM, SQ, IV	6 hours	May cause ataxia; *overdose* causes excitation; causes respiratory depression, auditory hypersensitivity, altered thermoregulation; metabolized by liver
Butorphanol	5	0.4–0.8 mg/kg IM, SQ, IV	3–6 hours	Analgesia for visceral pain lasts longer than for somatic pain
Buprenorphine	25–50	0.005–0.01 mg/kg IM, SQ, IV	6–8 hours	Agonist/antagonist; prolonged (>30 minutes) time from administration to onset of action; long duration; difficult to reverse with naloxone
Pentazocine	0.3	2–3 mg/kg IM	4–5 hours	Provides only visceral analgesia
Naloxone		0.04 mg/kg IM, IV; may be repeated as necessary	2 hours	Pure opiate antagonist; GABA-receptor antagonist

IM, intramuscularly; SQ, subcutaneously; IV, intravenously; GABA, gamma aminobutyric acid.
*Morphine is used as a standard of potency.

from gentle human contact such as talking and petting. Avoid excessive movement and treatments in patients recovering from a painful surgery (Fig. 20–17).

TECHNICIAN NOTE

When administering any of the NSAIDs, always be aware that they can cause gastric upset, vomiting, and ulceration.

When one is selecting an analgesic drug for the treatment of pain (Tables 20–4 through 20–8), animals should be divided into at least two categories: those with acute pain resulting from surgery and those experiencing chronic low-grade pain, frequently of musculoskeletal origin. Patients experiencing acute pain generally benefit the most from short-term opioid analgesics. When anxiety, as demonstrated by excessive vocalization, is involved with acute pain, low doses of tranquilizers may be added to opioid analgesics. Remember that tranquilizers alone have little or no analgesic effect. Patients with musculoskeletal pain often benefit from the use of one of the NSAIDs. In general, the most effective therapeutic approach is to begin with aspirin and then advance to one of the more potent NSAIDs such as naproxen or meclofenamic acid if aspirin is not effective. When administering any of the NSAIDs, always be aware that they can cause gastric upset, vomiting, and ulcer-

• Table 20–6 •

DRUG	**DOSE**	**FREQUENCY**	**COMMENTS**
Aspirin	10–25 mg/kg PO	8 hours	Induces gastric ulceration Decreases platelet aggregation
Phenylbutazone	10–25 mg/kg PO	8–12 hours	May cause agranulocytosis Induces gastric ulceration
Dipyrone	25 mg/kg IM, SQ	8–12 hours	Decreases prothrombin May cause agranulocytosis Causes seizures at high doses
Flunixin meglumine	0.5–1.0 mg/kg IM, IV	24 hours; 3-dose maximum	Induces gastric ulceration
Naproxen	3 mg/kg PO	24 hours	Induces gastric ulceration
Meclofenamic acid	1.1 mg/kg PO	24 hours	Induces gastric ulceration
Piroxicam	10 mg PO for dogs <15 kg; 20 mg PO for dogs >15 kg	24 hours	Induces gastric ulceration
Polysulfated glycosaminoglycans	5 mg/kg 1M	Weekly	

PO, orally; IM, intramuscularly; SQ, subcutaneously; IV, intravenously.

• Table 20–7 •

NONSTEROIDAL ANTI-INFLAMMATORY DRUGS USED IN CATS			
DRUG	**DOSE**	**FREQUENCY**	**COMMENTS**
Aspirin	10–20 mg/kg PO	36–48 hours	Slowly metabolized Analgesic, antipyretic Decreased platelet aggregation
Phenylbutazone	4–5 mg/kg PO	24–36 hours	May cause anorexia, vomiting, depression, death
Dipyrone	10–25 mg/kg IM, SQ	24 hours	Slowly metabolized; good antipyretic

PO, orally; IM, intramuscularly; SQ, subcutaneously.

ation. Patients with existing kidney disease may also experience a worsening of their condition when given NSAIDs.

Principles of analgesia in the cat should follow the same basic guidelines as for the dog, with several exceptions. Of the nonsteroidal drugs, aspirin is the best choice. When using aspirin in the cat, remember that cats metabolize the drug slowly. Aspirin given orally every other day is generally effective. Narcotics are effective in controlling acute pain in cats. Doses of narcotics should generally be lower than for the dog to avoid the excitatory effects sometimes observed with high doses.

TREATMENT OF PAIN IN HORSES

The relief of pain in horses with gastrointestinal or musculoskeletal pain is important both for the comfort of the patient and to minimize injury to attending personnel. Technical staff must be aware that analgesics may mask many important clinical signs including heart and respiratory rate that are used for monitoring colic patients or lameness associated with musculoskeletal injury. In both cases, worsening of the condition may occur in the face of improving clinical signs. Analgesic therapy should be tailored to each case based upon a thorough knowledge of the potency, mechanism of action, and drug side effects.

Analgesics in the Treatment of Colic

Colic produces many behavioral and cardiovascular changes that are frequently used to assess the severity and prognosis of the disease. The cause of pain associated with gastrointestinal injury is most frequently related to abdominal visceral distention, obstruction, and torsion, along with the release of inflammatory mediators such as histamine, serotonin, kinins, prostaglandins, and leukotrienes (Clark, 1992). Severe colic is capable of causing such extreme pain that both the horse and attending technical staff may be at risk of injury. NSAIDs, narcotics, and tranquilizers are all used to control pain associated with colic (Table 20–9). In experimental equine models, xylazine was found to produce the most pronounced visceral analgesia for the longest period of time (Kohn and Muir, 1988).

TECHNICIAN NOTE

In experimental equine models, xylazine was found to produce the most pronounced visceral analgesia for the longest period of time.

Visceral analgesia is immediate in onset after xylazine administration. Xylazine causes sedation characterized by lethargy, drooping and extension of the neck, and ataxia. Heart and respiratory rates are significantly depressed. Xylazine also depresses intestinal motility, which may contribute to postoperative ileus (Kohn and Muir, 1988). Butorphanol produces visceral

• Table 20–8 •

SUGGESTED POSTOPERATIVE ANALGESICS FOR DOGS AND CATS

Abdominal Surgery
Morphine
Butorphanol
Oxymorphone
Suggestions
- May add low doses of tranquilizers to opioids for additional sedation
- Opioids cause respiratory depression and are metabolized slowly in patients with liver disease

Thoracic Surgery
Intercostal nerve block with bupivicaine
Intrapleural nerve block with bupivicaine
Morphine
Butorphanol
Oxymorphone
Suggestions
- Use low doses of opioids with local nerve blocks for additional pain control
- May add low doses of tranquilizers for additional sedation
- Opioids cause respiratory depression; use with caution in patients with respiratory disease

Ophthalmic Surgery
Butorphanol
Oxymorphone
Suggestions
- May add low doses of tranquilizers for additional sedation

Orthopedic/Neurosurgery
Morphine
Butorphanol
Oxymorphone
Suggestions
- Butorphanol and morphine may not provide enough analgesia for severe postoperative pain
- May add low doses of tranquilizers for additional sedation
- By 24 hours after operation, NSAID may be tried in place of opioids; be alert for gastric ulceration

NSAID, nonsteroidal anti-inflammatory drug.

• Table 20–9 •

DRUGS USED TO PROVIDE VISCERAL ANALGESIA IN HORSES

DRUG	RECOMMENDED DOSE (mg/kg)
Narcotic agonists	
Morphine	0.02–0.04 IV
Meperidine	0.2–0.4 IV
Oxymorphone	0.01–0.02 IV
Mixed agonist/antagonists	
Butorphanol	0.02–0.05 IV
Pentazocine	0.4–0.8 IV
Nonsteroidal anti-inflammatories	
Ketoprofen	2 mg/kg IV
Flunixin meglumine	0.6–1.1 IV
Alpha$_2$ agonists	
Xylazine	0.3–0.5 IV
Detomidine	0.005–0.02 IV

IV, intravenously.

• Table 20–10 •

ANTI-INFLAMMATORY DRUGS USED IN HORSES

DRUG	RECOMMENDED DOSE (mg/kg)
Aspirin	15–100 PO, q12h
Flunixin meglumine	0.25–1.1 PO, IM, IV, q8–24h
Meclofenamic acid	2.2 PO, q24h
Naproxen	10 PO, q12h
Phenylbutazone	2–4 PO, q12–24h
Sodium hyaluronate	10–40 mg/joint intra-articularly q7d
Polysulfated glycosaminoglycans	250 mg/joint intra-articularly q7d 500 mg IM q5d

PO, orally; IM, intramuscularly; IV, intravenously.

analgesia and is second to xylazine in potency. The combination of xylazine (1.1 mg/kg IV) followed by butorphanol (0.1 mg/kg IV) produces excellent analgesia. Morphine, meperidine, and oxymorphone produce visceral analgesia that is highly variable and often inferior to that of xylazine and butorphanol. Pentazocine, nalbuphine, and NSAIDs, such as flunixin and dipyrone, did not produce significant analgesia in experimental colic models (Clark, 1992).

Analgesics for the Treatment of Musculoskeletal Pain

NSAIDs are extremely useful in the treatment of musculoskeletal pain in the horse (Table 20–10). This group of drugs provides analgesia when inflammation contributes significantly to pain. Examples include acute laminitis, joint sprains, severe muscle and tendon injuries, and chronic degenerative joint disease. The NSAID used most frequently in the horse is phenylbutazone. Drug actions and side effects for the nonsteroidal group in horses are similar to those described for the dog and cat.

TECHNICIAN NOTE

The NSAID used most frequently in the horse to control musculoskeletal pain is phenylbutazone.

A miscellaneous group of agents used for modifying the disease process in degenerative joint disease includes sodium hyaluronate (Hylartin V, Pharmacia; Equron, Solvay; Hyalovet, Fort Dodge Laboratories) and polysulfated glycosaminoglycans (PS-GAGs; Adequan, Luitpold Pharmaceuticals). The mechanism of action of these drugs is variable, but all are aimed at returning the synovial joint to normal. Individual responses are variable and dependent on the level of disease present. The intra-articular dose for hyaluronate is between 10 to 40 mg per joint. The dose may be repeated at weekly intervals. Polysul-

fated glycosaminoglycans are given at 250 mg per joint intra-articularly on a weekly basis. Alternatively, PS-GAGs may be given at 500 mg IM for 4 days for a total of seven treatments (May, 1992). The PS-GAGs have an advantage over hyaluronate in that they inhibit enzymes involved in cartilage degradation. Use of PS-GAGs is contraindicated in cases of infectious arthritis.

References

Boothe DM: The analgesic-antipyretic-antiinflammatory drugs. *In* Adams HR (editor): Veterinary Pharmacology and Therapeutics, 7th ed. Ames, Iowa State University Press, 1995, pp 432–449.
Branson KR, Gross ME, and Booth NH: Opioid agonists and antagonists. *In* Adams HR (editor): Veterinary Pharmacology and Therapeutics, 7th ed. Ames, Iowa State University Press, 1995, pp 274–310.
Clark ES: Pharmacologic management of colic. *In* Robinson NE (editor): Current Therapy in Equine Medicine, 3rd ed. Philadelphia, WB Saunders, 1992, pp 201–206.
Gross M and Booth NH: Tranquilizers. *In* Adams HR (editor): Veterinary Pharmacology and Therapeutics, 7th ed. Ames, Iowa State University Press, 1995, pp 311–357.
Guyton AC and Hall JE: Somatic sensations: II. Pain, headache, and thermal sensations. *In* Guyton AC and Hall JE (editors): Textbook of Medical Physiology, 9th ed. Philadelphia, WB Saunders, 1996, pp 609–620.
Insel PA: Analgesic-antipyretic and antiinflammatory agents and drugs employed in the treatment of gout. *In* Hardman JG, Limbird LE, Molinoff PB, et al (editors): Goodman and Gilman's The Pharmacologic Basis of Therapeutics, 9th ed. New York, McGraw-Hill, 1996, pp 617–658.
Kohn CW and Muir WW: Selected aspects of the clinical pharmacology of visceral analgesics and gut motility modifying drugs in the horse. J Vet Intern Med 2:85–91, 1988.
Longo F, Antefage A, Bayle R, et al: Efficacy of a nonsteroidal anti-inflammatory, ketofen 10% (ketoprofen) in the treatment of colic in horses. Equine Vet Sci 12:311–315, 1992.
May SA: Antiinflammatory agents. *In* Robinson NE (editor): Current Therapy in Equine Medicine, 3rd ed. Philadelphia, WB Saunders, 1992, pp 14–18.
McMurphy RM: Postoperative epidural analgesia. Vet Clin North Am Small Anim Pract 23:703–716, 1993.
Popilskis S, Kohn D, Sanchez JA, et al: Epidural vs. intramuscular oxymorphone analgesia after thoracotomy in dogs. Vet Surg 20:462, 1991.
Short CE: Pain, analgesics and related medications. *In* Short CE (editor): Principles and Practice of Veterinary Anesthesia. Baltimore, Williams & Wilkins, 1987, pp 28–46.
Thompson SE and Johnson JM: Analgesia in dogs after intercostal thoracotomy: A comparison of morphine, selective intercostal nerve block and interpleural regional analgesia with bupivicaine. Vet Surg 20:73, 1991.

21 Equine Medical and Surgical Nursing

Rustin M. Moore • *Bonnie Rush Moore* • *Deborah L. Skaggs*

INTRODUCTION

The role of the veterinary technician in equine practice is to be a team member with a goal of providing efficient, quality health care for horses. A skilled, observant veterinary technician with equine-specific training is an invaluable resource in an equine hospital. These persons are relied upon to provide patient monitoring, treatment, surgical assistance, and client education. Providing veterinary care for horses is particularly cumbersome because they are large, fractious, and fragile animals. Skilled technical support with expertise in patient restraint, specialized instrumentation, and equine-specific disease is crucial for the equine clinician to provide quality intensive care or perform advanced techniques. Familiarity with equine behavior will allow the veterinary technician to recognize abnormal behavior and permit early recognition of colic, pain, neurological disease, and respiratory distress during patient monitoring. The technician is often the first to identify a change in patient status, and may save valuable time at a crucial turning point for therapeutic intervention. Familiarity with equine-specific surgical equipment will reduce surgical time and improve patient prognosis. Recognition of the unique layman's language in equine medicine and surgery will help the technician recognize the significance of the patient's historical data and physical examination findings. Equine technical support imparts a tangible contribution to the quality and efficiency of patient care in a hospital setting.

PHYSICAL EXAMINATION OF THE EQUINE PATIENT

Physical examination is an integral part of the diagnostic work-up of horses and is an important monitoring tool for ill horses.

Because veterinary technicians play an important role in the day-to-day monitoring of hospitalized patients, learning to perform a thorough and complete physical examination is vital (see Chapter 3). Safety of the handler, the examiner, and the patient is important to consider when performing a physical examination. It is important to record results of the physical examination in the medical record. The medical record is a legal document and provides the only record of the patient's progress or deterioration.

TECHNICIAN NOTE

Because veterinary technicians play an important role in the day-to-day monitoring of hospitalized patients, learning to perform a thorough and complete physical examination is vital.

Physical examination should begin with observation of the equine patient from a distance to assess attitude (bright and alert, depressed, demented, excitable, and so forth) and to assess the horse's respiratory effort. Sometimes horses with mild depression or mild abdominal pain may appear relatively normal when approached and examined. However, when observed from a distance, they may be more likely to demonstrate their true behavior. Signs of horses experiencing mild abdominal pain include pawing the ground with their front feet; kicking at their abdomen with their rear feet; looking at their flank or abdomen; curling their lip; playing in their water bucket; and lying down in sternal, lateral, or dorsal recumbency.

Examination of the stall can also give important clues. Evidence of disrupted stall bedding could be an indicator of the horse being cast (unable to stand because the horse lay down too close to the wall) or could be an indication that the horse has experienced colic (abdominal pain). This may be recognized as bare stall floor being exposed (paw marks) owing to pawing of bedding. The amount of feed and water in the stall can be an important indicator of the horse's appetite and water intake. The character and quantity of feces in the stall and observation of the horse's drinking and urination can also yield important information. The horse's general body condition should be noted. The ribs should be easily palpated, but should not be visible in a horse in ideal body condition. The horse's use and the physiological demands such as intense training, pregnancy, and lactation should be considered when assessing body condition.

Close inspection of the horse should include evaluation of the head, including the nostrils (nasal discharge, flared nostrils) and eyes (epiphora, blepharospasm). Horses with viral respiratory disease often have a serous nasal discharge. Horses with an infection of the frontal or maxillary sinuses or guttural pouches or horses with pneumonia may have a mucopurulent nasal discharge. Horses may have evidence of blood at the nostrils (epistaxis) with guttural pouch mycosis, ethmoid hematomas, and exercise-induced pulmonary hemorrhage. Epiphora may be associated with a primary ocular disease or may manifest secondary to a viral respiratory disease or occlusion of the nasolacrimal duct system. Blepharospasm ("squinting") is usually a sign of ocular pain and is commonly observed in horses with corneal ulceration and uveitis. Coughing is generally a sign of lower respiratory tract disease (pneumonia, chronic obstructive pulmonary disease [COPD]) and can be productive or nonproductive. The presence of inspiratory or expiratory noise usually reflects an obstructive disease of the upper respiratory tract (nostrils to trachea). Dyspnea (difficult breathing) is characterized by flared nostrils, cyanotic mucous membranes, and rapid and shallow thoracic excursions; this should be brought to the attention of the attending veterinary clinician immediately. Flared nostrils (Fig. 21–1) combined with the presence of hypertrophied external abdominal oblique musculature ("heave line") extending from the elbow toward the

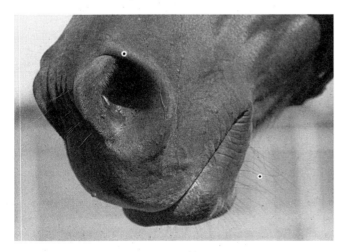

Figure 21-1. Flared nostrils on a horse with chronic obstructive pulmonary disease.

tuber coxae, and a forced expiration, usually signifies a horse with obstructive pulmonary disease.

Evaluation of the manner in which the horse ambulates in the stall can provide important information regarding the musculoskeletal system. Horses with laminitis (founder) often stand with their rear limbs camped underneath their torso and their front limbs extended in front of their torso in order to take weight off of the toe. These horses may ambulate in the stall, but are particularly painful when forced to turn. Horses with navicular disease may stand with the heels of the front feet elevated. Horses with severe unilateral limb lameness may stand with all their weight on the unaffected limb and may hold the affected limb in a slightly flexed position. Horses with laminitis, other causes of severe lameness, and rhabdomyolysis ("tying up") may spend long periods in sternal or lateral recumbency; these horses may develop decubital ulcers.

Monitoring of vital signs, including rectal temperature, heart rate (pulse), and respiratory rate is necessary. One must be careful when taking a horse's rectal temperature and take appropriate safety precautions to prevent self-injury. Some horses resent having their rectal temperature taken and will kick. The horse should be approached from the left side, standing as close to its body as possible. The handler should also be located on the left side of the horse. One should slowly work toward the rear of the horse, carefully raise the tail, and slowly insert a lubricated thermometer into the rectum. Some horses will clamp down their tail. Do not stand directly behind the horse when taking the temperature because a kick could cause serious injury or death. The thermometer should be attached to a string or piece of rubber tubing and an alligator clip so that it can be attached to the tail hairs, which will prevent it from dropping to the floor during defecation. The normal rectal temperature of adult horses is approximately 36° to 38.5°C (99° to 101°F). An increased rectal temperature usually indicates an infectious process somewhere in the body, but, hyperthermia can occur secondary to environmental conditions (hot, humid, poor ventilation), especially in anhidrotic (unable to sweat) horses. Hypothermia can occur, particularly in foals. The heart rate of adult horses should range from 25 to 50 beats per minute, and is generally from 30 to 40 beats per minute. The respiratory rate is generally 8 to 20 breaths per minute. The heart rate can be determined by auscultating the heart or by obtaining the pulse from the linguofacial or transverse facial arteries (Fig. 21–2). The heart rhythm should also be assessed during auscultation of the heart; second-degree atrioventricular block is a common arrhythmia in adult horses and usually is alleviated by exercise. Atrial fibrillation is characterized by an irregular cardiac rhythm and can be confirmed on an electrocardiogram by a rapid and irregular rate and absent P waves. Auscultation and percussion of the thoracic cavity is important to assess the status of the lower respiratory tract. Frequently, a rebreathing bag is used during auscultation of the lungs in adult horses to increase the depth of breathing (Fig. 21–3). Crackles and wheezes can be auscultated in horses with pneumonia. End-expiratory wheezes can often be heard in horses with COPD. The heart and lungs sounds can be muffled in horses with pleural effusion; frequently a fluid line can be identified by auscultation and percussion of the thorax.

Oral mucous membranes should be assessed for color, moistness, and capillary refill time after blanching. The oral mucous membranes should typically be light pink in color and be moist to the touch. The capillary refill time should be less

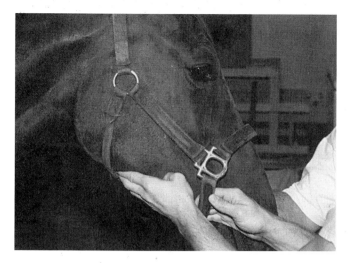

Figure 21-2. Determination of pulse rate and arterial pulse pressure through palpation of the facial artery.

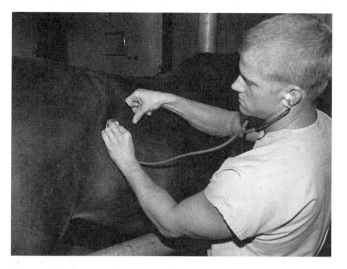

Figure 21-4. Auscultation and percussion of the abdominal cavity.

than 2 seconds. Cyanotic (whitish blue) mucous membranes often indicate hypoxemia (insufficient quantity of oxygen present in the blood) and are often observed in horses with respiratory disease. Dark-pink to bright-red mucous membranes are often observed in horses with endotoxemia. Dry, tacky mucous membranes often reflect volume depletion and are frequently observed in horses that are dehydrated or in shock.

Auscultation and percussion of the abdominal cavity (Fig. 21-4) should be performed carefully and thoroughly, especially in horses with diseases of the abdominal cavity (colic, diarrhea). The abdominal cavity is generally arbitrarily divided into right and left dorsal and ventral quadrants for purposes of auscultation and percussion. The degree of abdominal distention should be assessed and monitored. This can be performed by subjective visual observation or can be assessed more objectively by measuring abdominal circumference at a consistent site. This is especially useful in colicky foals with abdominal distention that are being monitored. A rectal examination is often considered an extension of the physical examination of horses with colic, diarrhea, or weight loss. This should only be

performed by a veterinarian in horses that are properly restrained (Fig. 21-5). Rectal trauma can be sustained during a rectal examination and can lead to a tear or perforation that is fatal.

TECHNICIAN NOTE

Because horses are unable to evacuate their stomach by vomiting, it is important that the technician become knowledgeable and proficient in nasogastric intubation to prevent a catastrophic rupture of the stomach.

Because ill horses are predisposed to develop laminitis, the digital pulse and hoof heat should be evaluated. The digital pulse can be palpated at the level of the fetlock over the abaxial surface of the sesamoid bones (Fig. 21-6). Normally, the pulse

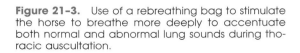

Figure 21-3. Use of a rebreathing bag to stimulate the horse to breathe more deeply to accentuate both normal and abnormal lung sounds during thoracic auscultation.

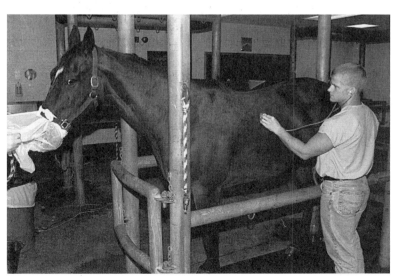

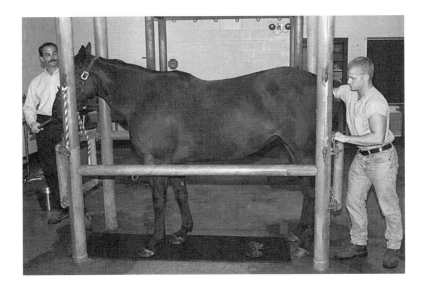

Figure 21-5. Rectal examination of a horse that is physically restrained with the use of stocks and a twitch.

can be palpated, but it should not be bounding. Although subjective, evaluation of hoof heat can be useful, particularly if there is a unilateral disease process. Hoof heat increases secondary to laminitis, sole abscess formation, and other infectious or inflammatory conditions of the foot. The digital pulse can increase subsequent to any disorder of the foot, but occurs commonly with laminitis, sole abscess, and third phalanx fractures.

Passage of a nasogastric tube is an essential part of the examination and treatment of horses with colic. Because horses are unable to evacuate their stomach by vomiting, it is important that the technician become knowledgeable and proficient in nasogastric intubation to prevent a catastrophic rupture of the stomach. The nasogastric tube can be passed by standing on the horse's left side and placing the right hand on the bridge of the nose to control movement of the horse's head (Fig. 21–7). The end of the nasogastric tube to be passed into the stomach should be held in the left hand and the opposite end of the tube should either be held in the mouth or draped around the neck of the person passing the tube. The thumb of the right hand is used to push the tube into the ventral meatus of the nasal passages. The tube should be advanced slowly through the nasal passages because if the tube briskly contacts the ethmoid turbinates, profuse bleeding can occur. As the nasogastric tube is advanced through the nasopharynx the neck should be flexed to facilitate swallowing of the tube. Once the horse swallows the tube the tube should be advanced. The person passing the tube should confirm that the tube is within the esophagus by obtaining negative pressure when sucking back on the tube, or by visually observing or manually palpating the tube within the esophagus on the left side of the neck above the jugular groove. After it has been confirmed that the tube is

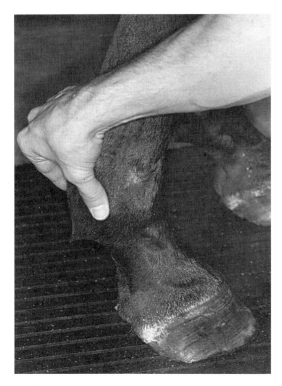

Figure 21-6. Location for palpation of digital pulse in a horse.

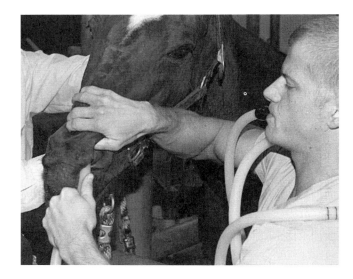

Figure 21-7. Nasogastric intubation in an adult horse.

within the esophagus, air should be blown through the tube to dilate the esophagus as the tube is being advanced into the stomach.

Once the tube is within the stomach it should be primed with water to obtain a siphon effect. The tube can be primed by pumping water or allowing water to flow by gravity through a funnel (Fig. 21–8). Once the tube is primed, the end of the tube should be lowered to allow stomach contents to flow; sometimes it is helpful to pull the tube out in small movements until flow becomes steady (Fig. 21–9). It is helpful to use a tube of as large a diameter as possible to facilitate removal of feed material from the stomach. It is also helpful to have several fenestrations along the end of the tube to encourage drainage if the end of the tube or some fenestrations become occluded with feed material. The quantity of fluid that is placed within the tube and stomach for priming should be subtracted from the total amount of fluid obtained to determine the net amount of reflux, which should be recorded in the medical record. This provides a monitoring tool for determining the magnitude of the intestinal obstruction and whether ileus (abnormal intestinal motility) is improving.

If no net reflux is obtained, then fluids or medications such as mineral oil (intestinal lubricant), magnesium sulfate (osmotic cathartic), dioctyl sodium succinate (surface-acting agent), psyllium hydrophilic muciloid (bulk laxative), bismuth subsalicylate (intestinal protectorant), and others can be administered through the nasogastric tube. Although the total capacity of the stomach of adult horses is large, no more than 6 to 8 liters should be administered at one time. In horses being administered oral fluids, 6 to 8 liters can be administered every 2 to 4 hours. In situations where net reflux is obtained or when fluids

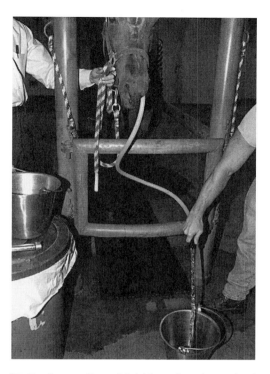

Figure 21-9. Evacuation of fluid from the stomach of a horse through a nasogastric tube.

are being administered via nasogastric tube, the tube can be secured in place with adhesive tape and tied to the halter (Fig. 21–10). Indwelling nasogastric tubes are not benign; horses with tubes that are kept in place for long periods can develop inflammation and ulceration of the pharynx and esophagus. Therefore, horses that salivate or chew excessively should be closely monitored because these horses are prone to develop esophageal ulceration. Nasogastric tubes can become fragmented, and the tube fragments could potentially cause gastrointestinal tract obstruction.

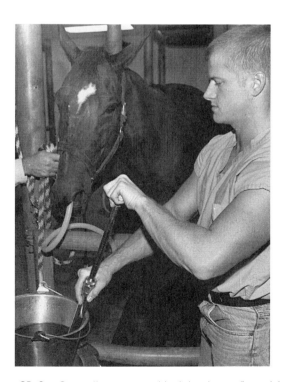

Figure 21-8. Once the nasogastric tube is confirmed to be within the stomach, the tube should be primed with water to initiate a siphon effect. This can be achieved by filling the tube with water, through the use of either a pump or gravity flow with a funnel.

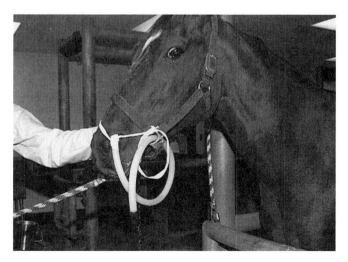

Figure 21-10. Technique for securing a nasogastric tube in the proper position. Adhesive tape can be applied to the tube and then tied to a securely fitting halter. This will help prevent dislodgement of the tube.

A similar method is used for nasogastric intubation in foals, but, a smaller-diameter, more pliable tube should be used. Indwelling tubes are often used for feeding sick foals; the end of the tube should be placed in the middle or distal esophagus rather than the stomach. When priming the tube with water or administering medication via a nasogastric tube in foals, the fluid should be administered with a funnel via gravity flow. It is often helpful to secure the tube to the foal's nostril with a tape butterfly and suture and to the foal's head with elastic tape (Elasticon Johnson & Johnson) placed over the bridge of the nose (Fig. 21–11).

The technician should be familiar with the normal range of vital signs in foals and the differences between adult horses. Temperature should range from 36° to 39°C (99° and 101.5°F). The heart rate varies considerably in foals within the first week of life; it is usually 40 to 80 beats per minute in the immediate postpartum period, increases to 120 to 150 beats per minute during the next several hours, and then stabilizes at approximately 80 to 100 beats per minute during the first week of life. The respiratory rate in the neonatal foal is approximately 60 to 80 breaths per minute in the immediate neonatal period and decreases to approximately 30 breaths per minute within 1 hour of birth. Thoracic auscultation is not a reliable indicator of lower respiratory disease in the foal; often only subtle abnormalities are detectable on auscultation, even in the presence of severe pulmonary disease. Physical examination of foals is similar to that of adult horses; however, there are several areas that need to be more closely evaluated in foals than in adult horses. The umbilicus should be observed and palpated for heat, pain, or swelling, which is an indicator of umbilical remnant disease; ultrasonography may help in further evaluation of umbilical remnant disease. All joints of foals should be evaluated and palpated on a daily basis; effusion (joint swelling) or periarticular swelling and heat are indicators of joint infection. See Neonatal Care for more information.

RESTRAINT OF THE EQUINE PATIENT

Proper restraint of the equine patient is important to protect the handler, examiner, and patient from injury or death (see Chap-

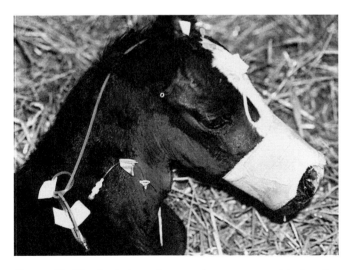

Figure 21–11. Technique for securing a nasogastric feeding tube in a foal. The tube is sutured to the nostril and the tube is secured to the maxilla with adhesive tape (Elasticon) placed circumferentially around the foal's muzzle.

ter 1). Both physical and chemical methods can be used to achieve proper restraint (see Chapter 1). The handler should always stand on the same side of the horse as the examiner. This is important because if the horse is anxious or fractious and is moving, the handler can turn its front end toward the examiner so that the rear limbs of the horse go away from the examiner. This will prevent injury that could occur secondary to the horse kicking the examiner. The handler should always lead the horse from its left side. The snap of the lead shank should be attached to the ring of the halter on the chin strap. A cotton or nylon lead shank can be used with or without a chain attached. The chain is useful when handling fractious or difficult horses. The chain portion of the shank can be placed over the bridge of the nose, under the chin, or over the gums to provide more secure control of some horses. This may be particularly necessary in stallions. The chain should be placed through the rings of the halter on the chin strap and on both sides of the halter, and then the snap attached to ring on the chin strap. Care must be taken when using the chain in this manner because many horses are not accustomed to this and may rear or resist handling.

TECHNICIAN NOTE

Proper restraint of the equine patient is important to protect the handler, examiner, and patient from injury or death.

Technicians are often involved in conducting lameness or neurological examinations of equine patients. When walking or jogging a horse, the handler should walk or jog along on the horse's left side and allow approximately 1 foot of shank between the right hand and the horse's head. This allows the horse to have some movement of its head which can be important when conducting a lameness examination. This also enables the handler to stay far enough away from the horse to prevent getting stepped on. The handler should not look back at the horse when walking or jogging because this often causes the horse to resist forward movement. The surface that the horse is being walked or jogged on is important. A hard surface such as concrete or asphalt allows one to better hear and sometimes better observe a subtle lameness, but, this kind of surface can cause damage to unshod hooves and can be slippery, particularly if wet. Therefore, caution must be taken when handling horses on this type of surface.

In a hospital setting, horses can be placed in stocks for performing many necessary procedures. Although this helps control the horse's movement, it is not the best method of restraining some horses. Some very anxious or fractious horses can actually cause more injury to themselves if placed in stocks. Therefore, the horse's temperament and level of training should be taken into consideration when contemplating the use of stocks for restraint. When placing a horse in stocks, both the front and rear gates should be opened and the handler should walk through from rear to front and allow the horse to follow. An assistant should close the gate behind the horse and secure it before the handler closes the gate at the front of the stocks. This will prevent the horse from suddenly backing out of the stocks before the rear gate can be closed. Many stocks have a

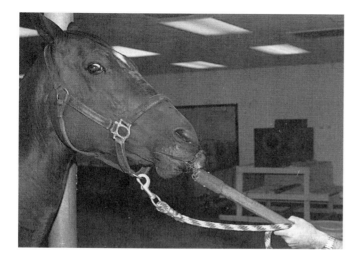

Figure 21-12. Technique for restraining a horse with a nose twitch.

set of crossties at the front. Many horses can be secured with crossties, but, they should not be used on fractious horses. Rather, the handler should remain at the horse's head. Horses should never be left unattended in stocks because they can easily become frightened or anxious and attempt escape. This can lead to severe injury, sometimes necessitating humane destruction.

A twitch can be used as the sole method of physical restraint or can be used in combination with other forms of physical or chemical restraint (Fig. 21–12). A chain or rope twitch can be placed over the horse's upper lip and tightened by rolling it toward the horse's poll. This should help prevent it from coming off the lip. The twitch should be placed on the nose from the side where the handler is standing. The restraining effects of a twitch have a limited period of effectiveness; therefore, the twitch should not be placed on the lip until immediately before it is needed. Some horses resist twitching, particularly if they have had it performed several times in the past. Other horses will tolerate it at first, but then start resisting it. If the procedure is lengthy, then taking the twitch off for a period may prevent the horse from becoming very anxious. It may be better to use chemical restraint in certain horses in which lengthy procedures are being performed. A hand can be used to twitch an ear or the skin in front of the scapula, which will provide variable degrees of physical restraint. When restraining horses for certain procedures such as nerve blocks during a lameness evaluation, one of the horse's limbs can be picked up and held off of the ground by an assistant. This often helps prevent the horse from lifting the limb that is being worked on.

Chemical restraint (sedation or tranquilization) is probably the most effective and safest form of restraint, but it can sometimes interfere with certain procedures. For example, sedation can alter the gait of horses and interfere with interpretation of a lameness or neurological examination. Some sedatives also have analgesic properties which could possibly alleviate or alter lameness. Sedation can also interfere with interpretation of an upper airway endoscopic examination. Because some sedatives have muscle-relaxing properties they can alter abduction and adduction of the arytenoid cartilages and can alter function of the epiglottis and soft palate. Therefore, if sedation is required during an endoscopic examination of the upper airway, then this should be taken into consideration when interpreting the endoscopic findings.

The most commonly used drugs for chemical restraint include alpha$_2$ agonists such as xylazine and detomidine, narcotic agonist/antagonists such as butorphanol, and phenothiazines such as acepromazine. These can be administered alone or in different combinations; they can be administered intravenously (IV) or intramuscularly (IM). Xylazine and detomidine are potent sedatives that have muscle-relaxing and analgesic properties. They provide marked visceral analgesia, which makes them effective in controlling pain associated with colic. The duration of effect depends upon the dose and the route of administration; xylazine lasts 20 to 30 minutes when administered IV. Detomidine is more potent and has a greater duration of effect; this can be beneficial in some instances, but can also cause problems because it can mask pain for an extended period. Butorphanol is best used in combination with one of the alpha$_2$ agonists or acepromazine. Acepromazine provides tranquilization, but no muscle relaxation or analgesia. It is frequently used in combination with other drugs. It can lead to marked hypotension and therefore should not be used in horses that are dehydrated or in shock. It can also cause permanent penile paralysis (paraphimosis) in stallions.

Foals are restrained differently from adult horses. Many foals have not been trained to be led by a halter; attempts at leading foals with a halter can lead to injury. Many times the foal can be moved by walking the mare to the desired location and allowing the foal to follow. This also works well when attempting to evaluate the foal's gait. It is probably best to have at least two and preferably three people when working on a foal. One person should handle the mare, one should restrain the foal, and the other should examine or treat the foal. Foals are probably best restrained by holding one arm around the lower portion of the foal's neck and grasping the tail at its base with the opposite hand (Fig. 21–13). Some foals tend to sink in the rear end if the handler tries to support them by holding too much tension on their tail. Therefore, the tail should be used as a handle to help control the foal's movement rather than as a method to support the foal's hindquarters. Foals should not

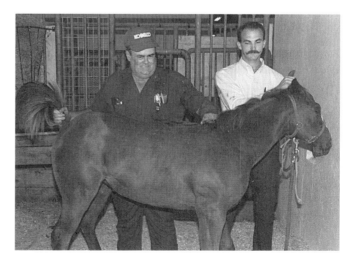

Figure 21-13. Technique for restraining a foal or weanling that is not halter broken.

be placed in stocks because the stocks are too large for their body size and foals are generally not trained to stand. A hand can be used to twitch an ear or the skin on the neck just rostrad to the scapula. Horsemen have many other effective methods of walking and restraining foals. Foals can be chemically restrained with tranquilizers or sedatives as with adult horses; the dose must be adjusted to body weight.

CARE OF HOSPITALIZED PATIENTS

In the equine hospital setting, veterinary technicians are often responsible for primary patient monitoring, administration of medications, general daily care of horses, and supervision of lay technical support. This section provides an overview of daily management of equine patients in the hospital setting.

Patient Monitoring

The level of patient monitoring required for a hospitalized horse will depend on the severity and nature of its disease. Horses hospitalized for elective surgery (castration, bone chip removal) require a thorough physical examination at presentation to ensure they are healthy surgical candidates. During hospitalization, elective patients usually require twice-daily monitoring of heart rate, temperature, respiratory rate, appetite, and fecal output. Horses with infectious disease or extensive traumatic injuries require antibiotic administration and patient monitoring every 6 hours. Colic (medical or surgical), diarrhea, or renal failure necessitates constant IV fluid administration and intensive care monitoring. Most will be monitored continuously or hourly for gastrointestinal motility, heart rate, abdominal pain, shock (capillary refill time), and laminitis. Recumbent foals are particularly fragile and labile. A 24-hour attendant is required to maintain an esophageal feeding tube, IV fluids, oxygen therapy, and sternal recumbent positioning. Additionally, the attendant will administer medications and monitor heart rate, temperature, character and rate of respiration, mental status, abdominal distention, and urinary output.

Patient monitoring forms are designed to identify trends in physical signs and patient treatment forms are designed to coordinate treatment periods when several individuals may be responsible for administering medications. Treatment sheets and monitoring forms may be combined for low-maintenance, elective patients (Fig. 21–14), but monitoring forms should be separate from treatment forms for intensive care patients (Fig. 21–15). A separate intensive care unit (ICU) flow sheet may be used to identify all treatments and monitoring periods for a particular patient (Fig. 21–16). The ICU flow sheets for all patients in the hospital may be assembled in a central area to allow one technician to easily identify treatment periods and thus coordinate efforts. It is important to recognize that monitoring and treatment forms are a permanent part of the medical record, which represents a legal document to record all events during hospitalization.

Horses with infectious, contagious diseases should be hospitalized in isolation facilities. The most common infectious diseases that require an isolation protocol are colitis (salmonellosis) and strangles (*Streptococcus equi*). Personnel should be supplied with disposable gloves, boots, and body suits to wear while attending to isolation cases, and a disinfectant foot dip should be used when entering and exiting the isolation area. Horses in isolation should not be walked in areas where other horses are grazing, and waste from the stall should be disposed of in an inaccessible area. If possible, personnel attending to isolation cases should not attend to foals or immunocompromised patients.

Recumbent horses are a particular challenge to manage effectively in a hospital setting. Neurological and musculoskeletal diseases are the most common problems resulting in recumbency in horses. Horses and foals that are recumbent will quickly develop pressure sores over the point of their hip (tuber coxae), elbows, and head (Fig. 21–17). Pressure sores rapidly become deep and may infect underlying bony structures. Additionally, recumbent horses may have decreased intestinal motility, failure to void urine, and are predisposed to developing colic. Recumbent horses should be deeply bedded on straw, placed on a padded mat, or placed on a waterbed to prevent development of pressure sores. Their position should be changed every 4 hours; multiple attendants are required to move an adult recumbent horse. A sling can only be used in horses that can support their own weight, but are too uncoordinated to remain standing (Fig. 21–18). The sling acts as a safety net to catch them when they stumble. Horses cannot be supported solely by the sling because of constriction of breathing and sling-induced pressure sores. Horses unable to urinate and defecate should have indwelling urinary catheters, and feces should be manually voided twice daily. Soft, laxative feeds such as fresh grass and bran mash should be offered to recumbent horses to prevent impaction. Rarely can recumbent adult horses be managed for more than 1 week without development of life-threatening complications (pneumonia, urinary tract infection, colic, pressure sores).

Feeding

Whenever possible, hospitalized patients should be offered feed similar to what they are fed at home. Sudden changes in diet can predispose horses to colic or diarrhea. In some instances, feeding must be specialized to accommodate the patient's disease. Horses with diarrhea should not be offered rich, calorie-dense feeds such as corn, barley, or alfalfa, which may exacerbate colitis. Grass hay, bran mash, and oats are the most appropriate feeds for horses with diarrhea. After colic surgery or medical resolution of colic, horses should be offered soft, laxative feeds such as bran mash, fresh grass, and small amounts of good-quality hay. Feed should be offered frequently in small quantities to horses with gastrointestinal tract disease rather than offering two large daily meals. Horses with allergic airway disease (heaves, COPD) should be offered water-soaked hay and dust-free grain. Horses with inappetence owing to infectious disease should be offered highly palatable, calorie-dense feeds to increase energy intake (see Chapter 27).

Therapeutics

Medication in tablet form is best administered to horses by crushing the pills with a mortar and pestle and mixing the powder with corn syrup, molasses, or applesauce. The resultant solution is sticky and palatable and can be placed directly in the horse's mouth with a syringe or placed over feed. The attendant must observe closely to ensure medication placed over feed is completely ingested.

Oral medications may also be administered via nasogastric intubation. The nasogastric tube is passed through the nasal

				EQUINE TREATMENT SHEET SID, BID, TID, and QID							

Date	T	P	R	Treatment	7AM	1PM	3PM	7PM	11PM	1AM

Person Administering Treatment Should Initial Box Under the Appropriate Time

Figure 21-14. Elective patient flow sheet for monitoring of patient's progress.

PATIENT PROBLEMS/POTENTIAL COMPLICATIONS:

Date   ICU DAY #

PAGE____ of ____   RESUS. CODE (circle) 0 1 2   WEIGHT____ (circle) lb/kg   WATER

RECORD OBSERVATIONS ON BACK TREATMENT PLAN	TIME:	DIET	FLUIDS	MONITORING 1	2	3	4	5	6	7	8	9	10
1) DIET:	9 am												
	10												
2) FLUIDS:	11												
	12												
	1 pm												
	2												
	3												
	4												
	5												
	6												
	7												
	8												
	9												
	10												
	11												
	12												
	1 am												
	2												
	3												
	4												
	5												
	6												
	7												
	8 am												

WARD_____ TECHNICIAN:_____ Phone:_____

CLINICIAN:_____ Beeper_____ Phone:_____

ICU DAILY RECORD

A

Figure 21-15. Treatment sheet for intensive care unit patients to identify treatments and administration schedule.

OBSERVATIONS & ASSESSMENTS: (eg. vomiting, stools, urinations, convulsions, procedures, and other events)

TIME	INITIALS	

B

Figure 21-15 *Continued*

passes into the esophagus and stomach. Proper placement of the nasogastric tube should be confirmed prior to administration of medications. The tube should be visualized as it passes through the cervical portion of the esophagus, negative pressure should be obtained when the examiner aspirates on the tube, and the aroma of stomach contents may be noted as gas escapes from the tube. Inadvertent administration of medication into the lung using an improperly placed nasogastric tube (in the trachea) can result in death of the horse.

Nonirritating, sterile solutions can be administered IM in horses. The volume of medication to be injected at a single IM site should not exceed 20 ml. Sites for IM injection include the semimembranosus or semitendinosus muscle and the musculature of the neck. The appropriate region for injection in the neck is above the cervical spine, cranial to the scapula, and below the nuchal ligament (Fig. 21–19). Owing to excessive postinjection swelling, the pectoral muscles are not recommended for IM injection. The gluteal muscles are not recommended for IM injection, because this region cannot effectively drain if an abscess forms at the injection site. In rare instances, postinjection abscesses in the gluteal muscles may drain into the abdominal cavity. Phenylbutazone, tetracycline, and thiamylal are irritating medications that should never be administered IM.

Intravenous medications may be administered directly into the jugular vein, using an 18-gauge, 1.5-inch needle. The jugular vein is most superficial and most distant from the carotid artery in the proximal one third of the neck. The needle should be seated in the jugular vein to the hub without the syringe attached to assure the needle has not been accidentally placed in the carotid artery. Blood flows continuously and slowly from an 18-gauge needle in the jugular vein, whereas blood spurts in a pulsatile manner from a needle placed in the carotid artery. Inadvertent intracarotid injection may result in seizure, coma, permanent neurological deficits, or death.

An IV catheter can be placed for repeated administration of IV medications or continuous IV fluid infusion. Intravenous catheters may be placed in the jugular, cephalic, and lateral thoracic (spur) veins in horses. Catheters should be placed aseptically and secured appropriately to prevent their dislodgment (Fig. 21–20). Teflon catheters are relatively irritating and should be replaced every 3 days. Silastic catheters can remain in the vein as long they are patent and show no signs of infection. Intravenous catheters should be monitored twice daily for heat, swelling, pain, patency, and positioning. Infection at the catheter site may occur in the subcutaneous tissue or within the vein (septic thrombophlebitis). Septic thrombophlebitis can be life-threatening in horses.

The ideal antibiotic is effective against a wide range of bacterial organisms (broad-spectrum), easy to administer, and nontoxic (see Chapter 25). Penicillin has good efficacy against common gram-positive pathogens in the horse (*Streptococcus zooepidemicus, S. equi*) and is relatively safe. It is frequently administered IM (procaine penicillin) and IV (potassium penicillin). Procaine penicillin should never be administered IV. Life-threatening anaphylactic reactions are reported with procaine penicillin administration and should be treated with epinephrine. Aminoglycoside antibiotics (gentamicin and amikacin sulfate) are efficacious against gram-negative pathogens, and can be administered IM or IV. These antibiotics are nephrotoxic and renal function should be monitored during the period of administration. Trimethoprim-sulfa antimicrobials have a moderate gram-positive and gram-negative spectrum, are administered orally, and are used for treatment of mild to moderate infection. Ceftiofur sodium has a good gram-positive and gram-negative spectrum, may be administered IM or IV, and is used for moderate to severe infection. Metronidazole is administered orally or per rectum to treat anaerobic bacterial infections. There are specific indications for administration of tetracycline, erythromycin, and rifampin in horses, but these antibiotics are not widely used owing to the risk of antibiotic-induced colitis. Chloramphenicol is used sparingly in horses because of the human health risk of idiosyncratic, fatal aplastic anemia after exposure during administration.

There are many analgesic medications available for horses. Phenylbutazone, ketoprofen, and flunixin meglumine are nonsteroidal anti-inflammatory drugs (NSAIDs) that provide mild to moderate pain relief without sedation or immunosuppression. The NSAIDs also reduce fever (antipyretic) and inflammation. Phenylbutazone is the most widely administered analgesic of horses and is most effective for treatment of musculoskeletal pain. Ketoprofen, meclofenamic acid, and naproxen are less commonly used drugs that provide mild to moderate analgesia for musculoskeletal pain. Flunixin meglumine is more effective

												EQUINE INTENSIVE MONITORING FORM

Date / Time	T	P	R	Digital Pulse	GI Motil	CRT	MM Color	PCV TP	Urine Feces	NG Reflux	Fluids	Comments pain, depression, etc.

Figure 21-16. Intensive care unit patient flow sheet for close monitoring of patient's condition. This helps readily identify trends that may indicate a deterioration in the patient's condition.

for soft tissue and visceral pain. In addition, flunixin meglumine may combat the effects of endotoxemia in horses with gastrointestinal tract disease. Xylazine and detomidine are alpha$_2$-agonist sedative analgesic medications, which provide immediate relief of moderate to marked pain with moderate to profound sedation. Xylazine provides 20 to 30 minutes of sedation and analgesia, whereas detomidine provides up to 1 hour of sedation and analgesia. Butorphanol is a narcotic agonist/antagonist

that provides up to 1 hour of sedation and analgesia for moderate to severe pain. Acepromazine has no analgesic properties, but provides moderate tranquilization. Caution should be used when administering acepromazine especially to horses with signs of shock, because it can cause hypotension. Additionally, caution should be used when administering acepromazine to stallions because it can lead to the development of persistent paraphimosis.

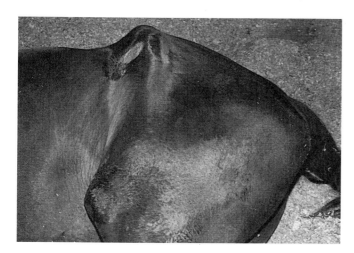

Figure 21-17. Pressure sores on a horse with chronic laminitis secondary to prolonged recumbency.

Corticosteroids have potent anti-inflammatory properties, and are administered for allergic airway disease, allergic skin conditions, immune-mediated disease, and joint inflammation. Corticosteroids are administered topically, orally, parenterally (IV or IM), and intra-articularly. Adverse effects of corticosteroid administration include immunosuppression, polyuria or polydypsia, poor hair coat, muscle wasting, poor wound healing, laminitis, and progression of degenerative joint disease. Therefore, corticosteroids are administered with caution in instances with specific indications for their use.

Dimethyl sulfoxide (DMSO) is a common anti-inflammatory drug used in horses to relieve swelling and edema associated with central nervous system trauma, traumatic musculoskeletal injuries, laminitis, and myositis. DMSO may be administered topically, orally, or IV, and the technician should wear gloves while handling the product. Rapid IV administration may result in hemolysis, hematuria, and sweating in horses.

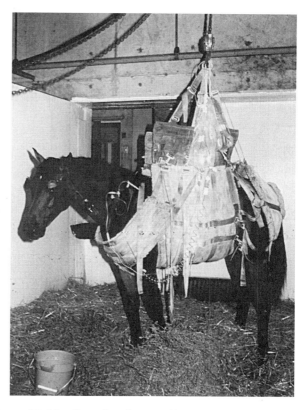

Figure 21-18. Use of a sling and hoist to provide some balance and support to an ataxic or weak horse.

ENDOSCOPY

Development of the fiberoptic endoscope has dramatically improved the diagnostic capabilities of the equine clinician. Endoscopy is used routinely in equine veterinary practice to evaluate the upper respiratory tract (nasal passages, sinuses, ethmoid turbinates, nasopharynx, guttural pouches, trachea, and bron-

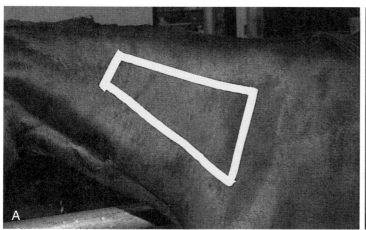
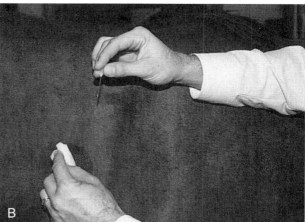

Figure 21-19. A, Location considered safe in the cervical region of horses for the administration of intramuscular injections. B, Technique for administering intramuscular injections; the skin should be cleansed and then swabbed with an alcohol-soaked gauze pad before insertion of the needle. The needle (1.5-inch) should be extend into its hub to deposit the medication deep within the muscle.

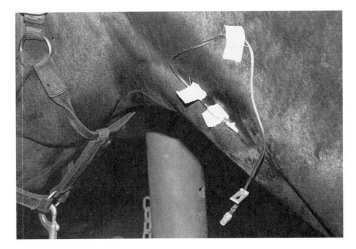

Figure 21-20. Technique for securing a catheter in the jugular vein of a horse.

chi), proximal gastrointestinal tract (esophagus, stomach, duodenum), distal gastrointestinal tract (rectum), and urogenital tract (uterus, urethra, urinary bladder). The endoscope is used most frequently for evaluating athletic horses with poor performance and those making respiratory noise. The endoscope can be used with horses standing (Fig. 21–21) or can be used with horses exercising on a high-speed treadmill. The latter enables the upper respiratory tract to be evaluated dynamically. The most common abnormalities detected in the upper respiratory tract include left laryngeal hemiplegia, dorsal displacement of the soft palate, epiglottic entrapment, arytenoid chondritis, and subepiglottic cysts. The endoscope can also be used to determine the source of mucopurulent nasal discharge or epistaxis. The most common source of mucopurulent nasal discharge is the lower airway; endoscopy would enable observation of this material in the trachea and bronchi. Other possible sources of discharge could be guttural pouch empyema or sinusitis. Horses with maxillary sinusitis often have mucopurulent discharge exiting the nasomaxillary opening into the nasal passages. Potential sources of epistaxis include ethmoid hematoma, guttural pouch mycosis, and exercise-induced pulmonary hemorrhage. The endoscope is also used to obtain a tracheal wash or bronchoalveolar lavage sample in horses with inflammatory or allergic lung disease.

The endoscope is useful for evaluating horses with esophageal obstruction (choke) to determine the location and cause of the obstruction. It is also useful for evaluating the integrity of the esophagus after resolution of the choke to determine if the mucosa is ulcerated, which could predispose the esophagus to forming a diverticulum or stricture. Development of the long endoscope (3 meters) has allowed examination of the stomach and duodenum in foals and adult horses for gastric and duodenal ulceration. Endoscopy has revealed that the incidence of gastric ulceration in adult performance horses is greater than previously suspected. This enables the clinician to document the presence and severity of ulceration and monitor the response to treatment.

The endoscope is often used to assess the integrity of the urethra and urinary bladder in horses with hematuria, stranguria, and pollakiuria. It may reveal erosive or neoplastic lesions in the urethra. Urinary bladder abnormalities that can be identified endoscopically include inflammatory and neoplastic diseases and cystic calculi. The endoscope has been used to assess the uterine lining for cysts and other pathologic conditions.

The technician is integrally involved in the care, use, and maintenance of the endoscope and associated equipment. There are specific instructions on the proper methods for cleaning and disinfecting the endoscope. It is important that the proper methods be followed to ensure that infectious agents such as *St. equi* is not transmitted from one patient to another and to prevent damage to the endoscope.

IMAGING TECHNIQUES

The veterinary technician in equine practice often participates in diagnostic imaging techniques. In some instances, the technician may be solely responsible for obtaining radiographic or scintigraphic images for interpretation by the veterinarian. It is important that the technician recognize good-quality images on the basis of technique and positioning, and understand indications for special radiographic studies. Additional information on imaging techniques may be found in Chapter 9.

Plain Film Radiography

Plain film radiography is used to identify disruption of bony structures such as fracture, osteochondrosis, osteomyelitis

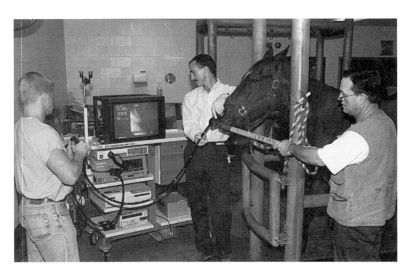

Figure 21-21. Use of endoscopy to evaluate the upper airway of a horse.

(bone infection), malalignment (luxation or subluxation), or degenerative joint disease (arthritis). If it is necessary to be near the horse when the x-ray examination is performed, lead aprons and gloves should be worn. Long-scale (low mAs, high kVp) techniques are used for plain film radiographic technique to preserve resolution of soft tissues and bone. Portable radiograph machines are typically used to image the carpus, hock, skull, and distal limbs in adult horses. The standard focal spot-to-film distance using portable radiographic units is 85 cm. To obtain detailed radiographs of the coffin and navicular bone, the horse's shoes should be removed and the frog should be packed with Play-doh. Portable radiograph units may also be used to image the thorax, abdomen, and cervical spine in neonatal and weanling foals. Large overhead radiograph units (1000 mA, 150 kV) are required to image the spine, thorax, elbow, shoulder, stifle, and hip in adult horses. The standard focal spot-to-film distance using overhead radiographic units is 100 cm. Radiographs of the thorax, cervical and thoracic spine, elbow, and stifle may be obtained in standing, sedated horses. However, high-quality radiographic imaging of the lumbar spine, shoulder, and hip usually requires general anesthesia. It is important to label the radiographs correctly with the name of the patient, the date of examination, the affected limb, and the radiographic marker used for orientation. Radiographic markers are generally used when performing radiographs of the limbs; the markers are placed externally on the radiographic cassette in a location that will either be lateral or dorsal to the limb.

TECHNICIAN NOTE

In some instances, the technician may be solely responsible for obtaining radiographic or scintigraphic images for interpretation by the veterinarian.

Contrast Radiography

Special radiographic techniques use a contrast agent to better define or outline lesions suspected clinically or radiographically, but not visualized on survey (plain film) radiographs. Positive contrast agents are most commonly used in equine radiography for investigation of puncture wounds or draining tracts (fistulogram), joints (arthrogram), bladder (cystogram), spinal cord (myelogram), and esophagus (barium swallow). Short-scale (high mAs, low kVp) techniques are used to highlight visualization of the contrast agent. Triiodinated, water-soluble contrast materials are used for the fistulogram, arthrogram, and cystogram. Nonionic, water-soluble, benzoic acid derivatives are used for myelographic examination, and oil-based barium solutions are used for evaluation of the gastrointestinal tract. The fistulogram is most commonly used to outline foreign bodies, a sequestrum (dead bone), and define the extent of a penetrating wound. A fistulogram can easily outline involvement or penetration of a synovial structure such as a joint or tendon sheath. Arthrograms allow a complete evaluation of articular cartilage integrity, synovial membrane proliferation, and joint capsule integrity. A surgical skin preparation is required prior to injection of sterile contrast agent into a joint. Positive contrast cystography can only be performed in foals

and is used to identify a tear in the bladder wall or persistent urachal remnants. Myelography is used to diagnose cervical stenotic myelopathy (wobbler's syndrome) wherein the cervical spine is malformed and narrowed, which compresses the spinal cord. Attenuation or obliteration of the contrast column is identified at vertebral sites where the cervical vertebrae are compressing the spinal cord. A barium swallow may be useful for investigating dysphagia, esophageal motility, esophageal integrity, and gastric emptying (foals only).

Ultrasound

Ultrasound examination is useful for investigating soft tissue structures and body cavities. The ultrasonic image is formed by ultrasound waves reflecting from tissue interfaces. The reflection of ultrasound waves is caused by the difference in acoustical impedance between tissues. Ultrasound can be used to investigate any soft tissue structure, solid organ, or swelling, but is most commonly used in horses to examine tendon, lung, heart, pleural space, abdominal organs, and reproductive tract. It is important to recognize that air impedes ultrasound penetration; therefore, investigation of gas-filled intestines and air-filled lung is unrewarding. Tendon ultrasound allows the examiner to identify and monitor core lesions, tears, and fibrosis of the tendons during the healing process (Fig. 21–22). Ultrasound examination of the heart is termed *echocardiography* and is used to identify congenital defects, valvular disease, and congestive heart failure. Ultrasound examination of the thorax is particularly useful in horses with pleuropneumonia to identify the location, depth, and character of pleural fluid. Identification of free gas, fibrin, or highly cellular fluid within the pleural space using ultrasound examination is a poor prognostic indicator in horses with pleuropneumonia. Pulmonary abscesses can only be identified if they communicate with the pleural space; deep pulmonary abscesses cannot be visualized because air in the lungs impedes ultrasound penetration. Abdominal ultrasound in foals is used to identify ruptured bladder, infected umbilical structures, and gastrointestinal intussusception (telescoping of the bowel). In adult horses, abdominal ultrasound is used predominately to investigate solid visceral organs such as the liver, kidney, and spleen. Reproductive ultrasound examination is used to identify the appropriate time for breeding, follicular development, early pregnancy diagnosis (15 days), twins, and metritis (septic fluid accumulation in the uterus).

Nuclear Scintigraphy

Nuclear scintigraphy (bone scan) is performed by injecting a radioactive isotope IV and monitoring its distribution in the bones and soft tissue of the limbs. Technetium 99m is the most commonly used radioactive isotope. Technetium is combined with phosphate compounds which localize within bone after IV administration. Localization of phosphate-labeled technetium is identified using a gamma camera. Bony uptake of phosphate-labeled technetium is greater in regions of high bone turnover or increased blood flow. Areas of increased uptake are termed "hot spots," and are usually indicative of an abnormality or disease process. Nuclear scintigraphy is indicated in horses with obscure, unlocalized lameness (using local anesthesia) and localized lameness with normal radiographic examination. Hot spots may identify nondisplaced fractures or stressed or

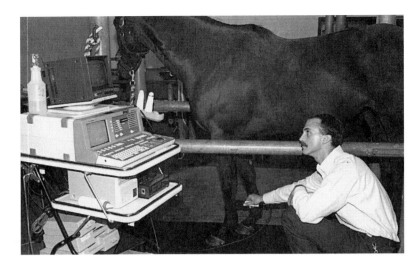

Figure 21-22. Use of ultrasonography to evaluate tendon injury in a horse with suspected flexor tendinitis.

damaged bone. Nuclear scintigraphic examination is quickly performed on an entire limb or multiple limbs, whereas radiographic examination of an entire limb is cost- and time-prohibitive. In instances of unlocalized lameness, a plain film radiographic examination should be performed after nuclear scintigraphy to identify bony abnormalities. Serial nuclear scintigraphic imaging should be performed in horses with normal plain film radiographic examination to monitor progression and healing of the injury.

A white blood cell scan can be performed to identify occult infection. In this procedure, the patient's white blood cells are isolated from a blood sample (60 ml), and labelled with technetium 99m. These technetium-labeled white blood cells are injected back into the patient and the patient is scanned with a gamma camera. The white blood cells travel to a focus of infection and create a hot spot detectable with the gamma camera. This technique may be used to identify a tooth root abscess, osteomyelitis (infected bone), or an intra-abdominal abscess.

CLINICAL PATHOLOGY

Clinicopathologic testing provides important information for the veterinarian to identify functional impairment of an organ system, confirm a clinical diagnosis, assess response to therapy, and formulate a prognosis. There are many species differences in the range of normal values for many common clinicopathologic tests. Additionally, there are species-specific idiosyncracies in the characteristic response to disease and the significance of abnormal findings. This section concentrates solely on equine-specific alterations in clinicopathologic valves in health and disease (also see Chapter 5).

Serum Chemistry

A serum chemistry panel provides specific information pertaining to the liver, kidney, muscle, and serum electrolyte concentrations. The serum sample should be drawn into a tube without anticoagulant (red-top tube) and submitted to the laboratory. If there will be more than 1-hour delay in submission, the tube should be centrifuged, serum removed from the clot, and stored in the refrigerator. Delayed sample submission without centrifuging produces artificially low serum glucose and

high serum potassium concentrations. Horses have high serum bilirubin compared to other species, and serum bilirubin concentrations will increase dramatically if feed is withheld for more than 24 hours. Fasting hyperbilirubinemia in horses is a normal physiological response and is not indicative of liver disease. Most species develop low serum albumin with chronic liver disease owing to decreased production; however, horses maintain production of albumin even with marked impairment of liver function. Reliable indicators of liver dysfunction in horses are high serum gamma glutamyltransferase (GGT) activity and serum bile acid concentrations, and low blood urea nitrogen (BUN) concentrations. In most species, renal failure produces low serum calcium and high serum phosphorus concentrations. Horses are obligate calcium excretors and chronic renal failure often produces a marked increase in serum calcium concentration. Reliable indicators of renal failure in horses include high serum creatinine and BUN, and electrolyte abnormalities, including low sodium and chloride and high potassium and calcium. The large colon of horses exchanges a vast amount of electrolytes and fluids on a daily basis. Horses with colonic inflammation may develop marked electrolyte abnormalities prior to development of diarrhea. Low serum sodium, chloride, and potassium in horses with abdominal pain or depression often indicate loss of electrolytes into the lumen of the colon and impending diarrhea. Serum creatine phosphokinase is an indicator of muscle damage in all species. Horses have large muscle masses in comparison to ruminants and small animals. Moderate increases in serum creatine phosphokinase (two to four times normal) readily occur in horses following prolonged transport, prolonged recumbency, exercise in an unconditioned horse, or rolling owing to abdominal pain. Moderate increases do not usually indicate primary muscle disease. Horses with primary muscle disease such as exertional rhabdomyolysis (tying up, azoturia, Monday morning sickness) have increases in serum creatine phosphokinase activity of up to 200 times normal values.

Hematology

A complete blood count (CBC) provides information pertaining to the red blood cell count, red cell morphology, total white blood cell count, differential white blood cell count (including neutrophils, lymphocytes, eosinophils, monocytes), white blood cell morphology, and fibrinogen concentration. Samples for CBC should be submitted in a tube with ethylenediaminetetraacetic acid (EDTA) anticoagulant (purple-top tube). Red blood cells are most easily quantified, using the packed cell volume (PCV); low PCV is indicative of anemia. Horses have a large muscular spleen that normally contains up to one third of the circulating red blood cell volume. With excitement and exercise, PCV in horses can increase by as much as 50% secondary to splenic contraction. Therefore, the resting PCV is highly variable and must be serially evaluated in excitable patients. Additionally, the response of the spleen to massive hemorrhage precludes use of the PCV to estimate the magnitude of blood loss for a least 24 hours. The normal range of PCV is dependent on breed. Hot-blooded breeds (Thoroughbreds, Arabians, quarter horses) have higher resting red blood cell counts, compared with cold-blooded breeds (ponies and draft horses).

Evaluation of the total and differential white blood cell count is important to identify the presence of infection. In most instances, bacterial infection will manifest as an increase in white blood cell count (leukocytosis) characterized by an increase in the number of mature neutrophils (mature neutrophilia). Fibrinogen is a coagulation factor and an acute-phase reactant in horses. The liver produces fibrinogen in response to bacterial infection and inflammation within 72 hours and fibrinogen concentrations remain increased until the infection is resolved.

Horses are particularly sensitive to circulating endotoxin released from the cell wall of gram-negative bacteria. Endotoxin causes margination and sequestration of white blood cells. Therefore, a profoundly low white blood cell count (leukopenia) characterized by low neutrophil count (neutropenia) and immature band neutrophils (left shift) is indicative of either gram-negative septicemia or gastrointestinal disease with mucosal absorption of gram-negative bacteria. High eosinophil counts (eosinophilia) are indicative of massive parasite infestation or possibly allergic diseases, and low lymphocyte counts (lymphopenia) are observed in horses with early viral infections.

Urinalysis

Urinalysis is essential for evaluation of primary renal disease. Urine can be collected as a voided sample or after catheterization of the bladder. Normal horse urine is usually alkaline (pH 7 to 9) and contains many calcium carbonate crystals. Alkaline urine usually produces a false-positive reaction for protein on urine dipsticks. Horses have a large number of mucous glands located within the renal pelvis; therefore, normal horse urine may appear very thick and mucoid. Normal horse urine may appear red or bloody in the snow, which often alarms novice horse owners. Truly red urine is abnormal and results from the presence of frank blood (primary urinary tract disease), hemoglobin (hemolytic anemia), or myoglobin (myositis). Differentiation of these sources of red urine requires special testing of urine and serum samples. Urine specific gravity and urinary electrolyte excretion ratios should be obtained to investigate primary renal function. Urine specific gravity indicates the ability of the kidney to concentrate urine, and normal values in resting horses should be 1.020 to 1.035. Urinary electrolyte excretion ratios indicate the ability of the kidney to conserve electrolytes. Identification of white blood cells and bacteria are indicative of a urinary tract infection.

Evaluation of Body Fluids

Evaluation of cerebrospinal, synovial (joint), and abdominal cavity fluid provides important information pertaining to inflammation, infection, or neoplasia within that particular body cavity. These body fluids are analyzed for total protein, total cell count, differential cell count, and bacterial culture.

Any form of neurological disease in horses constitutes an indication for cerebrospinal fluid (CSF) analysis. Cerebrospinal fluid is collected in standing, sedated horses with spinal cord disease from the lumbosacral space using a 6-inch, 18-gauge spinal needle. In horses with brain and brain stem disease, CSF is collected in anesthetized horses from the atlanto-occipital space using a 3-inch, 18-gauge spinal needle. Normal total cell counts are less than five cells per microliter (predominately lymphocytes), and normal total protein is variable depending on the laboratory, but is usually less than 80 mg/dl (higher than in other species). Abnormalities in protein and cell counts can identify an inflammatory, infectious, or neoplastic process, but results of CSF analysis are often nonspecific. Antibody to the causative agents of several equine neurological diseases (rabies, protozoal myelitis, herpes myelitis, equine encephalomyelitis) can be detected in CSF, which provides specific information regarding the cause of neurological signs. Complications associated with CSF tap include iatrogenic (operator-induced) spinal cord trauma and introduction of bacteria into the central nervous system.

Joint effusion, pain, or heat is an indication for arthrocentesis (joint tap) in horses. Synovial fluid is obtained by needle aspiration of almost any joint on the limbs of horses. Prior to needle aspiration, the hair must be clipped and a sterile preparation must be performed over the joint. Normal synovial fluid is highly viscous and will string 2 to 3 cm between your fingers before breaking. Normal synovial fluid is clear, yellow in color, and does not clot. Normal total protein is less than 2 g/dl and the normal cell count is less than 300/μl (less than 10% neutrophils). Analysis of synovial fluid can differentiate between synovial inflammation and infection. Bacterial culture of synovial fluid can identify the offending bacteria in horses with septic arthritis. Complications associated with arthrocentesis include iatrogenic septic arthritis and trauma to joint structures.

Abdominal pain, abnormal rectal examination, abdominal distention, and fever of unknown origin are indications for abdominocentesis in horses. Abdominal fluid is obtained by placing an 18-gauge, 1.5-inch needle into the peritoneal space of the ventral abdomen (Fig. 21–23). The needle should be placed one hand's-breadth behind the sternum, off the midline to the right of the horse (to avoid the spleen). If a 1.5-inch needle is insufficient to reach the peritoneal cavity, a teat cannula or female dog urinary catheter may be used. The use of a teat cannula is more invasive and increases the risk of traumatic bowel rupture. Normal abdominal fluid total protein is less than 2.5 mg/dl, and normal total cell count is less than 5000/μl (50% neutrophils). Analysis of abdominal fluid can identify devitalized bowel in horses with acute abdominal pain (colic), abdominal abscess, or tumor in horses with a mass in the abdomen identified via rectal palpation, and ruptured bladder in foals with abdominal distention. Complications of abdominocentesis include traumatic bowel rupture, intra-abdominal hemorrhage from trauma to the spleen, and iatrogenic septic peritonitis.

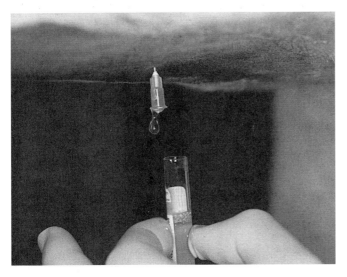

Figure 21-23. Technique for performing abdominocentesis in a horse.

Bacterial Culture and Susceptibility Testing

The veterinary technician often plays an important role in bacteriological testing of specimens collected from patients with infectious diseases (see Chapter 8). Specimens (blood, joint fluid, abdominal fluid, urine, wound exudate, infected bone, and so forth) are frequently collected from horses with infectious diseases for culture. Following proper procedures during collection and transport of these specimens to the laboratory for culture and susceptibility testing improves the chances of growing the causative organism. There are specific guidelines that should be followed for collection and transport of different types of specimens. For example, blood is usually placed in a special enhancement medium immediately after collection for transport to the laboratory. Likewise, there are special methods for collection and transport of samples submitted for aerobic and anaerobic culture. Identifying the causative agent in an infectious process and determining its *in vitro* susceptibility pattern to antibiotics is often critical in choosing the appropriate antibiotic regimen. Therefore, the technician contributes greatly to the successful outcome of equine patients with infectious diseases. Fecal samples are often submitted for *Salmonella* cultures from horses with diarrhea; it is usually recommended to take daily fecal cultures for 5 consecutive days; if no salmonellae are isolated from these five samples, then one can be reasonably confident that they are not shedding *Salmonella*.

PREVENTIVE HEALTH CARE

The equine veterinary technician may be a valuable resource for client education in areas of general horse care, vaccination programs, deworming protocols, and interstate shipment guidelines. Specific information in these areas will be dependent on geographic location. The technician and veterinarian should prepare standard recommendations that are appropriate for their region and clientele.

Vaccination

Vaccination plays a crucial role in equine management programs in preventing and controlling infectious disease within a

herd. Appropriate vaccination protocols will differ among horses depending on geographic location, age, use, and reproductive status. All horses should be vaccinated against influenza, rhinopneumonitis, encephalitis, tetanus, and rabies (see Chapter 14). The frequency of vaccination for these five diseases is dependent on age and reproductive status. Geographic and epidemiological circumstances dictate indications for administering vaccines to protect horses from botulism, strangles, equine viral arteritis, and Potomac horse fever. Initial vaccination schedules for naive horses should be administered according to manufacturer recommendations.

> **TECHNICIAN NOTE**
>
> The equine veterinary technician may be a valuable resource for client education in areas of general horse care, vaccination programs, deworming protocols, and interstate shipment guidelines.

Vaccinations are administered either subcutaneously or IM, depending on manufacturer instructions. Vaccinations are frequently given in the neck musculature; however, local inflammatory reactions may make the horse reluctant to lower or raise its head. The impact of local reactions can be reduced by administering vaccines deep in the semimembranous and semitendinosus muscles. Administration of vaccines into the pectoral or gluteal muscles is not recommended in horses.

Influenza is a highly contagious respiratory disease in horses and is characterized by fever, cough, and depression. Currently available influenza vaccines do not provide consistent protection from influenza virus challenge, but vaccination programs do reduce the incidence of disease within the herd and the severity and duration of disease in individual horses. Sedentary adult horses, not exposed to other horses, are at moderate risk of contracting influenza and should be vaccinated twice a year. Young horses and horses engaged in performance activities (racing, showing, training) are at high risk of contracting influenza because of their exposure to other horses and should be vaccinated every 3 months. Broodmares should be vaccinated against influenza in the 10th month of pregnancy to ensure adequate colostral transfer of antibody against influenza for the foal. Some horses may suffer a transient systemic reaction characterized by fever, inappetence, and depression several days after influenza vaccination. Therefore, vaccinations should be administered 7 to 10 days before a performance event.

Equine herpesvirus (the causative agent of rhinopneumonitis) is a highly contagious virus which produces respiratory disease, abortion, and neurological disease in horses. Protection against respiratory disease following equine herpesvirus vaccination is inconsistent and relatively short-lived. Sedentary adult horses, not exposed to other horses, should be vaccinated twice a year, whereas young horses and horses engaged in performance activities should be vaccinated every 3 months. Inactivated univalent vaccines should be administered to broodmares during the third, fifth, seventh, and ninth month of pregnancy to prevent abortion. Although 100% protection against abortion is not achieved, the incidence of equine herpesvirus abortion is significantly reduced by institution of this vaccination program. None of the current vaccines claim to provide protection against the neurological form (ascending paralysis) of herpesvirus in horses.

There are three forms of viral equine encephalomyelitis: eastern, western, and Venezuelan. The viral equine encephalitides produce rapidly progressive, highly fatal neurological disease in horses. Mosquitoes transmit the infection to horses; therefore, disease incidence is seasonal in most geographic regions. Vaccines for eastern and western equine encephalomyelitis are highly efficacious. Clinical disease in vaccinated horses is rare. All horses in the United States should be vaccinated against eastern and western equine encephalomyelitis virus in the spring. Horses that live in southern states with a year-round mosquito season should be vaccinated in the fall in addition to the spring vaccination. Broodmares should be vaccinated in the 10th month of gestation to ensure adequate colostral antibody protection for the foal. Vaccination against Venezuelan equine encephalomyelitis is not routinely recommended because the disease has not been reported recently in the United States and does not currently pose a threat to the U.S. horse population.

Tetanus is a highly fatal neurological disease in horses. It is characterized by a stiff, stilted gait, hyperexcitability, seizure, and coma. The causal organism is ubiquitous in the environment. The most common portals of entry for disease in horses include a subsolar abscess, penetrating wound, and infected IM injection site. Tetanus toxoid (inactivated) is a safe and efficacious vaccine for preventing clinical disease. Healthy horses without risk factors should be vaccinated for tetanus annually. Horses that acquire penetrating wounds, subsolar abscesses, or require surgery (colic and castration) should receive a booster vaccine if the most recent vaccination was administered more than 3 months before this incident. Unvaccinated horses at high risk of development of tetanus (wounds, subsolar abscess, surgery) should receive tetanus antitoxin, in addition to tetanus toxoid, to provide immediate protection against disease. Tetanus antitoxin is associated with fatal serum hepatitis, and administration should be limited to cases at high risk of disease.

Rabies is a rapidly progressive, fatal neurological disease in horses. Although the incidence of rabies is low, equine infection does represent a human health hazard. The most likely source of infection in horses is the bite of a rabid wild animal. Skunks, foxes, raccoons, and bats are the most common reservoirs in North America. Horses should be vaccinated against rabies on an annual basis starting at 3 months of age. Vaccinated horses that have been exposed to a rabid animal should be revaccinated promptly and observed for 90 days. Unvaccinated horses with a known rabies exposure should be observed for 6 months and should not be vaccinated.

Botulism is a rapidly progressive, fatal neurological disease in horses characterized by profound weakness, muscle fasciculations, and dysphagia (inability to swallow). The causal organism produces a neurotoxin which may gain entry to the body by colonizing the intestinal tract (foals), infected wounds, or contaminating feedstuffs. Colonization of the intestinal tract in foals occurs in particular geographic regions of the United States, especially Pennsylvania, Ohio, and Kentucky. Foals in endemic regions may be protected by vaccination of mares with botulism toxoid prior to foaling.

Strangles is a highly contagious, respiratory disease of horses caused by *Streptococcus equi*. The disease is characterized by abscess formation of the submandibular and retropharyngeal lymph nodes. Although strangles is common in young horses, vaccination is not routinely recommended. Vaccination provides incomplete, short-term protection against infection, whereas natural disease provides protection against infection for approximately 10 years. Additionally, currently available vaccines are commonly associated with swelling and abscess formation at the injection site and immune-mediated reactions (purpura hemorrhagica). Therefore, routine vaccination should be limited to herds with endemic clinical disease and rapid turnover of horses.

Equine viral arteritis is a contagious viral disease which produces limb swelling, abortion, and respiratory disease in horses. Stallions can develop a persistent infection in their reproductive tract which they readily transmit to mares during breeding. The vaccine for equine viral arteritis is approved for use in stallions and nonpregnant mares under the supervision of the U.S. Department of Agriculture (USDA). Pregnant mares should not be vaccinated for equine viral arteritis. Vaccination induces seropositivity and may interfere with testing requirements for export.

Potomac horse fever is caused by *Ehrlichia risticii* and produces diarrhea, fever, abortion, and laminitis. The mode of transmission is unknown, but suspected to involve an insect vector. Geographically, clinical disease is observed predominantly in states east of the Mississippi. Two inactivated bacterins are commercially available and should be administered to horses living in or traveling to endemic regions of the United States. Vaccination should be timed to precede the months (March through October) of peak disease incidence.

Systemic reactions may occasionally occur after vaccine administration. Anaphylaxis is a life-threatening systemic reaction which produces cardiovascular shock and respiratory distress. Anaphylaxis should be treated immediately with epinephrine. Local reactions characterized by swelling, heat, and pain are more common and are generally self-limiting. Administration of NSAIDs may speed recovery of local swellings, fever, and pain associated with vaccination. Fatal local reactions are rare, and are associated with infection of the injection site with clostridial organisms (malignant edema).

Deworming

Internal parasite control is an essential part of an effective preventive medicine program for all horses and is especially beneficial in young horses (see Chapter 6). Effective internal parasite control will allow young horses to grow to their full potential and will reduce the incidence of colic in horses of any age. An effective internal parasite control program should be directed at control of ascarids (large roundworms), small strongyles, large strongyles, and bots. Adult ascarids predominately affect young horses, live within the lumen of the intestinal tract, and may produce colic. Ascarid larvae migrate through the lungs and may produce parasitic pneumonia. The larvae of large strongyles migrate through the vascular system of the intestinal tract, and may reduce blood flow and cause colic. Bot larvae attach to the stomach wall creating inflammation, irritation, and potentially obstruction. Small strongyles migrate through the intestinal wall, which impairs nutrient absorption and creates inflammation. Small strongyles are particularly difficult to control because they have developed resistance to many of the commercially available anthelmintics. Small strongyle resistance to ivermectin, pyrantel pamoate, and oxibendazole is not currently recognized.

The frequency of anthelmintic administration is dependent on geographic location. In the northern United States, a seasonal deworming program can be used wherein dewormer is administered from March through November at 6- to 8-week intervals. A boticide should be administered after the first frost in the northern United States and Canada. In the southern United States, dewormer should be administered year-round at 6- to 8-week intervals. Foals should be dewormed beginning at 8 weeks of age. Properly administered paste dewormers have efficacy equal to tube deworming.

Daily administration of pyrantel tartrate is effective in controlling small strongyles, large strongyles, and ascarids. This product is added to the feed daily and kills larvae before their migration. A boticide (ivermectin) must also be administered in the fall of the year, in addition to daily administration of pyrantel tartrate. Daily deworming is more expensive than interval deworming.

Dental Care

Dental care is an important but frequently neglected part of health maintenance programs for horses. Regardless of age, the teeth of all horses should be examined annually. Dental problems may interfere with mastication, contribute to systemic infection, and cause chronic weight loss. Abnormal eating habits such as dropping grain, excessive salivation, dropping feed boluses (quidding), or tilting of the head during mastication are indications of dental problems. Thorough examination of the oral cavity often requires sedation, a flashlight, and a mouth speculum (gag). The frequency of routine dental care is dependent on the age and occlusal anatomy of the individual horse. Normal horses have three pairs of incisors, three pairs of premolars (second, third, and fourth premolars), and three pairs of molars on each arcade. Males usually have canine teeth, whereas females usually do not. Some horses will have "wolf teeth," which are remnants of the upper first premolar. Wolf teeth are small, round teeth adjacent to the second premolar (first cheek tooth). They often interfere with the bit and require removal between 12 and 18 months of age. Wolf teeth can be removed in standing, sedated horses.

Horses have hippsodontic dentition, meaning their teeth continue to elongate and wear throughout their lives. Therefore, dental surfaces that are not opposed by the adjacent arcade owing to abnormal anatomy, malalignment, or malocclusion develop sharp, protruding enamel surfaces called "points" and "hooks." The upper arcade of normal horses is wider than the lower arcade, therefore, points develop on the buccal (cheek) surface of the upper arcade and the lingual (tongue) surface of the lower arcade. Often the upper arcade is shifted rostrally (with respect to the lower arcade), and hooks will develop on the rostral surface of the first premolar on the upper arcade and the caudal surface of the last molar on the lower arcade. Dental hooks and points can cause erosion and ulceration of the tongue and cheek, dropping feed, and weight loss. Most hooks and points can be removed by floating (rasping) the teeth with dental floats (Fig. 21–24). Large hooks may be removed using molar cutters. Many of the severe, often untreatable malocclusions and wear abnormalities seen in older horses can be prevented by regular dental care.

The most common malocclusive disorder in horses is parrot mouth or prognathism, and there is likely a heritable component to this disorder. Prognathism is characterized as an unsoundness in horses and results in difficult prehension of food and dental hooks on the first premolar (upper) and last molar (lower). Dental examination should be performed every 6 months in horses with prognathism.

Horses with an infected tooth root typically present with malodorous nasal discharge. The tooth roots of the last four teeth on the upper arcade are located within the maxillary sinus; therefore infected teeth result in secondary sinusitis. The affected tooth can be identified by skull radiographs, and the fourth premolar and first molar are most commonly involved. Removal of the affected tooth is the only effective treatment approach. Teeth generally cannot be removed from the oral cavity. Rather, teeth are repelled from their roots via an incision into the maxillary sinus or trephination in the maxilla or mandible (under general anesthesia) and driven into the oral cavity for removal.

Young horses (2 to 3 years) may retain deciduous caps after eruption of the permanent teeth. Retained caps can produce ulcerations on the cheeks, inadequate mastication, and dropping of feed, and should be removed if retained for more than a few months. Retained caps can be removed in standing, sedated horses.

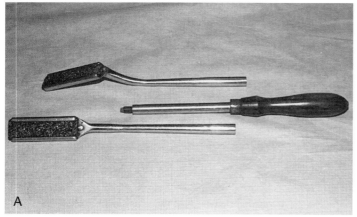
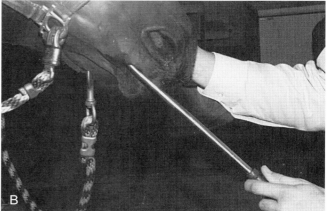

Figure 21–24. A, Tooth floats used to file off the enamel points of the upper and lower cheek teeth of horses. B, Technique for floating teeth in a horse.

Equine Infectious Anemia

Equine infectious anemia (EIA) is a viral disease of horses that results in anemia, fever, and weight loss. The disease is transmitted by biting flies, and once infected, horses become permanent carriers of the disease. Horses must have a negative (Coggins) test for EIA within 1 year for issuance of health certificates for interstate travel, international travel, show, and sale. A USDA-accredited veterinarian must draw blood for testing and provide a detailed description of the horse on specified forms. The health certificate for interstate travel cannot be issued until the negative test is returned from a state or federally recognized laboratory. Horses that are not traveling or sold should still be tested on a yearly basis. If a positive test is obtained, the entire herd is quarantined until all horses on the premises are tested (usually 60 days). Only the state veterinarian can release the quarantine. Because horses that test positive for EIA are persistent carriers, they serve as a reservoir of infection for all horses they contact. Therefore, infected horses must be quarantined for life (greater than 200 yards from other horses) or euthanized. The veterinary technician may be involved in collection of blood, completing submission forms, and sending samples for EIA testing under the direct supervision of the attending veterinarian.

SELECTED MEDICAL DISEASES

Equine Respiratory Diseases

Strangles is a common, highly contagious respiratory disease of horses caused by the bacterial pathogen *S. equi.* Typically, strangles produces swelling and abscesses of the submandibular and retropharyngeal lymph nodes. Affected horses have fever, depression, poor appetite, and painful swellings under the mandible. The abscesses under the mandible enlarge, rupture, and drain a large volume of purulent exudate. Horses may develop abscesses within the guttural pouch, thorax, abdomen, and central nervous system. Development of abscess in abnormal locations is termed "bastard strangles." These cases are particularly difficult to treat successfully. Horses with complicated cases of strangles should be treated with antibiotics, and *S. equi* is typically sensitive to penicillin. Horses with strangles should be maintained under strict isolation protocol. Recovered horses remain contagious and represent a threat to susceptible horses for approximately 6 weeks after recovering from clinical disease.

Influenza is a highly contagious viral respiratory disease in horses characterized by a temperature of 40°C (104°F), cough, and depression. The incubation period is short (2 to 3 days) and horses remain ill for 3 to 4 days. Equine influenza virus is transmitted through a herd via aerosolization of virus during coughing. The virus damages the clearance mechanisms in the lung, and predisposes horses to bacterial pneumonia. Horses should be rested for a minimum of 3 weeks after recovery from viral respiratory disease. Currently available influenza vaccines do not provide consistent protection from influenza virus challenge; however, vaccination programs do decrease the incidence of disease within the herd, and the severity and duration of disease in individual horses.

Equine herpesvirus is a highly contagious virus which produces respiratory disease, abortion, and neurological disease (ascending paralysis) in horses. The clinical signs of respiratory disease caused by equine herpesvirus is indistinguishable from equine influenza. The incubation period is longer (2 to 10 days), and horses may remain ill for 4 to 5 days. Equine herpesvirus is transmitted through the herd by aerosol transmission, respiratory secretions, and fomite transmission. Protection against respiratory disease following equine herpesvirus vaccination is inconsistent and relatively short-lived. Abortion secondary to equine herpesvirus occurs in the 7th to 11th month of gestation, and the mare does not appear sick at the time of abortion. Although 100% protection against abortion is not achieved, the incidence of equine herpesvirus abortion is significantly reduced by institution of a vaccination program. Ascending paralysis is the least common manifestation of equine herpesvirus infection. Affected horses demonstrate signs of incoordination, inability to urinate, and poor tail tone. Recovery from neurological diseases is prolonged (2 to 3 months) and horses may not return to completely normal neurological function. None of the currently available vaccines claim to provide protection against the neurological form of herpesvirus in horses.

Equine viral arteritis is a contagious viral disease that produces limb swelling, conjunctivitis, abortion, and respiratory disease in horses. Limb swelling is painful and results from vasculitis (inflammation of blood vessels). Stallions infected after puberty develop a persistent infection in their accessory sex glands (ampullae), and transmit the viral infection to mares during breeding. Abortion can occur at any point during gestation and results from viral damage to the blood vessels of the placenta. The vaccine for equine viral arteritis is approved for use in stallions and nonpregnant mares under the supervision of the USDA. Pregnant mares should not be vaccinated against equine viral arteritis.

Chronic obstructive pulmonary disease (COPD, heaves) is an allergic airway disease which produces narrowing of small airways (bronchoconstriction) and excessive mucus production. The clinical signs of COPD are cough, nasal discharge, flared nostrils, increased respiratory rate, and increased respiratory effort. The severity of clinical signs may range from exercise intolerance to severe respiratory distress (dyspnea) at rest. Most affected horses are allergic to the molds present in hay and straw. Ideally, horses should be maintained at pasture and hay should be removed as the source of roughage in the diet. A similar form of this disease is observed in horses during the summer months in the southern United States. Summer pasture–associated obstructive pulmonary disease (SPAOPD) usually occurs from June to September and is associated with horses' access to molds on the pasture. Horses cannot be "cured" of COPD or SPAOPD, but the diseases can often be controlled with appropriate management practices. Changing the environment to remove offending allergens is the single most important principle in the treatment of COPD and SPAOPD. Medical therapy of horses with COPD or SPAOPD may be intermittently necessary in moderate to severely affected horses, and consists of corticosteroids to reduce inflammation and bronchodilator therapy to relax small airways.

The guttural pouches are two, large symmetrical dilations of the eustachian tube that are present in all Equidae. They are located just above the pharynx and larynx, and can be accessed during endoscopic examination through small openings in the dorsal lateral nasopharynx. The internal and external carotid arteries and several cranial nerves travel superficially under the surface of the guttural pouch lining and are vulnerable to damage from pathologic conditions. The purpose of the guttural pouches may be to lower the temperature of the blood that is traveling to the brain (internal and external carotid arteries) during exercise. Bacterial infection of the guttural pouch is termed *guttural pouch empyema* and is often associated with strangles. Fungal infection of the guttural pouch is termed *guttural pouch mycosis* and the causative agent is often *Aspergillus* sp. The fungal plaque usually forms over the internal carotid artery, adjacent to nerves that control swallowing. Horses may have life-threatening blood loss from rupture of the internal carotid artery or dysphagia from damage to the nerves. Accumulation of air in the guttural pouches (guttural pouch tympany) occurs in foals and weanlings and is usually associated with an abnormality of the opening to the pouches. It can occur unilaterally or bilaterally and is characterized by a fluctuant nonpainful swelling in the throatlatch region. Guttural pouch empyema is characterized by accumulation of mucopurulent material in the pouches, which is often secondary to retropharyngeal lymph node abscess formation from a streptococcal infection.

Gastrointestinal Disease

"Choke" refers to obstruction of the esophagus. Chronic dental disease and retained deciduous caps are common predisposing conditions for development of choke. The esophagus is usually obstructed by grain or hay and most horses will continue to attempt to eat despite their inability to swallow. Clinical signs include anxiety, gagging, and feed and saliva coming from the nostrils. The obstruction can be visualized via endoscopic examination, and in most instances can be relieved by manipulation and hydropulsion using a nasogastric tube. Horses must be heavily sedated to lower their head during manipulation of the nasogastric tube to prevent water and feed from entering the trachea. Aspiration pneumonia is a significant complication and must be addressed in all cases. Esophageal stricture or rupture is a less common complication, and occurs in horses with circumferential damage to the esophageal mucosa.

Young horses are particularly prone to development of gastric ulceration. Stress, high-grain diet, musculoskeletal pain, and administration of NSAIDs are common predisposing factors. Clinical signs of gastric ulceration are bruxism (grinding teeth), hypersalivation, and abdominal pain after eating. Foals with gastric ulceration will often lie still in dorsal recumbency with their forelimbs over their head or extended out straight. Human antiulcer medications such as histamine H_2 blockers, intestinal protectorants, and hydrogen ion pump blockers are used to treat gastric ulceration in horses. Most equine facilities administer prophylactic antiulcer therapy to hospitalized foals because of the stressful environment.

Colitis in horses can result in rapid, life-threatening fluid loss (hypovolemia), shock, endotoxemia, electrolyte loss, and acid-base imbalance as a result of diarrhea. Some horses may develop hypovolemic shock and electrolyte imbalance before the appearance of diarrhea. In addition to diarrhea, clinical signs of colitis include depression, inappetence, abdominal pain, tachycardia (increased heart rate), injected (brick-red) mucous membranes, and prolonged capillary refill time. Etiologic agents that produce life-threatening diarrhea in horses include *Salmonella, Clostridium,* and *Ehrlichia risticii.* Horses with diarrhea should be considered contagious and maintained under isolation protocol. Intravenous fluid therapy is crucial to support the cardiovascular system, replace fluid losses, and correct electrolyte and acid-base imbalance. Complications of colitis

include laminitis (founder), cardiovascular collapse, cardiac arrhythmias, and thrombophlebitis.

Phenylbutazone toxicosis in horses can produce renal insufficiency and oral, gastric, and colonic ulceration in horses. The colonic ulcers occur in the right dorsal colon and are the most difficult aspect of phenylbutazone toxicity to treat. Colonic ulcers secondary to phenylbutazone toxicity can produce abdominal pain, marked protein loss, melena (blood in manure), peritonitis, colonic stricture, or colonic rupture. Dehydration and excessive dosages are the most important predisposing factors for development of phenylbutazone toxicosis.

Neurological Disease

The five most common disorders of the spinal cord include cervical stenotic myelopathy (wobbles), equine protozoal myelitis, equine herpesvirus myelitis (rhinopneumonitis), equine degenerative myeloencephalopathy, and vertebral fracture. Damage to the spinal cord produces spinal ataxia (incoordination of the limbs without abnormalities of the brain and brain stem). Diagnostic aids which help to differentiate these diseases include neurological examination, cervical radiographic examination, myelographic examination, and CSF analysis. CSF can be obtained at the lumbosacral space in standing, sedated horses, and at the atlanto-occipital space in anesthetized horses. CSF travels from cranial to caudal. Therefore, CSF should be obtained at the lumbosacral space in horses with spinal cord disease and at the atlanto-occipital space in horses with brain and brain stem disease.

Cervical stenotic myelopathy is a manifestation of developmental orthopedic disease characterized by compression of the cervical spinal cord by malformed or unstable cervical vertebrae. Males are affected four times more frequently than females, and Thoroughbreds appear to be predisposed. Clinical signs of symmetrical incoordination usually begin between 6 months and 3 years of age. The hindlimbs are usually more severely affected than the forelimbs. Likelihood of disease is determined by plain film cervical radiographs, and the diagnosis is confirmed by myelographic examination. Surgical stabilization improves the neurological status of some patients.

Equine protozoal myelitis (EPM) is the most common cause of spinal ataxia in the United States. Horses are dead-end, aberrant hosts of the protozoan parasite *Sarcocystis neurona (Sarcocystis falcatula).* Opossums are the primary hosts of this parasite, and horses are likely infected via fecal-oral transmission. Birds are the secondary hosts, and do not appear to be infectious for horses. The clinical signs of EPM are directly referable to the location of the organism in the central nervous system. Therefore, EPM should be considered in any horse demonstrating neurological signs. Most horses with EPM (85%) demonstrate signs referable to spinal cord damage. Diagnosis is confirmed by identification of antibody to the organism in CSF. Treatment consists of administration of two antibiotics that inhibit folic acid metabolism: sulfadiazine and pyrimethamine. The average treatment period is approximately 120 days, and the prognosis for return to normal neurological function is 60%. Folic acid should be administered to prevent development of anemia during treatment.

Equine herpesvirus can produce respiratory disease, abortion, and neurological disease in horses. The neurological form is characterized by ascending paralysis with the hindlimbs more severely affected than the forelimbs. Horses often demonstrate urinary incontinence, poor tail tone, and penile prolapse. Diagnosis is confirmed by cytological analysis of CSF. Administration of corticosteroids may improve recovery if administered early in the disease process. Prognosis for return to normal neurological function is approximately 80%.

Equine degenerative myelopathy results in symmetrical spinal ataxia with both the forelimbs and hindlimbs equally affected. Clinical signs appear between 6 months and 2 years of age, and the disease appears to be familial in some breeds. There is no definitive antemortem diagnostic test, and diagnosis is usually made on the basis of the neurological examination, CSF analysis, cervical radiographs, and myelographic examination. Dietary supplementation with vitamin E may prevent progression of disease and may result in improvement in clinical signs in some instances. The prognosis for return to normal neurological function is poor.

The most consistent clinical sign associated with *vertebral fracture* is pain. The cervical vertebrae, caudal thoracic vertebrae, and thoracolumbar junction are the most common sites of vertebral fracture. Cervical vertebral fracture results in tetraparesis (weakness of all four limbs), whereas fracture of the thoracic and lumbar vertebrae produces paraparesis (weakness of hindlimbs) or paraplegia (paralysis of hindlimbs). Diagnosis is confirmed by plain film radiography. If the fracture is nondisplaced, nuclear scintigraphy may aid in identification of the fracture site. Surgical correction may be attempted for fractures of the cervical vertebrae, but repair of thoracic or lumbar vertebrae is not attempted.

The four most common disorders of the brain and brain stem in horses are rabies, equine viral encephalitis (eastern, western, and Venezuelan), leukoencephalomalacia (moldy corn toxicity), and head trauma. Damage to the cerebrum may produce altered mentation, altered states of consciousness, head-pressing, and seizure. Damage to the brain stem may potentially damage the cranial nerves which control the muscles of facial expression, facial sensation, mastication, swallowing, balance, vision, taste, and ocular position. Brain stem lesions also produce incoordination of the limbs and altered breathing patterns. Diagnostic aids for evaluation of horses with cerebral or brain stem dysfunction include CSF analysis and skull radiographs.

Rabies is a zoonotic infection (infectious to man) and is universally fatal (see Chapter 7). Horses usually acquire the infection by a bite wound from a rabid skunk, fox, or bat. Clinical signs are highly variable, but often begin as fever, hindlimb ataxia, and hyperesthesia (hyperresponsive to touch). Neurological signs rapidly progress to involve the brain and brain stem. The average duration of neurological signs prior to death is approximately 3 days. Diagnosis is confirmed by fluorescent antibody stain of brain tissue. Humans handling potentially rabid horses should avoid contact with saliva, wear gloves, and avoid contact with CSF. Individuals with occupational exposure to livestock and wildlife should undergo prophylactic rabies vaccination series. Postexposure rabies vaccination should be administered to humans contacting rabid animals.

The *equine viral encephalitides*, eastern, western, and Venezuelan, are transmitted to horses by mosquitos. Clinical signs include profound depression, fever, and multiple cranial nerve abnormalities, and mortality is extremely high. Treatment consists of supportive care to provide fluids, nutrition, and a clean, dry environment. The prognosis is poor, and recovery to normal neurological function in surviving horses is rare. Diagnosis is confirmed by mouse inoculation. The viral encephalitides can be prevented by yearly vaccination, 1 month before mosquito season. In southern regions of the United States, vaccinations should be administered twice a year.

Equine leukoencephalomalacia (moldy corn toxicity) is caused by ingestion of a fungal toxin produced by *Fusarium moniliform*. This mold has a predilection for moldy corn, and affected kernels are usually pink to brown. The fungal toxin produces liquefactive necrosis of the cerebral cortex, and clinical signs include profound depression, head-pressing, altered states of consciousness, incoordination, and aimless wandering. Treatment consists of supportive care, and the prognosis for recovery is poor. Horses often die within 24 hours of manifesting neurological signs.

Horses acquire two types of skull fractures depending on the nature of their traumatic injury. Horses that suffer frontal impact with a solid object develop depression fractures of the frontal and parietal bones. The common neurological signs observed in horses with this type of fracture are referable to cerebral damage and include depression, seizure, stupor, and aimless wandering. Horses that flip over backward develop fractures of the petrous temporal bone, and the junction of the basisphenoid and basioccipital bone. Neurological signs associated with these fractures include abnormalities of balance, incoordination of limbs, nystagmus (rhythmic eye movement), abnormal respiratory patterns, and coma. Diagnosis is confirmed by radiographic examination of the skull. Treatment consists of supportive care and anti-inflammatory therapy (corticosteroids and DMSO). Surgical decompression of frontal and parietal fractures may improve the neurological status of some horses.

Dermatologic Disease

Equine dermatophytosis (ringworm) is a fungal infection of the superficial layer of skin. The fungi commonly involved are *Trichophyton* and *Microsporum* species. Transmission of the fungal infection is by direct contact between affected animals, and younger animals (less than 4 years old) are more likely to be affected. Infected areas of skin have a bull's-eye appearance with circular patches of hair loss with a circle of inflammation at the periphery of the lesion. Diagnosis is confirmed by fungal culture on commercially available dermatophyte culture medium. Although the infection is usually self-limiting, application of topical antifungal drugs will speed recovery.

Dermatophilosis (rain scald, rain rot) is a common bacterial infection caused by *Dermatophilus congolensis* that produces crusting lesions over the topline. The crusts can be pulled out with a tuft of hair, and the remaining lesion is a glistening, yellow crater. The organisms readily colonize wet, macerated skin, and therefore the disease is common in the winter and spring. An impression smear of the tuft should be stained with Wright's stain, and organisms are identified as a double chain of cocci with a "railroad track" appearance. The organisms are usually easily cultured, and form an applesauce-like colony on specialized growth medium. Affected horses should be bathed with an iodine-based shampoo, and placed in a dry environment. Administration of penicillin will speed recovery in severely affected horses.

Culicoides hypersensitivity is a syndrome characterized by mane and tail rubbing whereby affected horses develop an allergic pruritic skin condition secondary to the bite of *Culi-*

coides flies. The classic body regions affected include face, ears, mane, withers, rump, and tail. The dermatitis usually begins as a seasonal condition, but its severity and duration increase as the horse ages. Pruritus usually is noted during the fly season, but will vary in length depending on geographic location. The condition is diagnosed by correlating the historical findings of seasonal pruritus with physical evidence of self-mutilation, especially in the mane and tail areas. Intradermal skin testing can be useful in confirming the diagnosis. Treatment involves reducing insect exposure and concomitant use of anti-inflammatory medication. Because *Culicoides* breeds in stagnant waters, affected horses should be moved from proximity to ponds, lakes, or irrigation canals. Water troughs and barrels should be cleaned frequently and the water kept fresh to prevent use as breeding sites by the flies. Because *Culicoides* feeds primarily at dusk, night, and dawn, horses should be kept stabled during these times. Stabling is most effective if the doors and windows can be closed and if the stall is lined with a fine-mesh screen. Frequent application of insecticide to the screen may also be useful. Ceiling fans help reduce exposure because *Culicoides* cannot fly well in brisk breezes. Application of insecticides and repellents are a necessary part of disease control. The most effective products are those containing pyrethrins with synergists and repellents. Frequent bathing not only decreases scale and crust but also seems to decrease pruritus. Corticosteroid therapy may be required in some horses to control the pruritus.

Equine sarcoid is a benign, locally invasive tumor of skin, and is the most common tumor in horses. These tumors produce either raised, hairless lesions with a corrugated surface that often bleed when traumatized, known as a fibroblastic sarcoid, or a flattened form known as a verrucous sarcoid. The cause of sarcoid is unknown, but a viral cause is suspected. Surgical resection, cryotherapy (freezing), laser therapy, immunotherapy (intralesional mycobacterial cell wall extract), radiotherapy (iridium 191), and chemotherapy (intralesional cisplatin) are accepted treatment modalities with variable success. It is difficult to predict response to a given treatment modality, and combination therapy is often necessary.

Melanomas are relatively common skin tumors that develop particularly in gray horses. They occur most commonly in the perineal region, but can occur on other areas of the body. Melanomas appear as darkly pigmented nodules in the skin. They are usually benign, but tend to progress and can cause mechanical problems such as interfering with defecation. Most clinicians believe it is better not to attempt surgical removal unless they are located in an area that interferes with tack or they are so large that they interfere with normal body functions. These tumors often become more aggressive following unsuccessful attempts at complete surgical removal. Administration of cimetidine has been reported to be effective in some horses in causing reduction in size or resolution of melanomas, but, it does not seem to be effective in all horses. Once the cimetidine is discontinued, the tumors usually enlarge.

Ophthalmologic Disease

Anterior uveitis (moon blindness, periodic ophthalmia) is the most common cause of blindness in horses. Affected horses suffer episodes of intraocular inflammation characterized by blepharospasm, corneal edema, and hypopyon (exudate in the anterior chamber). Over time, the episodes become more frequent and severe, and produce permanent ocular lesions, in-cluding retinal degeneration, cataracts, synechiae (adhesions in the anterior chamber), and low ocular pressure. The disease may be unilateral or bilateral. Anterior uveitis is classified as an unsoundness in horses, which constitutes failure during prepurchase and insurance examinations. Anterior uveitis cannot be cured, but can be controlled in some instances with chronic anti-inflammatory therapy (phenylbutazone, aspirin). Acute episodes are treated with atropine and anti-inflammatory therapy (flunixin meglumine, phenylbutazone, aspirin, or corticosteroids). Although many factors have been implicated (heredity, parasites, leptospirosis), the cause of uveitis is unknown. Horses with end-stage uveitis are blind and have very small, collapsed, ocular globes (phthisis bulbi).

Corneal ulceration commonly results from ocular trauma. Corneal ulceration can be detected by application of fluorescein dye to the surface of the eye. Defects in the corneal surface will stain an apple-green color. Corneal ulceration in most horses responds readily without complications to administration of topical antibacterial ointment (bacitracin, neomycin, polymyxin B). In some instances, the ulcer will be colonized by *Pseudomonas* or *Aspergillus* species. These organisms produce collagenase, which destroys the cornea and creates a "melting" corneal ulcer. These ulcers are rapidly progressive and prone to uveal prolapse or ocular rupture. Frequent antibiotic dosage regimens may require placement of a subpalpebral lavage system, wherein polyethylene tubing is placed into the eyelid and exits the conjunctiva dorsal to the globe. The port of the tubing can be braided into the horse's mane which facilitates frequent dosing for a painful eye. Aggressive topical antibacterial therapy may be successful, but, suturing a conjunctival pedicle flap to provide blood supply to the affected area may be necessary to save the globe in some instances. Deep, melting corneal ulcers often heal with a fibrous scar which may impair vision in the future.

Neonatal Care

The normal gestation period of mares ranges from 320 to 360 days. As a mare approaches parturition, the udder begins to enlarge ("bagging up") and may leak small amounts of colostrum which dries over the ends of the teats ("waxing"). Increasing calcium and magnesium concentrations in milk correspond to impending (less than 24 hours) parturition, and can be detected using commercially available "foal predictor" kits. Parturition occurs in three stages. Stage 1 is under voluntary control of the mare (within 24 hours), and is characterized by positioning of the fetus in the birth canal. External signs of stage 1 labor include restlessness, sweating, pacing, inappetence, and raising the tail. The onset of stage 2 labor is signaled by rupture of the chorioallantoic membrane and release of allantoic fluid (breaking water). Delivery of the foal should be complete within 20 to 40 minutes of the onset of stage 2 labor. The third stage of labor begins after expulsion of the foal and is defined by expulsion of the fetoplacental membranes. Fetoplacental membranes should be passed within 2 hours of expulsion of the foal. Retained placenta (failure to pass fetal membranes within 3 hours of delivery) is an emergency in mares and may result in toxic metritis and laminitis. After parturition, the umbilicus is dipped in an iodine or chlorhexidine solution, foals are examined for developmental anomalies and traumatic injury, the mare's reproductive tract is examined for traumatic injury, and the placenta is inspected for completeness and evidence of thickening or infection.

Normal foals should stand and suckle within 2 hours of parturition. It is important for the foal to ingest the colostrum ("first milk") produced by the mare. Colostrum contains immunoglobulins and other factors which provide protection against infection. Foals are born without immunoglobulin in their blood, and the immunoglobulin in colostrum represents the only form of immune protection (passive transfer of immunity). The immunoglobulin in colostrum is absorbed intact by the intestinal tract for the first 18 hours of life. After that time, the intestinal tract will no longer absorb the large immunoglobulin proteins (gut closure). If a foal does not receive adequate colostrum it is termed "failure of passive transfer." Failure of passive transfer can occur with failure to suckle, premature gut closure, failure of the dam to produce good-quality colostrum, and leakage of colostrum prior to parturition, and is the single most important predisposing factor for development of life-threatening neonatal infections. Adequate transfer of immunity should be assessed at 18 to 24 hours of life, using a commercially available foal immunoglobulin G (IgG) test kit, such as the enzyme immunoassay (CITE, IDEXX Laboratories) for semiquantitative measurement of IgG concentration in serum, plasma, or whole blood. This test is frequently performed by the veterinary technician. If the foal has not received adequate colostrum, it should be supplemented by IV plasma transfusion, using either commercial hyperimmune plasma or plasma collected from an appropriate donor.

Normal foals suckle 25 to 30 times per day, ingest 20% of their body weight in milk, and gain 4.4 to 6.0 kg (2.0 to 2.5 lbs) per day. Foals are particularly fragile, and failure to suckle is the first sign of disease. Neonatal septicemia and neonatal maladjustment syndrome are the most common life-threatening diseases of foals. The most common cause of neonatal septicemia is failure of passive transfer, and the umbilicus is a common portal of entry (navel ill). Clinical signs include depression, fever, tachycardia, injected mucous membranes, respiratory distress, shock, hypothermia, and coma. If untreated, neonatal septicemia usually results in death of the foal. Septic arthritis (joint ill) is a common sequela to neonatal septicemia which may produce permanent damage to the joint cartilage. Neonatal maladjustment syndrome (dummy foal) occurs secondary to low blood oxygen concentrations in late gestation (insufficient placentation), during parturition (dystocia), or immediately after birth (premature cord rupture, failure to rupture placental membranes). Foals may be born abnormal or may develop neurological abnormalities within 24 hours after birth. The range of neurological abnormalities includes failure to suckle, hyperresponsiveness, depression, bizarre vocalization (barkers), failure to recognize the dam, stupor, coma, and seizures. The neurological signs result from hemorrhage and edema in the brain and brain stem. Less common causes of neonatal distress include ruptured bladder, neonatal isoerythrolysis (hemolysis due to incompatible blood type with mare), and pulmonary insufficiency due to prematurity (failure to produce surfactant).

Recumbent neonatal foals require intensive supportive care consisting of a 24-hour attendant, constant IV infusion system, nutritional supplementation, oxygen supplementation, and accessible blood gas and electrolyte analyzers. Recumbent foals are placed on a foal bed, which is designed to allow the attendant to care for the foal from one side, and the mare to access the foal from the other. Foals should be maintained in sternal recumbency to prevent collapse of the down lung, allowing maximal ventilation. Foals must be kept clean and dry, and their position should be changed every 4 hours. Recumbent foals are prone to corneal ulceration; therefore, triple antibiotic ointment or artificial tears should be placed in their eyes every 4 hours. Heart rate, respiratory rate and character, temperature, mucous membrane character, capillary refill time, abdominal distention, and gastrointestinal motility should be monitored every 2 hours. Urinary and fecal output should be recorded. Arterial blood gas, PCV, total protein, serum electrolyte, and serum glucose concentrations should be determined every 4 to 8 hours depending on the severity of the disease. Palpation of the umbilicus and joints should be performed daily.

Intravenous fluid therapy is necessary to support the cardiovascular system, correct electrolyte abnormalities, and maintain acid-base balance. Bactericidal antibiotics with a broad spectrum of activity against gram-negative organisms should be used to prevent and treat bacterial infection in foals. Foals readily develop gastric ulceration under conditions of stress, and therefore prophylactic antiulcer medication is administered to all foals in intensive care. Nutritional support can be provided by feeding the mare's milk using a small nasoesophageal feeding tube. The mare should be hand-milked every 2 hours, but, if the mare does not produce sufficient milk to meet the nutritional requirements of the foal, equine milk replacers may be used. Total parenteral nutrition (TPN—IV nutritional support) may be necessary in foals with poor gastrointestinal motility and primary gastrointestinal disease. TPN requires a dedicated IV catheter and a constant infusion pump. Most recumbent foals demonstrate some degree of respiratory insufficiency. Oxygen can be supplemented to the foal using nasal insufflation with 100% oxygen at 4 to 8 liters/minute. If nasal insufflation is inadequate, the foal may require mechanical ventilation to ensure adequate oxygenation. Mechanical ventilation requires nasotracheal or endotracheal intubation and positive pressure ventilation. Pulmonary function can be monitored using serial arterial blood gas evaluation, obtained from the greater metatarsal artery.

✏️ **TECHNICIAN NOTE**

Regardless of the primary disease process, neonatal intensive care is a daunting task. The veterinary technician attending to the recumbent foal must be diligent, thorough, aseptic, and observant.

Regardless of the primary disease process, neonatal intensive care is a daunting task. The veterinary technician attending to the recumbent foal must be diligent, thorough, aseptic, and observant. Deterioration in patient status occurs rapidly and without warning. Meticulous patient care and monitoring will allow rapid correction of the therapeutic plan, which often determines the final outcome for neonatal foals.

Dystocia

Dystocia means difficult birth and is relatively uncommon in horses, compared with cattle. However, when dystocia occurs in mares it is usually a serious problem. Because parturition is rapid in horses, and the expulsive efforts of the mare are violent, veterinary obstetrical manipulations are difficult and exhausting. Care must be taken at all times not to injure the reproductive tract of the mare. There are many causes of dystocia in the mare, but the most frequent is abnormal presentation, especially when either the head or limbs, or both, are deviated. Because the neck of the foal is relatively long, it can easily become twisted. Sometimes the foal may come hindfeet first (rare), or if the hindfeet are retained, the tail comes first. This latter situation is true breech position. Transverse presentation is also rare in mares. Other occasional causes of dystocia include an excessively large fetus or fetal monsters (such as hydrocephalus). An anatomical or physiological abnormality in the mare herself may cause dystocia. For example, a mare that has sustained a pelvic fracture can develop callus formation, which impairs the shape and size of the birth canal. Another cause of dystocia is torsion of the uterus. This may occur during gestation, particularly during the last trimester.

Dystocia in mares is corrected using a variety of methods, depending upon the cause of the dystocia, the status of the foal, and the condition of the mare. Sometimes the dystocia can be corrected by manipulating fetal position or presentation with the mare standing, with or without the use of sedation or an epidural anesthetic. Placement of a nasotracheal tube will prevent the mare from exerting an abdominal press and will relieve straining. Sometimes, a short-acting anesthetic protocol combined with rolling the mare on her back or hoisting her hindlimbs is enough to relieve the dystocia and provide the veterinarian with enough relaxation in the mare to deliver the fetus. Fetotomy is sometimes performed to relieve dystocia, particularly if the fetus is dead. Fetotomy is a process in which a dead foal is cut into pieces while in the uterus and removed. Caution must be taken while performing a fetotomy to prevent serious injury to the reproductive tract of the mare.

✎ **TECHNICIAN NOTE**

Most cesarean sections are performed in the mare with general anesthesia. Generally, time is critical for saving the foal and for the overall health and well-being of the mare. The technician must be prepared for the surgery and have necessary equipment, personnel, and drugs ready for reviving the foal if necessary.

Most cesarean sections are performed in the mare with general anesthesia. Generally a cesarean section is performed though a caudal ventral midline or flank incision in mares. Time is usually critical for saving the foal and for the overall health and well-being of the mare. The technician must be prepared for the surgery and have necessary equipment, personnel, and drugs ready for reviving the foal if necessary. The same instruments that are used for colic surgery are often used for cesarean section, but additional instruments may be necessary. If the foal is alive, the technician or other personnel need to be prepared and equipped to revive it. The foal will usually be depressed from the effects of general anesthesia and may need vigorous

rubbing and drying. Oxygen should be available, as well as heat lamps and a nasotracheal tube and Ambu bag to ventilate the foal. Forceps to clamp the umbilicus should be readily available if excessive bleeding occurs. A suction device to remove mucus and stomach contents should be attended to by the technician or other personnel. The technician should be cognizant and attentive to the needs of the surgeon during this time even though the foal is requiring assistance.

A piece of straw inserted in the nostril is one of the most practical methods of initiating respiratory movements in a newborn foal. The foal's neck should be extended to help assure a patent airway. The foal should be vigorously dried because fluid will conduct heat away from the animal, resulting in hypothermia and a weak foal. The foal can be resuscitated with the self-inflating nonrebreathing Ambu bag. Air can be delivered through a cone-shaped face mask similar to the one used to induce anesthesia in small animals. The mask must fit tightly over the nostrils and mouth. Mouth-to-nose ventilation may be performed and is done by covering one nostril, closing the mouth, and blowing in the opposite nostril. A few short breaths are all that is usually required. Overinflation can obviously cause permanent damage to the lungs. Frequently, the veterinarian may order IV fluids, respiratory stimulants, and drugs to support the cardiovascular system. The foal should be kept warm (not hot) with heat lamps, circulating warm-water pads, and blankets. The next important thing is to ensure that the foal consumes or is administered an adequate amount of colostrum to provide passive immunity to infectious agents during the first few weeks of life.

Surgery of the Female Caudal Reproductive Tract

Perineal surgery is relatively common in equine practice. Primiparous mares develop rectovaginal and cervical lacerations during foaling. Abnormal perineal conformation can lead to reproductive unsoundness. Mares with abnormal conformation can develop pneumovagina or pneumouterus secondary to aspirating air into the reproductive tract. They also can develop vesicovaginal reflux in which urine pools in the cranial vaginal cavity; this can drain into the uterus during estrus when the cervix is opened, leading to endometrial inflammation. Most surgical procedures to correct these caudal reproductive tract abnormalities are performed in standing mares that have been sedated and a caudal epidural anesthesia is performed.

A caudal epidural anesthesia is performed after clipping the hair over the tail head and aseptically preparing the skin. An 18-gauge 1.5-inch needle is inserted through the skin between the last sacral and first coccygeal vertebrae or between the first and second coccygeal vertebrae and advanced (Fig. 21–25). The correct location can be confirmed by checking to see if local anesthetic placed in the hub of the needle is drawn into the epidural space. Once the correct location has been identified, the local anesthetic is injected. The most commonly used agents for horses are lidocaine, carbocaine, or xylazine. A caudal epidural anesthetic will desensitize the perineal region. Because horses will also become incoordinated in their rearlimbs following the procedure, care should be taken when moving them until the effects of the anesthetic dissipate.

There are several surgical procedures for correcting caudal reproductive tract abnormalities. The most important factor in the eventual success of repairing a rectovaginal tear is that the

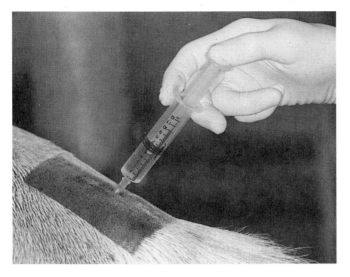

Figure 21-25. Technique for performing a caudal epidural between the first and second coccygeal vertebrae in a horse with an 18-gauge, 1.5-inch needle.

mare's feces be made soft (cow patty consistency) and kept soft for 30 days after surgery. This decreases the straining and tension placed on the repaired rectal shelf. The most effective method for getting the feces soft is to remove hay and other coarse roughage from the diet and feeding the mare on lush pasture or a complete pelleted feed. Administration of mineral oil or magnesium sulfate to the diet also help soften the feces.

The most commonly formed perineal surgery is Caslick's operation. This is performed in many fillies on the racetrack and in mares with poor vulvar conformation to prevent pneumovagina and fecal contamination of the vagina, respectively. This procedure is usually performed with sedation and local anesthetic infiltration of the edge of the vulva. The edges of the dorsal vulvar labia are incised and then sutured, using a continuous suture pattern. The closure is extended down to the level of the pelvic floor. The suture should not be any lower than this because it may interfere with urination and contribute to urine pooling.

Urogenital Tract Surgery

Urinary calculi occur infrequently in horses. Urinary calculi in horses are usually composed of calcium carbonate and have a spicular appearance. These calculi may develop in the kidney or urinary bladder. Small-diameter calculi can be passed during normal urination and go unnoticed. Clinical signs of urinary calculi include straining to urinate (stranguria), pollakiuria (frequent urination), and hematuria (bloody urine). Horses that develop renal calculi will develop signs of abdominal discomfort when the stones become lodged in the ureter. Additionally, cystic (urinary bladder) calculi that become lodged in the urethra in male horses cause an inability to urinate and subsequent abdominal pain. Urinary calculi can be diagnosed based upon clinical signs, urinalysis, palpation of the urinary bladder per rectum, and endoscopic evaluation of the urethra and urinary bladder. Occasionally, a calculus can be palpated in the proximal urethra of male horses at the level of the ischial arch. There are several techniques and certain instruments available for removing urinary tract calculi.

Foals commonly develop diseases of the umbilical remnants, including infection (navel ill) in the umbilical arteries, veins, and urachus. These foals often become depressed, inappetant, and febrile. Many foals also develop secondary septicemia and septic arthritis. *Umbilical remnant infection* may be diagnosed based upon clinical signs of swelling, heat, or drainage in the umbilical area. However, foals can have infection within these structures and be normal on palpation. Transabdominal ultrasonography is also helpful in diagnosing diseases of the umbilical structures. Foals with umbilical remnant infection require treatment with broad-spectrum antibiotics; many of these foals require surgical removal of the affected structures. Surgery for umbilical remnant disease involves a similar approach and instrumentation as for repairing an umbilical hernia. It is necessary to proceed with caution, and have suction available and ready while dissecting the umbilical structures, to prevent contamination of the abdominal cavity.

Patent urachus is a condition wherein foals dribble urine from the umbilicus because a patent canal between the urachus and urinary bladder is present at birth or develops in the postnatal period. Because those that develop in the postnatal period often occur secondary to an infectious process, it is imperative to rule out umbilical remnant infection and systemic infectious disease. Foals with a patent urachus may be treated nonsurgically by applying an irritant such as betadine solution or using silver nitrate sticks on the external surface of the urachus to promote scarification and closure. This is probably most effective in those foals that have a patent urachus at birth. Foals that do not respond to this treatment or those that have an infectious process occurring in the umbilical remnants should have an umbilical remnant resection.

Castration is one of the most commonly performed surgeries in horses. It is usually performed in the field and does not require extensive surgical facilities or instrumentation. Although under most circumstances castration is performed under short-acting IV general anesthesia, it can be performed in the standing horse with heavy sedation and infiltration of a local anesthetic into the scrotum and spermatic cord. The most common drugs for castration under IV anesthesia include xylazine-ketamine or xylazine-thiobarbiturate; both can be used with or without guaifenesin. It is important to document that both testicles have descended into the scrotum before commencing with castration in the field. One needs to be prepared for a more extensive surgery requiring entrance into the abdominal cavity (as in a retained testicle); this needs to be planned for because it often takes more time than a routine castration. If both testicles cannot be palpated in the scrotum, then the testicle may be located intra-abdominally, in the inguinal canal or immediately outside the external inguinal ring. A horse with a testicle located outside the abdominal cavity, but not within the scrotum, is referred to as a "high flanker." If the testicle cannot be palpated in the scrotum, then sedation may relax the horse and the cremaster muscle and allow the examiner to palpate the testicle or a portion of it. If the testicle still cannot be palpated after sedation, then a rectal examination with or without ultrasonography may help confirm the location of the testicle. Involvement of the veterinary technician for castration includes general restraint, handling, administering and monitoring anesthesia, preparation of the surgical site, and preparation of instruments.

Castration is usually performed with the horse in lateral recumbency with the upper rear limb pulled forward and tied around the horse's neck. Castration involves making an incision

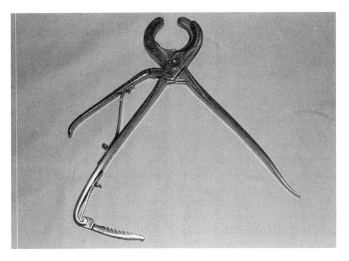

Figure 21-26. Emasculators used to crush and cut the spermatic cord of horses during castration.

over each testicle parallel to the median raphe through the skin and subcutaneous tissue. The testicles are removed by crushing and cutting the spermatic cord proximal to the testicle and epididymis using emasculators (Fig. 21–26). The emasculators should be placed on the spermatic cord so the cord is crushed on the side toward the body wall and cut on the side toward the scrotum (Fig. 21–27). There are numerous types of emasculators and each surgeon may have an individual preference. The entire spermatic cord may be crushed and cut simultaneously with the tunic (closed castration) or the tunica albuginea may be opened and the emasculators can be applied to the vascular structures separately (opened castration); this is often done in aged stallions that have an excessively large-diameter spermatic cord. The spermatic cord should be examined after the emasculator is removed to make sure there is no bleeding. The skin incisions are stretched manually to promote drainage.

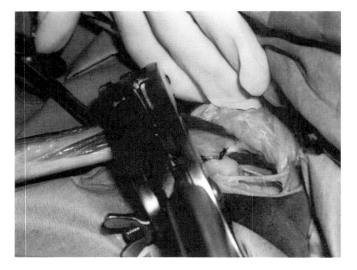

Figure 21-27. Use of emasculators during castration of a horse. The emasculators are placed around the spermatic cord so that the nut on the emasculators is located toward the testicle; this will ensure that the spermatic cord is crushed toward the body side and the cord is cut toward the testicle side.

Postoperative care usually includes strict stall confinement for 24 hours and then controlled exercise (hand walking) once or twice daily for 1 to 2 weeks to promote drainage, prevent excessive swelling, and prevent or reduce stiffness and soreness. The horse should be monitored closely during the first day after surgery for signs of excessive hemorrhage, evisceration of intestine or omentum (herniation), or excessive swelling.

If the testicle has not descended (cryptorchidism), then surgery is more involved and requires anesthesia of longer duration. Cryptorchidectomy (removal of cryptorchid testicle) also requires the surgeon to use a different surgical technique than for routine castration. The testicle can be approached through various incisions, but, an approach through the inguinal ring is most often used. A sponge forceps is used to grasp the structures that lead to the scrotum (gubernaculum) and the testicle is extracted from the inguinal canal. In some horses the testicle cannot be retrieved in this manner and the surgeon must manually explore the inguinal canal or caudal abdominal cavity. Once the testicle is retrieved, it is removed using a similar technique as described for routine castration. Following removal of the retained testicle, the other one is removed in a routine manner. Occasionally, horses have both testicles retained.

It is believed that cryptorchid horses are more at risk for evisceration after surgery. To prevent this, some surgeons may elect to temporarily pack a length of gauze soaked in sterile saline or an antiseptic into the subcutaneous areas of the inguinal canal. The gauze packing is held in place with large sutures in the skin, and is usually removed in 24 to 72 hours. Other surgeons place interrupted absorbable sutures in the external inguinal ring.

Ovariectomy is performed in mares with diseased ovaries, mares with normal reproductive tracts for use as teaser mares, and in some mares used as performance horses that have unacceptable behavior associated with estrus. An ovariectomy can be performed unilaterally or bilaterally depending upon the reason for the procedure. Diseased ovaries are usually enlarged and require removal through an incision in the ventral body wall (caudal midline or diagonal paramedian) or the flank. The most common cause of ovarian disease necessitating removal is neoplasia; the most common types of ovarian neoplasia include granulosa theca cell tumors and teratomas. Mares with granulosa theca cell tumors often display abnormal behavior such as anestrus, persistent estrus or nymphomania, or stallion-like behavior. Ovarian tumors and other diseases are diagnosed by clinical signs, palpation findings per rectum, and transrectal ultrasonography. Nondiseased ovaries of normal size can usually be removed through a flank incision or via an incision in the vaginal wall (colpotomy) in standing sedated mares with either local anesthetic infiltration in the body wall or a caudal epidural anesthetic. Hemostasis of the ovarian pedicle is provided either by transfixing with multiple sutures, application of an automatic stapling device, or crushing with a chain ecraseur. Complications include hemorrhage, abdominal pain, myositis, and others related to anesthesia and abdominal surgery.

Hernia Repair

Herniation of omentum or abdominal viscera through the abdominal wall can occur with an umbilical hernia, inguinal (scrotal) hernia, or incisional hernia. *Umbilical hernias* are usually congenital and are relatively common in foals. Small hernias may close spontaneously as the foal grows, whereas others require surgical intervention. Umbilical hernias can be repaired using several different methods. Generally, the body wall is closed with either interrupted or continuous absorbable suture. Some surgeons open the peritoneum (open herniorrhaphy) and others leave the peritoneum intact (closed herniorrhaphy). If an umbilical hernia is large or it has not closed by several months of age, then it should probably be surgically repaired. The owner should be instructed to manually reduce hernial contents at least daily; if at any time the hernia cannot be reduced, then it should be evaluated immediately by a veterinarian. If intestine becomes incarcerated in the hernia, then vascular compromise can occur leading to ischemic injury.

Inguinal or *scrotal hernias* can occur in horses of any age, but newborn foals and adult breeding stallions are probably the most commonly affected. Frequently, the herniated contents do not become incarcerated and can be easily reduced. The hernia should be reduced at least daily in foals because intestine could become incarcerated, which would necessitate emergency surgery. Sometimes, these hernias will spontaneously resolve in foals, but, many foals require surgical repair. Because the tissues are friable in foals, successful surgical repair can be difficult. Scrotal hernias in adult horses most commonly occur in stallions shortly after breeding. In most instances, the herniated structure(s) becomes incarcerated (not reducible), which necessitates immediate surgery. Incarceration of intestine within the scrotum will result in a large, firm, and cold scrotum on the affected side secondary to compromised testicular blood flow. The blood supply to the intestine also becomes compromised, resulting in ischemic injury. Generally, the testicle on the affected side is removed and the affected segment of intestine often requires resection. This necessitates preparation of the horse for inguinal and ventral midline surgery.

Acquired *body wall herniation* occurs in horses subsequent to trauma and following surgery. Blunt trauma such as a kick can lead to disruption of the body wall musculature. Body wall hernias occur secondary to abdominal incisions; these occur more frequently in horses that develop incisional infection or other complicating factors. Small body wall hernias can be repaired primarily by suturing. Larger body wall defects require the use of mesh implants. It is critical that there be no residual incisional infection present at the time of mesh herniorrhaphy and that aseptic technique is followed during placement of the mesh.

Musculoskeletal Diseases

Laminitis (founder) is a serious, often life-threatening disease of horses. It involves ischemic necrosis and inflammation of the sensitive laminae of the feet. It often involves both front feet or all four feet. However, it can occur in only one fore- or rearfoot if there is a severe lameness in the opposite limb. The cause of laminitis is unknown, but horses with serious infectious or inflammatory diseases resulting in endotoxemia, such as ischemic or inflammatory bowel disease, pleuropneumonia, septic metritis, and grain overload, are predisposed. Certain medications such as corticosteroids have also been incriminated as a potential cause of laminitis. Laminitis occurs almost exclusively in adult horses; it rarely occurs in horses less than 1 year of age.

Acute laminitis occurs in the initial stages of the disease, resulting in extreme pain and reluctance to move. Horses often have increased heat in the hooves and have a pronounced or bounding digital pulse. They are reluctant to walk, turn, or allow their feet to be picked up. They stand with a characteristic stance with their rear legs camped underneath their torso and their front feet camped out in front. Chronic laminitis occurs when, because of degeneration of the sensitive laminae on the coffin bone (distal phalanx), the dorsal laminar attachments to the insensitive laminae of the hoof detach and the coffin bone rotates. In severe chronic laminitis, the rotated coffin bone may protrude through the sole of the foot. A lateral radiograph of the foot is usually required to determine whether coffin bone rotation has occurred (Fig. 21–28). In more severe cases, all laminar attachments may be detached and the coffin bone is displaced distally within the hoof wall. Horses that have distal displacement of the coffin bone develop a characteristic depression at the coronary band, and are termed "sinkers." Horses with chronic laminitis develop characteristic concentric rings on the hooves as well as an abnormal shape of the hooves.

The main focus of treatment of horses with laminitis involves reducing inflammation and providing analgesia with anti-inflammatory drugs (phenylbutazone), promoting digital blood flow with vasodilator drugs (acepromazine or isoxuprine), and mechanically supporting the distal phalanx by providing frog support (frog pads or heart bar shoes). Nursing care is also an important component of the therapeutic regimen, particularly in chronic laminitis. Because laminitis is extremely painful horses often spend long periods of time lying down. This necessitates care of decubital ulcers. Additionally, they often develop subsolar abscesses which require daily soaking and bandaging. The prognosis for return of the horse to athletic competition depends upon the occurrence and severity of rotation or sinkage of the coffin bone. Most horses that have appreciable rotation do not return to athletic function. The prognosis for horses that develop distal displacement of the coffin bone is poor.

Rhabdomyolysis (myositis, tying up, azoturia, Monday morning sickness) is an acute inflammatory disease of muscle. It can be initiated by exertion or by a change in either the diet or the amount of exercise. It is characterized by a stiff, stilted gait with firm or hard muscles. The most commonly affected muscles are those of the rear limb and back. Severely affected horses may be reluctant to move and some may become recumbent and be unable to rise. Affected horses are often anxious, sweat excessively, and have elevated heart and respiratory rates and body temperature. Horses often have dark, discolored urine secondary to myoglobinuria. Confirmation of this disease is often based on increased serum muscle enzyme (creatine phosphokinase, aspartate aminotransferase) concentrations. Treatment involves exercise restriction, diet modification, IV fluid therapy, NSAIDs (phenylbutazone, flunixin meglumine), muscle relaxants, and tranquilization.

Bog spavin is a term used to describe the accumulation of synovial fluid (effusion) in the tarsocrural joint of the hock. Fluid can accumulate secondary to osteochondrosis, synovitis, and arthritis. Degenerative joint disease (arthritis) is a common performance-limiting condition of horses and can affect numerous joints. *Bone spavin* refers to arthritis in the distal intertarsal and tarsometatarsal joints of the hock. *High* and *low ringbone* refer to arthritis in the proximal interphalangeal (pastern) and distal interphalangeal (coffin) joints, respectively. *Osselets* is a term to describe arthritis in the metacarpal or metatarsophalangeal (fetlock) joints.

Tendinitis (bowed tendons) is an injury involving primarily the superficial digital flexor tendon and occasionally the deep

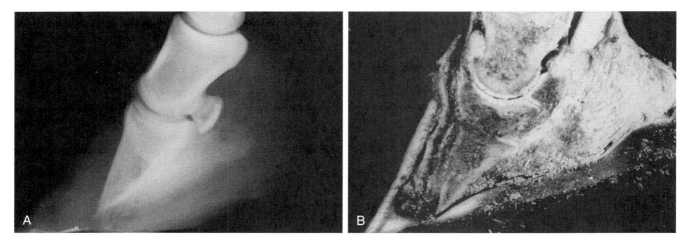

Figure 21-28. A, Lateral radiograph of the front foot of a horse with laminitis that has evidence of coffin bone rotation. B, Gross pathological photograph of a sagittal section of the front foot of a horse with laminitis that has undergone coffin bone rotation.

digital flexor tendon of the front limbs. This injury is usually sustained secondary to racing or other strenuous activity. There are different degrees of tendinitis ranging from mild edema and inflammation, tendon fiber separation, and tendon fiber tearing or disruption. When tendon fibers tear the result is hemorrhage and inflammatory debris accumulating in a cavity within the tendon, which is known as a core lesion. Treatment of tendinitis includes hydrotherapy, NSAIDs, support bandages, topical anti-inflammatory agents (sweats, poultices), and exercise restriction or controlled exercise. There are several surgical procedures that have been used to either treat tendinitis or prevent its recurrence. The most commonly performed surgery is tendon splitting, which evacuates the core lesion and allows more rapid vascularization and healing of the area. The prognosis for return to athletic function is dependent upon the severity of the injury; some horses with severe core lesions can return to athletic function if given appropriate treatment and time for convalescence.

Osteochondrosis is a form of developmental orthopedic disease in which the articular cartilage and underlying subchondral bone do not develop appropriately. This can result in the formation of osteochondritis dissecans (cartilage flaps), osteochondral fragments, cartilage erosion, and subchondral bone cysts. These abnormalities often manifest as joint effusion and lameness when young horses are first put into strenuous exercise. Many of these lesions are amenable to treatment via arthroscopy, resulting in the horse returning to athletic function.

Subsolar abscess is a common cause of severe lameness. Horses usually will not bear weight on the limb. There is palpable heat in the hoof and a bounding digital pulse similar to that in a horse with laminitis. However, the difference is that subsolar abscesses usually occur only in one foot. Pain can be localized by applying focal pressure to the sole with hoof testers. Occasionally, purulent debris will accumulate and migrate, and an area breaks open at the coronary band and drains (gravel). Treatment involves paring out the sole until the abscess is located to provide drainage. The foot should be kept bandaged to keep it dry and clean. The affected foot can be soaked daily in a solution of betadine and magnesium sulfate (Epsom salts) and then rebandaged. The horse should be administered analgesics (phenylbutazone) for a few days. Appro-

priate tetanus prophylaxis should be administered. The foot needs to be protected from dirt and debris until the area fills in with granulation tissue and is covered with cornified tissue.

Septic arthritis is a common occurrence in adult horses secondary to iatrogenic inoculation of joints during arthrocentesis or joint surgery or subsequent to traumatic joint injuries. It occurs commonly in foals subsequent to hematogenous spread from a focus of infection such as the umbilicus (navel ill), lungs (pneumonia), or intestinal tract (enteritis). The cornerstone of treatment of septic arthritis includes broad-spectrum antibiotics administered systemically, intra-articular antibiotics, NSAIDs, and joint drainage and lavage.

Horses frequently sustain severe musculoskeletal injuries such as long bone fractures or disruption of tendons or ligaments. These injuries often require stabilization with the use of bandages, splints, or casts prior to transport to a referral hospital. Successful stabilization of these injuries and safety of transport are important considerations in the outcome of these cases. Most severe injuries should be bandaged and splinted or casted to a level at least one joint above the injury. A heavy Robert Jones bandage should be applied and then rigid splints placed on the lateral and either the dorsal or palmar aspects of the limb to provide appropriate support. Splints can be made out of rigid materials such as wood, steel, or aluminum. The splints should not be excessively heavy or bulky, but must provide appropriate support. Horses with phalangeal fractures can be casted with their distal limb in flexion or can be placed in a commercially available device such as a Kimsey splint (Fig. 21–29). Horses with limb injuries should be hauled in a trailer with partitions to provide some support for them to balance themselves. The head should be tied loosely enough to enable the horse to use the head and neck for balance. Horses with front limb injuries should be transported with their head toward the rear of the trailer and those with rear limb injuries should be transported with their head toward the front of the trailer.

SURGERY OF THE EQUINE PATIENT
Preoperative Preparation of the Equine Patient

Numerous procedures are required in preparation of the equine patient for anesthesia and surgery. Many, if not all of these

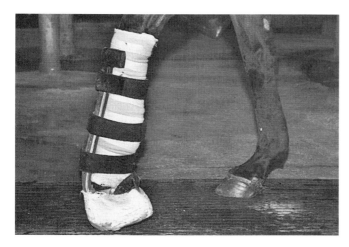

Figure 21-29. Use of Kimsey splint to stabilize fractures or joint subluxations in the lower limb of horses.

procedures, involve the veterinary technician. It is probably wise that a checklist be developed that the technician can use to make sure all procedures are performed. This is particularly helpful in a hospital where more than one technician is working on the same case. Because of the dense hair coat of horses, thorough grooming is necessary. This may include simply brushing or currying the horse's coat or it may require that the horse be bathed. The aim of grooming is to remove as much loose hair, dander, and dirt from the horse's body as possible, thereby keeping such material out of the operating room. If the horse is shod, the shoes are generally removed prior to surgery to prevent injury to the horse during recovery from anesthesia or damaging the recovery stall flooring. The horse's feet need to be picked out and cleaned. One of the main responsibilities of the technician will be to clip a wide area of hair in the vicinity of the surgery site prior to anesthetic induction. If the surgery will be performed on a limb, then the hair can be clipped the day before surgery and the limb can be cleaned and a bandage placed to keep the site clean. The final aseptic preparation is performed once the horse is under anesthesia. Clipping the hair and cleaning the surgery site prior to anesthetic induction will reduce anesthesia time.

TECHNICIAN NOTE

Numerous procedures are required in preparation of the equine patient for anesthesia and surgery. Many, if not all of these procedures, involve the veterinary technician. It is probably wise that a checklist be developed that the technician can use to make sure all procedures are performed. This is particularly helpful in a hospital where more than one technician is working on the same case.

It is important that the technician consult the clinician as to the exact site that should be clipped. Areas of the mane and tail should be clipped only under special circumstances. Most

owners are adamant that these areas should not be clipped for cosmetic purposes. The hair of the mane and tail takes months to years to grow out, and unnecessarily clipping these areas may cause needless delay in a show horse's convalescence. The location of the skin incision and the appropriate part of the horse to clip before surgery can usually be found in equine surgical textbooks. However, because of variation among surgeons, the technician should always consult the individual surgeon prior to clipping the patient.

Unlike ruminants and small animals, horses do not regurgitate or vomit. Adult horses are generally held off feed for approximately 12 hours to allow time for emptying of the stomach, which may allow the horse to ventilate more easily. Horses are generally provided water during this time. Young foals that are still nursing are generally not held off feed prior to anesthesia, but, if they are it is usually only for 1 to 2 hours. A complete physical examination should be performed, including auscultation of the heart and lungs. In adult horses, a rebreathing bag may need to be used to increase the respiratory effort enough to hear air moving through the lung fields. An electrocardiogram should be run if there is any evidence of an abnormal heart rhythm detected during auscultation. Preoperative blood work usually includes a CBC and fibrinogen determination. Some clinicians also perform a chemistry profile depending on the age and health of the horse.

Prior to general anesthesia, an IV catheter is placed in one of the jugular veins. The anesthetic agents for induction are administered through the catheter. Some anesthetic agents (thiobarbiturates) and perioperative medications (phenylbutazone) are irritating if injected perivascularly. Therefore, it is imperative that the catheter be placed into the vein and appropriately secured. Catheter placement can be performed by the clinician or by the technician under the supervision of the clinician. Perioperative medications such as antibiotics and NSAIDs are usually administered prior to anesthetic induction. However, if an infectious process is suspected, then it may be opted to start antibiotics after a sample has been obtained at surgery for culture and susceptibility testing. In this case, the medication can be administered during anesthesia or after recovery; this will be dependent upon the medication and the condition of the patient while under anesthesia. Because horses are generally intubated with an endotracheal tube through the oral cavity, it is important that the mouth be thoroughly washed out prior to anesthetic induction; this will reduce the chance that feed material will be carried into the airway during intubation. Once the horse is intubated, the cuff should be inflated to prevent saliva and other materials from draining into the lower airway and leading to aspiration pneumonia.

Intraoperative Nursing

The technician should consult with the surgeon regarding which instruments will be required. In a hospital where there is more than one technician and several surgeons, a card system that has the necessary instruments listed for each surgical procedure should be used. This will allow the technician to know the different requirements of individual surgeons. One of the common differences among surgeons is the type of suture material they choose to close wounds. The technician must learn to adapt to these individual preferences. It is recommended that the technician have all the available instruments close to the surgery. Even if the instrument is used infrequently, it is better to have it nearby rather than waste time looking for it once it is needed. Time-wasting activities lead to prolonged anesthetic time, which could lead to increased morbidity or mortality. Correctly labeled radiographs are essential for most limb surgery. The radiographs should be placed on a radiographic view box in the operating room. The technician should have available gloves, gowns, and drapes and all other supplies that are anticipated to be used. In some lower limb surgeries, an Esmarch bandage (Latex Rubber Bandage/Tourner Wrap, Smiths & Nephew Richards) and tourniquet are used to assist with hemostasis during surgery (Fig. 21–30). An Esmarch bandage is a flat, gum-rubber elastic bandage that is wrapped around the limb in a spiral fashion from distal to proximal to a point above the surgical site. At this point an inflatable tourniquet is applied and secured. The aim of the Esmarch bandage is to force blood out of the limb while the tourniquet prevents blood from entering into the site. The Esmarch bandage is removed after the tourniquet is fully inflated. The use of an Esmarch bandage and tourniquet enables the surgeon to operate in a bloodless field and results in a shorter surgery time. Following surgery, a pressure bandage is applied and the tourniquet is released.

The technician must help ensure that the patient is properly padded. Because of their body weight, horses are prone to myositis (muscle damage) that can be life-threatening. The pressure of the horse's body and the hypotension that can occur during anesthesia can result in hypoperfusion of the muscles. If this condition is prolonged, the muscles can undergo metabolic change, resulting in extreme soreness and pain. In severe cases, muscle pigment (myoglobin) is released into the blood stream and excreted in the urine (coffee-colored urine); the pigment can lead to kidney damage. The first sign that muscle damage has occurred during anesthesia is manifested during recovery. Usually, the front or rear limb, or both, on the side the horse is lying on will be most commonly affected. However, the uppermost limb or any limb in a horse in dorsal recumbency can be involved. The horse may be unable to bear weight on the limb. If a forelimb is involved, the horse will drag the limb in a flexed position and will be unable to bear weight; this is associated with triceps damage. If the hindlimb is involved, the horse may knuckle in the lower joints and walk on the dorsal aspect of the fetlock, and the limb will collapse as the horse tries to bear weight. Most horses show some improvement over the first few days, but, some horses are unable to rise. Management of a postoperative recumbent patient presents a number of problems to clinicians and technicians. Appropriate padding materials are an inflatable waterbed, semi-inflated tire inner tubes under the shoulder and hip, dunnage bags, or foam rubber pads.

The patient and the surgery site must be positioned so it is comfortable to the surgeon and safe for the patient. This will help ensure that the surgeon does not become fatigued or frustrated, and a subsequent compromise in technique does not occur. It is not wise to overextend, overflex, abduct, or adduct the limbs because of potential complications of myopathy and neuropathy.

Aseptic preparation of the surgery site, surgical instruments, and the surgeon is imperative to a successful and uncomplicated surgery. It is the responsibility of all personnel involved to maintain asepsis, but, the technician(s) should assume primary responsibility for ensuring that the surgical site is properly prepared and the instruments are properly sterilized and packaged. The technician must be cognizant of all activities in preparation for surgery and during the surgical procedure. If a technician observes a break in aseptic technique it should be brought to the attention of the surgeon so the problem can be remedied. The techniques involved in sterilization of surgical instruments and supplies, and aseptic preparation of the surgery site are covered in Chapter 17.

Postoperative Nursing

Technicians play a vital role in the postoperative care of the equine patient. Although veterinary clinicians are responsible

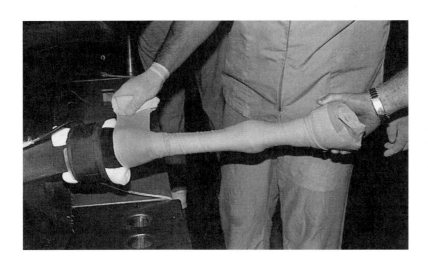

Figure 21–30. Application of an Esmarch bandage and tourniquet on the limb of a horse. The uninflated tourniquet is placed around the limb just proximal to the carpus. An Esmarch bandage is placed tightly around the limb beginning at the foot and extended to the level of the tourniquet. The tourniquet is then inflated, and the Esmarch bandage is removed.

for the patients' care, technicians are often primarily involved with postoperative monitoring, administering medications, changing bandages, grooming, and other tasks required on postoperative patients. Monitoring of the postoperative patient is similar to previously discussed patient monitoring. Although all body systems should be evaluated, the important things to consider in the postoperative patient are the presence and magnitude of postoperative pain, whether the patient is febrile, and whether there are any signs of infection (swelling, erythema, heat, or pain) at the incision site. The postoperative patient should be examined for any complications such as pneumonia, diarrhea, jugular vein thrombophlebitis, or laminitis.

TECHNICIAN NOTE

Technicians play a vital role in the postoperative care of the equine patient. Although veterinary clinicians are responsible for the patients' care, technicians are often primarily involved with postoperative monitoring, administering medications, changing bandages, grooming, and other tasks required on postoperative patients.

Technicians are generally responsible for administering medications postoperatively. This may involve giving antibiotics or NSAIDs orally, IV, or IM. Many horses that undergo surgery have an IV catheter that is often used in the postoperative period to administer perioperative antibiotics. The duration of antibiotic therapy is dependent upon clinician preference and the type and severity of the underlying disease process. Many horses are administered NSAIDs in the postoperative period for their anti-inflammatory and analgesic properties.

Horses undergoing limb surgery generally have a bandage placed on the limb at the conclusion of surgery prior to recovery from anesthesia. The limbs are often kept bandaged until the skin sutures are removed 10 to 14 days postoperatively. The bandages should probably be changed every 2 to 3 days initially or more frequently if they become wet or soiled from the outside or if wound drainage soaks through from the inside. There are several types of materials used for limb bandages in horses and several methods of application (see Chapter 19). In general, a sterile nonadherent material is usually placed directly against the incision and held in place with sterile, soft roll gauze (Kling, Johnson & Johnson). The next layer of the bandage is usually a sterile, soft combine that covers the circumference of the limb for the entire distance of the bandage, which is also held in place with soft roll gauze. This layer can be skipped if the outer bandage that is placed is a thick, sterile combine material. Next, a thick layer of rolled cotton, sheet cottons, or combine material is placed on the limb and secured with soft roll gauze. An Ace bandage or Elastikon (Johnson & Johnson), or Vetwrap (Animal Care Products/3M), can be used as the final layer of the bandage. Elasticon is useful for securing the top of the bandage to the skin above it and the bottom of the bandage to the foot below. This helps seal the bandage and prevent debris from getting between the skin and the bandage. All layers of the bandage should be applied in the same direction (dorsal to palmar or plantar) and with even tension; this should help prevent constriction of the tendons in the metacarpal or metatarsal area and subsequent tendinitis (bandage bow). When the bandages are changed postoperatively the incision should be examined for swelling, heat, exudate, and pain on palpation. The exudate should be removed, the wound gently cleaned, and the bandage reapplied. If there has been an appreciable change in the horse's gait or in the incision from the last bandage change, this should be brought to the immediate attention of the clinician.

Colic

Colic is a general term used to describe abdominal pain; many diseases can result in abdominal pain or signs that mimic abdominal pain. Diseases of the gastrointestinal tract are the most common causes of abdominal pain in horses. Owing to the anatomy and physiology of the gastrointestinal tract and the fact horses suffer from varying degrees of parasitic infestations (e.g., *Strongylus vulgaris*), horses are more predisposed to colic than are most other animals. It is one of the most common and important diseases of horses and is one in which the veterinary technician plays a vital role in assisting in the diagnosis and both medical and surgical treatment. The technician is also intimately involved in the daily monitoring and treatment of horses with colic.

The typical cause of colic in horses is an obstruction to flow of ingesta and gas in the gastrointestinal tract, causing intestinal distention, stretching of the intestinal wall, and tension on the mesentery, all of which lead to pain which is manifested in a variety of behavioral signs. Not all signs of abdominal pain are attributable to intestinal obstruction. For example, a mare that is near parturition will show similar signs owing to uterine contractions. A horse with an obstruction of the urinary tract (urethral calculus) may also show signs of abdominal pain. Although it is important that the veterinary technician recognize signs of colic, the diagnosis of the actual cause of colic is the responsibility of the veterinarian. There are various signs of abdominal pain displayed by horses with different types and magnitudes of colic; however, certain signs are common to most. Mild signs of colic include inappetence, stretching more frequently than normal, yawning, and looking at the flank. Other signs include playing with water or frequent urination. More obvious signs of colic include pawing the ground, stamping the feet, walking the stall, kicking the abdomen, and violent rolling. Some horses will actually sit like a dog or roll into dorsal recumbency to relieve the pain. Horses with colic often sweat profusely, have an increased heart and respiratory rates, and have congested mucous membranes.

The causes of gastrointestinal tract–related colic include volvulus (twisting of the intestine), intestinal incarceration, impactions of feed material or foreign bodies, obstruction due to enteroliths (stones that form in the intestinal tract), parasitic infections, displacement of the intestine, tympany (primary gas distention), and inflammatory bowel disease (anterior enteritis, enterocolitis). Volvulus can occur in numerous portions of the intestinal tract, but it most commonly occurs in the small intestine and large colon. The small intestine frequently becomes incarcerated (entrapped) in numerous sites such as the inguinal ring, epiploic foramen, mesenteric rent, and a diaphragmatic hernia. Intestinal incarceration and volvulus result in obstruction of the intestinal lumen and occlusion of the intestinal blood vessels resulting in intestinal distention and ischemic necrosis of the bowel wall. Therefore, these horses display severe abdominal pain and usually develop signs of shock owing to absorption of endotoxin through devitalized bowel. These horses require emergency abdominal exploration with correction of the volvulus or reduction of the incarceration; depending upon the duration and magnitude of the disease, the affected segment of intestine often requires resection. Because of the anatomy of the gastrointestinal tract, horses are predisposed to large-intestinal displacement. Large-colon displacement results in luminal obstruction, but no vascular occlusion. Therefore, these horses develop mild to severe abdominal pain depending upon the magnitude of the luminal distention, but do not develop intestinal ischemia. Treatment usually involves surgical correction. However, one particular type of large colon displacement (entrapment of the large colon in the nephrosplenic space) is sometimes correctable by rolling the horse under general anesthesia.

Horses develop impactions in the ileum, cecum, and large and small colon. Many of these horses can be treated medically with IV or oral fluids, lubricants (mineral oil), cathartics (magnesium sulfate), and analgesics. Other horses with intestinal impactions require surgery to evacuate the intestinal contents to prevent rupture. Intestinal contents are usually evacuated through an incision in the bowel wall (enterotomy) and the lumen is lavaged to remove as much of the contents as possible. The enterotomy incision is then sutured. Intestinal obstruction can occur secondary to an enterolith lodging in a segment of the large intestine that has a reduced diameter (pelvic flexure, transverse colon, small colon). Enterolithiasis results from mineral deposition that forms around a nidus within the intestinal tract. Sometimes horses pass numerous small-diameter stones in the feces, whereas larger-diameter stones may develop and obstruct the lumen; these larger-diameter stones frequently cause abdominal pain secondary to luminal distention and require removal through an enterotomy. Horses can develop intestinal obstruction secondary to ingestion of foreign bodies; young curious horses are most commonly affected and the most common type of foreign bodies are fibrous (nylon rope or string, hay netting, feed sacks, rubber fencing, and hair). Occasionally, a horse will be able to pass these fibrous foreign bodies, but often surgery is required to remove the foreign body and relieve the intestinal obstruction.

Although parasite-related causes of colic are less common now than in the past because of the development of effective anthelmintic drugs and management strategies, they still represent a possible cause of colic, especially on farms with poor preventive medicine programs. Larvae of *Strongylus vulgaris* (blood sucking worms) migrate through the mesenteric arteries causing arteritis; this can lead to thromboembolic colic wherein segments of the intestine become infarcted. Ascarids (*Parascaris equorum*) usually cause a problem in young horses. The problem usually arises after deworming a heavily infested foal when a large number of adult ascarids die and obstruct the intestinal lumen (ascarid impaction). The best way to prevent this is to begin effective deworming programs early in the foal's life or to use a dewormer that is not especially effective in a heavily infested foal. Once the ascarid impaction occurs, the most effective treatment is evacuation of the worms via an enterotomy. Tapeworm (*Anoplocephala perfoliata*) infestation has been anecdotally related to cecocolic and ileocecal intussusception and to development of cecal impactions. These parasites are frequently identified in the cecal lumen in horses with these conditions, but no cause-and-effect relationship has been confirmed. The most effective treatment regimen for tapeworms is twice the recommended dose of pyrantel pamoate. Small strongyles are probably the most important intestinal parasite in horses because of their resistance to benzimidazole anthelmintics. Infestation with small strongyles can cause poor doing, weight loss, diarrhea, and colic (see Chapter 6).

Horses with inflammatory bowel disease often have signs of abdominal pain, fever, increased heart and respiratory rates, congested mucous membranes, diarrhea, and nasogastric reflux. These horses are usually best treated with IV fluids, gastric decompression, administration of intestinal protectorants, antibiotics, analgesics, and anti-inflammatory drugs.

The prognosis for horses with colic is dependent upon the type of abnormality and its magnitude and duration. In general, horses with simple obstruction (no compromise in blood flow) of the intestinal tract (impaction, enterolith, displacement, tympany) have a good prognosis for survival with appropriate medical or surgical treatment. Horses with strangulating obstruction (compromised blood flow) of the intestinal tract (volvulus, incarceration, intussusception) have a more guarded prognosis, but some of these horses will survive and be functional if treated early and appropriately. The prognosis for horses with parasitic and inflammatory bowel diseases is dependent upon the severity and duration before treatment and the development of life-threatening complications, such as laminitis.

The veterinarian will conduct a thorough examination and perform several diagnostic procedures in an attempt to arrive at an accurate diagnosis of the cause of colic. Most of these procedures will either directly or indirectly involve the veterinary technician. Such procedures include a rectal examination, nasogastric intubation, abdominocentesis and abdominal fluid analysis, collection of blood for CBC and chemistry profile, transabdominal ultrasonography, urinalysis, fecal floatation for intestinal parasites, and fecal cultures for *Salmonella*. The technician may be involved in organizing the instruments and supplies for performing these procedures or actually participating in the procedures.

The veterinary technician will be intricately involved in both medical and surgical treatment of horses with colic. Medical treatment is usually appropriate for impactions, tympany, and spasmodic colic, whereas surgical treatment is necessary for intestinal volvulus and incarceration, enterolithiasis, fibrous foreign body obstruction, and intestinal displacements. Fortunately, most horses with colic respond to conservative treatment such as analgesic, anti-inflammatory or antispasmodic drugs; intestinal lubricants or cathartics; IV or oral fluids; restriction of feed; and controlled exercise. It is only a small percentage of horses with colic that require surgery. Sometimes surgery is necessary to arrive at an accurate diagnosis. Abdominal surgery is a major undertaking and requires a full team to perform it in an effective and efficient manner.

Abdominal Surgery

Adult horses and foals frequently undergo abdominal surgery for gastrointestinal and urogenital tract disease. Although a flank incision in a standing, sedated horse is sometimes used for horses with colic or other abdominal disease, the most common approach to the abdominal cavity is through a ventral midline incision with the horse under general anesthesia and positioned in dorsal recumbency (Fig. 21–31). Because most horses with colic requiring surgery will be operated on under general anesthesia, the veterinary technician will be involved in the preparation of the horse for surgery. This will include placing a catheter, administering perioperative medications, passage of a nasogastric tube, washing out the mouth, clipping the hair, preparing the anesthetics, aseptically preparing the incision site, and opening surgical packs at the time of surgery. Most colic patients can be clipped prior to anesthesia, but if the horse is in severe pain it may be done after anesthetic induction for the safety of the horse and personnel. The hair should be clipped from rostral to the xiphoid area to the udder or preputial area and to the flank folds on either side; clipped hair and other debris can be removed with a vacuum. The incision site (ventral midline) may be shaved to remove the hair remaining after clipping, and the clipped area is then aseptically prepared. The incision is draped with four small drapes or towels and then a large, water-impermeable drape is placed that covers the entire horse. The incision is usually made from the umbilicus rostrally toward the xiphoid until the necessary exposure is achieved, but, the incision can be extended caudal to the umbilicus. This is particularly necessary for urogenital tract surgery such as a cystotomy for removal of cystic calculi. Once the incision is made, a thorough exploration is usually performed depending upon the reason for surgery. Once the abnormality is identified it is corrected. Suction is often necessary to decompress gas from the gastrointestinal tract or aspirate fluid such as urine from the bladder during a cystotomy.

There are numerous surgical techniques and manipulations that the veterinarian may perform at the time of abdominal surgery. They are too numerous to describe here, and the

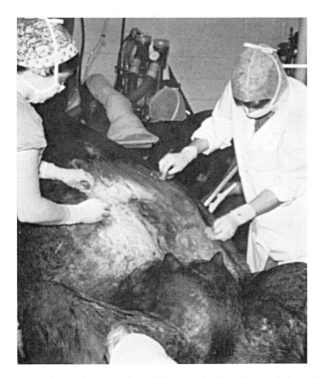

Figure 21–31. Preparation of the ventral abdominal area for abdominal surgery in a horse with colic that is under general anesthesia in dorsal recumbency.

veterinary technician will become familiar with them through instruction and experience. Many specialized instruments are required for abdominal surgery (see Chapter 16). One group of instruments that has become increasingly popular with veterinary surgeons for use in equine abdominal surgery is gastrointestinal stapling equipment. The technician must become familiar with the different instruments and cartridges. Intestinal resection and anastomosis often requires specialized instruments and supplies.

Once the cause of colic has been corrected and the horse has recovered from anesthesia, the veterinary technician becomes even more closely involved with patient management. Horses usually require administration of IV fluids, antibiotics, anti-inflammatory drugs, and other medications in the postoperative period. The veterinary technician usually administers or oversees administration of these medications. The technician may also be involved in nasogastric intubation, blood collection, IV catheterization, and changing bandages. Additionally, the technician will often be responsible for feeding and watering, exercising, grooming, and monitoring the horse.

Arthroscopic Surgery

Arthroscopy is commonly performed for the diagnosis and treatment of joint disease. It is commonly performed for removing osteochondral chip fractures, treating cartilaginous and bony abnormalities associated with osteochondrosis, treating septic arthritis, and evaluating causes of joint lameness that have no definitive radiographic abnormalities. Depending upon the joint being evaluated and the type and location of the lesion, the horse may be positioned in dorsal or lateral recumbency. It is necessary to have the radiographs on a view box in the operating room so the surgeon can evaluate them intraoperatively. During arthroscopy the technique of triangulation is used whereby the lesion forms one corner of the triangle and the arthroscope and surgical instruments serve as the other two corners of the triangle. Generally, the arthroscope is placed in the joint on the side opposite the lesion and the surgical instrument is placed in the joint on the same side as the lesion. The portal for placement of the arthroscope is usually made by making a small (1 cm) incision in the skin and subcutaneous tissue and then using a sharp trocar to advance the arthroscopic canula through the fibrous joint capsule and synovial lining. Once the canula has penetrated the joint cavity, the sharp trocar is replaced with a blunt obturator to pass the canula across the joint; this prevents iatrogenic damage to the cartilage. The skin incisions are usually made before joint distention in the carpus, but after joint distention in other joints. The joint is distended with sterile polyionic fluid to facilitate placement of the arthroscope. Once the arthroscope is in place the joint is evaluated; once the lesion is identified the most appropriate location for the instrument portal is determined by using a needle to triangulate the lesion with the arthroscope. Once the appropriate location for the instrument portal is identified, the instrument portal is made with a scalpel blade (no. 11 or 15). The appropriate instrument is placed into the joint. The instruments commonly used in arthroscopy include a blunt probe for palpating intra-articular structures, rongeurs for removing osteochondral fragments, and curettes for debriding diseased cartilage and bone. A fenestrated canula is often used at the end of surgery to facilitate removal of cartilage and bone debris via lavage.

Motorized equipment is available and is sometimes necessary for debridement of large areas of diseased bone.

The surgeon uses specific instruments for arthroscopy and these may vary depending upon the joint involved and the individual surgeon's preference. Generally, there will be a standardized set of arthroscopy instruments that are packaged together. Instruments are steam sterilized, but if they are to be used on more than one case per day, they are sterilized with a cold sterilization solution prior to each use. Following sterilization, the instruments are packed in a sterile stainless steel pan, which is later used to rinse disinfecting solution off the arthroscopy instruments. One of the most important and most expensive instruments is the arthroscope; it should be handled carefully to prevent damage. Additional items necessary are a sterile needle (usually 18-gauge) and syringe, which are used for distending the joint. During arthroscopic surgery, the joint is kept distended with sterile physiological solution; this solution is usually delivered with a pump through a sterile IV set.

Many hospitals perform arthroscopy, using a video camera so that the entire procedure can be viewed on a television screen (Fig. 21–32). This causes less strain on the surgeon's eye, makes the procedure more educational for surgery assistants and technical staff, provides an opportunity to videotape the procedure, and probably allows the procedure to be performed with fewer breaks in aseptic technique. To provide the intense light required to illuminate the inside of the joint, a fiberoptic light source and light cable are required. It is essential that the technician be familiar with the assembly and function of the arthroscopic equipment, and the proper care, cleaning, and disinfecting of the instruments. The arthroscopy instruments are disinfected using a.cold sterilization solution such as activated dialdehyde (Cidex, Surgikos); the instruments, arthroscope, and light cables are soaked for a minimum of 10 minutes. One should read the manufacturer's recommendations regarding the time required for disinfecting. To avoid delays, the instruments can be placed in the sterilizing solution at the start of anesthesia. This will also ensure adequate sterilization time. Before using the instruments, the instruments are transferred sterilely into an empty sterile tray. The instruments are then rinsed with sterile saline to remove the sterilization solution.

After the surgical site has been aseptically prepared and draped, and the instruments removed from the sterilizing solution, the technician will be responsible for attaching the fiberoptic cable to its light source. The system that delivers the fluid to distend the joint must also be connected to the appropriate fluid source. Once the system is connected to the fluid source, the surgeon must run fluid through the system to flush all air bubbles out of the tubing so they do not enter the joint. Electric fluid pumps are generally used to maintain joint distention; these may be manually or pressure controlled.

Following surgery, all specialized arthroscopy equipment and instruments need to be cleaned. The arthroscope lens should be examined for scratches and the video camera dried carefully. If several arthroscopy surgeries are scheduled for the day, then the instruments are placed in the cold sterilization solution in preparation for the next surgery.

Orthopedic Surgery

Orthopedic surgery has become more common in horses. Athletic horses develop numerous orthopedic conditions that are amenable to surgical correction. Historically, fractures of long bones in adult horses were considered irreparable. However, with advanced techniques and stronger surgical implants many of these injuries are potentially correctable. Certain bony fractures are amenable to surgical correction, using bone screws that are placed in lag fashion to stabilize the fracture by creating compression of the bone fragments (Fig. 21–33). Although developing an understanding of the principles of lag screw fixation and the instrumentation involved will help the equine technician in preparing instruments and assisting with surgery, this area is beyond the scope of this book. Major fractures of long bones in horses are best repaired with screws and bone plates to prevent movement at the fracture site while the bone heals under rigid fixation. Although aseptic technique is imperative for all surgical procedures, it is crucial to the overall success of orthopedic surgery in horses. If bony infection develops, it can lead to instability of the implants and fixation failure, which often necessitates euthanasia. It is the responsibility of all personnel to follow aseptic protocol. The technician should strive to maintain asepsis by monitoring the activities of all personnel involved in surgery. Orthopedic surgery requires the use of several specialized instruments and implants; because many of these surgeries are performed on an emergency basis, it is imperative that the technician make sure instruments are avail-

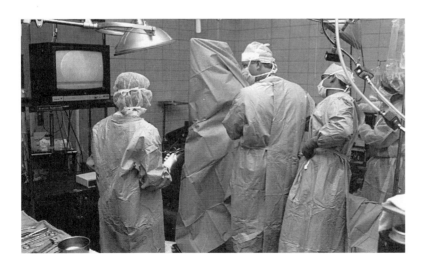

Figure 21-32. Use of arthroscopy for evaluating joint disease in horses. The arthroscope is inserted into the joint and attached to a camera that projects the image on a television screen for easy viewing by the surgeon and other personnel.

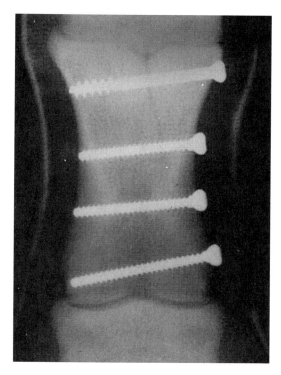

Figure 21-33. A proximal phalanx fracture in a horse is repaired with cortical bone screws placed in lag fashion to compress the fracture line.

able and ready for use. Many orthopedic injuries that are surgically repaired require the use of external coaptation (cast) for anesthetic recovery or for longer periods postoperatively (see Chapter 19). Therefore, the technician should anticipate this need and have the appropriate materials available at the conclusion of surgery. The technician may also be needed to assist with anesthetic recovery of the orthopedic equine patient.

Postoperative monitoring of the orthopedic patient is vital for early detection of potential problems. It is particularly important to observe how the horse is using the affected limb in the stall; any dramatic change in use of the limb may signal an impending problem (infection or cast sores). The cast should also be monitored for heat, odor, or exudate, which would indicate the development of cast sores. The most common locations for sores to develop in association with a half-limb cast is at the proximal, dorsal aspect of the metacarpus or metatarsus, the palmar or plantar aspect of the fetlock over the sesamoid bones, and over the heel bulbs. Bandages need to be changed frequently and the incision sites should be monitored for swelling, erythema, and discharge. Drains are commonly used in orthopedic surgery following repair of a long bone. Drains can be useful in preventing seroma formation, but they can serve as potential routes for inoculation of the surgery site. Therefore, it is important to maintain these drains sterile by keeping a clean, sterile bandage on the leg. This may require changing the bandage more frequently than once daily.

Upper Respiratory Tract Surgery

Abnormalities of the upper respiratory tract can be performance-limiting to athletic horses and, if severe, can also be life-threatening. Many of the obstructive diseases of the upper respiratory tract are amenable to surgical correction. The most common of these are left laryngeal hemiplegia, epiglottic entrapment, dorsal displacement of the soft palate, and arytenoid chondritis. Others are subepiglottic cysts, guttural pouch empyema, guttural pouch tympany, and guttural pouch mycosis.

Left laryngeal hemiplegia ("roarer") is a condition resulting in paralysis of the left arytenoid cartilage, which prevents it from being abducted during inspiration. This results in the arytenoid collapsing and being pulled into the airway secondary to the negative pressure that is generated during inspiration. The cause of this condition is unknown, but it results in a recurrent laryngeal neuropathy. Because this nerve normally provides innervation to the major abductor muscle of the arytenoid cartilage, the cricoarytenoideus dorsalis, a neuropathy results in muscle atrophy and an inability to abduct the arytenoid. As the name implies, this condition occurs almost exclusively on the left side (95%); it is believed that this is related to the longer length of the nerve on the left side and the fact it may become damaged from the vibrations as it courses around the aortic arch. This condition is diagnosed using endoscopy at rest or during exercise on a high-speed treadmill; the left arytenoid cartilage is not fully abducted during inspiration, and in severe cases actually collapses into the airway. Horses with this condition make a characteristic inspiratory noise (roaring) and develop exercise intolerance. Surgical treatment is a prosthetic laryngoplasty, which involves placing a suture between the cricoid cartilage and the muscular process of the arytenoid cartilage to mimic the action of the cricoarytenoideus dorsalis and abduct the arytenoid cartilage (tieback). The laryngeal ventricles (saccules) are also everted and resected (ventriculectomy or sacculectomy) through either a ventral laryngotomy or by use of an endoscopically guided laser. Approximately 70% of horses treated with a prosthetic laryngoplasty and sacculectomy return to athletic function. Most horses will continue to make some noise, and in some the noise may not improve. The laryngotomy incision is usually left open to heal by second intention. This requires daily cleaning with gauze sponges with saline or water followed by application of petrolatum to the skin around the incision and on the mandible and neck to prevent skin scald from the drainage. It usually takes approximately 3 weeks for the incision to heal. Some clinicians partially close the incision which reportedly shortens the time required to heal.

Epiglottic entrapment is a condition where the aryepiglottic membrane that extends from the arytenoid cartilage to the ventral surface of the epiglottis hypertrophies and rolls upward to envelope the rostral and abaxial portions of the epiglottis. Normally, the epiglottis should have a serrated edge and a distinct vascular pattern present on the dorsal surface. When the epiglottis becomes entrapped, the serrated edge and vascular pattern can no longer be seen. The shape or outline of the epiglottis can still be observed (unlike that seen with a dorsal displacement of the soft palate), but the tip appears more rounded and the abaxial surface is smooth rather that serrated. In more chronic cases, the tip of the epiglottis may become ulcerated. The cause of epiglottic entrapment is unknown, but it is believed these horses have an instability between the caudal edge of the soft palate and the epiglottis and that the aryepiglottic membrane hypertrophies and makes the epiglottis more rigid. Epiglottic entrapment can be intermittent or permanent. Some horses can continue to perform athletically with an entrapped epiglottis, but it does appear to affect performance in most horses. Treatment of epiglottic entrapment includes transecting the aryepiglottic membrane to release the epiglottis. This can be done using several techniques. First it can be performed with a hooked bistoury placed through the nasal passages in a standing sedated horse with or without endoscopic guidance; care must be taken to prevent trauma to other structures and to prevent laceration of the soft palate. Second it can be performed in an anesthetized horse with a mouth speculum by manually guiding a hooked bistoury and transecting the membrane on midline. Third, it can be performed using an endoscopically guided laser in a standing sedated horse. Finally, in more severe or chronic recurring cases the aryepiglottic membrane can be resected through a ventral laryngotomy. The prognosis for return to athletic performance is good, but, entrapment can reoccur. Some of these horses may develop dorsal displacement of the soft palate after the entrapment is released. Horses that have the entrapment released using the hooked bistoury or laser can generally resume training in a few days, whereas those treated via resection through a laryngotomy require approximately 3 weeks before resuming training.

Dorsal displacement of the soft palate (DDSP) is generally a dynamic obstructive disease of the upper respiratory tract that occurs during exercise. Normally, the soft palate remains ventral to the epiglottis. However, if the epiglottis is small or flaccid or the caudal edge of the soft palate is flaccid, the soft palate can become displaced dorsal to the epiglottis during strenuous exercise. The cause of this condition is unknown, but it is believed the factors listed above predispose the palate to become displaced during inspiration when negative pressure is generated in the upper airway. This condition usually is intermittent, occurring during strenuous exercise and dissipating once exercise has stopped and the horse swallows. Because horses are obligate nasal breathers, dorsal displacement of the soft palate interferes with the horse's breathing. Horses with DDSP usually make a characteristic gurgling or snoring type of noise, which will dissipate as soon as they swallow and replace the palate into its normal position. Treatment options for a horse with DDSP include placing a cloth or leather tie on the horse's tongue and pulling the tongue rostrad and tying the tongue to the mandible in the interdental space. The epiglottis, tongue, and sternothyrohyoideus muscles are attached to the hyoid apparatus. Because the tongue is attached at the rostral aspect of the hyoid apparatus and the sternothyrohyoideus muscles are attached at its caudal aspect, a tongue tie prevents caudal retraction of the hyoid apparatus, including the epiglottis. This seems to help approximately 50% of horses with DDSP because it prevents caudal retraction of the epiglottis and maintains normal epiglottic-palate alignment. Because of its noninvasive nature, the tongue tie is generally the first thing attempted in horses with DDSP. If this does not work, a section of the sternothyrohyoideus muscles can be resected in the midcervical region; this also prevents caudal retraction of the hyoid apparatus. This myectomy procedure helps in approximately 50% of horses with DDSP that fail to respond to a tongue tie. If this procedure does not work, then the caudal margin of the soft palate can be resected (staphylectomy). There are two theories as to why this may help prevent DDSP. First, it is believed the caudal edge of the palate becomes more fibrous as it heals with scar tissue; this makes the caudal edge more rigid and therefore more resistant to displacement. The other theory is, if the palate does displace, then it enables the palate to be replaced more easily. Regardless of the mechanism it seems that it helps prevent DDSP in approximately half of the horses that do not respond to the tongue tie or myectomy.

Arytenoid chondritis is an inflammatory, degenerative condition of the arytenoid cartilages resulting in a proliferative mass on one or both arytenoids. This usually results in an obstructive disease of the upper airway with signs similar to the conditions described earlier. These cartilages are usually enlarged and more fibrous than normal, which prevents effectively being treated with a tieback. The treatment of choice is to remove the affected arytenoid cartilage through a ventral laryngotomy. Because of the time required for dissection in the laryngeal region during an arytenoidectomy, a tracheotomy is usually performed in the middle or proximal trachea to provide a mechanism for ventilation during anesthesia. The tracheotomy can be performed either before anesthetic induction or once the horse is anesthetized. These horses are prone to upper airway obstruction postoperatively and need to be closely monitored. The tracheotomy tube is usually left in place, at least for a couple of days, until it is believed the horse has an airway of adequate diameter for breathing. It is imperative that these horses be monitored closely while the tracheotomy tube is in place to make sure it does not become dislodged or obstructed with mucus or other discharge. The laryngotomy and tracheotomy sites require daily cleaning and application of petrolatum on the skin around the incisions. Both of these incisions will heal by second intention in approximately 3 weeks.

Bacterial infection of the guttural pouch (empyema) usually is a sequela to strangles or retropharyngeal lymph node abscesses. Clinical signs include swelling in the throatlatch region and a bilateral mucopurulent nasal discharge. Horses with guttural pouch empyema can be treated conservatively with antibiotics and guttural pouch lavage; this may be effective in many horses that are treated early in the course of the disease. However, in more chronic cases the mucopurulent material becomes inspissated and forms gelatinous concretions (chondroids) that lie in the floor of the guttural pouches. Resolution of empyema requires removal of the chondroids and chronic effective drainage can usually only be achieved with surgical drainage. Several approaches are reported for surgical drainage of the guttural pouches, but the most common surgical approach for guttural pouch empyema is the modified Whitehouse technique; the incision is made in the skin on the ventrum of the throat region just axial to the linguofacial vein and is followed by blunt dissection into the pouch. The guttural pouch is lavaged intraoperatively. Indwelling catheters can be placed into the guttural pouches in standing sedated horses under endoscopic guidance; these catheters enable frequent lavage of the pouches. The guttural pouches should not be lavaged with irritating solutions because of the proximity of blood vessels and nerves coursing through the area. The incision is managed similarly to a laryngotomy or tracheotomy incision.

Guttural pouch tympany is an accumulation of air in the guttural pouches; this occurs in foals and weanlings and is usually associated with an abnormality of the opening to the pouches. It can occur on one or both sides and is characterized by a fluctuant nonpainful swelling in the throatlatch region. If unilateral guttural pouch tympany is present, then it is usually treated by surgically creating an opening in the septum between the left and right pouches; this is usually approached through an incision in Viborg's triangle on the affected side. If bilateral tympany is present, then creating an opening in the septum will not effectively drain the two sides. Therefore, the opening

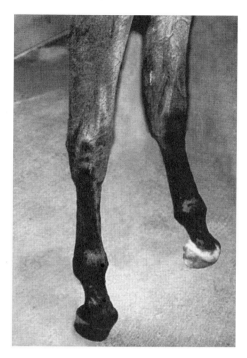

Figure 21-34. Severe flexural deformity of the distal interphalangeal (coffin) joint of both front limbs in a weanling horse.

to one or both of the guttural pouches is surgically revised through a Viborg's triangle approach. Surgical revision of the guttural pouch opening may be performed on only one side with creation of an opening in the septum to enable both pouches to evacuate the air through one opening.

Guttural pouch mycosis can be life-threatening. Fungal plaques form in the lining of the guttural pouches; if the plaques involve vascular structures such as the internal carotid artery, then severe fatal hemorrhage can occur. Fatal hemorrhage is often preceded by several episodes of substantial epistaxis. However, once the diagnosis is made, surgery should not be delayed. The most accepted method of surgical treatment involves either direct ligation or use of a balloon-tipped catheter to occlude either the internal carotid artery, external carotid artery, or both depending on which vessels are affected. Both the internal and external carotid arteries can be ligated unilaterally with no untoward effects. The major potential complication of external carotid artery occlusion is blindness. Once the affected vessels are ligated the fungal infection is treated by lavage of the guttural pouches and instillation of antifungal medication into the pouch via indwelling catheters or via the endoscope.

Surgical Musculoskeletal Diseases

Flexural and angular limb deformities (crooked legs) are abnormalities of the limbs that arise from abnormal development of bones and musculotendinous structures in the limbs. Flexural limb deformities result in overflexion of certain joints. There are three main manifestations of flexural limb deformities in horses. These can be present at birth or develop during the first few months or years of life. Carpal flexural deformities result in the front limbs being flexed or buckled forward at the carpus.

This may range from mild deformity to a severe deformity that prevents the foal from standing. Mild to moderate cases are often amenable to treatment with controlled exercise combined with application of bandages and splints that extend from the ground to the elbow or tube casts that extend from just above the fetlock to the middle portion of the antebrachium. Tube or sleeve casts are useful, because by not encasing the foot, the foal is able to weight-load the limb, which helps prevent excessive laxity of the tendons. Intravenous administration of oxytetracycline may be beneficial to help relax the musculotendinous structures. The second type involves flexural deformity of the distal interphalangeal (coffin) joint, which results in a characteristic clubfoot-shaped hoof (Fig. 21–34). This often is first noticed when the foal is a few months of age and can progress to the point the foal walks on the toe or the dorsum of the hoof wall. Mild to moderate cases (those in which the foot has not passed the vertical plane) often respond to corrective trimming (lower heel) and application of an extended toe shoe, which helps to stretch out the deep digital flexor tendon. More advanced cases usually require surgical transection of the inferior check ligament, which lengthens the deep digital flexor musculotendinous unit.

The third type of flexural deformity involves the metacarpophalangeal joint and is characterized by an increased steepness to the pastern and fetlock (Fig. 21–35). This usually begins to develop around 1 year of age, but may occur as late as 2 years. It can progress until the horse knuckles over at the fetlock. This condition, commonly occurs in rapidly growing heavily muscled horses such as 1- to 2-year-old quarter horses. Conservative treatment involves controlled exercise, dietary management (balanced minerals, low energy and protein), management of pain (arising from osteochondrosis or physitis) with NSAIDs, and application of bandages and splints that extend from the ground to the elbow. More severely affected

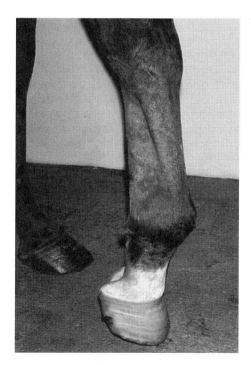

Figure 21-35. A flexural deformity of the metacarpophalangeal (fetlock) joint of a yearling horse.

horses or those that do not respond to conservative treatment may be successfully treated surgically by performing a superior check or inferior check ligament desmotomy, or both, depending upon whether the superficial digital flexor or deep digital flexor tendons or both, are involved.

Angular limb deformities are deformities that develop in the appendicular skeleton in a medial-to-lateral direction. These deviations can be present at birth or develop during the first few months of life. Mild deformities may self-correct, others may persist but not worsen, and others may become more severe with time. These deformities are named in reference to the joint involved and the direction of the deviation. The most common deviation is carpal valgus, where the limb distal to the carpus deviates laterally (Fig. 21–36). Other common deviations include fetlock varus, where the limb distal to the fetlock deviates medially (Fig. 21–37), and tarsal valgus. These deviations can occur because of disproportionate growth of bone on either side of the growth plate, incompletely ossified cuboidal bones in the carpus and tarsus, or ligamentous laxity. The deviations in foals with incompletely ossified cuboidal bones or ligamentous laxity can usually be manually straightened, whereas those with disproportionate growth at the physis cannot.

Treatment of mild to moderate angular deviations may include stall rest with controlled exercise, depending upon the age of the foal. Successful surgical procedures have been developed to treat moderate to severe deformities. Transection and elevation of the periosteum near the affected growth plate on the concave (short) side of the limb will stimulate more rapid bone growth, which usually leads to correction of the disproportionate growth. Periosteal transection and elevation can be repeated in 4 to 6 weeks if the deformity has not been

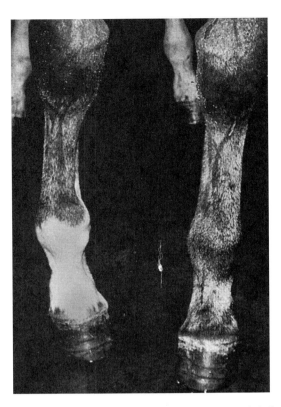

Figure 21-37. A varus deformity of the right front fetlock in a foal.

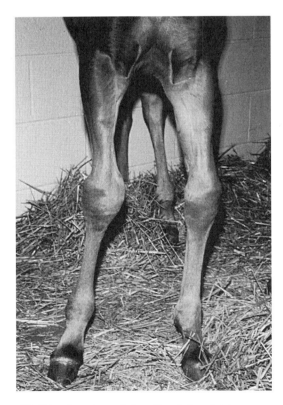

Figure 21-36. A valgus deformity of the right carpus and a varus deformity of the left carpus in a foal.

completely corrected. The deformities do not overcorrect with this procedure. In more severe deformities or in older foals with less growth potential, bone growth on the convex (long) side of the bone can be slowed by performing transphyseal bridging. This is usually performed by placing a screw on either side of the growth plate and then tightening a figure-of-eight wire around the screw heads to provide compression of the growth plate. Use of transphyseal bridging can lead to correction of more severe deformities, but it is imperative that these implants be removed at the correct time to prevent overcorrection leading to the opposite type of deformity.

EMERGENCY SITUATIONS AND PROCEDURES

Several emergency situations can arise that necessitate immediate action on the part of a technician or clinician to prevent

---

TECHNICIAN NOTE

Several emergency situations can arise that necessitate immediate action on the part of a technician or clinician to prevent death of a horse. One of the most common emergency situations is the development of upper airway obstruction leading to dyspnea. Obstructive diseases involving the nasal passages, nasopharynx, and larynx can be alleviated by a tracheotomy.

death of a horse. One of the most common emergency situations is the development of upper airway obstruction leading to dyspnea. Obstructive diseases involving the nasal passages, nasopharynx, and larynx can be alleviated by a tracheotomy. A tracheotomy is generally performed at the junction of the middle and proximal thirds of the neck on the ventral midline. An incision is made on the ventral cervical midline through the skin, subcutaneous tissue, and cutaneous colli muscle parallel to the trachea. The paired sternothyrohyoideus muscles are then split on midline to expose the tracheal rings. The membrane between two adjacent rings is then cut with a scalpel on the ventral surface for a distance of approximately one-half the circumference of the tracheal rings. Care should be taken not to cut the tracheal rings and not to cut vital structures adjacent to the trachea (carotid artery, recurrent laryngeal nerve, jugular vein). Many times the tracheotomy must be performed on an extremely anxious horse or after the horse has collapsed from insufficient oxygen. Therefore, one should be careful not to get into a situation where injury occurs.

Veterinary technicians should become familiar and comfortable with the dosages and indications for drugs commonly used in emergency situations. A list of drugs and doses along with the drugs and syringes should be kept readily available in several locations throughout the hospital. These can be prepared in small emergency packs.

> **TECHNICIAN NOTE**
>
> Veterinary technicians should become familiar and comfortable with the dosages and indications for drugs commonly used in emergency situations. A list of drugs and doses along with the drugs and syringes should be kept readily available in several locations throughout the hospital.

Occasionally, horses develop reactions to certain drugs. These may be anaphylactic reactions resulting in shock or death or allergic-type reactions resulting in skin wheals. Horses may develop a reaction to procaine penicillin, which usually results in a anaphylactoid reaction. These horses usually require treatment with corticosteroids and epinephrine. They may recover or die subsequent to pulmonary edema. Horses often develop skin wheals in response to drugs or environmental allergens. The drugs that most commonly cause these wheals in horses are NSAIDs and trimethoprim-sulfa antibiotics.

Intracarotid injection of drugs can cause seizure-like activity. This can be life-threatening to the horse and is potentially injurious to the handler and other personnel in the vicinity. The chance for this can be minimized by using an 18-gauge needle that is unattached from the syringe and directed down the jugular vein. Normally, if the needle is in the jugular vein blood will slowly ooze out of the needle hub only if the jugular vein is occluded. If the carotid artery is inadvertently entered with the needle, then blood will exit in a pulsatile manner. If this occurs, do not inject the medication. The needle should be removed and compression should be applied to decrease hematoma formation. The needle should be reinserted into a different location using the same technique.

ANESTHESIA FOR THE EQUINE PATIENT

> **TECHNICIAN NOTE**
>
> The veterinary technician may be directly or indirectly involved in anesthesia of horses. Frequently, the technician is primarily responsible for all aspects of anesthesia, including selection of induction and maintenance anesthetic agents, instrumentation, monitoring, and recovery of patients.

The veterinary technician may be directly or indirectly involved in anesthesia of horses. Frequently, the technician is primarily responsible for all aspects of anesthesia, including selection of induction and maintenance anesthetic agents, instrumentation, monitoring, and recovery of patients. It is important that the technician be familiar with the properties and recommended doses of the anesthetic agents being administered, and the equipment (ventilator, blood pressure monitor, anesthetic machine, and so forth) being used (see Chapter 15). Numerous complications can arise, and it is important that the technician be familiar with the methods of treating these complications, including the correct drugs and doses for treating hypotension and cardiac arrhythmias. Because it is important to maintain mean arterial blood pressure at 70 mm Hg or greater to help prevent myopathies and neuropathies, blood pressure should be monitored via an indirect or direct method. Hypotension is usually treated by reducing the depth of anesthesia and increasing the rate of administration of IV fluids and vasoactive drugs, such as dobutamine, dopamine, or phenylephrine. It is important to monitor how well the horse is being oxygenated and ventilated during anesthesia; this can be done most effectively by monitoring arterial blood gases. The technician should monitor recovery from anesthesia and be prepared for any potential complications.

Recommended Reading

Auer JA (editor): Equine Surgery. Philadelphia, WB Saunders, 1992.

Koterba AM, Drummond WH, and Kosch PC (editors): Equine Clinical Neonatology. Philadelphia, Lea & Febiger, 1990.

Robinson NE (editor): Current Therapy in Equine Medicine, 2nd ed. Philadelphia, WB Saunders, 1987.

Robinson NE (editor): Current Therapy in Equine Medicine, 3rd ed. Philadelphia, WB Saunders, 1991.

White NA and Moore JN (editors): Current Practice of Equine Surgery. Philadelphia, JB Lippincott, 1990.

22 Food Animal Medicine and Surgery

Margaret L. Cebra • *Christopher K. Cebra*

INTRODUCTION

The food animal industry encompasses a wide variety of animal species and economic functions. Domestic food animal species include cattle, sheep, goats, llamas, alpacas, and pigs. The major functions of food animals include food and fiber production and providing genetic stock. Although the trend in the food animal industry has shifted from small farms toward intensively managed, large production systems, a knowledge of the medical and surgical problems of individual food animals is the basis of effective herd health and production management.

Veterinary technicians play a vital role in food animal practice. They work closely with veterinarians to restrain and handle animals for examination, collect samples for diagnostic testing, and treat sick animals. Other functions of veterinary technicians include preparing equipment and animals for surgical or diagnostic procedures, assisting the veterinarian in performing diagnostic and surgical procedures, and preparing animal health and production records, written reports, and financial statements to the animal producer. In addition, the technician is responsible for stocking equipment, pharmaceuticals, biologics, and supplies used by the veterinarian. A technician who is well trained, competent, and efficient can enhance the success and efficiency of the veterinary service provided to the food animal producer. The more knowledgeable the veterinary technician is about the diseases and procedures performed, the better he or she can anticipate the needs of the veterinarian.

The purpose of this chapter is to acquaint the veterinary technician with common medical and surgical problems of food animals. The chapter has been organized by organ system using a problem-oriented approach. Because the principles of surgery and medicine are the same for all species, the various food animal species are discussed together, unless a unique feature of a specific animal warrants special mention. Emphasis has been placed on those diseases and procedures that are commonly encountered in food animal practice and with which the veterinary technician should be familiar.

HEAD LESIONS

Infectious keratoconjunctivitis (pinkeye) is caused by *Moraxella bovis* in cattle and *Mycoplasma* spp. or *Chlamydia* in small ruminants. Bacteria may be spread by flies or through direct contact. In cattle, the lesion often starts as a central corneal opacity, which helps differentiate this lesion from viral conjunctivitis (Fig. 22–1). In small ruminants, the lesion start as conjunctivitis and spreads to the cornea. Photophobia, ocular reddening, and discharge are commonly seen. Systemic or subconjunctival antibiotics are used to treat affected animals, and fly control is important to prevent new cases.

Oral and nasal vesicular or ulcerative lesions are common in ruminants and swine with a variety of viral diseases. Some of these are accompanied by conjunctivitis, diarrhea, abortion, and coronary band lesions and should be investigated due to the significant effect on a herd. Soremouth (orf) is a less severe disease that is common and transient in small ruminant neonates (Fig. 22–2). Morbidity is due to the pain caused by the mouth lesions and teat lesions on the dams. Basic supportive care is essential for animals that cannot eat.

Facial swelling is a common complaint due to its visibility. To determine the cause, careful palpation of the swollen area is necessary. Hard masses suggest that bony structures are affected, whereas softer, moveable masses suggest that the lesion is primarily within the soft tissue. The causes of bony swelling include displaced or healing fractures, osteomyelitis (lumpy jaw, actinomycosis [most common in cattle]), tooth root

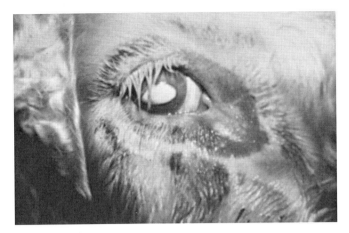

Figure 22-1. Cow with infectious bovine keratoconjunctivitis (pinkeye) with a large central corneal opacity.

abscesses (most common in camelids and pigs), and bony tumors (rare in all species) (Fig. 22–3). Causes of soft tissue swelling include snake or insect bite, cellulitis or lymphadenitis (actinobacillosis in cattle or corynebacterial caseous lymphadenitis in small ruminants), foreign body reactions, lymphoma or other soft tissue tumors, or salivary mucocoele (Fig. 22–4). Bony lesions also may lead to inflammation and draining tracts in the adjacent soft tissue.

Other clinical information may aid in arriving at a diagnosis. A fracture or tooth root abscess frequently causes the animal pain on mastication. Dysphagia, quidding, or weight loss may be seen, although camelids with a tooth root abscess rarely show evidence of oral pain. Malalignment of teeth secondary to osteomyelitis or a tumor also may cause painful trauma to soft tissue. Radiographs are helpful in differentiating the causes of bony swelling but are not always practical. They are espe-

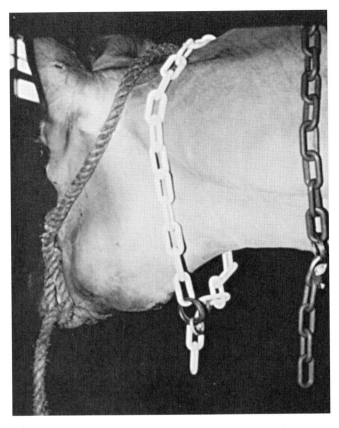

Figure 22-3. A bony mass on the mandible of a cow with actinomycosis (lumpy jaw).

cially useful in differentiating osteomyelitis from a tooth root abscess. Gram stains or cultures of discharges or aspirates may help determine a bacterial etiology. Biopsy is necessary to definitively diagnose a tumor.

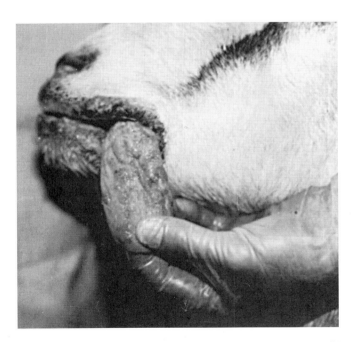

Figure 22-2. Goat with contagious ecthyma (orf, soremouth) with ulcerative and proliferative lesions on the lips and tongue.

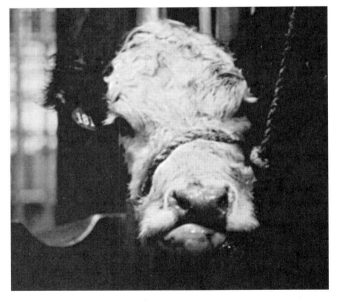

Figure 22-4. Calf with actinobacillosis (wooden tongue). The enlarged tongue protrudes from the calf's mouth.

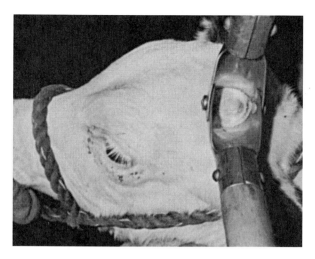

Figure 22-5. Dehorning a calf with a Barnes scoop dehorner.

There usually is a surgical and medical option to treat all facial swellings. Fractures may be repaired surgically, whereas infected bone may be curetted, abscessed teeth removed, tumors debulked, and abscesses drained. Due to the size of most food animals, surgical repair of mandibular fractures is uncommon, although external fixation is useful to reduce displaced fractures. Curettage of osteomyelitis also is uncommon, because surgery does not significantly improve the prognosis, and fractures may result. Repulsion of abscessed teeth is facilitated through a sinus flap or trephine hole. Drainage from abscesses may be facilitated by lancing. This is best achieved by clipping and surgically preparing a site over the softest, most ventral part of the swelling, using a hypodermic needle to establish the purulent nature of the material within the mass, and then opening a large hole with a scalpel blade into the center of the mass.

Medical treatment also can be very effective. Mandibular osteomyelitis in cattle may be treated successfully with a month-long course of antibiotics if the lesion is not too extensive. Camelids with tooth root abscesses appear to respond satisfactorily to a similar regimen of antibiotics without surgery. Because bacteremia with metastasis of infection may occur in cattle with tooth root abscesses, medical treatment of this lesion may be inferior to removal of the tooth. Lymphadenitis and cellulitis may be treated with a combination of antibiotics and sodium or potassium iodide; the iodide salt reduces inflammation, which allows better penetration of the antibiotic into the lesion. Prognosis is poor for caseous lymphadenitis in small ruminants because internal abscesses often are present.

Simple management changes may be necessary. If multiple animals in a herd are affected by bony or soft tissue infection of the mouth, the feed should be checked for grass awns or foxtails. If quidding is noted, providing the animal with soft feed will help it maintain weight. This is especially useful for healing fractures.

Tooth Trimming

Male llamas and pigs may develop prominent canine teeth, which can cause injury to others. Annual trimming of these teeth is recommended. This may be accomplished with the animal under heavy sedation or general anesthesia. A piece of obstetric wire is placed around the tooth above the gumline, and the tooth is sawed off.

Dehorning

Except for polled breeds, most ruminants of either sex will develop horns. Horn buds can be palpated toward the back of the skull within the first weeks of life. Although favored by some for their appearance, horns can be dangerous weapons. Removal or destruction of the horn buds early in life is easier and less traumatic than the removal of a fully developed horn (Fig. 22–5).

Sensation to the horn comes from the cornual nerve in cattle. This may be blocked by infiltrating the area midway between the horn base and the lateral canthus of the eye with a local anesthetic agent. Goats and older cattle have additional innervation and may require a ring block around the base of each horn. Horn buds may be burned with a hot iron or removed with a scoop or gouge (Fig. 22–6). Burning is best done on animals less than 1 month old, whereas the scoop or gouge may be used on any horn that fits within their lumen. In adult animals, a skin incision may be made around the horn base, and the horn is then cut off with a wire or hand saw. Regardless of the technique, it is important to remember that the horn is produced by the germinal epithelium around the horn base, and this tissue must be destroyed or removed to prevent regrowth. Extreme care must be taken when dehorning small ruminants because their poorly developed frontal sinus often leaves the brain cavity in direct contact with the horn base.

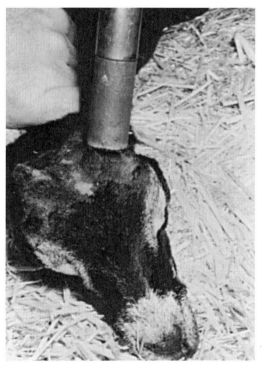

Figure 22-6. Disbudding a kid by burning with an electric dehorning iron.

RESPIRATORY DISEASE

Respiratory problems in food animals are commonly infectious and can be divided into upper and lower respiratory tract disorders depending on whether the pharynx, larynx or trachea (upper) or lungs (lower) are primarily involved. Assessment of the respiratory system involves auscultation and percussion of the thorax as well as ancillary tests such as transtracheal wash and bronchoalveolar lavage.

Transtracheal Wash

Both percutaneous and endoscope-guided sampling may be done. In both cases, the animal should be adequately restrained, preferably standing with the head and neck extended. For endoscope-guided sampling, a double-sheathed catheter should be used. The trachea can be visualized with the endoscope and positioned with the tip of the endoscope near a pocket of fluid if present. The catheter or tubing is passed into the trachea, and 20 ml of sterile saline is flushed into the trachea and followed by rapid aspiration. For percutaneous sampling, the ventral midcervical area is clipped, surgically prepared, and infiltrated with local anesthetic. One sterile hand is used to grasp the trachea while a 1-cm longitudinal scalpel incision is made over the trachea. Tracheal rings should be palpated and an area between rings identified. A stab incision is made into the lumen of the trachea between rings with a 9-gauge bleeding trocar (bevel directed down) while continuing to stabilize the trachea with the other hand. Sterile, polypropylene tubing (90 cm) is passed into the trachea at least 15 cm. Once the tubing is within the trachea, the trocar is removed, leaving the tubing in place. Sterile physiologic saline (30 mL for a cow) is injected via a 15-gauge needle that is placed in the end of the tubing. Immediately afterward, the saline wash is aspirated using the same or a different sterile syringe. From 5 to 10 mL of saline wash is sufficient for analysis. The sample is placed in a tube with EDTA for cytology or transported in the syringe or onto transport media for culture.

Upper Respiratory Disease

Causes of upper respiratory tract infections include viral and bacterial agents. Common viruses include infectious bovine rhinotracheitis (IBR), bovine viral diarrhea (BVD), and malignant catarrhal fever (MCF) for cattle; border disease in sheep; and influenza (paramyxovirus) in swine. Common clinical signs include fever (often up to 41°C with MCF), conjunctivitis, rhinitis, tracheitis, oral and nasal erosions and ulcers, listlessness, coughing, and dyspnea (Figs. 22–7 and 22–8). BVD and border disease are also associated with reproductive and gastrointestinal diseases, whereas MCF often causes corneal opacification. Typically, the viruses facilitate bacterial invasion of the lungs by damaging the respiratory defense mechanisms. Recovery from acute viral infection is often rapid if not complicated by bronchopneumonia. Diagnosis for all viral respiratory diseases consists of viral isolation from nasal swabs (IBR, influenza) or white blood cells (BVD, border disease, MCF) or serologic testing. Treatment consists of supportive care and prophylactic antibiotics. Control is based on vaccination for IBR, BVD, and swine influenza, (see Chapter 14).

Probably one of the most common causes of bacterial upper airway disease in cattle between 3 to 18 months old is

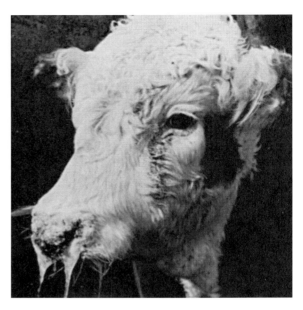

Figure 22-7. Mucopurulent oculonasal discharge in a calf with respiratory disease.

necrotic laryngitis (calf diphtheria). It is an acute-to-chronic infection of the laryngeal mucosa and cartilage. Damaged mucosa allows invasion of *Fusobacterium necrophorum*. Signs include acute onset of moist, painful cough; inspiratory dyspnea with loud stridor and open-mouthed breathing; hypersalivation; anorexia; depression; fever; bilateral nasal discharge; fetid breath; ill-thrift; and death. Mild pressure to the larynx causes cough, pain, marked dyspnea, and stridor. Aspiration pneumonia may develop. Diagnosis can be confirmed by endoscopy or laryngoscopy. Treatment consists of long-term antibiotic administration, anti-inflammatory agents, or surgical removal of the diseased arytenoids through a ventral approach.

Atrophic rhinitis is a multifactorial disease complex in pigs caused by toxigenic *Bordetella bronchiseptica* and *Pasteurella multocida*. The disease is characterized by turbinate atrophy

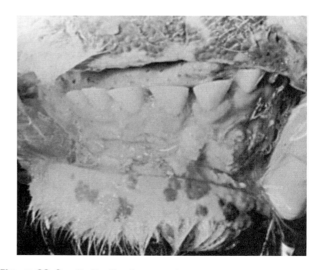

Figure 22-8. Calf with ulcers and erosions of the gums associated with bovine virus diarrhea (BVD).

and nasal deviation. Treatment includes antimicrobial therapy of sows, piglets, and weaners. Poor environmental conditions contribute to increased incidence and severity of atrophic rhinitis (e.g., poor ventilation, overcrowding, and temperature extremes).

Lower Respiratory Disease

Some of the more common causes of viral pneumonia in cattle include parainfluenza 3 (PI-3) and bovine respiratory syncytial virus (BRSV). PI-3 causes respiratory disease in cattle and sheep. Uncomplicated disease is usually mild, often asymptomatic. BRSV infection occurs in calves less than 6 months of age. Clinically, calves have pneumonic signs, and subcutaneous emphysema is sporadically reported. Animals affected with either virus often succumb to secondary bacterial pneumonia due to impaired clearance of organisms from the lungs. Diagnosis is confirmed by viral isolation from nasal mucosa (PI-3) or tracheal or bronchial secretions (BRSV) collected early in the disease process or by serologic testing. Prevention is through vaccination, which reduces the severity of disease but does not prevent infection. Immunity to natural infection with BRSV does not prevent reinfection.

In small ruminants, there are three retroviral causes of pneumonia. These include two nononcogenic retroviruses, ovine progressive pneumonia (OPP) and caprine arthritis and encephalitis virus (CAE), and pulmonary carcinoma or adenomatosis. OPP causes chronic pneumonia in sheep and can also occur in goats, whereas CAE causes interstitial pneumonia in goats only. Both OPP and CAE have long incubation periods and insidious, progressive clinical disease courses. Small ruminants rarely show signs before 2 years of age. Several syndromes can occur for both OPP and CAE, of which respiratory disease is only one. Clinical signs include weight loss; listlessness, with progression to exercise intolerance; dyspnea, often without pyrexia; and death within 18 months. Routes of transmission for OPP and CAE include lactogenic (through nursing) and vertical (rarely). Diagnosis is by serology, clinical signs, and histopathology. Control measures are directed at identification of infected animals with serologic testing and depopulation. Newborn lambs and kids should be separated from seropositive ewes and does immediately after birth before colostral ingestion. The lambs and kids should be fed pooled seronegative colostrum.

Pulmonary carcinoma is a contagious neoplastic disease of adult sheep characterized by insidious, progressive weakness, dyspnea, nasal discharge, and death. Transmission is horizontal and by inhalation. Diagnosis is based on typical signs and histopathologic lesions. There is no specific treatment for any of these viral infections, but antibiotics and anti-inflammatory agents may temporarily improve the quality of life.

Coronavirus has been identified as a cause of pneumonia in cows and pigs. The virus is antigenically related to the organism associated with gastrointestinal disease in both species but causes bronchointerstitial pneumonia in naive animals. Pseudorabies virus (PRV) causes pneumonia or upper repiratory tract infection in grower-finisher pigs. Signs are nonspecific and referable to the respiratory system. Morbidity is usually high, but mortality is low, with recovery often within 10 days. PRV persists in infected swine and is actively shed during periods of stress. Transmission may occur during mating, transplacentally, or through aerosol.

Porcine respiratory and reproductive syndrome (PRRS) is associated with respiratory distress in sows. Pigs have increased susceptibility to bacterial causes of pneumonia. Nursing pigs develop rapid abdominal breathing and a characteristic "thumping" sound on auscultation. Mortality may be as high as 50% in some litters. Infected finishing pigs may exhibit rapid breathing, dyspnea, rough hair coat, and poor growth. Reproductive problems have also been associated with PRRS.

The primary bacteria responsible for producing acute fibrinous bronchopneumonia in ruminants is *Pasteurella haemolytica,* whereas chronic pneumonia in ruminants and pigs is often caused by *P. multocida. P. haemolytica* is part of the normal nasal flora but present in the lungs only when causing pneumonia. Management, environmental, and infectious stressors may facilitate *Pasteurella* spp. infections. *P. haemolytica* can cause pneumonia independent of viral or other bacterial agents; however, viral agents, such as IBR, BRSV, and PI-3, and bacteria such as *Mycoplasma bovis* increase susceptibility to challenge with *P. haemolytica. Haemophilus somnus* and *H. parasuis* can cause conjunctivitis, tracheitis, pleuritis, suppurative bronchopneumonia, pericarditis, arthritis, and meningoencephalitis in cattle and pigs, respectively. The respiratory form is seen in feedlot calves and nursing, nursery, and finishing pigs. The route of transmission is unknown. Mycoplasma are small bacteria lacking a cell wall. *M. bovis* causes cuffing pneumonia and alveolitis. *M. dispar* and *Ureaplasma* spp. are probably associated with respiratory disease in calves. Transmission occurs through direct contact, exposure to droplets or fomites, discharge from nose or eyes, and aerosolization. Diagnosis of bacterial pneumonia is by culture of tracheal or bronchial secretions. Treatment consists of antibiotics and anti-inflammatory agents. Vaccines are available for most of the bacterial agents; however, efficacy is not completely satisfactory.

Many simple pneumonias in calves, pigs, and adult cattle are syndromes involving one or more infectious agents, environmental and management stressors, and a susceptible host. Enzootic pneumonia of calves is commonly diagnosed in housed calves from 2 to 6 months of age. The syndrome in pigs often occurs during the growing and finishing stages. Adult cattle with respiratory disease complex (shipping fever) often manifest clinical signs within 2 weeks of arrival at a feedlot. Several different pathogens have been implicated in all three syndromes with combinations of organisms common. Viral agents often associated with enzootic pneumonia of calves include PI-3, BRSV, BVD virus, IBR, and several adenoviruses. For adult shipping fever, IBR, BVD, PI-3, and BRSV are often implicated. *P. haemolytica* is the most significant cause of shipping fever, although *P. multocida* and *H. somnus* are sometimes involved. For enzootic pneumonia of calves, common bacterial agents include the same three agents in addition to *Mycoplasma* spp., *Actinomyces pyogenes,* and *Salmonella* spp. Common agents for enzootic pneumonia of swine include *Mycoplasma hyopneumoniae* (primarily) and *P. multocida.*

Clinical signs for all three syndromes range from subclinical to acute and fulminating to chronic. Signs include ill-thrift with poor weight gain, prolonged recumbency, listlessness, persistent and dry hacking cough, intermittent fever, dehydration, and a history of recurrent episodes of mild pneumonia that tend to become refractory to therapy. Wheezes and crackles may be auscultable. Radiographically, there often is evidence of atelectasis and consolidation of cranioventral lung lobes.

Diagnosis for all three syndromes can best be achieved by

a postmortem examination, premortem serologic testing, and culture of lung or tracheal secretions from the most severely affected animals. Treatment is largely supportive, consisting of appropriate antibiotics for bacterial pathogens, fluids, anti-inflammatory agents, and oxygen as needed. The most successful cases will be those that are recognized and treated early before irreversible damage to the lung and growth potential of the animal occurs. Management considerations for avoidance of these syndromes emphasize colostral management for calves, nutritional support for pigs and older cattle, good-quality housing facilities (air quality, ventilation, low population density), preconditioning for older cattle (processing before marketing), and appropriate vaccination programs.

Acute bovine pulmonary emphysema and edema is a non-febrile, noninfectious respiratory distress syndrome of adult beef cattle that usually occurs in the fall. It occurs in cattle grazing on alfalfa, rape, kale, or turnip tops. Clinical signs include dyspnea and crackles and wheezes on auscultation. Mortality of affected cattle may approach 50%. Treatment is primarily supportive in addition to removal of the animals from affected pastures. Prevention involves gradual introduction to lush pasture, ionophores such as monensin and lasalocid, and prophylactic oral antibiotics.

Parasites such as *Ascaris suum, Dictyocaulus viviparus, Dictyocaulus filaria, Protostrongylus rufescens,* and *Muellerius capillaris* can cause inflammation in the lungs with resultant eosinophilic or granulomatous pulmonary infiltrates in food animals. All except *A. suum* primarily invade the pulmonary system, whereas larvae from *A. suum* migrate through the lungs, causing inflammation and impaired resistance to secondary infectious pathogens. Diagnosis can be made by detection of larvae in the feces or eggs in respiratory secretions. Anthelmintic administration is usually effective in keeping parasite burdens low or nonexistent (see Chapter 5).

TECHNICIAN NOTE

The importance of viruses in respiratory disease in food animals primarily resides in their ability to act synergistically to facilitate bacterial invasion.

CARDIOVASCULAR DISEASE

Heart disease, in general, is uncommon in food animals. Endocarditis is an often undiagnosed cause of cardiac disease in food animals. It is usually caused by bacteria that gain entrance through damaged valvular surfaces by hematogenous spread. Common infectious causes in cattle include *Actinomyces pyogenes* and alpha-hemolytic *Streptococcus.* In sheep and pigs, the common causative organisms are *Erysipelothrix rhusiopathiae, Streptococcus* spp., and *Escherichia coli.* In cattle, the tricuspid valve is most commonly affected, although multiple valves can be involved.

A systolic cardiac murmur is the most specific physical examination finding in food animals with this condition. However, affected animals may show nonspecific signs such as constant or intermittent fever, anorexia, respiratory signs, weight loss, exercise intolerance, diarrhea, or sudden death. Dairy cows may have decreased milk production. There may

be evidence of heart failure if the condition is severe or long-standing (peripheral edema, severe dyspnea, jugular pulses, or distention). Isolation of pathogens on blood culture, auscultation of a murmur, and echocardiographic evidence of a vegetative lesion on a cardiac valve are highly suggestive of bacterial endocarditis.

TECHNICIAN NOTE

Signs of congestive heart failure in food animals include submandibular edema, jugular distention and pulsation, dyspnea, and ascites.

Treatment of bacterial endocarditis involves long-term administration of antimicrobials (4 to 6 weeks); penicillin is often chosen. Adjunctive treatments include furosemide (diuretic) and oxygen therapy if there is evidence of congestive heart failure or pulmonary compromise, respectively. The prognosis is poor to guarded with post-treatment relapses common due to the inability of the antimicrobials to reach the site of infection and thrombogenic properties of the exposed heart valve leaflet. If an animal has evidence of congestive heart failure on initial evaluation, treatment response is often poor; consequently, treatment may not be economically justifiable.

Traumatic reticulopericarditis (*hardware disease*) resulting from penetration of the pericardium by ingested foreign objects such as a wire or nail is a common cause of pericarditis in cattle. Nontraumatic pericarditis in cattle may be caused by *Pasteurella* spp., *Clostridium* spp., and *Haemophilus* spp. In sheep and pigs, *Pasteurella* spp. and *Mycoplasma* spp. are common causes of pericarditis. *Staphylococcus aureus* and *Streptococcus* spp. are other causes in sheep and pigs, respectively. In all species, inflammation of the pericardium causes hyperemia and deposition of fibrinous exudate, followed by effusion. The animal may show nonspecific signs such as fever, anorexia, depression, or weight loss. More specific signs may include tachycardia, friction rubs, muffled heart sounds, and absent lung sounds in the ventral thorax on thoracic auscultation. Splashing sounds are heard frequently during thoracic auscultation due to accumulation of gas and liquid in the pericardium (*washing machine murmur*). If congestive heart failure develops, the animal may develop peripheral edema, jugular venous distention and pulsation, and dyspnea (Fig. 22–9). Cattle with traumatic reticulopericarditis may exhibit cranial abdominal pain (see discussion of gastrointestinal problems).

Echocardiography can be used to confirm the diagnosis of pericarditis. There will be evidence of an echo-free space between the two pericardial layers that is suggestive of fluid accumulation. Electrocardiograms and thoracic radiographs may be helpful, although often they are not. Treatment often is unrewarding and usually is directed toward salvage or short-term survival. Pericardial drainage with lavage and culturing may be used both diagnostically and therapeutically. Broad-spectrum antimicrobial and anti-inflammatory agents are important for systemic use. Surgical removal of the foreign body in cattle with traumatic reticulopericarditis through a rumenotomy site or release of the effusion through pericardiectomy has been attempted with varying success. A common long-term sequela of pericarditis is the formation of pericardial adhesions,

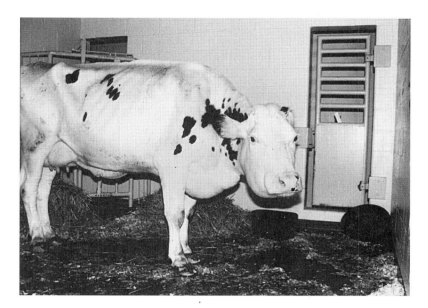

Figure 22-9. Cow with congestive heart failure, showing rough haircoat and edema of the ventrum and brisket.

causing complete attachment of the pericardium to the epicardium. As a result of restriction of cardiac movement, congestive heart failure develops.

Pulmonary hypertension (*brisket disease*) can develop in susceptible cattle with prolonged exposure to high altitudes (more than 1800 m [6000 ft] above sea level). Goats and sheep are reported to be susceptible but less so than cattle. Pigs, llamas, and alpacas are resistant. The low oxygen tension at these altitudes causes hypoxic vasoconstriction of the pulmonary arteries, leading to increased pulmonary vascular resistance and hypertension. Pressure overload of the right ventricle results in cardiac hypertrophy, dilation, and failure. The disease is reversible in the early stages by moving the animal to a lower altitude.

The most common presenting clinical sign is subcutaneous edema of the brisket, ventral thorax, or submandibular area. Cattle often show dyspnea, tachypnea, chronic cough, or weight loss. A cardiac murmur may be ausculted, caused by either tricuspid valve insufficiency or pulmonic valve compromise. Genetic predispositions are seen in some herds. Ingestion of locoweed can also predispose cattle to right heart failure at high altitudes by causing toxic myocardial damage. Other factors, such as myocardial dystrophy, anemia, cold, pulmonary disease, or hypoproteinemia, may exacerbate the primary cardiac dysfunction.

Diagnostic tests that aid in the diagnosis of pulmonary hypertension and cardiomegaly include measurement of pulmonary arterial pressures and echocardiography. Mean pulmonary arterial pressures of more than 35 mm Hg are suggestive of high altitude disease. Echocardiography may reveal right heart enlargement or valvular problems. The disease can be controlled by removing susceptible animals from the high altitude and preventing locoweed ingestion. Lung disease may need to be treated with oxygen therapy. Heart failure responds poorly to treatment; however, it may be controlled with digoxin and diuretics such as furosemide.

Congenital heart defects occur uncommonly in all food animal species; the prevalence is highest in cattle. In some defects, heredity appears to play a role. Defects can occur alone or in combination. The most commonly reported heart defect in cattle and sheep is a ventricular septal defect (VSD). In pigs, dysplasia of the tricuspid valve and atrial septal defects are more common than VSDs. Congenital cardiac defects allow for the mixing of oxygenated and reduced oxygenated blood through aberrant circuits between the pulmonary and systemic circulations. Clinical signs include heart murmur, exercise intolerance, cyanosis at rest or with exertion, lethargy, poor growth, weakness, or acute death. Often, the defect produces signs at birth and causes severe illness or death within the first few weeks of life. If adequate compensation occurs, signs may appear later in life and manifest as stunted growth due to reduced cardiac output, congestive heart failure, systemic infections due to cardiac dysfunction, or sudden death from severe cardiac arrhythmias. Diagnosis is best achieved by auscultation of a characteristic heart murmur and direct visualization of the defect and blood flow pattern with M-mode echocardiography and Doppler. Treatment is generally nonrewarding.

Atrial fibrillation is the most common arrhythmia of food animals. Cattle with atrial fibrillation often are asymptomatic at rest or have signs referrable to the source of the dysrhythmia. Gastrointestinal disease, hypocalcemia, foot rot, and pneumonia can lead to atrial fibrillation in cattle; anorexia and decreased milk production may occur as a result. Auscultation reveals an irregularly irregular heartbeat. The heart rate may be slow, normal, or rapid. The diagnosis can be confirmed with an electrocardiogram. Therapy is directed at correcting the underlying problem. Usually, the arrhythmia will resolve on its own within 5 days of treatment of the underlying problem. Quinidine can be used to convert atrial fibrillation to normal sinus rhythm in ruminants; it must be given slowly in intravenous fluids in cattle with constant monitoring. Diarrhea and depression are common side effects. If arrhythmias develop, the infusion should be discontinued. Therapy should be discontinued after the infusion, regardless of whether conversion has occurred. It should also be stopped as soon as conversion occurs.

GASTROINTESTINAL DISEASES
General Mechanisms of Disease

Ruminants use foregut microbial fermentation to extract nutrients from plant material. Regurgitation and repeated chewing are used to break down fibrous material and expose nutrients to the rumen bacteria and protozoa. Products of fermentation include organic acids and gas. The organic acids, which make rumen fluid acidic, are absorbed through the gastric or intestinal wall and are used by the animal for energy, whereas gas is eructated. Accumulation of either of these products in the rumen can be detrimental to the animal. Organized ruminoreticular contraction cycles, which are important for normal digestion, also prevent accumulation of acids and gas by stimulating outflow of ingesta, enhancing absorption of acids, and expelling gas. Camelids have similar gastrointestinal function, although the morphology of the gastric compartments is different. On the other hand, pigs are monogastric but have a well-developed cecum for fermentation in the caudal gastrointestinal tract.

Proper ruminoreticular (foregut) function is dependent on the physiologic well-being of the ruminant, as well as the continuous intake of appropriate feed. In that regard, auscultation for motility and palpation of the fill and consistency of the rumen are valuable tools in assessing the health of the ruminant. In addition, because the rumen is the biggest contributor to abdominal volume in the nonpregnant ruminant, size changes of the rumen often are mirrored by the abdominal contour.

Dysfunction of the rumen can be classified as hypomotility, shrinkage, gas distention, or fluid distention. Shrinkage is due to decreased feed or water intake and is not a primary disease. Ruminal hypomotility or stasis can be caused by lack of feed intake, rumen overdistention, gastric hyperacidity, systemic disease, and emotional stress. Hypomotility often is accompanied by a decreased fluid content in the rumen, which inappropriately is referred to as *rumen impaction*. Hypomotility is best addressed through treatment for the primary disease. Oral electrolyte fluids, liquified feed, or gastric fluid from a healthy cow (transfaunation) may be beneficial in increasing the function of a static rumen, but mineral oil and laxatives seldom are helpful.

A thorough physical examination is necessary to determine the cause and importance of abdominal distention. Gas accumulation typically results in dorsal distention and can cause a hyperresonant area or *ping* detectable by simultaneous auscultation and percussion (Fig. 22–10). Fluid accumulation typically

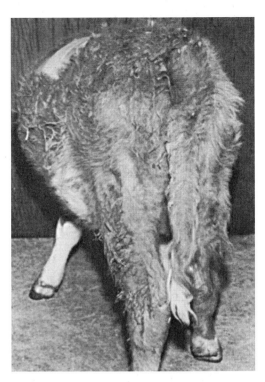

Figure 22-11. Ruminal gas distention (bloat) in the dorsal left paralumbar fossa of a cow.

causes ventral distention and can cause a "splashy" area detectable by simultaneous auscultation and ballotment. Transrectal palpation for distended abdominal viscera may aid in identification of the disorder. Distention of the rumen is most visible on the left side of the abdomen. A large, fluid-filled rumen is L shaped, with bilateral ventral distention and left-sided dorsal distention. Enlargement of the abomasum, cecum, or multiple loops of small intestine leads to distention of the right flank and possibly secondary rumen stasis, fluid accumulation, and left flank distention. Problems in the urogenital system also may lead to ventral abdominal distention.

> **✎ TECHNICIAN NOTE**
>
> Simultaneous ballotment and percussion of the abdomen (*pinging*) of a ruminant can help localize sites of fluid and gas accumulation.

Distention of the rumen with gas (*bloat*) can occur as a result of stasis, failure to eructate, overproduction of gas, or production of gas trapped in a stable foam. Gas distention of the rumen is important because it inhibits normal motility and prevents expansion of the lungs (Fig. 22–11). Gas produced by fermentation usually is free but may be trapped in foam (*frothy bloat*) if a proteinaceous feedstuff, particularly a legume hay, is being fed. If respiration is unaffected and the skin over the rumen is not tightly stretched, emergency treatment is not necessary. An orogastric tube may be passed to release free gas, and the animal should be observed for progression of signs. If

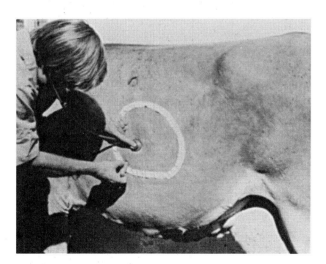

Figure 22-10. Auscultation and percussion of the left flank. The tape outlines the area of resonance associated with left abomasal displacement.

frothy bloat is suspected, a detergent (poloxalene) or mineral oil should be given orally to destabilize the foam. If the distention is impairing the animal's ability to breathe, an aggressive attempt should be made to relieve the distention: a larger-bore stomach tube may be passed, or a fistula may be made through the dorsal left paralumbar fossa into the rumen. A temporary fistula can be made with a large-gauge hypodermic needle or trochar, but a surgical fistula will decrease abdominal contamination and provide longer relief.

Fluid distention of abdominal viscera occurs as a result of regurgitation from a distal site (*internal vomition*), physical or functional outflow obstruction, or fluid shifts secondary to the accumulation of osmotic particles. Thus, fluid distention can occur as a primary problem or secondary to another disorder. Excess ruminal fluid inhibits eructation by causing the lower esophageal sphincter to spasm, leading to secondary gas distention. Unlike gas distention, fluid distention rarely is correctable by passage of an orogastric tube.

Specific Gastrointestinal Diseases

Overingestion of rapidly fermentable feed (carbohydrate engorgement, grain overload) results in the production of large quantities of gas and osmotically active organic acids in the rumen. Body water follows the osmotic gradient into the rumen, resulting in a "splashy," ventrally distended rumen and decreased circulatory volume. Gas accumulation leads to dorsal ruminal distention. Circulatory shock and absorption of acid into the systemic circulation lead to systemic acidosis and depression.

Treatment goals include relieving the gas and fluid distention of the rumen, reducing production and absorption of acid, and correcting systemic fluid and acid-base derangements. These goals can be accomplished through orogastric intubation with a large-bore (Kingman) stomach tube, ruminal lavage with cold water, rumenotomy to remove feed material, oral alkalinizing agents (magnesium oxide, sulfate, or hydroxide), oral mineral oil to promote gastrointestinal transit, and systemic alkalinizing fluid treatment. Secondary metabolic and infectious diseases may occur and are best treated prophylactically with thiamine and penicillin. Not all treatments are required for all animals.

Perforation of the reticulum by a metallic foreign body (hardware disease) can lead to peritonitis with possible extension into the pleural and pericardial cavities. Pain and secondary infection lead to anorexia, a drop in milk production, and cranial abdominal pain. The cow may resist ventroflexion when manual pressure is applied to the thoracic spine or may grunt when pressure is applied to the xiphoid region. Cattle with chronic hardware disease may develop weight loss, recurrent fever, and rumen distention. Retrieval of the foreign body through a rumenotomy may be beneficial if the lesion is recent. With more long-standing lesions, medical treatment with a rumen magnet and systemic antibiotics gives similar results to surgery. Due to the possibility of diffuse peritonitis and pericarditis, the prognosis for hardware disease is guarded to poor.

The abomasum of ruminants is similar to the acid-secreting stomach of monogastrics, and the lower intestinal tract is also very similar to that of other mammals. The greater curvature of the bovine abomasum has a loose omental attachment, making this organ very mobile. When filled with gas, the abomasum may displace dorsally on either side of the abdomen. Left or right abomasal displacement is most common in dairy cows and leads to anorexia, decreased milk production, and distinctive pings on abdominal auscultation and percussion. *Ketosis* (excess ketone production) is a frequent sequella to abomasal displacement because the milk production of the cow does not drop as quickly as energy intake. *Volvulus* (twisting of the bowel) of a displaced abomasum can lead to compromise of the blood supply, regurgitation of hydrochloric acid-rich fluid into the rumen, and a rapid decline in clinical condition. Surgical correction of right abomasal displacement or volvulus can be done through a right paralumbar or paramedian incision. Left abomasal displacement can also be corrected surgically through a left paralumbar incision or percutaneously through the right paramedian area. Percutaneous fixation is not recommended for right abomasal displacements due to the inability to determine whether volvulus of the organ has occurred.

A variety of other surgical gastrointestinal lesions can occur, including intraluminal obstruction, intussusception, volvulus, and entrapment. Intraluminal obstruction is most common in pet pigs, which are prone to ingest foreign bodies, and in camelids. Clinical pathology data as well as good physical and rectal examinations are helpful in identifying these lesions. Abdominal ultrasonographic and radiographic examinations may be useful in animals too small for rectal examination. Depression, abdominal distention, colic, tenesmus, and failure to defecate may be seen. Ruminants and camelids may sequester a large volume of fluid in the forestomach (internal vomition), making the obstruction less apparent, whereas pigs often vomit with obstruction. Disease signs and metabolic compromise are related to the location, nature, and duration of the lesion. The more cranial and complete the obstruction, the more likely gastric fluid is to be refluxed, with concomitant development of systemic dehydration and hypochloremic metabolic alkalosis. This can also develop with time with complete distal obstructions.

These metabolic abnormalities result in dry mucus membranes, prolonged tenting of skin, forestomach distention, and depression. Strangulating lesions tend to cause a rapid decline in clinical condition, whereas nonstrangulating lesions often have a slower onset of signs. With slower onset, greater metabolic derangement can occur. Intestinal distention places pressure on mesenteric stretch receptors, causing colic; this does not occur with most gastric lesions. Exploratory laparotomy is necessary to accurately identify and correct most obstructive lesions.

TECHNICIAN NOTE

Proximal gastrointestinal obstruction is associated with metabolic derangements without colic signs, whereas distal obstruction causes few metabolic derangements but frequent colic signs.

Paralumbar Laparotomy

A cow is best restrained while standing in a chute, although surgery can be performed with head restraint only. Small ruminants, pigs, and camelids are best restrained in lateral recumbency. The area bordered cranially by the last rib space, dor-

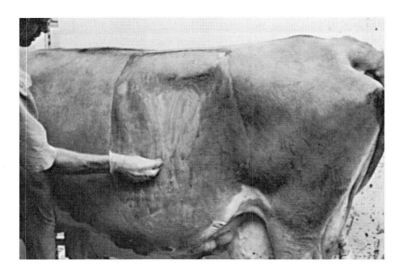

Figure 22-12. Preparation of the flank of a cow for aseptic surgery. The area has been clipped.

sally by midline, and caudally by the tuber coxae should be clipped and cleaned with antiseptic solutions (Fig. 22–12). The ventral border of the prepared site varies but is usually one half to two thirds of the way down the lateral abdominal wall. Regional (proximal or distal paravertebral block) or local (line or inverted L block) anesthesia is used. General anesthesia or a combination of physical restraint, sedation, and local anesthesia may be used for animals in lateral recumbency. The left flank is used for rumenotomy, cesarean section, and repair of left abomasal displacement, especially when it is suspected that the abomasum may be adhered to the left abdominal wall. The right flank is used for most abomasal or intestinal disorders and some cesarean sections (Fig. 22–13).

The skin and external abdominal oblique muscle are sharply incised, whereas the fibers of the internal oblique muscle may be incised or bluntly separated (*gridded*). The transversus muscle and peritoneum are sharply incised with a scalpel or Metzenbaum scissors, with care taken to not perforate abdominal viscera. After surgical repair, the internal abdominal layers are closed individually from ventral to dorsal with a

simple continuous pattern using large-diameter chromic gut suture. The skin is closed using a synthetic suture (No. 0 to 3 multifilament nylon) dorsal to ventral with a Ford interlocking pattern. Usually, the ventral part of the skin incision is closed with several simple interrupted or cruciate stitches; these will be removed should excessive fluid build up at the incision site after surgery.

Ventral Paramedian or Midline Laparotomy

The cow must be restrained in dorsal recumbency. Although certain chutes are adaptable to this task, most practitioners will use hobbles to extend the legs forward and backward and a halter for head restraint. Sedation often is necessary, and a casting rope may be used to make a cow recumbent (see Chapter 1). The area between the ribs cranially and the lateral abdominal (*milk*) veins should be clipped and cleaned with antiseptics. General or local anesthesia may be used. The umbilicus is the caudal extent of the incision for cranial abdominal surgery, and the udder is the caudal extent for caudal abdomi-

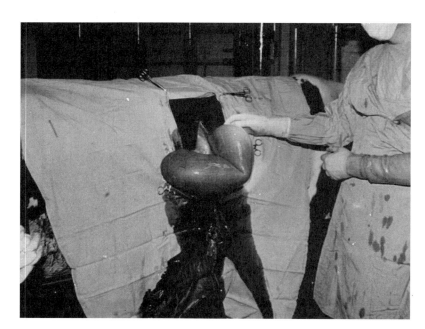

Figure 22-13. Dilated cecum exteriorized from the abdomen of a cow during standing right paralumbar laparotomy. The cow is restrained in a metal chute.

nal surgery. A right paramedian incision (8 cm to the right of midline and from 10 to 20 cm caudal to the sternum) is used for abomasal problems, whereas a midline or paramedian incision between the udder and umbilicus may be used for cesarean sections. For a ventral midline laparotomy, the skin, linea alba, and peritoneum are sharply incised. For a ventral paramedian laparotomy, the skin, ventral rectus sheath, rectus abdominis muscle, dorsal rectus sheath, and peritoneum are sharply incised. After the surgical procedure, the dorsal rectus sheath and rectus muscle are closed with large-gauge chromic gut in a simple continuous pattern, incorporating seromuscular bites from the lateral greater curvature of the abomasum (2 cm lateral to the omental attachment) if abomasopexy is desired. The linea alba or ventral rectus sheath is the holding layer and thus responsible for bearing the weight of the abdominal viscera. Therefore, simple interrupted or cruciate stitches or short chains of continuous suture should be used. Large-diameter chromic gut or absorbable synthetic suture material should be used. Subcutaneous tissue should be apposed carefully because fluid accumulates easily in dead space around ventral incisions. The skin is closed with large-diameter suture material. Although nonabsorbable suture is desired for skin closure, subsequent removal may not be possible in all management settings.

Diarrhea in Juveniles and Adults

Diarrhea in juvenile and adult ruminants and pigs can be caused by a variety of digestive disorders due to the passage of osmotically active, undigested feed into the lower gastrointestinal tract and altered intestinal motility. Cattle often have very loose feces, whereas species that normally pass pelleted feces are noted to have softer, less-formed stool. In contrast to neonatal diarrhea, most diarrhea in juveniles and adults is not accompanied by systemic signs, is self-limiting, and does not require treatment. However, diarrhea may result in reduced milk production or growth, and because severe acute infectious enterocolitis can be life threatening at any age, animals displaying diarrhea with signs of systemic disease should be examined and treated. Morbidity occurs due to fluid and electrolyte loss, bowel inflammation, systemic toxemia, and possibly viremia or bacteremia.

Several viruses cause fever and acute ulcerative enteritis and range in severity from the relatively benign winter dysentery to the more severe bluetongue, BVD, and MCF. Abortion and birth defects may also be seen. Careful examination of the mucosal surfaces of the mouth, eye, and nose for characteristic erosive lesions plus an evaluation of fecal, tissue, and blood samples by a veterinary diagnostic laboratory may aid in identification of the etiologic agent in herd outbreaks. Supportive treatment consisting of replacement fluids, anti-inflammatory agents, and prophylactic antibiotic drugs may be useful in individual animals.

Acute bacterial enteritis is uncommon, except in neonates and pigs. Epizootics of severe hemorrhagic diarrhea often are attributable to *Salmonella* spp., which may be introduced by rodents, contaminated feed, or asymptomatic carrier animals. Juvenile small ruminants and calves are susceptible to enterotoxemia (caused by *Clostridium perfringens*), which may be fatal before diarrhea is apparent due to gut wall necrosis and toxemia. Weanling and feeder pigs are very susceptible to hemorrhagic enteritis due to *Serpulina (Treponema) hyodysenteria*. Secondary bacterial infection in juvenile swine with proliferative

ileitis, which is caused by an unidentified organism, also may result in severe hemorrhagic or necrotizing enteritis. Individual animals are managed best with fluids, antibiotics and anti-inflammatory agents, whereas medicated water or feed may be used for large groups of animals. Specific vaccines and antitoxins are available to prevent or treat some of these disorders. With herd outbreaks, identification of the etiologic agent and management changes to prevent new cases are recommended.

Coccidiosis is the most common cause of diarrhea in juvenile ruminants. Although the diarrhea often is hemorrhagic, the affected animals usually are bright unless dehydration becomes severe. Tenesmus and neurologic disease also may be seen with coccidiosis. Fecal examination for oocysts usually is diagnostic. Effective control consists of management changes to decrease fecal contamination of feed and water plus treatment of all contact animals with a coccidiostatic or coccidiocidal drug (see Chapter 6).

Gastrointestinal parasitism may be a significant problem in ruminants on grass (strongyles) and pigs on dirt (ascarids). Blood-sucking abomasal worms in ruminants can cause poor weight gain or weight loss, diarrhea, anemia, hypoproteinemia, and death. Migrating ascarids in pigs can cause poor weight gain, diarrhea, and liver condemnation at slaughter. Fecal examination for ova may be diagnostic but also may be negative, as many of the clinical symptoms are caused by immature worms. Although worm burden may be controlled in part with anthelmintic drugs, pasture or pen sanitation and rotation also can be effective.

Chronic diarrhea often is impossible to treat due to permanent changes in the bowel wall. Johne's disease is a granulomatous disease of the ileocecal region of cattle and, rarely, other ruminants or camelids caused by *Mycobacterium paratuberculosis;* it leads to a protein-losing enteropathy. Animals are thought to become infected with the organism when young but often show clinical signs in early adulthood.

In addition to chronic diarrhea, affected animals often display weight loss, hypoproteinemia, and submandibular or brisket edema (Fig. 22–14). A similar wasting syndrome may be seen in swine with the chronic form of proliferative ileitis. Removal of young from their dams, sanitation, and pasteurization of colostrum are recommended to prevent the spread of Johne's disease. These diseases must be differentiated from

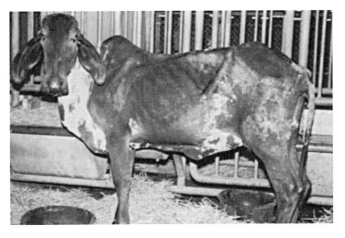

Figure 22-14. Severe emaciation in a Brahman cow with Johne's disease.

noninfectious causes of chronic diarrhea, including parasitism, inflammatory bowel disease, and copper deficiency, which are treatable and have a different herd significance.

LOCOMOTOR DISORDERS

Lameness in food animals is one of the most common complaints requiring veterinary attention. Bovine veterinarians or producers who deal with a high volume of lameness disorders will find it worthwhile to invest in a hydraulic table to place the cow in lateral recumbency for examination and treatment. The table allows superior restraint of the animal and the simultaneous examination of all four feet. If this option is unavailable, the head of the cow should be restrained adequately, and the affected leg should be elevated with straw bales or rope for examination. Sheep can be tipped up on their rear, whereas goats tend to struggle with this means of restraint. Llamas can be trained to allow foot handling, whereas pet pigs can be suspended in a sling to gain access to their feet. If necessary, tranquilizers may be used in all species to facilitate inspection of the affected leg.

The foot is the most common site of lameness. The normal ruminant or porcine foot consists of two digits, each of which ends in a horny hoof. A white line is found on the cranial, axial, and abaxial aspects of the bottom of each digit, where the sections of horn formed by the coriums of the sole and wall meet. The caudal portion of the weight-bearing surface is the heel bulb, which is separated by a line of demarcation from the horn of the sole. The heel bulb is covered by softer horn than the sole and is more prominent in pigs than in ruminants. Front claws bear more weight and usually have a greater solar surface area, being more ovoid than the thinner hind claws. The angle between the dorsal wall and coronary band should be approximately 55 degrees. Weight should be borne on the abaxial wall. The camelid foot is unique; the weight-bearing bottom of the middle phalanx is covered by a keratinized digital pad. The horny claw extends from the cranial surface of the pad and normally is not weight bearing.

Because most food animals are not broken to lead, lameness examination involves careful observation of the stance and gait of the animal. Animals will shift their weight to spare sore feet or digits. Lameness is most common in the lateral digit of the hind foot and may cause the animal to stand with a base-wide stance. Hindlimb lameness may cause the animal to shift its weight forward, lowering the head and giving the elbows an abducted appearance. The medial digit often is affected in forelimb lameness and may cause the animal to stand with a base-narrow stance or, in severe cases, the animal may stand with forelegs crossed or walk on its carpi (Fig. 22–15). Forelimb lameness may cause the animal to shift its weight backward, raising the head and giving the hocks an adducted appearance. Occasionally, the medial digit of the hind leg or lateral digit of the foreleg is involved.

Horn Lesions

Lameness may be attributable simply to excessive horn growth. In some cases of chronic lameness, overgrowth of a specific region may reflect decreased wear, as the animal adapts its gait to spare a painful region. Overgrowth of horn is seen most commonly as elongated toes, excessive abaxial wall, or thickening of the heel. Overgrowth of the toes will increase the

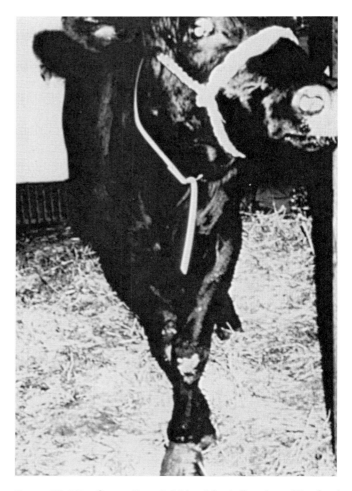

Figure 22–15. Cow with painful front feet. Crossing of the front feet is common when both medial claws are painful.

angle between the dorsal wall and coronary band and may cause the animal to bear weight on the soft tissue of the heel. Overgrowth of the abaxial walls may cause splaying of the digits and trauma to the interdigital space. Hard flooring (concrete) will exacerbate the effects of hoof overgrowth by forcing the digits into an abnormal position.

Laminitis (pododermatitis aseptica diffusa) in cattle rarely receives the attention that the disease does in horses, in part because acute clinical laminitis is rare. In contrast, subclinical laminitis is a common and important contributor to several of the hoof abnormalities of bovine lameness. Inflammation or engorgement of the horn-forming corium leads to a form of compartmental syndrome, in which the swollen corium is compressed between the pedal bone and hoof wall. Resultant damage to the corium leads to the production of abnormal, discolored horn.

The primary lesion of laminitis is not visible, but the consequences are easily seen. Partial rotation and sinking of the pedal bone can contribute to white line or toe lesions and sole hemorrhage or ulcers, respectively. Complete cessation of sole formation, followed by resumption, can lead to the formation of a double sole. Abnormal horn production by the corium of the wall can lead to horizontal fissures or laminitic rings (*hardship grooves*). By measuring the distance from the coronary band to the laminitic ring, the timing of the laminitic event can be estimated (normal wall growth is about 0.5 cm per month). Laminitic lesions of the sole commonly become apparent 2 to 3 months after the insult, which often occurs in the early postparturient period. Bacterial invasion along the laminae may lead to heel horn erosion.

Predisposing factors to laminitis are thought to include heel conformation, high-energy diets (acidosis), disease (histamine and endotoxin), lack of exercise, high protein or barley diets, concrete flooring, calving, and poorly bedded stalls (increased time standing). Gradual acclimation of an animal to a new ration or housing facility may decrease the incidence of laminitic events.

Pododermatitis circumscripta (*sole* or *Rusterholz ulcer*) is the result of damage to the corium at the sole-heel junction and may be a local form of laminitis. Hemorrhage causes discoloration of the horn as well as separation of the horn from the laminae. This weakened area ulcerates with wear and subsequently fills with granulation tissue. Secondary infection can occur, and deeper structures (most importantly, the deep flexor tendon and navicular bursa) can be affected.

Pododermatitis septica is infection and abscess formation within the horn or between the sole or wall horn and the corium. If ventral drainage is impaired, these infections often track dorsally to break out at the coronary band or heel. Laminitis predisposes to development of pododermatitis septica by allowing for soft horn formation, cracks, and white line separation. Trauma also may cause separation of the sole from the wall and deep inoculation of bacteria. These lesions are very painful and often can be localized with hoof testers. Although found in all species of hoofstock, pododermatitis septica is the most common horn lesion associated with lameness in pigs (*porcine foot rot*).

Vertical and horizontal wall cracks are common findings and occasionally associated with lameness. Cracks form when abnormal (postlaminitis) or excessively dry horn is subjected to pressure. Overgrown toes contribute by increasing leverage on the weakened area. Lameness is uncommon unless the crack becomes full thickness through the horn or reaches the coronary band. In cases of severe lameness, secondary infection of the underlying soft tissue is likely. Vertical cracks that reach the coronary band may lead to abnormal (*corkscrew*) hoof growth.

When lameness involves the horn, corrective trimming should be performed. Excessive and separated horn should be removed. Large nippers or grinders may be used to remove large sections of horn, and knives and sanders may be used to prepare the final surface. The abaxial wall should be weight bearing, with the sole, heel, and axial wall trimmed to form a concave surface.

Dissecting tracts into the hoof should be excavated and flushed with antiseptic solutions. Subsolar lesions should be opened to allow drainage, and excessive granulation tissue should be trimmed. Partial hoof wall resections may increase drainage from lesions that track along the wall. Deep cracks may be excavated with a rotary grinding tool, and vertical cracks may be held together with wire to prevent extension of the lesion. Wall growth is slower in bulls and older animals, and bulls have proportionally less foot surface area for their weight, so care must be taken to not remove excessive horn from these animals. In many cases, a growing period of new hoof together with one or more trimmings is necessary to obtain a normal hoof.

If lameness can be localized to one digit, increased comfort and soundness of the animal can be achieved by supporting the sound digit of that hoof. This is done by trimming and grooving the horn of the sound digit and attaching an appropriately sized wooden, rubber, or plastic block or slipper to the sole with a cement. These usually come off or wear down after several weeks and rarely need to be removed. Open wounds may be protected with a bandage, which protects the wound, absorbs exudates, prevents drying of tissue, holds medications, and aids in hemostasis. In a clean environment, some lesions heal faster without a bandage.

Bacterial infection of horn lesions may extend into deeper tissue structures; these include joints, bones, tendons, and bursae. Rupture of the deep flexor tendon causes the toe to point up, whereas damage to other structures often results in severe lameness, swelling of the digit, and lack of response to conservative treatment. Such animals require radical debridement of lesions as well as antibiotic and anti-inflammatory treatment.

Minor surgical procedures (debridement, digit amputation) are facilitated through the use of local or regional anesthesia. Local anesthesia involves infiltration of the soft tissue around the lesion. Regional anesthesia of the entire foot is achieved by the injection of 20 ml of lidocaine into a superficial vein (Fig. 22–16). A tourniquet should be placed, and the skin around the vein should be clipped and disinfected before the intravenous block is attempted (see Chapter 15). Tourniquets also are useful in minimizing hemorrhage during surgical procedures.

Soft Tissue Lesions

Digital dermatitis often causes only mild lameness, especially of the hind limb, which may be unnoticeable if bilateral. The

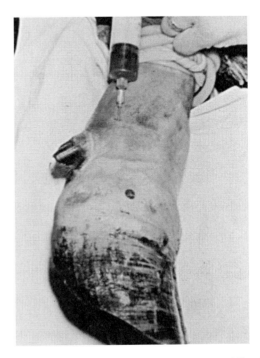

Figure 22–16. Local intravenous anesthesia of the bovine foot. The tourniquet, which is placed proximal to the injection site, aids in palpation of the vein and distribution of the anesthetic agent.

etiology appears to be multifactorial, with poor hygiene and infectious agents (especially spirochetes) implicated, and is most common in heifers entering the milking herd. The lesion is circumscribed and partially or completely alopecic and begins as an erosion or ulcer. With time, the ulcer fills with granulation tissue (*strawberry-like*) or proliferative projections (*papillomas* or *warts*). Lesions most commonly occur at the plantar or dorsal commissure but also occur at the skin-horn junction of the heel and other sites. Some lesions regress spontaneously.

Interdigital dermatitis (*contagious foot rot, ovine foot rot*) is the most common cause of lameness in sheep; it also occurs in other hoofstock species. *Dichelobacter* (formerly *Bacteroides*) *nodosus* is the contagious, causative agent, whereas *Fusobacterium necrophorum* can coinvade, causing necrosis. These same organisms are thought to cause digital pad ulcers and lameness in llamas. Spirochetes also may play a role, suggesting a relationship between this disease and digital dermatitis. The lesion usually starts on the interdigital skin, and animals may be sensitive to interdigital palpation, even if no lesion is visible (Fig. 22–17). With progression, a malodorous, necrotic break in the skin is formed, and deeper tissues may become infected. If the coronary band (either axial and abaxial) is affected, wall or heel separation can follow. A vaccine against *Dichelobacter* exists in some countries.

Interdigital hyperplasia (corn/fibroma) is a proliferation of fibrous tissue that protrudes into the interdigital space (Fig. 22–18). Chronic irritation of the region secondary to interdigital dermatitis, hoof conformation (excessive axial sole), and housing surface probably contribute. Laxity of the distal interphalangeal (cruciate) ligaments also may allow excessive splaying of the digits and increase the risk of trauma to the interdigital space. Pain appears to increase with the size and degree of ulceration or infection of the mass.

Interdigital phlegmon (*bovine foot rot*) occurs when *F. necrophorum* and *Porphyromonas asaccharolytica* (formerly *Bacteroides melaninogenicus*) act synergistically to penetrate the epidermis and cause cellulitis. Although *Dichelobacter* is more important with interdigital dermatitis, the pathogenicity of *Fusobacterium* may dictate the severity of interdigital phlegmon. The lesion starts as a generalized soft tissue swelling

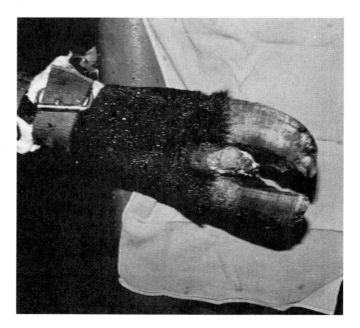

Figure 22–18. Interdigital hyperplasia (fibroma) on the foot of a cow.

in the interdigital space or heel bulb. Subsequent necrosis can lead to a splitting of the epidermis and an appearance similar to interdigital dermatitis. Deeper structures can be affected, and lameness can be severe. Because both interdigital dermatitis and phlegmon can be contagious, separation of diseased animals may be helpful.

The treatment of soft tissue lesions follows a general course: the foot should be cleaned thoroughly. Necrotic or proliferative (fibroma, proliferative dermatitis) soft tissue lesions should be debrided or resected. Granulation tissue must be debrided with care near the dorsal coronary band, due to the proximity of the joint capsule. Open soft tissue wounds may be treated with foot baths (10% zinc sulfate, 10% copper sulfate, or 5% formalin), topical disinfectants, or antibiotics, whereas systemic antibiotic therapy should be used if there is evidence of deep infection. Because most bacteria that affect the foot are anaerobic, penicillin-class antibiotics usually are effective.

Bandages may be used for open wounds, and the digits should be bandaged together if the lesion is in the interdigital space. If excessive laxity and splaying of the digits are contributing to trauma to the interdigital space, the toes may be wired together. Hoof lesions that may have contributed to soft tissue damage should be addressed through corrective hoof trimming and balancing. Management practices that promote soft tissue trauma or prolonged contact between the foot and manure or mud should be addressed, whereas routine footbaths are useful in decreasing the incidence and severity of interdigital infections. Because the disinfectants in footbaths are toxic, animals should not be allowed to drink the solutions.

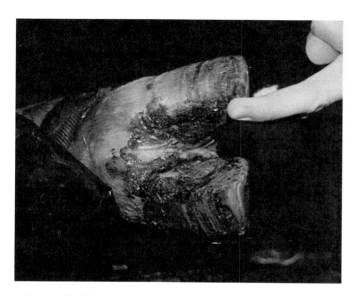

Figure 22–17. Interdigital dermatitis on the foot of a cow.

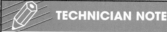
TECHNICIAN NOTE

The source of most lameness in food animals is the foot.

Ischemic Lesions

Ischemic (*decreased blood supply*) lesions of the foot can occur due to *fescue foot,* ergotism, or frostbite. With ergotism, *Claviceps* spp. fungi invade the seeds of cereal and pasture grasses and produce ergot alkaloids. After ingestion, these cause arteriolar vascular spasms, which lead to ischemia. Nervous signs and agalactia also can be caused by the same or different toxins produced by the fungus. Fescue foot is a similar disease associated with tall fescue grass in cool seasons. A toxic agent produced by a fungus (not *Claviceps*) is the most likely cause. Signs with both syndromes occur days to weeks after exposure and are seen in the extremities (legs, ear tips, tail, nose), with hind legs being the most common site. Lameness and pain are noted, with swelling and erythema from the fetlock to the coronary band. If the ischemia is severe and prolonged, a line of demarcation may be seen between healthy and affected tissues. Both syndromes are exacerbated by cold weather. Treatment consists of removing the source of toxin, avoiding cold, and enhancing circulation (hydrotherapy, hot packs). Protective salves and bandages may be helpful if the skin sloughs.

Frostbite also affects the extremities, especially of young animals. Such animals frequently have another disease condition that limits their activity. The upper hind leg is not tucked under the body in sternal recumbency and thus is the most common limb affected. Teat ends of dairy animals also can be affected, if sanitizing liquids are not dried off before exposure to cold. Clinical signs and treatment of frostbite resemble those of ergotism.

Skeletal Lesions

Septic arthritis, physitis, and osteomyelitis can be the result of direct inoculation through a wound, hematogenous seeding, or extension of infection from adjacent tissues. The larger joints are most commonly affected in septic arthritis, whereas osteomyelitis often affects long bones or vertebrae. Hematogenous origin of infection is most common in the young and often results in multiple sites being affected. Common clinical signs include lameness, joint distention, soft tissue swelling, pain on palpation, and warmth. Vertebral body osteomyelitis may lead to compression of spinal nerves or the spinal cord and can cause neurologic deficits.

Radiographs are useful in localizing and determining the extent of the lesion. Radiographic lesions include an increase or a decrease in the joint space, subchondral or medullary bone lysis, and periosteal bone reaction. Synovial fluid from infected joints contains high concentrations of protein and inflammatory cells.

Treatment consists of systemic antibiotics, nonsteroidal anti-inflammatory agents, and removal of any septic focus (umbilicus). Joints may be lavaged with several liters of sterile isotonic fluids through an arthroscope or multiple large-bore hypodermic needles introduced into the affected joint space. If there are large fibrin deposits or proliferative synovium, an arthrotomy may be performed to establish drainage. Osteomyelitis or physitis may be treated with long courses of antibiotics with good bone penetration, but if there is a sequestrum or severe bone involvement, local curettage and infiltration of antibiotics may be necessary. A culture of synovial fluid or affected bone is useful in determining the appropriate antibiotic.

Digit Amputation

If the structures within the hoof are severely damaged, especially with digital osteoarthritis, amputation of the affected digit may provide the fastest and most satisfactory resolution of clinical signs. The hair should be clipped to the fetlock, and the region should be surgically prepared. After local or regional anesthesia is achieved, an incision is made through the skin from the interdigital space axially to the level of the proximal interphalangeal joint of the affected digit abaxially. Instead of completing the skin incision, the abaxial skin may be dissected off the digit before amputation and used to close the wound, but this is not recommended if infected structures are left on the proximal stump. A wire saw is then used to excise the affected digit, using the skin incision as a guide. Care must be taken to remain below the fetlock joint. After amputation, the support structures of the remaining digit on that foot often break down due to increased weight load, although this may not occur for 1 year or longer.

Viral arthropathies are very common in adult sheep and goats from flocks harboring the ovine progressive pneumonia (Maedi) or caprine arthritis-encephalitis viruses, respectively. Affected adults typically have enlarged joints; they may also display chronic weight loss and respiratory disease. Lambs and kids may display weakness at birth or neurologic signs that develop over the first few months of life, with high mortality. Treatment of the individual animal is symptomatic and palliative. More important are management changes that can be made to prevent further spread of the viruses; these include serologic testing of all animals, with isolation or culling of seropositive stock or contact animals (sires). Colostrum is thought to be the major source of infection, so neonates should be separated from dams at birth and fed colostrum from seronegative dams or colostrum that has been pasteurized.

Fractures are managed as in other species, except that a poor prognosis must be given for upper limb lesions in larger animals. Economic constraints often restrict the use of internal fixation, leading to extensive use of casts, splints, and transfixation pins. Food animal species usually tolerate casts well, form exuberant callus, and are able to spend large amounts of time recumbent, contributing to the success of external fixation techniques. A block placed on the sole of the sound claw greatly increases soundness if the fracture is below the fetlock. Adequate footing and confinement are essential during the healing process.

Peripheral Neuropathies

The radial nerve is necessary to extend the elbow, and the femoral nerve is used to extend the stifle. Both may be damaged by excessive traction on the calf during a difficult birthing (*obstetric paralysis of the calf*) and result in an inability to support weight on the affected leg. The sciatic and obturator nerves are most commonly damaged in the dam during birthing because both course through the pelvic canal (*obstetric paralysis of the dam*). The obturator nerve is necessary for adduction of the hind limb, especially if the animal is on poor footing, whereas the sciatic nerve is important for extension of the hip and flexion of the stifle and affects the lower hind leg through two major branches: the peroneal nerve (extension of the foot) and the tibial nerve (flexion of the foot). The peroneal branch is most commonly affected during birthing. The sciatic and tibial nerves can also be damaged by intramuscular injections given in the gluteal muscle region and on the craniolateral border of the semitendinosus muscle, respectively. Numerous nerves, including the radial, peroneal, and tibial, may also be damaged by pressure during extended periods of recumbency.

Drug treatment for peripheral nerve trauma includes corticosteroids in the acute stage, nonsteroidal anti-inflammatory agents, and dimethylsulfoxide. Of equal or greater importance is supportive care, including making food and water easily accessible, slinging or hoisting the animal, good footing, and frequent rolling of the animal to prevent additional pressure damage to nerves and muscles. Smaller animals may benefit from physical therapy in a flotation tank, an option that is also available for cattle.

Myopathy

Any cause of excessive recumbency can lead to *downer syndrome*. This is a combination of nerve and muscle damage that tends to perpetuate the recumbency. The most common causes of recumbency are peripheral neuropathy, hypocalcemia, and severe musculoskeletal lesions. Myoglobinuria occurs with excessive muscle necrosis and can lead to renal damage; therefore, adequate hydration of down animals is very important. Otherwise, treatment is similar to that recommended for peripheral neuropathy.

Tick paralysis is a myopathy that mimics peripheral neuropathy in that muscles are flaccid and neurologic reflexes are absent. The paralysis usually starts with hindlimb ataxia but progresses craniad. Death can result from respiratory paralysis or aspiration pneumonia. Geographic and seasonal factors are important in judging the likelihood of tick paralysis. Although affected animals frequently are covered with ticks, one engorged female tick can secrete sufficient toxin to affect a large animal. Therefore, in addition to downer animal care and topical or systemic acaricidal drugs, an earnest effort must be made to remove all ticks. Most animals will recover within 24 hours of removal of the tick.

Nutritional muscular dystrophy (*white muscle disease*) is a polysystemic disease caused by a deficiency in vitamin E or selenium. The disease is seen most commonly in juveniles born of dams fed deficient diets. Because these two compounds are important antioxidants, their deficiency leads to the greatest problems in metabolically active tissues such as skeletal or cardiac muscle and often follows periods of increased muscular exertion. In severe cases, myocardial damage leads to dyspnea or sudden death; this is most common form in swine. The more common syndrome in ruminants is that of swollen, painful muscles; stiffness; and weakness due to skeletal muscle involvement. Characteristic necropsy lesions include pale skeletal muscle and pale myocardial foci, although in pigs with sudden death, focal hemorrhage is seen in the cardiac muscle. Laboratory analyses for vitamin E and selenium status aid in the diagnosis. Treatment of clinical animals with injectable vitamin E and selenium compounds may be successful, although ultimately ration analysis and dietary modification are necessary.

A variety of anaerobic clostridial organisms can cause myonecrosis and cellulitis (*blackleg, malignant edema*), especially in muscle damaged by rough handling, injections, or other trauma. The organisms may reach the site either hematogenously or through a wound. Clostridial myositis causes lameness with swollen, hot, painful muscles; fever; systemic toxemia; and sudden death. Although subcutaneous emphysema around the lesion is a hallmark sign in cattle, this is a less common finding in other species. A foul-smelling, serous fluid or gas is found when the lesion is opened or aspirated. Due to the extensive damage and toxemia, the prognosis is poor. Affected muscles can be treated by opening and cleansing the area to disrupt the anaerobic environment. Systemic penicillin and supportive care also may be beneficial. The diseases are endemic in some areas. Although information on efficacy is lacking, improved hygiene, vaccines, and management changes to avoid muscle damage may be useful in preventing these diseases.

Clostridial Neurotoxicities

Tetanus is caused by a central nervous system toxin elaborated by *Clostridium tetani* and results in generalized or localized hypertonia of skeletal muscles. Cattle are less susceptible than small ruminants. The source of infection is often the uterus for adult cattle (occurring as sequelae to metritis and retained fetal membranes) or a wound for small ruminants and pigs (caused by castration, disbudding, tail docking). Clinical signs of tetanus include stiff gait, prolapse of the third eyelid, hyperesthesia, bloat, trismus (*lockjaw*), dysphagia, and death due to asphyxiation (Fig. 22–19). Diagnosis is often made on the basis of clinical signs and positive culture of an infected uterus or wound.

Treatment consists of high doses of parenteral and local procaine penicillin, tetanus antitoxin, and nursing care, which includes housing animals in dark, quiet, well-bedded stalls and provision of adequate nutrition and fluids. Prognosis is usually good for cattle and more guarded for small ruminants. Prevention is best achieved by vaccination and improving management practices. Sheep and goats are regularly vaccinated, whereas cattle rarely need to be.

Botulism is a fatal, progressive disease of voluntary muscles resulting in flaccid paralysis. Ruminants are more susceptible than pigs. The neurotoxin acts peripherally at nerve endings and is elaborated by *Clostridium botulinum*. The source of the toxin for animals is usually a dead animal or decaying plant material. Clinical signs include reduced tongue tone, dysphagia, ataxia, ptosis, flaccid paralysis, and death. Diagnosis is often presumptive because it is difficult to grow the organism or isolate the toxin from gut contents of the animal or the feed source. Treatment is symptomatic and includes efforts to eliminate the toxin from the gut via ruminal lavage and purgatives and procaine penicillin. Polyvalent serum containing antibotulinum toxin antibodies is available and may be useful in subacute cases before the toxin is bound to nerve endings. Control measures consist mainly of good husbandry and disposal of carcasses.

BLOOD-BORNE DISEASES

Anaplasmosis occurs in cattle, sheep, and goats. It is a subclinical disease in sheep and goats. In cattle, however, it causes severe debilitation, anemia, and jaundice or abortion in adult cattle and neonatal weakness. The disease is caused by rickettsial bacteria, *Anaplasma marginale, A. centrale,* or *A. caudatam* in cattle and wild ruminants and *A. ovis* in sheep and goats. The organisms are blood borne. Mechanical transmission occurs via insect vectors, particularly ticks, or contaminated blood products. Morbidity is high during outbreaks, but mortal-

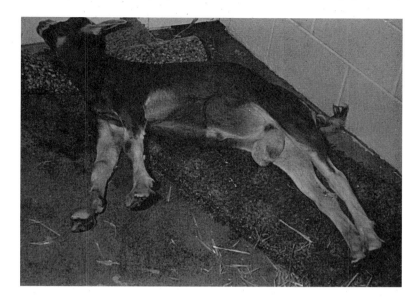

Figure 22-19. Goat with extensor rigidity caused by tetanus.

ity varies widely and increases with the age of the affected animal. Bison are naturally resistant to infection. Once infected, the food animal remains a carrier for many years. Clinical findings in cattle include fever, hemolytic anemia, jaundice, abortion, severe dyspnea, and death. Goats may occasionally succumb to a similar anemic syndrome. Diagnosis depends on serologic testing and the presence of insect vectors. Treatment consists of antibiotic administration and supportive care, including blood transfusions. Vaccines are available and are thought to be effective.

Eperythrozoonosis occurs in pigs, cattle, sheep, and llamas. The causative agent is *Eperythrozoon* spp., a rickettsia that parasitizes red blood cells. Disease is particularly important in pigs and immunocompromised llamas. Latent infections can occur in deer, elk, and goats. In swine, *E. suis* causes acute hemolytic anemia in stressed feeder pigs. Reproductive failure, weakness, and poor weight gain also may be seen in pigs of other ages. In cattle and sheep, *E. wenyoni* and *E. ovis* infections, respectively, often are subclinical but may cause ill-thrift, reproductive problems, and edema. Transmission is thought to occur through insect vectors or blood products. Diagnosis can be made by evaluation of a blood smear and positive identification of the organism on the periphery of red blood cell membranes or serologic testing. Treatment consists of antibiotics and blood transfusions if necessary.

URINARY DISORDERS

Urinary tract obstruction is the most common ailment of the urinary system in ruminants and pot-bellied pigs, as well as the most common cause of colic in many ruminant species. Castrated males are especially susceptible, although the condition also occurs in intact males and, rarely, females. Early clinical signs include colic, dysuria, and stranguria. Later signs may include anorexia, depression, death, or subcutaneous or abdominal swelling subsequent to a urethral or bladder rupture (*water belly*). Sites of obstruction, in order of occurrence, include the urethral process (small ruminants only), distal sigmoid flexure, pelvic urethra, and trigone (neck) of the bladder (Fig. 22–20). Struvite calculi are most common in animals fed high-grain diets (feedlots), whereas carbonate calculi are most com-

mon overall. Silicate calculi may be seen in range animals in certain geographic areas. In most cases, multiple stones occlude the urethra, and still more are found in the bladder.

> **TECHNICIAN NOTE**
> Urethral obstruction is the major cause of colic in many food animal species.

Optimal treatment often is dictated by the intended use of the animal. For feedlot animals, incising the ventral skin over a subcutaneous rupture site or dissecting out the sigmoid flexure and incising the urethra proximal to the obstruction will lead to resolution of the uremia and enable marketing of the animal. Amputation of the urethral process may lead to resolution of the obstruction in small ruminants, although this often is temporary. Attempts to clear the obstruction through retrograde catheterization rarely are successful because of the urethral diverticulum, and reobstruction is common.

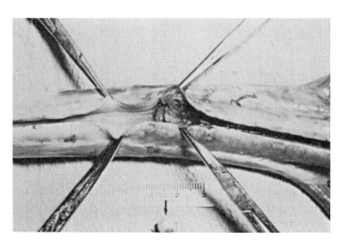

Figure 22-20. Obstruction of the urethra by a calculus in a steer with a corresponding mucosal lesion.

Surgical options available for long-term correction of the obstruction include cystotomy, perineal urethrostomy, or both. Perineal urethrostomy may be performed with the animal under general, local, or regional (epidural) anesthesia and thus can be performed on animals of any size. Postoperative urethral strictures or reobstructions are common, especially in small ruminants or pigs. Preservation of breeding ability in males also precludes permanent perineal urethrostomy.

Perineal Urethrostomy

The procedure may be done with the animal standing or in lateral recumbency, with use of one of the above forms of anesthesia. The area behind the scrotum or scrotal remnant is clipped and surgically prepared. A midline incision is made over the distal sigmoid flexure, which then is dissected free of subcutaneous tissues, transected, and exteriorized. Care must be taken to transect the penis proximal to the attachment of the retractor muscles or, alternatively, the distal stump should be amputated. The skin is closed around the protruding proximal penile stump, which is directed caudad, and the visible urethra is split longitudinally (Fig. 22–21). Urine scald of the medial thigh is common after this procedure. Possible preservation of breeding ability may be achieved by performing a urethrotomy and removing any visible stones without anchoring or transecting the penis. In this case, the wound is left to close spontaneously once distal flow of urine is achieved.

Cystotomy

Cystotomy requires general anesthesia and is accomplished through a caudal ventral midline incision (see midline laparotomy section). The bladder is identified and exteriorized. A 2- to 4-cm incision is made into the bladder. Cystotomy allows for removal of all calculi from the bladder and normograde catheterization (passing the catheter from the bladder out to the end of the urethra) of the urethra to test patency. Distal obstruction or urethral spasms may prevent catheterization and are potential indications for performance of a perineal urethrostomy. The bladder incision is closed in two inverting layers and the abdomen is closed routinely.

Combining cystotomy with perineal urethrostomy has

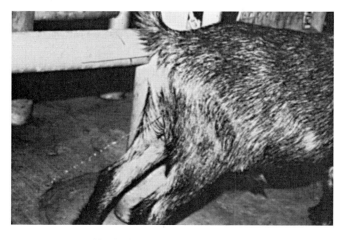

Figure 22–21. Healed perineal urethrostomy in a male goat. The goat is able to direct urine caudad.

given the best results in small ruminants, which rapidly reobstruct with urethrostomy alone. Conversely, recent evidence suggests that longer survival is attained by performing a tube cystotomy without urethrostomy in small ruminants, even if the distal urethra is left obstructed. This involves placing a bulb tip catheter through the body wall into the bladder during laparotomy. Temporary diversion of urine flow allows the urethra to relax and stones to pass. The catheter is removed after patency of the distal urethra is established, which may take several weeks. By performing this procedure without urethrostomy, postoperative urethral stricture is uncommon.

Medical management of other contact animals is recommended if there is a herd problem of urinary tract obstruction. Increasing dietary salt to 4% of the ration will increase water intake and urine volume, flushing small stones out of the bladder. Dietary ammonium salts acidify the urine and decrease formation of phosphate and carbonate stones. Ultimately, dietary modification is recommended to decrease formation of the specific type of stone.

Although cystitis and pyelonephritis (inflammation of kidney) occur sporadically in ruminants, these diseases are common in pigs, especially those kept in confinement. The two most common bacterial isolates are *Eubacterium* (formerly *Corynebacterium*) *suis* and *E. coli,* although many bacteria and the kidney worm *Stephanurus dentatus* also cause a similar disease. Clinical signs include repeat breeding, anorexia, pyuria or hematuria, fever, weight loss, and death. Although ascending infection after heavy fecal contamination of the perineum is blamed for the high incidence of this disorder in housed pigs, venereal transmission of *E. suis* from carrier males also can occur. Gross appearance of the urine often is sufficient to make a diagnosis, although bacteriologic culture of urine is useful in confirming the etiologic agent if there is a herd problem. Penicillin and ampicillin have good efficacy against *Eubacterium,* but a different antibiotic should be used if the infection is caused by a Gram-negative organism.

REPRODUCTIVE DISORDERS

The major causes of dystocia are fetal-maternal size mismatch and fetal malpresentation. In animals with multiple fetuses (commonly pigs, sheep, and goats), malpresentation can be complicated by simultaneous entry of more than one fetus into the birth canal.

Early intervention is the key to successful resolution of dystocia. Multiparous animals should be able to deliver a fetus within 30 minutes of the onset of abdominal contractions, whereas in primiparous animals this should occur within 1 hour. If possible, examination of the animal with dystocia should begin with transrectal palpation for uterine torsion and presentation of the fetus or fetuses. If uterine torsion is not present, the dam's tail should be tied, the external vulva cleaned with surgical scrub, and vaginal examination performed. Epidural anesthesia may help reduce maternal straining during the vaginal examination or correction of a malpresentation, but this will also reduce maternal effort when the fetus is being delivered (Fig. 22–22).

The fetus should be positioned so both hind legs or the fore legs with the head are within the birth canal. To correct a flexed leg, the hoof should be directed caudomedially while the carpus or hock is directed craniolaterally until the leg can be extended. Adequate lubrication and traction should be used

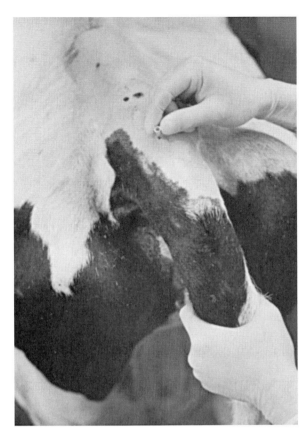

Figure 22-22. Epidural anesthesia in a cow. A 1.5-inch needle is placed into the epidural space between the first two coccygeal vertebrae.

to deliver the fetus. If there is inadequate space in the birth canal to deliver the fetus, cesarean section or fetotomy should be performed. Neonates delivered after dystocia require more care than do those delivered normally.

Endometritis and retained fetal membranes are common problems in cattle, especially after induced or difficult parturition. Although such cattle typically have a fetid uterine discharge, they often are not clinically ill. Many treatments have been recommended for such cattle; however, it is generally accepted that intrauterine therapy is unnecessary, if not detrimental. Intramuscular prostaglandin injections may speed resolution of the condition, although this also is controversial. Oxytocin may be beneficial immediately postpartum but has decreasing efficacy after the first 24 hours. Cattle that demonstrate clinical signs, including fever, depression, and anorexia, should be treated aggressively because deeper layers of the uterus may be infected and fatal bacteremia or toxemia can occur. Systemic antibiotic treatment and lavage of the uterus with fluids to remove inflammatory debris may be beneficial for animals with systemic disease signs. Attempts to manually remove the placenta usually are not warranted. Small ruminants, pigs, and camelids are more susceptible to developing systemic disease signs with retained fetal membranes and therefore should be treated aggressively with antibiotics and oxytocin.

Postpartum straining and uterine inertia may allow prolapse of the uterus. This condition is easily recognized in ruminants by the presence of the caruncles on the inverted uterine

tissue (Fig. 22–23). Dystocia and hypocalcemia are important risk factors. To replace the uterus, epidural anesthesia should be administered and the prolapsed tissue should be cleaned. The cow may be left standing or restrained in dorsal recumbency with the hind legs extended caudad (*frog-legged*). When possible, the cow should be positioned with the hindquarters higher than the forequarters, so gravity aids in replacement of the uterus. Elevation of the prolapsed uterus on a board or towel also will aid in replacement. Using firm pressure with the flat of the hands, the uterus must be worked back into the vagina. Once replaced, the horns should be palpated to ensure they are fully everted. A pursestring suture of umbilical tape may be placed in the subcutaneous tissue of the vulva to prevent recurrence of the prolapse.

> **✎ TECHNICIAN NOTE**
>
> Tetanus prophylaxis should be considered when treating uterine infections in small ruminants.

In contrast, prolapse of the vagina usually occurs in pregnant animals in which increased abdominal pressure and increased recumbency contribute (Fig. 22–24). Short tail docking, hereditary factors, respiratory disease, estrogen-containing feeds, and obesity also contribute to prolapse. Vaginal prolapse usually is progressive during gestation and often will occur in that animal during subsequent pregnancies. Due to the progressive and possibly hereditary nature of this disorder, removal of the animal and its offspring from the breeding program should be considered. To treat, the prolapsed tissue should be cleaned and gently replaced with the animal under epidural anesthesia. Vaginal prolapse is very prone to recurrence despite the use of a vulvar pursestring suture or specialized retaining paddle. Epidural anesthesia with alcohol can be used to decrease straining for a longer period but should be reserved for animals that will be culled.

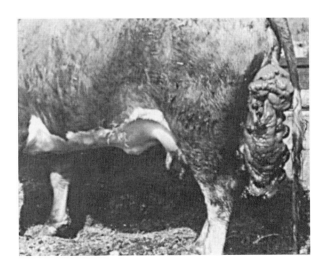

Figure 22-23. Complete uterine prolapse in a cow after calving, showing caruncles on the uterine wall.

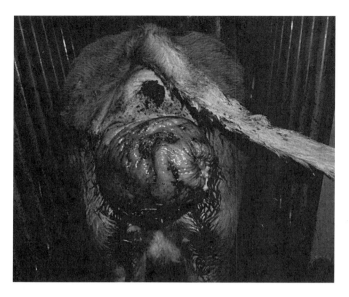

Figure 22-24. Cow with vaginal prolapse. The cow is restrained in a metal chute.

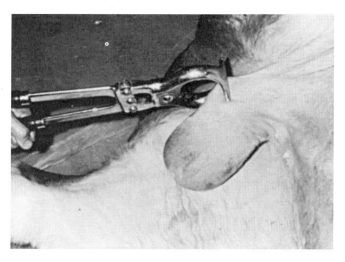

Figure 22-26. Closed castration with an emasculator. The two sides of the scrotum are crushed individually, with care taken to incorporate the spermatic cord in each crush.

Castration

Male ruminants have a pendulous scrotum, which allows easy access and good drainage. Castration usually can be performed without anesthesia if the animal is restrained adequately. To perform a surgical castration, the bottom third of the scrotal skin is removed. Each testicle is pulled out, a crushing clamp or emasculator is applied as high on the cord as possible, and the testicle is removed (Fig. 22–25). The duration of the crush depends on the size of the animal. Because field castration is not a sterile procedure, the scrotal incision should be left open to drain, and antibiotic treatment may be indicated.

During fly season, nonsurgical castration may be preferred. This can be performed adequately on young ruminants with an elastrator band (up to 2 weeks of age) or a Burdizzo clamp (up to 2 months of age), taking care that both testicles are completely below the level of the crush (Fig. 22–26). Prophylactic vaccination against clostridial diseases, including tetanus, is recommended. Other procedures, such as dehorning and tail-docking, may be performed at the same time.

Pigs and camelids do not have a pendulous scrotum but may be treated with surgical castration similar to ruminants and horses. Owners of pet pigs or camelids may prefer general anesthesia and a closed wound for castration. In those cases, the testicles should be removed using sterile technique through a prescrotal incision (similar to a canine castration), which then is closed.

DISEASES OF THE UDDER

Mastitis is the leading cause of lost income among dairy herds through treatment costs, decreased production, discard of affected milk, and premature culling of affected animals. Mastitis also is important in nondairy animals because maternal discomfort or decreased milk production may adversely affect the growth or health of nursing young. In rare cases, mastitis can be directly life threatening to the cow.

Several specialized diagnostic tests are used to diagnose mastitis. Strip-cup examination involves spraying some milk from each quarter individually onto a black surface to look for aggregations of cells (*clots* or *gargot*), one sign of clinical masti-

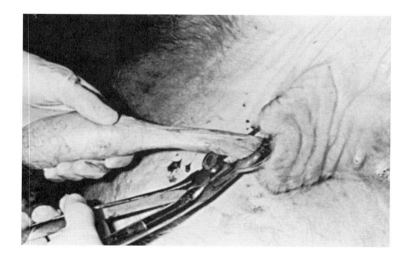

Figure 22-25. Open castration with an emasculator. The bottom of the scrotum has been removed with a scalpel blade.

tis. The California Mastitis Test (CMT) involves mixing a small amount of milk from each quarter with a detergent. Detergent lysis of cell membranes allows aggregation of nucleic acids, causing a gel to form in the mixture. This test is useful for diagnosing subclinical mastitis or specific forms of mastitis in which clot formation is uncommon. A milk sample may be collected in a sterile tube for bacteriologic culture after the teat end has been cleaned with alcohol.

> **TECHNICIAN NOTE**
>
> Because most mastitis is subclinical, prevention rather than treatment is the primary concern of dairy producers.

S. aureus and *Streptococcus agalactiae* are commonly referred to as contagious organisms of mastitis because the main reservoir for infection is the infected gland of one cow, and the organism is spread to other cows during milking. Other streptococcal organisms (collectively referred to as *S. non-agalactiae*) are common environmental contaminants and cause mastitis after successful penetration of the teat cistern. Although invasion may occur in a contaminated environment, especially if the cow spends excessive time recumbent (seen with periparturient paresis, lameness, and inadequate stalls), these organisms usually contaminate the skin and gain access to the gland during milking.

Mastitis caused by Gram-positive organisms can be clinical or subclinical and due to bacterial attachment, invasion, and exotoxin release and the resultant inflammatory response. Often, cattle will have repeated bouts of clinical mastitis punctuating times of apparent normalcy. Subclinical mastitis results in decreased production and quality of milk and may only be detectable through CMT examination. Clinical mastitis results in visible milk clot formation and possibly reddening, warmth, and pain in the affected quarter. Systemic signs usually are absent, although the cow may display mild fever and an awkward gait. Rarely, peracute gangrenous mastitis can be caused by *S. aureus*.

There are many intramammary antibiotic preparations for the treatment of mastitis caused by Gram-positive bacteria. In fact, systemic antibiotics probably are more efficacious, and many animals will clear the infection without treatment. Stripping of affected glands to remove debris and bacteria may be beneficial and is facilitated by the use of oxytocin. Proper hygiene during milking and separation of affected animals will reduce the incidence of all types of mastitis. Identification and segregation of animals with mastitis, antibiotic treatment of dry animals, and culling of persistently infected animals will help reduce herd incidence. In cases of chronic, nonresponsive mastitis, chemical destruction of the gland by injection through the teat end of formalin or chlorhexidine solution may be the best treatment option.

Mastitis caused by coliform organisms is potentially life threatening. The organisms are found in the environment and gain access to the gland in a similar fashion to *S. non-agalactiae*. Once in the gland, coliform organisms multiply rapidly and invoke a strong cellular immune response. Unlike Gram-positive organisms, coliform bacteria release endotoxin during periods of rapid growth or destruction. Endotoxin triggers a cascade of endogenous inflammatory mediator release, which increases local blood flow, vascular permeability, and immune cell activity. Locally, the udder often is warm and erythematous, and the milk is replaced by a characteristic watery secretion. Clots are not always seen with coliform mastitis, but the secretion usually yields a very positive result on CMT due to the large numbers of bacteria and neutrophils.

Severe coliform mastitis resembles other diseases characterized by systemic endotoxemia or generalized weakness, making examination of the udder essential in such cows. Characteristically, there is tachycardia, tachypnea, anorexia, ruminal atony, and evidence of dehydration. Fever is an inconsistent finding. Treatment of coliform mastitis involves decreasing the effects of endotoxin. Frequent stripping out of the affected quarter will remove endotoxin and bacteria from the gland, whereas nonsteroidal anti-inflammatory agents and oral or intravenous fluids will help combat the endotoxemia. Intramammary antibiotics are of limited value and should not be used in place of stripping. Systemic antibiotics may be of value in animals with severe, protracted disease. Vaccination with a Gram-negative mutant bacterin appears to decrease the clinical signs of coliform mastitis.

Trauma to the teat end may allow invasion by *Actinomyces pyogenes* and lead to abscess formation in the gland. The characteristic secretion from the gland is thick and foul smelling. Similar to basic abscess management, adequate drainage, in this case through amputation of the distal teat end, may be necessary to resolve the infection. The affected quarter is highly unlikely to return to normal production, so chemical destruction of the gland also may be indicated to speed resolution of the infection.

> **TECHNICIAN NOTE**
>
> Due to concerns over the presence of drugs and chemicals in our food supply, food animal veterinarians and producers must carefully adhere to guidelines concerning withdrawal times and extralabel use of drugs.

Teat lacerations potentially threaten the future production of a milking animal through mastitis or loss of the quarter. Trauma may also predispose the quarter to destruction by *A. pyogenes*. Surgical repair of lacerations is only necessary if the wound extends into the streak canal. In such a case, fine suture should be used to close the mucosa, submucosa, and skin in separate layers. A cannula or piece of tubing may be sutured into the streak canal to prevent stricture formation and allow milk to drain past the wound. Machine milking is less traumatic than hand milking and should be used during the recovery period. If possible, the injury should be repaired during the nonlactation period.

METABOLIC DISEASE

Hypocalcemia (*milk fever, parturient paresis*) is the most common of all metabolic diseases of dairy cattle and also occurs in sheep, goats, and pigs. It occurs when homeostatic mechanisms to mobilize calcium from bone or absorption from the gut fail to replace calcium lost from the plasma into milk at the onset of lactation or into the fetus during late gestation. Lactational hypocalcemia is most common in older dairy cows, particularly Channel Island breeds, and dairy goats. Ewes and pigs more frequently develop the problem during late gestation. Pigs fed a heavy concentrate ration with insufficient calcium supplementation can also develop clinical hypocalcemia.

Clinical signs vary depending on the severity of hypocalcemia. Signs often occur within 96 hours of delivery or within the last couple of weeks of gestation, although 7% of cases occur at other times associated with disease-induced anorexia. Signs range from mild excitement, tetany, and hyperesthesia to flaccid paralysis, loss of consciousness, and death. Sheep, goats, and pigs more frequently exhibit tetany than flaccid paralysis. If chronic calcium deficiency occurs, growing pigs may develop osteodystrophia fibrosa, whereas sows develop slipped femoral heads. Sheep often display dental maldevelopment. Other nonspecific signs of chronic calcium deficiency in food animals include poor growth, inappetence, stiffness, pathologic fractures, loss of condition, reduced milk production, and reduced fertility.

Treatment of acute hypocalcemia consists of slow intravenous or subcutaneous administration of calcium gluconate. Although subcutaneous administration is safer, intravenous administration often is necessary in severely affected animals. Products containing phosphorus also may be beneficial in hypocalcemic ruminants because many often have concurrent hypophosphatemia. Response to treatment often is rapid. Good footing and nursing care also are important to prevent recumbency-induced muscular and neurologic damage. Preventative measures in dairy cows include efforts to increase calcium mobilization during the dry period through dietary manipulation, including the feeding of high anionic salts during the dry period or reducing calcium in the diet in the last 2 weeks of gestation. Injections of vitamin D_3 at specific times during gestation also are reported to be beneficial.

✎ TECHNICIAN NOTE

Diagnosis of hypocalcemia is based on clinical signs and rapid response to treatment. Blood analysis can confirm the diagnosis only retrospectively.

Hypomagnesemia (*grass tetany, grass staggers, transport tetany*) occurs most commonly in lactating beef cows but can occur in dairy cows, pigs, sheep, and goats under certain management conditions. It occurs commonly in ruminants on rapidly growing grass pastures, winter wheat, or other cereal crops. Cattle and sheep that are transported long distances or ruminants or recently weaned pigs fed marginally low-magnesium diets are susceptible to hypomagnesemia. Affected ruminants often are hypocalcemic as well as hypomagnesemic. Clinical signs relate to the role of magnesium in neuromuscular conduction. Ruminants frequently exhibit tetany, muscle fasciculations, excitability, aggression, seizures, and convulsions. Signs of hypocalcemia also may be present. Pigs may show weakness of

the pasterns, particularly in the forelegs, causing backward bowing of the legs, sickled hocks, hyperirritability, arched back, reluctance to stand, and tetany. Death ensues if treatment is not given.

Treatment consists of subcutaneous administration of magnesium sulfate or mixtures of calcium, magnesium, phosphorus, and potassium, followed by oral magnesium oxide. Clinical signs often resolve quickly with treatment. Prevention consists of feeding magnesium supplements to animals maintained on pastures low in magnesium or concentrates low in magnesium and minimizing contact with lush, green, young pastures.

Ketosis, hepatic lipidosis, and fatty liver are all conditions associated with negative energy balance in ruminants. Ruminants typically exist in a state of low glucose availability. They have adapted to use lipids for energy, but with severe or prolonged negative energy balance, there can be clinical complications associated with the mobilization of peripheral fat stores in the form of fatty acids for energy. Some fat is incompletely oxidized by the liver to ketone bodies. These can be utilized for energy, but excessive ketones spill into the urine and milk.

Causes of negative energy balance include late pregnancy, heavy lactation, anorexia, and concurrent disease. Clinical ketosis (*acetonemia*) occurs typically in early lactation cows and often is accompanied by persistent hypoglycemia. Spontaneous recovery may occur as cows reduce their milk production to match energy intake. Hepatic lipidosis (*fatty liver*) occurs when the transport of fat to the liver overwhelms the ability of the liver to export or metabolize fat.

Pregnancy toxemia shares many metabolic similarities with ketosis. It occurs in sheep, goats, and cows with multiple fetuses or in advanced pregnancy. Unlike postpartum ketosis and fatty liver, pregnancy toxemia is irreversible without aggressive treatment due to the inability of the affected ruminant to decrease energy flow to the fetus. It also can result in hepatic lipidosis. Mortality is associated with severe dehydration and acidosis. Camelids may develop hyperlipemia and ketonuria in late gestation in response to inadequate energy intake. When faced with severe metabolic stress, camelids convert excess fatty acids to triglycerides and incorporate them in lipoproteins that are poorly cleared by peripheral tissues.

Clinical signs of clinical ketosis, pregnancy toxemia, and fatty liver are indistinguishable and include depression, lethargy, decreased milk production, anorexia, and possible neurologic signs such as excessive salivation, excitement, blindness, and head pressing. Diagnosis may be aided by measurement of serum glucose concentration and urine or milk dipstick for ketone bodies.

The major goal of therapy for these metabolic diseases is to reestablish normal appetite and energy balance and interrupt the destructive feedback loop of fuel utilization. Elective abortion, cesarean section, or induced parturition can be considered for pregnancy toxemia and hyperlipemia in camelids. Restoration of normal energy metabolism involves restoring normal blood glucose and ketone body levels. Therapeutics include intravenous fluids supplemented with glucose, oral glucose precursors such as propylene glycol and glycerol, glucocorticoids, insulin, and niacin. Often, ruminants with severe clinical ketosis and hyperlipemia are refractory to treatment.

Polioencephalomalacia (*polio*) is a noninfectious disease of ruminants characterized by cerebrocortical necrosis. Clinical signs are referrable to the central nervous system and include blindness, depression, incoordination, recumbency, convulsions, and death. Polio has been associated with improper diets such as certain milk replacers, high carbohydrates (leading to rumen acidosis), selenium toxicosis and deficiency, poisonous plants, mycotoxins, cobalt deficiency, and sulfate toxicity. Regardless of the cause, the disease is responsive to thiamine treatment during the early stages. Although thiamine deficiency has been postulated as the cause of this disease, this has not been demonstrated. Thiamine is important in cerebral energy metabolism, and the responsiveness of the syndrome to thiamine treatment suggests that the common pathogenesis involves impaired cerebral energy metabolism.

Definitive diagnosis of polio is based on postmortem evidence of cerebrocortical necrosis. Presumptive diagnosis can be achieved by measurement of erythrocyte or tissue thiamine levels, ruminal thiaminase activity, or erythrocyte transketolase activity. Responsiveness to thiamine supplementation is supportive but not conclusive of the diagnosis. Treatment consists of parenteral thiamine supplementation, dietary modification, and possibly rumen transfaunation.

NEONATAL PROBLEMS

Youngstock are an important commodity for many ruminant producers. Lambs, piglets, crias, kids, and calves represent the marketable commercial product for their respective producers, as well as the genetic stock for future generations. Care and treatment of the neonate can be divided into several topics: management in the immediate postpartum period, colostral considerations, differentials for the weak neonate, general treatment approach for neonates, and other specific problems, such as diarrhea, sepsis, and congenital defects.

During parturition, the newborn experiences severe stress, temperature changes, and oxygen deprivation. These stresses trigger elevations in catecholamine and cortisol levels that stimulate the newborn to adapt to extrauterine life. Adaptation to extrauterine life is a dynamic process. Fetal organs must adjust to autonomous function in an aerobic environment. Some adaptive changes must be made immediately, such as adjusting to air breathing, whereas others are more gradual, such as development of a competent immune system.

Management of the neonate immediately postpartum consists of facilitating the many physiologic changes occurring at that time. At birth, physical stimulation and oxygen debt encourage the newborn to develop rhythmic, productive respirations. Surfactant is produced in the lungs under the influence of cortisol and helps reduce alveolar surface tension. Fetal lung fluid is gradually absorbed, and alveoli are cleared to enable oxygen absorption. The producer or technician can facilitate adaptation of the respiratory system of the neonate by manually rubbing and stimulating the newborn, clearing fluid from the nasal and oral cavities manually or with suction, positioning the animal in sternal recumbency, and providing intranasal oxygen if necessary. With the first few respiratory efforts, the pulmonary vascular resistance in the neonate declines and the systemic vascular resistance increases comparatively. As a result, the cardiovascular system switches from fetal circulation, which is centered on the umbilicus, to the adult system of circulation, which is centered on the lungs. Cardiovascular fetal shunts such as the foramen ovale and ductus arteriosus close gradually.

The producer and technician can facilitate these cardiovascular changes by providing oxygen as necessary and encouraging the neonate to move around and breathe well.

At birth, the neonate leaves a temperature-controlled environment (the uterus) and enters an environment with a wide range of temperature extremes. Immediately, the neonate starts to lose body heat. The neonate attempts to compensate for heat loss by nonshivering and shivering thermogenesis. Physical activity increases thermogenesis and can be encouraged by the producer and technician. Provision of external heat via blankets, hot water bottles, or heat lamps can enable the neonate to maintain body heat without as much energy and effort on its part. Glycogen is the major energy source for thermogenesis and is depleted quickly. The producer and technician can replace depleted glucose by quickly providing the neonate with high-quality, warm colostrum.

TECHNICIAN NOTE

Basic neonatal care includes cauterization of umbilical remnants, application of suction or manual clearance of air passages, and vigorous rubbing to warm, dry, and stimulate the neonate.

The neonatal food animal is exposed to infectious agents at birth but has limited endogenous immune capabilities. Unlike carnivores, which receive maternal antibodies in utero, the neonatal artiodactylid relies on colostral ingestion to receive maternal immunoglobulins (*passive transfer*). Ability of the neonate to absorb colostral antibodies decreases with time; therefore, it is important that appropriate amounts of high-quality colostrum be offered postnatally to the newborn in a timely fashion. The quality of the colostrum depends on the age and breed of the dam from which it is obtained (older animals are better), postpartum time during which it is collected (early postpartum is best), storage (stable when frozen), and source (same farm is better than from elsewhere). Ideally, the neonate should receive at least 10% of its body weight of high-quality colostrum within the first 12 hours of birth. Frequent, small feedings are best (every 2 hours if possible). The best absorption occurs if the neonate suckles the dam; however, the amount consumed cannot be regulated. Bottle feeding is better than orogastric administration via an esophageal feeder, but the latter ensures that the entire quantity reaches the gut for absorption.

Colostrum can be qualitatively assessed by use of a colostrometer, which provides a crude estimation of the specific gravity of the liquid (excellent, specific gravity of more than 1.047). Good-quality colostrum is only one part of the procedure to ensure adequate immune protection of the neonate; the other part is the absorptive capacity of the neonate, which can be reduced by hypoxemia. Techniques for assessment of neonatal immunoglobulin absorption vary in cost, ease of use, availability, and quantity measured. They include refractometry for total plasma solids, precipitation and coagulation tests (zinc sulfate, sodium sulfite, glutaraldehyde), latex agglutination, and radial immunodiffusion. Not all of these tests measure the same serum component, and they must be interpreted in light of their limitations. To determine the success of passive transfer, one of these tests should be performed at approximately 24 hours of age to allow maximal time for colostral ingestion and absorption. Determination of passive transfer of immunoglobulin status of the neonate by any of these methods provides only a rough assessment of disease resistance.

There are several important problems or differentials to consider when evaluating a weak, unthrifty neonate. One of the most common is hypoxemia or perinatal asphyxia. Dystocia or prematurity contributes to these problems. An important sequella of hypoxemia and asphyxia is widespread organ damage or malfunction. The neonate usually shows neurologic signs, including the inability to maintain sternal recumbency or to stand, poor suckle reflex, hyperventilation followed by reduced respiratory efforts, and dull demeanor.

Hypoxemia can be diagnosed definitively by arterial blood gas analysis. Suspected hypoxemia should be treated by efforts to improve aeration of the lungs. Intranasal oxygen may be sufficient to correct this problem, but in some cases intubation and use of an Ambu bag or a ventilator may be required if poor ventilation is suspected. Fluid support may help correct lactic acidosis caused by tissue hypoxia. The use of epinephrine during ventilatory support may be beneficial.

Two other common differentials to consider for a weak neonate are hypoglycemia and hypothermia. These two problems are common if the food animal is born in the field during cold and/or damp weather and does not get dry or nurse quickly. Septicemia also can cause hypoglycemia in the later, advanced stages of the disease. Hypoglycemia and hypothermia can be diagnosed by a rectal body temperature reading for the latter and measurement of blood glucose concentrations for the former. Treatment for hypothermia consists of using towels or a hair dryer to help dry the neonate; provision of blankets, hot water bottles, or a heat lamp; provision of shelter away from adverse weather conditions; and the administration of warm isotonic fluids parenterally or warm colostrum orally. Treatment of hypoglycemia consists of fluids with glucose added and provision of warm colostrum orally.

Prenatal or postnatal infections may result in a weak neonate. The neonatal food animal may not show signs of disease for several days to weeks. Signs may be localized to a particular organ system, such as the lungs, gastrointestinal tract, umbilicus, or joints, or manifest as more widespread and generalized disease, such as diffuse septicemia. The umbilicus may serve as a wick to draw infection from the environment; therefore, cauterization of the umbilical remnants at birth with iodine solutions may decrease infection entering the neonate through that route.

The major predisposing factor for the development of neonatal septicemia is failure of the neonate to acquire adequate passive immunity from colostrum. Causative organisms are those residing in the environment of the neonate and frequently include Gram-negative bacteria. Clinical signs of septicemia are nonspecific and include weakness, depression, and reluctance or inability to stand and suckle; neurologic dysfunction; and ophthalmologic abnormalities. Fever and diarrhea are inconsistently observed. Confirmation of septicemia depends on isolation of the causative bacterial organism from the blood. Because blood culture results are unavailable for several days, diagnosis often is based on clinical signs and ruling out other causes of the weak neonate.

Treatment for localized infection depends on the site but consists of antibiotics, anti-inflammatory agents, and possibly local wound management. Therapeutic aims for generalized septicemia are directed toward decreasing bacterial numbers, decreasing the effects of endotoxemia, improving the immune status of the neonate, and supportive care. Specific treatment includes antibiotics selected on the basis of bacterial identification and susceptibility patterns, anti-inflammatory agents, intravenous fluids, and species-specific plasma or whole blood.

Another common cause of a weak neonate is infectious diarrhea. Morbidity and mortality result from dehydration and acidosis caused by fluid and electrolyte losses rather than gut damage itself. Diarrhea in neonatal food animals results from a complex interaction among etiologic, immunologic, and husbandry factors. Diarrheal disease often occurs under conditions of overcrowding and poor sanitation. Common etiologies in calves, pigs, goats, and sheep include *E. coli;* rotavirus and coronavirus; coccidia such as *Cryptosporidium* spp., *Isospora,* or *Eimeria;* and *Clostridium perfringens*. Pigs and calves also may have diarrhea caused by *Enterococcus durans*. Uncommonly, *Salmonella* spp. can cause diarrhea in neonates but often causes septicemia due to absorption of the organism into the bloodstream through the damaged gut.

The enteric viruses and *Cryptosporidium* spp. infect the cells lining the intestinal tract and thereby interfere with digestion and absorption of milk. One unique feature of the life cycle of *Cryptosporidium* is its potential for autoinfection due to recycling merozoites or sporozoites within the gut (see Chapter 5). Thus, relapses after apparent cure are common. *E. coli* causes diarrhea by secreting a toxin that causes hypersecretion of water and electrolytes by the intestinal lining cells. Septicemic colibacillosis may occur if the bacteria enter the bloodstream through the damaged gut. These bacteria, as well as *Salmonella* spp. and *Cryptosporidium* spp., have zoonotic potential. Enterotoxemia caused by *C. perfringens* causes high mortality due to vascular effects of the exotoxin elaborated. Bovine virus diarrhea is an uncommon cause of diarrhea in neonatal calves. Congenital defects are another manifestation of BVD infection. Historically, older cows on the farm may also have diarrhea.

All of these causes of infectious diarrhea result in dehydration, depression, gastrointestinal atony, and weakness in addition to diarrhea in the neonatal food animal. Sometimes, the animal dies before diarrhea is observed, due to *C. perfringens* or *Salmonella*. In such cases, bloat, fever, colic, and anorexia may be the only clinical signs. Treatment for neonatal diarrhea involves replacement of fluid and electrolyte losses. Oral fluids may suffice if the neonate is still suckling. However, intravenous administration is required if the animal is poorly responsive or inappetant. Physical examination, blood gas, and serum biochemical panel can aid in evaluation of the calf and direct appropriate bicarbonate, electrolyte, and fluid supplementation.

Replacement fluids should consist of a balanced electrolyte mixture with amounts estimated based on percentage dehydration, with the average calf requiring 2 to 6 liters. If bicarbonate deficits exceed the amounts provided in the polyionic fluids, supplemental sodium bicarbonate should be provided (mEq bicarbonate = body weight in kg × 0.6 × base deficit). If used, systemic administration of antibiotics is vastly superior to oral administration. Antibiotics may protect against secondary bacterial infections and septicemia, although their efficacy against the enteric pathogens per se is questionable. The neonate should be kept in a clean, warm, dry environment and be provided good nutritional support (continued milk feeding).

> **TECHNICIAN NOTE**
>
> With undifferentiated neonatal scours, maintenance of fluid and electrolyte balance is the major goal of treatment.

Prematurity or congenital defects may be responsible for weakness in food animals. Premature food animals adapt to extrauterine life more slowly than do full-term animals. Problems may include poor suckle reflex, hypoxemia and impaired ventilatory effort, inability to stand or thermoregulate, and/or abnormal mentation. Some of the problems resolve over time with supportive therapy. Because poor colostral absorption is a common sequella to prematurity, the premature neonate should be frequently offered good-quality colostrum or provided with plasma if necessary. Congenital defects can include any number of derangements that impair normal neonatal behavior and function. Depending on the severity of the problem, directed treatment or supportive care may be warranted.

A minimum data base may help to accurately evaluate a weak, unthrifty neonate and distinguish between problems. These tests include

1. A measurement of serum immunoglobulin to determine passive transfer of maternal antibodies
2. Complete blood count and plasma fibrinogen measurement to identify focal or widespread inflammation or infection
3. Arterial blood gas analysis to diagnose respiratory impairment
4. Aerobic and anaerobic blood cultures to identify causative organisms and direct antibiotic therapy
5. Serum chemistry panel to identify metabolic or organ dysfunction.

If the ruminant has signs specific to the gastrointestinal system (colic, abdominal distention, absence of feces), abdominal radiographs may be important. Method for collecting samples to run these tests are described in Chapter 10.

Other tests may be appropriate for identifying focal disease processes; these include thoracic radiographs for pneumonia, fecal culture or viral isolation for infectious causes of diarrhea, abdominal radiographs for gastrointestinal obstructions or congenital GI defects, joint tap for cytology and culture if joint distention is present, and ultrasound of the umbilical remnants if umbilical swelling, heat, or pain is present.

Even in the field without access to a clinical pathology laboratory, some of these tests can be performed to differentiate causes of weakness; these include a good physical examination with rectal temperature and auscultation of the chest, glucose dipstick using whole blood, and a field test for immunoglobulin estimation.

NEOPLASIA
Lymphoma

The bovine leukemia virus (BLV) is an oncogenic retrovirus spread through transmission of infected lymphocytes between animals. Hypodermic needles, rectal sleeves, dehorning and tatooing instruments, and semen may transmit the virus from one animal to another, making the veterinarian and technician important potential vectors. Although most new infections occur in calves, disease signs often take years to develop. Most infected cattle do not develop clinical disease, although many develop high peripheral blood lymphocyte counts. A small percentage of infected adult cattle develop multicentric lymphoma, with the lymph nodes, heart, uterus, abomasal wall, kidneys, and retrobulbar space being common sites of tumor formation. Clinical signs are variable, depending on the location of the masses, but include mass lesions, weight loss, melena, fever, and exophthalmia. Treatment usually is not economically feasible, and the disease is rapidly fatal. Although cattle are the primary host for BLV, other species may develop lymphoma after being infected with bovine blood products. Serologic tests can be used to identify infected animals, which may be culled from the herd. Thymic, cutaneous, and multicentric lymphomas also occur sporadically in juvenile cattle and camelids, swine, and small ruminants of all ages, but these neoplasms are not thought to have a contagious cause.

> **TECHNICIAN NOTE**
>
> Although serologic testing is useful for identifying retrovirus-infected animals, only a small portion of these animals will develop clinical disease.

Squamous Cell Carcinoma

Ocular squamous cell carcinoma is the most common malignancy in cattle in many parts of the world. Ultraviolet radiation

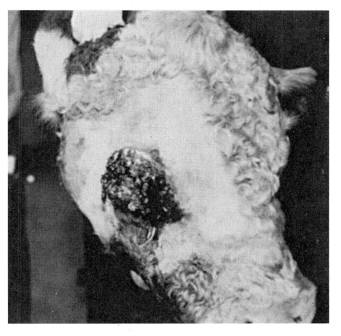

Figure 22-27. Advanced ocular squamous cell carcinoma (cancer eye) in Hereford bull.

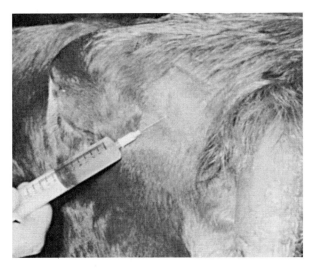

Figure 22-28. Corneal nerve block on a cow. The anesthetic agent is deposited subcutaneously, midway between the lateral canthus of the eye and the base of the horn.

(altitude) and unpigmented ocular membranes increase risk. Growths start as pale pink plaques, usually on the limbus, eyelid margin, or third eyelid, but can become large and papillomatous (Fig. 22–27). Early lesions may be treated with topical liquid nitrogen sprays or hyperthermia, whereas larger lesions or those that threaten to invade deep periorbital tissues should be removed by exenteration (occular removal). Metastasis of tumor to local lymph nodes is rare but can occur with long-standing lesions. Gastrointestinal and urinary tract squamous cell carcinomas also occur in ruminants and camelids and are thought to have a toxic etiology.

Exenteration

The skin around the eye is clipped and aseptically prepared. Regional anesthesia is achieved by infiltrating the retrobulbar space with a local anesthetic agent and blocking the auriculo-palpebral nerve at the lateral canthus of the eye (Fig. 22–28). The lids may be sutured or clamped together. An elliptical incision 1 cm from the lid margins is made around the eye. Subcutaneous and periorbital tissues are separated from the orbit by a combination of blunt and sharp dissection until the tissue behind the globe can be transected. All tumor tissue should be removed. The eye is removed, and the incision is closed with simple interrupted or cruciate sutures.

Recommended Reading

Howard JL: Current Veterinary Therapy: Food Animal Practice. 3. Philadelphia, Lea & Febiger, 1993.
Noordsy JL: Food Animal Surgery. 3rd ed. Trenton, NJ, Veterinary Learning Systems, 1994.
Radostits OM, Blood DC, and Gay CC: Veterinary Medicine: A Textbook of the Diseases of Cattle, Sheep, Pigs and Horses. 8th ed. Philadelphia, Bailliere Tindall, 1994.
Smith BP: Large Animal Internal Medicine. 2nd ed. St. Louis, Mosby, 1996.

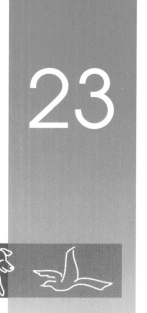

23 Birds, Reptiles, Ferrets, Rabbits, and Rodents

Thomas N. Tully, Jr.

INTRODUCTION

The veterinary medical field of exotic or nondomestic pet medicine is growing as the popularity of these animals increases (Fig. 23–1). Caged and aviary birds are now the third most common small animal pet. In a 1992 study, 5.7% of households in the United States owned a pet bird and 8.7% of the households owned pets other than a dog, cat, or pet bird (Wise and Yank, 1992). On the basis of the percentage of households with pet birds, the projected population of birds owned in 1991 was 11.7 million. This chapter discusses these species, with attention paid to individual requirements and emphasis placed on birds, ferrets, rabbits, and rodents. It is important to note that approximately 85% of the problems seen in exotic pet medicine result from lack of information on the part of pet stores, pet owners, veterinarians, and veterinary technicians. With increased veterinary and public education, all species covered in this chapter will have a greater chance of living long and healthy lives.

TECHNICIAN NOTE

Approximately 85% of the problems seen in exotic pet medicine result from lack of information on the part of pet stores, pet owners, veterinarians, and veterinary technicians.

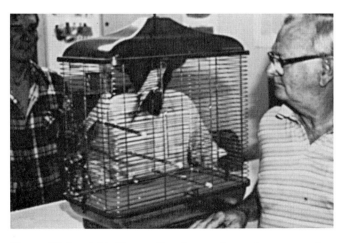

Figure 23-1. A bird is an attractive and popular companion.

RESTRAINT

A general rule regarding restraint should be noted: The best protection for both the handler and the patient is knowledge of the animal—its anatomy, its physiology, location and capabilities of its weapons, its strength, and its agility and speed, as well as its natural response to stress and escape. Minimal handling of all exotics is recommended and must be done efficiently, quietly, and confidently. The best method of learning restraint is by watching an experienced handler. It is often difficult to quantify the stress factor. The importance of fast, competent handling cannot be overemphasized. The exotic animal in a veterinary hospital is already stressed by the sights, sounds, smells, and temperatures of the strange environment. As a general rule, the more tame the animal, the better it will tolerate handling. However, do not underestimate the added stress of disease or injury. One should never attempt to learn handling on an exotic animal whose condition is already compromised by disease and trauma. One should always discuss the subject of handling and stress with the owner of an ill or traumatized nondomestic pet before handling begins. All treatment and testing material (such as culturettes and syringes for blood work-ups) must be in place before the animal is restrained to minimize stress. In some cases, the patient work-up must be done incrementally because of the patient's poor physical condition.

TECHNICIAN NOTE

One should always discuss the subject of handling and stress with the owner of an ill or traumatized nondomestic pet before handling begins.

BIRDS

The veterinary technician may, on occasion, be involved in telephone communication with clients. When clients call regarding avian patients, it is important to instruct owners in the following areas.

Ask the owners to bring the bird in its own cage if at all possible. They should not clean the cage, except to empty the water dish to prevent it from spilling during the trip. A good evaluation of the bird's environment is helpful to the veterinarian, and clean papers and a clean cage do not provide that information. All grit should be removed because some birds tend to gorge themselves on grit, particularly when ill. The cage should be covered with a towel or blanket to protect it from the weather, and the owner should be instructed to bring along any medication and vitamin supplements the bird is taking, as well as a sample of the food. Most avian telephone inquiries should be considered emergencies because of most owners' inability to note early signs of illness, the bird's inherent ability to mask clinical problems, and the rapid speed with which avian species succumb to disease.

Taking the Clinical History

The following is a suggested list of questions to ask the client regarding avian patients:

1. Chief complaint
2. Signalment (including the species, sex, and breed)
3. Origin—Where was the bird obtained? How long has it been owned?
4. Environment—What is the construction and design of the cage? Is it painted? If so, what type of paint has been used? What types of water and food bowls, substrate (newspaper, wood shavings, corn cob, and so forth), and types of perches are used? Where is the bird kept (indoors or outdoors)? In what room of the house (e.g., kitchen or garage where potential toxins may be located)? Is it close to a window? Are insecticides, household cleaners or other chemicals used around the house in the vicinity of the cage? Is the bird allowed out of the cage? If so, is it allowed to fly freely, and how well is it supervised?

5. Diet—What is the bird being fed (such as seed, fruits, vegetables, grain)? How often is the animal fed? Are vitamins and minerals added to the food? How often is the water changed? How is the food prepared and stored?
6. Appetite—Notes should be made regarding the bird's overall appetite and daily food consumption.
7. Feces—Questions regarding consistency, color, and number of droppings per day are all important. The client should be asked whether feces have been submitted for parasite evaluation previously.
8. Cagemates—Are there other animals in the collection in the same cage or in the household? If so, how many, what species and what degree of contact do they have with the patient? Does the owner maintain a quarantine policy?
9. Molting cycle—When has the bird gone through its last general molt, and are there any abnormalities in the feather coat or feather growth?
10. Overall attitude, behavior, including voice quality and changes in vocalization.
11. Previous medical history—Has the bird been ill before? Is there a history of disease in other pets in the house? If so, what illnesses have been diagnosed and treated in the past? Have they been to a veterinarian before?

Restraint Techniques for Psittacine Species

When holding and examining a psittacine patient, the medical team should avoid the strong beak, jaws, wings, and feet. The feet usually have sharp, pointed claws. The equipment needed to deal with these patients will include towels or drapes, perches, and nets. Gloves should never be used with psittacine birds. Gloves are not supple enough for the handlers to feel the patient within their grasp. Do not use gloves during stressful events with a pet bird because that bird will soon associate the shape of the human hand with negative experiences. The handler should first remove water bowls and perches from the cage. Room lights may be dimmed to take advantage of the bird's inability to rapidly accommodate to changes in lighting. The psittacine bird's primary weapon is the beak; therefore, the head should be promptly secured. This is best done by placing a towel or drape over the animal and securing the head through the towel (Fig. 23–2, *A* and *B*). A wooden perch may be used to give the bird something to bite on other than fingers. The bird cannot bite the catcher if it is chewing on the cage. Once the head is secured, the body is wrapped in the towel, the feet are held, and the bird is held against the holder's body to control the wings. The towel or drape may then be slowly removed from the patient's head for examination, keeping the towel around the wings to secure them from flapping.

TECHNICIAN NOTE

Gloves should never be used with psittacine birds.

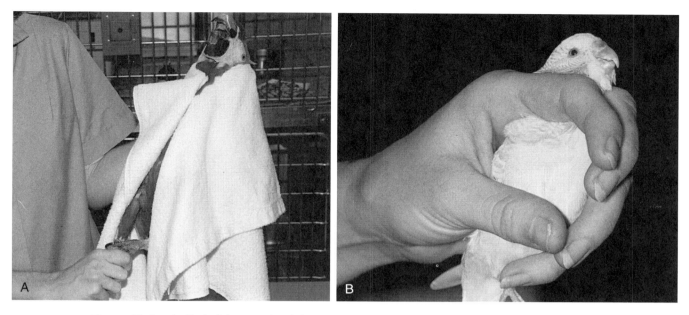

Figure 23-2. A, Restraint on a Scarlet macaw with the use of a towel and an Elizabethan handgrip. B, One-handed restraint techniques can be used for a budgerigar.

Restraint Techniques for Passerine Species

Canaries and finches are the most common passerine species seen in veterinary offices. These birds are easily stressed under normal conditions but are extremely sensitive when they are ill. Catching the patient for an examination must be done quickly and efficiently. To catch the passerine patient, all lights should be turned off and the cage door slowly lifted. Grab the patient with one hand and then turn on the lights. To hold the bird for examination, let the bird's head rest between the middle and index fingers while lying on its back. Do not put pressure on the breast or the patient may suffocate (Fig. 23–3).

Restraint Techniques for Raptorial Species

Birds of prey use their anatomic weapons in a different way. For them, it is of utmost importance to secure the talons. Although many raptors will bite, their jaws are not tremen-

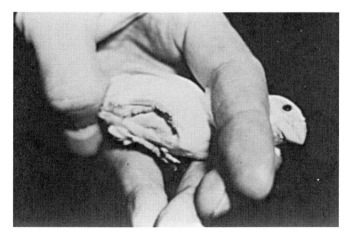

Figure 23-3. Proper technique for restraining a passerine for a physical examination.

dously strong, and they do little damage with the beak. The mouth is soft except close to the very point of the beak, which the birds use for tearing flesh. The wings should also be considered a weapon and should be properly secured. Equipment needed for restraining raptors includes towels or drapes, gloves of appropriate size and thickness, and hoods. To approach a bird of prey using gloves, the handler should be bent down low and approach quietly. Dimming the lights may be a disadvantage for examining a species that hunts at night. The handler should present as little threat as possible to the raptor. As the handler places one hand in front of his face, the second hand should be brought in low—toward the bird's feet. The upper hand should be held between the handler's face and the bird and may be used to distract the bird. The lower hand should quickly grasp the feet, trying to place the index finger between the bird's feet. The bird is then smoothly and quickly pulled up out of the cage or off the floor so that it does not beat its wings on any surfaces in the room. It is important to hold the bird away from objects, such as the examining table or cage. The bird can then be brought into a cradle position, the wings secured between the handler's arm and body, and hooded (Fig. 23–4). If hoods are not available, a towel may be draped over the bird's head; reducing visual and auditory stimuli will help to calm the bird significantly. An alternative approach to secure a bird of prey may be done with a towel or drape. Again, the handler approaches quietly and bent low, with the towel or drape spread in front with both hands. The handler moves in slowly until close enough to almost reach the bird, and then quickly—with the drape or towel used as a large glove—the bird is completely covered, with the handler's hands resting roughly on the bird's shoulders. It is important to avoid simply throwing the drape or towel, as the bird will be able to dodge it or move from under it. The bird is then pressed through the towel with enough pressure to make the bird push upward, using its legs on the ground. The technician's hands are then worked downward, alongside the wings, toward the legs, and the legs are grasped at the tarsometatarsus. Now, with

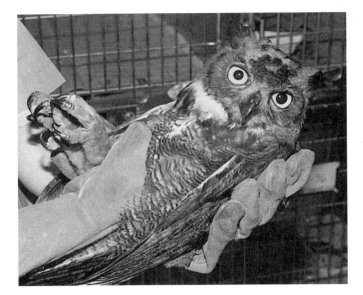

Figure 23–4. Restraint of a great-horned owl with the use of gloves. Emphasis is placed on restraint of the talons.

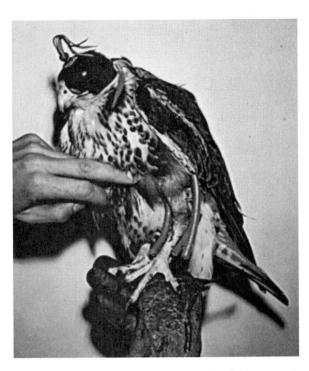

Figure 23–5. A falconer restrains a prairie falcon with hood and jesses for examination of an external fixator applied to a tibiotarsal fracture.

the bird still on the ground, its body covered by the towel and its feet secured, the bird is lifted up to the handler's body with the back adjacent to the handler's abdomen. The towel over the head may then be replaced by a hood. It is important never to release the feet of a bird of prey until someone else has secured them. When examining a bird of prey, one should use 1-inch white cloth tape to secure the talons. A 4- to 5-inch piece of tape wrapped around the closed foot will prevent accidents when these strong birds are being handled. If taloned, the legs must be fully extended before the talons can be removed. Birds of prey under the control of a falconer are a different story because the falconer is often adept at restraining the bird for a physical examination (Fig. 23–5).

TECHNICIAN NOTE

Equipment needed for restraining raptors includes towels or drapes, gloves of appropriate size and thickness, and hoods.

Sample Collection and Diagnostic Procedures Commonly Used in Birds

Diagnostic plans in avian species are no different from the clinical approach to other domestic pets. Evaluation of the stool is an important first step. The technician should become familiar with normal stool to determine differences between polyuria (excessive urine output) and diarrhea (change in the fecal consistency and amount) (Fig. 23–6). Fecal parasites may be detected on fresh smears with saline and a coverslip. This is the best method to check for protozoa, such as *Giardia*. Fecal flotations will bring some parasite ova to the surface, such as ascarids and *Capillaria*. Fecal sedimentation is an important procedure for the diagnosis of flukes, which are common in imported cockatoos and raptors. Fecal specimens that are Gram-stained are useful to determine the bacterial flora of the

digestive tract. Most cage bird species have predominantly gram-positive organisms inhabiting the digestive system. Fecal Gram stains are only a preliminary diagnostic test and should be followed up with bacterial culture.

TECHNICIAN NOTE

Most cage bird species have predominantly gram-positive organisms inhabiting the digestive system.

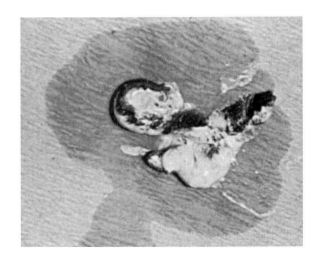

Figure 23–6. Normal psittacine stool. Note the dark solid feces, white solid urates, and liquid urine.

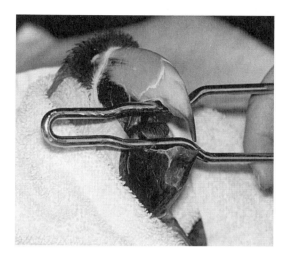

Figure 23-7. Oral examination demonstrating the use of a beak speculum on a macaw.

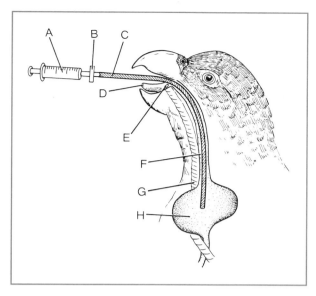

Figure 23-9. Proper tube placement for a crop wash or for tube feeding a bird. The bird's neck should be gently stretched. A, Syringe. B, Adapter if necessary. C, Tube. D, Tongue. E, Tracheal opening. F, Proximal esophagus. G, Trachea. H, Crop.

Cloacal Swab. A cloacal swab is often done on psittacine species to determine the bacterial flora of the lower gastrointestinal (GI) tract. A cotton swab is moistened, inserted into the cloaca and gently rotated. Cloacal swabs are useful for cytological evaluations, looking for inflammatory cells, such as heterophils. They may also be used for culture and sensitivity tests and *Chlamydia* or viral isolation.

Oral Examination and Crop Wash. The technician should become adept at assisting in the performance of oral examination and crop wash by the veterinarian. Good restraint technique is essential. An avian beak speculum is placed in the bird's mouth parallel to the commissure and then rotated to open the mouth (Fig. 23–7). A choanal culture should be taken when birds are exhibiting upper respiratory signs. The culturette is placed in the rostral area of the choana to prevent cross contamination with flora in the oral cavity (Fig. 23–8).

Another important diagnostic technique is the crop wash. The crop wash permits examination of the upper GI tract. A sterile or clean tube is passed through the mouth into the crop, or into the esophagus in those birds that do not have a crop. A

syringe of sterile saline is connected to the tube, and a simple flush is performed (Fig. 23–9). Tubes may be made of plastic, rubber, or metal, with a ball tip (Fig. 23–10). The crop wash is important for direct microscopic examination to check for protozoans, such as *Trichomonas* or yeast *(Candida albicans)*, using a wet mount technique. Slides may be prepared for cytologic examinations with Diff-Quick stains or Wright's stain, looking for inflammatory cells such as heterophils. A Gram stain is often done on crop wash samples from psittacine species, or the sample may be submitted for culture and sensitivity (see Color Plate 1, Part I in Chapter 5). A culturette may be passed into a bird's crop for culture and sensitivity diagnostics. Care must be taken so that the patient does not bite the culturettes and swallow it. Young psittacine species readily accept culturettes into the crop through normal feeding responses.

Passing a tube into the crop of the psittacine bird is an important technique to learn, because tube feeding is often necessary. The one rule of thumb to remember when using a

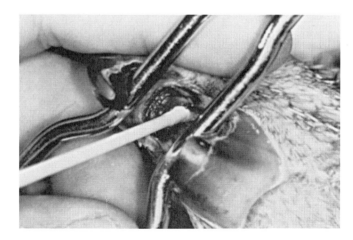

Figure 23-8. Culturette placement in the rostral aspect of the choana.

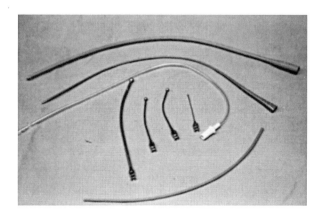

Figure 23-10. Various tubes used for tube feeding and crop washes.

tube for either feeding or a crop wash is to try to pick a tube with a diameter larger than the glottis. The glottis of the bird is located at the base of the tongue and is easy to visualize (see Fig. 23–9E). The tube may be passed into the crop easily by positioning the tube in the side of the bird's mouth (see Fig. 23–9). The tube is easily palpated through the wall of the crop and the skin. While doing a crop wash or tube feeding, the handler should watch the back of the bird's mouth to ensure that food or water does not begin to accumulate. If the crop is overfilled, the bird may aspirate. If the crop overfills, put the bird down and let it attempt to clear its airway. The bird itself has a better chance of clearing its airway than does the technician or veterinarian using cotton-tipped applicators. Never handle a bird after placing oral medication into the crop or filling the crop unless the bird is experiencing respiratory difficulty.

TECHNICIAN NOTE

The one rule of thumb to remember when using a tube for either feeding or a crop wash is to try to pick a tube with a diameter larger than the glottis.

Bloodwork. Bloodwork is an important part of the diagnostic examination in avian species. Venipuncture sites include the cutaneous ulnar vein, the right jugular vein, the medial metatarsal vein, and toenail clipping. Each has its own advantages and disadvantages, and the veterinarian and technician will tend to develop their own sites of preference, but the right jugular vein is the recommended site.

The right jugular vein is large and easily found in most birds on the right dorsolateral aspect of the neck. However, it is highly mobile and therefore difficult to immobilize. In most birds the right jugular vein is located in a featherless tract lateral to the trachea. With minimal practice and proper restraint, it becomes an easy procedure. An avian restraint board is recommended for blood collections from larger psittacine patients. Small psittacine and passerine patients can be handheld when blood is being drawn for diagnostic tests.

In general, the basilic vein is accessible but difficult to completely immobilize in the psittacine patient, due to the tremendous strength of the pectoral muscles (Fig. 23–11).

The medial metatarsal vein is easy to immobilize and secure, even on an awake and fractious patient. However, if large volumes of blood are to be collected, the medial metatarsal vein may not be a good choice in psittacine patients (Fig. 23–12).

Toenail clipping is available but is painful to the patient and often causes limping for several days following the procedure. It may result in a poor blood flow, low yield, and invalid results.

The blood may be collected in syringes, microhematocrit tubes, or blood collection tubes from the hub of the needle. A 3-ml syringe with a 26-gauge needle should be used in most avian patients. In extremely small psittacine and passerine patients a 1-ml syringe with a 30-gauge needle may be used. The technician should learn to proficiently perform a complete blood count (CBC) on avian blood.

Radiography. Radiography is an important diagnostic tool in avian patients. Typically, lateral and ventrodorsal views of the

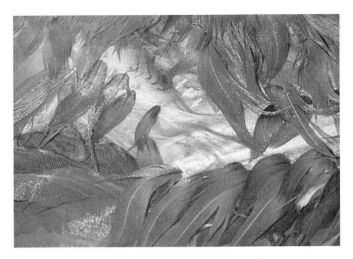

Figure 23–11. Location of the basilic vein (white arrows). Ventral view of humerus, radius, and ulna.

whole body or selected extremities may be taken (Fig. 23–13). Technique charts must be developed based on the equipment available. Contrast films may be made with standard contrast agents, including barium sulfate. Because good positioning and absence of motion are important to high-quality radiographs, it is generally recommended that all avian patients be sedated or anesthetized, except those who may be too ill (Fig. 23–14). Proper positioning is important and an avian restraint board is essential. Other diagnostic procedures, such as laparoscopy, endoscopy, tracheal or air sac washes, biopsies and cytological examinations, and bone marrow aspirates, may be performed on the patient. The technician's role may be to secure the animal with good restraint during these more sophisticated procedures.

Husbandry and Treatment in the Hospital

Generally speaking, drugs administered in the food or water will not reach adequate therapeutic levels. This is an unreliable

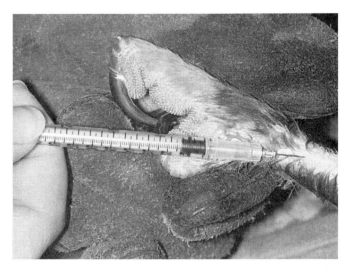

Figure 23–12. Intravenous injection using the medial metatarsal vein of a great-horned owl.

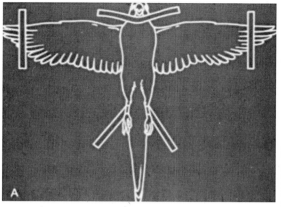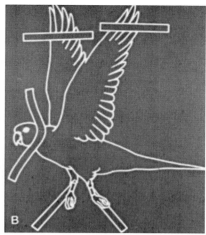

Figure 23-13. Positioning of a budgerigar for radiographs using masking tape: (A) ventrodorsal and (B) lateral positions.

way to administer medications because of the inconsistent intake of most birds. Direct oral absorption is inconsistent with tablets, but most liquid suspensions tend to work well. Injections of drugs into birds are best done in the large pectoral muscle mass. Drugs injected into the caudal half of the animal (such as the legs) may result in the drug's being absorbed into the bloodstream and shunted toward the kidneys by way of the renal portal system. Therefore, potentially nephrotoxic drugs, such as aminoglycosides, should never be administered by injection into the legs except in ostriches, emus, and rheas.

TECHNICIAN NOTE

Injections of drugs into birds are best done in the large pectoral muscle mass.

Two common procedures that the veterinary technician is often called on to perform are nail trims and wing clips. Figure 23–15 illustrates the proper technique for clipping the flight feathers of pet birds. Both wings should be clipped for a symmetrical effect. If only one wing is clipped, the bird cannot

control its flight and will become prone to injury. Wing clipping is flight restriction, not prevention. Find out what the owner wants to achieve through the wing clip and how the owner wants the wings to be clipped. No clipping technique will prevent the bird from flight.

Trimming nails in larger psittacines should be done with a dremel tool. For small psittacines and passerines, human nail clippers should be used. Cautery units can be used on the nails of birds of all sizes but work especially well on the smaller species (Fig. 23–16). Grinding the nails with a dremel tool cauterizes as it reduces the length (Fig. 23–17). Chemical cautery (as with silver nitrate sticks) should be ready for back-up, especially in younger psittacines.

Dietary management and nutritional support are particularly important in the compromised avian patient. Table 23–1 provides the basic feeding guidelines important in psittacine species and other seed eaters. It is important to remember to keep the cage as clean as possible. Food and water dishes

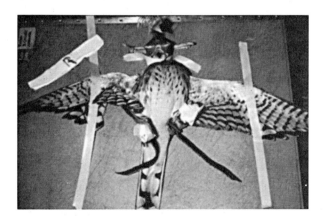

Figure 23-14. Ventrodorsal positioning of an American kestrel with the use of masking tape. Bird is sedated with ketamine. A hood decreases visual stimulation, and the talons are taped closed for safety.

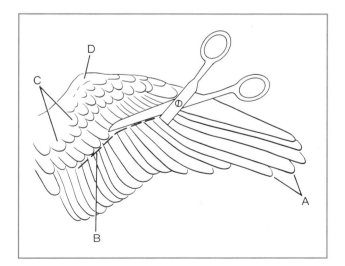

Figure 23-15. Dorsal view of extended wing showing the proper technique for wing clipping. Leaving the first three or four primary or flight feathers intact (A), the cutting line should be (B) underneath the overlying contour feathers (C) to maintain the appearance of the wing; (D), the wing is grasped firmly at the carpal joint.

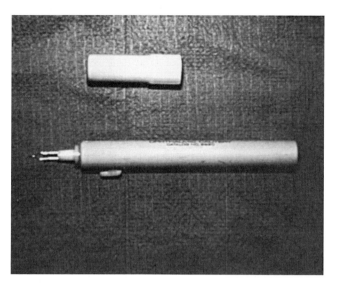

Figure 23-16. Electrocautery unit for trimming small birds' nails.

• Table 23–1 •

RECOMMENDED PSITTACINE DIET		
FOOD GROUP	**WHAT IT SUPPLIES**	**WHAT IT LACKS**
Cereals and grains 45%–50%	Proteins, fats, and B vitamins	Vitamins A, D, and K and calcium (high phosphorus)
Vegetables 45%–50%	Vitamins A and K, fiber, carbohydrates ± calcium	Protein, fats, vitamin D_3
Fruit Approximately 5%	Sugars, simple carbohydrates	Proteins, vitamins, and minerals
Meats (in combination with dairy products) about 5%	Proteins, fats, calcium	
Mineral supplements, e.g., cuttlebone, oyster shell, mineral blocks, or avian vitamins may be added to the above diets.		

should be cleaned at least daily and occasionally more often. Fresh fruits, vegetables, and meats should be left out only for short periods. Food consumption should be monitored closely. New foods should be introduced gradually, especially the pelleted avian diets. Some foods may provide the bird a source of activity during the ingestion process, such as peeling vegetables, fruits, and nuts. Tube feeding in psittacine birds is an important nursing procedure. Generally, a cereal-based product should be used, such as a number of baby avian formula products on the market. Tube feeding should begin with small amounts frequently, which are then slowly increased in volume and decreased in time interval. The bird should be weighed one or two times a day to chart weight gain. The crop should be monitored for prompt emptying, and the stools should be examined for consistency. The basal metabolic rate (BMR) may be calculated as a rough approximation of energy requirements. The normal BMR for a nonpasserine species, such as parrots, is approximately $79 \times BW$ (in kg). This should be doubled for

an ill bird. For passerine species, 130 times the body weight raised to the power of 0.7 should be used. For carnivorous birds such as raptors, a high-quality canned cat food such as Control Diet (Hill's Pet Products, Inc.) may be used to meet their energy requirements.

Hospital facilities should be appropriate for the species being housed. Bird cages should be in a separate room if possible to minimize the stress of sounds and sights of other species. Isolation of birds also prevents contamination of potentially pathogenic bacteria. For example, most psittacine birds have a predominantly gram-positive gut flora. Housing these birds near animals with gram-negative gut flora, such as dogs, cats, reptiles, and carnivorous birds, could result in gram-negative enteric infections. A visual barrier should be provided for the bird, such as a cage cover or hide box in the cage. Large parrots may do well in standard dog or cat cages. Alternatively, Plexiglas custom cages work well and are easily cleaned. Perches should be disposable or easily disinfected and sized according to the individual patient. An isolation area should be available for psittacosis suspects. Again, cleanliness is one of the most important details in the hospital.

Temperature control is important, particularly with sick birds. In general, birds will tolerate cold better than heat. Sudden changes in temperature and drafts should always be avoided. Sick birds have difficulty maintaining and regulating their own body temperature, as will birds with poor feather coats, oil-damaged feathers, or plucked feathers. Therefore, these should be kept warm but not hot. Temperatures between 80° and 90°F are best. The bird should be observed for signs of heat stress or shivering. An environmentally controlled cage or unit should be available for the intensive care avian patients.

Zoonoses and Common Clinical Problems

Avian patients can present a wide range of clinical diseases; however, their clinical signs are relatively limited. Therefore, a sick bird presented with signs of diarrhea, vomiting, or just not doing well should be considered as a potential source of *Chlamydia* infections. Those that have recently been through quarantine or pet shops and exposed to high numbers of other birds are most suspect.

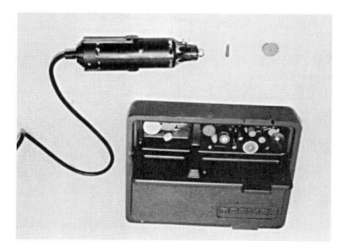

Figure 23-17. Motor tool for grinding larger birds' nails and grooming beaks.

Psittacosis is a disease transmissible to humans, caused by the bacterium *Chlamydia psittaci*. Those patients suspected of potentially being infected with *Chlamydia* should be treated with appropriate techniques. The bird should be isolated, gloves and masks should be used, and feces should be disposed of quickly and promptly. Transmission is primarily through fecal contamination. Psittacosis is a potentially fatal disease in humans as well as birds when not properly treated. Many wild birds may carry *Chlamydia* organisms without showing clinical signs. It is important that the veterinary technician working with birds become familiar with this disease.

Other clinical problems frequently encountered in a pet practice include lead poisoning, with signs of GI disturbance such as vomiting and diarrhea; gram-negative enteric infections, which generally cause diarrhea and vomiting; and upper respiratory infections, usually caused by a gram-negative bacteria.

REPTILES

It is estimated that there are 7.3 million pet reptiles in the United States. Although the number of pet reptiles do not match dog and cat populations, this is a significant population of animals that require veterinary health services. The diversity of reptile species maintained in captivity require owner education in health, nutritional, and environmental management. With excellent owner care, most reptile species live long, healthy lives. In many cases, it is the responsibility of the technician to handle and collect diagnostic samples and educate the owner about their captive reptile.

Once a veterinary hospital decides to treat reptiles, there are a few pieces of specialized equipment needed to provide an adequate hospital environment and aid the technician and veterinarian. Required medical equipment includes an electronic gram scale, an incubating heating pad, tuberculin and microliter syringes, exotic animal formulary (see Recommended Reading), microhematocrit tubes, snake sexing probes, and metal feeding tubes. Common materials used on turtle shell repair includes expoxy, resin, and Fiberglas patches. Surgical equipment used for reptiles but available in most exotic animal practices include a Dremal Moto Tool, stainless steel suture material, transparent surgical drapes, and a magnifying surgical headset.

Reptile housing equipment must be adaptable to the different species that may be hospitalized. Examples of hospital caging and equipment include fluorescent light tubes (regular and full spectrum), humidifier, Fiberglas cages, small aquaria with secure ventilated lids, heated room, or heat lamps and pads. To aid in capture and restraint, a snake hook, tongs, Plexiglas tubes, and pole snare should be available. As with other exotic species, proper restraint reduces stress to the client, animal, and health care personnel. Once a practice is properly equipped and personnel trained, interesting patients and cases will begin to receive quality health care.

The following is a list of questions to ask clients regarding reptile patients:

1. Chief complaint—Why does the owner want the pet examined?
2. Signalment (including the species as specifically as possible)—What is the age and sex of the animal, and how long have they owned the animal?
3. Origin—Where did the animal come from?

4. Environment—Factors such as cage design, construction materials, substrates, perches, or branches are of critical importance in determining the health of these species. Temperature and humidity, as well as photoperiod and exposure to sunlight or full-spectrum artificial light, may have a significant impact on the animal's health. The owner should be questioned as to where the cage is kept in the house, as well as the type of heat source used and the usual temperature gradient within the cage. For aquatic species, questions pertaining to water quality control, filter systems used, sources of water, and frequency of water change are important. It is also important to ask the owner about the types of cleaning agents and disinfectants being used and frequency.
5. Food—How often is food offered? How much is consumed? What is the source of the food? How is the food stored, and how it is presented to the animal?
6. Water—How often is the water cleaned or changed? How is it offered to the animal? If a water bowl is used, how large is it? For many species, it is important to offer water in a bowl large enough for the animal to completely submerge itself in.
7. Feces—How often does the animal defecate in relation to feeding? What are the color and consistency of the stool? Has the owner submitted a fecal sample previously for parasite evaluation?
8. Cagemates—Does the client have other animals in his or her collection or in the same cage? If so, what species are they, and where are they kept? Does the owner maintain a quarantine policy? If so, for how long?
9. What are the current attitude and behavior of the patient, and have there been any recent changes?
10. For lizards and snakes, how often does the animal shed? When was the last period of shedding or ecdysis?
11. Previous medical history—Has the animal been ill previously? If it has, it is important to get the owner to describe its illness and any treatments that were done. It is often helpful to include the attending veterinarian's name. Have other animals in the collection ever been ill?

Restraint Techniques for Reptiles

In handling reptiles, the veterinary technician should become as familiar as possible with anatomic and physiologic adaptations of reptiles. Several sources of information are found in the Recommended Reading list at the end of this chapter. Restraint of turtles or tortoises should be done carefully and with caution. Some species of turtles have long necks and a sharp powerful beak (rhamphotheca) that can inflict a serious bite to the unwary handler. Some turtles may be able to extend their head and neck nearly to the level of the hindlimbs, two thirds of the body length. Many are quick and therefore should be approached from the rear, with the tail and legs held securely. Simply covering the head, neck, and forelimbs with a cloth towel is usually adequate to prevent injury to the turtle and handler. To prevent an animal from walking during an examination, it may be placed on a broad-based object that will keep

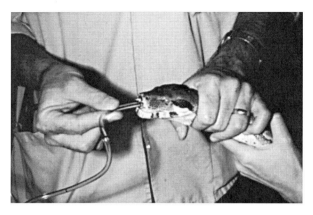

Figure 23-18. Restraint of a common boa constrictor and passage of a stomach tube.

the chelonian limbs from touching the examination table surface. The legs may be kept in place by wrapping the shell, with the legs inside, with an elastic bandage. To remove a turtle's head from the shell for examination, straight ovid delivery forceps may be used. Care must be taken using steady gentle traction without allowing the forceps to touch the eyes. The main force of the forceps' jaws is applied away from the shell and not onto the head (Frye, 1995).

Snakes are usually more difficult for the inexperienced handler. Equipment needed may include Plexiglas shields, Plexiglas tubes, tongs, canvas bags or drapes, snake hook, gas anesthetic machine, and plastic bags. Venomous reptiles are not recommended as pets and should be handled only by experienced snake handlers and veterinarians. The general approach to restrain any snake is to immobilize the head and grasp it firmly with the hands at the base of the skull (Fig. 23–18). Several methods may be used to immobilize the animal's head initially; a drape, piece of paper, or Plexiglas shield may be used to block the animal's vision while the hands grasp the animal behind the head. The Plexiglas shield can be held in one hand, pressing the head of the snake to the floor, while the other hand grasps the snake at the base of the skull

as the shield is slowly moved rostrally off the body. A snake hook may be used to pin the head to the floor. When a snake hook is used, a suitable soft and resilient padded surface is useful to help restrain the animal to prevent trauma. The hook is then replaced by a hand. In using a snake hook, it is possible to injure the reptile by applying too much pressure; therefore, only experienced technicians should use a snake hook on client's animals. Most snakes can be easily maintained through hand control at the base of the skull. A few snake species can autotomize their tails as a defense mechanism. Snakes should not be picked up by their tails to prevent skin loss (degloving injury) and autotomization.

> **✏ TECHNICIAN NOTE**
>
> Venomous reptiles are not recommended as pets and should be handled only by experienced snake handlers and veterinarians.

Plexiglas tubes may be used in conjunction with a hook or pole. The hook is used to guide the snake into the Plexiglas tube, and the tube should be of sufficiently small diameter to prevent the snake from turning around and coming back out of the tube. The aim is to get the snake to crawl up the tube; when it has reached the point of being halfway in the tube, the technician grasps the junction of the snake and the tube, trapping the animal's head within the tube. Plastic tubes are not generally recommended for many elapid snake species because of their ability to turn around and injure the handler.

For further restraint, a gas anesthetic unit may then be attached to the open end of the tube. The caudal half of the animal is accessible with this technique. Snakes may also be anesthetized by placing them in a plastic bag or box and filling the bag or box with anesthetic gases. They are then intubated and monitored on a gas anesthetic machine with intermittent ventilation (Fig. 23–19).

Snakes can be easily transported in canvas bags. When

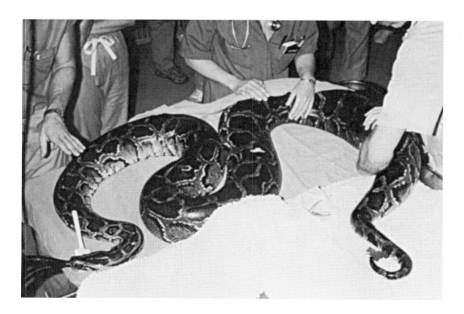

Figure 23-19. Intubation and anesthesia with isoflurane of a Burmese python for deep palpation. Anesthesia was induced by placing the snake inside a large plastic trash bag filled with isoflurane.

handling snakes, the body should always be supported, and large species should never be handled alone.

When working in a veterinary clinic, it is always important to remember to wash the hands well before handling reptiles, particularly if the previous patient was a rabbit or rodent—many snake's typical prey—because snakes attack primarily on the basis of smell.

> **TECHNICIAN NOTE**
>
> It is always important to remember to wash the hands well before handling reptiles, particularly if the previous patient was a rabbit or rodent—the snake's typical prey—because snakes attack primarily on the basis of smell.

Lizards and crocodilians may be restrained using a combination of experienced hands, snare poles, towels, drapes, nooses, or Plexiglas shields. All lizards will tend to bite, and some have strong jaws and sharp teeth. In addition, most lizards will use their claws and tails as weapons. The approach for small to medium-sized lizards is to attempt to block their vision with a towel or sheet of paper, make a quick grab around the shoulder girdle at the base of the skull with one hand, and then restrain the pelvic girdle with the other hand. The tail may then be tucked in against the body, under the arm (Fig. 23–20). For very small lizards, a noose made of fine fishing line at the end of a pole may be used. The noose is lowered over the animal's neck, and the pole is quickly lifted, with the noose tightened

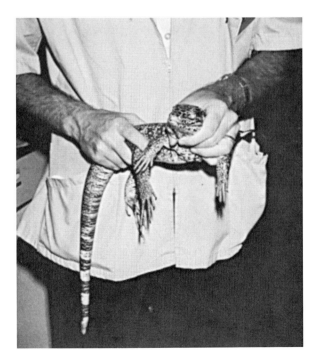

Figure 23–20. Proper restraint technique for a large lizard (tegu). One hand is placed firmly about the pelvis, and the other is about the shoulders and neck. The tail may be tucked beneath the elbow.

and the animal lifted by the neck. The animal should be restrained and removed from the noose as quickly as possible.

For large lizards and crocodilians, it is important to block the animal's vision and then quickly and safely immobilize the head and body simultaneously. This is best accomplished by grasping the animal at the base of the skull or neck with one or both hands and then sitting on the reptile. Two or more people are necessary, and the mouth should then be taped shut. A noose or rabies pole may be used to help control the mouth before attempting to restrain the head, legs, and tail. Crocodilians, most large lizards, and some chelonians can be immobilized for short periods of 20 to 30 seconds by application of gentle inward pressure on their closed eyes for a few moments. Many lizards have tails that detach during stress or trauma. Use extreme caution when grabbing any lizard or reptile by the tail.

> **TECHNICIAN NOTE**
>
> Many lizards have tails that detach during stress or trauma. Use extreme caution when grabbing any lizard or reptile by the tail.

Sample Collection and Diagnostic Procedures

Diagnostic approaches in reptiles are often similar to those of other small animal species.

Colonic Wash. Fecal samples may be collected and examined for GI parasites. A fresh sample should be examined under a wet mount, and fecal flotation and sedimentation should also be done. If a fecal sample is not available at the time of the examination, specimens may be collected by performing a colonic wash; this is done by passing a lubricated tube or catheter through the cloaca into the colon. A syringe of sterile saline is attached, and a typical flush is performed (Fig. 23–21). Samples may then be examined for parasites or parasite eggs or prepared for cytology or culture and sensitivity tests.

Bone Marrow. Large lizards, crocodilians, and some chelonians yield adequate bone marrow specimens from their femoral cavities (Frye, 1995). Bone marrow from turtles and tortoises may also be obtained by drilling a hole between the outer and inner layers of the bony shell and using a biopsy needle (Vim-Silverman, Becton-Dickinson Primary Care Diagnostics, Franklin Lakes, NJ) to obtain the sample (Frye, 1995). The hole should be patched with epoxy or acrylic resin (Frye, 1995). Snake bone marrow specimens may be obtained from the marrow cavities in their ribs.

Stomach Lavage. To examine the upper GI tract, especially for identification of cryptosporidiosis, a stomach wash is often performed. This procedure is well tolerated by most reptiles and is a quick and easy procedure in the clinic. A lubricated soft rubber catheter is advanced through the mouth into the stomach after premeasuring alongside the animal. A syringe containing sterile isotonic saline is attached to the catheter, and a simple flush is performed after agitating the stomach with

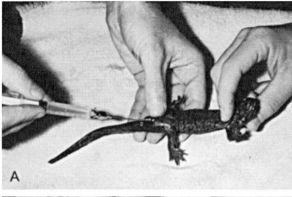

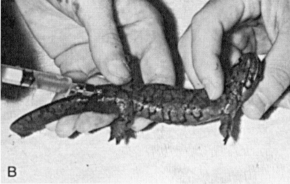

Figure 23-21. Colonic wash in a tiger salamander using (A) a metal ball-tipped gauge needle and (B) a syringe of warm, sterile saline.

external palpation. Samples obtained are used for direct microscopic examination for parasites, to prepare slides for cytology, or to perform Gram stains or culture and sensitivities.

Urine Samples. Urine samples may be collected from those species that produce a large volume of urine. Many turtles and lizards have urinary bladders. All reptiles have a cloaca into which the reproductive, GI, and urinary tracts empty. A routine urinalysis may be performed on fresh urine samples. A cystocentesis may be performed on turtles by advancing a needle cranial to the hind limb. Turtles will typically void when stressed; thus, simply handling them may yield a urine sample. Green-stained solid urates when rehydrated with saline may reveal amoebic cysts and/or fluke ova when examined under a microscope.

Blood Samples. Blood collection in reptiles varies considerably, depending on the species. Do not withdraw more blood than is necessary. If you are not sure of the volume needed, contact your diagnostic laboratory. Direct cardiocentesis and venipuncture using the ventral and lateral caudal veins, jugular, brachial, popliteal, periorbital, pterygopalatine, and dorsal post-occipital sinuses can be used depending on the species and size of the animal (Frye, 1995). Toenail clipping is not recommended for blood sample collection due to the inability to obtain reliable hematologic results from this site.

Venipuncture techniques in snakes depend on the experience of the handler. Sites that are often used include the caudal or coccygeal vein of the tail, cardiac puncture, and the ventral abdominal vein or palatine vessels. For any site, good restraint is necessary. For lizards, the caudal tail vein is often the most accessible; however, cardiac puncture and the ventral abdominal vein may also be used (Figs. 23–22 and 23–23). In turtles, large jugular veins are present and are easily used for venipuncture sites (Fig. 23–24).

In large crocodilians, turtles, and tortoises, the occipital sinus or the caudal vein of the tail may be used. The site chosen will depend on the veterinarian and the technician and their experience with that species. In small lizards, the peribulbar and retrobulbar plexi may be used for blood samples by inserting a heparinized microhematocrit tube between the eyelids and directing it to the inner edge of the orbit.[1] Rotating the tube will damage the plexis yielding enough blood to fill the collection device.

Radiography. Radiography often is useful to aid in the diagnosis of reptile patients. For many species, radiographs may be

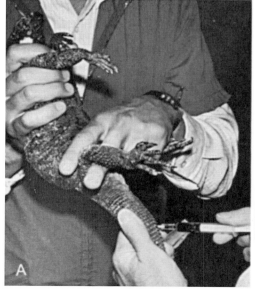

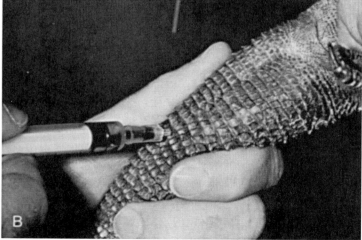

Figure 23-22. Restraint of a giant chuckwalla for venipuncture using the tail vein.

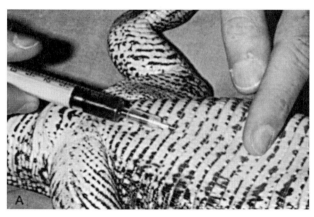
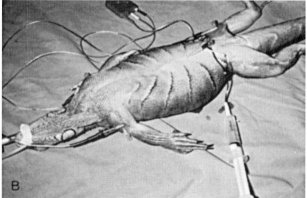

Figure 23-23. A, Venipuncture from the ventral abdominal vein from an anesthetized regu lizard. This is a blind technique. B, Intravenous catheter placed in ventral abdominal vein and ECG lead placement in an anesthetized common iguana.

taken on unsedated animals by restraining them in shallow boxes, acrylic tubes, or canvas bags. It is important to remember to take at least two views. With turtles, a third view—a frontal view—should also be taken. Contrast studies may be done, and barium sulfate is easily administered; however, gastrointestinal transit times are long, and it may take 1 week to complete a gastrointestinal barium study. Various other diagnostic procedures may be used, according to the preference of the veterinarian. The technician's knowledge of restraint and reptile behavior will aid in any immobilization process.

Husbandry in the Hospital. Reptiles are easily provided for in a hospital setting. It is important to remember that temperature and humidity are important because these animals are poikilothermic, that is, dependent on their environment to regulate their body temperature. A temperature gradient should be provided whenever possible by using a thermostat at each end of the cage resulting in a cooler and a warmer end. For most species, temperatures should not exceed 32°C (90°F) or dip below 24°C (75°F). It is important that hospitalized reptiles are maintained at the upper end of their temperature gradient during convalescence to aid in recovery. For many species, a variety of aquaria are sufficient for short-term hospitalization. Any substrate used should be one that is easily cleaned and

disinfected or disposable, such as newspaper. It is important to house reptiles separately from psittacine birds, in particular, to avoid contamination of birds from the normal gram-negative flora of most reptiles. Cages should be provided with hide boxes or areas of seclusion, as well as perching for some species such as iguanas and some snakes.

TECHNICIAN NOTE

It is important that hospitalized reptiles are maintained at the upper end of their temperature gradient during convalescence to aid in recovery.

Tube feeding is an important technique for the veterinary technician to become adept at when handling reptiles. Tube feeding is easily accomplished, even by those without much experience with reptiles. A tube should be well lubricated and then passed the distance necessary to place it in the stomach. The glottis of reptiles is adjacent to the base of the tongue and is easily avoided. The glottis of snakes may actually be extended by the animal outside the mouth to accommodate large prey items. The tube is gently passed all the way to the stomach, and food is injected. Fluids may also be administered by this route. For patients that are anorectic, supplemental tube feeding may be accomplished by using a blended formula of food that is appropriate for the species being cared for. There are a number of dietary references for reptile species listed in Recommended Reading. It is imperative that the technician become familiar with proper reptile diets to maintain healthy animals and supplement sick patients.

Injections in reptiles are usually performed on the cranial half of the animal's body. This is due to the renal portal system that routes blood from the caudal third of the body through a capillary network into the kidneys before returning it to general circulation. It is important to remember not to give nephrotoxic drugs in the caudal third of the reptile's body. Injection sites are easily found in all reptile species, either in the forelimbs or in the epaxial musculature of the snake. Oral medications are

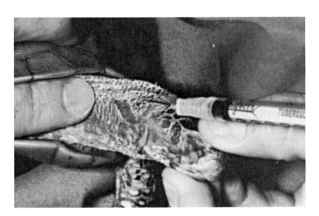

Figure 23-24. Jugular venipuncture in a box turtle. The jugular veins are located dorsally in the 10 and 2 o'clock positions.

easily given using a stomach tube. Liquids are preferred over tablets, which are not consistently absorbed.

Dietary requirements vary tremendously from species to species and may be an important factor in the disease of the patient. Dietary deficiencies are not commonly seen in snakes, which eat a whole-animal diet; however, a variety of dietary deficiencies are commonly seen in lizards, turtles, and crocodilians. One of the most common is metabolic bone disease. Metabolic bone disease is caused by inappropriately low calcium intake, low vitamin D$_3$ intake, or excessive phosphorus intake (Fig. 23–25). This may be prevented by suitable diets and exposing the animal to ultraviolet light, either naturally or artificially. It is essential that reptiles, especially lizards, have full-spectrum light available during normal daylight hours. Sunlight through glass is insufficient to prevent nutritional deficiencies. The animals with metabolic bone disease must be treated very gently because the bones are subject to pathologic fractures. Vitamin A deficiency is commonly seen in turtles and tortoises and usually manifests itself by overgrown beak, palpebral edema, and conjunctivitis. This underscores the importance of thoroughly researching the dietary history of the reptile patient.

TECHNICIAN NOTE

It is essential that reptiles, especially lizards, have full-spectrum light available during normal daylight hours.

Skin. There are clinical dermatologic diseases noted in reptilian species as in other animals. Proper diagnostic techniques are needed to identify the problem to implement the appropriate treatment.

Skin specimens may be cultured for bacterial and fungal organisms. For fungal identification, DTM fungal growth medium and/or Sabouraud's culture media may be used. Bacterial organisms may be isolated on blood agar or subcultured in thioglycholate-containing medium. Samples for skin culture may be taken using cotton-tipped culturettes or by using pieces of the affected skin, scales, or dermal scutes.

Feces. Fecal material can be very useful in diagnosing parasite infestations, bacterial infections, pancreatic enzyme levels, and

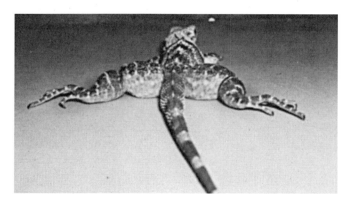

Figure 23–25. Metabolic bone disease in a lizard due to an improper diet.

the presence of blood in the gastrointestinal tract. The fecal specimen should be as fresh as possible. If a fresh voided sample is not available, then fecal material may be removed from the terminal alimentary tract by gentle palpation or by the insertion of a fecal extractor or cotton-tipped applicator stick through the cloacal vent (Frye, 1995). The aid of a warm water enema may stimulate defecation in difficult cases.

Sputum. To obtain a sample of sputum, insert a cotton-tipped applicator into the discharge. Roll the sample applicator across a microscope slide, add a drop of coloring agent, apply a coverslip, and examine for parasite ova (Frye, 1995). Common parasites diagnosed in sputum samples are *Rhabdias* spp., *Entomelas* spp., and *Strongyloides stercoralis*. When handling diagnostic samples, proper hygiene is essential because of the zoonotic potential of many animal diseases and parasites.

Zoonoses and Common Clinical Problems

The technician should be aware of some common zoonotic infections and clinical problems (see Chapter 7).

Most reptiles carry a variety of gram-negative enteric bacteria. This may include such species as *Salmonella* spp., *Arizona* spp., *Klebsiella* spp., and *Providentia* spp. Many of these may cause infection in people as well as in other animals. It is therefore important to keep the reptile separate and to maintain a high standard of sanitation when working with these animals.

Bites from reptiles should be treated as potentially severe infections. Wounds should be thoroughly scrubbed out, and medical attention should be sought.

FERRETS

Ferrets have been gaining in popularity over the past decade. Elective surgery (ovarohysterectomies and neutering) is common in these animals. As ferrets are seen with increasing frequency in veterinarians' offices, it is imperative that technicians become familiar with these pets.

Restraining a ferret is sometimes difficult. Ferrets belong to the family group that includes weasels, and as such, are quick, agile animals and possess a sharp set of teeth. The ferret's primary weapons are its teeth, and when threatened, it will not hesitate to bite. Ferrets that are hand raised, however, do make docile pets in the right circumstances. As with all animals in the veterinary clinic, proper precautions should be taken when restraining ferrets.

Primary restraint for a ferret is to secure the head and forelegs by gripping the animal with one hand behind the neck and around the shoulders (Fig. 23–26). The other hand is used to support the bottom of the animal. For the highly aggressive ferret, a towel or drape may be placed over the animal to occlude its vision and the animal's head, neck, and shoulders grasped through the drape or towel. The handler may want to use gloves. Remember, it is not good for any pet animal to associate negative experiences with gloved hands. Once the animal is restrained in this method, the handler may alter the grip on the head to perform a thorough physical examination and other diagnostic techniques.

For obtaining sample collections of blood, physical restraint alone is not often adequate. Blood samples are drawn from either the jugular vein, the cranial vena cava, or the cephalic vein. To draw samples of blood from these sites, the

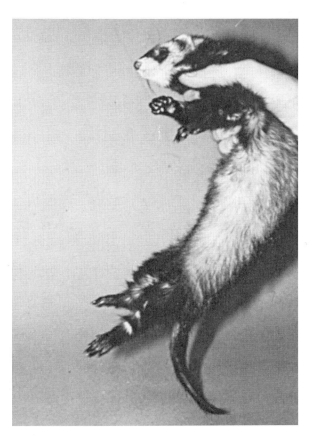

Figure 23-26. Proper restraint of a ferret with the head and forelegs secured. The other hand should be placed to support the bottom of the animal.

animal's head must be securely restrained and grasped around the neck with thumb and fingers resting on the mandibles. To position an animal for jugular venipuncture, it is often best to stretch the animal out, using the other hand grasping the hind limbs. The ferret's thick skin and subcutaneous fat make blood collection from the jugular vein difficult. To draw adequate blood samples, however, anesthesia or sedation is commonly employed, especially from the cranial vena cava (Fig. 23–27). Ketamine hydrochloride or gas anesthetic agents such as halo-

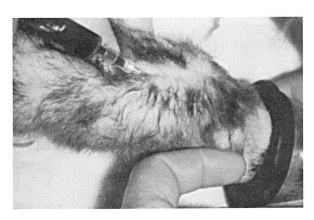

Figure 23-27. Jugular venipuncture of an anesthetized ferret with its head in an anesthetic mask to the right.

thane or isoflurane may be used. When using gas anesthetics in ferrets, it is easiest to place them in an induction chamber, such as a Plexiglas box, to which the anesthetic machine is then attached. The animal may be removed from this chamber as soon as it loses the ability to right itself. Anesthesia may then be continued with the use of a face mask. Sample collection on the anesthetized animal is much easier, safer, and less stressful to the animal. Urine may be obtained by cystocentesis since the bladder is easily palpated. If desired, for prolonged anesthesia, ferrets are easily intubated with small standard endotracheal tubes or Cole tubes.

Strategies for treating ferrets in the clinic revolve around the handler's ability to restrain the animal and perform the treatment in the most efficient and quickest manner possible. For giving drugs, dairy products and sweets are useful in bribing animals and in hiding medications. Most ferrets will do almost anything for yogurt or ice cream. Liquid medications are much easier to administer than pills.

A potentially fatal common clinical problem of the ferret is estrogen toxicity in females due to prolonged estrus. Female ferrets are induced ovulators and occasionally will not cycle out of heat unless bred. These animals then become severely anemic and thrombocytopenic due to the toxic effects of estrogen on the bone marrow. Ferrets often present with signs of lethargy, dyspnea, petechial hemorrhages, vomiting, and diarrhea. This is best treated by prevention and client education. Female ferrets not intended for breeding should be spayed.

Clinical signs similar to those of prolonged estrus, hair loss and swollen vulva, may be due to adrenal hyperplasia. Female ferrets that have been spayed at an early age are extremely susceptible to this clinical condition. An adrenal hyperplasia work-up should be performed on an older spayed female ferret exhibiting signs of vulvar swelling. Adrenal hyperplasia can be treated by a partial adrenalectomy and/or administration of therapeutic agents. Response to therapy and surgery has been varied.

Ferrets are susceptible to human influenza, and therefore clients should be counseled that when members of the family have influenza the ferret should not be handled. Human influenza in a ferret must be differentiated from canine distemper and bacterial pneumonia, to which ferrets are also susceptible. Both present with similar signs of respiratory disease: nasal and ocular discharges, coughing, and sneezing. The ferret with influenza will, in most cases, get over the infection on its own in 5 to 10 days. Topical antihistamines and decongestants may be of benefit. The nonvaccinated ferret will not survive a canine distemper infection, and signs usually progress to severe dyspnea, anorexia, and sometimes involvement of the central nervous system.

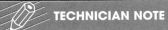

TECHNICIAN NOTE

A potentially fatal common clinical problem of the ferret is estrogen toxicity in females due to prolonged estrus.

Parasites are a problem that must be understood by the ferret owner. Heartworm prevention is required in animals maintained in an outdoor enclosure or exposed to mosquitos.

Fleas commonly plague ferrets, even if maintained within a household setting. Feline flea control products are generally safe to use on flea-infected animals (see Chapter 6).

Ferrets are also fond of chewing on things, preferably soft rubbery objects, and, as such, should be watched closely for foreign body ingestion. A ferret that presents with signs of anorexia should be considered as having a potential GI obstruction. There are also many reports of various neoplastic diseases in ferrets, including insulinomas, osteomas, lymphosarcomas, and fibrosarcomas. If a ferret presents depressed or moribund, a blood serum glucose test should be performed because of common hypoglycemia.

Ferrets should be vaccinated for canine distemper with a chick embryo cell line product. A distemper vaccine approved for ferrets is manufactured and recommended. Under no circumstances should a canine distemper vaccine of ferret cell origin be used. The animal should be revaccinated according to the schedule used for dogs (see Chapter 14). Ferrets are not susceptible to feline panleukopenia and therefore need not be vaccinated. Other preventive medicine measures regarding ferrets include good dental care and surveillance for GI parasites. Ferrets are strict carnivores and, as such, should be fed a strict carnivore diet. The Purina Company does make a ferret chow. If this is not available, a high-quality cat food may be used. Although this may be slightly low in protein requirements for the pregnant or lactating ferret, few problems have been reported in ferrets on high-quality cat food diets.

> **TECHNICIAN NOTE**
>
> Ferrets should never be vaccinated against canine distemper using a vaccine of ferret cell origin.

The zoonotic disease of primary importance in ferrets is rabies. Although ferrets are potential carriers, their indoor lifestyle makes exposure very unlikely. Only one case of a rabid ferret that bit a human has been documented, and this was an animal that had escaped from its owner. Ferrets should be vaccinated for rabies, using only a vaccine approved for use in ferrets.

RABBITS

The rabbit is not a rodent but rather a lagomorph of the family Leporidae. Rabbits may be housed indoors or outdoors and may be fed one of many commercial pelleted feeds. Rabbits come in many sizes, ranging from the Flemish Giant (6 to 7.5 kg) to the Dutch and Polish breeds (1 to 2 kg). If proper husbandry practices are maintained, a pet rabbit should live a long, healthy life (5 to 6 years). Rabbits are sensitive to extreme hot and cold conditions.

Rabbit restraint is important (Fig. 23–28). The most common cause of spinal fracture or dislocation is improper restraint. A rabbit should *never* be picked up, carried, or restrained by the ears. To carry a rabbit short distances, grasp the nape skin with one hand while supporting the rear legs with the other (Fig. 23–29). When walking long distances, the handler should conceal the head in the bend of the elbow while supporting

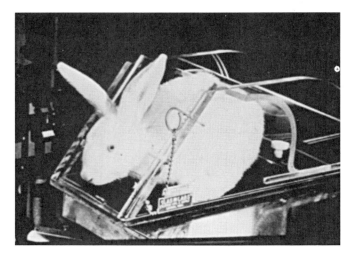

Figure 23–28. Rabbit in special restraint box.

the body with the forearm and grasping the flank with the opposite hand (Fig. 23–30). Small plastic pet carriers should be used when carrying rabbits long distances.

> **TECHNICIAN NOTE**
>
> A rabbit should *never* be picked up, carried, or restrained by the ears.

Rabbits defend themselves by using their long incisors to bite and by kicking with the hind legs. To sex the rabbit, stretching the perineum while the animal is in dorsal recumbency will reveal the anogenital area. Males have a round urethral opening; females have a slit opening.

The rabbit that is a candidate for anesthesia should have

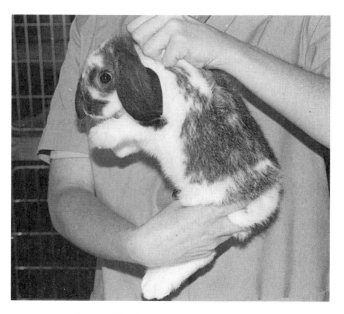

Figure 23–29. Proper rabbit restraint.

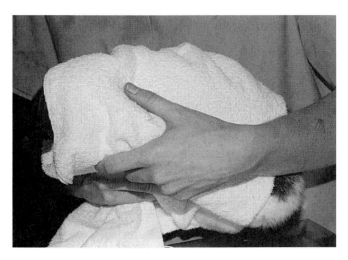

Figure 23-30. Technique for carrying a rabbit over short distances.

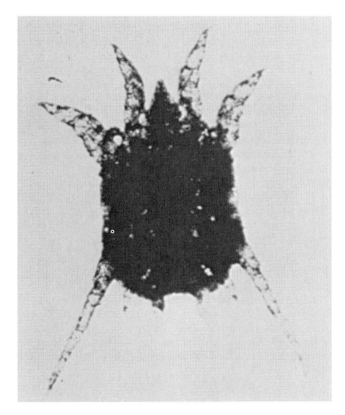

Figure 23-31. Microscopic view of *Psoroptes cuniculi,* the rabbit ear mite.

food withheld for 8 to 12 hours and be free from respiratory disease. Some strains of rabbits have atropinesterase, which inactivates atropine. Atropine may be given subcutaneously as a preanesthetic to decrease salivation. If a rabbit has atropinesterase, it may be necessary to increase the dose of atropine. Rabbits are seldom intubated during anesthesia because they rarely regurgitate and are difficult to intubate. Recommended endotracheal tubes in rabbits have inside diameters of 2.0 to 4.0 mm. A medium laryngoscope will aid in passing the tube into the rabbit's glottis to near the thoracic inlet. Do not use topical anesthetic in rabbits to prevent laryngospasm.

TECHNICIAN NOTE

Rabbits are seldom intubated during anesthesia because they rarely regurgitate and are difficult to intubate.

Injectable anesthetic agents used in rabbits include ketamine, xylazine, and acepromazine; isoflurane is the inhalation anesthetic of choice. The movement of the nictitating membrane over approximately one third of the cornea, a respiratory rate of 18 to 24 respirations per minute, abdominal musculature relaxation, and the loss of the ear, mouth, toe pinch, and palpebral reflexes indicate a suitable plane of surgical anesthesia in the rabbit.

By placing a rabbit in dorsal recumbency and gently stroking its ventrum, one causes hypnosis to occur. Hypnosis is a good restraint for injections and radiographic procedures.

To give intravenous injections to rabbits, the dorsal surface of the ear should be shaved to expose the marginal ear vein. Visibility of this vein will increase if alcohol is rubbed on the area. The marginal ear vein or central artery can also be used for bleeding. Cardiac puncture for blood collection should be used only under strict professional supervision and only as a last resort in the clinical setting.

Rabbits are affected by a number of infectious and parasitic organisms. A pet rabbit may be presented for hair loss due to self-trauma, nutritional deficiencies, bacterial dermatitis (*Pasteurella multocida, Pseudomonas aeruginosa, Staphylococcus aureus,* and *Fusobacterium*) or parasites (ear mite *Psoroptes cuniculi* [Figs. 23–31 and 23–32], fur mite *Cheyletiella parasitovorax,* and rabbit lice *Haemodipsus ventricosus*). Ulcerative lesions on the ventral surface of the rear hocks is usually due to poor husbandry or environmental pressures. Fungal organisms that have been noted to cause dermatopathies in rabbits are *Microsporum gypseum* and *Trichophyton mentagrophytes.*

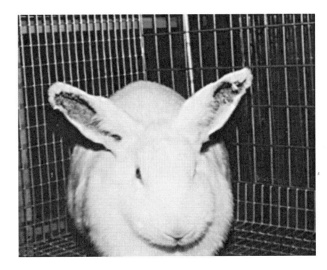

Figure 23-32. Rabbit exhibiting typical clinical signs of *Psoroptes cuniculi* infestation.

An anorexic pet should be examined for malocclusion, hair balls, trauma, dietary change, stress, or poor feed. Heat stress (stroke) is common when adequate cooling is not provided in the summer. Diarrhea may be caused by colibacillosis, rotavirus infections, *Clostridium* infections, mucoid enteropathy, antibiotic intake, and Tyzzer's disease *(Bacillus piliformis)*.

One of the main disease problems in rabbits is *Pasteurella multocida* infection (snuffles). Clinical signs include nasal discharge, torticollis, abscesses, conjunctivitis, and respiratory distress. Venereal spirochetosis should always be considered when rabbits are exhibiting infertility. *Eimeria steadia* is a hepatic coccidium that may affect attitude and eating habits.

Rabbits are territorial and fight when sexual maturity is reached or a male is placed in a female's cage for breeding. Neutering or ovariohysterectomy is recommended to prevent unwanted offspring.

RODENTS

Rodent species commonly presented to the veterinary hospital include guinea pigs, hamsters, gerbils, and, to a lesser extent, mice and rats. Although all of the animals listed above are rodents, each species has particular anatomical characteristics, dietary requirements and diseases.

Antibiotics in Rodents

Care must be taken when prescribing antibiotics to rodents. Guinea pigs, rabbits, and hamsters are extremely sensitive to penicillin antibiotics, which may cause severe intestinal flora changes; penicillins, streptomycin, and dihydrostreptomycin are drugs that may cause this problem. Tetracyclines work well in cases that require antibiotic therapy. An exotic animal formulary is essential to an exotic animal practice to obtain specific information and dosage.

TECHNICIAN NOTE

Guinea pigs, rabbits, and hamsters are extremely sensitive to penicillin antibiotics.

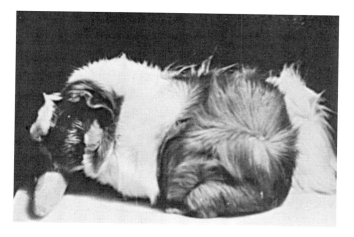

Figure 23-33. An Abyssinian guinea pig.

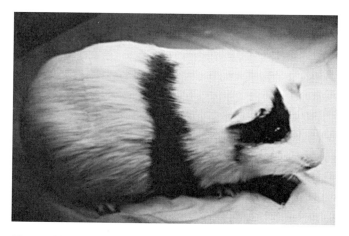

Figure 23-34. The English guinea pig, a common house pet.

Anesthetics in Rodents

Ketamine HCl, pentobarbital sodium, and thiamylal sodium are injectable anesthetics that may be used in rodents. Isoflurane is an acceptable gas anesthetic that provides quick induction and recovery while providing an adequate plane of anesthesia. Chapter 15 discusses anesthesiology.

Antiparasitic Agents in Rodents

Carbaryl powder, dichlorvos, and ivermectin can be used safely to treat ectoparasites. Dichlorvos, thiabendazole, and ivermectin are adequate to treat internal parasites. See Chapter 6 for additional information on parasitology.

Guinea Pig

The cavy, or guinea pig, is a rodent related to porcupines and chinchillas. Guinea pigs have a long gestation that leads to the birth of large, precocious young.

The most common guinea pig species kept as pets are the English or American, Abyssinian, and Peruvian long hair (Figs. 23–33 and 23–34).

The guinea pig has open-rooted teeth that may become maloccluded. The overgrown teeth will irritate the gingiva, causing excessive salivation (Fig. 23–35).

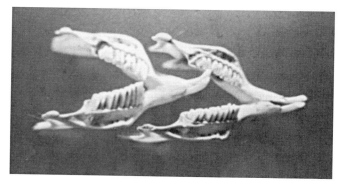

Figure 23-35. Examples of elongated premolars and molars from a guinea pig with malocclusion.

Although the female has only two vaginal mammary glands, it can successfully raise litters of three or more offspring.

A female that is bred past 7 or 8 months of age may have trouble separating the pubic symphysis. Fat pads may also occlude the pelvic canal, complicating parturition. These problems usually lead to dystocia and/or death. If the sow is experiencing dystocia, a cesarean retrieval of the young often yields excellent results. Food preferences are established within a few days after birth for the young. Hand-rearing of the young requires regular stimulation of defecation and urination as with most neonatal mammals. Females usually allow foster nursing of other young.

The pet cavy should be lifted with one hand supporting the dorsal thorax region and one hand under the hind quarters (Fig. 23–36). They rarely become excited or bite. Through their gentle nature, guinea pigs become conditioned to their surroundings and may have an adverse response to change. If a group is contained in an enclosure, subordinate animals may be traumatized (as by hair loss and bite wounds).

Foot pad dermatitis ulcers may develop on animals placed on wire. Metal, plastic, and glass make excellent habit cages. Substrate may be paper (shredded), wood shavings, or hay. Chewing their substrate is a vice commonly associated with an animal developing submandibular abscesses. Hard fibrous splinters penetrate the oral mucosa, inoculating the tissue with bacteria (usually *Streptococcus zooepidemicus*) that develop into abscesses. Changes in the substrate may be indicated to stop this problem, although it may be difficult to find an adequate alternative substrate, which must have absorptive qualities for the opaque, pale-yellow crystalline urine.

The feed and water are best placed in bowls that cannot be chewed (such as stainless steel and ceramic crocks). A vitamin C supplementation may be added to the water, such as Tang (General Foods Corp., White Plains, NY). The food should be a freshly milled complete guinea pig ration. Storage in a freezer or refrigerator will extend the life of the food. All food and water containers should be placed above the substrate to prevent soiling.

Unlike other pet rodents, guinea pigs require dietary vita-

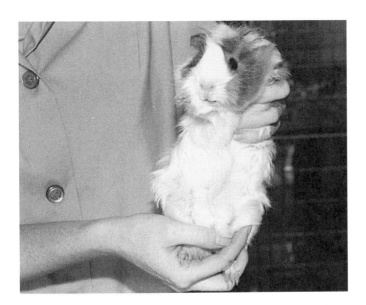

Figure 23–36. Proper restraint technique for a guinea pig.

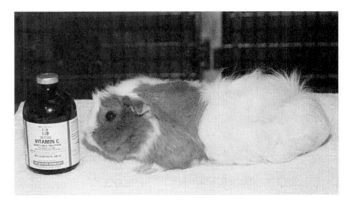

Figure 23–37. Vitamin C dietary supplementation is critical for maintenance of excellent health.

min C supplementation. Vitamin C is highly unstable in the feed, especially when exposed to heat. Old feed is one of the primary reasons that vitamin C deficiencies are seen (Fig. 23–37).

TECHNICIAN NOTE

Unlike other pet rodents, guinea pigs require dietary vitamin C supplementation.

The cavy require 0.5 mg/kg body weight dietary ascorbic acid per day because they lack L-gulonolactone oxidase. Guinea pigs *must* be fed species-specific food within 90 days of milling. Fruit and vegetable supplementation is discouraged because of the possibility of disturbing the normal gut bacterial flora.

To sex a guinea pig, the handler must observe the urethral orifice and anus. The male has no break in the ridge between the openings, whereas the female has a shallow U-shaped break.

One boar will service up to 10 sows beginning at 8 weeks of age. The sow becomes sexually mature around 5 to 6 weeks of age.

Gestation length is on the average 63 to 68 days, with litter size ranging from one to six precocious offspring.

Hamster

The golden hamster is a native of Syria and comes in many different color varieties. Cheek pouches that extend along the head and neck to the proximal dorsum of the back serve as a food transportation device (Fig. 23–38). Along the caudal lateral abdominal region lie the flank glands. A dark-brown patch of skin on each side delineates these sebaceous glands that are used to mark territory and in mating rituals.

Hamsters have a tendency to bite and are good at chewing through cage material. To accommodate the animal's physical nature, an exercise wheel should be placed in the cage.

Female hamsters often attack newly introduced males and females. Hamsters live, on the average, 18 to 24 months, with a gestation length of 16 days and offspring averaging five that wean in 20 to 25 days. If disturbed, the female may cannibalize

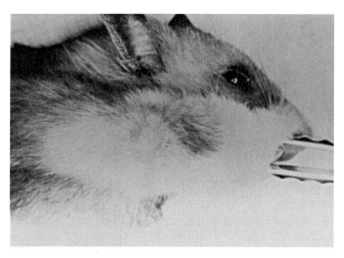

Figure 23-38. Hamster cheek pouches extended by forceps.

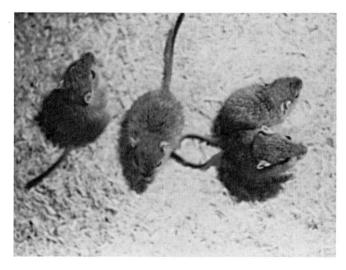

Figure 23-39. Young gerbils.

her litter or hide them in her cheek pouches. When the young are hidden in the cheek pouches, they may suffocate. Hamsters can be picked up by the nape skin at the base of the neck or by cupping the hands under the hind limbs.

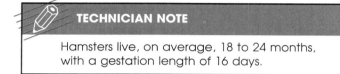

> ✎ **TECHNICIAN NOTE**
>
> Hamsters live, on average, 18 to 24 months, with a gestation length of 16 days.

There are a number of commercially available hamster habitats. An aquarium with a mesh top may be used to house a hamster, with hardwood shavings being the choice substrate. Aromatic shavings such as cedar or pine may cause ocular and respiratory irritation. Sipper bottles are perfect for water dispensing, and nonchewable bowls should be used for food containers or the food should be placed on the floor. All food and water access should be made available to the young.

Males have a greater anogenital distance than females. Hamsters may be mated monogamously or in a harem situation. Females with young should not be disturbed to prevent cannibalism and abandonment of the litter.

Wet tail is used as a general term to describe diarrhea in the hamster. Bacterial infections, cestodiasis, and antibiotic administration may also cause diarrhea in these rodents.

Zoonotic Diseases. Lymphocytic choriomeningitis, salmonellosis, and hymenolepid tapeworm infections are diseases that may be transferred from hamsters to man. Proper hygiene should be practiced after one has handled these animals.

Gerbil

The Mongolian gerbil is a popular pet native to Mongolia and Northeastern China. It is an active burrowing animal adapted to desert environments. Gerbils have a midventral pad consisting of sebaceous glands used in territorial marking.

The gerbil has a life span of 3.5 years, with a gestation length of 25 days without lactation and 24 to 48 days with

lactation. The litter sizes average five that wean in approximately 25 days (Fig. 23–39). Certain gerbil lines are prone to epileptiform seizure activity. Gerbils are friendly rodents that may be housed in hamster units (Fig. 23–40). These animals are good in escape methods; therefore, the cage should be designed to prevent chewing.

The gerbil's diet may be similar to that of the hamster, and water can be supplied in a sipper bottle. Sexing is accomplished by measuring the urogenital distance. The male has a much longer distance than the female. Males aid in the care of the young.

Gerbils commonly present with a nasal dermatitis caused by a bacterial infection initiated by their burrowing activity. Topical antibiotic treatment is recommended for resolution of this infection.

Tyzzer's disease may be diagnosed in gerbils and is caused by *Bacillus piliformis*. Dietary change and colibacillosis also cause diarrhea in these animals.

Mouse

Mice are small rodents that are commonly used in the research setting but make excellent small pets. They are territorial ani-

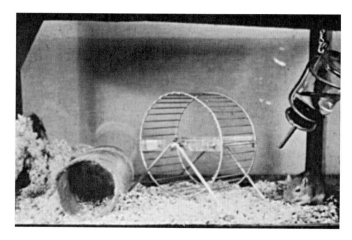

Figure 23-40. Typical small rodent cage containing gerbils.

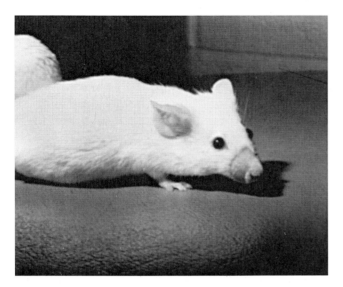

Figure 23–41. Trauma (cage mate–inflicted hair loss) on a mouse. This is commonly referred to as *barbering*.

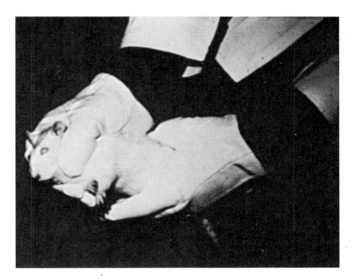

Figure 23–42. Proper restraint of a rat.

mals and quickly develop a hierarchy when placed in groups (Fig. 23–41). These small animals require small amounts of food and water but are escape prone and may develop an unpleasant odor.

Mice should be handled by grabbing the tail with one hand and the back of the neck with the other. Do not use excessive force when grabbing the tail because the skin may be damaged.

Housing should be similar to that of gerbils and hamsters. Hardwood shavings or chips are recommended instead of the aromatic softwood chips (cedar and pine) because of potential liver damage and epithelial damage.

Housing should be cleaned regularly to prevent odor and health problems. Pelleted rodent feed and fresh water in sipper bottles should be supplied free choice.

Male mice have a greater urogenital distance than females. Female mice become sexually mature at 50 days of age and are best bred in the harem scheme, with one male combined with two to six females.

Rat

Rats are clean and unassuming and can be trained to be good pets. These animals may live up to 3 years or longer and become sexually mature at 1½ to 2 months of age.

Restraint is best performed by grabbing the base of the tail and grabbing the animal behind the forelimbs (Fig. 23–42). Rats seldom bite, but caution must be used in a stressful situation.

 TECHNICIAN NOTE

Rats seldom bite, but caution must be used in a stressful situation.

Commercial rodent cages can be obtained for proper housing. Substrate should be similar to that of other rodents.

Males have a longer anogenital distance than females. The gestation length is 22 days, and nesting material should be provided prior to birth.

Although zoonotic diseases are rare in domestic rats, these animals can carry many diseases transmissible to man. These diseases include rat bite fever, *Yersinia pestis,* leptospirosis, *Streptococcus* spp., cestodiasis, and Korean hemorrhagic fever.

Recommended Reading

Boyer TH: A Practitioner's Guide to Reptilian Husbandry and Care. Lakewood, CO, American Animal Hospital Association, 1993.

Campbell TW: Avian Hematology and Cytology. 2nd ed. Ames, IA, Iowa State University Press, 1995.

Carpenter JW, Mashima TY and Rupiper DJ: Exotic Animal Formulary, Manhattan, KS, Greystone Publications, 1996.

Fox JG: Biology and Diseases of the Ferret. Philadelphia, Lea & Febiger, 1988.

Fudge AM (editor): Seminars in Avian and Exotic Pet Medicine. Philadelphia, WB Saunders (published quarterly).

Harkness JE and Wagner JE: The Biology and Medicine of Rabbits and Rodents. Philadelphia, Lea & Febiger, 1995.

Jacobson ER and Kollias GV Jr. (editors): Exotic Animals: Contemporary Issues in Small Animal Practice. New York, Churchill Livingstone, 1988.

Journal of Avian Medicine and Surgery. Lawrence, KS, Allen Press (published quarterly).

Journal of Small Exotic Animal Medicine. Valley Village, CA, Gray Publishing (published quarterly).

Journal of Zoo and Wildlife Medicine. American Association of Zoo Veterinarians, Lawrence, KS (published monthly).

Mader DR: Reptile Medicine and Surgery. Philadelphia, WB Saunders, 1996.

Mattison C: The Care of Reptiles and Amphibians in Captivity. New York, Sterling Publishing, 1990.

Ritchie BW, Harrison GJ and Harrison LR: Avian Medicine: Principles and Application. Lakeworth, FL, Wingers Publishing, 1994.

References

Frye FL: Reptile Clinicians Handbook. Malabar, FL, Krieger Publishing Co., 1995, pp. 70–100.

Wise JK and Yank JJ: Veterinary service market for companion animals. JAVMA 201:990–992, 1992.

24 Veterinary Oncology

Krista Dickinson • *Maura G. O'Brien* • *William S. Dernell*

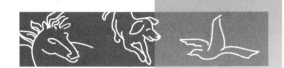

The treatment of cancer in pet animals has become an important field in veterinary medicine. As the quality of pet care has improved over recent years, dogs and cats are living extended lives, and there has been an associated rise in the prevalence of cancer in these animals. Clients have become increasingly aware of the health care needs of their pets and often seek veterinary care for preventative medicine or in the early stages of the disease. It is no longer acceptable practice to disregard seemingly benign lumps and bumps and hope they are not cancer. The four most dangerous words in veterinary oncology are, "Let's just watch it."

In response to the needs of an educated and dedicated clientele that seek improved health care for their pet, training programs have become established in the discipline of oncology. Trained veterinarians are providing expertise in university referral centers as well as private practice. Significant advances have been achieved by studying tumor behavior and response to treatment in spontaneously occurring tumors in animals. The contributions to both human and animal health that can be made in cancer therapy in animals are countless and can be rewarding to the veterinarians and technicians participating in these clinical research programs.

The recognition of the importance of the human-animal bond has also become apparent in veterinary medicine. The emotional aspect of treating cancer in animals cannot be ignored. Many clients have had past experience with cancer either in themselves or in family members or friends. Such experience makes these clients sensitized to the cancer affecting their pet. The veterinarian and technicians treating the cancer patient must be compassionate and recognize the emotional needs of the client as well as provide quality medical care to the animal.

As part of the veterinary health care team, the veterinary technician's role in providing appropriate case management, quality patient care, and client support is vital. Knowledge of the basic principles of oncology will help the technician to understand the diagnostic and therapeutic approach to cancer therapy and to become an active participant in the treatment of the cancer patient.

ONCOLOGY

Oncology is the study of cancer. In general, cancer is defined as an uncontrolled growth of cells on or within the body. This growth can cause clinical signs due to the (1) destruction of local tissue, (2) pain, inflammation, infection, or impairment of function of an organ secondary to the cancer, or (3) paraneoplastic syndromes associated with the cancer. Paraneoplastic syndromes are conditions that occur distant to the tumor itself, usually as a result of the various substances produced by the tumor (Table 24–1). Cancer is therefore not a single disease but rather a collection of hundreds of diseases that can affect all organ systems and tissues as well as various species and breeds. Other terms that have been commonly used to describe cancer include *tumor, neoplasm,* and *growth.*

Tumors can be either *benign* or *malignant.* Benign tumors are characterized by an unchecked growth of cells that do not destroy local tissues but can impair function by their presence. An example of this would be a dog with a large lipoma in the axilla, hindering its ability to use the front leg. Malignant tumors are characterized by an uncontrolled growth of abnormal cells that cause local tissue destruction and also have the potential for metastasis. *Metastasis* is the spread of cancer cells from the primary tumor to distant locations such as lung or liver. The

• Table 24–1 •

EXAMPLES OF PARANEOPLASTIC SYNDROMES AND ASSOCIATED TUMORS

Hypoglycemia

Hepatocellular carcinoma
Hepatoma
Islet cell carcinoma
Lymphoma
Hemangiosarcoma
Leiomyosarcoma
Oral melanoma

Hypercalcemia

Lymphoma
Anal sac apocrine gland
  adenocarcinoma
Parathyroid tumors
Thymoma
Mammary adenocarcinoma
Multiple myeloma

Disseminated intravascular coagulopathy

Hemangiosarcoma
Thyroid carcinoma
Others

Cancer cachexia

Multiple tumors

Leukopenia

Lymphoma
Multiple myeloma

Anemia

Multiple tumors

Hyperproteinemia

Multiple myeloma
Lymphoma

Thrombocytopenia

Lymphoma
Hemangiosarcoma
Fibrosarcoma
Mammary adenocarcinoma
Nasal carcinoma

Leukocytosis

Lymphoma
Multiple tumors

Gastric ulcers

Mast cell tumors

Adapted from Ogilvie GK: Paraneoplastic syndromes. *In* Withrow SJ and MacEwen EG (editors): Clinical Veterinary Oncology. Philadelphia, JB Lippincott, 1989, p. 30.

ated), with few mitotic figures in the nuclei (slow cell division), and exhibit minimal invasion of surrounding normal tissues. The cells in a similar tumor with a different grade may have poorly defined cell architecture (undifferentiated), exhibit numerous mitotic figures (rapid cell division), and appear to invade normal tissues. Unfortunately, most of these systems have been adapted from human pathology and do not always accurately represent the behavior of similar tumors in animals.

Tumors are staged according to their physical characteristics and the extent of tumor present. The World Health Organization's staging system is known as the TNM system and categorizes tumors according to the presence of tumor at the primary site (T), whether there is involvement of regional lymph nodes (N), and whether tumor is present as metastases at distant sites (M). Further divisions, represented as numbers following the T, N, or M, describe the size and extent of the tumor and evidence of any clinical signs of illness (e.g., "a" means healthy, "b" means sick).

The exact cause of cancer is not fully understood. Carcinogenesis is the process by which normal cells become transformed into neoplastic cells. The development of cancer is thought to be a multifactorial event. In general, two events must take place before cells transform: *initiation* and *promotion*. During the first event, initiation, it is thought that the cell is exposed to some agent that irreversibly alters the deoxyribonucleic acid (DNA). The promoting factors then appear to enhance replication of the transformed cell. Under appropriate

exact mechanism of metastasis is not fully understood and varies between tumor types. Basically, the metastatic process involves viable cancer cells leaving the primary tumor, entering the lymphatic and/or blood vessels, traveling to distant tissues, and then becoming reestablished and capable of growing in the tissue of the distant location.

Tumors can be categorized according to the tissue of origin and their histologic features (Table 24–2). Carcinomas arise from any epithelial tissue, including skin, mucous membranes, and organs such as liver, kidney, prostate, and so forth. Carcinomas generally spread through the lymphatic system. Sarcomas arise from the mesenchymal tissues (such as blood, cartilage, and bone) and generally spread by the circulatory system. A prefix on the tissue type indicates the specific tissue of origin. For example, osteosarcoma would be a sarcoma originating from bone. The suffix of a tumor generally indicates a benign or malignant condition, for example, fibroma (benign) versus fibrosarcoma (malignant). There are exceptions to this rule such as *melanoma, insulinoma,* and *thymoma,* which are all malignant tumors. More than 100 histologic types of cancer exist, and each may require special treatment and carry a different prognosis. It is also important to realize that the incidence and behavior of cancer in dogs versus cats is often quite different.

Additional methods to further classify tumors and to help in predicting the behavior of a tumor and the prognosis include the tumor's *grade* and *stage*. Established grading systems categorize tumors of the same histopathologic type according to shared histologic features. The cells in the tumor of one grade may have well-defined cellular architecture (well-differenti-

• Table 24–2 •

CLASSIFICATION OF TUMORS IN ANIMALS

TISSUE TYPE	BENIGN	MALIGNANT
Connective tissue		(Sarcomas)
Bone	Osteoma	Osteosarcoma
Cartilage	Chondroma	Chondrosarcoma
Fibrous tissue	Fibroma	Fibrosarcoma
Fat	Lipoma	Liposarcoma
Myxomatous tissue	Myxoma	Myxosarcoma
Muscle	Leiomyoma	Leiomyosarcoma
	Rhabdomyoma	Rhabdomyosarcoma
Vascular tissue	Lymphangioma	Lymphangiosarcoma
Hemolymphatic cells		Lymphomas
		Mast cell sarcomas
		Multiple myeloma
Epithelial tissue		(Carcinomas)
Skin		Squamous cell carcinoma
Glands	Adenomas	Adenocarcinomas
Sebaceous		
Sweat		
Ceruminous		
Epithelial lining tissue	Adenomas	Adenocarcinomas
Nasal		
Gastrointestinal		
Biliary tract		
Urinary tract		
Undifferentiated	—	Carcinomas and sarcomas
Mixed tissue types	Mammary gland adenomas	Mammary gland adenocarcinomas
		Mesenchymoma

Adapted from Dubielzig RR: Cancer pathology. *In* Withrow SJ and MacEwen EG (editors): Clinical Veterinary Oncology. Philadelphia, JB Lippincott, 1989, p. 19.

conditions, a single transformed malignant cell may multiply and become an invasive cancer. Carcinogenic influences may include genetic, hormonal, congenital, viral, nutritional, immunologic, traumatic, implantation, irradiation, or chemical factors. Unfortunately, determination of a simple cause-and-effect relationship between a carcinogen and tumor development and prevention of that relationship is rare. Cancer causation and subsequent prevention therefore remain a complicated issue.

The search for all the answers in cancer cause and therapy continues with the hope that each new development will bring oncologists closer to understanding tumor behavior, possible prevention, and options for treatment.

DIAGNOSTIC APPROACH IN THE CANCER PATIENT

Through early diagnosis and appropriate treatment of cancer, the prospects for cure and/or tumor control are greatly improved. A consistent diagnostic approach and biopsy are essential for establishing the correct diagnosis.

History, Physical Examination, and Minimum Data Base

The first step is taking an accurate history from the client and performing a complete physical examination. There is no diagnostic test that can equal the valuable information obtained from a complete history and physical examination. Knowledge of the signalment (age, breed, and sex) of an animal can help in the diagnosis of some tumors and may also help in determining a prognosis. Some types of tumors are known to occur more frequently in certain species or breeds, in either sex, at different ages, and at different anatomic sites. Most companion animals that develop cancer are 6 to 15 years old. It is important to remember that the age of the animal should not be a deterrent to aggressive treatment. The physiologic age, determined by evaluation of cardiovascular, renal, and hepatic function, is more important for predicting risks associated with therapy than is the chronologic age of an animal.

The history should include the owner's conception of the primary problem, clinical signs, duration of signs, any treatments given, and response to treatments. Other concurrent or past medical problems should also be elucidated.

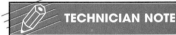

TECHNICIAN NOTE

Use the jugular vein for blood sampling to save peripheral veins for chemotherapy administration.

The physical examination should be thorough (see Chapter 3). All organ systems should be examined, not only to assess the primary problem but also to detect concurrent disease. Regional lymph nodes should be palpated for enlargement, especially those close to the cancer. Evidence of tumor extension beyond the primary site into lymph nodes or distant sites will aid in staging the extent of tumor. Any lumps or bumps detected on the body should be measured and their location recorded in the medical record.

A minimum data base generally consists of a complete blood count (CBC), serum chemistry diagnostic profile (profile), urinalysis (UA), and thoracic radiographs. All blood samples should be obtained through venipuncture of the jugular veins if possible. Peripheral veins should be spared in the event that repeated catheterization for anesthesia or chemotherapy administration is indicated.

The CBC is useful in assessing for the presence of any abnormal parameters in the red blood cells and white blood cells, as well as platelets. The biochemical profile will reveal abnormal values in electrolytes, liver enzymes, creatinine, blood urea nitrogen (BUN), and proteins. The UA helps to assess renal function and should be obtained by cystocentesis to evaluate the urine sediment for abnormalities that may otherwise be obscured by debris washed out of the urethra in a voided sample. The specific gravity of the urine should also be determined before the animal receives any fluid therapy because parenteral administration of fluids can lower the specific gravity. Additional diagnostic tests are available to further assess organ function if indicated by abnormalities detected by the minimum data base.

Radiography

Radiology plays an important role in the diagnosis and staging of cancer (see Chapter 9, Diagnostic Imaging). The lungs are a common site for development of metastases from certain malignant tumors. To accurately evaluate all lung fields for metastatic nodules, radiographs should be obtained when the animal is in right lateral *and* left lateral recumbency, as well as in a ventrodorsal position. Views in two planes are mandatory for all radiographic examinations in order to localize the lesion. The use of the additional lateral view improves examination of both lung fields by allowing the "up" lung to be expanded and filled with air, thereby enhancing the radiographic appearance of any nodule that may be present. Additional radiographs of the abdomen or other regions may be required if indicated by findings on the physical examination to determine the full extent of the disease.

Ultrasound can be used as a noninvasive method to examine the architecture of specific organs or masses found in the thoracic cavity or abdomen. Computed tomography (CT) scans, magnetic resonance imaging (MRI), and nuclear medicine are additional noninvasive diagnostic tools that are available at many universities and some private veterinary hospitals. Each provides methodology to assess inaccessible areas of the body or silent lesions and to help in staging the extent of the cancer and formulating treatment plans.

Cytology

Cytology is the study of individual cell morphology for the purpose of a diagnosis (see Chapter 5, Clinical Pathology). It is an effective screening tool and can help to differentiate neoplasia from inflammation or infection. Results of the cytological examination may then indicate the need for a biopsy to obtain more tissue to determine a diagnosis. Every lump or bump that is identified should be assessed by either cytological or histopathologic examination and not assumed to be benign because of its gross appearance. Collection of populations of cells can be obtained for microscopic examination, with minimal effort, from tissue masses, lymph nodes, bone marrow, or fluid in cysts or body cavities.

Adherence to the proper techniques used for obtaining and preparing these samples is important for accurate results. Failure to obtain sufficient cells or distortion of their architecture by poor processing will make diagnosis impossible. Tumors that are easily diagnosed by cytological examination are generally composed of cells that exfoliate, or shed easily, and can be processed onto glass slides with minimal distortion to their architecture (e.g., mast cell tumors, lymphoma, and histiocytomas).

Samples can easily be obtained by fine-needle aspirates of accessible soft tissue masses or fluid-filled spaces, by impression smears of small biopsy samples or ulcerated lesions, or by needle biopsy of bone marrow. These procedures can be performed quickly with minimal discomfort to the patient. Usually it is not necessary to anesthetize or sedate the patient.

Fine-Needle Aspiration

Samples for cytologic evaluation of cutaneous tissue masses and lymph nodes are obtained by fine-needle aspiration (FNA). Improvements in ultrasound and in fluoroscopically guided instrumentation have also allowed FNA to be used safely within body cavities. For external masses, a 6- or 12-ml syringe, 22- to 25-gauge needle, and clean glass slides, preferably with a frosted edge to indelibly label the slide, are needed to perform the procedure.

The lesion is swabbed with alcohol and stabilized between the clinician's fingers, and the needle is inserted into its center. The needle may be inserted with or without the syringe attached and several core samples obtained by redirecting the needle several times without exiting the skin (Fig. 24–1). Small portions of the needle contents are then squirted onto clean glass slides, and a second slide is used to smear the preparation.

Slides should be labeled with a permanent marker on the frosted edge of the slide before staining. Identification of the slides should include the client's name and identification number and location of the mass that was aspirated. The slides are then air-dried and fixed with appropriate stain. The most common stains available include Wright's stain, new methylene blue, and Romanovsky's stains such as Diff-Quick (American Scientific Products, McGraw Park, IL). Slides can be evaluated in your practice and/or sent to a qualified cytologist for evaluation. Remember that the results of cytology will be useful only if proper technique for sample preparation has been followed and clinical and historical information is complete and made available to the cytologist.

TECHNICIAN NOTE

Stain some of the prepared cytology slides for in-house review but save unstained (representative) slides for outside laboratory review.

Bone Marrow Aspirate

Evaluation of the cellular elements in the bone marrow is sometimes indicated when abnormalities exist in the erythrocytic, leukocytic, or thrombocytic cell lines in the peripheral

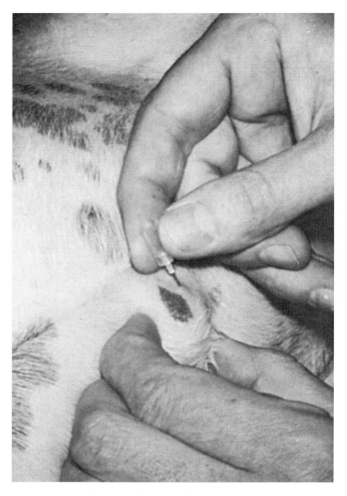

Figure 24–1. Fine-needle aspiration of a cutaneous mass. A 22-gauge needle is inserted into the center of a mass. The needle is redirected several times to obtain an adequate cellular sample. A syringe is then attached to the hub of the needle, and the contents are expelled onto clean glass slides.

blood. The bone marrow is also examined to determine the stage of certain tumors such as lymphoma, multiple myeloma, and mast cell tumors. The most common technique used to obtain a sample from the bone marrow is aspiration biopsy using 16- or 18-gauge bone marrow needle (see Chapter 5, Clinical Pathology). If this method fails to produce enough cells, a core sample can be obtained by means of a Jamshidi bone marrow biopsy needle (American Pharmaseal Co., Valencia, CA).

The optimal sites for biopsy of the bone marrow are the proximal humerus, iliac crest, and trochanteric fossa of the proximal femur. Most animals tolerate this procedure after infiltration of the overlying skin with a small amount of local anesthetic; other animals might require sedation.

Histopathology

Determining the histopathologic diagnosis is one of the most important steps in the overall diagnostic procedure. The results of a biopsy will determine the method of treatment and the prognosis and will often influence the owner's decision to treat.

It is crucial that every mass that is removed be submitted for histopathologic examination, regardless of its gross appearance.

A benefit of histopathology over cytology is that the pathologist is presented with more tissue that is not likely to be distorted by procurement and processing techniques. Individual tumors can exhibit cellular heterogeneity and consist of areas of necrosis, fibrosis, and inflammation as well as neoplastic cells. Because of this variable cellularity, entire masses or multiple representative sections of large tumors should be submitted for evaluation. All tissue samples are examined to determine cell type, histologic grade, and surgical margins.

Common methods used to biopsy tissue include (1) needle core biopsy, (2) incisional biopsy, and (3) excisional biopsy.

Needle Core Biopsy

Specialized needles provide a method to obtain multiple core samples of tissues through small, 1- to 2-mm skin incisions. The Tru-Cut needle (Travenol Laboratories, Deerfield, IL) is most commonly used for biopsy of cutaneous or subcutaneous masses. In addition, adaptations of this type of needle can be used for ultrasonically or fluoroscopically guided biopsy of tissues within body cavities. These needles obtain a 1- to 1.5-cm-long sliver of tissue approximately the same diameter as that of the lead in a pencil. The biopsy site is clipped and prepared for minor surgery. The mass is stabilized between the clinician's fingers, and a small incision (1 to 2 mm) is made in the skin. Local anesthetic infiltrated into the incision site renders sedation or anesthesia unnecessary in most cases. The needle is introduced and the sample is obtained (Fig. 24–2). The tissue is gently scraped off the needle blade and placed in 10% buffered neutral formalin. Impression smears of this tissue can also be made by gently rolling the sample out onto clean glass slides.

Samples of bone lesions can also be obtained by a closed, needle core biopsy in a similar manner. The animal is placed under general anesthesia for this procedure. Trephine bone biopsy instruments or Jamshidi bone marrow biopsy needle (American Pharmaseal Co., Valencia, CA) can be used for bone biopsy procedures. These instruments retrieve multiple core samples of the bone. Possible complications include pathologic fracture of an already weakened bone after biopsy. To minimize this risk, the smaller-gauge Jamshidi needle is preferred, and only one cortex of the bone is penetrated. It is possible to obtain multiple samples from the one cortical access site. The preparation of the biopsy site is as for any sterile minor surgery. To locate the lesion within the bone, one should have knowledge of normal anatomical landmarks, so as to avoid accidental penetration of nearby joints or major nerves and vessels. In addition, two radiographic views of the bone containing the lesion should be available.

Incisional Biopsy

Incisional biopsy consists of making a small skin incision and removing a wedge of tissue. It is useful for obtaining more tissue than by needle core biopsy, especially when the cancer cells are intermixed with abundant necrotic or inflammatory tissue. It is important to limit the size of the incision and to predetermine the placement of the incision, as in needle core biopsy.

Contamination of the biopsy tract with tumor cells is a potential complication with needle core biopsy and incisional biopsy. The biopsy should be obtained through a small incision, with minimal disruption of the surrounding tissue, and the incision should be along the same line as the surgical incision in order that the biopsy tract can be removed with the tumor.

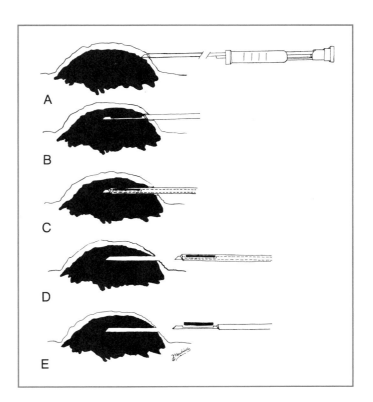

Figure 24-2. Mechanism of action of Tru-Cut biopsy needle used for typical nodular biopsy. A, With the instrument closed, the outer capsule is penetrated. A small skin incision is made with a No. 11 blade to allow insertion of the instrument. B, The outer cannula is fixed in place, and the inner cannula with specimen notch is thrust into the tumor. The tissue to be excised then protrudes into the notch. C, The inner cannula is now fixed, while the outer cannula is moved forward to cut off the biopsy specimen. D, The entire instrument is removed, with the tissue sample contained within. E, The inner cannula is pushed forward to expose the tissue in the specimen notch.

It would be best if the surgeon who will perform the definitive surgery also performs the biopsy or is available for consultation.

Excisional Biopsy

Excisional biopsy involves the complete removal of the mass for biopsy. Depending on the results of the histopathologic examination, this method of biopsy may be all that is required for diagnosis and treatment. A second surgery or adjuvant therapy may be indicated if the tissue margins are not free of tumor.

Biopsy Preparation

Once the biopsy is obtained, it should be handled gently so as not to distort the cellular architecture. Evaluation of the surgical margins is extremely important for determining the success of the removal of the tumor. The edges or surfaces of the resected tissue that need to be carefully evaluated for presence of tumor should be marked so that the pathologist can identify those sites. The use of India ink to "paint" selected margins has been shown to be extremely helpful in marking surgical margins (Rochat et al., 1992) (Fig. 24–3). Ink will not distort the tissue and can be used to mark the entire margin. The ink will be present as a peripheral black line when the tissue is examined under the microscope. If tumor cells are in contact with this ink-labeled margin, then tumor cells probably remain within the animal, indicating the need for further surgery or alternative treatment.

The tissue should then be placed in 10% buffered neutral formalin solution to be fixed. The ratio of formalin to tissue for initial fixation should be approximately 10:1. The tissue should be no thicker than 1 cm to allow penetration of the formalin. If it is thicker, it can be cut as is a loaf of bread to allow the formalin to penetrate, but one edge should be left intact so that the pathologist understands the original orientation of the mass (Fig. 24–4). Once the sample has been sufficiently fixed, it can be transferred to plastic bags (two, at least) or commercial mailers with less formalin (1:1 ratio) for transportation to the laboratory.

A detailed information sheet should accompany the sam-

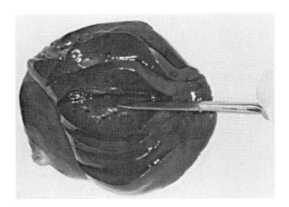

Figure 24–4. A large mass is sliced (loafed) into 1-cm sections. A 1-cm-thick base connecting all the slices is left to help orient the pathologist.

ple. Information that should be recorded includes the clinic and veterinarian's name, owner's name, pet's name, identification number, signalment, site of biopsy, and a brief but detailed clinical history including pertinent treatments and the suspected diagnosis. Any margins that need to be evaluated should be recorded as well. For some tumors, such as mast cell tumors, a histologic grade may also be requested to help predict the tumor behavior.

TECHNICIAN NOTE

For proper fixation, allow a fixative-to-tissue ratio of at least 10:1 and section samples no thicker than 1 cm.

The pathologist is responsible for identifying the tumor type and providing information regarding completeness of surgical margins and histologic grade. However, the pathologist is limited by the quality of the sample submitted and the amount of information provided. It is ultimately the responsibility of the attending clinician to assess whether the pathologist's diagnosis appropriately reflects the clinical presentation of the patient.

THERAPEUTIC OPTIONS

Once a diagnosis is made, the method of treatment is planned. The clinician, technician, and client should discuss the diagnosis and treatment options in terms of prognosis, benefits and complications associated with each treatment, and cost. The clinician should talk in terms that are understood by the client. Informational handouts are helpful to explain commonly performed procedures (e.g., amputation, mastectomies, care and monitoring of incisions and bandages). Handouts can also be used to explain the nature, method of action, timing of administration, and expected side effects of common chemotherapy drugs.

In oncology, the treatment options generally include surgery, chemotherapy, and/or radiation therapy. The use of a single or multimodality protocol is determined for each case.

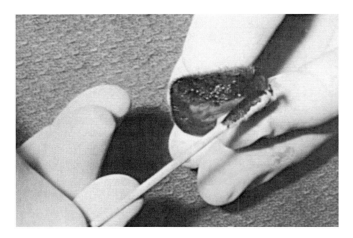

Figure 24–3. The cut edge of a resected mass is painted with India ink to mark the surgical margin. The ink is allowed to dry (1 to 2 minutes) before the mass is placed into 10% neutral buffered formalin.

Surgery

Traditionally, surgery has been the treatment of choice for most types of cancer. It is the best method for removing solitary masses, but its benefits are limited by wide resections that can damage important normal structures or by the extension of tumor to distant sites (metastasis). In such instances, combining surgery with other modalities (adjuvant therapy) or using other modalities in place of surgery is necessary. The oncological surgeon must understand all the potential options for therapy to provide the best care.

Surgical resection of malignant cancer requires an aggressive approach. For the surgery to be successful, the tumor must be removed completely with a minimum of cosmetic and functional loss to the patient. An attempt is made to avoid entering the tumor and exposing the surgical field to tumor cells. Tumor cells released in this manner may implant in the wound and result in local recurrence. Instead, the resection should occur in the normal tissues surrounding the mass. Extensive surgical resections and prolonged surgery times in animals that may be debilitated from the cancer or concurrent disease require careful perioperative planning and monitoring to avoid complications.

It is the responsibility of the clinician and technician to make sure the patient has had a complete presurgical work-up and that the surgical team is aware of any conditions that may complicate anesthesia, surgery, or recovery. The anesthetic protocol must be tailored to the needs of the individual patient. It is best to perform major surgeries early in the day for the animal to receive adequate monitoring in the recovery period. The preparation for surgery should include clipping wide areas for extensive resections, thorough surgical scrubs, and perhaps the use of perioperative antibiotics if prolonged surgery or potential contamination during surgery is anticipated. The benefits of intravenous fluids and regional analgesics (epidural anesthesia, local anesthesia in regional nerves) and the parenteral use of analgesic agents provide for an improved recovery in most patients (see Chapter 20, Pain Management).

Another type of surgery used in treating cancer is cryosurgery. This involves the use of a cold source (usually liquid nitrogen) to freeze superficial cancers usually less than 2 cm in diameter. The tissue then undergoes a period of sloughing before healing. Discoloration or loss of hair may be permanent. This technique is useful for small, superficial lesions, such as eyelid, skin, and anal masses. A disadvantage of cryosurgery is that the completeness of tumor removal cannot be determined because there is no tissue to submit for margin evaluation.

The goal of surgery may be curative or palliative. Palliative surgery is offered when the tumor is resected in order to improve the animal's quality of life, despite metastasis or poor long-term prognosis. An example would be a dog that presents with an ulcerated or painful mass (e.g., mammary gland tumor, osteosarcoma) that has metastasized, but the metastatic lesions are not causing clinical signs. Removal of the mass improves the dog's quality of life until the metastatic disease progresses.

Chemotherapy

Chemotherapy means the treatment of disease by chemical agents. Most people associate chemotherapy with cancer therapy, but in reality all drug therapy (even antibiotics) constitute chemotherapy.

The drugs for cancer therapy are categorized into groups based on their mechanism of action. The majority of these drugs are by nature cytotoxic, and the target is generally the DNA or the protective cellular membrane of the cancer cell. Drugs that disrupt DNA will often target cells that exhibit rapid cell turnover (as in neoplastic cells). Unfortunately, these drugs can also be harmful to normal cells with high cell turnover, such as the cells within the gastrointestinal tract, the bone marrow, and hair follicles.

The dose and timing of administration of each agent are predetermined to achieve maximum cancer cell destruction while at the same time minimizing the damage to normal cells. Dosages are generally based on the surface area of the body (meter squared). A meter-squared dosing chart can be found in Chapter 25 for both dogs and cats. Neutropenia is often the dose-limiting toxicity, and the interval between doses is determined by the response time the bone marrow requires to replenish the leukocyte population.

Antineoplastic drugs at therapeutic doses have the potential to be teratogenic (malforming), mutagenic (chromosomal damaging), and carcinogenic (cancer inducing). The risks from chronic low-dose exposure are unknown, and no safe level of exposure has been identified. The Occupational Safety and Health Administration (OSHA) in February 1994, with the revision of the Hazard Communication Standard, requires by law that employees must be protected from all occupational health hazards, including chemotherapeutics, that are now deemed hazardous drugs (HDs). The veterinary community must recognize, promote, and instate policies and procedures that facilitate the safe mixing, handling, and administration of these agents. A fume hood should be used when mixing chemotherapy agents.

 TECHNICIAN NOTE

Protective gloves, mask, and clothing, as well as appropriate handling precautions, in the work space must be standard protocol when handling antineoplastic drugs.

There are many important nursing considerations in regard to the administration of cytotoxic drugs (Table 24–3). Veterinary professionals must become knowledgeable and skillful in using these antineoplastic agents because many clients want to treat their pets' cancer. Drug toxicities such as myelosuppression (Table 24–4), extravasation (Table 24–5), anaphylaxis (Table 24–6), and problems with personal exposure are well documented. Other toxicities may include alopecia, gastrointestinal upset, cystitis, cardiac toxicity, and/or neurotoxicity. Taking the necessary precautions to minimize these risks to the patient and personnel is vital. References to veterinary literature are necessary to devise appropriate hospital policies for the dosing, mixing, handling, and administration of these drugs (see Recommended Reading).

After each treatment, the patient should be monitored for signs of toxicities. Clients should be given detailed handouts describing known toxicities for each agent. If any abnormalities are detected by the hospital staff or the client, the animal should be reevaluated. If these drugs are administered properly and the client is educated as to the risks, the toxicities can be

• Table 24–3 •

NURSING CONSIDERATIONS FOR THE ADMINISTRATION OF CHEMOTHERAPEUTIC AGENTS		
CONCERNS BEFORE DRUG ADMINISTRATION	**CONCERNS DURING DRUG ADMINISTRATION**	**CONCERNS AFTER DRUG ADMINISTRATION**
Admitting	Extravasation of drug	Latent anaphylaxis
Patient status	Anaphylactic reaction	Nadir toxicities
History since last chemotherapy	Patient comfort	Medications
Physical examination		*Documentation*
Appropriate blood work submitted		Chemotherapy flow sheet
Treatment Plan		Treatment plan
Verification		Client information handouts
Patient, drug/dosage, blood work		
Appropriate catheterization		
Necessary equipment assembled		
Vein selection		
Aseptic technique/absolute clean stick		
Venous challenge with saline bolus		
before and after drug		
administration		
Appropriate protective equipment for		
person mixing and/or administering		
the drug and patient restrainer		
Knowledge of drug toxicities		
Emergency protocols established		
Treatment of extravasation		
Treatment of anaphylaxis		
Treatment of chemical spill		
Client informed of potential toxicities		

From Dickinson K: Unpublished data. Comparative Oncology Unit, Colorado State University Veterinary Teaching Hospital, May 1996.

minimized and the patient can maintain a good quality of life during therapy. The incidence of serious toxicities for most commonly used drugs or protocols should not occur in more than 5% of the cases treated.

Radiation Therapy

Ionizing radiation can also be used for cancer therapy. Radiation causes cell death by disrupting the DNA of the cell or destroying important biological molecules required by the cell. Cell death occurs as a result of the failure of injured cells to repair themselves and/or the inability of subsequent cell generations to divide. Currently, more than 30 radiation therapy facilities are available in the United States to treat animals with cancer.

• Table 24–4 •

MYELOSUPPRESSIVE CHEMOTHERAPEUTIC DRUGS COMMONLY USED IN VETERINARY MEDICINE		
HIGHLY MYELOSUPPRESSIVE	**MODERATELY MYELOSUPPRESSIVE**	**MILDLY MYELOSUPPRESSIVE**
Doxorubicin	Melphalan	L-Asparaginase
Vinblastine	Chlorambucil	Vincristine
Cyclophosphamide	5-Fluorouracil	Bleomycin
Actinomycin D	Methotrexate	Corticosteroids
Carboplatin	Cisplatin	

Adapted from Ogilvie GK and Moore AS. Managing the Veterinary Cancer Patient: A Practical Manual. Trenton, Veterinary Learning Systems, 1995.

Radiation therapy can be used as a single therapy or in combination with surgery, chemotherapy, and hyperthermia. Routine protocols consist of giving multiple doses (fractions) daily on a Monday, Wednesday, and Friday schedule or a Monday through Friday schedule for approximately 15 fractions. Because radiation targets DNA, like chemotherapy, it is most effective in controlling cells with rapid cell turnover. Subsequently, the side effects from radiation therapy are seen in normal tissues with high cell turnover and located in the irradiated field.

TECHNICIAN NOTE

The use of oil-based topical creams should be avoided, and self-trauma should be prevented when dealing with acute radiation dermatitis.

The radiation effects observed are divided into acute and long-term effects. Acute effects are seen during the end stages of actual therapy and, although they may require additional nursing care, are temporary. Late effects develop months to years after treatment and usually involve permanent changes such as necrosis or fibrosis of normal tissues.

Acute effects observed with irradiation of oral or nasal tumors results in mucositis of the oral cavity. Tea or warm water flushes can sooth oral mucositis. Irradiation of skin will induce a desquamative dermatitis or loss of the superficial

• Table 24–5 •

CHEMOTHERAPEUTIC DRUGS THAT ARE CLASSIFIED AS VESICANT/IRRITANT AGENTS

VESICANT		IRRITANT	
Generic Name	**Brand or Other Name**	**Generic Name**	**Brand or Other Name**
Dactinomycin	Actinomycin D	Carmustine	BCNU
Daunorubicin	Cerubidine	Cisplatin	Platinol
Doxorubicin	Adriamycin	Dacarbazine	DTIC
Epirubicin	—	5-Fluorouracil	5-FU
Vinblastine	Velban	Etoposide	VP-16
Vincristine	Oncovin	Mitoxantrone	Novantrone

Definition of terminology used for some chemotherapy agents:
Vesicant—An agent capable of causing tissue destruction and/or necrosis on extravasation at injection site
Irritant—An agent capable of causing pain, inflammation, and blotches at injection site
Extravasation—Leakage of a drug into subcutaneous tissue capable of causing pain, necrosis, and/or tissue sloughing
Antidote—Treatment plan for a specific drug extravasation

Adapted from Cancer Chemotherapy Guidelines: Module—Recommendations for the Management of Vesicant Extravasation, Hypersensitivity and Anaphylaxis. Oncology Nursing Society, 1992.

layers of the epidermis. Both conditions will resolve in 2 to 3 weeks with attention to local hygiene and use of analgesics if needed. The use of oil-based topical creams should be avoided, and self-trauma such as licking should be prevented. Hair loss or change in color may be permanent. The owner must be warned of these effects along with the potential benefits of radiation therapy before treatment.

EUTHANASIA

Unfortunately, cancer therapy does not always result in a cure. In some cases, the best the client and clinician can hope for is a long disease-free interval and a good quality of life. Euthanasia is an important component of pet cancer management. The choice of euthanasia for a pet may be the option chosen by the client at the time the cancer is diagnosed or after therapy has been instituted. In either situation, it is a difficult decision to be made and one that the client should be comfortable with and

decide on after careful consideration of all available treatment options.

The veterinarian and technician must be available to provide all the medical information as well as the emotional support and compassion the client and patient deserve. Many times this support comes from the technical staff. Clients often feel inhibited when talking to the clinician but can sometimes talk more freely with a nurse or receptionist. Technicians need to be aware of the important role they play in veterinary medicine, not only in providing the treatment for the patient but also in supporting the needs of the client. Good communication and compassion are as important as the treatment in cancer therapy and inherent to its success (see Chapter 29).

Reference

Rochat MC, Mann FA, Pace LW, et al.: Identification of surgical biopsy borders by use of India ink. J Am Vet Med Assoc 201:873–878, 1992.

• Table 24–6 •

HYPERSENSITIVITY POTENTIAL OF CHEMOTHERAPEUTIC DRUGS

HIGHEST REPORTED INCIDENCE*	CASE REPORTS
L-Asparaginase	Etoposide (VP-16)
Taxol	Methotrexate
Cisplatin	Cytarabine
Melphalan (intravenous)	Cyclophosphamide
Anthracycline antibiotics	Chlorambucil
(doxorubicin, daunorubicin)	5-Fluorouracil
	Mitoxantrone
	Bleomycin
	Dacarbazine (DTIC)
	Vinca alkaloids
	(vincristine, vinblastine)

*Reports of >5% incidence in the literature.
Adapted from Cancer Chemotherapy Guidelines: Module—Recommendations for the Management of Vesicant Extravasation, Hypersensitivity and Anaphylaxis. Pittsburgh, Oncology Nursing Society, 1992.

Recommended Reading

Cancer Chemotherapy Guidelines: Modules 1–5, Recommendations for Cancer Chemotherapy. Pittsburgh, Oncology Nursing Society, 1992.
Couto CG: Management of complications of cancer chemotherapy. Vet Clin North Am Small Anim Pract 4:1037–1053, 1990.
Dickinson KL and Ogilvie GK: The safe handling and administration of chemotherapeutic agents in veterinary medicine. *In* Kirk RW and Bonagura JD (editors): Current Veterinary Therapy VII. Philadelphia, WB Saunders, 1995, pp. 475–478.
Ogilvie GK and Moore AS: Managing the Veterinary Cancer Patient: A Practical Manual. Trenton, Veterinary Learning Systems, 1995.
Ringlein JW: Principles of oncology nursing and safe handling of chemotherapeutic agents. *In* Skeel RT (editor): Handbook of Cancer Chemotherapy. Boston, Little, Brown & Co., 1987.
U.S. Department of Labor, Occupational Safety and Health Administration. Hazard Communication Standard. 29 CFR 1910.1200, as amended February 9, 1994.
U.S. Department of Labor, Occupational Safety and Health Administration Instruction CPL 2–2.20B CH-4, Directorate of Technical Support, Chapter 21; Controlling Occupational Exposure to Hazardous Drugs, 1995.
Withrow SJ and MacEwen EG: Small Animal Clinical Oncology. 2nd ed. Philadelphia, WB Saunders, 1996.

Ziegfeld CR (editor): Core Curriculum for Oncology Nursing. Philadelphia, WB Saunders, 1987.

Organizations for Cancer Information and Treatment

Veterinary

Veterinary Cancer Society
c/o Dr. Richard E. Weller
Developmental Toxicology Section
Batelle, Pacific Northwest Labs
P7-52, P.O. Box 999
Richland, WA 99352

Human

American Cancer Society
1825 Connecticut Avenue N.W.
Suite 315
Washington, DC 20009

National Cancer Institute
Executive Plaza North
6130 Executive Blvd. MSC 7405
Bethesda, MD 20892-7405
Cancerfax Information Telephone Number
1-800-624-7890

American Cancer Society

25 Pharmacology and Pharmacy

Marvene Augustus

In most practices, the technician shares the responsibility of administering drugs, which can range from the simplest chewable tablet to a gaseous anesthetic. As new drugs and strategies are applied to veterinary care, the role of the technician becomes increasingly sophisticated. The technician must have some knowledge regarding the mechanisms of drug actions and therapeutic uses and potential side effects. Verification that the drug and dosage are correct is a major responsibility of the technician. For this reason, the technician should be familiar with the dosage forms of drugs, able to recognize common medications, and translate drug dosages into the appropriate number of tablets or volume of drug for the individual patient.

This chapter is intended to provide the technician with a minimal basic knowledge of drugs, including the calculation of dosages; drug laws; and drug inventory control. Anesthetic agents and drugs used in the treatment of cancer are discussed in Chapters 15 and 24. There are several good books dedicated entirely to the subject of veterinary drugs; *Drugs in Veterinary Practice* (Spinelli and Enos, 1978) was written primarily for veterinary technicians and should prove helpful for those with a greater interest in veterinary therapeutics.

GENERAL PRINCIPLES

Definitions

A *drug* is defined as any chemical agent that affects living processes; these agents may be used to prevent, diagnose, or treat diseases. *Pharmacology* is a broad term defined as the study of drugs. Aspects of pharmacology include the history and source of drugs *(pharmacognosy)*; physical and chemical properties of drugs and effects and actions of drugs on living organisms *(pharmacodynamics)*; characteristic ability of living organisms to absorb, distribute, metabolize, and excrete drugs *(pharmacokinetics)*; and therapeutic uses of drugs *(pharmacotherapeutics)*.

 TECHNICIAN NOTE

Drugs do not create functions in tissues or organs; they can only modify or alter those that already exist.

Generally, use of the term *pharmacology* is limited to the study of the action of drugs on living systems to produce biological effects. Drugs do not create functions in a tissue or organ but instead modify or alter existing ones.

PRINCIPLES RELATING TO DRUG ACTION

Pharmacokinetic factors of a drug (absorption, distribution, metabolism, and excretion) will determine how the drug enters the body, reaches the site of action, and is removed from the body.

Drug Absorption

For drugs to exert an effect, they must reach their site of action *(target tissue)*. For some drugs, a simple topical application accomplishes this. Most drugs, however, must cross several barriers of cell membranes to produce the desired action. Cell membranes also must be crossed for the subsequent deactivation and elimination of the drug from the body. *Absorption* is defined as the uptake of substances into or across tissues.

Drugs with systemic actions that are administered orally must cross the gastrointestinal lining of the stomach or small intestine to be effective. Absorption of drugs from the gastrointestinal tract will be influenced by several factors. To pass through the membrane lining of the gastrointestinal tract, a drug must dissolve to some degree in oil *(lipid soluble)* because the membranes contain a high concentration of lipid (fat). Ionic *(charged)* forms of drugs do not easily pass through these membranes, whereas the nonionic forms of drugs pass more easily. Most drugs are weakly acidic or basic and have some lipid-soluble properties. The stomach is a highly acidic environment. The weakly basic drugs that are highly ionized (charged) in the acidic stomach will not be readily absorbed until they are farther down the digestive tract in the small intestine, because it is basic in nature. In the small intestine, the weakly basic drugs exist in an un-ionized form, which permits easier transport across the lipid membrane. Drugs that are weak acids are un-ionized in the acidic stomach and diffused more easily through the lipid membrane. They are rapidly absorbed from the stomach and therefore expected to exert their action more quickly than a weakly basic drug. Most drugs with poor lipid solubility cannot pass through cell membranes. Drugs such as the antimicrobial aminoglycosides (e.g., gentamicin) have poor lipid solubility and therefore are inadequately absorbed and ineffective after oral administration.

Stomach contents may inactivate or trap certain drugs. The volume of stomach contents also may delay absorption, thus delaying action. In ruminants, one is confronted not only with slow absorption from dilution but also with the effect of the action of the ruminal microorganisms on certain susceptible agents. Common drugs of plant origin, such as digoxin and atropine, are ineffective in the ruminant when administered orally because of digestive microorganisms.

Drugs that require injection *subcutaneously* or *intramuscularly* must be absorbed from the injection site to exert their action. The subcutaneous route is appropriate for small drug volumes (less than 1 ml) and drugs intended to be absorbed slowly. Due to the limited blood flow, subcutaneous drug administration results in a more sporadic absorption compared with those injected intramuscularly. Insulin and heparin are examples of drugs that are administered subcutaneously. In animals that are highly dehydrated, there is a restricted blood flow at body surfaces, so subcutaneous administration is not usually recommended.

Intramuscular injection is appropriate when a larger volume of drug must be administered. Absorption from the intramuscular site is faster than that from subcutaneous sites because muscles are better supplied with blood vessels than the skin. Procaine penicillin is an example of a drug to be injected in the muscle.

Absorption from the subcutaneous or intramuscular site can be hastened by applying heat or massage to the site to accelerate the blood flow. Conversely, absorption can be slowed by applying ice packs at the injection site to decrease blood flow.

Drugs that are introduced into the vascular system *(intravenous)* will not go through an absorption phase. These drugs are placed directly into the plasma compartment and take effect immediately.

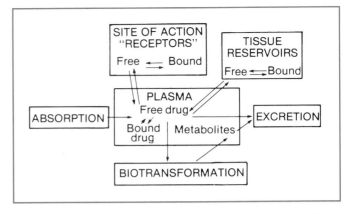

Figure 25-1. Schematic depicting fate of drug on administration.

Figure 25–1 depicts the distribution of drugs after administration. Drug concentration is a dynamic process that continually varies at different sites until it is virtually all excreted. Generally, another dose is administered before the complete removal of the previous dose, so the effective tissue levels *(site of action)* may be maintained. High lipid solubility and low protein binding are favorable characteristics indicative of the ability of a drug to diffuse through membranes. Drug transport into tissues involves passage through lipid-containing membranes. Diffusion is a difficult process for water-soluble compounds.

Most drugs in the blood stream bind in varying degrees to plasma proteins such as albumin. Only the unbound drug *(free drug)*, which may be as little as 10%, is available to diffuse into tissues and produce biological effects. As a rule, drugs bound to albumin or other proteins remain in the blood because these proteins do not diffuse through capillary walls. Drug binding to albumin is a reversible process. Protein binding serves as a reservoir site because the drug becomes available as the plasma concentration of the free drug is reduced. An equilibrium is maintained at all times between protein bound and free drug in the blood. A common form of drug interaction occurs when a second drug has a stronger affinity for the plasma protein. The first drug is replaced and becomes free to exert its effects in a greater concentration at its site of action.

Accumulation of drugs may occur in various body compartments, such as fat, muscle, liver, and so forth, prolonging the effects of the drug as it is released from these storage sites. The potential of a drug to accumulate at these different sites will vary greatly among drugs, depending on their physiochemical properties. For example, a highly lipid-soluble drug, such as thiopental, will accumulate in body fat; this accounts for the slow recovery of obese dogs from barbiturate anesthetics compared with leaner dogs, such as the greyhound.

Although all the aforementioned distribution sites of a drug are important, the amount of drug reaching its site of action is of primary concern. The place at which a drug interacts with cellular components to exert its effect is called a *receptor*. There are numerous receptor sites throughout the body. Some sites are specific for certain drugs, whereas others are general and may respond or interact with several types of drugs.

The ability of a drug to bind to a specific receptor determines the biological activity of the drug. The interaction of a

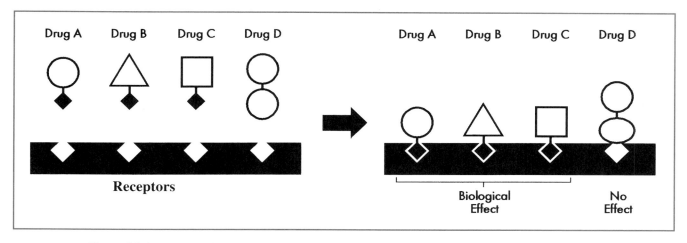

Figure 25-2. Lock-and-key fit between drugs and receptors through which they act. The drug and site on receptor must have definite shapes that conform to each other to bind and produce biological response.

drug with a specific receptor is similar to a lock-and-key fit (Fig. 25–2). Only a certain critical portion of the drug is usually involved in binding with the receptor. Drugs that have similar critical portions but differ in other parts of the biological molecule might be expected to have similar biological activity.

A drug, in interacting with its receptor, may mimic the action of a natural body substance *(transmitter)*. For example, acetylcholine is a natural transmitter that is secreted at terminal nerve endings, causing muscle contraction. A drug (bethanechol chloride) that is chemically similar to acetylcholine produces similar effects. Such drugs that directly produce the normal function of the receptor are termed *agonists*.

Drug Metabolism

For free drugs to be removed *(cleared)* from the blood, they must be excreted directly without change or metabolized *(biotransformed)*. *Biotransformation* is the ability of a living organism to modify the chemical structure of drugs so that they are no longer active *(inactive metabolites)*. The liver is the principal organ responsible for biotransformation, but some of the activity may occur in the kidneys, brain, lungs, small intestine, and other organs.

Simple changes in the drug molecule, such as the removal or addition of certain atoms, may completely inactivate the drug. Through the mammalian enzyme system, potentially toxic compounds are changed into water-soluble compounds, which are more easily eliminated from the body by the kidneys. One means of removing many of the lipid-soluble drugs is through *conjugation*. This process involves the attachment of various endogenous substances to the drug. An example is the attachment of glucuronic acid to aspirin. After conjugation, the aspirin complex is much more water soluble, making it more readily excreted by the kidney. Cats are deficient in the enzymes required to conjugate drugs with glucuronic acid. This accounts for the relatively longer action of certain drugs in cats compared with most other mammalian species that do not have this deficiency.

Other common biotransformations of drugs by the liver include *hydroxylation* and *acetylation*. Biotransformation often inactivates drugs, but it does not always produce inactive prod-

ucts. Drugs such as codeine, diazepam, and amitriptyline are changed by the liver into metabolites that also exert a pharmacological effect. These are called *active metabolites.*

In older animals or animals with hepatic disease, the ability of the liver to biotransform drugs may be impaired. Newborns less than 30 to 60 days of age are generally not capable of metabolizing many drugs because their liver enzyme system is not yet fully developed. To avoid drug toxicity, it might be necessary to reduce the drug dosage, increase the interval between doses, or switch to a drug that is not metabolized by the liver.

A few drugs are administered in an inactive form and do not become active until they are biotransformed by the liver; these are called *pro drugs*. For example, the angiotensin-converting enzyme (ACE) inhibitor enalapril must be converted by the liver to enalaprilat before it will exert any biological activity.

Bacteria may carry out some biotransformation within the colon. This process may limit absorption of the drug from the bowel after oral administration, or it may help to eliminate drugs from the blood after parenteral administration.

Excretion

Most drugs or their metabolites are eliminated *(excreted)* by the kidney, although some drugs may be removed via the bowel or lungs or in some other minor way in limited amounts. The removal of drugs from the blood by the kidney is somewhat complex and will vary from drug to drug. One route of elimination involves the liver and kidney. Biotransformation of drugs by the liver tends to form more polar compounds, which can be more efficiently excreted by the kidneys. For example, the drug chloramphenicol is changed by the liver to chloramphenicol glucuronide. In this form, the drug cannot be reabsorbed via the kidney tubules from the urine back into the blood and therefore is excreted in the urine.

The pH of the urine will also influence excretion of drugs. Urine pH is normally basic, so drugs that are weakly acidic will exist in the ionized state and be more readily excreted. The weakly basic drugs will be in an un-ionized state and more apt to be reabsorbed back from the urine. For example, the elimination of aspirin, a weak acid, is enhanced in a more basic urine. The reverse is true of weak bases in an acidic urine. Ammonium chloride can be used to produce a more acidic urine, and sodium bicarbonate can be used to produce a basic urine.

Some drugs are not extensively metabolized by any organ in the body and are excreted unchanged in the urine. Some are excreted through passive diffusion into the glomerular fluid and are not reabsorbed to any significant degree and therefore enter the urine. Other drugs are actively secreted by specific systems in the renal tubules, which lead to more rapid drug elimination.

Drugs that are excreted by the kidney will accumulate in the body when there is a loss of kidney function. Creatinine (a natural waste product) levels in the blood are sometimes measured to determine the extent of renal damage so the dose of various drugs can be adjusted accordingly. Kidney function declines with age, even in the healthy animal. Elderly animals may show a reduced ability to excrete drugs in their urine. Certain drugs, such as the aminoglycosides, may directly damage the kidney *(nephrotoxic)* and ultimately interfere with their own excretion.

Another route of drug excretion involves uptake by the liver, release into the bile, and elimination in the feces. Drugs in the bile enter the small intestine, in which they may be reabsorbed into the blood, returned to the liver, and secreted again into the bile. This process is called *enterohepatic circulation.* The drugs that are reabsorbed and resecreted will persist in the body much longer than the drugs that remain in the lumen of the intestine and pass out with the feces.

> **✎ TECHNICIAN NOTE**
>
> Pharmacokinetic factors include absorption (how the drug enters the body), distribution (how the drug reaches the target tissue organs), metabolism (how the drug is chemically altered), and excretion (how the drug is removed from the body).

ROUTES OF ADMINISTRATION

Several methods are available for administering drugs to animals. Each route of administration has advantages and disadvantages. The route selected will depend on a number of factors, including (1) the patient's size, disease state, temperament, and unique species characteristics; (2) the characteristics and commercial formulation of the drug; and (3) the expertise *and* knowledge of the individual administering the drug. The cost of drugs should be a factor in the selection of a route of administration when all other clinical factors have been considered.

Oral Administration

Oral administration is one of the most convenient methods used by clients and animal health personnel for giving drugs. Tablets and capsules are fairly economical and provide accurate and uniform doses. Oral liquids offer some convenience, but the amount of active ingredient administered may vary from dose to dose, depending on measurement or the animal's acceptance. Administration of oral liquids by force in cats usually results in an undesirable salivary gag reflex episode. Oral paste

forms for horses and food-producing animals have gained popularity because of their ease in administration. The acceptance of oral granules and powders, although variable among animals, offers convenience for dosing larger species. Drugs formulated for mixing in the animal's drinking water are least desirable because water consumption is highly variable and unpredictable. However, when dealing with large numbers of sick animals in flocks or herds, the use of water mixes may be the only economical and feasible method of treatment. For small birds, medicated drinking water is sometimes used to avoid that stress that occurs with other methods.

> **✎ TECHNICIAN NOTE**
>
> Factors affecting routes of administration include physical characteristics and temperament of the animal, clinical state of the animal, characteristics and formulation of the drug, expertise in drug administration, and costs.

Absorption of drugs administered orally depends on a number of factors. Even when accurate doses are given, the actual amount of drug absorbed may vary, altering the expected therapeutic response. Most medications that can be administered orally can also be administered via feeding tube. It is preferred to give liquids by tube; however, some solid medications can be finely crushed and mixed with sufficient liquid to ensure complete passage of the drug into the stomach. Before administration of any drug via tube, make sure the tube is correctly placed.

Parenteral Administration

Parenteral administration of drugs is usually accomplished by subcutaneous, intramuscular, intradermal (Fig. 25–3), or intravenous injections. Each requires sterile technique to reduce the possibility of introducing infection into the animal (see Chapter 10).

An *intradermal injection* is made just below the outer layer of skin *(epidermis).* This route of administration is used for allergy testing and giving local anesthetics. The volume of drug injected is small, usually less than 0.5 ml.

Subcutaneous injections are common in veterinary medicine because they are less painful to the animal and are easily administered. Some drugs cannot be given in this way because tissue irritation or sloughing may occur. Many vaccines are given subcutaneously, but some require intramuscular injection to produce the desired immune response.

Increased risks are inherent in the intramuscular administration of drugs. One must ensure the drug will not be injected into a vein or an artery by accident. The potential also exists for injecting the drug in or near a major nerve fiber, which could cause paralysis. One must have knowledge of the location of major nerves to avoid accidental damage.

When giving drugs subcutaneously or intramuscularly, only a limited amount can be administered at the injection site. Multiple sites may be used for some preparations, but the absorption may be more erratic.

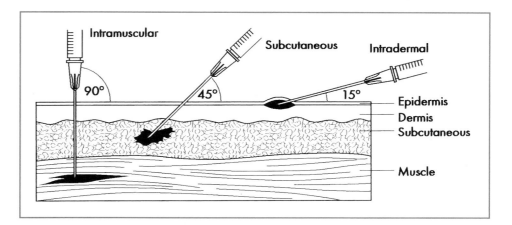

Figure 25-3. Comparison of angle of injection and location of medication deposit for intramuscular, subcutaneous, and intradermal injections.

The absorption from an intramuscular or a subcutaneous injection site is primarily through simple diffusion. A number of factors will influence the rate of diffusion from the site. Of primary importance is capillary circulation in the area. Because circulation is limited at subcutaneous sites, compared with intramuscular sites, one would expect slower absorption and longer action for drugs given subcutaneously.

Label directions should be followed regarding route of administration when administering drugs by injection. There may be a few exceptions for preparations with which sufficient experience exists for administration by routes other than those stated on the label. In most cases, however, there is a definite reason why the recommended route is stated. For example, antibiotics given by subcutaneous injection may not produce adequate blood levels to destroy microorganisms.

For intravenous administration, one must not only know the location of the larger veins that are used but also possess some skill in placement of the needle or catheter within these blood vessels. An immediate effect can be obtained from drugs administered intravenously without the delay of absorption encountered with other administrative routes. This route may also be used when larger volumes are required. Even certain irritating compounds can be given intravenously if they are given slowly, allowing adequate blood dilution.

Although intravenous administration has advantages, it also has risks. Highly irritating drugs, such as phenylbutazone, sodium thiopental, triple sulfa, and so forth, can severely damage blood vessels and surrounding tissue if injected outside of the vein *(perivascularly)*. Injecting certain drugs too rapidly may lead to untoward effects, including circulatory collapse and death.

Intravenous administration of drugs avoids the side effects caused by intramuscular or subcutaneous injection. Errors made with intravenous administration can be serious, even fatal, because the medications take effect quickly.

The technician should be aware there are several other important methods for introducing drugs into the body. Most, however, produce their effects locally at the site. Examples of other routes include topical (both skin and mucous membrane), intrathecal (into the spinal fluid), intraperitoneal, rectal, and inhalation.

DOSAGE FORMS

To administer drugs through the various routes, manufacturers have produced products in different formulations to accomplish the desired effect. For oral administration, there are not only traditional tablets and capsules but also chewable, flavored tablets to encourage animal acceptance and ease in owner administration. Oral liquids for human use may not be readily received by animals because of an undesirable flavor or high alcohol content. Liquids specifically flavored and designed for dogs and cats reduce stress for both client and patient during administration.

Many drugs cannot be administered orally to horses by their owners because of a disagreeable taste or odor. Some crushed tablets and powders can be mixed with molasses or other suitable compounds and then mixed with the animal's grain ration. Veterinary drug manufacturers have formulated granules and pellets for ease in oral administration. Oral paste forms, although somewhat more expensive, have gained popularity because of convenience to the owner and receptiveness of the animal.

Injectable drugs are frequently available in solutions or suspensions ready for use. Special buffers to maintain pH or absence of oxygen are required because of the instability of some components. Instability of some drugs may require a dry lyophilized powder be mixed with a diluent *(reconstituted)* such as sterile water or saline just before use.

Some vials of drugs in solution are designed for single use only because the preparation may not have a preservative or the drug is highly susceptible to oxygen in the air. Certain vaccines or intravenous products may advise in their labeling that unused portions be discarded.

A variety of other dosage forms exist for use in veterinary medicine, such as ophthalmic ointments, solutions, or suspensions; topical sprays, creams, ointments, and lotions; and otic drops. Most are designed for a local effect, although occasionally there may be sufficient absorption from the application site to produce a systemic side effect. The transdermal patch is an example of a drug formulation designed for local application to produce systemic results.

Intrauterine administration of some antibacterials is not uncommon in mares, cows, and other breeding stock. Antibiotics are also formulated for intramammary infusion in milk-producing animals. Some of these products are used to prevent *(prophylactic)* infections at the end of the milking period only. These agents are designated for use in dry cows and usually have a longer duration of action. Other mastitis preparations are for use in lactating cows to treat an infection during the milking period. Milk must be discarded during the treatment period and for a time after the last treatment. The withdrawal

Acetylcholine → parasympathetic

Epinephrine → sympathetic
"fight or flight"

time (usually 36 to 72 hours) will vary with the drug and formulation and is stated on the product label.

NEUROPHARMACOLOGY

Many different classes of drugs affect the nervous system, even though they are used for a variety of therapeutic uses. Some drugs will cause a direct effect, and others will alter functions of the nervous system as a side effect. The *central nervous system* includes the brain and spinal cord. Its function is to monitor, convey, and process signals from receptors throughout the body.

Neurons (nerve cells) relay information from the central nervous system to the rest of the body. They use neurotransmitters (NTs) to contact neurons and other cells. A *neurotransmitter* is a chemical substance released from the axon terminal of a presynaptic neuron or excitation *(stimulation)*, which diffuses across the synaptic cleft to either excite or inhibit the target cell *(receptor)*. Most neurons make only one kind of NT. The receptor recognizes only one specific NT and initiates a cellular response to it. The binding of the NT to its receptor is reversible. The stimulation of the cell is terminated when the NT is degraded or removed away for the receptor.

The nervous system is divided according to general function. The two primary divisions of the central nervous system are the *autonomic nervous system* or involuntary system and the *somatic* (motor) *nervous system* or voluntary system. The somatic system initiates muscle contraction by both conscious and unconscious control. The autonomic system innervates involuntary activities of the body. Although both systems have efferent fibers leading from the central nervous system, the focus of this discussion is on those of the autonomic nervous system.

AUTONOMIC NERVOUS SYSTEM

The role of the *autonomic nervous system* is to monitor and control internal body functions such as digestive processes, blood volume, cardiac output, kidney function, and so forth.

For impulse transmission to occur between nerves or between nerves and effector sites (e.g., muscles, glands, organs), a small amount of an NT must be released by the efferent nerve (Fig. 25–4). Two major NTs exist in mammals: *acetylcholine*

(ACh) and *norepinephrine* (NE). ACh is released into the synapse. ACh that diffuses into opposing membranes is degraded into acetate and choline by the membrane-bound enzyme acetyl cholinesterase. ACh that diffuses into the blood is degraded by nonspecific cholinesterases in the blood and tissues. NE is also deactivated by enzymes, but *reuptake* of NE by the nerve that released it occurs as well and the NT is again stored in the granules.

The autonomic nervous system is subdivided into the *sympathetic* and *parasympathetic* nervous systems. Both divisions commonly act on a given organ, but they produce opposite responses. NE is the predominant NT in the sympathetic system, and ACh is the principal NT of the parasympathetic system. ACh is also the transmitter substance found at the ganglia and at the neuromuscular junction in the somatic nervous system (Table 25–1).

Within the sympathetic nervous system, at least three different types of receptors exist (alpha, beta$_1$, and beta$_2$), with others being postulated. All of these receptors may be found within the same effector tissue, and response to the transmitter will therefore vary, depending in large part on the type of receptor that is predominant at the site as well as on the amount of transmitter substance present. The general response of various effector tissue to normal sympathetic and parasympathetic stimulation is listed in Table 25–2. This antagonism allows full control of organ function according to bodily requirements. It should be noted that sympathetic response is a *fight-or-flight* response in that the animal's heart rate increases, bronchioles are dilated for better ventilation, and blood vessels to the heart and skeletal muscles dilate to increase blood supply. In the parasympathetic response the heart rate slows, bronchioles constrict to restrict airways, and blood vessels constrict in the heart and skeletal muscle.

Drugs affecting the autonomic nervous system may mimic or block all or selected effects of the NT, or they may alter the synthesis, storage, release or degradation, and uptake of the transmitter. The classification of these drugs is difficult, not only because there are so many different types of action possible but also because most drugs possess more than one specific action. Drugs are generally classified based on their primary or predominant action.

Cholinomimetic (cholinergic or parasympathomimetic) *agents* are drugs that mimic the stimulatory effects of ACh. Cholinomimetic drugs can be further divided into muscarinic

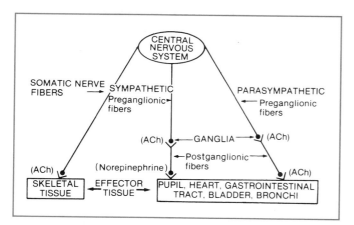

Figure 25–4. Schematic of efferent fibers showing sites of neurohumoral transmitters.

• Table 25–1 •

CHARACTERISTICS OF CHOLINERGIC (ACh) TRANSMISSION SITES		
SITE	**STIMULATED BY**	**RESPONSE BLOCKED BY**
Ganglionic (both sympathetic and parasympathetic)	ACh + nicotine	Hexamethonium, tetraethylammonium chloride
Postganglionic (parasympathetic primarily)	ACh + muscarine	Atropine and related belladonna alkaloids
Neuromuscular (somatic and skeletal muscle)	ACh + nicotine	*d*-Tubocurarine, gallamine

• Table 25–2 •

A PARTIAL LISTING OF GENERAL RESPONSES SEEN AT EFFECTOR SITES

EFFECTOR TISSUE	SYMPATHETIC STIMULATION (DOMINANT RECEPTOR TYPE)	PARA-SYMPATHETIC STIMULATION
Pupil	Dilated	Constricted
Glands		
Salivary	Scanty viscous secretion	Copious secretion (watery)
Gastrointestinal tract	—	Increased
Bronchioles	Dilated	Constricted
Heart		
Rate	Accelerated	Slowed
Contractile force	Increased	Decreased
Blood vessels		
Muscle (skeletal)	Dilated	—
Heart	Dilated	—
Skin	Constricted	Dilated
Gastrointestinal tract		
Muscle wall	↓ Peristalsis and tone	↑ Peristalsis and tone
Sphincter	↑ Tone	↓ Tone
Urinary bladder		
Wall	Relaxed	Contracted
Sphincter	Contracted	Relaxed

and nicotinic (see Table 25–1) agents. Receptor sites that are found to be postganglionic in the effector tissue may be stimulated by a naturally occurring alkaloid, *muscarine.* Most other ACh receptor sites, including end-plates of muscle, may be stimulated by *nicotine. Anticholinergic* (cholinergic blocking or parasympatholytic) *agents* are those that are capable of blocking ACh effects. They can also be subdivided according to the site or sites blocked.

Sympathomimetic (adrenergic) *agents* and *sympatholytic* (adrenergic blocking) *agents* are those drugs that mimic or block, respectively, the effects of NE. These agents also are further classified by the particular receptor that they stimulate or block.

AUTONOMIC DRUGS

Cholinomimetic Agents

ACh is not effective systemically as a drug because it is rapidly *hydrolyzed* by the enzyme acetyl cholinesterase at the receptor site. Only an ACh ophthalmic formulation is available for immediate constriction of the pupil during eye surgery.

Bethanechol is similar in structure to ACh and mimics much of its pharmacological action. Bethanechol is sufficiently different from ACh in that it can resist hydrolysis by the cholinesterase enzymes; therefore, it is a fairly long-acting drug. Bethanechol is available in injectable and oral tablet forms. It is used as a smooth muscle stimulant. When given orally, indications for bethanechol use include gastric atony or stasis and urinary retention when there is no obstruction.

Adverse reactions to bethanechol in small animals are mild and may include vomiting, diarrhea, salivation, and anorexia. Arrhythmias, hypotension, and asthma are most likely to occur in overdosage.

Several drugs are able to bind with the cholinesterase enzyme, preventing it from breaking down ACh. This not only allows ACh to act longer but also creates increased concentrations, resulting in exaggerated effects. These agents are toxic (some related compounds were used as nerve gases in World War II), and their therapeutic usefulness is limited to a few unique medical problems. In veterinary medicine, the use of cholinesterase inhibitors is primarily for treatment of parasites—both internal and external. (These parasitic anticholinesterase compounds are discussed later in this chapter and in Chapter 6).

Cholinesterase inhibitors (anticholinesterases) are divided into three groups on the basis of reversibility: (1) truly reversible (short-acting, 5 minutes), edrophonium chloride; (2) reversible (long-acting, 30 minutes to 4 hours), physostigmine and neostigmine; and (3) irreversible, organophosphates and ecothiophate iodide.

Edrophonium chloride is a drug used to diagnose myasthenia gravis, a disease of the nerves and muscles that is characterized by weakness and marked fatigue of skeletal muscles. Edrophonium chloride induces an immediate improvement, although it is of very short duration. The longer-acting agents *physostigmine, pyridostigmine*, and *neostigmine* are used to treat the disease in humans. Myasthenia gravis is a disease with a poor prognosis. It is a condition that is very expensive to treat; therefore, treatment is rare in veterinary medicine.

A common veterinary use of injectable neostigmine is in the treatment of ruminal atony or gut stasis. Neostigmine is relatively short acting (2 to 4 hours), but its stimulatory effects may be beneficial in returning the rumen and gastrointestinal tract to normal peristaltic activity after surgery. This agent is sometimes employed to treat urinary retention because of its stimulatory effects on smooth muscle in the urinary bladder.

Neostigmine and physostigmine can also be used to treat atropine intoxication and to reverse the effects of certain neuromuscular blocking agents (e.g., tubocurarine, gallamine, and pancuronium) used during surgery.

TECHNICIAN NOTE

> Neostigmine and physostigmine may be used to treat atropine intoxication and reverse the effects of some neuromuscular blocking agents.

Symptoms of overdose of the anticholinesterase agents include gastrointestinal effects (nausea, vomiting, and diarrhea), salivation, sweating, respiratory effects (increased bronchial secretions, bronchospasms, and pulmonary edema), ophthalmic effects (miosis, blurred vision, and lacrimation), cardiovascular effects (bradycardia or tachycardia, hypotension, cardiac arrest), muscle cramps, and weakness.

Other cholinesterase inhibitors are available only as ophthalmic preparations to treat glaucoma. Glaucoma is a disease complex that is characterized chiefly by an increase in intraocular pressure that may lead to blindness if left untreated. The anticholinesterase agents reduce the intraocular pressure by lowering the resistance to outflow of the aqueous humor.

Anticholinergics

As mentioned previously, *nicotinic* receptors are predominant at the end-plates of skeletal muscle and autonomic ganglia. *Muscarinic* receptors are predominant in smooth muscle, heart, and glands. Some drugs have the capability of stimulating both types of receptors to varying degrees, whereas other drugs are capable of blocking both sites in varying degrees. Furthermore, some drugs may block the nicotinic effects at the skeletal muscle and not at the autonomic ganglia.

Drugs that inhibit the action of ACh at the muscarinic sites (antimuscarinic drugs) are used widely in veterinary medicine; the most popular drug in this class is *atropine*. Atropine is a belladonna alkaloid found in nature and commonly incriminated in plant poisoning. Other belladonna alkaloids, such as homatropine and scopolamine, are commercially available and have a slight difference in action.

Because these drugs exhibit their usefulness in inhibiting the action of ACh by competing at a number of sites, their potential for correcting a disorder or altering a response is significant. One can rarely choose a single site for therapeutic action without concomitant side effects occurring at the other muscarinic sites. There have been numerous compounds synthesized in attempts to reduce certain unwanted actions and enhance desired effects. The success of such efforts has been limited, depending somewhat on the unique response of the individual patient.

The significant responses that are seen with therapeutic doses of atropine and related drugs are nearly the opposite of parasympathetic stimulation (see Table 25–2). The pharmacological effects of atropine are dose related. Low doses will produce decreased salivation and bronchial secretions. Dilation of the pupil and increased intraocular pressure and heart rate are experienced with moderate systemic doses. High doses decrease motility and tone of the gastrointestinal and urinary tracts.

The antimuscarinic drugs are frequently used before and during surgery in small animals to reduce or prevent secretions of the respiratory tract and to reduce *bradycardia* (decreased heart rate). Atropine and its analogs have been used in combination with other drugs to treat diarrhea (see later discussion on antidiarrheals).

> ✎ **TECHNICIAN NOTE**
>
> Anticholinergics increase intraocular pressure and are contraindicated in certain types of glaucoma.

Atropine is indicated in eye examinations and some ophthalmic surgery in which dilation of the pupil is desired. Atropine is long acting; therefore, some of the shorter-acting *mydriatics* (dilating agents), such as tropicamide, are used. One of the most important uses of antimuscarinic drugs is to block spasms of the small ciliary eye muscles, thereby alleviating the associated pain.

Another significant use of atropine is as an antidote for organophosphates and other anticholinesterases found in many insecticides or parasiticides. Muscarine toxicity from poisonous mushrooms is also treated with atropine.

Atropine must be used with caution because of the potential side effects, which are merely extensions of the pharmacological effects. Some clinicians believe atropine is contraindicated in the horse except for life-threatening organophosphate toxicity because the decreased peristaltic activity in the lengthy gut of the horse leads to gas and toxin complications. Atropine can increase ocular pressure and is therefore *contraindicated* in the treatment of animals with certain types of glaucoma.

Neuromuscular Blockers

Neuromuscular blockers (NMBs) act at the junction of the nerve and skeletal muscle to paralyze skeletal muscle. These compounds are classified according to their onset and duration of action. Some of the more popular agents are d-*tubocurarine, succinylcholine, gallamine*, and *pancuronium*. Newer agents used in veterinary medicine are *vecuronium* and *atracurium*.

Some NMBs have been used in darts to capture animals, but they are dangerous because respiratory paralysis occurs. The main clinical use of NMBs is an adjuvant in surgical anesthesia to obtain relaxation of skeletal muscle, particularly of the abdominal wall, and in orthopedic surgery. These agents are selectively used in veterinary medicine. *Guaiafenesin*, another type of muscle relaxant, is commonly used in equine and bovine surgery. Symptoms of NMB overdose include increased risks of hypotension, histamine release, and prolonged muscle blockade.

Sympathomimetics

The *sympathetic nervous system* is extensively involved in regulating a number of body functions, including heart rate, blood pressure, bronchial airway tone, body temperature, carbohydrate and fatty acid metabolism, and appetite. Although NE is the primary transmitter substance, *epinephrine* is released from the adrenal gland when an animal is stressed through physical, psychological, or other stimulatory means.

Because the NE molecule can be modified extensively and still possess some type of stimulatory properties, numerous agents are commercially available. Manufacturers seek a molecule that produces a desired response and eliminates or reduces all the other adrenergic effects. NE possesses only alpha effects and has limited therapeutic use in the treatment of certain hypotensive shock conditions.

Epinephrine has several therapeutic applications in veterinary medicine, although the actual frequency of use is limited. Clinical applications include use for (1) allergic reactions, often life saving in the face of shock; (2) bronchospasm, provides rapid relief; (3) cardiac effects, sometimes used in specific heart disorders; (4) local hemostasis, may be used in dilute solutions (1:100,000 to 1:20,000) to control surgical bleeding in highly vascular tissue; and (5) prolongation of the effects of local anesthetics, even though there may be undesirable systemic effects from epinephrine if overused.

Isoproterenol, which has few alpha effects but powerful beta effects, is useful as a bronchodilator in respiratory disorders and as a cardiac stimulant in certain heart conditions.

A synthetic catecholamine gaining increased popularity in treatment of heart disorders involving depressed contractility is *dobutamine*. In therapeutic doses, the drug directly stimulates beta$_1$ receptors, resulting in cardiac stimulation with only a slight decrease in peripheral resistance, but it has little effect on beta$_2$- or alpha-adrenergic receptors.

Epinephrine and NE are not available in oral forms because both are destroyed by stomach acid. In addition, both drugs are relatively short acting when given by injection.

Isoproterenol is available in many preparations for humans that are designed for inhalation use or as tablets for under the tongue *(sublingual)*. Only the short-acting injectable form has application in veterinary medicine.

Epinephrine and *phenylephrine hydrochloride* are also commercially available as ophthalmic preparations. They cause the pupil to dilate, but unlike atropine, they directly stimulate those muscles of the eye controlled by sympathetic nerves. This mydriatic effect is useful in selective cases of glaucoma as well as in ophthalmic examinations.

Symptoms of toxicity include arrhythmias, pulmonary edema, dyspnea, vomiting, headache, and sharp rises in systolic, diastolic, and venous blood pressures.

Sympatholytics

Many chemicals interfere with the function of the sympathetic nervous system. Some agents act by interfering with the synthesis, storage, and release of the transmitter substance. Others interfere with the ability of receptors to interact effectively with NTs. Some blocking agents are specific in their action; for example, prazosin hydrochloride is specific in blocking the alpha receptors. Other agents (e.g., the phenothiazine tranquilizers [e.g., *acepromazine*]) are more general in their action, blocking alpha and beta$_1$ receptors.

The alpha-adrenergic–blocking agents cause vasodilatation and are used mainly in animals for lowering blood pressure or improving blood flow in certain vascular diseases. An older, popular drug, *phenoxybenzamine hydrochloride*, which is used to dilate blood vessels and lower blood pressure, is being replaced by newer drugs, such as *prazosin*. Other hypotensive drugs, such as *hydralazine hydrochloride*, act directly on the vascular smooth muscle to cause relaxation.

Phentolamine, an expensive, injectable alpha blocker, is used to diagnose adrenal gland tumors and during surgery to control abnormally high blood pressure. Adverse effects seen with use of alpha$_1$-adrenergic–blocking agents include first-dose syncope, transient lethargy and dizziness, nausea, vomiting, diarrhea, and constipation.

Beta-adrenergic–blocking agents are therapeutically useful as antihypertensive agents and in the treatment of certain heart arrhythmias. *Propranolol* and *atenolol* are products used in humans that are gaining popularity in veterinary medicine.

Betaxolol and *timolol* are two beta-adrenergic–blocking agents that are widely used in veterinary ophthalmology. After topical application to the eye, each reduces both elevated and normal intraocular pressure with or without glaucoma. Overuse of beta-adrenergic–blocking agents results in symptoms of hypotension, bradycardia, bronchospasms, depressed consciousness to seizures, hypoglycemia, respiratory depression, and atrioventricular block.

Tranquilizers (Ataractics)

Tranquilizers are drugs that act on the central nervous system to produce a calmness of mind or detached serenity without loss of consciousness or marked depression. Their use in veterinary medicine is to modify the behavior of the animal to make it more manageable or less responsive to external stimulation.

Phenothiazines

Phenothiazine was originally used in veterinary medicine as an anthelmintic. Derivatives of the drug (chlorpromazine, acepromazine and promazine) have been synthesized to enhance the sedative effects of phenothiazine. Some of the derivatives are used as antihypertensive agents because they exhibit peripheral alpha-adrenergic–blocking activity and cause vasodilatation. The exact mechanism of action for sedation is unknown, but phenothiazines block postsynaptic dopamine receptors. These drugs have found usefulness as antihistamines, antiemetics, and anti–motion sickness agents.

The phenothiazine tranquilizers are used as preanesthetics by "taking the edge off the animal" and enhancing or prolonging the effects of certain anesthetics. Some side effects to be aware of when administering the phenothiazines include a drop in blood pressure, paralysis of the retractor penis muscle in horses, and lowering of the seizure threshold in dogs.

Alpha$_2$ Agonists

Although *xylazine* and *detomidine* in the strictest sense may not be classified as tranquilizers, their sedative and analgesic properties are useful for chemical restraint, especially in the horse. Detomidine is approved for use only in the horse and has little application in other species. It appears to differ slightly from xylazine by producing greater analgesia and sedation. Although it is dose dependent, the duration of action of detomidine is longer than xylazine.

Both xylazine and detomidine are commonly used in combination with other sedatives, tranquilizers, and anesthetic agents. The effects of these drugs in combination are greatly potentiated and must be used with caution. Common side effects seen in the horse include muscle tremors, heart block, bradycardia, respiratory changes, sweating, and penile prolapse.

Xylazine is used widely in cattle, although it is not currently approved by the Food and Drug Administration (FDA) for use in food-producing animals. The popularity in ruminants results from its excellent anesthetic properties. Ruminants are sensitive to xylazine, requiring approximately one-tenth the dose (based on body weight) as is used in horses. Adverse effects in cattle include ruminal atony, intestinal stasis, salivation, diarrhea, bloating, and regurgitation with aspiration pneumonia.

TECHNICIAN NOTE

Yohimbine, an alpha$_2$-adrenergic antagonist, competitively blocks and antagonizes bradycardia and central nervous system and respiratory depression caused by xylazine.

Although xylazine is approved for the management of hyperexcitable behavior in the cat and dog, it is not widely used in these species. Vomiting is a common side effect seen in the cat, and xylazine is frequently used as an emetic when this effect is desired (e.g., emptying stomach before surgery).

Yohimbine is an alpha$_2$-adrenergic receptor antagonist that competitively blocks and antagonizes central nervous system depression or sedation and the bradycardia and respiratory depression caused by xylazine.

Anticonvulsants

Of the several different causes of *seizures* (convulsions) in dogs, only about two thirds can be controlled by the various anticonvulsant drugs. *Diazepam* may be the most popular (Valium) injectable drug for use during seizures or in other emergency situations. This benzodiazepine agent depresses the subcortical levels of the central nervous system, thus exhibiting sedative, skeletal muscle relaxant, and anticonvulsant properties. Diazepam is relatively short acting (30 minutes to 2½ hours). *Phenobarbital sodium* is also available for injection when a longer effect (4 to 6 hours) is required.

Adverse effects seen with diazepam use include muscle fasciculations, weakness, and ataxia in the horse at sedative doses; irritability, possible development of hepatic failure, and aberrant demeanor in cats; and central nervous system excitement in the dog.

Phenobarbital is a barbiturate with central nervous system effects. The mechanism of action of this group of drugs is not quite understood, but they have been shown to inhibit the release of ACh, NE, and glutamate. Phenobarbital tends to depress motor activity without causing excessive sedation, which makes it a good anticonvulsant agent. One major side effect of this drug is dose-dependent respiratory depression.

fix: epilepsy also

An effective and inexpensive agent used to treat epilepsy (status epilepticus) and seizures caused by acute encephalitis or meningitis in dogs is *oral phenobarbital*. For some cases that are uncontrolled by phenobarbital, oral administration of potassium bromide has been effective. (Potassium bromide is not available in a commercial formulation. Authorization may be obtained from the FDA to compound preparations for treatment of refractory cases.)

Analgesics, Antipyretics, and Anti-inflammatory Agents

Analgesics are agents that alleviate pain. Although local as well as general anesthetics inhibit the sensory perception of pain, analgesics are generally considered to increase the threshold of pain in the pain perception areas of the brain. Antiprostaglandins (e.g., aspirin and flunixin) inhibit the biosynthesis of these natural pain-producing substances and are also considered analgesics.

Opioid Analgesics

The naturally occurring narcotics (e.g., morphine and codeine) as well as synthetic narcotics (e.g., oxymorphone and meperidine) are the most potent analgesics. These agents stimulate the *mu*-opioid receptor and are thought to have some activity at the *delta*-opioid receptor. Although these addictive agents are used for severe postsurgical or post-trauma pain in dogs and horses, their more common use is as an anesthetic or preanesthetic agent.

The pharmacological effects differ somewhat among the various narcotics, but most will produce the following:

1. Central nervous system depression in the dog, monkey, and human
2. Central nervous system stimulation (excitement) in the cat and horse
3. Cough sedation in the dog and human
4. Respiratory depression (panting may initially be seen)
5. Increased tone of intestinal smooth muscle, causing constipation

The effects of these drugs are reversed by narcotic antagonists, such as naloxone.

Unfortunately, the action of narcotic analgesics is fairly short in the dog and the horse (2 to 4 hours). Gut stasis in the horse is also a concern when considering the use of the opioid analgesics. Because the opioid analgesics have questionable efficacy in the ruminant, their use in veterinary medicine is limited.

The agonist activity of *butorphanol* is thought to be exerted at the *kappa* and *sigma* receptors. Butorphanol, a morphine congener, has shown promise in dogs as a longer-acting (4 to 8 hours) analgesic. Butorphanol is used in horses as an effective analgesic, although its stimulatory effects must be suppressed by the concurrent use of depressant drugs such as xylazine. Butorphanol is also approved by the FDA as an antitussive in dogs. Adverse effects seen in the dog include sedation (occasionally) and anorexia or diarrhea (rarely). Transient ataxia and sedation may occur in the horse.

Gaining popularity in veterinary medicine for pain relating to surgery is the use of *fentanyl*. Fentanyl shares the actions of the opioid agonists; the same precautions should apply. One advantage of using the transdermal patch system for pain management is that continual analgesia is provided for about 72 hours.

Hydrocodone bitartrate is a phenanthrene-derivative opioid agonist that is used in veterinary medicine mainly as an antitussive agent.

Opioid Antagonists

The opioid antagonists reverse the pharmacological effects of the narcotics. Naloxone, which was discovered in 1960, appears to be the only true antagonist because it possesses no other apparent pharmacological effect.

Although narcotic antagonists are used commonly in human addicts to reverse overdoses of self-administered narcotics, their principal use in veterinary medicine is to reverse the sedative and quieting effects of analgesics used for temporary restraint. Dogs receiving narcotic sedation for minor procedures (e.g., radiographs or suture removal) are easily "reversed" with naloxone; the animal is almost immediately alert. The duration of action of naloxone is shorter than that of most narcotics, and generally the effects of the unmetabolized analgesic are inadequate to cause the animal to return to its sedated state.

Corticosteroids

Corticosteroids are extremely active compounds that have numerous pharmacological effects on all organ systems. They are valuable in the treatment of certain conditions; however, there

Naloxone reverses narcotics

are significant risks when one considers the potential adverse effects.

Because corticosteroids are naturally occurring body substances (cortisol is derived from the adrenal gland), one indication for the use of steroids would be replacement therapy to correct a deficiency. Such a deficiency is relatively rare. Most steroids used in veterinary medicine are given for their anti-inflammatory effect; the mechanism for the anti-inflammatory is complex. They suppress the tissue swelling and pain that normally follow injury. Because inflammation is common in a variety of diseases, there is extensive use, perhaps overuse, of these agents.

Steroids also possess anti-immunological effects, altering the immune response of the body. They are therefore used in certain allergic diseases because they reduce the hypersensitive and allergic reactions of the patient. Immunizations generally should not be given during corticosteroid therapy because of the potential for inadequate immune response.

TECHNICIAN NOTE

Immunizations should not be given during corticosteroid therapy due to the potential for inadequate immune response.

Common side effects seen with the long-term use of steroids include (1) gastrointestinal bleeding; (2) increased susceptibility to infections or wounds that will not heal; (3) potassium loss, causing irregular heart beats, muscle cramps, and weaknesses; (4) sodium and water retention (edema or ascites); (5) muscle weakness resulting from protein breakdown; and (6) behavioral changes.

Steroids are found in various dosage forms, including ophthalmic, otic, topical, injection, and oral. It should be noted that long-term use of these steroids as ophthalmic or topical agents may lead to some of the systemic toxic effects previously mentioned.

Dexamethasone is one of the most popular steroids used in veterinary medicine; it is fairly long acting (more than 48 hours). *Prednisone* is another very popular agent. These agents are commercially available in injectable, oral tablet, and liquid forms. *Prednisolone*, which is used interchangeably with prednisone, is available in tablet, ophthalmic, and injectable forms. *Triamcinolone* and *betamethasone* are also used extensively in veterinary medicine.

Nonsteroidal Anti-inflammatory Drugs

To avoid side effects inherent to steroids, other agents possessing anti-inflammatory action have been synthesized. *Phenylbutazone*, one of the original members of this group of compounds, remains one of the most widely used agents in equine medicine. Phenylbutazone is not frequently used in small animals, although there is label claim for use in dogs. Dogs metabolize phenylbutazone rapidly, which makes it difficult to maintain therapeutic levels of the drug. Cats metabolize the drug slowly and thus become prone to its toxic effects.

Flunixin has gained popularity not only for its anti-inflammatory effects but also for its ability to reduce gastrointesti-

nal pain in horses and ruminants. Although not approved for food-producing animals, flunixin appears to be the best analgesic available for ruminants, providing relatively long, effective relief.

TECHNICIAN NOTE

Phenylbutazone may be toxic to cats due to the slow metabolism of the drug.

Ketoprofen is a proprionic acid derivative structurally related to ibuprofen and naproxen. It is a relatively new nonsteroidal anti-inflammatory drug and has been approved for use in the horse to alleviate inflammation and pain associated with skeletal muscular disorders.

Oral administration of the nonsteroidal anti-inflammatory drugs is apparently irritating to the gastrointestinal tract and may cause ulceration in the mouth, stomach, or intestine. Most nonsteroidal anti-inflammatory drugs used in human medicine are not used in small animal practice because dogs are prone to gastrointestinal tract side effects. Blood dyscrasis is reported in several species receiving phenylbutazone. The drug has the potential for reducing the effects of other drugs metabolized by the liver because it increases the hepatic microsomal enzymes necessary to deactivate these drugs.

Diuretic and Cardiovascular Drugs

Fluid and electrolyte imbalances and their treatment are discussed in Chapter 12. The function of the kidney and its role in maintaining proper fluid volume and electrolyte concentration are also mentioned. Blood is initially filtered in the kidney, and most of the filtrate is reabsorbed from the kidney tubules back into the blood. Most diuretic drugs affect the reabsorption process, preventing the reabsorption of some sodium and water from the filtrate. As a result, urinary output and sodium excretion are increased.

Diuretics

Diuretic drugs are used primarily to relieve edema associated with diseases of the kidney, heart, or liver. Although there are numerous diuretic agents, *furosemide* appears to be the most routinely used diuretic in veterinary medicine. It is commercially available in convenient forms for oral and injectable administration in small and large animals. Besides being potent and effective in most cases, furosemide is rapid acting and usually produces diuresis within 5 minutes when given intravenously.

Furosemide can cause a "wasting" of potassium, so serum potassium levels should be monitored for animals that take furosemide.

Occasionally, when renal blood flow is inadequate because of trauma or shock, furosemide or similar diuretics are ineffective in altering tubular reabsorption. In such cases, an osmotic diuretic such as *mannitol*, which is poorly absorbed from the glomerular filtrate, is used to produce diuresis. Animals that have been hit by cars may be likely candidates to receive mannitol.

Cardiac Glycosides

Cardiac drugs are probably the most potent and hazardous group of drugs used in medicine because of their effects on such a vital organ. Any carelessness in calculations, administration, or observation of the patient may lead to death. The dosage for these drugs should be individualized through frequent and careful monitoring to ensure the desired therapeutic response and avoid or minimize toxic effects.

The heart performs a relatively simple function (to circulate the blood), and it is essential to life. The heart consists primarily of muscle (myocardium), valves, and some specialized impulse-conducting nodes and fibers. Even though the heart has the ability to compensate for certain defects, disorders left untreated reduce the quality of life with severe disability, leading to premature death.

Significantly severe defects in the valves can only be treated surgically. Medical therapy is available for the treatment of a weakened myocardium and conductance disorders *(arrhythmias)*.

The normal healthy heart can increase its output readily when demands, such as increased exercise, are placed on it. This increased cardiac output is a result of either an increased heart rate or an increase in the volume of blood pumped per beat (stroke volume), but usually it is a combination of both. Heart muscle weakened with age does not contract as fully and therefore leads to reduced output. Because the body cannot tolerate much decrease in cardiac output, the heart rate will increase slightly and the heart will become enlarged because the myocardium will thicken in an attempt to improve contractility. *Congestive heart failure* is the condition of an enlarged heart with poor myocardium contractility.

Various glycosides found in the leaf of the plant digitalis have been found to be useful in the treatment of congestive heart failure. *Digitoxin* and *digoxin* are two of the glycosides that are commonly used in veterinary medicine, with the latter being more popular. The cardiac glycosides are unique in that they not only improve the contractility of the myocardium but also reduce the demand of the heart for energy and oxygen. These drugs also decrease the conduction of certain impulses within the heart and therefore decrease the heart rate. Glycosides are used for treatment of atrial fibrillation, an arrhythmic disorder of the heart.

✎ **TECHNICIAN NOTE**

Concomitant therapy of diuretics and cardiac glycosides may invoke low serum potassium levels, making animals more prone to digoxin toxicity.

Although the cardiac glycosides are effective by injection in horses and cattle, and to some extent orally in horses, it is not feasible to use these drugs to treat congestive heart failure because of the chronic nature of the disease. These drugs are commonly used in dogs and cats. There is adequate absorption of digoxin from the gastrointestinal tract in these species; however, it may differ somewhat among animals and can be influenced by feeding times.

 Digoxin dosing is very critical. Toxic effects of the cardiac glycosides are seen at doses close to the therapeutic dose and therefore complicate its use. Owners should be aware of signs of toxicity, which include vomiting, diarrhea, loss of appetite, and depression. Associated with these symptoms are a decreased heart rate and drug-induced arrhythmias.

Animals that are concurrently using a diuretic may have low serum potassium levels and are more susceptible to digoxin toxicity.

Further complications to digoxin therapy are animals with reduced liver or kidney function, as is common to the older animal. Good client compliance and close monitoring are essential in digoxin therapy because of toxicity possibilities. The drug is available as oral tablet, oral liquid, and injection.

Antiarrhythmic Drugs

Arrhythmias of the heart fall into several categories and require skilled clinicians and electronic instrumentation for proper diagnosis and treatment. Some minor cardiac arrhythmias are likely to correct themselves and may be left untreated. The use of antiarrhythmic drugs in veterinary medicine is usually limited to treatment of those arrhythmias that are life threatening and require immediate attention.

Calcium channel blockers provide the veterinarian with an efficacious weapon in the treatment of certain cardiovascular disorders. This group of drugs has a low incidence of side effects. Of the numerous agents, *diltiazem* has surfaced as the most commonly used agent to treat supraventricular tachyarrhythmias in dogs and cats. It also is used in the treatment of hypertrophic cardiomyopathy in cats. Diltiazem acts as an antihypertensive agent through arteriolar dilation, but the benefit of this action is not fully known.

Three older commonly used antiarrhythmic drugs are *quinidine, procainamide,* and *lidocaine.* Only their more ordinary uses are mentioned because detailed discussion is beyond the scope of this chapter.

Quinidine is used in horses and large dogs for the treatment of supraventricular and ventricular arrhythmias. Other uses include treatment of atrial fibrillation and atrial flutters. Procainamide is related chemically to procaine, and it is used in the treatment of ventricular extrasystoles and tachycardia, atrial arrhythmias, ectopic contraction and tachycardia, flutter, and fibrillation. Lidocaine, although used primarily as a local anesthetic, has therapeutic application in the treatment of ventricular tachyarrhythmias. Clinical monitoring and electronic evaluations should accompany the use of these drugs.

All antiarrhythmic drugs are toxic to the heart and may produce their own serious arrhythmias. In addition, in the horse, quinidine can produce urticarial wheals, gastrointestinal disturbances (e.g., anorexia, colic, and diarrhea), erythema, and edema of nasal mucosa with dyspnea and laminitis. Signs of quinidine toxicity in the dog include vomiting, depression, incoordination, and convulsions. Procainamide toxicities are exemplified in dogs by a loss of appetite, vomiting, and serious immunological reactions with long-term use. A serious decrease in blood pressure may also occur when procainamide is given intravenously. Lidocaine is not effective orally and has brief action when given intravenously. In large doses, lidocaine can produce a drop in blood pressure.

Angiotensin-Converting Enzyme Inhibitors

ACE inhibitors prevent the conversion of angiotensin I to angiotensin II (a potent vasoconstrictor). The drugs compete with angiotensin I for the active site of ACE. In veterinary medicine, this group of drugs is primarily used to treat canine congestive heart failure. *Captopril* was the first agent in this class to be commercially available. Treatment presented risks such as renal failure. Other ACE inhibitors have been synthesized; they are *pro drugs* because they require a functioning liver to convert them to the active metabolite. *Enalapril* is commercially available with label indication for use in veterinary medicine. Other ACE inhibitors that are in use, although experience is limited, are *benazepril hydrochloride* and *ramipril*.

The side effect profile of the second generation of ACE inhibitors has improved, and the dosing schedule is one or two times a day, which should improve client compliance.

AGENTS USED TO TREAT PARASITISM

Treatment of Internal Parasitism

Anthelmintics (wormers) are an extremely important group of drugs in veterinary medicine. The presence of internal parasites in an animal can shorten its life span or reduce the quality of life. It can contribute to considerable economic loss in food-producing animals. Although there are several different parasites capable of infecting each species, most parasite infections can be effectively prevented or treated with proper care and medication. Current anthelmintics are much improved because they are more effective in eradicating the parasite and less toxic to the host. In addition, some dosage forms such as pastes or chewable tablets are available. These formulations are much more easily administered, which reduces stress to the animal and client.

There are a vast number of anthelmintics currently available; however, this discussion is limited to a select, popular few. A parasite treatment summary chart and specific parasite information are given in Chapter 6.

Piperazine

Piperazine is an older, safe drug used for the eradication of roundworms (ascarids) in dogs, cats, horses, swine, and poultry. Because most of the newer anthelmintics are either more efficacious against ascarids than piperazine or have a broader spectrum of anthelmintic activity, piperazine has lost much of its popularity. Once commercially available as a single-ingredient product for large animal use, it is more frequently found in combination with other anthelmintics to broaden the spectrum or increase efficacy. Piperazine salts block neuromuscular transmission of the nematode, resulting in paralysis of the nematode in the gastrointestinal tract and passive removal from the body by peristalsis. Piperazine is considered to be a safe drug to use, even during pregnancy and concurrent gastroenteritis.

Benzimidazoles

Benzimidazoles are a large class of anthelmintics. They inhibit the enzyme fumarate reductase and thereby interfere with parasitic carbohydrate metabolism. *Thiabendazole, oxibendazole, mebendazole, albendazole, parbendazole, fenbendazole, cambendazole,* and *oxfendazole* are safe and effective agents against several gastrointestinal parasites. They are formulated primarily for large animals to eradicate strongyles, pinworms, and ascarids in the horse and roundworms as well as several other parasites in cattle, sheep, and goats. Albendazole is also active against liver flukes. Fenbendazole and mebendazole are available for use in small animals to eradicate roundworms, hookworms, whipworms, and some tapeworms, although neither is effective for the common *Dipylidium* tapeworm. Adverse effects are not usually seen at recommended doses of benzimidazoles.

Organophosphates

Trichlorfon, coumaphos, and *dichlorvos* are a group of agents that bind irreversibly to cholinesterase in the parasite, leading to ACh "poisoning" of the parasite. These drugs would also be toxic to the host, but they are selectively formulated to be poorly absorbed from the gastrointestinal tract of the animal. Precautions must be taken so animals dewormed with organophosphates are not exposed to other organophosphates, cholinesterase inhibitors, pesticides, or muscle relaxants, such as succinylcholine, until a few days after treatment. Organophosphates should be used only on the species indicated on the product label because the agents are toxic and specially formulated for the safety of each species. In addition, there is potential danger to humans in administration of these products.

Common toxic signs of organophosphate poisoning (e.g., widespread parasympathetic stimulation) include miosis, salivation, breathing difficulties, vomiting, defecation, and muscle fasciculation. *Atropine* is used as a specific treatment to block the muscarinic effects. *Pralidoxime* (2-PAM) is an expensive product for humans and may be used in severe cases to reactivate the cholinesterase enzyme.

> **TECHNICIAN NOTE**
>
> Atropine is the antidote for organophosphate poisoning. Pralidoxime (2-PAM) is used to reactivate the cholinesterase enzyme.

The organophosphates are fairly effective in treatment of a number of principal parasites in horses, cattle, swine, sheep, dogs, and cats. With the potential toxicity of the organophosphates, many are being replaced with safer agents.

Tetrahydropyrimidines

Pyrantel and *morantel* are two drugs in the tetrahydropyrimidine class. These drugs act as cholinergic agonists and depolarize neuromuscular junctions. Morantel is a newer analog of pyrantel that is apparently safer and more effective in sheep and cattle than is pyrantel. Pyrantel is widely used in horses for the treatment of ascarids, strongyles, and pinworms. In dogs, pyrantel is used in the prevention and treatment of hookworms and ascarids. In general, the pyrantel products are safe and nontoxic to all species at the recommended therapeutic dose. There is no contraindication for use of these agents with other cholinergic drugs. Tetrahydropyrimidines are effective against the adult nematode but not active against larval forms.

Imidazothiazoles

Febantel is approved by the FDA for use in the horse to treat most of the common equine parasites except bots. Apparently, it is also effective against gastrointestinal parasites in a number of species, although it is not commonly used. This drug is reported to be safe and may be used in pregnant mares.

Levamisole has broad anthelmintic activity in a large number of hosts, including sheep, cattle, pigs, horses, chickens, dogs, and cats. Use and FDA approval are limited primarily to food-producing animals. Levamisole was used investigationally as a microfilaricide in heartworm infections of dogs when no other agents were commercially available. It causes neuromuscular depolarization. Although levamisole is relatively safe, some signs of toxicity occur similar to those of organophosphate poisoning. The toxic doses are only one or two times the therapeutic dose. Muzzle foam may be seen in ruminants after oral administration, but it usually disappears within a few hours. Transitory excitement has been seen in horses after treatment.

Thenium Closylate

Thenium closylate is used specifically for the treatment of canine hookworms, although it is moderately effective against canine ascarids. Approximately 10% of dogs vomit after treatment, but this does not affect the action of the drug if emesis occurs more than 2 hours after treatment. Fasting is not recommended. Because fat in the diet facilitates undesirable absorption of this product, thenium cylosate should not be given to small suckling or recently weaned puppies still receiving milk. There have been a few unexplainable sudden deaths after treatment, which has somewhat limited use. Thenium closylate is no longer available in a commercial formulation.

The Ivermectins

The *ivermectins* enhance the release of gamma-aminobutyric acid (GABA), which paralyzes nematodes by blocking neurotransmission at excitatory motor neurons. Ivermectin has demonstrated effectiveness in a number of species against a wide variety of internal and external parasites. In cattle, swine, sheep, and goats, ivermectin is used to treat infestation by numerous gastrointestinal roundworms, lung worms, cattle grubs (cattle only), sucking lice, and mites.

The paste and oral liquid forms of ivermectin have been approved for treatment of infestations by large and small strongyles, pinworms, and bots, as well as for other equine parasite infestations. It is also approved for the treatment of ascaridiasis, although for some stages it may be less effective than desirable.

TECHNICIAN NOTE

Most collie breeds are inherently sensitive to ivermectin toxicities.

Ivermectin has been approved for use in dogs only for heartworm prevention (see below); however, it has also been used at higher doses for treatment of other canine parasite infestations, including scabies. In certain dogs (most collie breeds) that are inherently sensitive to ivermectin, toxicities, sometimes fatal, have occurred with higher doses. Except for these unique toxicities, ivermectin has proved to be safe in other breeds and species when given at therapeutic doses.

Handwritten margin note: ↑ dose for tx of scabies in dogs

AGENTS USED IN HEARTWORM TREATMENT AND PREVENTION

There is considerable risk involved in the treatment of heartworms; therefore, the AVMA Council on Veterinary Service (1973) established guidelines suggesting that first adult heartworms and then the microfilariae be eliminated. Heartworm disease is primarily seen in dogs; however, cats may also become infected. Dogs subject to infestation or reinfestation must be found free of microfilariae and adult heartworms before being placed on a preventive heartworm regimen.

An agent introduced into the market for treatment of adult heartworm disease caused by immature to mature adult infections is *melarsomine dihydrochloride* (Immiticide, Merial Ltd.), an organic arsenic agent. Dogs are at risk for post-treatment pulmonary thromboembolism; therefore, they should be exercise-restricted after treatment. The site of administration is critical for this drug, and it should be given only by deep intramuscular injection into the epaxial muscle. Adverse reactions observed with melarsomine dihydrochloride treatment include abdominal hemorrhage and pain, discolored urine, hematuria, tachypnea, disorientation, restlessness, and icterus. *Dimercaprol* (BAL) is an antidote for arsenic toxicity and may reduce signs of toxicity in overdoses. Coadministration of BAL may reduce the efficacy of melarsomine dihydrochloride.

TECHNICIAN NOTE

Thiacetarsamide and melarsomine overdosages may show signs of arsenic toxicity. BAL is the antidote for arsenics.

Microfilariae ingested by mosquitoes from infected animals molt in the mosquitoes and are then introduced back into other dogs when another blood meal is taken. It is these reintroduced microfilariae that molt again into larvae and become adult heartworms. Drugs used for heartworm prevention, such as *diethylcarbamazine* (DEC), *ivermectin*, and *milbemycin*, act by killing the tissue-migrating larvae. To review the heartworm life cycle, see Chapter 6.

Milbemycin (Interceptor, Novartis) and ivermectin (Heartgard and Heartgard Plus, Merial Ltd.) are available as once-a-month heartworm preventatives. Milbemycin and Heartgard Plus have the added protection against adult hookworms caused by *Ancylostoma caninum*. Ivermectin toxicities (although rarely observed at the low-dose heartworm preventative level) unique to collies and collie-mix breeds are not seen with milbemycin.

DEC should be administered daily at the beginning of mosquito season and continued for 2 months after the season is over. If ivermectin or milbemycin is used, it should be given within 1 month of the initial exposure and then monthly. The final dose is given within 30 days of the last exposure. If more than 45 days elapses between doses, animals should be retested for heartworm before restoration of preventive therapy. In mild climates in which mosquitoes prevail year-round, prophylactic treatment must be administered for the lifetime of the dog.

Although relatively nontoxic at the low dose used for heartworm prevention, DEC is somewhat irritating to the gastric mucosa. Oral administration is therefore recommended immedi-

↗ DEC

ately after a meal to reduce nausea and vomiting. These adverse effects are usually seen only with the higher doses of DEC that are sometimes used to treat ascarids.

Anticestodal Drugs

Anticestodal drugs kill and/or facilitate expulsion of tapeworms. The original drugs used were agents that temporarily paralyzed the tapeworms, causing them to lose their attachment to the gastrointestinal tract. Even when these drugs contained purgative properties or were given with harsh laxatives, reattachment of a number of tapeworms was likely to occur. This treatment was stressful to the host because its ineffectiveness required repeated dosing. Newer drugs, although more expensive, kill the tapeworm.

When *praziquantel* (Droncit, Bayer) became commercially available for veterinary use, it soon replaced most other anticestodal drugs on the market because of its efficacy, limited toxicity, and wide margin of safety. It is quickly absorbed from the gastrointestinal tract after oral administration and can also be given by injection. Its distribution throughout the body makes praziquantel unique in that it is effective against various stages of tapeworm development, including the adult stage. In addition, it is nontoxic, with a wide margin of safety. The cost of praziquantel is the only factor discouraging the further development and expanded use of this drug in species other than dogs and cats.

The more recently introduced *epsiprantel* (Cestex, Pfizer Animal Health) has also proved to be safe and effective. Unlike praziquantel, only trace levels of epsiprantel are absorbed after oral administration, and it remains at the site of action within the gastrointestinal tract. This drug exerts its action directly on the tapeworm.

Drugs Used to Treat Giardiasis

Giardia canis is a protozoan that may produce chronic diarrhea in dogs. Treatment with *metronidazole* is usually effective. In general, the toxicity is low, with few adverse effects reported during or after the 5-day treatment period. ✗

Giardiasis is also found in cats, but clinically it is usually not a problem (its diarrhea-producing role is not known). For treatment in the cat, metronidazole is given in a dosage regimen similar to that used for dogs. The margin of safety in cats is much narrower, and overdosing must be avoided; several deaths have been reported.

Recent investigations show that giardia with presenting diarrhea may be successfully treated with an alternating 7-day on/7-day off regimen of *fenbendazole*. The manufacturer of fenbendazole (Panacur, Hoechst) has not made label claim to this indication.

External Parasite Treatment

Chlorinated Hydrocarbons

Various *chlorinated hydrocarbon compounds* (e.g., *lindane, toxaphene,* and *methoxychlor*) were once popular and marketed in several different formulations for a variety of uses in a number of species. Most compounds were effective and possess rapid knockdown capability, with some having residual effects for several days. The long-lasting residual properties posed a

threat as environmental hazards, and as a result, many of these products have been banned. Other efficacious but less-endangering agents have been made available. Although the degree of toxicity will vary among the various chlorinated hydrocarbons, they should all be treated with caution and used as advised on the container label. Some diluted aqueous suspensions and powders may be applied directly to livestock. Signs of toxicity include vomiting, weakness, and other central nervous system effects, such as tremors, incoordination, convulsions, coma, and respiratory failure. Young, debilitated, or lean animals are more susceptible to the toxic effects. There is no specific antidote for chlorinated hydrocarbon toxicity. The animal should be removed from further exposure and given supportive treatment such as barbiturates to control seizures if necessary.

Organophosphates

Although *organophosphates* are the same class of drugs mentioned previously for treatment of intestinal parasites, these agents (*ronnel, coumaphos, trichlorfon, fenthion,* and *malathion*) are formulated specifically for the treatment of external parasites. As with chlorinated hydrocarbons, a number of preparations exist, such as sprays, dips, foggers, pour-ons, and pest strips. These compounds have good insect killing ability, but residual effects are related to the vehicle used to apply the agent. Topical application of these preparations permits significant absorption through the skin to produce signs of toxicity. Signs and treatment of toxicity are the same as those mentioned in the discussion on internal parasitism treatment. Persons applying these agents should avoid getting them in their eyes or on their skin. The use of disposable gloves and eye protection is recommended. Prolonged breathing of spray mists should also be avoided.

Pyrethrins

Pyrethrum flowers (chrysanthemums) have been used as insecticides for centuries, with the first powdered formulation being introduced in the United States in 1855. Before the advent of DDT, the annual importation of pyrethrins reached 18 million lb. Use dropped dramatically with the development of chlorinated hydrocarbons and organophosphates, but pyrethrins have gained in popularity. They are reported to be nontoxic to mammals as well as having little effect on the environment. Some toxicity has occurred in cats.

Pyrethrins are marketed in numerous formulations for convenient use. Most have chemicals, such as piperonyl butoxide, added to potentiate their killing power. Also, microencapsulation has significantly increased the residual activity of these compounds that were known initially for their quick "knockdown" effect.

Permethrin, a synthetic pyrethroid, is formulated and used similarly to the natural pyrethrins. Little can be found in the literature to compare the potency, toxicity, and environmental impact between the natural and synthetic agents.

Miscellaneous Agents

Several manufacturers have marketed new once-a-month flea control products. *Lufenuron* (Program, Novartis) is a benzoylphenyl-urea derivative classified as an insect development inhibitor. The product does not kill adult fleas but instead safely and effectively controls flea populations by breaking the life cycle at the egg stage. Preexisting flea populations may continue to develop and emerge after flea treatment, so noticeable control may not be seen for several weeks after dosing. Lufenuron is available in tablet formulation for dogs and oral liquid formulation for cats over 6 weeks of age.

Imidacloprid (Advantage, Bayer Animal Health) is a flea adulticide formulated for topical application. It is classified as a nitroguanidine and acts as a NT blocker in the insect. Imidacloprid will kill fleas within 1 day of treatment. The disadvantage with this product is shampooing may shorten the duration of flea protection. The product is considered safe for dogs and cats over 4 months of age.

Fipronil (Frontline, Merial Ltd.) is classified as a phenylpyrazole and acts as a GABA inhibitor. It is a topical formulation for control of fleas by killing adult fleas. The manufacturer has also made product label claims for killing all stages of brown dog ticks, American dog ticks, lone star ticks, and deer ticks. After application, the animal can be handled immediately and shampooed the following day. Fipronil is safe for dogs and cats 8 weeks of age and older.

ANTIMICROBIAL AGENTS

Initially, *antibiotics* (antimicrobials) were defined as substances produced by microorganisms, which in low concentrations destroy or inhibit growth of other species of microorganisms. Many of these substances may be produced totally or in part through chemical synthesis. Because antibiotics have the potential to cure life-threatening infections, they are one of the most popular and useful groups of drugs in veterinary medicine.

It is important to know the characteristics and uses of the various antibiotics and have a proper understanding of the principles of antibiotic therapy *(chemotherapy)*. It is beyond the scope of this chapter to present a thorough discussion of chemotherapy; however, some basic principles are discussed. Not all microorganisms are harmful or disease-producing *(pathogenic)*. Many bacteria normally found in the gastrointestinal tract, mucous membranes, and skin are helpful to their host. They compete with invading harmful pathogens and keep them from proliferating, thereby preventing progression to a disease state.

Each antibiotic is effective against specific groups of microorganisms. Some antibiotics are *bactericidal* (destroy bacteria), and some are *bacteriostatic* (inhibit growth); some may be both, depending on the concentration of the antibiotic (Table 25–3). The various species of bacteria that are affected by the antibiotic are known as the *spectrum*. Broad-spectrum antibiotics are those that are effective against a wide range of microorganisms.

For an antibiotic to be effective, it must be able to reach the site of infection in a sufficient concentration to exert its effect on the microorganism. In addition, the antibiotic concentration must be maintained or reached frequently over a period of time to completely destroy all bacteria or inhibit bacteria growth and provide time for the natural defense mechanisms of the body to eradicate the pathogen.

The length of antibiotic therapy may vary, depending on such factors as the site of infection, the microorganism, and the duration of infection. When antibiotics are prescribed, the treatment is usually for a minimum of 5 days. Although improvement may be seen with inadequate antibiotic therapy, it is an unwise practice. Microorganisms exposed to subtherapeutic antibiotic levels may develop resistance to that particular antibiotic, which will then be ineffective even when given at high doses. Bacteria not only can develop resistance to several antibiotics but also can pass resistance on to other species of bacteria. Multiple antibiotic-resistant bacteria are also a serious problem if resistance is developed in a hospital or clinic. *Nosocomial* (originating in hospitals) *infections* from resistant bacteria can be treated with only the most potent and expensive antibiotics. Nosocomial infections are discussed in Chapter 7.

The choice of antibiotic is obviously critical to successful therapy. The microorganism must be sensitive to the antibiotic chosen. A sample from the site of infection (blood, urine, tissue) should be collected for culture and antibiotic sensitivity testing to determine the causative organism and the effective antibiotics (see Chapter 7). This is not always economically feasible, so a potentially effective antibiotic is frequently just chosen. Administered antibiotics that are not effective may actually worsen the disease by destroying nonpathogenic bacteria that are actively competing with the pathogen. Even when antibiotics are effective against the suspected pathogen, destruction of the nonharmful bacterial flora may allow a second pathogen to manifest and proliferate.

Ideally, it is desirable to choose an antibiotic that is effective only against the identified pathogen. Even the narrow-spectrum antibiotics are effective against a number of types of bacteria, both pathogenic and nonpathogenic. In selecting an antibiotic, one tries to choose an agent that is most likely to be effective against the pathogen and least likely to disturb normal, nonpathogenic bacteria. Indiscriminate use of broad-spectrum antibiotics eventually leads to resistant strains, ineffective antibiotic use, and expensive, perplexing therapeutic problems.

Penicillins

The discovery of penicillin in 1929 and its subsequent clinical use in 1940 represent one of the most significant advances in all of medical history. Penicillin dramatically changed the outcome of many life-threatening infections. Since its discovery, the basic penicillin molecule (Fig. 25–5) has been continuously manipulated and changed to produce a number of improved penicillins with unique characteristics.

Penicillin G (benzylpenicillin), the first clinically used penicillin, is still used extensively in large animals in its procaine salt form. *Procaine penicillin G* is poorly soluble and is released slowly from its site of injection, providing adequate penicillin levels to allow once-daily dosing. However, twice-daily dosing is usually recommended. Penicillin G is effective when given

• Table 25–3 •

ANTIBACTERIAL ACTION AT USUAL SERUM CONCENTRATIONS	
BACTERIOSTATIC	**BACTERICIDAL**
Chloramphenicol	Penicillin
Tetracyclines	Aminoglycosides
Erythromycin	Cephalosporins
Sulfonamides	Trimethoprim-sulfa combinations
Lincomycin	Quinolones

A = beta-lactam ring
B = thiazolidine ring
X = salt formation site
R = side chain site

Figure 25–5. Penicillin nucleus.

orally, but high doses must be administered, because only approximately one fourth of it is absorbed from the gastrointestinal tract. Most of the antibiotic given orally is destroyed by stomach acid, so it should *not* be given directly after feeding, when stomach acid is greatest.

Penicillin acts by blocking bacterial cell wall synthesis in the final stages of replication. Without a cell wall, the bacteria swell and cannot function properly, and some *lysis* (rupturing) may occur. New infections in their high log growth phase are therefore most susceptible to penicillin. Penicillin has no direct effect on mammalian cells because they do not have cell walls.

One method of classification of bacteria is to determine their tendency to absorb dye (gentian violet) into their cell wall. Those absorbing stain are referred to as gram-positive (dark-blue cell walls), and those that do not absorb the stain are known as Gram-negative (light-pink cell walls) (Table 25–4). Penicillin G is effective against most of the gram-positive microorganisms, including many of the streptococcal and staphylococcal species. Some staphylococcal species have the ability to produce penicillinase, an enzyme that hydrolyzes the lactam ring and thus renders the penicillin inactive. At high doses, penicillin G is effective against a few gram-negative species.

One alteration of the penicillin molecule was to make it more resistant to hydrolysis by stomach acid. Another improvement was to prepare penicillins that are resistant to the action of penicillinase. (*Clavamox* [Pfizer Animal Health] is a combination product containing amoxicillin and a specific beta-lactamase inhibitor, potassium clavulanate.) Table 25–5 provides some comparisons among various commercially available penicillins. From side-chain alterations of the molecule emerged penicillins that are effective against a wide variety of microorganisms. Some of the penicillins available for human use have a broad

• Table 25–4 •

COMMON ANIMAL PATHOGENS	
GRAM-POSITIVE ORGANISMS	**GRAM-NEGATIVE ORGANISMS**
Streptococcus spp.	*Escherichia coli*
Staphylococcus spp.	*Proteus* spp.
Clostridium perfringens	*Pseudomonas* spp.
Corynebacterium spp.	*Klebsiella* spp.
	Salmonella spp.
	Brucella
	Vibrio
	Pasteurella spp.

spectrum of activity and are our most important potent antibiotics for use against many gram-negative organisms that may be resistant to most other antibiotics. These penicillins are expensive and should be held in reserve and used when other agents are ineffective.

In general, the penicillins are safe. Allergic reactions, such as skin rashes, fever, urticaria, salivation, cutaneous edema, and other hypersensitivities, may occur and lead to justifiable concern.

Aminoglycosides *G* −

Aminoglycosides *(streptomycin, neomycin, kanamycin, amikacin, and gentamicin)* have a fairly broad spectrum but are used primarily for their activity against gram-negative organisms. Aminoglycosides are not adequately absorbed when administered orally, but they may be used orally for intestinal tract infections or "sterilization" of the gastrointestinal tract before surgery. Aminoglycosides exert their action by interfering with bacteria protein synthesis. Although toxicity may vary among agents, all are potentially *ototoxic* (affecting hearing balance) as well as *nephrotoxic* (renal toxicity). Neuromuscular blockage is also an adverse effect that is manifested by apnea and progressive paralysis of skeletal muscle. When aminoglycosides are administered to animals with preexisting renal damage, the patient must be closely monitored because the potential for toxicity is much greater.

✎ TECHNICIAN NOTE

All aminoglycosides are potentially ototoxic and nephrotoxic and cause neuromuscular blockade.

Resistance, toxicity, and expense are major considerations in the selection of these agents. Resistance demonstrated by organisms may be to a particular aminoglycoside or, commonly, to several within this class of drugs (cross-resistance).

Dihydrostreptomycin, one of the first in this class to be discovered, is no longer commercially available even in the once popular combination with procaine penicillin. Most microorganisms were either resistant or readily developed a resistance to dihydrostreptomycin. Streptomycin is available as a product for humans and may be substituted as the agent of choice for some sensitive pathogens such as *Bacteroides nodosus.*

Neomycin is nephrotoxic and therefore finds its use primarily in topical or ophthalmic preparations. Kanamycin, gentamicin, and amikacin are commercially available as veterinary products. Other aminoglycosides, although expensive products for humans, are finding use in veterinary medicine for highly resistant organisms that are not susceptible to other antibiotics.

Aminoglycosides are frequently used simultaneously with some of the newer penicillins or cephalosporins to treat stubborn Gram-negative infections. Because the combinations are more effective than the use of either agent alone, the activity of the combination is called *synergism.* The use of aminoglycosides and chloramphenicol together is contraindicated because

• Table 25–5 •

		RESIST PENICILLINASE	
PENICILLIN	**ACID STABLE**	**HYDROLYSIS**	**SPECTRUM, COMMENTS**
Penicillin G	No	No	Mostly gram-positive
Penicillin V	Yes	No	Mostly gram-positive, less effective than penicillin G against some species
Procaine penicillin G	NA*	No	Same as penicillin G
Dicloxacillin, oxacillin	Yes	Yes	Mostly gram-positive
Ampicillin, hetacillin	Yes	No	Mostly gram-positive plus *Escherichia coli, Proteus mirabilis,* and a few other gram-negative organisms
Amoxicillin	Yes	No	Spectrum similar to ampicillin, better absorbed
Carbenicillin	Yes†	No	Gram-positive plus several gram-negative, including *Pseudomonas aeruginosa* (oral form effective only in urinary tract infections)
Azlocillin, mezlocillin, piperacillin	NA	No	Broadest-spectrum penicillins effective against most gram-negative organisms, including *Klebsiella* spp.

* NA: Not applicable (no oral forms)
† Indanyl sodium salt for oral use

it is an *antagonistic* combination, resulting in decreased antibacterial action.

Cephalosporins

Cephalosporins *(cephalexin, cefadroxil, cephradine, cephapirin,* and *ceftiofur)* are somewhat chemically similar (Fig. 25–6) to the penicillins and share a similar mechanism of action and spectrum. Although some resistance exists to the cephalosporins, they are not destroyed by penicillinase-producing bacteria.

The cephalosporins are subclassified primarily by spectrum into first, second, and third generations. Only minor differences exist in the spectrum of the first generation; all are effective against most gram-positive bacteria and several gram-negative species. The second generation has a somewhat broader spectrum, displaying activity against most clostridial species. Although *Pseudomonas aeruginosa* is not susceptible to the first- or second-generation cephalosporins, it may be treated with the third-generation cephalosporins. Severe infections, such as *Pseudomonas* infection, are usually treated with a combination of antibiotics to ensure eradication and limit the possibility of developing resistance.

The cost of the cephalosporins limits their use in veterinary medicine. Even with the availability of veterinary cephalosporin and generic products for humans, cost remains a major concern when considering second- and third-generation cephalosporins. *Ceftiofur* (Naxcel, Pharmacia and Upjohn) is approved for use in cattle, horses, swine, dogs, and chickens.

The cephalosporins have a low incidence of adverse effects. Chronic use of excessively large doses may lead to some complications similar to those of other antibiotics, including possible allergic reactions or overgrowth of nonsusceptible bacteria or fungi, leading to intestinal pain, bloating, and diarrhea.

Quinolones

This relatively new class of antibiotics is finding extensive use in veterinary medicine for treatment of a wide variety of organisms, including *P. aeruginosa. Enrofloxacin* (Baytril, Bayer) is approved primarily for urinary, skin, and respiratory infections in dogs and cats, but it is also being used to treat bone and other infections in several additional species.

Enrofloxacin seems to be well tolerated, and few side effects have been noted in animals. It is contraindicated in puppies during the rapid growth phase because it can induce abnormal cartilage formation, leading to weakness or lameness. This potential adverse effect discourages the use of enrofloxacin in other young animals as well as in adult horses.

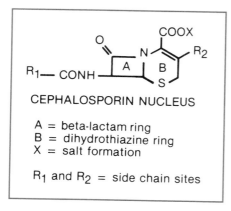

Figure 25–6. Cephalosporin nucleus.

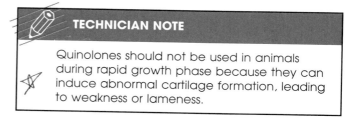

TECHNICIAN NOTE

Quinolones should not be used in animals during rapid growth phase because they can induce abnormal cartilage formation, leading to weakness or lameness.

Although bacterial resistance to enrofloxacin is not yet common, indiscriminate use to treat routine infections is likely to produce resistant strains, making this very valuable drug worthless.

Chloramphenicol

Chloramphenicol use in humans is limited to a few specific infections because of a rare but potentially fatal occurrence of irreversible aplastic anemia. Even personnel who handle and administer chloramphenicol to animals should use care, avoiding direct contact with the drug. Although some blood dyscrasias have been seen in animals, particularly in neonates, the condition is usually reversible by withdrawal of the drug.

Chloramphenicol has been a popular, important antibiotic in veterinary medicine. To some extent, newer, safer, and more effective antibiotics have replaced it. Although chloramphenicol is bacteriostatic, it has a fairly broad spectrum of activity. It is rapidly distributed to most body compartments and tissues in adequate therapeutic concentrations. A small amount of chloramphenicol is excreted unchanged in the urine, but most undergoes biotransformation in the liver to the inactive glucuronide conjugate.

> **TECHNICIAN NOTE**
>
> Chloramphenicol may cause blood dyscrasias. Personnel who handle and administer the drug should avoid direct contact.

Adverse effects include blood dyscrasias (as previously mentioned), anorexia, diarrhea, vomiting, and depression, as well as other rare but somewhat severe effects. Chloramphenicol in combination with other antibiotics is usually contraindicated. In addition, chloramphenicol interacts with several specific drugs or groups of drugs, including anticonvulsants, penicillins, phenylbutazone, and lincomycin.

Tetracyclines

Oxytetracycline and *tetracycline* are used practically interchangeably because of a similarity in spectrum and pharmacological properties. One tetracycline available for human use, *doxycycline*, has gained acceptance for use in small animals. It requires less frequent dosing and penetrates the central nervous system better than other tetracyclines.

These bacteriostatic agents affect the vital protein synthesis of the microorganism. Although the tetracyclines possess a relatively broad spectrum of activity, the development of resistant organisms has been a factor limiting their use. Through more judicious use of these agents, less-resistant strains are being encountered.

The absorption of tetracyclines from the gastrointestinal tract is adequate but is decreased in the presence of food, milk, or antacids. Some injectable preparations use propylene glycol as a solvent and are not recommended for intramuscular use because they are painful. When given intravenously, the tetracycline must be injected slowly because the solvent and drug may exert a blocking effect on the heart, causing the animal to temporarily collapse. Other injectable preparations contain povidone or similar agents, which reduce intramuscular irritation

and eliminate the cardiac problem. The intramuscular product formulated for extended action must not be given intravenously.

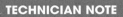

> **TECHNICIAN NOTE**
>
> Tetracyclines form complexes with calcium in developing bones and teeth and should not be given to young animals. The absorption of tetracyclines is decreased in the presence of milk, food, and antacids. Out-of-date or improperly stored tetracyclines should never be administered because they form nephrotoxic products.

→ cause yellow teeth

Tetracyclines are relatively inexpensive and widely used, especially in food animals. The tetracyclines are also commonly used at low levels as a livestock feed additive to increase weight gain and decrease liver abscesses. This practice promotes the development of resistant strains of bacteria, rendering the tetracycline useless for treatment even when given at therapeutic levels.

Although popular, the tetracyclines have toxicities. A common toxicity is the intestinal problems associated with disruption of the natural intestinal flora, including the possibility of superinfection by resistant organisms. Hypersensitivity reactions of rashes, fever, and liver damage may also occur with use of tetracyclines. The tetracyclines form complexes with calcium in developing bones and teeth; they should not be given to pregnant or young animals because tooth discoloration, increases in dental caries, and temporary suppression in bone growth may occur.

Although outdated products are never recommended, outdated or improperly stored tetracycline should never be used because the degradation products are actually toxic to the kidneys.

Miscellaneous Antibiotics

Erythromycin and *tylosin* are classified as macrolide antibiotics because of their high molecular weight. Their spectrum of activity is similar to that of penicillin; therefore, they are commonly used instead of penicillin against penicillinase-producing microbes. Erythromycin does not alter intestinal flora extensively, but gastrointestinal effects such as vomiting and diarrhea have been observed.

> **TECHNICIAN NOTE**
>
> Tilmicosin should be administered only by subcutaneous or intramuscular routes.

Tilmicosin is a macrolide used to treat bovine respiratory diseases, including those caused by *Mycoplasma*. A distinct advantage of tilmicosin is the long half-life, which allows a single-dose treatment. Tilmicosin must be administered only by subcutaneous or intramuscular routes because intravenously dosing has been fatal. Deaths have been reported after the use of tilmicosin in swine, horses, and nonhuman primates. The drug must be handled with extreme caution and administered in accordance with the detailed label instructions.

Lincomycin has a spectrum of activity similar to erythromycin and is particularly effective against *Staphylococcus* and *Streptococcus* spp. It has been useful when resistant strains or hypersensitivities to other antibiotics exist. Favorable results have been reported in the treatment of bone infections and various skin disorders (pyoderma) with lincomycin. The drug is concentrated and excreted in the bile. Lincomycin causes severe intestinal flora disturbances in horses, hamsters, and rabbits, so it should be avoided in these species.

Other Antimicrobial Agents

In addition to the antibiotics discussed, other chemical agents exist that are effective against certain strains of microorganisms. The *sulfa* drugs were the first antimicrobial agents to be used systemically in the treatment of bacterial infections.

Sulfonamides

Numerous sulfonamides *(sulfamethazine, sulfadiazine,* and *sulfadimethoxine)* have been formulated, and many have been used clinically since their initial clinical use in 1932. Although their value and use have declined with the discovery of newer antibiotics, a few sulfonamides remain useful for certain conditions. These agents are relatively inexpensive, which make them attractive for use in large animals for herd or flock treatment. The sulfonamides are particularly useful in the treatment of various infections of the respiratory system and urinary tract, bacterial diarrhea, foot rot, and coccidial infections. Unfortunately, bacterial resistance to the sulfonamides limits their effectiveness. A toxicity seen with the original sulfonamides was crystalluria, a condition in which the sulfa drug formed insoluble crystals in the urine, causing renal damage. Because the solubility of one sulfonamide is independent of other sulfonamides, the formulation of *triple sulfa* was developed to avert crystalluria. More soluble sulfonamides are also available, thereby further reducing concern. It is important that animals receiving sulfonamide have adequate water available.

The intravenous preparations of sulfonamides have a high (basic) pH and are therefore damaging to tissue when inadvertently given perivascularly. In addition, the intravenous preparations should be given slowly to avoid acute toxicity demonstrated by central nervous system effects, such as salivation, vomiting, diarrhea, weakness, ataxia, and convulsions.

Trimethoprim-Sulfonamide Combinations

A popular, effective antibacterial that is being used in veterinary medicine today is a combination product of one part *trimethoprim* and five parts *sulfadiazine* or *sulfamethoxazole. Ormethoprim with sulfadimethoxine* is a comparable combination with similar use and actions. These combinations block two essential sequential steps in the replication process of the bacteria, resulting in a synergistic antibacterial action. The combinations are effective against a wide range of organisms but not *Pseudomonas.*

Undesirable side effects seen with these combinations are infrequent. Although vomiting may occur, diarrhea is seldom

seen. Animals that are deficient in folic acid may be prone to develop blood disorders, as has been reported in humans.

Nitrofurans

The nitrofurans *(nitrofurazone, nitrofurantoin,* and *furazolidone)* have been replaced, to a great extent, by newer, more effective, and safer antibacterials. These synthetic agents have a fairly broad spectrum of activity, but they are not effective against *Pseudomonas.*

Although nitrofurazone and furazolidone are not absorbed from the gastrointestinal tract, they were once widely used orally in food animals to treat intestinal bacterial disorders. Except for topical application, their use in food animals is now strictly forbidden by the FDA because of their potential carcinogenicity.

Nitrofurantoin is sufficiently absorbed to have some use in small animals in the treatment of urinary tract infections. Nausea and vomiting, which are common adverse effects, can be reduced by administering nitrofurantoin with food or using the macrocrystal human preparations.

Antifungal Agents

There are numerous agents available to treat fungal infections of the skin *(dermatomycosis). Griseofulvin* is an antibiotic that is administered orally; it has no antibacterial activity but inhibits the growth of various skin fungi. It is an expensive product and is not usually the first-line choice unless the infection is widespread. Common topical agents found in creams, lotions, sprays, and other forms include *miconazole, tolnaftate, undecylenic acid, iodine compound, nystatin, various dyes,* and *phenolic compounds.*

The treatment of systemic fungal infections (e.g., cryptococcosis, blastomycosis, and histoplasmosis) is usually expensive, requiring lengthy treatment with limited success. *Amphotericin B,* an antibiotic used for various fungal infections, is toxic, causing kidney and liver damage, central nervous system abnormalities, and so on.

TECHNICIAN NOTE

Amphotericin B causes liver and kidney damage and central nervous system abnormalities.

A newer formulation of amphotericin B in a lipid complex suspension (Abelcet, Liposome, Inc.) eliminates some toxic effects experienced with the original solution. *Nystatin,* another antibiotic, is relatively nontoxic but has a narrow spectrum of activity. *Ketoconazole,* an expensive antifungal agent, has proven to be effective against a variety of fungal infections. Ketoconazole causes *hepatotoxicity* (liver damage), so liver enzymes should be monitored during therapy. *Itraconazole* is a newer agent that is efficacious against a variety of fungal infections. It is less hepatotoxic than ketoconazole and more expensive.

HORMONES AND SYNTHETIC SUBSTITUTES

Hormones are substances that are produced and secreted by glands and carried by the blood, producing an effect on a target organ. A number of hormones are secreted by several different glands. Our discussion is limited to the most clinically significant.

Thyroid Preparations

The thyroid gland is controlled primarily by the amount of *thyroid-stimulating hormone* released from the pituitary gland. When stimulated, the thyroid gland releases thyroid hormones consisting primarily of *thyroxine*. Because the thyroid hormones affect the metabolism of carbohydrates, protein, and fats, thyroid-deficient (hypothyroid) animals show signs of lethargy, reduced alertness, increased body weight, poor hair coat, and other related signs. Insufficient amounts of iodine in the diet can result in inadequate production of thyroid hormones. Such hormone deficiencies can be treated with desiccated thyroid because it is effective orally. *Sodium levothyroxine* (Synthroid, Knoll Pharmaceutical and Soloxine, Daniels Pharmaceuticals) may be the most popular agent for the treatment of hypothyroidism. *Sodium liothyronine* (Cytomel, SmithKline Beecham), the other active component of desiccated thyroid, is also available commercially.

Feline hyperthyroidism is treated with *methimazole* (Tapazole, Lilly). It interferes with iodine incorporation into tyrosyl residues of thyroglobulin, thereby inhibiting the synthesis of thyroid hormones.

Insulin

Insulin is normally produced and released by islet cells of the pancreas. This hormone is necessary to facilitate the use of food by the body, especially sugar. Insulin enhances the absorption of glucose in most cells of the body. Animals with inadequate insulin will have abnormally high blood glucose levels (hyperglycemia) and other associated metabolic disorders. Insulin injection (regular Iletin) is a solution of dissolved insulin crystals, which accounts for its immediate action and short duration. There are other insulin preparations that are intermediate acting (approximately 24 hours) to long acting (approximately 36 hours). Isophane insulin suspension (NPH), an intermediate-acting insulin, tends to be the most widely used in small animal medicine.

With the emergence of recombinant products (e.g., Humulin, Lilly), it may be difficult to obtain insulin of animal origin. Animals that were originally administered insulin from animal sources may need to have dose adjustments if switched to recombinant products. Any change in insulin should be made cautiously and under the medical supervision of the veterinarian.

Overdoses of insulin produce hypoglycemia, which if severe can lead to coma and death. Treatment of hypoglycemia consists of administration of intravenous dextrose.

Oxytocin

Oxytocin is a hormone released at the end of pregnancy to stimulate uterine contractions during parturition and induce milk letdown. The synthetically produced oxytocin is beneficial during delayed parturition or for aiding milk letdown.

Prostaglandins

Although *prostaglandins* (PGs) were discovered in 1935, it has only been since the 1980s that these substances have been extensively studied and developed. PGs are found in many mammalian tissues and have been shown to have a wide variety of effects on a number of body systems, including the central nervous, cardiovascular, urinary, gastrointestinal, and reproductive systems. Commercially available PGs such as *dinoprost* and *cloprostenol* are used because of their effects on the reproductive system.

In cattle, PGs can be used to regulate the heat cycle so breeding and consequent calving times for a herd can be planned. PGs are also approved by the FDA to abort feedlot heifers. For certain conditions in mares, PGs can effectively restore the normal heat cycle so the animals can be bred.

Because these agents are abortifacients, they should not be handled by pregnant women. Bronchospasm is another serious adverse effect in animals and humans that may occur as a result of contact with the product. Consequently, PGs should not be handled by asthmatics or used on animals with respiratory diseases.

GASTROINTESTINAL DRUGS
Antiemetics

Certain species, such as horses, rabbits, and rodents, are unable to vomit, but protracted vomiting may become a problem in dogs, cats, and other species.

The vomiting reflex may be stimulated through at least four different pathways. For example, chemical substances in the blood (bacterial toxins or certain drugs) may mediate vomiting via the chemoreceptor trigger zone (CTZ) pathway (medulla of brain). Vomiting arising from movement of the head (motion sickness) is transmitted through another pathway (cortex of the brain). In selecting an antiemetic agent, it is desirable to know the underlying cause of vomiting and the pathway involved because some antiemetic drugs are specific in their site of action. Vomiting may be a symptom of a disease state, so initial attention should be directed to treatment of the primary disease.

Although independent of their antihistaminic activity, a few of the antihistamines (e.g., *dimenhydrinate, cyclizine,* and *meclizine*) and *scopolamine* are effective in preventing vomiting induced by motion sickness. The principal side effect of the antihistamine is drowsiness, which may be desirable in pets that are traveling.

A number of phenothiazine tranquilizers (e.g., *chlorpromazine, prochlorperazine,* and *triflupromazine*) are classified as broad-spectrum antiemetics that control vomiting by blocking the CTZ at low doses and at the emetic center (in the medulla of the brain) at higher doses. Although these agents have the potential of producing a number of adverse effects, the risk of toxicity is low because of the low dose and short duration of therapy. Some potent broad-spectrum, human antiemetics (e.g., *haloperidol* and *metoclopramide*) are finding use in veterinary medicine.

Metoclopramide is a unique pharmacological agent. Besides its potent antiemetic property, especially in drug-induced emesis (e.g., cancer chemotherapy), metoclopramide is a peristaltic stimulant that increases gut motility. It has been used for gastric stasis in a number of species, including horses and cattle.

In addition, to facilitate radiological examination of stomach or small intestine, metoclopramide may be used to stimulate gastric emptying and intestinal transit of barium in cases in which delayed emptying interferes. Reflux esophagitis in dogs and cats has been treated with metoclopramide.

Cisapride (Propulsid, Janssen) is not classified as an emetic; however, its use is increasing as an equine gastrointestinal prokinetic agent (increases motility) in reflux conditions.

Emetics

Agents to induce vomiting are used clinically as a rapid means of eliminating certain poisons or to remove food from the stomach before induction of general anesthesia. A once common emetic used in veterinary medicine is *apomorphine*. Although still commercially available, it is extremely expensive and difficult to obtain. Apomorphine stimulates the CTZ and may be administered orally, intramuscularly, intravenously, or via the conjunctival sac of the eye. Because apomorphine depresses the emetic center, repeated dosing is not recommended when the initial dose is ineffective. Apomorphine should not be given to cats because it produces extreme excitement. *Xylazine*, a sedative analgesic, can be used as an emetic because of the routine vomiting it produces in the cat.

Ipecac, once used commonly in cats and occasionally in dogs, has the disadvantage of having to be administered via stomach tube because of taste. In addition, its effects may be somewhat sporadic. Some toxic effects, including death, may be induced with ipecac in cats. However, ipecac syrup remains a popular, convenient emetic for children for the removal of accidentally ingested noncorrosive poison.

Antidiarrheal Agents

Diarrhea, like vomiting, may be only a symptom of an underlying problem. Ideally, it is best to identify the specific problem and correct it. Current trends are not to slow the gut but to allow it to remain active to remove any present toxins or irritants. Most small animals with diarrhea recover regardless of therapy. Persistent diarrhea not only may be offensive to pet owners but also may require supportive treatment, such as electrolyte and fluid replacement. Anticholinergics, such as the various belladonna alkaloids *(atropine, homatropine,* and *scopolamine)*, have historically been used to treat diarrhea. Although *peristalsis* (propulsive intestinal contractions) is reduced, a minimal antidiarrheal effect results. The value of anticholinergic use is questionable because they have adverse effects such as increased heart rate, dryness of mouth, and diarrhea from gut paralysis.

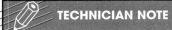

TECHNICIAN NOTE

Atropine should never be used in horses except as an antidote to life-threatening organophosphate poisoning.

Opiates, including opium tincture, morphine, codeine, and similar derivatives, such as diphenoxylate, are unique in that they increase rhythmic segmentation contraction, which resists intestinal flow and decreases peristalsis. In addition, the opiates increase the tone of various sphincters and valves in the gastrointestinal tract, which further delays movement of the contents. The commercial product *diphenoxylate* (Lomotil, Searle), which is available with only a small amount of atropine, is effective in treating diarrhea in dogs.

The use of antidiarrheal opiates in cats is controversial because this species may react with excitatory behavior. Opiate antidiarrheals should be used with caution in patients with head injuries or increased intracranial pressures and acute abdominal conditions, such as colic, because the opiates may obscure diagnosis or clinical course of the condition. Opiate antidiarrheals should be used with extreme caution in patients with hepatic disease and central nervous system symptoms of hepatic encephalopathy because hepatic coma may result.

The use of opiates in animals with acute diarrhea that may be bacterially induced may enhance bacterial proliferation, delay the disappearance of the microbe from the feces, and prolong the febrile state. Acute overdoses of the opiate antidiarrheals could result in central nervous, cardiovascular, or respiratory system toxicity.

An over-the-counter combination suspension of *kaolin* and *pectin* is widely used in human medicine. Kaolin is thought to act as an adsorbent, binding toxins and bacteria and rendering them somewhat harmless. It also serves as a protectant because it coats the gastrointestinal tract. Pectin may also have some adsorbent and protectant properties. The kaolin-pectin mixtures are difficult to administer to animals because of poor palatability and the volume required per dose. Even though tablets are available, the number of tablets required to be effective makes treatment of large dogs expensive and cumbersome. Kaolin-pectin mixtures have been used to treat diarrhea in horses with varying degrees of results.

Another over-the-counter preparation that is extensively used in veterinary medicine is the human product *loperamide*. Loperamide is a synthetic piperidine derivative that slows intestinal motility through a direct effect on the nerve endings and/or intramural ganglia of the intestinal wall. In animals, loperamide does not have analgesic activity, even in extremely high doses. Loperamide is available in tablet, capsule, and oral liquid formulations.

Bismuth subsalicylate is thought to have weak antibacterial properties as well as being a protectant and antiendotoxic. Popular thought suggests the compound is cleaved in the small intestine into bismuth carbonate and salicylate. The bismuth carbonate is responsible for the protective, antiendotoxic, and weak antibacterial properties. The salicylate component has antiprostaglandin activity, which may contribute to its effectiveness and reduce symptoms associated with secretory diarrhea. In humans, the preparation is used for other gastrointestinal symptoms (e.g., indigestion, cramps, and gas pain) and in the treatment and prophylaxis of traveler's diarrhea.

Cathartics (Laxatives)

There are relatively few clinical reasons to use cathartics in veterinary medicine. Occasionally, an older animal may have constipation, but usually alteration of the diet will correct the problem. Another indication might be for the treatment of hair balls in cats. After bowel or anal surgery, stool softeners may reduce stress at the surgery site until healing takes place. Cathartics as well as enemas may also be used before gastrointestinal tract radiographic examinations, proctoscopy, or elective surgery. One of the most legitimate uses of cathartics is in treating food animals and horses with overingestion of concentrated carbohydrates, such as grain. There are a few other unique circumstances in which the use of cathartics is appropriate; however, one is discouraged from overuse because it leads to dependence.

Cathartics increase the motility of the bowel by directly stimulating the smooth muscle or indirectly activating receptors through increased bulk. The irritant laxatives, which directly increase bowel motility, include (1) *emodin*, found in cascara sagrada, aloe, and senna; (2) *sodium ricinoleate*, a digestive end product of castor oil; and (3) *danthron*, a synthetic compound. Bulk-producing cathartics include (1) indigestible materials, such as psyllium seed (Metamucil, Searle), methyl cellulose, mineral oil, and white petrolatum, which not only increase bulk but also lubricate and soften the fecal mass; (2) saline cathartics, such as magnesium sulfate, sodium sulfate, magnesium oxide, and phosphate salts, which draw water into the bowel; and (3) stool softeners, such as docusate sodium and dioctyl calcium sulfosuccinate (Surfak, Hoechst), which are surface active agents like soap that increase bulk through water retention and lubricate and soften the fecal mass.

The cathartics as a group are relatively safe for short-term use, although some may be harsh and cause cramping and diarrhea. Chronic use of the petrolatum-type cathartics may lead to deficiencies in fat-soluble vitamins because of absorption interference.

Ulcer Management Drugs

Gastric ulceration and subsequent blood loss appear to be related to acid damage commonly associated with high doses of corticosteroids or nonsteroidal anti-inflammatory drugs (NSAIDs) as well as with certain medical disorders. Several methods are available for treatment and prevention.

Antacids were initially used, but required round-the-clock administration every 2 to 3 hours to truly be effective. A major advancement in human medicine for ulcer management was the introduction of cimetidine, a histamine$_2$ receptor antagonist. Although these agents are not approved for veterinary use, cimetidine, ranitidine, and others are being used to block the acid-producing effects of histamine on the gastric parietal cells.

Sucralfate in an acid environment forms an ulcer-adherent complex providing a protective, Band-Aid–like barrier for the damaged mucosa. Sucralfate also inhibits pepsin activity.

Omeprazole is an agent that acts directly on the parietal cell, blocking acid secretion. *Misoprostol* not only blocks gastric acid secretion but also appears to enhance natural gastromucosal defense mechanisms.

CALCULATIONS

The first step in solving any calculation problem is to express all quantities in the same system of units. If *strengths* (concentrations) of solution are given in percentages, they must be converted to g/100 ml.

Calculating the Strength of a Drug Solution

The following basic equation is used to calculate the concentration of a liquid dosage form:

Concentration (g/ml) = mass (g) ÷ volume (ml)

If you know any two of these quantities, the third can be found.

Example 1: What is the strength of a 1-liter solution containing 50 g of drug?
You know:
1. Volume of solution (1 liter = 1000 ml)
2. Mass of drug (50 g)
Solution:
Substitute all known quantities in the equation. Solve for the unknown.

Concentration (g/ml) = 50 g ÷ 1000 ml = 5 g ÷ 100 ml
× 100% = 5% solution

Manipulation of this equation is frequently used to find the quantity (mass) of a given volume of drug solution at a known concentration:

Mass (g) = volume (ml) × concentration (g/ml)

Example 2: How much drug is needed to prepare 4 oz of a 2% solution?
You know:
1. Volume of solution (4 oz = 120 ml)
2. Concentration of solution (2% = 2 g/100 ml)
Solution:
Substitute all known quantities in the equation. Solve for the unknown.

Mass (g) = 120 ml × 2 g/100 ml = 2.4 g

The original equation is also used to find out the total volume of drug solution that can be prepared at a desired concentration with a given quantity of drug:

Volume (ml) = mass (g) ÷ concentration (g/ml)

Example 3: How much of a 10% solution can be prepared with 15 g of drug?
You know:
1. Concentration of desired solution (10% = 10 g/100 ml)
2. Mass of drug (15 g)
Solution:
Substitute all known quantities in the equation. Solve for the unknown.

Volume (ml) = 15 g ÷ 10 g/100 ml = 150 ml

Calculating the Strength of Diluted Solutions

A basic equation can be used to solve problems for dilution stock (concentrated) solutions. (You can never make a more concentrated [stronger] solution from a diluted [weaker] solution without adding pure drug):

Concentration of desired solution × volume of desired
solution = concentration of stock × volume of stock

If you know any three of these quantities, you can solve for the unknown.

Example 4: Prepare 2 quarts of a 1:1000 solution from a 20% solution.

You know:

1. Concentration of desired solution (1:1000 = 1 g/1000 ml)
2. Volume of desired solution (2 qt = approximately 2000 ml)
3. Concentration of stock (20% = 20 g/100 ml)

Solution:

Substitute all known quantities in the equation. Solve for the unknown.

Volume of stock solution (ml) = 1 g/1000 ml × 2000 ml
÷ 20 g/100 ml = 10 ml

Example 5: How much of a 1% solution can be prepared from 6 ml of a 5% solution?

You know:

1. Concentration of desired solution (1% = 1 g/100 ml)
2. Volume of stock (6 ml)
3. Concentration of stock (5% = 5 g/100 ml)

Solution:

Substitute all known quantities in the equation. Solve for the unknown.

Volume of desired solution (ml) = 5 g/100 ml × 6 ml
÷ 1 g/100 ml = 30 ml

Calculating Drug Dosages

A drug dosage is expressed as units or mass of drug per body weight (BW) of the patient. The usual dosage for human drugs is based on the ideal BW of 140 lb (70 kg). There is no ideal BW in veterinary medicine because of the variety of species and breeds of animals. The usual drug dose for animals is based on BW expressed in lb or kg.

The following equation is used for calculating the quantity of drug to be administered based on BW:

BW × dosage ÷ concentration of drug
= volume of drug (dose)

Example 6: An 88-lb dog is to receive a drug dosage of 25 mg/kg of BW. How many milliliters of the supplied drug at 50 mg/ml are required?

You know:

1. Drug dosage (25 mg/kg of BW)
2. Animal's body weight (88 lb = 40 kg)
3. Concentration of drug solution (50 mg/ml)

Solution:

Substitute all known quantities in the equation. Solve for the unknown.

Volume of drug = 40 kg × 25 mg/kg ÷ 50 mg/ml
= 20 ml (dose)

The dosage of highly toxic drugs such as *antineoplastic* (anticancer) agents are calculated on the basis of body surface area (BSA). BSAs are difficult to calculate. Nomograms and charts (Table 25–6) have been constructed to help relate BW to BSA. BSA is expressed in *square meters*.

To determine dosage based on BSA, modification of the previous equation will enable this:

BSA (m²) × drug dosage ÷ concentration of drug
= volume of drug

• Table 25–6 •

CONVERSION TABLES FOR WEIGHT (kg) TO BODY SURFACE AREA (m²)					
DOGS				CATS	
kg	m²	kg	m²	kg	m²
0.5	0.06	33	1.03	2.0	0.159
1	0.10	34	1.05	2.5	0.184
2	0.15	35	1.07	3.0	0.208
3	0.20	36	1.09	3.5	0.231
4	0.25	37	1.11	4.0	0.252
5	0.29	38	1.13	4.5	0.273
6	0.33	39	1.15	5.0	0.292
7	0.36	40	1.17	5.5	0.311
8	0.40	41	1.19	6.0	0.330
9	0.43	42	1.21	6.5	0.348
10	0.46	43	1.23	7.0	0.366
11	0.49	44	1.25	7.5	0.383
12	0.52	45	1.26	8.0	0.400
13	0.55	46	1.28	8.5	0.416
14	0.58	47	1.30	9.0	0.432
15	0.60	48	1.32	9.5	0.449
16	0.63	49	1.34	10	0.464
17	0.66	50	1.36		
18	0.69	52	1.41		
19	0.71	54	1.44		
20	0.74	56	1.48		
21	0.76	58	1.51		
22	0.78	60	1.55		
23	0.81	62	1.58		
24	0.83	64	1.62		
25	0.85	66	1.65		
26	0.88	68	1.68		
27	0.90	70	1.72		
28	0.92	72	1.75		
29	0.94	74	1.78		
30	0.96	76	1.81		
31	0.99	78	1.84		
32	1.01	80	1.88		

Example 7: A 44-lb dog is to receive a dosage of 0.2 mg/m². What volume of a drug should be given at a concentration of 1 mg/ml?

You know:

1. BSA (44 lb = 20 kg = 0.74 m²)
2. Drug dosage (0.2 mg/m²)
3. Concentration of drug solution (1 mg/ml)

Solution:

Substitute all known quantities in the equation. Solve for the unknown:

Volume of drug solution = 0.74 m² × 0.2 mg/m² ÷ 1 mg/ml
= 0.148 ml

Calculating Infusion Rates

Many drugs must be administered intravenously by slow infusion rather than as a rapid bolus injection. Large volumes of fluids are also given by intravenous infusion. Disposable intravenous sets and infusion pumps are used to deliver intravenous fluids at a steady rate over a period of time.

Calculations of infusion rates can be found by using the following equation:

Rate (drops/min) = drops/ml calibrated ÷ 60 min/hr × total volume to be administered ÷ total hr of infusion

Example 8: If 500 ml of a solution is to be infused over 6 hours, what is the correct infusion rate if the set delivers 10 drops/ml?
You know:
1. Drops/min calibration of intravenous set (10 drops/ml)
2. Volume to be infused (500 ml)
3. Infusion time (6 hours)
Solution:
Substitute all known quantities in the equation. Solve for the unknown.

Rate (drops/min) = 10 drops/ml ÷ 60 min/hr × 500 ml ÷ 6 hr = 13.89 drops/min

INVENTORY CONTROL

The maintenance of an active working inventory requires both planning and continuous monitoring. Failure to keep abreast of use and needs results in shortage, inefficient use of time, increased costs, and added stress. The time invested to sustain appropriate levels of stock is therefore beneficial to the overall operations of the practice.

Veterinary technicians who demonstrate interest in an active inventory may find themselves acquiring an increasing role in inventory control and maintenance. Assuming this additional responsibility not only increases employee value in the practice but also adds to job satisfaction.

Ideally, the quantities of each item stocked should be as small as possible without running out between reasonable ordering periods. Because it is worse to have a shortage of certain items than to have extra, most practices lean toward a higher inventory than actually required. Inventory turnover (the number of times per year an item is bought and sold) should be at least four to six times per year. Some items, such as pet food, may turn over 12 to 14 times per year. With the assistance of a computer, monitoring of daily usage, and keeping helpful records, the average turnover rate can usually be increased. The higher the turnover, the lower the investment in the item. Ordering of drugs can become a full-time duty if care is not given to organization and planning.

Inventory Maintenance

The primary disadvantage of having a large inventory is the expense of having working capital tied up in drugs and supplies. A large inventory makes switching to equivalent products difficult, even at a cheaper price. There is great potential for product outdates, breakage, spoilage, and obsolescence when the inventory is large. Some states have an inventory tax that provides added incentive for keeping working stock to a minimum.

Occasionally, there is some justification for increasing the purchase of certain products. The "savings" claimed through many of the "deals" offered by vendors should be approached with caution. Unless one can accurately predict the use of certain products, quantity buying is difficult to justify. To partici-

pate in most marketing promotions, a significant financial commitment is usually required. Before entering into these agreements, one should truly determine whether the products offered are desirable and will be used within a reasonable period and whether the "savings" really merit the capital commitment.

Processing small orders is costly because the time commitment required to process the order is not much different than that of a larger order with several items. One is justified in increasing quantities on these small orders, especially if the items are inexpensive, to reduce ordering frequency and cost of acquisition. Some vendors charge handling fees if the total order is below a minimal required dollar amount or volume.

Availability of replacement goods is a factor that will affect the inventory turnover. With some items, one may be able to accurately predict monthly use and maintain a few weeks' supply. Unfortunately, the use of most items cannot be readily anticipated, which results in larger inventory requirement, especially if delivery time cannot be predicted.

Procurement
Veterinary Suppliers

One may purchase supplies through veterinary wholesale suppliers (distributors) or directly from manufacturers. Distributors may specialize in one class of items, such as surgical supplies or bulk pharmaceuticals. Some wholesale suppliers may offer a complete line of products, ranging from buckets to gas machines.

One advantage in dealing with wholesalers is the ability to reduce the number of small orders that would be required in purchasing from several individual vendors. A few manufacturers only sell their products directly to veterinarians rather than distributors. *The Veterinary Pharmaceuticals and Biologicals* (Veterinary Medicine Publishing, 1997) and the *Compendium of Veterinary Products* (North American Compendiums Inc., 1997) offer a fairly complete reference to veterinary pharmaceutical companies and their product lines.

Veterinary Clinics

It is an excellent idea to establish and maintain a good working relationship with another clinic in the area. In a crisis situation, you can "borrow" items from that clinic to see you through the emergency. Borrowing seldom used items in an emergency is encouraged rather than stocking them. However, your practice is expected to order the item and return it. Thus, inventory of seldom-used items is maintained elsewhere and record keeping is not necessary. Purchasing some items from another practice may be helpful, especially for expensive short-dated items.

In England, several large buying groups have been established by some practices to increase their purchasing power and decrease costs. Buying groups are being organized in the United States.

Pharmacies and Drug Wholesalers

Using the services of a retail pharmacy is nearly essential to the practice of quality veterinary medicine. Veterinarians have need for various human products that are not obtainable through veterinary suppliers. Retail pharmacies may not stock many injectable products, but they can help with most ophthalmic and oral products and some topical preparations. In some locations, a human drug wholesaler may deal directly with the small, individual practitioner. Most, however, do not welcome these small accounts and will serve only as distributor for hospitals and pharmacies. The veterinary practitioner must make arrangements with pharmacists to obtain human products for clinic or client use. Most pharmacists welcome this opportunity to serve the veterinarian.

Human Hospitals and Hospital Suppliers

A local human hospital may be a valuable resource for the veterinary clinic. Federal laws restrict hospitals with special buying privileges from selling to anyone outside their institution. As a result, it may be difficult for veterinarians and their clients to obtain some of the more potent, expensive, or rarely used medical supplies, except in an emergency. Human hospital contacts should be made to determine the local availability of drugs and supplies. The hospital's library and clinical laboratory may also provide some welcomed assistance.

Local hospital suppliers will stock items such as syringes, needles, cotton balls, tongue depressors, and other disposable supplies. Although veterinarians do not routinely purchase from the local supplier, do not overlook them as an immediate source in times of shortages.

Other Sources of Suppliers

In addition to bulk chemicals, major chemical suppliers will stock glassware, balances, disposable beakers, brushes, carboys, and other laboratory and clinic supplies and equipment that would be useful in a veterinary practice. Most of these suppliers are located in metropolitan areas and have addresses and telephone numbers listed in the telephone directory.

Numerous mail order suppliers exist that provide not only pharmaceuticals but also a wide variety of veterinary products and equipment. The quality of products and service may vary greatly among these outlets. Of major concern are return policies for handling inferior or unacceptable items.

Feed stores and lay veterinary drug outlets can be used for an occasional urgently needed item. One may at times also want to take advantage of certain specials offered through these suppliers.

ORGANIZING THE PHARMACY

Whether planning a major hospital complex or rearranging a small portion of one hospital, a comprehensive list should be prepared of all activities conducted in the pharmacy. Activities related to the pharmacy include storage (refrigeration, security), ordering, receiving, clean up, dispensing, withdrawal and administration of medication, compounding and manufacturing, product information, and so forth. In the design, the location of each activity must be determined, and each activity should be coordinated with other areas when required. Although most areas will be multifunctional, some activities may be unique and have their own special requirements.

A detailed list of functions pertaining specifically to the pharmacy inventory should include:

1. *Ordering* requires a telephone, desk, file, and calculator.

2. *Receiving* should be near an outside door and requires temporary counter or floor space.

3. *Returns* require space for holding broken items, outdated, and damaged items.

4. *Storage* areas must be adequate for working and back-up (such as refrigeration for perishable items and security for volatile hazardous bulk materials).

5. *Pricing* involves the use of a computer or price book, markup schemes, records, and a collection of material safety data sheets (MSDS) for all products. An MSDS is required for all products potentially hazardous to workers. Detailed information is available in Chapter 36.

In addition, consideration should be given to the movement of items to areas of use or dispensing. Monitoring of inventory levels of all items is a much needed function to be able to have an adequate supply at demand without shortages.

ARRANGEMENT OF INVENTORY

Working inventory should be placed on shelves in an organized fashion. One method is to arrange items by dosage form. Categories would include:

1. Oral solids (tablets and capsules)
2. Oral liquids
3. Oral miscellaneous (boluses, powders, pastes)
4. External liquids
5. External miscellaneous (sprays, powders, ointments, creams)
6. Ophthalmics (ointments, suspensions, solutions)
7. Otics
8. Small-volume injectables
9. Large-volume injectables
10. Mastitis preparations
11. Miscellaneous, such as chemicals for compounding

Each section should be further arranged, perhaps by generic name, brand name, or the more common name used by individuals in the practice. One may wish to make exceptions for items that are popular, but they should be limited.

A different type of arrangement would be to group items by their most common therapeutic use. Classification would be similar to that in the discussion of drugs found in the first portion of this chapter.

1. Anesthetics
2. Tranquilizers
3. Anticonvulsants
4. Analgesics
5. Anti-inflammatories
6. Cardiovascular drugs
7. Fluids and electrolytes
8. Diuretics
9. Parasiticides
10. Antibiotics
11. Other antibacterials
12. Antineoplastics
13. Hormones and related substances
14. Gastrointestinal drugs
15. Vitamins

Each drug class could then be further divided into more specific uses, such as gastrointestinal drugs into antiemetics, emetics, antidiarrheals, and so forth. Some classes may have only two or three items. Disadvantages of using this system are the poor use of shelf space and the possibility of gallon jugs ending up next to ampules.

Another arrangement is to group items by company or vendor. This method may be acceptable for backup stock because it is helpful when preparing orders. In an active inventory, there may be poor use of shelf space. Perhaps the greatest disadvantage is trying to recall the last supplier for rarely used items. Another disadvantage is purchasing generic items from multiple vendors, which may lead to multiple locations of the same item and duplicate stock.

Pharmacy organization is desirable and has advantages, primarily by assisting each individual in locating items. The best method of organizing stock is probably a combination of the various arrangements above. Each practice should design its own method. In addition to the methods listed, placement of selected items in areas where they are frequently used should be considered.

DRUG LAWS

Federal Laws

Although the Food, Drug and Cosmetic Act of 1938 has been amended numerous times, it is still the basic federal law governing drugs in the United States. This law assures the public that drugs have been prepared through approved manufacturing standards and are safe as well as effective for the claims made. The Durham-Humphrey Amendment (1951) restricted the availability of certain drugs to prescription through licensed practitioners. This class of drugs, referred to as prescription drugs or *legend drugs*, is deemed unsafe for lay medication, even with clear and precise label directions.

Veterinary labeled drugs bear the legend, "Caution: Federal law restricts this drug to use by or on the order of a licensed veterinarian." Human labeled drugs bear the legend, "Caution: Federal law prohibits dispensing without a prescription." Nonprescription or *over-the-counter* drugs may be sold directly to clients but must bear extensive labeling, which includes warnings as well as instructions for proper use.

State Laws

Most state pharmacy laws are primarily concerned with the distribution of drugs within the state. These laws specify who is authorized to prescribe and dispense legend drugs, the licensing of outlets, records required, and certain processing standards.

Because state laws are unique to each state, it is the responsibility of those practicing veterinary medicine to know the laws that apply to them. State laws work in conjunction with federal laws. Sometimes state laws are more restrictive than federal laws; in such cases, one should comply with the stricter law. Most states have regulations governing dispensing practitioners, although these regulations are directed primarily toward physicians. Two important concerns that veterinary clinics should address regarding dispensing of drugs are proper labeling and dispensing records.

Labeling requirements vary between states but may include (1) name, address, and telephone number of clinic, (2) name of client, (3) species of animal, (4) date, (5) prescribing veterinarian, (6) adequate directions for proper administration of medication, (7) name of medication, and (8) prescription transaction number (optional). Auxiliary labels may also be required to caution or inform the client. Examples include "Shake well," "Keep refrigerated," "Do not use after [date]," "Poison," "External use only," and "For veterinary use only."

The ultimate responsibility for any medication dispensed through a veterinary practice lies with the authorizing veterinarian. In some states, the technician may be allowed to assist the veterinarian by typing labels, counting or pouring, attaching labels, and pricing. The technician *should not issue or refill medications without the veterinarian's approval.* For most medications, this would be in violation of the federal law.

Readily retrievable dispensing records may be required by some states to safeguard public health. Accidental ingestion of prescription drugs by animals and small children is not uncommon. Proper records can provide attending physicians with the name and the amount of medication dispensed so appropriate treatment can be provided.

The federal Poison Prevention Packaging Act passed in 1970 requires pharmacists and physicians to dispense medications intended for oral human use in childproof containers. Although this act does not apply directly to veterinary drugs, use of childproof containers is considered "state of the art." Veterinary clinics failing to use such a safeguard would be highly vulnerable to legal action in a case of accidental poisoning.

Controlled Substances

The Controlled Substances Act of 1970 was passed to reduce drug abuse by defining certain legal and illegal acts regarding substances of high abuse potential. It is established and authorized the Drug Enforcement Administration (DEA) to enforce this law. The law is designed to provide an approved means for proper manufacture, distribution, dispensing, and use of controlled substances through licensing of legitimate handlers of these drugs. This "closed" system has been effective in reducing widespread diversion of these drugs into the illicit market. Controlled substances are classified into five categories (schedules) according to their use or abuse potential (Table 25–7).

All veterinarians using these drugs in the course of their practice are required to have a DEA license number. Those who engage in administering or dispensing controlled substances in Schedules II, III, IV, and V are required to keep records of such transactions for 2 years. Receiving records or reports of controlled substances received must also be kept for 2 years. Some states, such as Louisiana, require records to be kept for a period of 5 years.

In addition, practitioners who handle controlled substances are required to take an initial inventory at the opening of business of all controlled substances. Biannual inventories are required after the initial inventory. Records for receipts and dispensing of Schedule II substances must be kept separate from all other records. Records for substances in Schedules III, IV, and V may be kept separate or incorporated with records for other drug items. When schedule III, IV, and V drugs are

• Table 25–7 •

SCHEDULE OF CONTROLLED SUBSTANCES

SCHEDULE	ABUSE POTENTIAL	DISPENSING LIMITS	DISTRIBUTION RESTRICTIONS	SCHEDULE EXAMPLES	COMMENTS
I	High	Research use only	DEA form 222 required	LSD, heroin	No accepted medical use
II	High	Requires written prescription, no refills	DEA form 222 required	Oxymorphone, sodium pentobarbital injection	Abuse may lead to severe dependence
III	Less than I and II	Oral or written, refills up to five times within 6 mo	DEA registration number	Hycodan, Tylenol with codeine, anabolic steroids	Abuse may lead to moderate dependence
IV	Low	Oral or written, refills up to five times within 6 mo	DEA registration number	Diazepam, phenobarbital	Abuse may lead to limited dependence
V	Low	No DEA limits	DEA registration number	Lomotil, Robitussin AC	Lowest potential for abuse

incorporated with other drugs they should be identified with a red "C" in the lower righthand corner of the record. All controlled substance records must be "readily retrievable."

It is best that those persons responsible for handling controlled substances be familiar not only with federal laws governing them but also with state laws, which may be more strict. Agencies such as the State Board of Pharmacy or the local DEA office are quite helpful in answering questions concerning compliance.

The law states that, "A practitioner who has controlled substances stored in his office or clinic must keep these drugs in a securely locked, substantially constructed cabinet or safe." A secure area is usually interpreted as a double-locked container that cannot be picked up and moved. Examples would be a locked metal box stored inside a floor safe or an attached locked wall cabinet. The responsibility for access to controlled substances should be restricted to only one or two persons in the clinic practice. Practitioners experiencing theft or significant loss of controlled substances must report such loss to the DEA Regional Office and the local police department when the loss is discovered.

The state of Colorado developed and published an excellent, comprehensive set of guidelines for the proper handling of controlled substances in a veterinary practice. These guidelines were "deregionalized" and included in the Appendix of *Veterinary Drug Handbook 1992*. Some of the material incorporated into the guidelines was obtained from a government publication entitled the *Physician's Manual: An Information*

Outline on the Controlled Substances 1970. This government manual may be obtained free by request from the following:

U.S. Department of Justice
Drug Enforcement Administration
1465 "I" Street, N.W.
Washington, D.C. 20537

References

Plumb DC: Veterinary Drug Handbook. 2nd ed. White Bear Lake, MN, PharmaVet Publishing, 1995.
Spinelli JS and Enos LR: Drugs in Veterinary Practice. Minneapolis, MN, Alpha Editions, Division of Burgess Publishing Co., 1978.

Recommended Reading

Adams HR (editor): Veterinary Pharmacology and Therapeutics. 7th ed. Ames, IA, Iowa State University Press, 1995.
Compendium of Veterinary Products. Port Huron, MI, North American Compendium, 1997.
Hardman JG, Gilman AG, Limbird LE, Molinoff PB and Ruddon R: The Pharmacological Basis of Therapeutics. 9th ed. New York, McGraw-Hill, Health Professions Division, 1996.
Kirk RW and Bonagura JD: Current Veterinary Therapy XII: Small Animal Practice, Philadelphia, W. B. Saunders, 1995.
Upson DW: Upson's Handbook of Clinical Veterinary Pharmacology. 3rd ed. Manhattan, KS, Dan Duson Enterprises, 1988.
USP DI: Drug Information for the Health Care Provider. 16th ed. Rockville, MD, USPC, 1996.
Veterinary Pharmaceutical and Biologicals. 11th ed. Lenexa, KS, Veterinary Medicine Publishing Co., 1997.

26 Companion Animal Clinical Nutrition

Stephen W. Crane • *Sheila R. Grosdidier*

The professionalism and knowledge displayed by the veterinary technician strongly complement the veterinarian's provision of nutritional information to clients. Information most commonly sought is what to feed and how to feed. Education of the owner before a patient's discharge is important at transitional feeding periods, that is, when foods are being changed. Nutritional assessment and specialized feeding for anorectic and hospitalized patients represent another major role for the technician.

In addition, nearly every veterinary practice dispenses dietary animal foods, and many provide well-animal pet foods. The technician will be seen as a source of authoritative advice and a complement to the veterinarian's recommendations.

This chapter defines nutrients and their use, distinguishes nutrients from ingredients, and suggests nutrient intake levels for pets, horses, and livestock. Determination of food dosage for pet animals, true feeding costs (cents per calorie or cents per day), and quality assessment guidelines for horse forages and prepared animal foods are also discussed. A summary of companion animal clinical nutrition familiarizes the reader with dietary therapy. Basic assisted feeding techniques for hospitalized animals are also described.

OVERVIEW OF NUTRITIONAL OBJECTIVES AND PRINCIPLES

Nutritional goals differ sharply between agricultural and companion animals. As in human nutrition, the goal of feeding pets is to maximize the length and quality of life by reducing food intake risk factors that work against wellness (Morris et al., 1987). The other aspect of well-pet nutrition is to elect nutrient intake patterns consistent with current physiological need. Feeding an adult dog for maintenance, instead of as a puppy,

is one example. Feeding the horse for its maintenance requirement plus its work level is another skill in matching nutrient provision to requirements.

ENERGY-PRODUCING NUTRIENTS

> **TECHNICIAN NOTE**
>
> A nutrient is any substance ingested to support life and may be classified as an energy-producing nutrient or a non–energy-producing nutrient.

A nutrient is any substance ingested to support life and may be classified as an energy-producing nutrient or a non-energy-producing nutrient. Energy-producing nutrients are sugars, amino acids, and fatty acids. While nutritionally different, each possesses a common availability and structure of hydrocarbon, making them suitable as metabolic "fuels." Digestion, assimilation, and metabolism of nutrients produce the chemical energy for the "fire of life" (Fig. 26–1). The energy released from metabolism of food fuels deposits in chemical bonds that are held in a ready-to-use form in storage molecules (adenosine triphosphate [ATP]). The storage molecules are the source of energy for cell maintenance, reproduction, repair, heat production, muscle contraction, and the synthesis of new tissue.

Carbohydrates: Sugars, Starches, and Fibers

Carbohydrate is a general biochemical classification that includes sugars, starches, and fibers. Sugars are numerous and

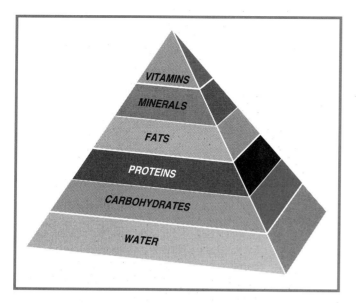

Figure 26–1. Six basic classes of nutrients are important for life sustenance.

include monosaccharides and disaccharides and more complicated sugar molecules. Multiple sugars can bond and link to form complex sugar polymers. Polymerized sugars are the starches and fibers. The starch or fiber type depends on sugar species and type of polymer linkages (see Carbohydrates). Glucose (a monosaccharide blood sugar) and lactose (a disaccharide milk sugar) are two important animal sugars. Glycogen is an animal-specific starch and can quickly depolymerize to release its glucose content. Glycogen storage in the body is limited.

In the plant kingdom, starches and fibers are numerous and diverse. Feed grain starches are an energy source of fundamental importance to animals. Cellulose and other fiber are structural elements of grass, plants, and wood. Mammals lack fiber-degrading enzyme systems, so fiber is not digestible by the monogastric mammal; however, fiber is digestible by bacteria and protozoan microbes in the rumen and cecum of herbivorous animals. Short-chain fatty acids result from fiber digestion, and these are transformable to glucose. Fiber thus serves as a major energy source for grazing animals. Debates over the environmental impacts and costs of cattle grazing and feedlot finishing sometimes ignore the creation of high-quality animal-source protein from inedible plant tissues. In monogastrics, fiber reduces digestibility and effective caloric density yet maintains dry matter bulk. This effect finds applications in reducing

caloric density for weight control foods. Some metabolic and gastrointestinal (GI) tract transit disorders also respond to fiber therapy (Blaxter et al., 1990; Dimski, 1992).

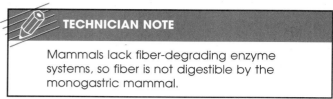

TECHNICIAN NOTE

Mammals lack fiber-degrading enzyme systems, so fiber is not digestible by the monogastric mammal.

Lipids, Fatty Acids, Fats, and Oils

Fatty acids are building block components of vegetable and animal fats. The type and distribution of constituent fatty acids determine the physical, nutritional, and biological characteristics of the fat or oil. Lipids have one to three molecules of fatty acids, are highly digestible, and have twice the caloric density of a similar quantity of carbohydrate or protein. Fat imparts significant food flavor that often improves its acceptability and palatability. Fat also facilitates digestion and assimilation of fat-soluble vitamins (A, D, E, and K). The technician will see literature referring to types of fatty acids. The length of the carbon chain *backbone* identifies a fatty acid as *long-chain, medium-chain,* or *short-chain.* Short-chain fatty acids (1 to 8 carbon atoms in length) from rumen fluids and gases are important sources of energy, but their distribution ratio can be unbalanced by rapidly changed roughage:concentrate ratios in feeds. Long-chain fatty acids (12 to 20+ carbon units) are the most common components of dietary fats and oils.

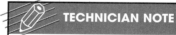

TECHNICIAN NOTE

The length of the carbon chain *backbone* identifies a fatty acid as *long-chain, medium-chain,* or *short-chain.*

The degree of hydrogen saturation (numbers of hydrogen atoms per carbon atoms) is variable, and *saturated, unsaturated,* or *polyunsaturated* denotes hydrogen content. A high quantity of unsaturated or polyunsaturated fatty acid distribution usually yields the oil form of a lipid at room temperature. More saturated fatty acid content produces fats with a higher melting point. Positioning of double-bond carbon to carbon linkages within the fatty acid leads to further subclassifications. *Omega 6* and *omega 3* fatty acids designate some of these positioning features. The ratio of omega 6 to omega 3 distribution has different biological effects in several body systems and

---

CARBOHYDRATES

Soluble	Insoluble
Starches	Pectin
Sugars	Lignin
	Cellulose
	Mucilage
	Gum
	Guar gum

ESSENTIAL FATTY ACIDS

Cats	Dogs
Linoleic	Linoleic
Linolenic	Linolenic
Arachidonic	

ESSENTIAL AMINO ACIDS

Arginine
Histidine
Isoleucine
Leucine
Lysine
Methionine
Phenylalanine
Threonine
Tryptophan
Valine
Taurine (essential in cats only)

FOOD DIGESTIBILITY

Grams of nutrients absorbed − grams of nutrients passed = food digestibility

---

FOOD UTILIZATION

Grams of nutrients eaten − grams of nutrients lost = food utilization

---

has increasingly important therapeutic applications in clinical nutrition (Bauer et al., 1989; Campbell, 1992) (see Essential Fatty Acids).

Amino Acids and Protein

> **TECHNICIAN NOTE**
>
> Amino acids are the building blocks for plant and animal protein.

Amino acids are the building blocks for plant and animal protein. Gastric and intestinal digestion subdivides protein into progressively smaller peptide units. The peptides undergo further digestion to yield the amino acids that are assimilated. The amino acid pool is then available for protein synthesis. The turnover and depletion of the pool determine the current amino acid requirement. Growth and lactation increase requirements more than maintenance and exertional work or exercise.

Amino Acids as Energy Sources

Amino acids can serve as energy nutrients as well as the synthesis substrate for new protein. Any amino acid intake beyond withdrawal from the circulating pool is metabolized into energy. This is because there is no way to "store" extra amino acids from excess dietary protein as new viscera or muscle. Conversion of extra amino acids into energy is a several-step process. Removal of the amino (nitrogen-containing) group from the hydrocarbon skeleton of the amino acid is the first step. The conversion of the hydrocarbon skeleton into ATP, CO_2, and water is the second step. The nitrogen content must be eliminated as the third step. In addition to being "expensive energy," the metabolism of excess amino acids increases liver and kidney processing and excretory requirements for the urea and organic acid waste by-products.

BIOLOGICAL VALUE

$$\text{Biological value} = \frac{\text{Grams retained}}{\text{Grams absorbed}} \times 100$$

Essential Amino Acids

All 22 amino acids are necessary for synthesis of new protein. As the body synthesizes 12 amino acids, an *essential* amino acid is one requiring supply from oral intake (see Essential Amino Acids). The quantity and distribution of essential amino acids in a protein are important features determining a protein's biological quality. All proteins are not of equal worth, and an ideal protein contains the exact essential amino acid distribution profile to meet a specific requirement (Schaeffer et al., 1989; Van Horn, 1991). When profiles are not ideal (the case in practical diets), a higher protein digestibility and a higher biological quality of protein better fulfill amino acid requirements with more efficiency and lower total nitrogen content than a low-quality protein (see Biological Value, Food Digestibility, and Food Utilization). A "limiting" amino acid is one cause of a decreased protein quality. When an otherwise high biological value protein has a missing essential amino acid and, therefore, a more limited quality, the full potential of the biological value of the protein is restored when the limiting acid is added. This is one reason why mixed animal and plant protein sources are often complementary to each other in food formulation.

Amino Acids as Emergency Fuels

Amino acids can produce energy during starvation or other negative energy balance situations. As starch and fatty acid stores are depleted, amino acids mobilize from skeletal muscle and visceral proteins to provide glucose for energy. *Gluconeogenesis* (chemical breakdown of protein for glucose) is a valuable survival mechanism but "wastes" vital circulating and structural proteins. Loss of muscle mass and strength is a common clinical observation during anorexia and illness/injury, and muscle atrophy is a fundamental signal to the technician that protein is supplying energy.

Protein Requirements

Clients often inquire about the "best" protein intake for animals. Crude protein quantity (on the label) is the usual concern, and clients assume that "more is better." However, a "high protein number" is not always the defining criterion for food quality. Chemical analysis for crude protein measures only total nitrogen content. The essential-to-nonessential amino acid profile, protein digestibility, and amino acid bioavailability are neither measured nor stated. Lower quantities of a higher biological quality protein usually represent a higher-quality food and a more appropriate nutritional objective.

In cats, gluconeogenic amino acids are a major source of energy, and cats are specifically adapted to high protein intake (Morris and Rogers, 1989). Herbivores evolved eating seasonal grasses and plants and have rumen or cecal microbes capable of synthesizing a portion of the amino acid requirement (Simons and Hand, 1993).

NON–ENERGY-PRODUCING NUTRIENTS

Oxygen and Water

Oxygen is an indirect *nutrient* because it permits the "burn" of the energy-producing substrates. If oxygen is the most limiting of all nutrients, water is the most important of the orally ingested nutrients. Water quality issues matter greatly to animals. In horse husbandry, the provision of an accessible and potable water supply is a fundamental issue (Carson, 1993). Dehydration from heavy sweat and prolonged work can be compensated for in animals by periodically watering them while they are working if that is possible. Frozen water can result in dehydration of animals, and a functioning stock tank heater or ice-breaking is needed for livestock and horses under conditions of prolonged freezing weather. Dehydration is a common and frequently major clinical problem in sick patients unwilling or unable to eat and drink.

TECHNICIAN NOTE

If oxygen is the most limiting of all nutrients, water is the most important of the orally ingested nutrients.

Minerals

Macro and *micro* describe two mineral intake levels. Calcium, phosphorus, magnesium, sodium, potassium, chlorine, and sulfur are dietary macrominerals (Table 26–1). Macrominerals are constituents of bone and structural proteins, and they participate as cofactors and catalysts in many biochemical reactions. When minerals circulate as ionized cation or anion electrolytes, they participate in osmotic fluid balance, nerve conduction, muscle contraction, blood clotting, blood pH buffering, and numerous other physiological processes (Table 26–2).

Food provision of the macrominerals is expressed as parts

• Table 26–1 •

MINERAL CATEGORIES					
MACROMINERALS*		**MICROMINERALS†**			
Salt (sodium chloride)	NaCl	Zinc	Zn	Copper	Cu
Potassium	K+	Selenium	Se	Iron	Fe
Phosphorus	P	Manganese	Mn	Silicon	Si
Magnesium	Mg²⁺	Iodine	I	Molybdenum	Mo
Calcium	Ca²⁺	Fluorine	F	Cobalt	Co
Sulfur	S	Chromium	Cr		

*Measured in mg/kg.
†Measured in ppm or μg.

per hundred (percent). Deficiency of macromineral intake produces serious clinical effects, but these are uncommon with proper feeding of appropriate foods. Deficiency most frequently follows anorexia, starvation, or poor-quality food. Excess macromineral intake results from supplementation or poorer-quality foods high in mineral-containing ingredients, such as meat and bone meal. Owner supplementation leads to excess total intake when a food is already adequate in macrominerals. The technician most commonly encounters this situation among well-intentioned, but uninformed, purebred animal hobbyists. For example, when adequate calcium and vitamin D in foal or puppy foods are supplemented for "support" of rapid skeletal growth, a resulting hypercalcemia may actually inhibit normal bone growth and cartilage maturation.

Microminerals

TECHNICIAN NOTE

Important microminerals or ``trace'' minerals are iron, zinc, manganese, copper, iodine, and selenium.

Important microminerals or "trace" minerals are iron, manganese, copper, iodine, and selenium. Dietary requirements for these minerals are in parts per million (mg/kg) instead of the percent levels for macrominerals. Hemoglobin, thyroxin, and many enzymes and cofactors contain micromineral constituents. Trace mineral deficiency and intoxication syndromes are potentially important in all species. Iron-deficient intake and chronic blood loss lead to depleted iron stores. Trace mineral deficiency can also result from bioavailability reductions from a competitive inhibition of assimilation. High calcium and/or phytate content may reduce bioavailability of zinc, copper, and other minerals, and zinc-responsive dermatoses are seen in hogs and dogs fed inferior, high-mineral foods.

Vitamins

Vitamin (from *vital amine*) describes essential dietary cofactors that participate in many biochemical reactions. Vitamins have both common and chemical names. Vitamins are classified as fat soluble (A, D, E, and K) or water soluble (all B and C), based on water solubility and route of excretion. Vitamins are not energy nutrients, and intake in excess of requirements does not improve performance. However, vitamins are often ascribed mystical performance enhancement values, and the "more-is-better" philosophy is frequently encountered. In the world of performance athletes, in which vitamin megatherapy is routinely encountered, abusive oversupplementation levels of fat-soluble vitamins may lead to hypervitaminosis syndromes (Table 26–3).

Nutrients Versus Ingredients

The terms *nutrient, ingredient, formula,* and *nutrient profile* are easily confused and sometimes used interchangeably. *Nutrients* are fundamental energy and metabolic substrates and cofactors such as lysine, glucose, or zinc. *Ingredients* are the

• Table 26–2 •

MINERAL FUNCTIONS AND EFFECTS OF DEFICIENCY AND EXCESS

MINERAL	FUNCTION	DEFICIENCY	EXCESS
Calcium	Constituent of bone and teeth, blood clotting, myocardial function, nerve transmission, membrane permeability	Decreased growth, decreased appetite, decreased bone mineralization, lameness, spontaneous fractures, loose teeth, tetany, convulsions, rickets (osteomalacia: adults)	Decreased feed efficiency and intake, nephrosis, Ca^{2+} urate stones, lameness, enlarged costochondral junctions
Phosphorus	Constituent of bone and teeth, muscle formation, fat, carbohydrates and protein metabolism, phospholipids and energy production, reproduction	Decreased appetite, decreased feed efficiency, decreased growth, dull hair coat, decreased fertility, spontaneous fractures, rickets	Bone loss, urinary calculi, decreased weight gain, decreased feed intake, calcification of soft tissues, secondary hyperparathyroidism
Potassium	Muscle contractility, transmission of nerve impulses, acid-base imbalance, osmotic balance, enzyme cofactor (energy transfer)	Anorexia, decreased growth, lethargy, locomotive problems, hypokalemia, heart and kidney lesions, emaciation	Rare
Sodium chloride	Osmotic pressure, acid-base balance, transmission of nerve impulses, nutrient uptake, waste excretion, water metabolism	Inability to maintain water balance, decreased growth, anorexia, fatigue, exhaustion, dryness/loss of hair	Occurs only if there is inadequate nonsaline, good-quality water available; causes thirst, pruritus, constipation, seizures and death; chronic amounts may induce hypertension, resulting in increased heart and renal diseases
Magnesium	Component of bone, intercellular fluids, neuromuscular transmission, active component of several enzymes, carbohydrate and lipid metabolism	Muscular weakness, hyperirritability, convulsions, anorexia, vomiting, decreased mineralization of bone, decreased body weight, calcification of aorta	Urinary calculi
Iron	Enzyme constituent: activation of O_2 (oxidases, oxygenases), O_2 transport (hemoglobin, myoglobin)	Anemia, rough hair coat, listless, decreased growth	Anorexia, weight loss, decreased serum albumin
Zinc	Constituent or activator of 200 known enzymes (nucleic acid metabolism, protein synthesis, carbohydrate metabolism), skin and wound healing, immune response, fetal development, growth rate	Anorexia, decreased growth, alopecia, parakeratosis, impaired reproduction, vomiting, hair depigmentation, conjunctivitis	Relatively atoxic. Reported cases in Zn toxicity from consumption of die-cast Zn nuts
Copper	Component of several enzymes (i.e., oxidases), catalyst in hemoglobin formation, cardiac function, cellular respiration, connective tissue development, pigmentation, bone formation, myelin formation, immune function	Anemia, decreased growth, hair depigmentation, bone lesions, neuromuscular, enzootic ataxia, aortic rupture, reproductive failure	Hepatitis, increased liver enzymes
Manganese	Component and activator of enzymes (glycosyl transferases), lipid and carbohydrate metabolism, bone development (organic matrix), reproduction, cell membrane integrity (mitochondria)	Decreased growth (rare in dogs and cats)	Relatively toxic
Selenium	Constituent of glutathione peroxidase and iodothyronine-5'-deiodinase, immune function, reproduction	Muscular dystrophy, reproductive failure, decreased feed intake, subcutaneous edema, renal mineralization	Vomiting spasms, staggered gait, salivation, decreased appetite, dyspnea, "garlicky" breath
Iodine	Constituent of thyroxine and triiodothyronine	Goiter, fetal resorption, rough hair coat, enlarged thyroid glands, alopecia, apathy, myxedema, lethargy	Similar to deficiency, decreased appetite, listlessness, rough hair coat, decreased immunity, decreased weight gain, goiter, fever
Boron	Regulates parathormone action, influences metabolism of Ca^{2+}, P, Mg^{2+}, and cholecalciferol	Decreased growth, decreased hematocrit, hemoglobin, and alkaline phosphate	Similar to deficiency. 150–200 ppm maximum tolerated level

Information provided by Dr. Karen Wedekind, Mark Morris Institute, Topeka.

• Table 26–3 •

VITAMINS			
VITAMIN	**FUNCTION**	**DEFICIENCY**	**TOXICITY**
Vitamin A	Component of visual proteins, differentiation of epithelial cells, spermatogenesis, immune function, bone resorption	Anorexia, retarded growth, poor hair coat, weakness, increased cerebrospinal fluid pressure, eye disorders, aspermatogenesis, fetal resorption	Cervical spondylosis (cat), retarded growth, anorexia, erythema, large bone fractures
Vitamin D	Ca^{2+} and P homeostasis, bone mineralization and resorption, insulin synthesis, immune function	Rickets, osteoporosis, osteomalacia	Hypercalcemia, calcinosis, lameness, anorexia
Vitamin E	Biological antioxidant, maintains membrane integrity	Sterility (males), steatitis, anorexia, dermatosis, immunodeficiency, myopathy	Minimally toxic, increased clotting time reversed with vitamin K
Vitamin K	Allows blood clotting protein formation	Prolonged clotting time, hemorrhage, hypoprothrombinemia	Minimally toxic, anemia (dogs), none described in cats
Vitamin B complex	Multiple metabolic reactions, component of energy-producing biochemical reactions that produce energy and allow proper function of tissues and organs	Retarded growth, diarrhea, emaciation, ataxia, anemia, dermatitis	Low toxicity, except niacin in the cat, which can cause convulsions and death
Vitamin C	Synthesized from D-glucose in dogs and cats; synthesis of collagen proteins and carnitine, enhances iron absorption	Deficiency symptoms have not been described in normal dogs and cats	None described in dogs and cats
Choline	Component of membranes, neurotransmitter	Fatty liver (puppies), thymus atrophy, decreased growth rate, anorexia	None described in cats or dogs
Vitamin-like nutrient L-carnitine	Synthesized from the amino acid lysine, transports long-chain fatty acids into the cell	Hyperlipidemia, cardiomyopathy, muscle asthenia	None described in cats and dogs

Courtesy of Chris Cowell, Mark Morris Institute, Topeka.

materials used to manufacture a finished feed. The *formula* selects and apportions ingredients. The *nutrient profile* describes the resulting quantitative distribution of the individual nutrients within the finished formula. These definitions are important in client education efforts when nutrient profile becomes confused with ingredients. In particular, some pet food advertising focuses on the presence of a particular ingredient as a brand point of difference. However, at the absorptive surface of the small intestinal mucosa, the ingredient of origin for a digested nutrient is immaterial.

TECHNICIAN NOTE

Nutrients are fundamental energy and metabolic substrates and cofactors such as lysine, glucose, or zinc. *Ingredients* are the materials used to manufacture a finished feed.

Additives and Preservatives

Additives are nonenergy, non-nutrient components added to protect nutrient stability or enhance acceptability. Clients sometimes question additives and preservatives from the standpoint of necessity and food safety. The technician will need an opinion on the subject of natural versus synthetic additives in particular.

Colors, flavors, palatability enhancement digests, emulsifying agents, stabilizers, thickeners, and dough conditioners are examples of additives. Preservation of the nutrient profile is an important need achieved by both physical and chemical means. Dehydration is an important form of food preservation as seen in dried meats, dry pet food, and dry hay. Drying can protect nutrients for months. Canned pet foods involve the use of heat sterilization, an anaerobic environment, and a physical vacuum as a preservative and antioxidant system. Chemical preservatives are additives that retard oxidation, discoloration, or spoilage.

Organic acids or inorganic salts, such as common table salt, have preservative effect through their antimicrobic activity (salted meats). Humectants are a preservative additive that binds water to inhibit mold and fungal growth. Chemicals that inhibit oxygen's destruction of vulnerable bonds are antioxidants. These agents primarily protect fatty acids and fat-soluble vitamins from rancid oxidation and loss of potency. Over the food's shelf life, a significant percentage of an antioxidant is "consumed" doing its job. Additives protect product quality and have good safety records based on years of application in animal agriculture and in pets (Mumma et al., 1986). One may question the need for coloring additives.

ESTIMATING ANIMALS' ENERGY REQUIREMENTS

Energy requirement estimates are used to calculate feeding quantity. There are several predictive equations for energy requirements based on the animal's species and physiological requirements. The maintenance energy requirement is simply the calories needed to maintain neutral weight for the animal's current activity and environment. This number is a range affected by several activity and environmental factors (Fig. 26–2). Work, lactation, and growth further modify energy requirements, and such multiples over maintenance are sometimes called production energy requirements.

Predictive equations are useful, but judging the body composition and condition is the key issue for energy balance assessment. The guideline for maintenance energy requirements is simply "To feel but not see the ribs" in a scheme of Body Condition Scoring (BCS) (Table 26–4).

COMPANION ANIMAL NUTRITION

Feeding Dogs

Dogs are highly social pack animals and cooperative team hunters. Wild-type feeding is both hierarchical and competitive with intrapack feeding order maintained by the alpha dominant animal. Food intake in wild canids is distinctly omnivorous, although pet food advertising emphasizes the carnivorous aspects of intake ("meatier is better"). Wild dogs eat intestines and intestinal contents of herbivorous prey, as well as organs and flesh. Many domesticated dogs will eat vegetables, grains and pastas, meat, processed foods, various dairy products, and even fruit. Dental and digestive anatomy and nutritional bio-

chemistry further document the dog as omnivorous, and it is fair to say domesticated dogs can adapt well to a varied dietary intake (Morris and Rogers, 1989). However, when domesticated dogs eat grass and/or feces, owners complain that the pet is not behaving as a carnivore. Although such ingestive behavior is natural, behavior modification (e.g., the use of cayenne pepper sauce on the feces) may reduce the objectionable activity.

Canine Pediatric Nutrition

Puppies usually nurse soon after birth. Postsurgical nursing of the canine who has undergone cesarean section specifically notes colostrum production by the dam and intake by puppies before discharge from the hospital. Colostrum provides fluid for vital postpartum circulatory expansion and maternal immunity factors (globulin antibodies) for absorption by the intestine. Most puppies are healthy and are capable and active in nursing. Most mothers are lactating well and attentive to the litter; therefore, no assistance is needed from the technician or owner. The possible exception is in extremely small, toy-breed puppies for whom frequent, assisted hand-feeding for several weeks after birth may be needed to preclude hypothermia and hypoglycemia. When there is concern about lactation, a quick indicator for quality and quantity, in addition to examining the milk itself, is to weigh the puppies. A normal growth rate for puppies is 2 to 4 g/day/kg of anticipated adult weight. Weight gain below this rate accompanied by restless hungry-seeming puppies is a sign of feeding distress.

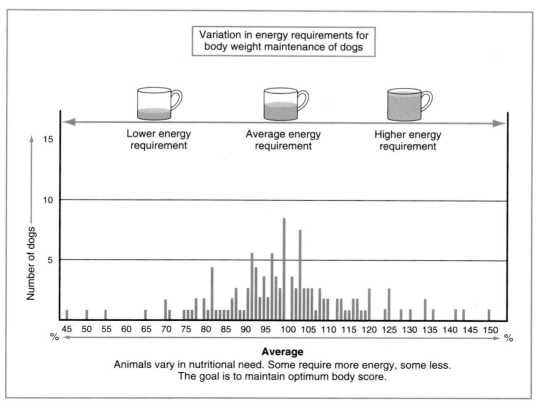

Figure 26-2. Variation in canine energy requirements.

• Table 26-4 •

	ENERGY	PROTEIN	FAT	FIBER	CALCIUM	PHOSPHORUS	SODIUM
	Kcal ME/g						
LIFE STAGE				**% Dry Matter**			
Dog							
Growth/reproduction	4.0–5.0	28–35	15–30	5 max	1.0–1.8	0.8–1.4	0.3–0.5
Large-breed growth	3.5–4.0	28–35	8–15	10 max	0.9–1.2	0.8–1.2	0.3–0.5
Adult maintenance	3.5–4.5	15–28	5–20	5 max	0.5–0.9	0.2–0.8	0.1–0.4
Obesity prone	3.0–3.5	15–28	5–15	5–17	0.5–0.9	0.2–0.8	0.1–0.4
High energy	>4.5	17–30	20 min	5 max	0.5–0.9	0.2–0.9	0.1–0.5
Geriatric	3.5–4.5	15–20	5–15	10 max	0.2–0.6	0.2–0.6	0.1–0.3
Cat							
Growth/reproduction	4.0–5.0	35–50	18–35	5 max	1.0–1.6	0.8–1.4	0.3–0.6
Adult maintenance	4.0–5.0	30–45	10–30	5 max	0.5–1.0	0.3–0.8	0.2–0.6
Obesity prone	3.3–3.8	30–45	8–17	5–15	0.5–1.0	0.3–0.8	0.2–0.6
Geriatric*	3.5–4.5	30–45	10–25	10 max	0.6–1.0	0.3–0.7	0.2–0.5

Nutrients are expressed as % dry matter. Energy is expressed as Kcal Me per gram dry matter.
*Older cats require frequent body condition scoring. Feed intake adjustment may be required to maintain a (3) body condition as some older cats tend to be heavy and others tend to lose weight.

Average Caloric Content of Pet Foods
Dog food (generic, private label, and popular)
Dry	350 Kcal/cup
Soft-moist	275 Kcal/cup
Canned	500 Kcal/15-oz can

Cat food (generic, private label, and popular)
Dry	300 Kcal/cup
Soft-moist	250 Kcal/cup
Canned	180 Kcal/6.5-oz can

Raising Orphan Puppies

Neonatal puppies unable to nurse require a canine milk replacer formula. Canine milk is higher in protein and lower in lactose than bovine milk, so water, not cow's milk, should be used to mix formula. The orphan formula dose is initially 15% of the puppy's weight per day divided into several doses. Food dose adequacy is usually announced by the puppy's becoming content and going to sleep after feeding. Assisted feeding of neonates is by feeding syringe and a flexible, rubber feeding tube (Fig. 26–3A). If there is adequate nursing vigor, one may substitute a pet nurser system (Fig. 26–3B). At litter discharge from the hospital, the technician should pretest flow rate from all nipples dispensed and give explicit instructions for sanitation and formula mixing. When the puppy reaches 2 to 3 weeks of age, the food dose approximates 25% of the body weight divided into four to six daily feedings.

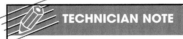

TECHNICIAN NOTE

The orphan formula dose is initially 15% of the puppy's body weight per day divided into several doses.

Weaning Puppies

Peak lactation occurs at 4 weeks, and weaning concludes at 6 to 8 weeks. Begin introducing puppies to semisolid gruel made

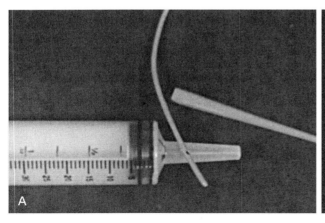

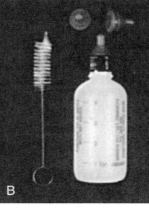

Figure 26-3. A, Orphan puppies and kittens are raised on species-specific milk replacer. Tube gavage with flexible feeding tube and a catheter-tip syringe is an easy and safe technique in neonatal puppies and kittens. B, Pet nursers are used in neonates with adequate sucking vigor. Always test the flow and temperature of formula in advance and sanitize equipment between uses.

OBESITY-PRONE DOG BREEDS

Beagle
Labrador
Sheltie
Cocker spaniel
Golden retriever
Cairn terrier
Scottish terrier
Dachshund
Bassett hound

from 2 parts of water to 1 part of a high-quality, dry, canine growth/lactation pet food. Three weeks of age is a suitable time to introduce a semisolid gruel, except for toy breeds and weak animals. Mash the mixture with a fork, and place the gruel in a shallow pan. Gruel ingestion inevitably follows a play period and begins acclimating the puppies to intake of particulate solids. At 5 weeks of age, puppies are reducing their intake of mother's milk and consuming significant amounts of gruel. The ratio of water can be reduced as the puppies approach total weaning onto dry or moist foods.

Feeding Growing Dogs

Absolute and relative nutritional requirements change rapidly during a puppy's growth. Rate of growth, as well as final adult

FEEDING DO'S

- Provide fresh water
- Feed for control of calorie intake
- Feed for ideal weight and individuality
- Feel but do not see the ribs
- Provide a consistent food and ritualize the time and place of feeding
- Use life-stage feeding concepts by correlating diet to pet's life stage
- Feed treats with nutrient profile and caloric density considerations

FEEDING DONT'S

- Provide stagnant or frozen water
- Allow excess calories
- Feed obesity-prone dogs on an *ad libitum* basis
- Rotate flavors or brands on a frequent basis
- Make rapid transitions
- Use growth/lactation diets for adult maintenance
- Supplement a balanced/high-quality diet
- Allow competitive eating

size, is obviously and dramatically different between various dog breeds. Most growing puppies eat four or five times daily during the postweaning period, but meal frequency declines as gastrointestinal capacity increases. The quantity of food can be determined in several ways, and Figure 26–4 demonstrates some model calculations for establishing a food dose. The methods of feeding puppies require specific consideration. The *ad libitum* (ad-lib) feeding method permits excess nutrient intake in many puppies. When the puppy overconsumes energy and calcium, developmental bone disease may surface (Kallfelz, 1989B). This is especially evident in the rapidly growing members of the large and giant breeds. Unfortunately, some growth-type pet foods contain excessive calcium even at appropriate levels of dry matter intake (Kallfelz, 1989A, 1989B). Energy overconsumption, by itself, was studied in two groups of labrador retriever puppies (Kealy et al., 1992). One group ate ad-lib, and the second group was limited to 75% of the ad-lib quantity. Serial pelvic radiography for 2 years showed significant reductions in hip laxity in the meal-limited group. To help control the risk to normal orthopedic development of large-breed and giant puppies, a specific nutrient profile has been developed to control the potential overconsumption of energy and macro-minerals while supplying growth levels of protein and vitamins.

"Roly-poly" puppies also risk current and future obesity. The technician should emphasize the risk of juvenile overfeeding as a part of the client education program. This is especially true when the animal is a member (or cross breed) of obesity-prone breeds (see Obesity-Prone Dog Breeds).

Feeding Adult Dogs

A primary objective in feeding the adult dog is finding the energy requirement and food dose that maintains neutral energy balance (see Fig. 26–4). In adult dogs, ad-lib feeding is less labor intensive for animal colonies and kennels. Late detection of anorexia and timid animals not having adequate intake are potential problems with this method. When dogs are individually penned or can eat from self-feeders, these problems are eliminated.

Individual meal feeding is best whenever possible (Figs. 26–5 to 26–7). In the time-restricted method, feed from one to three times daily with an ad-lib consumption for 10 to 15 minutes. If the dog consistently leaves a little food in its dish and also maintains an ideal body condition, the conclusion must be that the animal is self-regulating its food intake at its energy requirement. Time-restricted feeding works well for many dogs and their owners; however, some dogs ravenously overeat during the allotted time. In dogs that overeat, try volume-restricted meal feeding by serving a calculated food dose. To determine the daily volume, divide the energy requirement by the food's caloric density. Then feed one half to one third of the daily volumes two or three times per day. An average caloric density guideline for pet foods is listed (see Table 26–4). Other aids for food dose calculations are suggested feeding amounts on labels, food dose calculators, and technical information from manufacturers (see Feeding Do's and Feeding Don'ts). Maintenance pet food is recommended for the average house pet.

It should also be recommended that table scraps be eliminated or used in moderation (10% or less). Fat trimmings quickly unbalance a base diet and lead to "finicky" behavior and predisposition to obesity. Avoid feeding animal bones be-

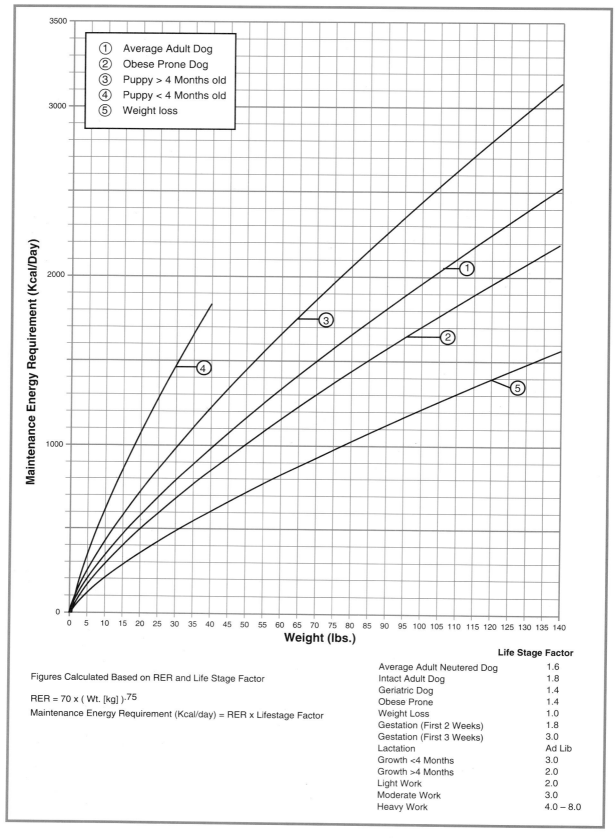

Figures Calculated Based on RER and Life Stage Factor

$RER = 70 \times (\ Wt.\ [kg]\ )^{.75}$

Maintenance Energy Requirement (Kcal/day) = RER x Lifestage Factor

	Life Stage Factor
Average Adult Neutered Dog	1.6
Intact Adult Dog	1.8
Geriatric Dog	1.4
Obese Prone	1.4
Weight Loss	1.0
Gestation (First 2 Weeks)	1.8
Gestation (First 3 Weeks)	3.0
Lactation	Ad Lib
Growth <4 Months	3.0
Growth >4 Months	2.0
Light Work	2.0
Moderate Work	3.0
Heavy Work	4.0 – 8.0

Figure 26-4. Canine daily energy requirements.

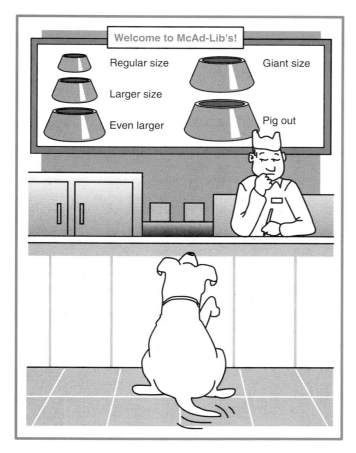

Figure 26-5. ''Ad-lib'' feeding means an excess of food, at all times, for self-feeding.

cause sharp fragments may wedge between teeth or lacerate the esophagus. Nylon bones and chew toys are safe substitutes for natural bones. Table 26–4 lists guidelines for assessing pet foods used in life-stage feeding.

> ✏ **TECHNICIAN NOTE**
>
> Avoid feeding animal bones because sharp fragments may wedge between teeth or lacerate the esophagus. Nylon bones and chew toys are safe substitutes for natural bones.

Feeding Adult Dogs with Increased Energy Needs

Increased energy is important in working dogs and stressed animals. Supply extra energy by using pet foods of increased caloric density and digestibility. This permits dry matter intake and gastric fill to remain at familiar, nonexcessive levels. Increasing the quantity and/or frequency of a regular food is a secondary option.

The technician can provide a high-quality client service by reminding hunting dog owners to aerobically condition animals before extensive field work. Aerobic training before work con-

ditions the muscles and cardiovascular system and induces enzyme changes in the muscle that allow more efficient use of fatty acids as muscle fuel. The aerobic use of fatty acids spares the rate of consumption of muscle glycogen and can increase the interval to exhaustion.

When aerobic conditioning begins, convert the dog(s) to the more calorie-dense food and suggest feeding the majority of daily calories after completion of training to help prevent hunting dog hypoglycemia. Unfortunately, the more obvious feeding recommendation would seem to be the reverse—feeding before work. However, insulin release follows glucose assimilation after the meal's digestion, allowing a high rate of glucose transfer into the cells. If the animal simultaneously begins hard work, the combination of the two glucose-consuming activities may precipitate hypoglycemia. If animals show consistent signs of hunting dog hypoglycemia, even after conditioning, they may be fed 10% to 15% of the daily calorie dose as a light feeding at 2-hour intervals during work. Clients should also be reminded of the importance of adequate water intake throughout the work period.

Feeding During Pregnancy and Lactation

Early and mid-term pregnancy is a nutritional "non-event," but requirements increase modestly during the last third of gestation. Recommend a growth/lactation formula to meet the increased requirements. Lactation markedly increases energy, protein, and mineral requirements. After whelping, the bitch

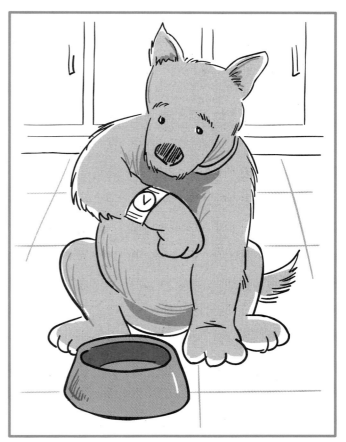

Figure 26-6. ''Time-controlled'' feeding provides an unrestricted food quantity in a 10-minute period.

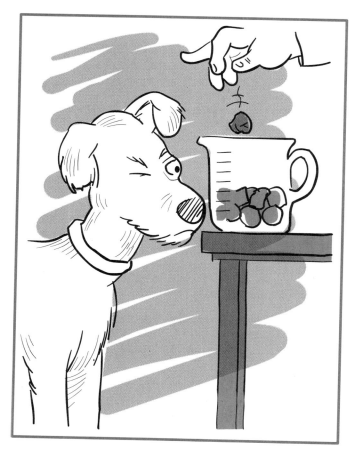

Figure 26-7. ''Portions-controlled'' feeding involves the measurement of pet food and providing it in a quantity that maintains optimum body condition.

returns to her regular body weight and eats to service increased needs (Fig. 26–8). Expect food intake to rise rapidly by 50% the first week and by 200% to 400% by the fourth week of lactation. This level of demand is equivalent to those of heavily pulling sled dogs, and the loss of fat and even muscle is common during lactation. This potential underfeeding situation can be helped by allowing ad-lib intake of a high-quality growth/lactation pet food. Supplements are *not* needed for normal animals when high-quality pet foods are used.

> ✎ **TECHNICIAN NOTE**
>
> Expect food intake to rise rapidly by 50% the first week and by 200% to 400% by the fourth week of lactation.

Weaning the Litter

Food intake should be terminated for 24 hours to help the bitch slow and stop her milk production. The food intake can be resumed using maintenance foods at one third of the customary maintenance level. On the second day, use two thirds feeding and full intake on day three. When lactation quickly dries from acute calorie deprivation, the bitch will more readily reject the puppies' attempts to continue to nurse.

Obesity-Prone Animals

Definition and Causes of Obesity

Malnutrition of obesity is at epidemic proportions. Canine obesity estimates are 30%, with feline obesity as high as 40% (MacEwen, 1992; Sloth, 1992). Obesity means body composition with a ratio of too much fat to lean tissue. (*Overweight* is not always an accurate measurement for *overfat.*) There are several known causes for obesity, and as a confidant of the owner, the technician is vital in the crusade to prevent and treat this epidemic.

> ✎ **TECHNICIAN NOTE**
>
> Canine obesity estimates are 30%, with feline obesity as high as 40%.

One cause for obesity-prone animals is overfeeding when young. A positive calorie balance during juvenile growth induces increased numbers of fat cells (hyperplasia) (Hand et al.,

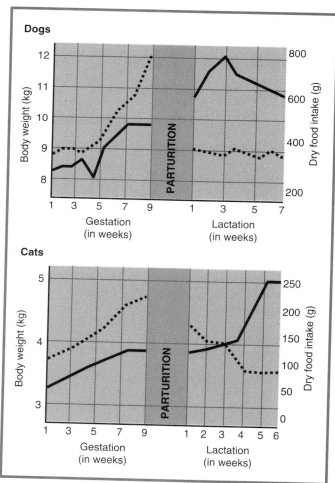

Figure 26–8. The pattern of normal weight gain during gestation and loss in the postpartum and lactation periods differs between the cat and dog.

1989). Once formed, these fat cells are present for life and have minimal volumes of triglyceride content below which they cannot shrink (Crane, 1991). Therefore, a lifelong predisposition for excess weight develops. Needless adipocyte hyperplasia is prevented by using meal feeding for puppies, kittens, and foals. A second cause of obesity is genetic predisposition. Several lines of evidence establish genetic inheritance as influential on the resting metabolic rate (Crane, 1991). This means "easy keepers" with less food intake required.

Third, a declining lean body mass and declining activity level are part of the normal aging process. Decreases in energy requirements may be considered in a geriatric feeding program (Markham and Hodgkins, 1989). However, some older pets may also become thin.

Fourth, animals may overeat just because they like the high palatability of the food. Volume-restricted meal feeding and control of the intake of treats will be needed when this situation is identified.

Fifth, multi-animal households or other group-feeding situations may provoke competitive eating. The control measures are volume-restricted feeding and separation of the competitive animals by time and/or place of feeding. Most owners can "engineer" these circumstances with a little thought and coaching.

Sixth, surgical neutering of males and females deregulates satiety and increases the desire to feed. One may suggest less calorically dense foods concurrent with postneuter suture removal. This seems especially prudent in obesity-prone breeds of dogs (Edney and Smith, 1986).

Diagnosis and Treatment of Obesity

One can assess the quantity of the patient's fat by examining the subcutaneous deposits visually and by palpation over the ribs, groin, and tail head. Radiographs of the abdomen and thorax will also reveal fat accumulations. Weighing only indirectly measures body composition. But using ideal weight tables for purebred animals is useful (Hand et al., 1989). Body condition scoring (Fig. 26–9) is a visual and useful method for combining various assessment criteria into an opinion regarding the pet's body composition and relative fatness. Obesity is best prevented but can be treated by caloric restriction and exercise. Specific treatment requires teamwork among the owner, the veterinarian, and the technician.

Weight control is rarely as easy as it sounds, but long-term success in weight reduction can be achieved in practice (MacEwen, 1992). However, success is precious, and some practices focus most strongly on identifying those clients most able or most likely to be educated and motivated. In monitoring any treatment program, the veterinary technician is of fundamental importance as educator and cheerleader. Part of the dietary management program is building awareness of extraneous contributions of calories such as treats, including both human snack foods and commercial pet treats (see Tables 26–5 and 26–6).

Feeding the Geriatric Animal

The definition of *geriatric*, as it pertains to the dog, is not precise because of breed variability in the natural life span and because "miles as well as years" influence the "wear-and-tear" of physiological aging. As a generality, toy and small-sized breeds are "geriatric" at 7 years, medium-sized dogs at 6 years, and large and giant breeds as early as 5 years of age.

Loss of reserve capacity of organ function (eyes to bones) is universal with the normal aging change. Chronic progressive renal disease, due to aging changes alone, is of high incidence in dogs and cats (Markham and Hodgkins, 1989). There is no proven cause for or prophylactic strategy against the scourge of renal aging. However, the progressive loss of renal reserve ultimately reduces the animal's capability to excrete phosphorus, urea, and other waste by-products of protein metabolism. Controlling excesses of intake during the geriatric period does no harm even in the absence of clinical signs of renal failure. Therefore, the recommendation to restrict excessive protein, phosphorus, and sodium seems medically prudent.

In renal failure, the veterinarian will prescribe specific intake restrictions of protein, phosphorus, sodium, and, perhaps, other measures to control hyperphosphatemia (Polzin et al., 1989). Cats have elevated potassium requirements during renal insufficiency and renal failure (Fettman, 1989). Many animals with renal insufficiency and failure will be in their geriatric period of life.

Calorie control may begin or be continued in older animals. On the other hand, other older animals may have inadequate calories due to systemic illness, dental or oral pain, failing sight and smell, or progression of "finicky" tastes or fixed food addictions. Blanket feeding recommendations based solely on age are unwise without consideration of the individual. Pet foods specifically intended for "seniors" emphasize moderate energy density with good palatability and reductions of some excess nutrients, as found in all-purpose pet foods.

Feeding Cats

Cats are not "small dogs" and are physically, physiologically, and behaviorally adapted as solo-hunting, carnivorous predators. Use of amino acids as important energy sources translates into cats having twice the protein requirement of the more omnivorous dog. The percentage of total dietary calories originating from an ideal protein source (biological value of 100%) is 8% in adult cats but 4% in adult dogs. Other feline specific requirements include taurine as an 11th essential amino acid (McDonald et al., 1984). Animal origin types and/or sources of vitamin A, niacin, pyridoxine, and arachidonic acid (a fatty acid) are other feline-specific requirements. Feeding dog food to cats for convenience or economy is ill advised. If the technician encounters this dietary history, the veterinarian should be alerted for educational intervention. Figure 26–10 summarizes energy requirements for cats in differing life stages and lifestyles.

Feeding Kittens and Adult Cats

One must confirm adequate colostrum intake for all kittens. Like puppies, the orphan kitten can be raised by tube gavage or nurser administration of queen's milk replacer. Kittens are weaned later than puppies—generally at 7 to 9 weeks. Growth-sustaining kitten foods are then meal-fed twice to three times daily until the kitten is 10 months of age.

As adults, feral cats have "nibbling" eating patterns as they hunt mice and other small animals most of the night and part of the day. Nibbling minimizes the effect of the postprandial alkaline tide—a physiological event that alkalinizes the urine

BODY CONDITION SCORING SYSTEM

Body condition assessment will assist the veterinary technician in determining if the puppy or kitten is growing appropriately and if the correct amount of food is being offered. Proper growth can reduce risk for obesity and growth related skeletal disease.

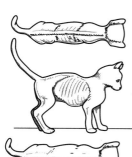

1. VERY THIN

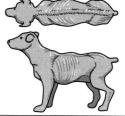

The ribs are easily palpable with no fat cover. The tailbase* has a prominent raised bony structure with no tissue between the skin and bone. The bone prominences are easily felt with no overlying fat. In animals over six months, there is a severe abdominal tuck when viewed from the side and an accentuated hourglass shape when viewed from above.

2. UNDERWEIGHT

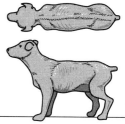

The ribs are easily palpable with minimal fat cover. The tailbase* has a raised bony structure with little tissue between the skin and bone. The bony prominences are easily felt with minimal overlying fat. In animals over six months, there is an abdominal tuck when viewed from the side and a marked hourglass shape when viewed from above.

3. IDEAL

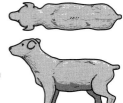

The ribs are palpable with a slight fat cover. The tailbase* has a smooth contour or some thickening and the bony structures are palpable under a thin layer of fat between the skin and the bone. The bony prominences are easily felt with a slight amount of overlying fat. In animals over six months, there is an abdominal tuck when viewed from the side and a well proportioned lumbar waist when viewed from above.

4. OVERWEIGHT

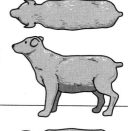

The ribs are difficult to feel with moderate fat cover. The tailbase* has some thickening with moderate amounts of tissue between the skin and bone. The bony structures can still be felt. The bony prominences are covered by a moderate layer of fat. In animals over six months, there is little or no abdominal tuck or waist when viewed from above. Abdominal fat apron present in cats.

5. OBESE

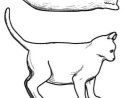

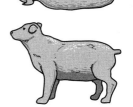

The ribs are very difficult to feel under a thick fat cover. The tailbase* appears thickened and is difficult to feel under a prominent layer of fat. The bony prominences are covered by a moderate to thick layer of fat. In animals over six months, there is a pendulous ventral bulge and no waist when viewed from the side. The back is markedly broadened when viewed from above. Marked abdominal fat apron present in cats.

*Tailbase evaluation is done only in dogs.

Figure 26–9. Body conditioning scoring system.

• Table 26–5 •

NUTRIENT CHARACTERISTICS OF HUMAN SNACK FOODS*						
FOOD	SERVING SIZE	Kcal/SERVING	Kcal/g	PROTEIN (g)	FAT (g)	Na⁺†
Cow's milk (3.5%)	1 c = 244 g	150	0.6	8	8	122/81
Whole egg (boiled)	1 egg = 50 g	79	1.6	6.1	5.6	69/87
Ice cream (vanilla, 10% fat)	1 c = 133 g	266	2.0	4.8	14.3	116/43
American cheese	1 oz	93	3.3	5.6	7	337/362
Cottage cheese (low fat, 2%)	1 c = 226 g	203	0.9	31	4.4	918/452
Jell-O	1 c = 280 g	162	0.6	3.2	0	108/67
Hot dog	8/lb = 57 g	180	3.2	6.9	16.3	585/325
Bologna (beef)	1 slice = 23 g	72	3.1	2.8	6.6	226/313
Big Mac	1 sand = 200 g	570	2.9	24.6	35	979/172
Peanut butter (smooth)	2 tbsp = 32 g	188	5.9	9	5.4	234/124
Popcorn (w/butter)	3 c = 37 g	192	5.2	2.8	11.5	273/142
Corn chips	1 oz	153	5.5	1.7	8.8	218/142
Potato chips	1 oz	148	5.3	1.8	10.1	133/90
Pretzels	1 oz	110	3.9	3.0	1.2	543/493

*Metabolizable energy for humans. All values from Pennington JAT: Food Values of Portions Commonly Used. 15th ed. New York, Harper & Row, 1989.
†Na⁺ content per serving/Na⁺ content per 100 Kcal.

after meal feeding. This may help to protect against urinary crystalluria, but twice-daily meal feeding is practical and works well for indoor cats.

A consistent feeding product and schedule should be recommended during adult maintenance. Decreased finickiness results from this approach, but flavor rotation is a perspective of some owners in response to the large number of cat food flavors present on supermarket shelves. Flavor rotation is unnecessary for variety, and a transient "newness" factor increases food intake when the new flavor is introduced. The result is the owner's perception of doing the cat a "favor" (expressed as increased intake). However, weight homeostasis may be upset by frequent flavor rotation.

Commercial feline treats are usually clones of dry cat food (see Table 26–6). As such, they are appropriate for treating when given in moderation and dietary restriction is not needed. Some cat owners prefer "natural" treats such as raw or cooked poultry necks, oxtails, or liver. Although little harm results from the use of such treats in moderation, finicky behavior and nutritional imbalance are potential hazards. Liver contains an inverted Ca:P ratio (1:17), and potentially toxic levels of vitamin A (hypervitaminosis A) can occur with long-term use (Goldman, 1992).

Feeding Cats in Gestation and Lactation

There are significant differences in food intake between the bitch and the queen during the initial stages of lactation (see Fig. 26–8). The queen apparently will forgo postpartum hunting to attend her kittens. As a solitary hunter, she hunts less and uses the body fat stored during gestation to support her lactation. The practical significance is that clients may question low food consumption in their new mother cat. Such clients are advised that the queen will eat heavily, as expected, by the third week of lactation.

Feline Lower Urinary Tract Disease (FLUTD)

Domestic cats evolved from desert-adapted ancestors. Urine specific gravity greater than 1.070 indicates excellent ability to concentrate dissolved urinary solutes as a water conservation

mechanism. High solute concentration may favor formation of urinary crystals (crystalluria). Specific minerals dissolve into solution or precipitate as solids at specific urine pH levels. Controlling urine pH to reduce crystalluria requires a knowledge of the crystal to be inhibited. This is because struvite and oxalate, the two most common stones, form most readily in alkaline and acidic urine, respectively.

It is an oversimplification to state that controlling urine solutes of magnesium or pH always controls FLUTD. This is because the FLUTD syndrome is multifactorial, and not all causative agents or combinations of contributory factors are presently known. The possibility that cats may have a low-grade interstitial cystitis that is exacerbated by stress is one of several theories regarding the cause of this frustrating clinical problem. However, maintaining a physiological urine acidity (pH 6.2 to 6.4) and controlling magnesium intake to non-excessive levels are prudent risk control measures for struvite crystalluria.

TECHNICIAN NOTE

The FLUTD syndrome is multifactorial, and not all causative agents or combinations of contributory factors are presently known.

PET FOOD ASSESSMENT

Many clients ask for recommendations about food form, specific brand information, and differences between brands. Some owners will inquire about the suitability of home cooking, feeding from the table, and using high percentages of table scraps. Although various home-made foods can be suitable for maintenance, most practices recommend commercial pet foods. The nutrient content, safety, and overall quality of commercial foods are good (Ogilvie and Vail, 1992).

Complete and balanced pet food is fundamental to suitability and quality, whether home-made or commercially prepared. A *complete* food contains all nutrients in a bioavailable form.

• Table 26–6 •

TREAT	MANUFACTURER	WEIGHT (g/treat)	CALORIES (Kcal ME)	PROTEIN (g)	FAT (g)	FIBER (g)	CALCIUM (mg)	P (mg)	Ca²⁺:P	SODIUM (mg)	MAGNESIUM (mg)
Dog Treats											
Milkbone (small)	Nabisco	5	17	1.1	0.3	0.14	71	54	1:1.3	21	7
Beggin Strips Orginal Bacon Flavor	Purina	10.3	29	1.7	0.6	0.14	44	49	1:0.9	65	11
Bonz	Purina	20.4	66	3.1	1.3	0.33	241	155	1:1.6	53	24
Purina Biscuits	Purina	10.2	37	2.5	1.3	0.24	114	106	1:1.1	29	21
Meaty Bone (medium)	Heinz	18.2	64	2.3	1.8	0.42	8	55	1:0.2	116	20
100% Natural Treats	Heinz	7.6	26	1.3	0.5	0.11	17	49	1:0.3	41	15
Snausages (beef flavor chewy sauce)	Heinz	6.6	17	1.5	0.6	0.05	61	46	1:1.3	44	7
Pup-Peroni Jerky Snack Sticks	Heinz	6.6	21	1.8	1	0.11	55	44	1:1.2	73	7
Original Jerky Treats	Heinz	6.8	22	2	1.3	0.11	35	35	1:1	140	7
Fiber Formula Biscuits (medium)	Stewart	10.1	26	1.5	0.3	1.73	63	37	1:1.7	7.3	NA
Science Diet (adult maintenance)	Hill's	5	17	1.1	0.5	0.28	29	29	1:1	11	3.8
Science Diet (light)	Hill's	5	14	0.8	0.3	0.6	29	29	1:1	11	6.6
Science Diet (senior)	Hill's	5	17	0.8	0.4	0.41	29	27	1:1	7	4.5
Cat Treats											
Pounce	Heinz	1.5	3.7	0.32	0.13	0.01	13.5	11.3	1:1.2	9.2	1.2
Whisker Lickin's (Kluckers)	Purina	1.05	3	0.32	0.12	0.01	9	10.7	1:0.84	6.2	0.7

From Clinical Nutrition (Crane and Grosdidier).

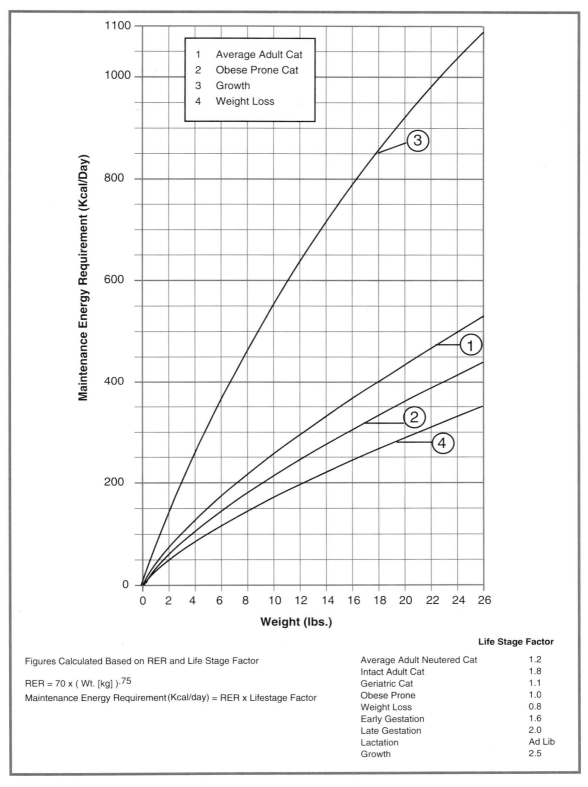

Figures Calculated Based on RER and Life Stage Factor

$RER = 70 \times (Wt. [kg])^{.75}$

Maintenance Energy Requirement (Kcal/day) = RER x Lifestage Factor

	Life Stage Factor
Average Adult Neutered Cat	1.2
Intact Adult Cat	1.8
Geriatric Cat	1.1
Obese Prone	1.0
Weight Loss	0.8
Early Gestation	1.6
Late Gestation	2.0
Lactation	Ad Lib
Growth	2.5

Figure 26-10. Feline daily energy requirements.

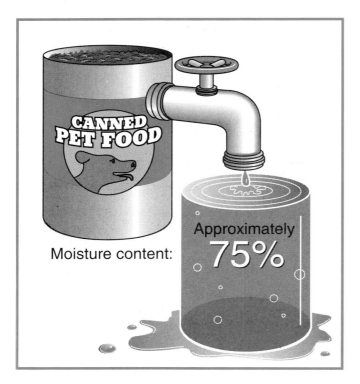

Figure 26–11. Moisture content in canned pet food.

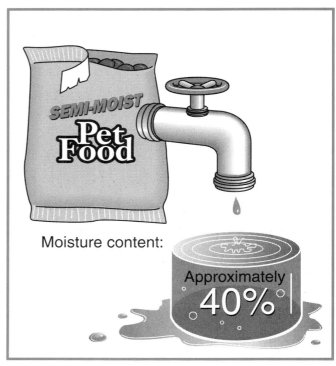

Figure 26–12. Moisture content in semimoist pet food.

Balanced means that nutrient concentrations are proportioned to total energy density. In combining these two definitions, the animal fulfills all nutrient requirements when consuming its energy requirement if it consumes a complete and balanced food. If non-energy nutrient requirements can be met in this fashion, feeding becomes as easy as calculating energy requirements. However, *balance* is a relative term, and two foods can be stated to be balanced with very different nutrient profiles. This situation occurs because official guidelines for energy requirements are published as ranges or a minimum number. Therefore, any nutrient value within the range or above the minimum can be said to be balanced.

A second general assessment is whether a pet food is specific purpose or all purpose. Formulations noting different nutritional requirements for growth, maintenance, reproduction, hard physical exertion, and the senior life stage are specific-purpose foods, and the nutrient profile can be more sharply focused to the specific need. All-purpose products, by definition, accommodate all physiological situations. Because all-purpose foods support puppy growth and lactation, they can be fed to all animals with no one needing to explain their proper use. Thus, all-purpose foods are commonly sold in mass market settings, including the generic, private label, and popular brands. This includes many pet foods perceived as specific for adult maintenance because there is no reference to "puppy" on the label.

Dry Matter Nutrient Content; Forms of Pet Food

Nutrient concentration is expressed *as is* or on a *dry matter* basis. Using dry matter removes the confusing effects of differing moisture levels (Figs. 26–11 to 26–14). The veterinary

technician most frequently needs to convert an as-is (with moisture) to a dry-matter basis (moisture removed). The example calculates protein on a dry-matter basis for a canned and dry pet food.

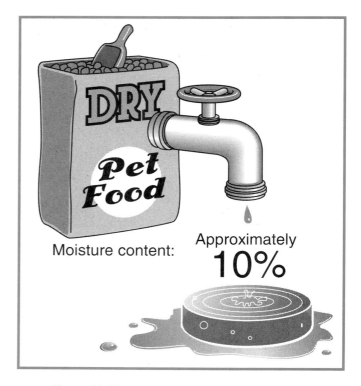

Figure 26–13. Moisture content in dry pet food.

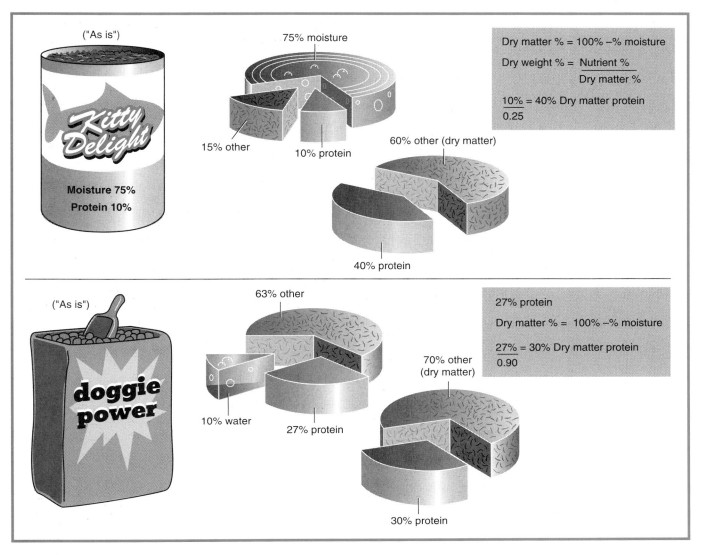

Figure 26-14. Dry matter analysis.

Differing moisture content characterizes four different pet food forms. New owners are often interested in pet food form when making food selection for a new pet.

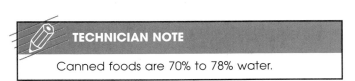

TECHNICIAN NOTE

Canned foods are 70% to 78% water.

Canned foods are 70% to 78% water and have three appearance forms—a ration loaf, an "all-meat" appearance, and processed meats and flours bound into a jellied matrix by gums or alginates. The high palatability of high-quality canned foods results from high content of water, protein, fat, and the inherent flavor of animal source tissues. Moist foods are expensive on a per-calorie basis, as fresh and frozen meat and by-product ingredients are more costly than equivalent meals and flours. In addition, the can's total dry matter (where the nutrients are) is diluted with water and the package is costly. These features

have major implications for the overall cost of feeding over time.

Questions arise regarding the use of moist foods as a combination mixer with dry foods. This is an acceptable practice and the compromise some owners seek in the trade-off between higher palatability at lower cost. As the ratio of moist food increases in a mix, the palatability and percentage of fat and protein calories usually increase as well. Finally, some owners use "gourmet" pet food as desserts or treats.

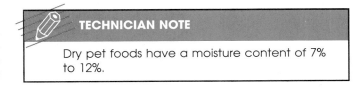

TECHNICIAN NOTE

Dry pet foods have a moisture content of 7% to 12%.

Dry pet foods have a moisture content of 7% to 12%. In making dry pet food, dry ingredients are mixed and moistened into a dough. The dough is kneaded, cooked, and extruded into an air-expanded particle. These steps are equivalent to the baking of bread. Although dry pet foods have less average palatability than the canned form, they have the advantage of lowest *true cost* when compared with canned foods (Fig. 26–15). There are also significant differences between the true costs of feeding dry foods and the impression that foods that are "expensive" on a cost-per-pound basis may actually be more economical (Fig. 26–16). Dry pet foods are the predominating source of calories in North America because of convenience and cost and are the only form suitable for ad-lib feeding.

Neither dry foods nor hard baked treats replace regular dental prophylaxis. Furthermore, clean teeth are found in dogs eating canned food and calculus-encrusted teeth occur in dogs eating dry food.

Water may be added to improve the acceptability/palatability of a dry pet food. The addition of water is the objective in dry pet foods that feature a self-originating "gravy." If more palatability is required for a dry food, use a moist food or canned palatability enhancement mixer. Several factors influence the acceptability and palatability of pet foods (see Palatability Factors).

TECHNICIAN NOTE

Semimoist foods have a 30% to 35% water content.

Semimoist foods have a 30% to 35% water content. This pet food form had considerable popularity in the 1970s but

---

EXAMPLE

Mrs. Wilson is discussing her cost of feeding concern over the diet of Rollo, her 10 lb Domestic Shorthair cat. The pet owner's intention is to obtain the best diet at the lowest cost. You have been discussing with her the nutrient profile needed for Rollo and now you will share with her a cost analysis comparing the moist food she is currently feeding (Diet A) and the dry diet you have recommended (Diet B).

CANNED FOOD VS DRY (Diet A) (Diet B)	A	Units	B
Cost per can	35	Cents	
Size of can (oz)	3	oz	
Cost per ounce	12	Cents	
Cans per day	2.5	Cans	
Cost per bag		Dollars	16.60
Size of bag		Pounds	10.00
Cost per ounce		Cents	3.80
Ounces fed per day		oz	4.30
Cost per day	88	Cents	16.40
Price difference	+437%		
15 year lifetime feeding cost	4818.00	Dollars	897.90

Figure 26–15. Cost of feeding on a per-day basis is a better measure of value than the unit cost of the can or package.

EXAMPLE

During your discussion with Mrs. Johnson about the nutritional needs of her dog, Peaches, a 22 lb mixed breed dog, she expresses concern regarding the cost of the diet (Diet B) recommended versus the current diet (Diet A) she is feeding. She says that if you can get the cost in line with what she is now feeding, she will follow your recommendation. So, you proceed in making the following calculation.

STEP	DESCRIPTION	Diet A	UNIT	Diet B
A	Cost per 40 lb bag	16.00	Dollars	31.50
B	Cost per pound of diet (A/40)	.40	Cents	.79
C	Cost per ounce (B/16)	2.5	Cents	5
D	oz/cup (by weight)	3.5	oz	3.0
E	Feeding amounts in ounces/day	17.5	oz	7.5
F	Days bag will last 640 (oz/E)	37	Days	85
G	Cost per day (C X E)	44	Cents	37
H	Cost per year (G X 365)	161	Dollars	135

Figure 26–16. Cost of daily feeding.

---

has declined in the 1990s. An intermediate moisture level and sweetness produce palatability between that found in canned and dry forms. Humectant preservatives and cellophane wrapping allow reasonable shelf life. Semimoist foods have readily available soluble sugars and simple carbohydrate sources and are not recommended in diabetics or other animals in which blood sugar control needs to be regulated.

When the dry and semimoist forms are mixed, a hybrid form of "soft-dry" results. The advantages of the dry food are enhanced by the extended palatability from the semimoist fraction. Many owners are interested in the volume and firmness of feces their pet excretes. Cat owners will be concerned with odor, and dog owners will be concerned with ease of clean up. The quantity and texture characteristics of feces relate to the amount of dry matter eaten and its digestibility (Fig. 26–17).

Market Categories

Understanding market objectives for a product may assist with some aspects of pet food quality assessment. Generic (white label) and private label (a grocery chain's own brand) foods are made at contract feed mills using least-cost formulation methods. Market emphasis is low cost. Nationally advertised and distributed (popular) brands predominate in grocery stores.

PALATABILITY FACTORS

Moisture
Odor
Fat/protein levels
Temperature
Texture
Cats: Shape (dry food)
     Acidity

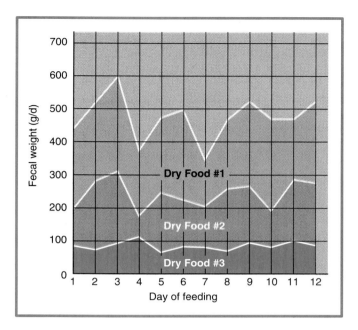

Figure 26-17. Increased digestibility and caloric density have an inverse relationship to fecal volume. Food 1 was a lower-energy food and produced voluminous stool volume with difficult clean-up characteristics. Food 3 featured high digestibility and was energy dense, and stool clean-up was quick and nonmessy.

These foods are also least-cost formulated and are marketed for their high palatability and anthropomorphic appeal. Flavor, shape, color, ingredient, and brand name proliferation characterize these products, allowing them to engage the largest amount of shelf-facing.

Premium pet foods are often sold in veterinary hospitals and pet shops. Fixed, specific formulations and high-quality ingredients characterize this category. Although differences in nutritional philosophy may be noted between different manufacturers, these brands are consistent in the overall objective of emphasizing a philosophy of optimum nutrition.

Dog and Cat Treats and Supplements

Treating is an enjoyable aspect of the human–companion animal bond. Treats include almost anything in the owner's kitchen from the "healthy" to items high in salt and calories (see Tables 26–5 and 26–6). Because treats are a potentially substantial source of calories and protein, it is important to inquire about treat intake if a patient's disease requires regulation of dietary intake. Diabetes mellitus, urolithiasis, obesity, cardiac failure, and renal failure are a few clinical examples.

Supplements and treats are not interchangeable terms, concepts, or products. A supplement adds something to improve a nutrient profile or to treat deficiency. When used to correct a diagnosed deficiency, supplements have a therapeutic role. More commonly, however, they affect the balance of an otherwise adequate food intake or create an unnecessary excess. When foods are of poor quality, the use of supplements probably will not correct the fundamental reasons for quality deficits. Nutritionally and economically, the prudent choice is to use a higher-quality food and skip attempts to supplement a poor product into adequacy.

Reading Pet Food Labels

Label information and ingredient description are controlled by the Association of American Feed Control Officials (AAFCO). Pet food labels must contain the net weight, product designator (e.g., "cat food"); maker or distributor; a list of guaranteed analyses for crude protein, fat, fiber, and moisture; a list of ingredients; and a nutritional adequacy statement (Fig. 26–18). Many labels contain much more information, such as feeding instructions.

There is considerable information regarding food quality and a few potential pitfalls requiring awareness when reading labels. The first is that guaranteed analysis states only maxima and minima. As feed labels are a legal contract between manufacturer and consumer, the guaranteed nutrient levels are conservative and may be far different from the actual analysis. Instead of using the numbers from guaranteed analysis, one can find a better source of data on nutrient content in the typical or average analysis supplied by a manufacturer. Furthermore, the ingredient list descends by weight as the ingredients were added on the as-is basis. This often means water-containing ingredients list high in the ingredient ordering when a dry ingredient actually predominates on a dry-matter basis.

Nutritional Adequacy Statement

The nutritional adequacy statement may be as simple as *totally nutritious* or *complete and balanced* or the statement may be more elaborate. The technician should interpret the method used to determine the nutritional adequacy statement. The statement "meets or exceeds NRC guidelines" (or similar wording) indicates only a laboratory analysis for a minimal chemical content. Such testing is not an animal feeding performance trial and says nothing about adequacy, bioavailability, or excesses.

The "AAFCO Protocol Feeding Test" statement (see Fig. 26–18), however, indicates that a representative product was used in animal feeding tests and performed at a defined level. Thus, the consumer knows that living animals have been test-fed, and the technician should recommend products with the AAFCO rather than the NRC statement when there is a choice. A nutritional adequacy statement is not needed on treats or dietary management foods intended to be used within the context of a professional diagnosis and relationship.

The Percentage Rules

The designator and modifying wording on pet food labels contain considerable information regarding content of the named ingredient in a product. According to AAFCO rules, when a label statement identifies only one ingredient, at least 70% of the total product will consist of that named ingredient (e.g., beef). When modifying words accompany the named ingredient, the amount of the named ingredient that must be present declines to 10% (chicken *dinner,* fish *entree,* liver *stew,* and so forth). When a named ingredient is modified by the word "with" (e.g., with beef), the total portion of the named ingredient declines to 3%. When the term *flavor* is used (e.g., cheese flavor), the named flavor must be "detectable" only by the animal. The designator *food* ("dog food") means that there are no rules regarding minimal content of ingredients. Indirectly, the technician may gather further quality information about a product through understanding these nuances of pet food labeling.

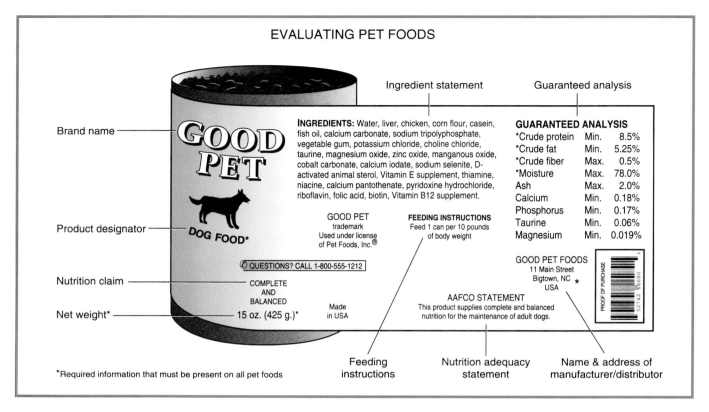

EVALUATING PET FOODS

Brand name

Product designator

Nutrition claim

Net weight*

GOOD PET

DOG FOOD*

© QUESTIONS? CALL 1-800-555-1212

COMPLETE
AND
BALANCED

15 oz. (425 g.)*   Made
in USA

Ingredient statement

INGREDIENTS: Water, liver, chicken, corn flour, casein, fish oil, calcium carbonate, sodium tripolyphosphate, vegetable gum, potassium chloride, choline chloride, taurine, magnesium oxide, manganous oxide, cobalt carbonate, calcium iodate, sodium selenite, D-activated animal sterol, Vitamin E supplement, thiamine, niacine, calcium pantothenate, pyridoxine hydrochloride, riboflavin, folic acid, biotin, Vitamin B12 supplement.

GOOD PET
trademark
Used under license
of Pet Foods, Inc.®

FEEDING INSTRUCTIONS
Feed 1 can per 10 pounds
of body weight

Guaranteed analysis

GUARANTEED ANALYSIS
*Crude protein	Min.	8.5%
*Crude fat	Min.	5.25%
*Crude fiber	Max.	0.5%
*Moisture	Max.	78.0%
Ash	Max.	2.0%
Calcium	Min.	0.18%
Phosphorus	Min.	0.17%
Taurine	Min.	0.06%
Magnesium	Min.	0.019%

GOOD PET FOODS
11 Main Street
Bigtown, NC ★
USA

PROOF OF PURCHASE

52742 65680

AAFCO STATEMENT
This product supplies complete and balanced
nutrition for the maintenance of adult dogs.

Feeding
instructions

Nutrition adequacy
statement

Name & address of
manufacturer/distributor

*Required information that must be present on all pet foods

Figure 26–18. A pet food label is the contract between the manufacturer and the consumer. Labels provide information required by law and may have optional information such as feeding directions.

Technician's Role

The technician is in a position to assess pet food and livestock food quality by far better means than reading even the most informative of labels. That method is the direct assessment of an animal's performance. Feeding performance in daily use defines the real "gold standard" of quality assessment.

Feeding Costs for Dog and Cat Foods

There are substantial variations in actual daily feeding costs (see Figs. 26–15 and 26–16). When cost comparisons are calculated, a pet food perceived as "expensive" may actually be cheaper on the per-calorie and actual feeding cost basis. Unfortunately, unit price comparison rather than feeding cost information influences the purchasing decision.

COMPANION ANIMAL CLINICAL NUTRITION

"Thy food is thy remedy."
HIPPOCRATES

Clinical nutrition is a veterinary medical subspecialty with the objective of modifying the cause, progression, or end-stage effects of illness by applying specific nutrient profiles. The application of prophylactic or therapeutic dietary management is the expression of this objective. Purpose-specific dietary management has a long history of efficacy, but the use of altered nutrient profiles should be justified by professional diagnosis, judgment, and monitoring (Bella, 1989).

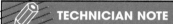

TECHNICIAN NOTE

When cost comparisons are calculated, a pet food perceived as "expensive" may actually be cheaper on the per-calorie and actual feeding cost basis.

Numerous nutrient profiles support various prophylactic and therapeutic applications in small animal patients. Examples are as follows: high protein/low carbohydrate; high protein/fat/micronutrient; low protein/high nonprotein calorie; low fiber/high digestibility; fiber enhanced; low sodium; very low sodium; low mineral; low fat/high fiber/low calorie; low copper; and restricted/novel protein sources. Specific effects on urine acidification or alkalization and restriction of urinary solutes such as magnesium are attained from specific formulations. Meat-free, soy-free, lactose-free, corn- and wheat gluten–free, and additive-free nutrient profiles are available in various commercially available products. Nutrient control objectives are fulfilled with either hospital-formulated/owner-cooked feedings or commercially prepared formulas. Table 26–7 summarizes objectives and nutrient profile for selected applications. Table 26–8 is a diary for use in taking food intake histories at home for animals with food hypersensitivity.

Feeding Hospitalized Small Animal Patients

Medical-surgical malnutrition is a major clinical problem for patients unable or unwilling to eat. To complicate the food

• Table 26–7 •

SUMMARY OF SMALL ANIMAL CLINICAL NUTRITION[1]

DISEASE	OBJECTIVES	CONSIDERATIONS	PRODUCT*	COMMENTS
Allergy, food				
Dog	Reduce antigen ingestion.	Novel protein source Reduce total protein. Simplify food. Distilled H_2O	Prescription Diet Canine d/d	6-week trial period Avoid antigen intake in treats.

Cat		Same as dog except
		  Control Mg^{2+} intake.
		  Provide taurine.
		  Control urine pH.
			Prescription Diet
			Feline d/d	

Anemia	Support RBC production.	↑ Iron, cobalt, and copper ↑ B complex vitamins ↑ Protein	Prescription Diet Canine p/d Feline p/d	
Anorexia	Prevent protein/calorie malnutrition. Stimulate appetite.	Establish fluid/electrolyte balance. Acid-base balance ↑ Protein and fat ↑ Micronutrients	Prescription Diet Feline/Canine a/d Canine p/d Feline p/d	Cat foods are suitable dog foods in acute care settings.
Ascites	Reduce fluid retention.	Restrict Na^+.	Prescription Diet Canine h/d, k/d Feline h/d, k/d	h/d = marked Na^+ restriction k/d = moderate Na^+ restriction
Bone loss and fracture healing	Correct deficiency of energy and protein.	Maintain hydration. ↑ Protein ↑ Energy Avoid supplementation.	Prescription Diet Canine p/d Feline p/d	Extra dietary calcium does not increase rate of fracture healing.
Colitis	Normalize GI motility. Rebalance microflora. Provide local healing factors.	Feed small meals: 3-6 times/day. Control dietary antigens. Vary levels of dietary fiber.	Prescription Diet Canine w/d, i/d, d/d Feline w/d, d/d	
Constipation	Normalize GI motility. Maintain stool water. Maintain stool bulk.	>10% fiber	Prescription Diet Canine w/d Feline w/d	No table scraps or bones Increase exercise. Cats: Keep litter box clean.
Copper storage disease	Restrict copper intake.	<1.2 mg copper/100 g dry diet	Prescription Diet Canine u/d	No table scraps or treats
Debilitation	Replete tissue, plasma, and nutrients.	↑ Protein ↑ Fat ↑ Macronutrients and micronutrients	Prescription Diet Canine a/d Feline a/d	Assist feed if needed.
Diabetes mellitus	Even rate of glucose absorption Consistent caloric intake	>10% fiber ↓ Soluble carbohydrates	Prescription Diet Canine w/d Feline w/d	Weigh animal frequently and note in medical record.
Acute diarrhea	Normalize GI tract motility and secretion.	Withhold food for 1-2 days. Feed small amounts: 3-6 times/ day. ↓ Fiber ↓ Sugar ↑ Digestibility	Prescription Diet Canine i/d Feline c/d	Electrolyte disturbances and dehydration are common.
Eclampsia	Provide Ca^{2+}/P in correct quantity and ratio pre partum.	High digestibility of diet Balanced minerals/vitamins	Prescription Diet Canine p/d Feline p/d	Avoid supplementation.
Flatulence	Decrease aerophagia Avoid food fermentation	Avoid milk or milk products. Feed small meals: 3-6 times/day. ↑ Caloric density	Prescription Diet Canine i/d Feline c/d	Feed in a flat, open dish. Avoid vitamin supplementation. Separate competitive eaters.
Gastric dilatation/ bloat (postoperative)	Prevent gastric distention	Avoid exercise before and after feeding. ↑ Digestibility of diet Small frequent feedings	Prescription Diet Canine i/d	Diet form or type is *NOT* related to risk of occurrence or recurrence.
Heart failure Dogs	Control Na^+ retention	↓ Na^+ intake Maintain energy and protein intake. ↑ B complex vitamins ↓ Na^+ intake	Prescription Diet Canine h/d	Prescription Diet k/d has moderate Na^+ restrictions.
Cats		↑ Taurine Control Mg^{2+} levels.	Prescription Diet Feline h/d	Avoid high Na^+ treats and water (see Table 26-5).

Table continued on following page

• Table 26–7 •

SUMMARY OF SMALL ANIMAL CLINICAL NUTRITION[1] *Continued*

DISEASE	OBJECTIVES	CONSIDERATIONS	PRODUCT*	COMMENTS
Hyperlipidemia	Control fat intake.	↑ Fiber intake ↓ Fat intake Limit sugars.	Prescription Diet Canine w/d Feline w/d	Common in schnauzers Consider fat in treats, scraps, and supplements.
Hyperthyroidism Cats	Support increased energy need.	↑ Energy intake ↑ Vitamins and minerals ↑ Protein	Prescription Diet Feline a/d	
Liver disease (fat tolerant)	Reduce protein metabolism. Maintain liver glycogen. Prevent ammonia toxicity.	↑ Digestible energy Protein restriction High biological value proteins Control Na⁺ intake.	Prescription Diet Canine k/d Feline k/d	May feed small meals (4–6 times/day).
Lymphangiectasia	Decrease dietary fat.	↓ Intake of long-chain triglycerides Control protein levels. Consider medium-chain triglycerides.	Prescription Diet Canine w/d or r/d	Medium-chain triglyceride oils and powder can increase caloric density.
Obesity	Maintain intake of all nutrients except energy.	↓ Energy digestibility Replace digestible calories with indigestible fiber. Increase bulk to control hunger.	Prescription Diet Canine r/d Feline r/d	Requires professional advice and teamwork with veterinary technician and client.
Oral disease: gingivitis (gum inflammation), periodontitis (loss of tooth attachment)	Control accumulation of plaque, stains, and calculus.	Mechanical cleansing of dental enamel	Prescription Diet Canine +/d Feline +/d	
Vomiting	Minimize gastric secretion. GI rest	↑ Digestibility ↑ Caloric density	Prescription Diet Canine i/d	Frequent, small meals
Acute pancreatitis (recovery phase)	Control pancreas secretions.	↓ Fat ↑ Digestibility Feed small meals: 3–6 times/daily.	Prescription Diet Canine i/d Feline w/d	Frequent, small meals
Pancreatic exocrine insufficiency	Reduce requirements for digestive enzymes.	↓ Fiber ↓ Fat Highly digestible carbohydrates ↑ Caloric density	Prescription Diet Canine i/d	Pancreatic enzymes complement highly digestible food.
Regurgitation	Decrease gastric acid secretion. Maintain caloric intake.	Low bulk Slurry of half food and half water for 72 hours	Prescription Diet Canine i/d Feline c/d	Elevate the food bowl. Try different food texture.
Renal failure Dogs	Reduce signs of uremia	↓ Protein (↑ biological value of protein)	Prescription Diet Canine k/d	Small meals several (4–6) times/day Conversion to a protein-restricted diet may take 7–10 days.
	Reduce signs of uremia.	↑ Nonprotein calories ↓ Phosphorus and sodium Increase B complex vitamins.		
Cats		↓ Protein ↑ Biological value of protein ↓ P, Ca²⁺, and Na⁺ Control Mg²⁺	Prescription Diet Feline k/d	
Canine urolithiasis (struvite): Treatment	↑ Urine volume ↓ Urine pH Restrict Mg²⁺, NH₄⁺, PO₄.	↓ Protein ↓ PO₄, Mg²⁺ ↑ Na⁺ ↓ Urine pH (5.9–6.1)	Prescription Diet Canine s/d	Evaluate and treat urinary tract infection. Average duration of stone dissolution is 36 days; follow-up via radiography.
Canine urolithiasis (struvite): Prevention	Maintain physiological level of urinary solutes and urine pH.	Control protein excess ↓ Ca²⁺, P, Ma²⁺ ↓ Sodium mildly ↓ Urine pH (6.2–6.4)	Prescription Diet Canine c/d	Monitor urine sediment for crystalluria and infection.
Canine urolithiasis (ammonium urate): Prevention		↓ Protein ↑ Nonprotein calories ↓ Nucleic acids ↓ Ca²⁺, P, Mg²⁺, Na⁺ Urine pH (6.7–7.0)	Prescription Diet Canine u/d	Drugs plus diet may be successful treatment. Monitor urinary crystalluria. Prevention may require long-term drug treatment.

• Table 26–7 •

SUMMARY OF SMALL ANIMAL CLINICAL NUTRITION[1] *Continued*				
DISEASE	**OBJECTIVES**	**CONSIDERATIONS**	**PRODUCT***	**COMMENTS**
Canine urolithiasis (calcium oxalate and cystine): Prevention	↓ Urinary concentration of calcium oxalate or cystine	↓ Protein ↑ Nonprotein calories ↓ Ca²⁺, P, Na⁺, Mg²⁺ ↑ Urine pH (6.7–7.0)	Prescription Diet Canine u/d	Treatment by surgical removal Prevention by dietary management ± drugs
Feline urolithiasis (struvite): Treatment	↑ Urine volume ↓ Urine pH (5.9–6.1) Restrict Mg²⁺, Ca²⁺, PO₄.	↑ Caloric density ↓ P and Ca²⁺ Mg²⁺ >20 mg/100 Kcal ↑ Na⁺ Urine pH (6.2–6.4)	Prescription Diet Feline s/d	Dissolution is complete 1 month after negative radiographs. Recurrence is high if prevention is not implemented.
Feline urolithiasis (struvite): Prevention	Maintain physiological levels of urinary solutes and urine pH.	Mg²⁺ >20 mg/100 Kcal (0.1% DMB) ↓ P ↑ Caloric density Urine pH (6.2–6.4)	Prescription Diet Feline c/d	In obesity, use calorie-restricted diets that maintain urine pH 6.2–6.4 (Prescription Diet w/d is suggested).
Feline urolithiasis (calcium oxalate): Prevention	↑ Urine volume ↓ Urinary Ca²⁺, oxalate ↑ Urine pH	↓ Protein ↑ Nonprotein calories ↓ P, Ca²⁺, Na⁺ Mg²⁺ <20 mg/100 Kcal	Prescription Diet Feline k/d	Monitor urinary crystalluria.

Nutrients in table are expressed on a dry weight basis.
*Other North American commercial brands include Cadillac, CNM (Pro·Visions; Purina), Hi Tor, Neura, Protocol, VMD, Vet's Choice (Nature's Recipe), Eukanuba (Iams); and Pedigree/Whiskas (Mars).

deficit, hypermetabolic energy requirements often follow significant illness or injury (Chandler et al., 1992). A state of "accelerated starvation" and lean tissue catabolism follows protein-calorie malnutrition (Crowe, 1986A). Decreased immune function, delayed wound healing (rate and strength), loss of muscle and visceral mass, delayed general recovery, and increased mortality all result from protein calorie malnutrition (Crane, 1989) (see Benefits of Nutrient Provision on the Debilitated Animal). The veterinary technician is a critical interface in daily cage-side nutritional management. A "wait-until-ready-to-eat" passivity is not beneficial, and no patient has yet been starved into wellness (Armstrong, 1992; Armstrong et al., 1990; Bright and Burrows, 1988; Chandler et al., 1992; Crane, 1995; Crowe, 1986B; Labato, 1992). Even when the patient is overweight, an acute hospitalization is not the setting for weight reduction.

BENEFITS OF NUTRIENT PROVISION IN THE DEBILITATED ANIMAL

Protein
- Helps maintain lean and visceral body mass
- Provides amino acids for anabolism
- Promotes wound healing
- Enhances immune function
- Provides a source of fuel for muscle

Carbohydrates
- Helps provide a source of fuel for energy
- Helps reduce protein catabolism

Fats
- Provides essential fatty acids
- Modulates immune function
- Provides concentrated energy source
- Promotes wound healing
- Provides anti-inflammatory effects

Vitamins and Minerals
- Enhances cellular and humoral immunity
- Enhances the ability to taste and smell
- Provides antioxidants

TECHNICIAN NOTE

The veterinary technician is a critical interface in daily cage-side nutritional management.

Patient Selection for Assisted Feeding

The technician frequently uses *subjective global assessment* (SGA) to determine nutritional status. SGA considers the dietary history, the body's condition scoring system (see Fig. 26–9), and the current morbidity index of the illness or injury. Body scoring is done by physical examination, with 0 = cachexia and 5 = obese. Albumin, globulin, and other "markers" for malnutrition decline with energy deprivation and protein-calorie malnutrition. However, these objective indicators change too slowly to be functional prognosticators, and the use of SGA permits functional, early clinical conclusion of "nutrient depletion and negative nitrogen balance" (Armstrong, 1992; Labato, 1992). The most important outlook for the hospital is an awareness of the critical "need to feed" and the need to do so

• Table 26–8 •

DAY	DATE	FOOD OFFERED	FOOD CONSUMED	OTHER ITEMS INGESTED*	CLINICAL SIGNS (scale 0–5 and comments)†	FECES (scale 1–5 and comments)‡	OTHER OBSERVATIONS
1							
2							
3							
4							
5							
6							
7							
8							
9							
↑ (Continue 10 through 58) ↓							
59							
60							

DIARY FOR DIETARY ELIMINATION TRIAL

* Other Items Ingested	† Clinical Signs	‡ Feces Assessment
List other ingested items, such as • Rawhide chews • Chewable vitamin supplements • Chewable heartworm prevention tablet • Commercial treats or snacks • Fatty acid supplements • Table scraps • Fresh food • Access to other food sources (e.g., dog eating cat food or cat eating an animal it has captured outdoors)	• 0 = No clinical signs • 5 = Severe clinical signs of • Itching (scratching, rubbing face, chewing, licking, head shaking) • Hair loss • Skin lesions (scabs, scales, bleeding, red skin, pimples)	1 = Liquid feces that have lost all form 2 = Soft feces with no form 3 = Soft feces that form a pile 4 = Mixture of soft and firm feces with a cylindrical shape 5 = Firm feces with a cylindrical shape Presence of mucus or fresh blood Number of bowel movements per day

early. These steps reduce catabolism and improve responses to virtually all other therapy.

Indications for nutritional support include recent weight loss of more than 10%, absent or poor food intake for more than 2 days, presentation of acute illness or injury with a high trauma index, acute muscle wasting, and heavy GI or urinary system losses of protein or electrolytes. The technician assesses daily needs and progress in conversation with the veterinarian and by the daily patient progress notes. The trauma index, the patient's desire and ability to eat, and response to therapy can all rapidly change.

Enteral Versus Parenteral Feeding

Total parenteral nutrition (TPN) is a complete intravenous nutrition technique whose objective is complete bypass of the seriously impaired GI tract. Parenteral nutrition technique is the controlled infusion of special feeding fluids of concentrated dextrose, amino acids, special fat emulsions, and micronutrients. Maintaining enterocyte function is important to reduce TPN complications of bowel atrophy and bacterial translocation across the intestine into the circulation (bacteremia). Even during TPN, partial enteral intake supports the enterocyte cells of the small intestinal mucosa (Allen and Hand, 1992).

Enteral feeding is more physiological, safer, and cheaper than parenteral nutrition. Therefore, feeding by mouth or tube is used if the GI tract can absorb nutrients (Abood and Buffington, 1991; Armstrong, 1992). Contraindications to enteral nutritional feeding are the need for complete GI secretory rest and a high risk of aspirating vomitus.

Methods of Assisted Enteral Feeding

Coax feeding, appetite stimulation with drugs, forced oral feeding, and various tube administration techniques are four separate enteral feeding methods. These techniques are reviewed in Table 26–9. The benefits of nutrient provision in the debilitated animal are presented in the previous boxed information.

TECHNICIAN NOTE

Total parenteral nutrition (TPN) is a complete intravenous nutrition technique whose objective is complete bypass of the seriously impaired GI tract.

The technician must carefully monitor all assisted feeding methods for the stress associated with restraint and monitor all feeding tubes for mechanical blockage or kinking. This is a critical monitoring obligation for small-bore tubes. Water is flushed through the tube to clear debris after each feeding. Capping the tube prevents air from entering the catheterized viscus between uses. It is preferable for the same person to feed, as this may allow quicker notation of flow and resistance changes in the tube.

It is also important to monitor GI tolerance during the refeeding of the animal. The objectives of repletion feeding may be at odds with the patient's best interests when serious vomiting and diarrhea follow feeding.

Steps in Enteral Alimentation Calculations and Food Selection

1. Calculate resting energy requirement (RER) as:
   RER = 70 (body weight in kg)$^{0.75}$
2. Factor the RER to obtain the illness/infection/injury energy requirement (IER). (Multiply RER × Trauma Index.) An IER of 1.2- to 1.5-fold that of RER is commonly used for many critical care applications (Armstrong, 1992; Chandler et al., 1992; Crowe, 1986A) (Figs. 26–19 to 26–21).
3. Consider the distribution of fuel sources among protein, carbohydrate, and fat. Dogs receiving more than 16% of energy from protein (protein calories) and cats receiving more than 24% protein calories recovered well when human liquid enteral products were enterally supplied (cats were supplemented with

casein-based protein sources) (Abood and Buffington, 1992). However, these protein levels are considered minimal, and higher levels may be prudent (Donoghue, 1989).

4. Consider physical form and other nutritional characteristics before the final selection of feeding products. Note that oral calorie paste supplements are extremely deficient in protein and that meat baby foods are neither complete nor balanced. Five percent dextrose does not provide adequate calorie concentrations and is devoid of protein. Table 26–10 summarizes the nutrient profile of selected enteral products used in small animal patients.
5. Establish the food dose, administration rate, and feeding schedule. A conservative rate of patient refeeding is needed after prolonged anorexia or GI disease. Controlling the size and frequency of the per feeding dose by giving small frequent feedings can be a critical factor in improving patient tolerance. Calorie and volume intake at IER levels may require a 3-day transition period.

FEEDING PET BIRDS

Avian nutrient needs are diverse, and the technician may variously accommodate insectivorous, frugivorous (fruit eating), nectivorous, carnivorous, seed eating, and omnivorous species of birds. The origins and ecological niche of common pet birds vary greatly. For example, the common budgerigar is a desert-adapted bird, whereas many parrots are acclimated to rainforest environments. When one considers the range of canaries, finches, parakeets, cockatiels, lovebirds, conures, macaws, and various parrots and cockatoos, a dangerous generalization would be that they all "eat seeds." Unfortunately, the knowledge of nutrient requirements and wild-type feeding behaviors is incomplete for some species.

The history for the pet bird should include the amount of free flight (if any), water intake, and brand and type of avian pet food provided. If birds eat from the owner's kitchen, note the general distribution of food types. Question the use of

HAND-FEEDING HATCHLINGS

Schedule
- Birth: Every 2 to 3 hours
- 3 Weeks: Four times a day
- 4 Weeks: Three times a day

Food Dose
- Distend crop
- Fill again when empty

Diet
- Liquid slurry of 25% dry matter (250 g of dry food powder and 750 g of water)

Commercial Formulas
Ground Primate Biscuits
Homemade Diets

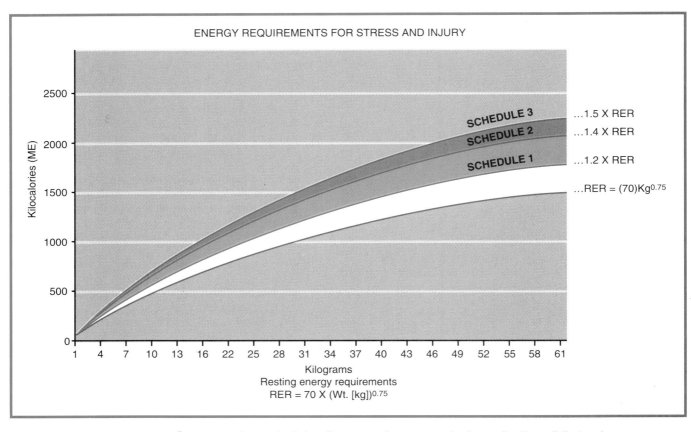

Figure 26-19. Energy requirements during illness vary in response to the patient's activity level and stress index. Schedules 1 through 3 suggest caloric intakes for resting convalescing animals with minor (1) through major (3) disease/injury stress.

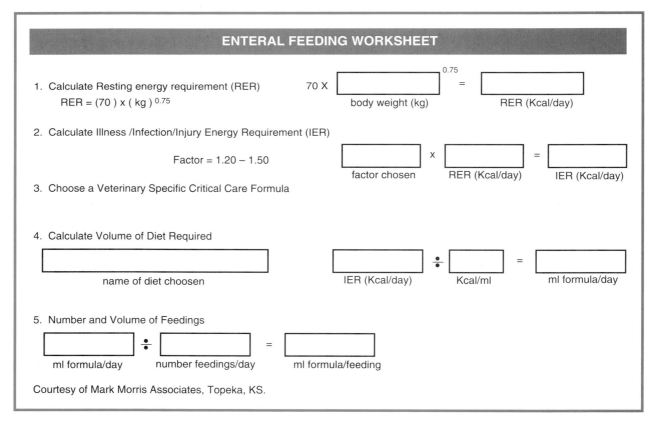

Figure 26-20. Calculations for the daily food dose are done by dividing the patient's Kcal requirement (see Fig. 26-19) by the Kcal/ml energy content of the food (see Table 26-10). The daily amount (milliliters) of food is usually divided into small portions that are given frequently.

• Table 26–9 •

OPTIONS IN ENTERAL FEEDING

FEEDING METHOD	OBJECTIVE	TECHNIQUE	ADVANTAGE	DISADVANTAGE
Owner hand feeding	Overcome partial anorexia	Hospital visit; bring favorite foods	Familiarity with food preferences should be explored	No effect in full anorexia
Temptation	Overcome partial anorexia	Use an unfamiliar food of high odor	New odor may stimulate food exploration	No effect in full anorexia
Force feeding pet foods	Overcome partial anorexia	Bolus of canned food; mouth held to force swallowing	Food is complete and balanced	High handling stress Probably limited calorie intake
Forced feeding (calorie pastes)	Overcome partial anorexia	Administer flavored pastes from tube	Moderate handling stress	Pastes not complete food Limited calorie intake Severe protein restriction
Assisted feeding	Achieve full calorie intake Overcome partial anorexia	Oral syringing of specific formula	User and patient friendly Moderate handling stress High calorie intake Food given at rate for comfortable swallowing	Learned aversion if nauseous
Orogastric	Achieve full calorie intake	Intubate esophagus/ stomach	Rapid administration No tube clogging Best for short-term use	High handling stress Intolerance to repeated feedings
Nasoesophageal	Bypass oral cavity and swallowing Achieve full caloric intake	Indwell 6–10 Fr. tube in nostril	Ease of intermediate use	Sedation/topical anesthesia Nonparticulate, liquid food only
Pharyngostomy	Bypass oral cavity and swallowing Achieve full caloric intake	Indwell 16–28 Fr. tube in pharynx	None	General anesthesia required Mechanical interference with laryngeal function Possible gagging and vomiting Possible esophagitis
Esophagostomy	Bypass oral cavity pharyn, and swallowing Achieve full caloric intake	12–18 Fr. tube in left lateral cervical esophagus	Easy to maintain and install Easy to "eat around the tube" Minimal risk of esophageal stricture	
Gastrostomy	Bypass proximal GI tract for full or partial caloric intake	16–28 Fr. tube placement at laparotomy Percutaneous endoscopic placement Nonendoscopic placement	Well-tolerated long term Effective and efficient	General anesthesia required Gastrocutaneous fistula forms in 5 days Wait 24 hours to use
Gastroduodenostomy	Bypass stomach	Duodenum cannulated via tube gastrostomy	Achieve full caloric intake	Loss of mechanical and chemical phases of gastric digestion May require endoscopic equipment
Jejunostomy	Bypass stomach and duodenum	10 Fr. tube through submucosal tunnel Anchor bowel and tube to body wall	Achieve full or partial caloric intake Predigested diets required to maximize nutrient delivery and minimize digestive work	Water transfer to gut lumen may cause cramping and diarrhea

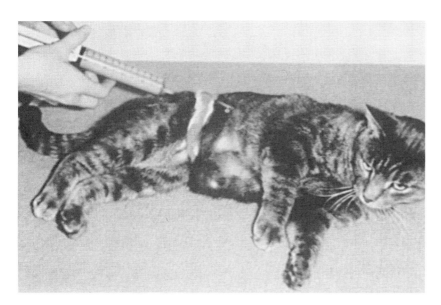

Figure 26–21. Feeding for convalescence, repletion, and recovery should extend past hospital discharge. This cat is anorectic and has received blended pet food by tube gastrostomy for 5 months. Most owners can be coached in food preparation for tube feeding techniques.

• Table 26–10 •

			ENERGY DISTRIBUTION		
PRODUCT	CALORIC CONTENT (Kcal/g)	PROTEIN CONTENT (g/100 Kcal)	% Protein Calories	% Fat Calories	% CHO Calories
COMPOSITION OF ENTERAL VETERINARY FORMULAE					
Veterinary Products (Canned)					
Prescription Diet					
Feline p/d*	0.9	9.3	37	56	7
Feline k/d†	0.9	4.4	21	67	13
Feline c/d†	0.6	8.9	33	52	15
Canine k/d†	0.6	3.1	13	49	39
Canine u/d†	0.7	1.9	8	48	45
Canine i/d†	0.6	5.9	24	31	45
Canine/Feline a/d	1.2	8.9	36	51	13
Purina CV Feline	1.4	8.7	34	48	18
Eukanuba Recovery Canine/Feline	2.0	7.8	31	54	15
Veterinary Products (Miscellaneous)					
Baby food (turkey)	1.0	14.6	58	42	0
CliniCare canine liquid	0.9	5.5	25	59	16
CliniCare feline liquid	0.8	8.6	36	84	16
CliniCare canine powder	0.9	6.0	24	64	12
CliniCare feline powder	0.8	9.1	36	53	11
NutriCal paste	4.6	0.3	1	62	37
Dyne liquid	5.2	0.7	3	74	23
Human Polymeric Foods					
Jevity	1.1	4.2	18	30	52
Pulmocare	1.5	4.3	17	55	28
Osmolite HN	1.1	4.4	17	30	53
Sustacal	1.0	6.8	24	21	55
Human Monomeric					
Peptemen	1.0	4.4	16	33	51
Supplement					
Promod (protein)	4.0	23.6	0	0	0
Casec (protein)	4.0	30.7	0	100	0
MCT oil (medium triglycerides)	47.7	0	0	100	0
Vegetable oil	8.5	0	0	100	0

*1/2 can (224 g) + 3/4 cup (170 ml) water.
†1/2 can (224 g) + 3/4 cup (170 ml) water.

treats, supplements, fresh foods, cuttlebone, and grit. Some seed mixes are supplemented with protein, vitamins, and minerals and are labeled as "fortified." If owners do not know whether seeds are fortified, one should request the label. The quantity of food consumption is often difficult to judge. This is true both in smaller passerines, which may go several days between seed cup refreshment, and in large psittacines, which frequently waste a sizable fraction of the food supplied. Food preferences and addictions are important to note, but many owners are unaware of an addiction until making an attempt to change the food. As with any other animal, direct observation of anorexia and body condition is important to physical diagnosis.

An increasing percentage of companion birds are being hand-raised in captivity. Breeder hatching and hand-feeding of baby birds increase socialization to humans and their value as pets. Hand-feeding baby birds permits the growing and weaning foods to be adjusted to intake requirements (Fig. 26–22). At "weaning," complete and balanced avian pet foods should be selected as the basis of feeding (Table 26–11). Some avicultural hobbyists and veterinarians recommend that mixed, fresh foods also be provided for nutritional diversity to complete foods or seeds (Fig. 26–23) (see Hand-Feeding Hatchlings, Nutritional Requirements, and Feed Diversity).

Nutritional Disease of Pet Birds

TECHNICIAN NOTE

Malnutrition of pet birds is common and potentially tragic.

Malnutrition of pet birds is common and potentially tragic. Obesity is common in pet birds but not as common as in mammalian pets. Lack of exercise (no flying) and high fractions of oil seeds are usually incriminated. Sunflower, safflower, other oil seeds, and peanuts are lipid rich and have a low protein

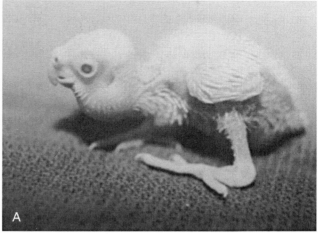

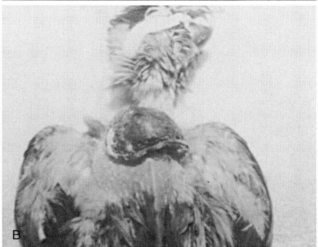

Figure 26–22. A, Hand-feeding formula to baby birds by cannula or tube must be gentle; esophagus perforation resulted from nongentle technique. (Courtesy of Dr. Jeffrey Jenkins.) B, A full-thickness crop burn resulted from overheated formula. Temperature of formula should never exceed 40°C (104°F), and microwave heating is hazardous because irregular warming may result in "hot spots." (Courtesy of Dr. Jeffrey Jenkins.)

content for their energy content. Seeds also lack vitamin A; epithelial distress is a sign of hypovitaminosis A (Fig. 26–24) (see Nutritional Deficiencies). The exceptional palatability of oil seeds commonly leads to addictions. Changing from seeds to complete foods may seem to be easy, although it might be difficult; fresh foods and/or specific transitional feeding products may be the "bridge" to complete avian diets. Protein,

• Table 26–11 •

	CANARY	BUDGERIGAR	COCKATIEL	CONURE	AMAZON/ AFRICAN GREY PARROT	MACAW/COCKATOO
SUGGESTED DIET FOR MAINTENANCE OF ADULT CAGED BIRDS						
Offer Daily						
Whole-grain bread cubes or primate biscuit	1/4 T	1/2 T	1 T	1½ T	2 T	4 T
Fresh dark green or yellow vegetables	1/2 T	1 T	2 T	4 T	3 T	1/2 c
Protein source (cheese, hard cooked eggs, egg, meat, mature legumes)	1/4 Size of pea	1/2 Size of pea	Size of pea	1/4 t	1/2 t	1 T
Dry seeds (two 15-min periods) (sunflower)	0	0	1 T	2 T	2 T	4 T
Small seeds (canary, niger, poppy, rape, millet, safflower, hemp)	Ad-lib	Ad-lib	Ad-lib	Ad-lib	Ad-lib	Ad-lib
2 to 3 Times Weekly						
Fruit (cantaloupe, apricot, apple)	1/8 t	1/8 t	1 t	1/12 Apple	1/12 Apple	1/6 Apple
Citrus fruit	0	0	0	1/12 Orange	1/12 Orange	1/6 Orange
Fresh corn on the cob	3 or 4 Kernels	1/8 Piece	1/4 Piece	1/2 Piece	1/2 Piece	1 Piece
Peanuts	0	0	0	1	2	4
Add Temporarily for New Birds						
Vitamin A (from 10,000 IU capsule)	1 Drop/week	2 Drops/week	3 Drops/week	1 Drop/day	1–2 Drops/day	4 Drops/day
Yogurt	Drop	Few drops	1/4 t	1/4 t	1/2 t	1
Always Available						
Calcium/mineral supplements (cuttlebone, mineral treat block, oyster shell, calcium lactate)						

Adapted from Harrison GJ and Harrison LR: Clinical Avian Medicine and Surgery. Philadelphia, W.B. Saunders, Table 2–1, p. 17.

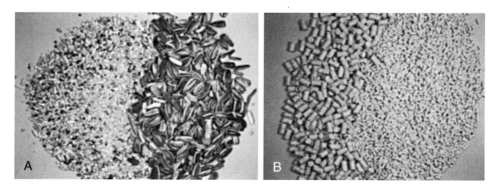

Figure 26–23. A, Seeds are an important part of many avian diets. However, high-oil seeds and nuts, such as sunflower seeds and peanuts, may cause addictions and nutritional imbalance. Oil seeds are deficient in protein relative to calorie content and have deficiency of calcium and micronutrients. B, Complete and balanced avian foods are available as fortified seed mixtures and extruded and pelleted foods.

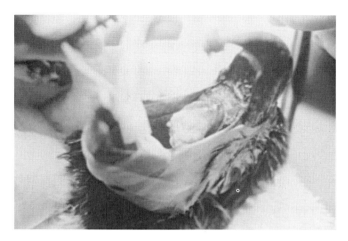

Figure 26–24. An abscess of a parrot's hard palate secondary to hypovitaminosis A. The vitamin A deficiency resulted from an exclusive intake of sunflower seeds. (Courtesy of Dr. Jeffrey Jenkins.)

vitamin, and mineral fortified mixtures may be given as an alternative.

Hypovitaminosis and hypervitaminosis D, hypovitaminosis E, calcium deficiency, and unbalanced Ca:P ratios are other common malnutritions. When a nutritional disease is clinically evident with physical signs, it is considered advanced. Specific drug and dietary therapy will be urgently needed. Vitamin A and other nutrients are more reliably given parenterally than by medicated water or food. Some patients benefit from enteral feeding by crop gavage. Place the feeding tube between the beak commissures (not beak tip), past the pharynx, and into the esophagus or crop. Palpate the tube in the crop to ascertain that the trachea has not been entered. Gentle technique and practice are necessary to ensure proper tube feeding.

Enteral feeding solutions for avian critical care will vary by species. For generally debilitated psittacines, use slurries of baby bird growth formula. These may be specifically supplemented according to the diagnosis. Raptorial species do well on a meat and organ tissue–based mammalian repletion formula such as Prescription Diet Canine/Feline a/d (Hill's, Inc.). Any formula should be freshly prepared, carefully strained, and warmed to a temperature not to exceed normal body temperature. Overheating foods may cause thermal burns to the esophagus or crop. Suggested gavage volumes in milliliters per feeding are as follows: budgerigars, 1 to 2; lovebirds, 2 to 3; cockatiels, 3 to 6; conures, 4 to 12; parrots, 15 to 35; cockatoos, 20 to 40; and macaws, 35 to 60. All equipment for feeding sick birds should be sanitized or sterilized between uses.

PRODUCTION ANIMAL NUTRITION

Equine Nutrients

Nutrients of concern for horses are water, energy, protein, calcium, phosphorus, and vitamin A. While all animals require access to good-quality water on an ad-lib basis, this is especially true for an animal capable of copious sweating (Carson, 1993). Hot, exhausted horses should rest and perhaps consume some hay while cooling. A waiting period of 30 minutes should occur before allowing water after heavy exercise.

Horses evolved eating grass and other range forages. Not surprisingly, grass and hays serve well as a foundation for feeding all horses. *Good-quality* grass or legume hay, free-choice water, calcium, phosphorus as needed, and trace mineralized salt are the only foods needed by the adult horse at maintenance.

> **TECHNICIAN NOTE**
>
> The role of grain and protein meal "concentrates" is to complement forages during periods of higher than maintenance nutrient demand.

The role of grain and protein meal "concentrates" is to complement forages during periods of higher than maintenance nutrient demand. Unfortunately, some horse feeding programs overlook quality forages and focus on elaborate programs of concentrate supplementation. The technician attending performance horses will also encounter a wide variety of owner- and trainer-selected supplements. These are diverse and may well match the current nutritional fad. Time-proven horse feeding programs emphasize simplicity and quality forage feeds.

Equine food dose calculations are based on the horse's weight, and an amount of feed per 100 lb of horse is a simple and frequently used method. Therefore, a horse weight tape is a simple and inexpensive tool worth having and using (Table 26–12). For example, a 6-year-old, 1000-lb light-breed gelding is at rest in a backyard paddock. The animal receives only 1 hour per week of light work. This horse is considered to be at "maintenance"—an activity requiring 1.5% of the horse's body weight (BW) per day as dry matter (Fig. 26–25). This means that 15 lb of a good-quality hay will suffice in addition to salt and water. If a 6-inch hay "flake" weighs 5 lb, then feeding three per day (one in the AM and two in the PM) can be suggested as a food dose. Table 26–13 summarizes different dry matter intake levels for various activity and physiological states (Fig. 26–26). As in small animals, equine overfeeding is a problem, and a routine portion of all horse evaluations is body condition assessment.

Some hays or hay/grain combinations need calcium and phosphorus supplementation. Most commonly, a source of phosphorus is added when a good legume hay is the sole source of nutrition. Powdered mineral supplements are often mixed with hay or loose rock salt and provided as part of the

• Table 26–12 •

ESTIMATING HORSE WEIGHT			
GIRTH CIRCUMFERENCE		BODY WEIGHT	
(in)	(cm)	(lb)	(kg)
64.5	163.8	800	363.6
67.5	171.5	900	409.1
70.5	179.1	1000	454.5
73.0	185.4	1100	500.0
75.5	191.8	1200	545.5
77.5	196.9	1300	590.9

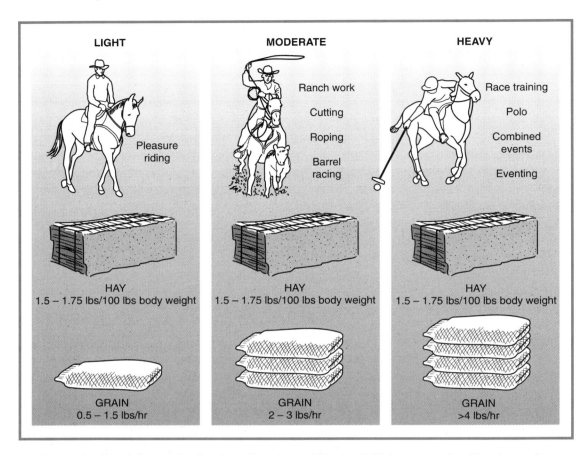

Figure 26–25. Adjusted feeding based on an activity level. Maintenance feed levels can be based per 100 pounds of weight. Supplemental feeding over maintenance should be based on the level and duration of work.

diet. Nutrient intake objectives and feeds to meet these are found in Table 26–14.

The microminerals zinc, manganese, iron, copper, cobalt, and sometimes iodine, found in "trace-mineralized" salt blocks, can also be provided ad-lib in a location protected from rain (Fig. 26–27).

TECHNICIAN NOTE

Routine horse feeding problems include overgrazed pastures, ingestion of sand and weeds, underfeeding due to poor-quality forage, too much grain, too fine a grind in pelleted feeds, various nutrient imbalances, and toxic supplementation.

Routine horse feeding problems include overgrazed pastures, ingestion of sand and weeds, underfeeding due to poor-quality forage, too much grain, too fine a grind in pelleted feeds, various nutrient imbalances, and toxic supplementation. Unfortunately, horses are not routinely or easily weighed in the typical setting, and changes in condition may be insidious. Accidental engorgement of grain may precipitate colic or founder with morbid or even tragic results.

Feeding Sick Horses

Hospitalized horses develop the same protein-calorie deficits, hypermetabolic stress, and catabolic wasting states as small animals. These have identical negative clinical effects, and early interventional feeding is vital in equine critical care. Major gastrointestinal tract (colic) surgery is especially challenging in the perioperative period. The animal needs a feed rich in protein, calories, and micronutrients but has reduced gastrointestinal motility (Ralston and Naylor, 1991). The veterinarian will focus closely on when gastrointestinal motility returns. Homogenized, moistened, alfalfa pellet mashes are high-protein, high-

• Table 26–13 •

BARNYARD METRICS	
VOLUME	**WEIGHT (lb)**
Hays	
Brome 6-in flake	4–5
Alfalfa 6-in flake	5–6
1 Quart	
Oats (whole)	1
Corn (whole)	1.7
Beet pulp	0.6
Bran	0.5

• Table 26–14 •

			VITAMINS AND	
AGE	**ENERGY**	**PROTEIN**	**MINERALS**	**COMMENTS**
Nursing foals	Supplement mare's milk if foal is very thin.	>16%	Ca²⁺ >0.85% P >0.5% Cu >25 mg/kg Vitamin A 50 IU/kg BW	At 2–3 months of age, begin 1 lb concentrate mixture/mo of age/day. Adequate Ca²⁺, P, trace minerals in grain mix If creep feeding, mix 50:50 chopped hay to grain. Wean at 4 months.
Weaning	Adequate to feel but not see the ribs	15%	Ca²⁺ 0.7% P 0.4% Vitamin A 50 IU/kg BW	Dry matter intake = 3% of BW Free-choice good roughage and trace mineral salt 1 lb concentrate mix/mo of age/day: 7–9 lb max
Yearling	Adequate to feel but not see the ribs	13%	Ca²⁺ 0.5% P 0.3% Vitamin A 50 IU/kg BW	Dry matter intake = 2.5% BW Free-choice good roughage, trace mineral salt 1 lb concentrate mix/mo of age/day: 7–9 lb max Feed as mature horse at 90% of mature weight.
Adult *Maintenance*	Adequate to feel but not see the ribs	8.5%	Ca²⁺ 0.3% P 0.2% Vitamin A 50 IU/kg BW	Dry matter = 1.5% BW 1½ to 1¾ lb roughage/100 lb BW Free-choice trace mineral salt
Adult *Working* *Light* (pleasure ride)	Add 0.5–1.5 lb of grain/hr of activity/day.	8.5%	Ca²⁺ 0.3% P 0.2% Vitamin A 50 IU/kg BW	Amortize grain supplement over the week.
Moderate (ranch work, roping, cutting, jumping, barrel racing)	Add 2–3 lb of grain/hr of activity/day.	8.5–10%	Ca²⁺ 0.3% P 0.2% Vitamin A 50 IU/kg BW	
Heavy (race training, polo)	Add 4 or more lb of grain/hr of activity/day.	8.5–10%	Ca²⁺ 0.3% P 0.2% Vitamin A 50 IU/kg BW	Dry matter = 1.75% BW
Adult reproduction *Mares*	Feed at maintenance until late pregnancy.	8.5%–10%		
Late pregnancy	Needs 20% more energy.	11%	Ca²⁺ 0.5% P 0.35% Vitamin A 50 IU/kg BW	Feed 1½ to 1¾ lb grass hays/100 lb BW with addition of ½ to ¾ lb grain or concentrate mix/100 lb BW Free-choice trace mineral salt–mineral Ca²⁺/P mix.
Last 3 weeks pregnancy	Needs 30% more energy.		Needs 100% more Ca²⁺ and P Vitamin A 60 IU/kg BW	1¾ to 2 lb legume hay/100 lb BW Free-choice trace mineral salt–mineral Ca²⁺/P mix
·Lactation	Allow 75% energy increase at peak lactation.	14%	Ca²⁺ 0.5% P 0.35% Vitamin A 60 IU/kg BW	Dry matter = 1.75%–2.0% BW free-choice grass hay Add 1½–2 lb/100 lb BW of concentrate. Add Ca²⁺/P mix and trace mineralized salt. At weaning: Stop concentrate; return to maintenance forage.
Stallions	Feed for maintenance.			

*Free-choice, potable water should be available at all times.

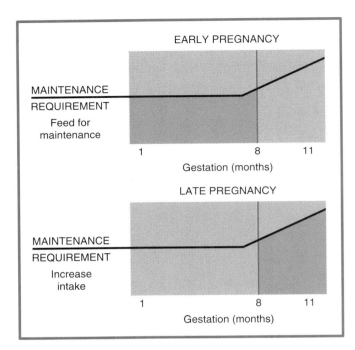

Figure 26–26. Early gestation is not "eating for two," and the mare should be fed for maintenance. In the last trimester of pregnancy, requirements increase for energy, protein, and minerals.

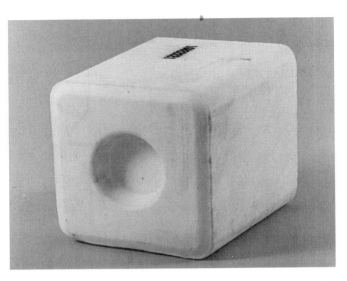

Figure 26–27. Additional sodium chloride and adequate intake of trace minerals can be provided with plain or trace mineralized salt blocks.

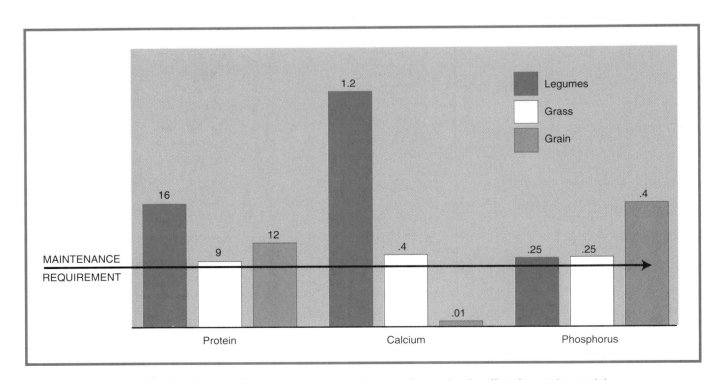

Figure 26–28. High-quality grass and legume hays, water, and salt suffice for equine maintenance. However, a source of supplemental phosphorus benefits some hay and can be provided as mineral mix.

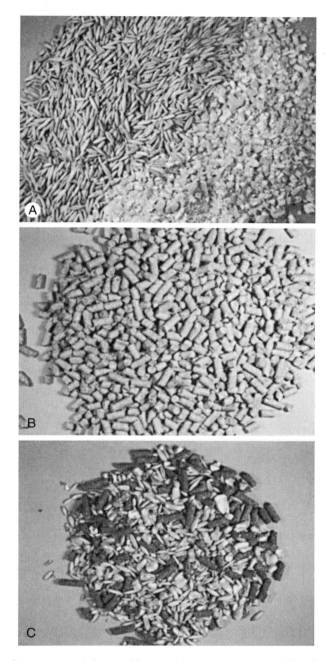

Figure 26–29. A, Grain and protein meal "concentrates" complement the forage foundation of equine feeds. Concentrates are needed when significantly extra energy or protein is required. Oats (left) and corn are two popular concentrate grains. On an equal volume basis, corn provides twice the energy of oats. This difference should be made clear to owners who usually feed by volume (coffee can) and may switch between the two grains. B, Pelleted horse foods are an expensive convenience but may lack the chewing or gastrointestinal fullness effects associated with long-stem roughage. Some horses chew or gnaw wood when consuming only complete foods. C, Complete horse feeds may be mixed from grain, forages, and mineral mixes and then pelleted or extruded. Complete feed can be used as a hay supplement or as the total diet when hay is unavailable.

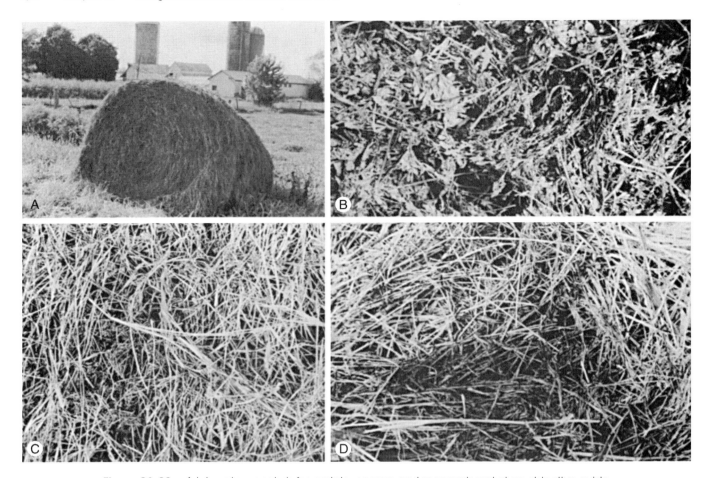

Figure 26–30. A laboratory analysis for protein, energy, and macromineral gives objective guidelines to forage quality and is available from agricultural extension services. Hay quality depends on the species of forage (legume versus grass), maturity, cutting number, curing, handling, storage (A), and age when fed. B, High-quality alfalfa hay is not overmature and has a high proportion of leaves to stems. Leaves contain two thirds of the energy and three fourths of the protein. Flexible, tender stems, light green color, and absence of molds and dust are seen in good legume hay. C, Poor-quality alfalfa hay has reduced leaf numbers and tough stems. Seed heads in a grass hay and flowers in alfalfa hay are indications of overmaturing at the time of cutting. D, A hay contaminated by mold (dark areas) is usually unpalatable and possibly dangerous.

energy, and nonirritating repletion formulas. These may be given as slurries through nasogastric tubes and are often enriched with nutriment modules. Liquid enteral formulas based on mare's milk replacer and commercial equine critical care formulas are available and well tolerated. These formulas should be given in small frequent feedings via indwelling nasogastric tubes.

Assessing Forages and Grains for Horses

The veterinary technician can assess the quality of water, of pastures, and hays (Fig. 26–28).

A feedbunk "rule" for horses is not to exceed a 50:50 ratio of concentrate to roughage. Oats and corn are the two most common feeds, and noting their relative energy content is important. Various horse grains, mixed concentrate supplements, and several totally complete extruded or pelleted horse feeds will be encountered on horse calls (Fig. 26–29). If horses consume only complete extruded or pelleted feeds, an issue may

be an adequate roughage intake. The sudden onset of fence chewing when only a complete pelleted food is used suggests the need for at least some long-stem or coarse chopped hay.

Forage quality varies greatly by soil quality, species of grass, season of year, rainfall, overgrazing, pasture rotation, weed control, and the presence of toxic weeds (Burrows and Case, 1993). Laboratory analysis of forages for moisture, energy, protein, fiber, and macrominerals is fundamental in assessing roughage nutrient content. Hay analysis is free (or inexpensive) from regional agriculture extension services. When hay analysis is unavailable, one can make some conclusions about hay quality from a physical inspection. Observe the leafiness and the leaf/stem ratio. This is important because two thirds of the energy and three fourths of the protein reside in leaves (Fig. 26–30). Smaller and more flexible stems suggest the correct maturity for grass and legume hays. Fully developed seed heads in grass hay and flowers in alfalfa mean overmaturity. Greenness (chlorophyll and beta-carotene), presence of weeds, mold, foreign material, rain damage, poor curing, and mechanical mishandling are other visual qualities to be checked in forage assessment. An additional discussion of feed analysis can be found in Chapter 27 (Concepts in Livestock Nutrition).

References

Abood SK and Buffington CA: Enteral feeding of dogs and cats: 51 cases (1989–1991). J Am Vet Med Assoc 201:621, 1992.

Abood SK and Buffington CA: Nutritional support of small animal patients and an improved technique for nasogastric intubation in dogs. J Am Vet Med Assoc 199:577–579, 1991.

Allen TA and Hand MS: Conditionally essential nutrients: antioxidant nutrients and glutamine. *In* Kirk RW and Bonagura JD (editors): Current Veterinary Therapy XI. Philadelphia, WB Saunders Co., 1992, pp 40–43.

Armstrong PJ: Enteral feeding of critically ill pets: the choices and techniques. Vet Med 87:900–909, 1992.

Armstrong PJ, Hand MS and Frederick GS: Enteral nutrition by tube. Vet Clin North Am (Sm Anim Pract) 20:235–276, 1990.

Bauer JE and Schenck PA: Nutritional management of hepatic disease. Vet Clin North Am (Sm Anim Pract) 19:522, 1989.

Bella JA: Principles of nutritional therapy for dogs and cats. Vet Tech 152:152–162, 1989.

Blaxter AC, Cripps PJ and Gruffydd-Jones TJ: Dietary fibre and post prandial hyperglycaemia in normal and diabetic dogs. J Small Anim Pract 31:229–233, 1990.

Bright RM and Burrows CF: Percutaneous endoscopic tube gastrostomy in dogs. Am J Vet Res 49:629–633, 1988.

Burrows GE and Case AA: Principal poisonous plants in the midwestern and eastern United States. *In* Howard JL (editor): Current Veterinary Therapy: Food Animal Practice 3. Philadelphia, WB Saunders Co., 1993, pp 349–352.

Campbell KL: Therapeutic indications for dietary lipids. *In* Kirk RW and Bonagura JD (editors): Current Veterinary Therapy XI. Philadelphia, WB Saunders Co., 1992, pp 36–39.

Carson TL: Water quality for livestock. *In* Howard JL (editor): Current Veterinary Therapy: Food Animal Practice 3. Philadelphia, WB Saunders Co., 1993, pp 375–376.

Chandler ML, Greco DS and Fettman MJ: Hypermetabolism in illness and injury. Compendium of Continuing Education 14:1284–1289, 1992.

Crane SW: Nutritional aspects of wound healing. Semin Vet Med Surg 4:263–267, 1989.

Crane SW: Occurrence and management of obesity in companion animals. J Small Anim Pract 32:275–282, 1991.

Crane SW: Perioperative nutritional support for the animal with cancer. Vet Clin North Am 25:63–76, 1995.

Crowe DT: Enteral nutrition for critically ill or injured patients (Part I). Compendium of Continuing Education 8:603–610, 1986A.

Crowe DT: Enteral nutrition for critically ill or injured patients (Part II). Compendium of Continuing Education 8:719–732, 1986B.

Dimski DS: Dietary fiber in the management of gastrointestinal disease. *In* Kirk RW and Bonagura JD (editors): Current Veterinary Therapy XI. Philadelphia, WB Saunders Co., 1992, pp 592–595.

Donoghue S: Nutritional support of hospitalized patients. Vet Clin North Am (Sm Anim Pract) 19:475–495, 1989.

Edney ATB and Smith PM: Study of obesity in visiting veterinary practices in the United Kingdom. Vet Rec 118:391–396, 1986.

Fettman MJ. Feline kaliopenic polymyopathy/nephropathy syndrome. Vet Clin North Am (Sm Anim Pract) 19:415–432, 1989.

Goldman AL: Hypervitaminosis A in a cat. J Am Vet Med Assoc 200:1970–1972, 1992.

Hand MS, Armstrong PJ and Allen TA: Obesity: occurrence, treatment and prevention. Vet Clin North Am 19:447–474, 1989.

Kallfelz FA: Evaluation and use of pet foods. Vet Clin North Am 19:397–402, 1989A.

Kallfelz FA: Overnutrition: An epidemic problem in pet animal practice? Vet Clin North Am 19:433–446, 1989B.

Kealy RD, Olsson SE, Monti KL et al.: Effects of limited food consumption on the incidence of hip dysplasia in growing dogs. J Am Vet Med Assoc 201:857–863, 1992.

Labato MA: Nutritional management of the critical care patient. *In* Kirk RW and Bonagura JD (editors): Current Veterinary Therapy XI. Philadelphia, WB Saunders Co., 1992, pp 117–125.

MacEwen EG: Obesity. *In* Kirk RW and Bonagura JD (editors): Current Veterinary Therapy XI. Philadelphia, WB Saunders Co., 1992, pp 313–321.

Markham RW and Hodgkins EM: Geriatric nutrition. Vet Clin North Am 19:165–181, 1989.

McDonald ML, Anderson BC, Rogers QR et al.: Essential fatty acid requirements of cats: pathology of essential fatty acid deficiency. Am J Vet Res 45:1310–1316, 1984.

Morris JG, and Rogers QR: Comparative aspects of nutrition and metabolism of dogs and cats. *In* Burger IH and Rivers JPW (editors): Nutrition of the Dog and Cat. Cambridge, England, Cambridge Press, 1989, pp 37–41.

Morris ML, Lewis LD and Hand MS: Small Animal Clinical Nutrition III. Topeka, Mark Morris Associates, 1987, pp 1–7.

Mumma RO, Rashaid KA, Shane BS et al.: Toxic and protective constituents in pet foods. Am J Vet Res 47:1633–1637, 1986.

Oetzel GR: Parturient paresis and hypocalcemia in ruminant livestock. Vet Clin North Am (Large Anim Pract) 4:351–363, 1988.

Ogilvie GK and Vail DM: Unique metabolic alterations associated with cancer cachexia in dogs. *In* Kirk RW and Bonagura JD (editors): Current Veterinary Therapy XI. Philadelphia, WB Saunders Co., 1992, pp 433–437.

Pennington JAT: Food Values of Portions Commonly Used. 15th ed. New York, Harper & Row, 1989.

Polzin DJ, Osborne CA, Adams LD et al.: Dietary management of canine and feline chronic renal failure. Vet Clin North Am 19:539–560, 1989.

Ralston SL and Naylor JM. Feeding sick horses. *In* Naylor JM and Ralston SL (editors): Large Animal Clinical Nutrition. St. Louis, Mosby–Year Book 1991, pp 432–445.

Schaeffer MC, Rogers QR and Morris JG: Protein in the nutrition of dogs and cats. *In* Burger IH and Rivers JPW (editors): Nutrition of the Dog and Cat. Cambridge, England, Cambridge University Press, 1989, pp 167–170.

Simons JC and Hand MS: Special dietary management in lactation and gestation. *In* Howard JL (editor): Current Veterinary Therapy: Food Animal Practice 3. Philadelphia, WB Saunders Co., 1993, pp 204–223.

Sloth C: Practical management of obesity in dogs and cats: J Small Anim Pract 33:178–182, 1992.

Van Horn HH: Protein nutrition and nonprotein nitrogen. *In* Naylor JM and Rolston SL (editors): Large Animal Clinical Nutrition. St. Louis, Mosby–Year Book, 1991, pp 31–33.

27 Concepts in Livestock Nutrition

Sheila R. Grosdidier • *William D. Schoenherr*

INTRODUCTION

Optimal nutrition has often been identified as the most expensive element in achieving full productivity and profitability in livestock (Ensminger, 1990). The veterinary technician must have a strong fundamental knowledge of nutrient needs and be able to identify potential for problems and increase the client's understanding of essential feeding philosophies. The client who has the greatest need for this type of information is not the large intensive livestock farmer who normally has feeds professionally formulated for optimum production. Most often, the questions will be from clients who run small operations, have family members raising livestock for 4-H or FFA projects, or possess a "hobby farm." With these needs in mind, this chapter focuses on common nutritional problems and sound principles to help the veterinary technician provide meaningful, relevant information.

Various nutritional disorders can be very similar to a vast array of diseases and may not be easily identified by the livestock producer as a nutritional disorder until the problem becomes chronic and additional assistance is sought. Therefore, it is essential to get a complete history, including a detailed feeding regimen, on any livestock patient who is exhibiting signs of illness.

Dramatic enhancements have occurred in large animal nutrition, including studies that have increased understanding of the specific nutrient needs of livestock to maximize the genetic potential for efficient production, successful breeding, and generation of high quality, lean meat. Future research will continue to improve our understanding of animal physiology and lead to improvements in livestock production (Table 27–1).

NUTRIENTS

Nutrients are ingested to support life. Livestock producers want to obtain the most desirable results from the nutrients their animals consume at an economical rate and with an advantageous financial return. Ingested nutrients are either retained by the animal or excreted in the urine and feces. Retained nutrients are used for a wide array of body functions, such as homeostasis, replenishment and development of tissues, reproduction, and milk, wool, and meat production.

Maintenance nutrient requirements (MNRs) are the levels of nutrients needed to sustain body weight without gain or loss. The MNR is the minimum level of dietary need; usually, the vast percentage of published requirements are higher than this standard. As a general rule, one half of consumed and absorbed nutrients are used to fulfill MNRs. Individual variation results in fluctuation from this standard; be sure to evaluate need against all information to achieve most accurate results.

> **TECHNICIAN NOTE**
>
> MNRs are the levels of nutrients needed to sustain body weight without gain or loss.

Digestion, the process of protein, carbohydrate, and fat breakdown into absorbable nutrients, is accomplished by both chemical and physical methods. It is essential to remember that it is not the alfalfa hay, corn, or oats that is actually used by the cells of livestock but rather the digested and absorbed nutrients, such as amino acids, sugars, fatty acids, minerals, and vitamins, that present at the cellular level. The quality, quantity, and cost of nutrients that can be provided by the feedstuff are of primary importance when choosing ingredients for farm animal feeding.

FEEDING PROBLEMS IN RUMINANTS

• Table 27-1 •

DISEASE	SYMPTOMS	CAUSE	PREVENTION	COMMENTS
Bloat	Distention of the left flank Then the right flank Hypersalivation Profuse burning ↑ Froth or gas accumulation in the rumen Respiratory distress Cyanosis Death	↑ Change in pasture with heavy fertilizer Genetics Bacterial overgrowth Overeating	Feed coarse grasses or dry forage before turnout to quick growing pastures Avoid straight pastures Keep stock on pasture continuously rather than sporadically Allow full access to water and salt	Watch legume exposure for all ruminants
Enterotoxemia (overeating disease)	Death is often the first symptom Circling Progressive weakness Head butting Convulsions	Often occurs in faster growing juveniles *Clostridium perfringens* Excess consumption of high-energy feeds or lush pasture or heavy milk supply	Vaccination with *Clostridium perfringens* type D for lambs and types C and D for breeding ewes	Primarily sheep and goats; sometimes cattle If outbreak occurs, consider enterotoxemia antiserum for 21-day protection in lambs
Fescue toxicosis (fescue foot)	↓ +/− Lameness Necrosis of tail end Milk production Abortion	↑ Change in parasitized animal ↑ In malnourished animal Endophyte fungus *Acremonium coerophbalum*	Avoid heavy parasitism and malnutrition Use fungus-free fescue seed for planting	Cattle and sheep mostly Highest occurrence in fall and winter in all fescue pasture
Grass tetany (hypomagnesemia)	Disorientation Paddling Convulsions Muscle twitching	Most common in cows 4 years and older ↑ Occurrence during early lactation in heavy milking cows Pastures with ↓ Mg²⁺ and ↑ K⁺ and ↓ Ca²⁺ availability	Start providing Mg²⁺ 30 days before high-risk times ↑ Mg²⁺ in lactating and older cows and ewes Highest risk spring, winter, and fall Molasses supplement with Mg²⁺ may be required	Stress from weather, movement, or environment ↑ Opportunity
Milk fever (parturition, paresis, or hypocalcemia)	↓ Appetite Nervous behavior Collapse Wrenching of head toward back	Postcalving in high producing cows ↓ Blood Ca²⁺	Feed ↑ P, ↓ Ca²⁺ 14 days before parturition Feed balanced Ca²⁺/P rations Vitamin D intake 1 week before parturition Avoid obesity	Watch Ca²⁺ and P levels in dry periods

Condition	Signs	Cause	Treatment/Prevention	Notes
Ketosis	Occurs: 14–50 Days after parturition in cattle; 2 Weeks before parturition in sheep; ↓ Milk production; ↓ Appetite; Sugary-acid breath; ↓ Body weight; Frequent urination; Trembling; Collapse	↑ Chances in multiple births with ewes and does; ↓ Rapid loss of body fat and low availability of carbohydrates in diet	Maintain lean body condition and excess fat; ↑ Energy intake before parturition and ↓ after parturition	Ewes at risk before lambing; Cows typically at risk after calving
Thiamine-deficiency polio	Decreased vision; Incoordination; Acute death; Excitable	Thiamine deficiency; Overgrazing; Feeding lambs in rich pasture	Cause not fully discovered; ↓ Grain intake while ↑ roughage quality, 1 week before; ↑ Animals intake of high-energy diets	Primarily feedlot and young cattle under 2 years old; Goats may be affected while nursing young
Rickets	In young animals, enlarged joints; Painful gait; Leg bowing	Incorrect Ca^{2+}, P, vitamin intake	Provide balanced Ca^{2+}, P, and vitamin D diets	
Urinary calculi; Urolithiasis; Water belly	Difficult urination; Bloody urine; Kicking at abdomen; Rupture of bladder	↑ Increase in feedlots; High K^+ consumption ↑P, ↓Ca^{2+}; Vitamin A deficiency; Excess silicate intake	Readily available water; Balance P/Ca^{2+} ratio; Avoid vitamin A deficiency; ↑ Salt availability; Balanced ratios	Males have ↑ risk
White muscle disease	Irregular gait; Hunched-back appearance; Heart irregularities; Death	Selenium deficiency; Geographic distribution ↓ Se in many areas of U.S. and Canada	↑ Se to dietary intake in known deficient areas	Most common in most rapidly growing individuals in flock or herd

From Naylor JM, et al.: Large Animal Clinical Nutrition. St. Louis, Mosby-Year Book, 1991; McDonald P, et al.: Animal Nutrition. New York, Longman Scientific and Technical, 1995; Maynard LA, et al.: Animal Nutrition, 7th Ed. New York, McGraw-Hill, 1979; and Ensminger ME, et al.: Feeds and Nutrition. Clovis, CA, Ensminger Publishing, 1990.

ELEMENTS THAT INFLUENCE NUTRIENT REQUIREMENTS OF LIVESTOCK

Body size	Behavior
Health status	Genetics
Stress	Reproductive status
Environment	Sex
Exercise	Breed

PROTEIN

Protein is the principal constituent of organs and soft tissues. It is constructed of building blocks called *amino acids* that are linked together in a chain. The arrangement of amino acids in the chain and the length of the chain are two factors that help to determine the composition of the protein. There are 10 essential and 12 nonessential amino acids. Essential amino acids must be supplied in the diet because the animal body cannot synthesize them fast enough to meet its requirement. The construction of amino acids involves nitrogen, carbon, oxygen, and sulfur. The deconstruction or deamination process results in the release of these elements into the body system and either the elimination from the body or the use as energy.

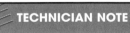

TECHNICIAN NOTE

Protein is a common component of plants, with highest constituency in the seed and leafy portions.

Animal feeds are identified often by crude protein content, but the measurement rarely illustrates the quality or utilization potential of the protein. A feed can possess a high protein content, yet the *biological value* of that protein is low. Protein biological value is the percentage of true absorbed protein that is available for productive body functions. Conceptually, it is the "amino acid grade card," as it defines the available amino acids. In general, proteins of animal origin have greater biological value than do proteins of plant origin. The higher the biological value, the better is the protein used for productive purposes. Protein quality is also measured as *protein efficiency ratio,* which is the number of grams of body weight gain per unit of protein consumed (McDonald, 1995).

Animal and plant proteins vary greatly in their distribution

PROTEIN ANALYSIS OF LIVESTOCK FEEDS

Pasture/grasslands	40.0%*
Corn	23.3%
Hay	12.2%
Grains/feeds	16.9%
Silage/miscellaneous	7.6%

*Varies significantly by season and pasture quality.
From the USDA Economic Research Service.

of amino acids and biological value. When combined in correct proportions with other protein (e.g., animal protein), proteins that individually have very poor biological value (e.g., corn) may yield a biological value similar to that of a single high-quality protein. The quality of proteins is dependent on disallowing overprocessing of feeds, overheating in storage, and form of the feed (Nash, 1985) (Fig. 27–1).

PROTEIN USE BY RUMINANTS

Rumen digestion facilitated by microbes has the ability to convert most feed protein into peptides and amino acids, many of which are further degraded into ammonia, organic acids, and carbon dioxide. The ammonia released on microbial degradation of feed protein will be removed from the rumen by absorption through the rumen wall or used by the microorganisms for synthesis of microbial protein. Microbial protein synthesized by the microorganisms results in a fairly constant protein quality supply to the lower digestive tract. The protein quality from moderate-to-poor feeds will usually be improved by rumen metabolism, whereas the opposite may occur with high-quality protein feeds. The rumen microbes also have the ability to convert nonprotein nitrogen sources into microbial protein. Typical nonprotein/nitrogen sources include urea, anhydrous ammonia, or free amino acids and are best used judiciously as excess or an imbalanced intake can be toxic (Church, 1984).

FATS

Fats provide dietary energy; serve as a source of heat, insulation, and protection for the animal body; and provide essential fatty acids. Fat has more energy per gram than all other nutrients—2.25 times more than protein or carbohydrates. Fats also aid the absorption of fat-soluble vitamins. Linoleic, linolenic, and arachidonic fatty acids are considered essential, even though linoleic acid is capable of being converted to arachidonic acid. However, the process to make these conversions is arduous and inefficient, and as such, arachidonic acid should be considered conditionally essential (McDonald, 1995).

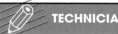

TECHNICIAN NOTE

Fat has more energy per gram than all other nutrients.

CARBOHYDRATES

Carbohydrates are the primary energy source in livestock rations. They are less expensive and more readily available than proteins or fats. Most feedstuffs of plant origin are high in carbohydrate content, especially cereal grains. Carbohydrates must be broken down into simple sugars for absorption from the digestive system. This requires digestive enzymes generated by the host or by microflora inhabiting the digestive system of the host. The carbohydrate-splitting enzymes are effective in splitting most complex carbohydrates into simple sugars except those with the beta linkage, as found in cellulose (fiber). Microflora in the rumen of ruminants and the cecum of some nonruminants, such as the horse or rabbit, produce an enzyme

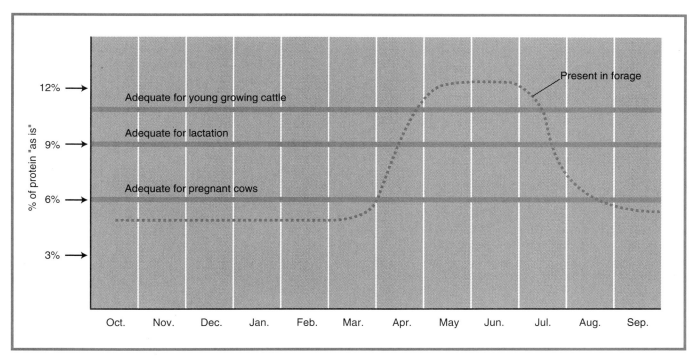

Figure 27-1. Nutrient content of forage varies with pasture quality and season.

CARBOHYDRATES

Energy sources:
 50–80% from DM* forages/grains
Categories of carbohydrates:
 1. Fiber-forages: structural carbohydrates, cellulose, hemicellulose
 2. Sugars: (molasses, growing plants) glucose, sucrose, fructose
 3. Starches: stored carbohydrates grains

*On a dry matter basis (DM).

---

so that these species can use large quantities of fiber for energy. Carbohydrates are commonly categorized into animal feeds as concentrates (grains, high starch compounds) and forages (grass hays, legumes). There are no minimum or maximum requirements for carbohydrates; rather, intake is defined in conjunction with energy need.

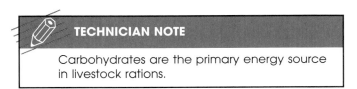

TECHNICIAN NOTE

Carbohydrates are the primary energy source in livestock rations.

Feedstuff Energy

The largest function of feed is to provide energy for body processes. Total digestible nutrients (TDNs), gross energy, di-gestible energy, metabolizable energy, and net energy are all different measures of feed energy value.

TDN is a general measure of the nutritive value of a feed. Digestibility coefficients are used to compute the content of total digestible nutrients. The usefulness of TDN as a measure of feed energy is limited in that it does not take into account energy losses in urine, combustible gases, and heat loss. The discrepancies can be large for forage-based feeds, as they tend to overestimate the energy available for productive purposes. TDN is expressed as a percentage of the ration or in units of weight and not as an actual caloric number.

Gross energy (GE) is the total energy potentially available in a feed consumed by an animal. All energy values used in the following scheme are expressed in kilocalories (kcal) or megacalories (Mcal) per unit of weight. During digestion and absorption, a portion of the GE escapes the body in the form of undigested food residue in the feces. Subtraction of the energy lost in the feces from the consumed GE accounts for energy that was digested and absorbed, or *digestible energy* (DE). The measurement of DE uses the same elements as TDN and gives similar energy values to feed. Energy that is digested and absorbed by the body is not used with 100% efficiency; a portion of the absorbed energy is lost in the urine and as combustible gases. Accounting for these energy losses leads to a step beyond DE or TDN, *metabolizable energy* (ME). The

---

ENERGY REQUIREMENTS

Variables
 Activity   Life stage
 Environment   Reproductive status
 Body size

energy values for ME are used widely in the formulation of equine and poultry feeds. One further refinement in this energy scheme is accounting for heat lost from the body during metabolism of the nutrients. *Net energy* (NE) represents the actual portion of energy available to the animal for use in maintaining body tissues or during pregnancy or lactation. NE values for swine and poultry have been developed and may be in widespread use by 2003.

MINERALS AND VITAMINS

Minerals and vitamins are needed in small amounts compared with other nutrients, but play integral roles in many metabolic processes. Minerals are divided into two categories: microminerals and macrominerals (Table 27–2). The list of minerals and vitamins and their functions are given in Tables 27–3, 27–4, and 27–5.

WATER

Water is the cheapest and most abundant nutrient. It makes up 65% to 85% of an animal's body weight at birth and 45% to 60% of body weight at maturity. Water is derived metabolically from the breakdown of organic nutrients in the animal tissues or drinking water or obtained from foodstuffs (Fig. 27–2). As the largest constituent of the animal, deprivation of water of only a few percentages of body weight is life threatening. Clean, fresh water should be readily available to maintain a zero water balance (Table 27–6).

TECHNICIAN NOTE

Water is the cheapest and most abundant nutrient.

DAIRY CATTLE

The dairy industry is successfully using many different production systems. Systems are based on geographical area and feedstuff availability. The traditional pasture system continues to be used in areas with readily available land, whereas dry lot systems are more popular in urban, suburban areas (Fig. 27–3).

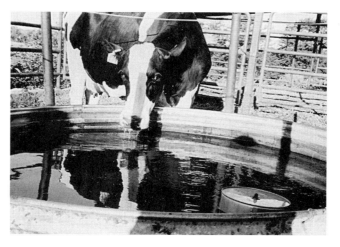
Figure 27-2. It is essential that fresh water is readily available to dairy cows to obtain maximum milk production. This watering system maintains an agitator to keep water from becoming stagnant.

Feeding, more than any other single factor, determines the productivity of lactating dairy cows. Feed represents about 50% of the total cost of milk production. Therefore, a good feeding program is necessary for profitable milk production. Nutrient requirements for lactation are large and often several times the MNR (Fig. 27–4, Tables 27–7, 27–8, and 27–9).

TECHNICIAN NOTE

Feed represents 50% of the total costs of milk production.

FACTORS AFFECTING WATER INTAKE

Dry matter intake	Environment
Reproductive status	Weight
Activity	Age
Type of feeding regimen	Rate of gain

THE IMPORTANCE OF WATER

- For digestion, absorption, and utilization of nutrients
- For production requirements
- Watering methods:
  Free water always available
  Twice-a-day watering
- Cleanliness:
  Water heaters must be supplied in winter to prevent freezing
  Troughs must always be kept clean

• Table 27–2 •

MINERAL CATEGORIES

MACROMINERALS*	MICROMINERALS†	
Salt (Sodium Chloride) (NaCl)	Zinc (Zn)	Copper (Cu)
Potassium (K⁺)	Selenium (Se)	Iron (Fe)
Phosphorus (P)	Manganese (Mn)	Silicon (Si)
Magnesium (Mg²⁺)	Iodine (I)	Molybdenum (Mo)
Calcium (Ca²⁺)	Fluorine (F)	Cobalt (Co)
Sulfur (S)	Chromium (Cr)	

*Measured in mg/kg.
†Measured in ppm or μg.

• Table 27–3 •

MACROMINERALS FOR FOOD ANIMALS

MINERALS	USE	TOXICITY	DEFICIENCY	SOURCES

Calcium	Nerve transmission
	Clotting cascade
	Cardiac function
	Muscle contraction
	Milk production
		Calcium kidney stones
		↑ Calcium deposition
		  into soft tissue
		↑ Blood calcium level
		↓ Absorption of Zn,
		  Mg^{2+}, Fe, Cu
			↓ Quality bone/teeth
			↓ Milk production
			Osteomalacia
			Osteoporosis
			Hypocalcemia
			(Tetany)
			Rickets
				Alfalfa
				Milk
				Fish by-products
				Soybean meal
				Bone meal
				Dicalcium phosphate
				  supplement

Phosphorus	Milk secretion
	Building muscle
	Teeth/bone development
	Acid-base balance
	Protein metabolism
		↓ Absorption Ca^{2+}
		Urinary stones if Ca^{2+} is
		  low
			Similar to Ca^{2+}
			Osteomalacia
			Rickets
			Hematuria
			Pica
			↓ Breeding capability
				Meat meals
				Soybean oil meal
				Wheat bran
				Bone meal
				Monosodium phosphate
				  supplement

Sodium	Muscle contraction
	Absorption of
	  carbohydrates
	Part of sweat and bile
	Osmotic pressure
	Acid-base balance
	Water balance
		↑ Toxicity with ↓ H_2O
		  intake
		Staggering
		Blindness
		Hypertension
		Neurological disorders
			↓ Breeding capability
			Cravings: urine drinking
			↓ Growth rate
			↓ Milk production
			Weight loss
			↓ Appetite
				Molasses
				Meat by-products
				Salt/mineral blocks
				Monosodium glutamate
				  supplement

Potassium	Heart function
	Insulin secretion
	Acid-base balance
	Muscle development
		↓ Heart rate
		↓ Mg^{2+} use
		Exaggerated when
		  ↓ Mg^{2+} and H_2O
		  restricted
			↓ Growth
			Excess NaCl depletes K
			Irregular gait
			Pica
			↓ Weight
				Molasses
				Forages
				Soy by-products
				Carrots
				Potassium gluconate
				  supplement

Chlorine	Water balance
	Osmotic pressure
	Acid-base balance
	HCl production in
	  stomach
		↑ When water is
		  restricted
		
		Rare
			↓ Appetite
			↓ Growth
			Alkalosis
			↓ Respiratory rate
			Muscle cramps
			Convulsions
				Alfalfa
				Meat meals
				Molasses
				Salt blocks (NaCl)
				Potassium chloride
				  supplement

Magnesium	Cellular energy metabolism Alkalinizer Nerve impulse relaxant Bone and teeth	Rare	↑ Grass tetany ↑ Body temperature Respiratory rate Hypersalivation Death	Meat/bone meal Molasses Wheat bran Alfalfa supplements

Sulfur	Carbohydrate metabolism
	Insulin production
	Hair and wool
	  production
		Hydrogen sulfide gas
		  production
			↓ Growth
			↓ Hair/wool production
				Meat meal
				Yeast
				Whey
				Supplements

• Table 27–4 •

MINERALS	USE	TOXICITY	DEFICIENCY	SOURCES
Zinc	Skin Hair Bone maintenance Synthesis of protein Development of reproductive organs	↓ Growth Anemia Bone changes ↑ Appetite Stiff gait	↓ Growth ↓ Appetite Bone irregularities ↓ Wound healing Wool and hair loss Parakeratosis	Meat meal Corn gluten or germ meal Wheat by-products supplements
Selenium	Vitamin and sparing tissue damage Fatty acid oxidation	Weight loss Blind staggers Lameness Anemia Paralysis	White muscle disease (sheep) Liver necrosis in pigs	Poultry/fish meals Wheat by-products Cereals Oil seed meals
Manganese	Bone/cartilage growth Clotting cascade Metabolism of nutrients	Nontoxic	↓ Growth Lameness Reproductive disorders	Wheat Grass/alfalfa/hay Corn Sorghum supplements

Iodine	Hormone production
	Influence growth
	Muscle tissue development
	Milk production
	Nutrient metabolism
		Horse:
		  Hyperparathyroidism
		  Goiter
		↓ Utilization of iodine
			↓ Hair quality
			↓ Growth
			Reproductive problems
			Abortion
				Molasses
				Meat/bone meal
				Oats
				Wheat
				Iodized salt
				Soybean meal

Fluorine	Bone Teeth	↓ Feed use ↓ Hair/wool quality Deformed teeth/bone	Rare	Fish meals Present in most foods
Chromium	Synthesis of some fatty acids ↑ Insulin use Stabilizes DNA and RNA	Rare	Hyperglycemia glucosuria ↓ Fat metabolism	Wheat Potatoes Corn Vegetable oil Supplements
Copper	Pigment of hair/wool Reproduction Skeletal structure Hemoglobin construction Absorption of iron	Although rare, sometimes seen in sheep ingestion of copper foot bath Gastroenteritis Hypersalivation ↓ Appetite Thirst	Swayback: Lambs ↓ Wool quality Lameness Anemia Diarrhea	Safflower oil Molasses Grass hays Cotton seeds Mineral mix
Iron	Hemoglobin production Muscle oxygenation Enzyme activation	Irregularity in red blood cell production Reproductive disorders	Anemia Pica Diarrhea ↓ Hair coat quality ↓ Iron in milk	Fish/meat meals Safflower Alfalfa Corn gluten meal Supplements
Silicon	Skeletal development	Calculi formation	Skeletal abnormalities	Meat by-products Grains
Molybdenum	Metabolism of fats, carbohydrates, and proteins Growth promotion Enamel production	Diarrhea ↓ Weight ↓ Hair quality ↓ Reproduction	Rare	Grass/alfalfa/hay Meat meal Corn Oats Wheat
Cobalt	Formation of vitamin B_{12}	Rare	↓ Skin/hair coat quality Abortion ↓ Milk ↓ Appetite	Soybean meal Meat/poultry meal Corn Wheat Molasses

• Table 27–5 •

VITAMINS FOR LIVESTOCK				
WATER SOLUBLE	**FUNCTION**	**TOXICITY**	**DEFICIENCY**	**SOURCES**
B Complex				
Biotin	Metabolism of carbohydrates, fats, and proteins Enzyme activities	No known toxicity	↓ Growth ↓ Hair quality Lameness ↓ Reproduction	Young grasses Safflower meal Soybean meal supplements
Thiamine (Vitamin B-1)	Coenzyme of energy metabolism Peripheral nerve function Maintenance assistance of appetite	No known toxicity	Heart irregularities ↓ Body temperature	Wheat Millet Oil seed meals Oats Supplements
Pyridoxine (Vitamin B-6)	Nitrogen metabolism Fat and carbohydrate metabolism	Nontoxic	Anorexia ↓ Growth Eye discharge Anemia	Green pastures Meat/fish meals Corn gluten meal Safflower meal Alfalfa
Cobalamin (Vitamin B-12)	Red blood cell formation Maintenance of nerve tissue DNA synthesis	Nontoxic	↓ Coordination (black legs: Pigs) ↓ Reproduction	Fish/meat meals Whey Brewer's yeast supplements
Niacin	Growth ↓ Cholesterol levels Release of energy from fats, proteins, and carbohydrates	Nontoxic	↓ Growth ↓ Appetite Diarrhea Unthriftiness	Wheat barley Yeast supplements
Folic Acid	Construction of hemoglobin Manipulation of protein Choline synthesis	Nontoxic	Anemia Diarrhea ↓ Growth	Soybean meal Alfalfa Wheat Meat/fish meal Supplement
Pantothenic Acid	Metabolism of fats, protein, and carbohydrates Hemoglobin production Maintain normal blood levels	Nontoxic	Neurological disorder Goose stepping (swine) ↓ Hair quality Enteritis	Wheat bran Alfalfa Safflower meal Supplements
Riboflavin (Vitamin B-2)	Metabolism of amino acids and fatty acids Retinal pigment Adrenal function	Nontoxic	↓ Growth Moon blindness (horses) Anemia Unthrifty ↓ Reproduction (swine)	Alfalfa Green pastures Sweet/white clover Supplements
Vitamin C	Absorption of iron Metabolism folic acid Antioxidant Teeth/bone integrity	Rare in food animals	↓ Wound healing Hemorrhage Enlarged joints Ulcerated gums	Green pastures Hay Potatoes

• Table 27–6 •

SPECIES	WEIGHT (lb)	CONSUMPTION (gallons/day)
WATER CONSUMPTION GUIDELINES		
Swine		
Pigs	30–125	0.3–2.0
Feeder pigs	126–200	2.0–3.2
Finisher pigs	201–250	3.2–4.0
Sow/boar maintenance	150–400	1.3–3.5
	401–600	3.5–5.2
Sow: late gestation	250–400	4.5–5.0
	401–600	5.0–7.5
Sow: lactation	250–400	5.5–6.5
	401–600	6.5–9.8
Sheep		
Lambs	20–50	0.4–0.6
Feeder lambs	50–110	0.5–1.4
Finisher lambs	111–125	1.4–1.8
Ewes: grain and hay intake*		
Maintenance	150–300	0.3–1.2
Lactation	150–300	0.5–2.4
Rams: grain and hay intake	150–300	0.3–2.0
Cattle		
Calves	100–200	1.2–2.5
	201–400	2.5–4.9
Developing steers/heifers	401–600	4.5–6.2
	601–800	6.0–8.2
	801–1000	8.0–9.8
Finishing steers		
Pasture	1001–1200	8.5–10.2
Maintenance	800–1000	3.6–4.6
	1001–1200	4.4–7.2
	1201–1400	5.0–7.2
	1401–1600	6.0–9.0
Cows: late gestation	800–1000	4.4–5.5
	1001–1200	5.3–6.6
	1201–1400	6.4–7.9
	1401–1600	7.7–9.5
Beef cows/heifer lactation	800–1000	6.7–15.6
	1001–1200	8.3–18.8
	1201–1400	10.0–21.8
	1401–1600	11.7–25.0
Dairy cow/heifer peak lactation†	800–1000	14.8–20.6
	1001–1201	18.5–24.3
	1201–1400	22.5–28.8
	1401–1600	28.0–32.2
	1601–1800	30.5–36.0

*Intake is influenced dramatically by factors found in table. Table is intended as a guide line.
†Dairy cattle intake varies on milk production more than beef cattle.

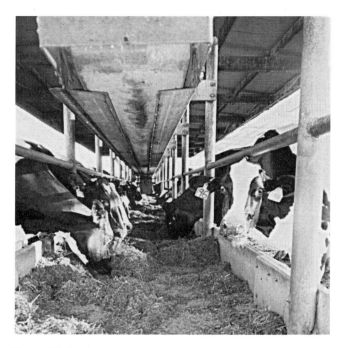

Figure 27–3. Large quantities of forage are ingested by dairy cows on a daily basis and are paramount to fulfillment of energy requirements.

If cows are allowed to consume all the forage they want, they will not have sufficient rumen capacity to consume enough concentrate to meet the energy requirements needed for lactation. In general, most dairy farmers try to feed forage at a rate of 1.75% of body weight. The concentrate fed with the forage will vary with the kind of forage offered (a high-protein concentrate will be needed with a low-protein forage) and the availability and cost of the feedstuffs. The concentrate provides more energy and usually is higher in protein than the forage.

Fat utilization varies with age, environment, and reproductive status. Fat intake during lactation can be 5% to 6% of total energy intake. Excessive dietary fat intake can negatively affect rumen microbial activity, depressing fiber utilization (Shirley, 1986).

Protein

Restriction of protein or energy during lactation can lead to reduced milk production and increased reproductive problems. Protein is supplied by the forage or concentrate and should be added at levels to ensure that minimum protein requirements are met (see Tables 27–7, 27–8, and 27–9).

Protein intake that exceeds the requirement is used as energy at a premium value. Protein is an expensive nutrient and is not an economical source of energy. Most cows are fed a high-protein legume hay, such as alfalfa, and grain, which should supply most or all of the protein needs during lactation. Nonprotein nitrogen supplied as urea also can be an effective feedstuff to supply protein equivalents in dairy rations.

Minerals and Vitamins

Milk is composed of 0.7% minerals on a dry weight basis. The average cow will lactate 140 lb of mineral as a portion of the

Energy

Carbohydrates (forage and concentrate) are the major energy source for lactation, followed by fats and proteins. Carbohydrates constitute 50% to 80% of energy on a dry matter basis of many forages and grains. Forages possess a significant fiber content that is broken down by the microbial population in the rumen and used as energy (Fig. 27–5).

Although the rumen capacity of the dairy cow is considerable, she cannot eat sufficient forage to meet her extensive nutrient needs during lactation. Estimated daily intake for forages is based on body weight and forage quality. A guide for estimating consumption of forage (dry matter basis) fed on a free-choice basis is in Tables 27–10 and 27–11.

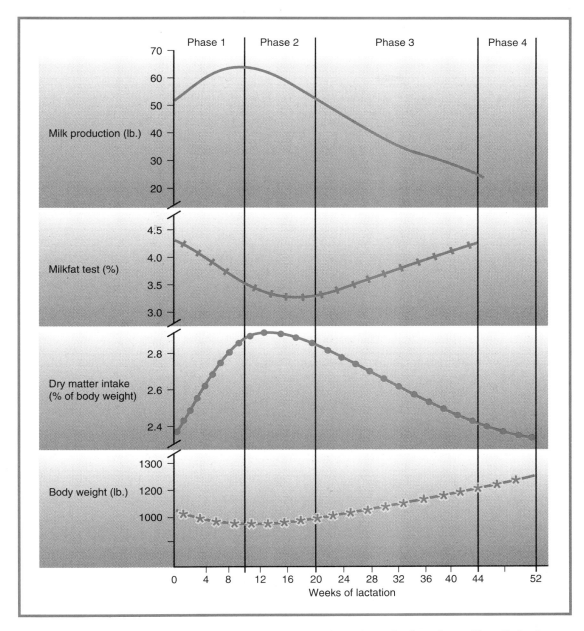

Figure 27–4. Milk production varies during a typical 52-week production phase. Disparity is also observed in milk fat content, dry matter intake requirements, and body weight.

milk produced per year. Balanced mineral intake is essential; mineral requirements for lactation are given in Tables 27–7, 27–8, and 27–9.

Rumen microorganisms can synthesize the water-soluble vitamins, whereas vitamin K is the only fat-soluble vitamin readily synthesized by microorganisms. The supplementation of water-soluble vitamins or vitamin K normally is not necessary in rations for ruminants.

Forages of good quality and properly harvested normally contain adequate levels of vitamin E and the precursor of vitamin A, carotene. Vitamin A is stored for extended periods in the body. Vitamin D is synthesized through ultraviolet radiation by the skin or added to a dairy ration as sun-cured forage or a vitamin supplement.

Although water-soluble vitamins are synthesized by the

rumen microflora, some evidence indicates that supplemental thiamine, choline, and niacin may be beneficial in cows undergoing heavy stress or various disease states. Daily requirements for vitamins for lactating dairy cows are found in Tables 27–7, 27–8, and 27–9.

DAIRY CALVES

Newborn calves require the mother's colostrum within the first 72 hours of life to acquire energy and maternal immunity from disease. Peak benefits of colostrum intake are realized within the first 24 hours post partum. Optimally, the first milking colostrum should be given to the calf at 10% to 12% of the calf's weight with at least one half administered within 4 to 6 hours after birth. Colostrum can be successfully frozen and

• Table 27–7 •

			MINERALS	
WEIGHT (lb)	**NE (Mcal*)**	**TOTAL CRUDE PROTEIN (%)**	**Ca²⁺**	**P**
200–399	6.4–11.5	16–18	15–18	9–15
400–599	11.5–15.4	12–16	18–23	13–15
600–799	15.4–19.5	12–14	23–24	15–17
800–999	19.5–23.9	12–14	24–26	17–18
1000–1199	23.9–28.4	12–14	26–28	18–19
1200–1399	28.4–33.8	12–14	28–30	19–21

DAILY FEEDING CONSIDERATIONS IN DEVELOPING FEMALE DAIRY CATTLE

*NE, net energy expressed in megacalories (Mcal).
   Ranges shown in table are to be used as guidelines recognizing that variations can occur due to breed, milk production levels, butter fat content, rate of gain, and lactation cycle.
   Ca²⁺/phosphorus ratio needs to be maintained from 0.43% to 0.66%; levels above 0.95% to 100% can result in decreased performance and metabolic abnormalities.

• Table 27–8 •

DAILY GUIDELINES FOR LACTATING DAIRY COWS

WEIGHT (lb)	**MILK YIELD (lb)**	**NE (Mcal)***	**TOTAL CRUDE PROTEIN (%)**	**MINERALS (g)**	
				Ca²⁺	**P**
800	15–45	13.1–21.6	12–16	40–77	25–49
	45–60	21.6–25.8	16–17	77–96	49–61
	61–75	25.8–34.0	16–18	96–115	61–78
1000	20–40	14.9–20.3	12–16	44–70	29–44
	41–70	20.3–25.6	16–18	70–114	44–73
	71–90	25.6–36.3	16–18	114–146	73–86
1200	20–40	17.0–23.7	12–16	50–81	33–52
	41–60	23.7–30.3	16–18	81–110	52–70
	61–80	30.3–37.0	16–18	110–139	70–87
1400	50–75	27.7–35.7	15–17	95–131	62–83
	76–100	35.7–43.7	16–18	131–165	83–104
	101–125	43.7–51.7	16–18	165–200	104–126
1600	60–90	31.0–40.0	15–17	108–146	69–92
	91–120	40.0–48.3	16–18	146–184	92–116
	121–150	48.3–57.0	16–18	184–221	116–137
1800	60–90	40.9–44.6	16–18	121–164	78–104
	91–120	44.6–54.4	16–18	164–207	104–131
	121–150	54.4–64.1	16–18	207–249	131–157

*NE, net energy measured in megacalories (Mcal).
   Mineral values assume that balance has been established. Variations occur with breed, lactation phase, milk yield, and age. This table is designed to be used only as a guideline. Feed to maintain body condition. Table assumes a 4% milk fat content of lactation.

• Table 27–9 •

DAILY NUTRIENT CONSIDERATIONS FOR DAIRY CATTLE						
WEIGHT (lb)	**ME* (Mcal)**	**TOTAL CRUDE PROTEIN (g)**	**MINERALS (g)**		**VITAMINS (1000 IU)**	
			Ca²⁺	**P**	**A**	**D**
*Females: *60 days before gestation*						
800–1000	13.8–16.4	850–925	24–30	16–18	30–35	12–14
1000–1200	16.4–19.2	925–1000	30–35	18–22	35–42	14–17
1200–1400	19.2–21.5	1000–1100	35–42	22–26	42–48	17–19
1400–1600	21.5–23.6	1100–1200	42–45	26–30	48–56	19–22
Dairy bulls					1000 IU	1000 IU
1000–1300	14.3–17.8	775–900				
1301–1500	17.8–19.7	900–1000	20–24	12–15	21.00–25.25	3.3–3.9
1501–1700	19.7–21.6	1000–1125	24–28	15–18	25.25–29.50	3.9–4.6
1701–1900	21.6–23.5	1125–1225	28–32	18–20	29.50–33.75	4.6–5.3
1901–2100	23.5–25.3	1225–1325	32–36	20–22	33.75–38.00	5.3–5.9
2101–2300	25.3–27.0	1325–1425	36–40	22–25	38.00–42.50	5.9–6.6
2301–2500	27.0–28.8	1425–1520	40–44	25–28	42.50–46.60	6.6–7.3
2501–2700	28.0–30.4	1520–1610	44–48	28–30	46.60–50.90	7.3–7.9
2701–2900	30.4–32.1	1610–1700	48–52	30–32	50.90–55.10	7.9–8.6

*ME, metabolizable energy measured in megacalories (Mcal).
Ranges shown in table are to be used as guidelines recognizing that variations can occur due to breed, milk production levels, butter fat content, rate of gain, and lactation cycle.
Ca²⁺/phosphorus ratio needs to be maintained from 0.43% to 0.66%; levels above 0.95% to 100% can result in decreased performance and metabolic abnormalities.

used at a later date as well as diluted equally with water should diarrhea occur due to the "richness" of the colostrum. The initial sucking of the calf will create a bypass of the rumen, allowing the milk to go directly into the abomasum. This ability will decrease as the calf ages and the rumen becomes functional.

Calves normally start on milk replacers and then are offered calf starters within the first week of life. Calf starter rations are commonly fed to about 3 months of age at a rate of 5 to 7 lb of calf starter per day. During the first week of life, a forage source should be added to diet selection as well as free-choice water. Calves are typically weaned at 4 to 8 weeks of age and accustomed to solid food.

BEEF CATTLE

Feeding represents almost three fourths of the cost of production of beef cattle (Neumann, 1977). Beef producers control their profitability by obtaining optimal nutrient intake with least cost feed formulation. Profitability hinges on the ability to balance utilization of resources, such as pasture and feedlot, with the production of high-quality finishing animals generated by the breeding herd. Beef production usually is divided into two primary areas: cow-calf production and finishing cattle.

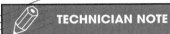

TECHNICIAN NOTE

Feeding represents 75% of the cost of beef cattle production.

COW-CALF PRODUCTION
Breeding Herd

A live calf from each cow each year should be the goal of the profitable cow-calf producer. Nutrition has a large impact on

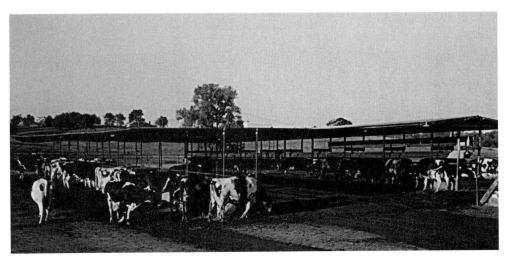

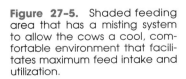

Figure 27–5. Shaded feeding area that has a misting system to allow the cows a cool, comfortable environment that facilitates maximum feed intake and utilization.

• Table 27–10 •

DRY MATTER INTAKE	
Dependent on	
Stage of lactation	Size of cow
Body condition	Milk production
Quality of feed	Feeding regimen
Environment	Age

the beef breeding herd. Cows gaining weight just before and during the breeding season have a shorter period between calving and the first estrus period and typically have higher conception rates.

Energy

Carbohydrates are the major energy source for beef cows, followed by proteins and fat. Forages commonly fed to beef cows possess a significant fiber content that is broken down by the microbial population in the rumen and used as energy.

TECHNICIAN NOTE

Carbohydrates are the major energy source for beef cows.

Feeding beef cows can be very economical because high-quality forage or pasture can supply all energy needs with no need for energy supplementation from grains or fats. In the summer, pasture normally will supply adequate energy for the cow. If pasture is inadequate, supplemental energy should be provided in the form of silage or hay. In the winter, pregnant cows are fed wintering rations (a combination of forages, grain, and a protein source supplemented with vitamins and minerals) to meet energy needs with minimal weight gain. Cows in good condition are more tolerant to the stresses of winter and require less maintenance energy per unit of weight than do cows in poor condition (Table 27–12).

Protein

Most pasture, silages, and forages contain adequate levels of protein to meet the needs of the breeding cow. If low-grade roughages (e.g., cobs, straw, and stalks) are fed over extended periods of time, the ration must be supplemented daily with 1

• Table 27–11 •

FORAGE QUALITY	
FORAGE QUALITY	DAILY INTAKE (% BODY WEIGHT)
Excellent	3.0
Good	2.5
Average	2.0
Fair	1.5
Poor	1.0

FEEDING CONSIDERATIONS FOR CALVES

Dairy calves
Days 1–3: Colostrum from dam
Days 4–7: Transition to milk replacer or other liquid feed, begin offering starter and free choice water
Days 5–84: Starter and free choice water through weaning, begin offering forage

Beef calves
Ensure calf nurses within 2 hours of birth to obtain vital colostrum
Ensure that calf continues to thrive and that cow does not show signs of mastitis or decreased milk production

Orphans
Can sometimes be grafted to another cow
Ensure that colostrum has been administered
Feed like dairy calves

to 1.5 lb of a 35% to 45% crude protein supplement. A review of deficiency and toxicity signs can be found in Table 27–13.

Minerals and Vitamins

Mineral supplementation will be necessary and is usually offered on a free-choice basis when animals are on pasture (Fig. 27–6). Trace-mineral salt blocks or granular salt are popular methods of offering minerals and salt to animals on pasture. Good-quality pasture and roughages are adequate in vitamins A and E with ample levels to meet the needs of breeding cows. Supplemental vitamin A should be provided when low-grade roughages or long-stored hays are used as a major source of energy in wintering rations. There are mineral mixes that contain a stabilized form of vitamin A.

TYPICAL GRAIN (NUTRITIONAL OVERVIEW)

20% (or less) protein
18% (or less) crude fiber
Variable moisture
85% (or less) carbohydrate
 6% (or less) fat
75–80% TDN (total digestible nutrients)

SIGNS OF UNDERNUTRITION

↓ Growth
↓ Hair/skin quality
  Skeletal irregularities
↓ Reproductive capabilities
↓ Immune function
  Death

• Table 27–12 •

DAILY NUTRIENT CONSIDERATIONS FOR BEEF CATTLE

WEIGHT (lb)	NET ENERGY NE (Mcal)	TOTAL PROTEIN (lb)	MINERALS (g) Ca²⁺	P
Growing/finishing*				
300–400	3.0–3.6	0.75–1.5	10–42	6–8
401–500	3.7–4.4	0.90–1.9	11–40	8–18
501–600	4.4–5.0	1.0–2.0	12–38	9–19
601–700	5.0–5.6	1.1–2.1	13–36	11–19
701–800	5.6–6.2	1.3–2.1	14–34	12–20
801–900	6.2–6.8	1.4–2.2	15–33	14–20
901–1000	6.8–7.3	1.5–2.3	16–37	16–22
1001–1100	7.3–7.5	1.6–2.3	19–35	18–23
1101–1200	7.5–7.8	1.7–2.4	20–34	20–24
1201–1300	7.8–8.4	1.8–2.4	20–32	20–24
Yearling heifers early to late gestation				
700–800	8.0–8.6	1.3–1.6	19–28	19–22
801–900	8.6–9.1	1.4–1.7	21–28	15–19
901–1000	9.1–9.8	1.5–1.7	20–23	14–20
1001–1100	9.8–10.3	1.5–1.7	23–25	18–20
1101–1200	10.3–10.8	1.6–1.8	25–27	20–21
1201–1300	10.8–11.4	1.6–1.8	26–28	21–23
1301–1400	11.4–12.0	1.8–2.0	26–28	23–24
Lactating cow/heifer				
800–900	10.0–14.0	2.0–2.4	23–35	19–20
901–1000	10.4–14.5	1.9–2.5	24–36	19–20
1001–1100	11.0–15.0	2.0–2.6	25–38	20–22
1101–1200	11.5–15.5	2.0–2.7	27–39	22–23
1201–1300	12.0–16.2	2.1–2.3	23–41	23–25
1301–1400	12.5–17.0	2.2–2.9	30–42	25–26
Breeding bulls				
1300–1500	9.3–10.3	2.0–2.2	23–31	22–25
1501–1700	10.3–11.3	1.7–2.2	23–31	22–25
1701–1900	11.3–12.3	2.0–2.2	26–29	26–29
1901–2100	12.3–13.3	2.0–2.3	27–33	27–33

*Assumes medium- to large-frame steers.

Values represent guidelines, and individual variations dictate the constant appraisal of body condition to ensure desirable results.

From National Research Council: Nutrient Requirements of Beef Cattle. 8th Ed. Washington, DC, National Academic Press, 1990.

Calves

The basic food for calves consists of the mother's milk plus access to pasture or forage fed to the cows. Many cow-calf producers offer calves a highly palatable creep feed to supply additional nutrients, leading to improved weaning weights and decreased weight loss by nursing cows. Creep-fed calves will weigh 30 to 50 extra pounds by weaning time. The greatest response to creep feeding is found when pasture is short or quality is poor. Beef calves generally are weaned at 7 to 8 months of age.

• Table 27–13 •

PROTEIN DEFICIENCY AND TOXICITY IN CATTLE

Deficiency
  ↓ Appetite
  Weight loss
  ↓ Growth
  ↓ Reproductive capability
  ↓ Milk production
Toxicity
  Ammonia: Avoid >40% excess protein or NPN intake

TECHNICIAN NOTE

Creep-fed calves can weigh 30 to 50 lb extra by weaning time.

Finishing Cattle

The *finishing* of cattle refers to the time in the growth phase of growing cattle when they are fed to produce beef that is desirable to the food consumer. Most finished cattle are between 1 and 2 years of age and weigh more than 1000 lb. The goal of the finishing feeding program is to maintain maximum feed intake and gain without causing digestive upsets (see Table 27–12).

Energy

High-energy diets are used to increase weight gain, improve the carcass characteristics, and decrease the cost of energy compared with diets high in fiber. Total dry feed intake commonly will be from 2% to 3% of the animal's body weight. The feed contains high levels of grains to supply readily available energy. Cattle fed these rations are more prone to develop digestive upset (rumen acidosis), founder, or liver abscesses and require more attention and management to avoid these problems.

Protein

Protein requirements (9% to 14%) are greatly affected by age, size of animal, and growth rate. Young cattle require higher levels of protein (as a percentage of the diet) than do older cattle. Protein sources cost more than feed grains, but experienced finishing cattle producers know that a protein deficiency is more expensive than a slight protein excess in the ration. When protein is deficient, energy is not well used, and performance suffers.

Supplemental protein for finishing cattle can be provided by natural protein sources or nonprotein nitrogen (e.g., urea). Nonprotein nitrogen sources are used most efficiently by cattle consuming relatively high levels of grain. A normal range of urea intake for many finishing rations is 0.10 to 0.15 lb per animal per day.

Minerals and Vitamins

Calcium is often added to the high-grain diets fed to finishing cattle. Generally, when forage (especially legumes) constitutes more than 25% of a finishing ration, additional calcium is not required. Grain contains adequate levels of phosphorus to meet the needs of finishing cattle. Finishing rations are balanced to contain a calcium-to-phosphorus ratio of 2:1 or higher. Salt is added to diets or fed on a free-choice basis to finishing cattle to meet the sodium requirement. The less forage that is formulated into the diet, the more need there is for trace mineral supplementation.

High-quality forages contain adequate amounts of vitamin A precursors and vitamin E. Generally, finishing rations are supplemented with 20,000 to 30,000 IU of vitamin A daily because they contain high levels of grain. Vitamins E and D are added to finishing rations when the feed ingredients are devoid

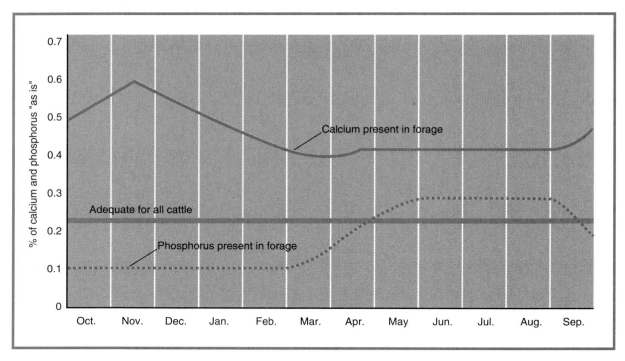

Figure 27-6. Calcium and phosphorus availability varies greatly during the seasons of the year and should be supplemented if inadequate amounts are present in livestock forage sources.

SALT USE IN CATTLE

Rule 1: Supply
   3–5 lb   Spring and summer/month
   1–1.5 lb   Fall and winter/month

Rule 2: Availability
   Make salt available at all times

Rule 3: Rotation
   Continue to rotate salt
   Manger throughout pasture

---

of these vitamins or the production practices merit their inclusion (see Table 27–12).

SHEEP

Feeding represents the single largest cost of production for all types of sheep operations. Sheep producers control their revenue by offering feeds that support optimum production, are cost-effective, and minimize nutritionally related problems. Sheep production is divided into two principal areas: the breeding flock and lamb production.

Breeding Flock

Ewes are the foundation of the sheep operation; they produce lambs and generate wool. These two cash crops can be influenced greatly by feeding management. The mature ewe (3 to 8 years of age) needs only sufficient feed to maintain her normal weight from the time her lambs were weaned until 15 weeks

(21-week gestation) into her next pregnancy, assuming not much weight was lost during lactation. Pasture is adequate to meet her nutrient needs during this period of production (see Figs. 27–1 and 27–6 for reviews of nutrient composition of pasture).

Energy

The energy requirements of the ewe are largely dependent on the stage of the reproductive cycle. During the first two thirds of the pregnancy, energy requirements are close to those required for MNR and good pasture or hays can supply all the energy needs (Table 27–14). In the last trimester, energy requirements increase, and forages must be supplemented with grains. Poor care during the last trimester of pregnancy leads to lambing problems, lower wool output, and depressed milk production. A common problem attributed to poor nutrition in ewes is lambing paralysis or ketosis. Feeding inadequate forages with little or no grain can create a deficiency of usable carbohydrates during the last trimester of pregnancy in ewes

---

COMMON SHEEP BREEDS

Wool Breeds	Meat Breeds	Combination Breeds
Rambouillet	Suffolk	Polypay
Merino	Dorset	Texel
Debouillet	Hampshire	Tunis
Columbia	Shropshire	Leicester
Targee	Southdown	Cheviot
	Oxford	

• Table 27–14 •

ADVANTAGES AND DISADVANTAGES OF PASTURE FEEDING LIVESTOCK

ADVANTAGES	DISADVANTAGES
• Provides exercise • Uses land unsuitable for other purposes • Decreases diseases transmitted through close contact with other animals • Decreases feed costs • Good quality pastures can provide quality feedstuffs	• Dependent on soil quality (deficiencies result in poorer quality pasture) • Large acreage often needed to support animal's energy requirements • Land may be made valuable for other uses

carrying twins or triplets and can lead to paralysis and coma in the mother (Fig. 27–7). Prevention is the least expensive route to avoid pregnancy disease in the breeding flock. Energy requirements are highest during lactation and proportional to the number of lambs the ewe is nursing.

TECHNICIAN NOTE

A common problem attributed to poor nutrition in ewes is lambing paralysis or ketosis.

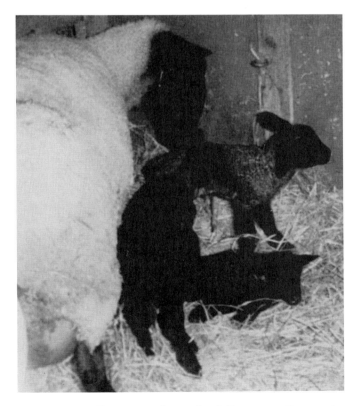

Figure 27–7. Energy requirements of the ewe will vary depending on the number of lambs she must nurse.

ENERGY INTAKE VARIABLES–SHEEP

Breed size	Age
Sex	Environment
Reproductive status	Stress
Weaning age	Shearing
Multiple birth	Forage quality

Protein

Adequate protein intake ensures good wool production and reproductive function. The most limiting amino acid for the maturation of wool is methionine; protein ingested by the breeding flock must contain adequate levels of this amino acid. Most pasture, silages, and forages contain adequate levels of protein and amino acids to meet the needs of the breeding flock. If low-grade roughages (e.g., cobs, straw, and stalks) are fed over extended periods of time, the ration must be supplemented daily with a protein supplement.

Minerals and Vitamins

Trace-mineral salt blocks and granular salt represent popular methods of offering minerals and salt to ewes on pasture. Sheep store copper quite well in various organs and tissues and develop toxicity symptoms to copper more rapidly than other

PROTEIN REQUIREMENTS–SHEEP

Variables
  Breed size
  Reproductive status
  Age
  Body condition
  Ratio of protein and energy
  Nonprotein nitrogen availability

NONPROTEIN NITROGEN USE IN SHEEP

Feeding guidelines
  Balance NPN within total nutritional profile
  Feed continuously after 3–6-week transition
  Avoid sporadic availability
  Nitrogen-to-sulfur ratio not more than 10:1
  Restrict use to not more than 1.0% dry matter, one third of total nitrogen ration as NPN
  Avoid excess intake and possible toxicity
  Watch NPN levels when coincided with high roughage intake

NPN, nonprotein nitrogen.
From Naylor JM, et al.: Large Animal Clinical Nutrition. St. Louis, Mosby–Year Book, 1991; McDonald P, et al.: Animal Nutrition. New York, Longman Scientific and Technical, 1995; Maynard LA, et al.: Animal Nutrition. 7th Ed. New York, McGraw-Hill, 1979; and Ensminger ME, et al.: Feeds and Nutrition. Clovis, CA. Ensminger Publishing, 1990.

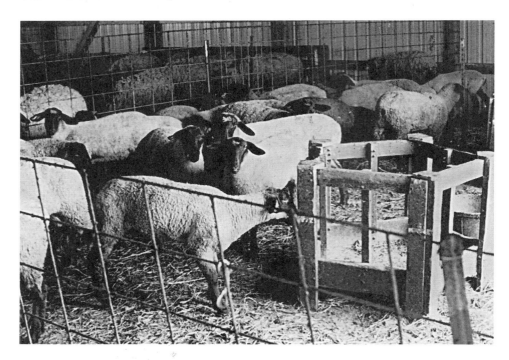

Figure 27-8. Optimal feed regimens in the grower-finisher lamb crop will provide excellent results.

livestock. Care should be taken to not expose sheep to high levels of copper in their trace-mineral source.

Good-quality pasture and roughages are adequate in vitamins A and E with ample levels to meet the needs of the breeding flock. Supplemental vitamin A should be provided when low-grade roughages or long-stored hays are used as a major source of energy in wintering rations.

Lambs

Lambs must be nursed with colostrum milk within the first hour after birth to improve survivability. Colostrum milk provides immunological protection and energy for the newborn lamb. The lamb must consume at least 6 to 8 oz of colostrum to receive immunological protection. Lambs are weaned successfully at eight weeks of age or earlier.

TECHNICIAN NOTE

Lambs must receive colostrum within the first hour after birth to receive immunological protection.

Lambs also can be successfully weaned from their mother at 1 day of age and offered a milk replacer (see Table 27–15). They should be weaned from the milk replacer at 3 to 4 weeks of age and transitioned to a high-quality, palatable solid feed. Postweaning rations (until lambs reach 50 lb) should be high-quality protein (16% to 20% crude protein), high energy, and well fortified with vitamins and minerals (Fig. 27–8).

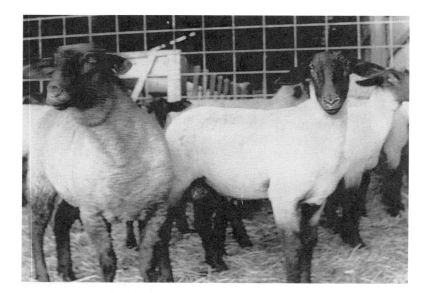

Figure 27-9. Growing-finishing lambs.

• Table 27–15 •

MILK REPLACEMENT: LAMBS

Optimal Requirement

25% to 30% fat
20% to 25% protein derived from milk product
<30% lactose derived from milk product

Feeding

Provide ration immediately
Ration should be 20% to 24% protein, high in vitamins and
    minerals, well-balanced and ground fine
Note: Avoid cow's milk (too high in lactose)

From Naylor JM, et al.: Large Animal Clinical Nutrition. St. Louis, Mosby–Year
Book, 1991; McDonald P, et al.: Animal Nutrition. New York, Longman Scientific
and Technical, 1995; Maynard LA, et al.: Animal Nutrition. 7th Ed. New York,
McGraw-Hill, 1979; and Ensminger ME, et al.: Feeds and Nutrition. Clovis, CA,
Ensminger Publishing, 1990.

Grower (50 to 85 lb) and finisher rations (more than 85 lb) for lambs are normally formulated to contain 15% to 16% and 13% to 14% protein, respectively. A simple ration of shelled corn, long alfalfa hay, and supplement (protein, calcium, vitamins, and trace minerals) can be fed to growing-finishing lambs (Fig. 27–9). Research does not clearly indicate the need for vitamin additions to rations for early lambs, but it has become a common practice to fortify the rations with vitamins A, D, and E (Table 27–16).

Large, fast-growing lambs are susceptible to overeating disease (enterotoxemia), which can cause death. This disease is caused by toxins produced by *Clostridium perfringens* and appears to be related to overeating by lambs of a ration high in grain (see Chapter 22). A vaccination with bacterin or toxoid can be used for lambs over 2 months of age and will virtually eliminate symptoms of overeating disease.

SWINE

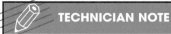

TECHNICIAN NOTE

Feed constitutes 60% to 70% of the cost of raising swine.

The swine industry has changed dramatically over the past 20 years. Most pigs are raised in confinement to reduce labor requirements for the owner and to improve the environment for the animal (Fig. 27–10). The genetic base of the swine industry has changed to a more prolific breeding herd and

• Table 27–16 •

DAILY NUTRITIONAL CONSIDERATIONS IN SHEEP

WEIGHT (lb)	ME (Kcal)*	DAILY CONSUMPTION (AS FED) (lb/day)	TOTAL CRUDE PROTEIN (lb/day)	MINERALS (G) Ca²⁺	P	VITAMINS A	E (IU)
Weaned Lambs to Finishing							
20–40	1.3–2.6	1.2–2.9	0.35–0.45	4.9–6.5	2.2–2.9	470	12
41–60	2.6–3.2	2.9–3.4	0.45–0.48	6.5–7.2	2.9–3.4	950	24
61–80	3.2–3.8	3.4–3.7	0.48–0.51	7.2–8.6	3.4–4.3	1400	21
81–100	3.8–4.0	3.7–4.1	0.51–0.53	8.6–9.4	4.3–4.8	2300	25
101–Finish	4.0–4.2	3.8–4.1	0.53	8.2–9.4	4.5–4.8	2800	25
Ewe Lambs							
Early							
80–100	2.9–3.0	3.4–3.7	0.35–0.36	5.2–5.5	2.7–2.8	3.0–3.1	21
101–120	3.0–3.1	3.7–3.9	0.35–0.36	5.2–5.5	2.8–3.0	3.1–3.4	22
121–140	3.1–3.2	3.7–3.9	0.35–0.36	5.5	3.0–3.3	3.4–3.7	24
141–160	3.1–3.3	3.9–4.1	0.35–0.36	5.5	3.3–3.4	3.4–3.7	26
Late							
80–101	5.0–5.4	3.7–3.9	0.41–0.44	6.4–7.8	5.0–5.4	3.1–3.9	22
101–120	5.4–5.8	3.0–4.1	0.44–0.45	7.8–8.1	5.4–5.8	3.9–4.3	24
121–140	5.8–6.2	4.1–4.4	0.45–0.48	8.1–8.2	5.8–6.2	4.3–4.7	26
141–160	6.2–6.3	4.4–4.7	0.46–0.48	8.1–8.2	6.2–6.3	4.3–4.7	27
Lactation						×1000 IU	
80–100	2.9–3.0	5.1–5.7	0.67–0.71	8.4–8.7	5.6–6.0	32	
101–120	3.0–3.1	5.7–6.1	0.71–0.74	8.7–9.0	6.0–6.4	34	
121–140	3.1–3.2	6.1–6.7	0.74–0.77	9.0–9.3	6.4–6.9	38	
Ewes: maintenance to early/mid							
110–130	2.4–2.6	2.4–2.9	0.21–0.27	2.0–3.2	1.8–2.5	21–25	18–20
131–150	2.6–2.7	2.5–3.1	0.27–0.29	2.5–3.5	2.4–2.9	25–32	20–21
151–170	2.7–2.9	2.9–3.7	0.29–0.31	2.8–3.8	2.4–3.3	32–36	21–22
171–190	2.9–3.1	3.0–3.9	0.31–0.33	2.9–3.9	2.8–3.4	36–40	22–24
Ewes late gestation last 30 days/lactation							
100–130	4.0–6.0	4.1–5.9	0.43–0.45	5.6–6.9	4.8–5.2	21–25	24–27
131–150	4.2–6.6	4.4–6.1	0.45–0.47	6.9–9.1	5.2–6.6	25–32	26–28
151–170	4.4–7.0	4.7–6.3	0.47–0.49	7.6–9.5	6.6–7.4	32–36	28–30
171–190	4.7–7.5	4.9–6.6	0.49–0.51	8.5–9.6	6.8–7.8	36–40	30–33

*ME, metabolizable energy is measured in megacalories (Mcal), which is equal to 1000 kilocalories.

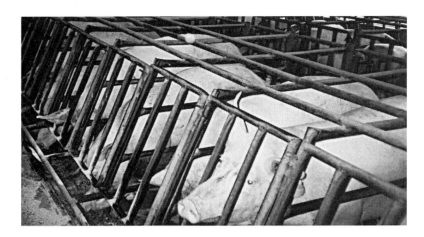

Figure 27-10. Sows are commonly kept in a farrowing containment pen to prevent injury to the piglets and ensure ready access to milk by the piglets.

better-muscled, faster-growing offspring. Feed still constitutes 60% to 70% of the cost of raising swine. Few swine are grazed on pasture; most are fed complete high-grain rations in self-feeders or are limit-fed if in the breeding herd. The production of pigs normally is divided into three distinct areas: the breeding herd, starter pigs, and growing-finishing pigs.

Breeding Herd

For profitable production of swine, the sows must be bred, gestate 114 days, nurse a litter for 21 to 35 days, rebreed within 10 days after weaning, and continue the cycle for 5 to 7 litters. Nutrition plays a key role in allowing this to occur, especially during lactation (Table 27–17).

Energy

After breeding and for the first two thirds of gestation, energy intake is limited to 6000 to 7000 kcal ME (metabolizable energy) per day. The total amount of feed is increased during the last third of gestation, providing 9000 to 10,000 kcal ME per day, which contributes additional energy to the developing fetuses during this last stage of gestation. Overfeeding energy during gestation has a direct negative impact on lactation feed intake, which can impair lactation performance.

In lactation, the goal of the swine producer is to encourage as much energy intake by the lactating female as possible (15,000 to 20,000 kcal ME per day). Sows are often fed twice per day to ensure fresh feed and improved energy intakes. Frequently, fat is added to the lactation ration to improve palatability and energy density. Sows peak in milk production between the second and third weeks of lactation, and they should be full-fed to support the production of milk. A rule of thumb for feeding lactating sows is to offer 4 to 5 lb of the base ration plus 1 additional pound for every pig nursing (Fig. 27–11).

> **TECHNICIAN NOTE**
>
> Sows are often fed twice daily to ensure adequate energy intake.

Protein

The protein requirements during gestation are relatively low (11% to 12% crude protein; .5 lb of protein per day). The development of the fetuses and reproductive tissue requires small amounts of protein each day.

During lactation, sows require higher levels of protein intake to support milk production (2 to 3 lb of protein per day), which is accomplished by feeding a ration with a higher protein

• Table 27–17 •

	COMPLETE FEED RATION CONSIDERATIONS IN SWINE		
STAGE WEIGHT	**PROTEIN (%)**	**COMPLETE RATION FED (lb)**	**COMMENTS**
Weanling pigs			
12–20 lb	20–24	Free feed	Use if weaned early and transitioning to solid feed
Starter pigs			
Up to 40 lb	18–20	Free feed	
Feeder/finisher pigs			
40 lb to 220–250 lb finishing weight	13–18	Free feed*	May be limited in feed after 125 lb
Gilts and sows			
Breeding/maintenance	12–16	4–6	Increase amount to maintain body condition and last
Gestation	12–16	4–6	month of gestation through weaning
Lactation	12–16	4–6	
Boars	12–16	4–7	Increase in breeding season

*See text on feeding methods.

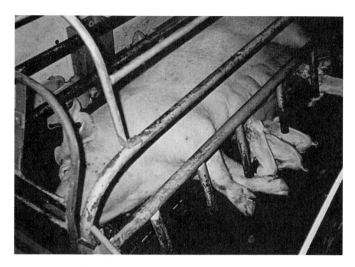

Figure 27-11. Sow nursing piglets in containment of pen.

content at a greater intake level. Sows not fed adequate levels of protein or energy during lactation will support milk production with loss of body tissue stores. Sows can lose more than 100 lb in weight during lactation if not fed proper amounts of energy or protein.

Minerals and Vitamins

Minerals and vitamins need to be supplemented throughout the life of pigs. The breeding herd is normally fed diets fortified with the minerals calcium, phosphorus, salt, zinc, iron, copper, iodine, selenium, and manganese. Calcium and phosphorus are kept in a balance of 1:1 to 2:1 for all stages of production. Low levels of calcium and phosphorus in the breeding herd rations can lead to fractures and lameness in the female.

Sow's milk is virtually devoid of iron, and anemia of nursing pigs will occur unless they are supplemented with another source of iron. The two most common ways to supply addition iron are (1) an injection of iron (150 to 200 mg) as iron dextran or other iron-carbohydrate complexes at 3 days of age and (2) an oral iron solution dosed at 3 days of age or swabbed onto the dam's udder several times during lactation.

The vitamins supplemented in breeding herd diets are the fat-soluble vitamins A, D, E, and K and the water-soluble vitamins thiamine, riboflavin, niacin, pantothenic acid, B_6, B_{12}, choline, biotin, and folic acid. Adequate additions of these vitamins ensure proper development of the fetus in gestation and milk production in lactation (Table 27–18).

TECHNICIAN NOTE

Sow's milk is devoid of iron, and nursing pigs will develop anemia unless they are supplemented with iron.

Starter Pigs

Pigs are commonly weaned at 3 to 5 weeks of age and remain in the starter phase until they weigh 40 to 50 lb (Fig. 27–12). The earlier the age at weaning, the more complex is the ration required to help in the transition from mother's milk to solid food. Starter diets (20% to 24% protein) are very complex and nutrient-dense complete feeds and therefore often purchased from a commercial feed manufacturer. The highest-quality ingredients are used to make starter diets and include milk products, fish meal, spray-dried blood products, oats, corn, and fat. Vitamin and mineral supplementation levels are high in starter diets. These feeds typically are pelleted and quite costly (see Table 27–17).

As the pig ages, the complexity and nutrient density of the starter ration decrease, leading to a lower-cost formula. In the last 2 or 3 weeks of the starter period, crude protein decreases to 18% to 20%, and the diet is often offered as a ground feed.

Growing-Finishing Pigs

Growing-finishing diets have been modified to complement the changes in the genetic base of modern swine. The leaner pigs require higher levels of protein and consume less energy than previous generations (Table 27–17).

Energy

Complete grower-finisher rations are based on cereal grains and frequently have fat added to increase caloric intake. Fibrous feed ingredients often are not used or are used sparingly to prevent depressions in caloric intake. Corn, wheat, sorghum, and barley are the more popular cereal grains used to supply energy and comprise 60% to 85% of the ration.

Protein

Contemporary swine nutrition does not concentrate on the protein content of feeds but on the amino acid levels. Lysine

---

IRON-DEFICIENCY ANEMIA IN SWINE

Prevention in baby pigs

Allow access to soil that has not been in contact with other pigs

Inject 100–200 mg iron before 72 hours of age

Paint sows teats lightly with iron solution periodically

Encourage prestarter ration creep feeding early

Provide iron supplementation in creep feeder

• Table 27–18 •

ORPHAN PIGLET FEEDING

Homemade Replacer
  32 oz whole cow's milk
  Water-soluble antibiotics
  1 raw egg
  16 oz half-and-half

Directions for Feeding Piglets
  Give 2 oz per feeding per piglet
  Every 3 hours
  Feed in a shallow, clean feeding pan
  Be sure that all piglets are eating
  Give iron supplementation as needed
  Start creep feeding at 7 days of age

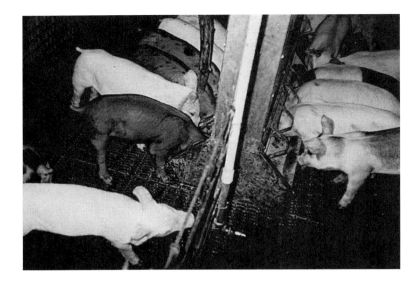

Figure 27-12. Grower-finisher pigs are fed large quantities of complete rations to obtain the most desirable carcass quality. Bottom left, pig is using an automatic watering system to fulfill water requirements at will.

typically is the first limiting amino acid in swine formulas. Amino acid levels decrease as a percentage of the diet throughout the growing-finishing phase.

Amino acid levels are matched to muscle growth throughout the growth period to maximize lean tissue growth. Underfeeding of amino acids depresses muscle deposition, and overfeeding amino acids leads to excess, which is costly.

Typical protein sources in growing-finishing diets are soybean meal, meat and bone meal, and synthetic amino acids. When protein sources are expensive, synthetic amino acids can replace a portion to the protein source with no loss in performance. The most commonly available synthetic amino acids are lysine, methionine, threonine, and tryptophan.

Minerals and Vitamins

Growing-finishing swine are fed diets fortified with the minerals calcium, phosphorus, salt, zinc, iron, copper, iodine, selenium, and manganese. Calcium and phosphorus are kept in a balance of 1:1 to 2:1 throughout this period. Deficiencies of phosphorus will depress growth performance as the animal grows.

Riboflavin, niacin, pantothenic acid, and vitamin B_{12} are the water-soluble vitamins most likely to be deficient in swine diets formulated with grains and plant protein. The fat-soluble vitamins A, D, E, and K also should be added to growing-finishing rations.

References

Church DC: Livestock Feeds and Feeding. Corvallis, OR, O and B Books, 1984, pp. 19–31, 89–93, 189–234.

Cunha TJ: Swine Feeding And Nutrition. New York, Academic Press, 1977, pp. 201–208.

Haresign DJ: Recent Developments of Pig Nutrition. London, Butterworth, 1985, pp. 368–386.

Jones DH, Wlson AD: Nutritive quality of forage. In Hacker ED: The Nutrition of Herbivores. Sydney, Australia, Academic Press, 1982, pp. 106–119.

Nash MJ: Crop Conservation and Storage. Oxford, Pergamon Press, 1985, pp. 85–101.

Naylor JM, Ralston SL: Large Animal Clinical Nutrition. St. Louis, MO, Mosby, 1991, pp. 21–42, 460–468, 267–274.

Additional Reading

Ensminger ME: Swine Science. Interstate Printers and Publishing, Danville, IL, 1990, pp. 416–441, 506–534.

Garmsworthy PC: Nutrition and Lactation in the Dairy Cow. University Press, London, 1988, pp. 246–254.

Kruesi WK: Sheep Raiser's Manual. Charlotte, VT, Williamson Publishing Co., 1985, pp. 23–26, 67–72, 90–111.

Linciciome DR: Sheep: Applied and Basic Research Information. Scottsdale, AZ, International Goat and Sheep Research, 1983, pp. 85–99.

Lloyd LE, Crampton EW, et al.: Fundementals of Nutrition. 3rd Ed. San Francisco, CA, WH Freeman and Sons, 1978, pp. 456–501.

Machlin LJ: Handbook of Vitamins. New York, Marcel Dekker, 1984, pp. 29–54.

Maynard LA, et al.: Animal Nutrition. 7th Ed. New York, McGraw-Hill 1979.

McDonald P, et al.: Animal Nutrition. 7th Ed. New York, Longman Scientific and Technical Publishing, 1995, pp. 91–134.

Menzies CS: United States Sheep and Goat Industry. Ames, IA, CAST Report, 1982, pp. 12–31.

Milk Facts. Washington, DC, Milk Industry Foundation

National Research Council: Nutrient Requirements for Beef Cattle. 8th Ed. Washington, DC, National Academic Press, 1990, pp. 12–45.

National Research Council: Nutrient Requirements for Dairy Cattle. 7th Ed. Washington, DC, National Academy Press, 1990, pp. 65–73.

National Research Council: Nutrient Requirements for Sheep. 6th Ed. Washington, DC, National Academy Press, 1988, pp. 45–60.

National Research Council: Nutrient Requirements for Swine. 6th Ed. Washington, DC, National Academic Press, 1989, pp. 78–98.

Neumann AL: Beef Cattle. New York, John Wiley and Sons, 1977, pp. 187–221.

Pond WG: Swine Production and Nutrition. Westport, CT, AVI Publishing, 1984, pp. 91–96.

Shirley RL: Nitrogen and Energy Nutrition of Ruminants. Orlando, FL, Academic Press, 1986, pp. 54–79.

Taylor RE: Beef Production and the Beef Industry. Minneapolis, MN, Burgess Publishing Co., 1984, pp. 389–404.

Tribble LG, Stansbury WF: Swine Report. Texas Technical University, Dallas, 1985.

Webster J: Calf Husbandry: Health and Welfare. London, Collins, 1984, pp. 71–78.

28 Euthanasia

Joseph Taboada

Old Dog

When the old dog had to die after long years full with love and honor,
When the weight of time grew wearying and she was content to have it finished,
I brought my old dog to our friend.
Old dog lay soft against me, old eyes already closed, waiting.
Our friend's hand was gentle on the weary body, with its ragged fur,
So gentle to find the frail small vein where death could enter.
DIFFICULT,
Old blood runs sluggish, old veins slackly resisting.
So patient, our friend, his knowing hands, all I can see through silent tears.
I watch capable strong hands lightly coaxing, and at last a small red flower blooms briefly in the crystal
*   before he eases the plunger in.*
Old dog only sighs very softly.
The weary heart slows and stops as the joyful spirit leaps free.
We wait a quiet minute, my tears dropping unheeded, into the soft fur.
Our friend withdraws, his gentle hands leaving old dog's cast-off body.
My head bowed over the weathered white mask for a moment before I let her lie by herself and draw the
*   blanket over her.*
I wish the old dog had made it easier for him.
To bring even a kindly death brings sadness.
He asked how many years she had, and I heard more than that in his voice.
I wish I could thank him for keeping zest in her years, for making a good end of them, for his capable
*   hands, for his gentle word, and caring heart.*
I took the old dog home, and laid her as if sleeping, wrapped in her worn blanket and sheltered deep in the
*   kindly silent earth.*

ANONYMOUS

Perhaps no single issue in veterinary medicine conjures up the range of emotion, ethical deliberation, and stress occasioned by euthanasia. There is a tremendous diversity of opinion and tolerance among veterinary professionals, both within the United States and abroad. Euthanasia was defined by the 1986 American Veterinary Medical Association (AVMA) Panel on Euthanasia as "the act of inducing painless death," but "the act" is only one small aspect of the larger issue facing the profession.

The word euthanasia is derived from the Greek root *Eu,* meaning good, and *thanatos,* referring to death. Few in the veterinary profession would argue that when used in the context of relieving suffering, the word runs counter to its Greek roots; however, as the word is currently defined, it also pertains to the killing of unwanted, abandoned, stray, or phenotypically undesired animals by the veterinary professionals with problems in balancing conflicting interests. It is not always in the common interest of the patient, client, and veterinarian that euthanasia is performed. Euthanasia is an emotionally charged issue, with members of the profession varying significantly in their acceptance of the practice and in their views as to its utility. On one hand, it might be viewed simply as "convenience killing," whereas on the other, it might be viewed as a means of furthering respect and love through the compassionate termination of hopeless suffering. No matter how one looks at it, the animal health professional may be caught in the middle, experiencing doubts, confusion, and moral questions over participation in the ending of an animal's life. It is an ethical dilemma that does not have an easy or even an absolutely right or wrong answer. It is an issue that all of us must wrestle with, individually and collectively.

TECHNICIAN NOTE

Euthanasia is an issue that all of us must wrestle with, individually and collectively.

THE DECISION

The decision to perform euthanasia is one of the most difficult decisions that the owner of a companion animal will ever have to face. Some owners may make the decision quickly because of financial constraints or fear of what the illness may eventually cause, others may never be able to make the decision, preferring to let their pet die naturally. The decision is often made more difficult by the fact that few pet owners have an adequate support group available that understands the bond that develops between an animal and the recipient of its unconditional love.

Most owners who elect to have euthanasia performed make the decision because they perceive that their pet's illness involves some degree of suffering. Suffering is difficult to define, and perceptions of animal suffering differ markedly between individuals and from case to case. The place the pet holds in the owner's family circle, how long the pet has been owned, the relationship between the pet and other loved ones, the financial resources available to the owner, and the disease process afflicting the pet are other factors that most owners take into consideration when trying to make the decision.

The veterinary team (veterinarian, veterinary technician, and animal health care providers) can play an important role in the decision-making process. The veterinary staff often serves as a sounding board for the client who is trying to make the decision. We can help with the decision by approaching the subject professionally with compassion and respect. The most important help that the team can give is the providing of information. What the owner can expect from the disease process, what treatments are available, the prognosis with and without treatment, and what costs are involved are all questions that should be answered by the veterinarian. The veterinary technician can play a vital role as a client resource by answering questions about euthanasia. How euthanasia is performed, whether the animal will feel pain, how long the procedure will take, and what happens to the body afterward are all areas that a technician may be asked to address.

TECHNICIAN NOTE

We as veterinary professionals can help clients with euthanasia decisions by approaching the subject professionally with compassion and respect.

When interacting with an owner considering euthanasia, the veterinary professional should go to great lengths to lay out all the options available while being careful not to make the decision for the client. Too many veterinary professionals make judgments as to the "value" of an animal (both monetary and personal) that only the owner can make. Questions such as "What would you do if he were your animal?" are difficult to address and perhaps best answered by urging the client to verbalize what he or she sees as the pros and cons of each choice. In doing this, it may become obvious that the client has already made the decision and is looking for support or validation. The client may feel guilt, anger, sadness, depression, pain, and helplessness during the decision-making process and after euthanasia has been performed (see Chapter 29). The veterinary professional can help by assuring the owner that these feelings are normal, and indeed expected, and by assuring the client that he is not alone in the pain that he is feeling.

Once an informed decision has been made, it should be supported, even if it may not have been the decision that the veterinarian or veterinary staff would have made. Pet owners are sensitive to the actions of hospital personnel, and for this reason it is extremely important that persons interacting with the client or handling the animal in the presence of the owner be supportive, gentle, and empathetic.

AS THE END DRAWS NEAR: THE BEGINNING OF THE END

The death of a pet can be a devastating experience that can drastically affect the relationship between client and veterinarian. As many as 40% of clients change veterinarians after a pet has died. This number probably approaches 100% if euthanasia is handled in a manner that causes the client to perceive a lack of care, concern, or respect on the part of the veterinarian or other staff members. On the other hand, much can be done to foster a long-lasting relationship through the professional and compassionate handling of a euthanasia. It is often true that the client who loudly sings the praises of a veterinarian and his staff is not the owner of an animal saved through long hours of hard work and outstanding medical care but rather the owner who was treated with compassion, care, and concern at and around the time of the loss of a pet.

TECHNICIAN NOTE

Many clients change veterinarians after the death of a pet, especially if euthanasia is handled without the utmost of care and respect.

Preparations for pet loss should begin as soon as it becomes apparent that death is a possibility. The veterinarian will often discuss euthanasia with a client early so that he understands that it is an available option. However, it is important to discuss all of the other medical or surgical options first. Euthanasia should not be presented in such a manner that it is either completely discounted or viewed as the only reasonable course. Remember that the initial reaction of a client receiving bad news is often denial or feelings of numbness or shock. It is important to allow time for this initial reaction to fade and for the entire family to be given time to discuss the various options before allowing the client to make such a difficult and important decision.

While discussing options with the client, the veterinarian should use alternative jargon terms for euthanasia such as *put to sleep, put down, put away, humanely destroy, rock, shoot,* and so forth only when their meaning is understood by all individuals involved. Confusion will result from the use of a term such as *put to sleep* when talking to a companion animal owner who perceives the phrase to refer to anesthesia instead of euthanasia. Children are especially confused by the term *put to sleep* and may be afraid that they might die when going to sleep at night. Whatever term is used to describe the act of euthanasia, it is important that it be fully understood by all parties involved.

Once the decision has been made to have an animal undergo euthanasia, there are many choices that a client must make. When and where should the euthanasia take place? Should they or other family members be present during the euthanasia? What is to happen to the body after euthanasia? Should a necropsy examination be allowed? What special method, if any, will they use to memorialize the pet? It is best to discuss these concerns thoroughly in advance so that everyone understands precisely the wishes of the client.

The client, together with the veterinarian, should decide who will be present during the euthanasia. This is sometimes a difficult decision for both the client and the veterinarian. Some veterinarians do not offer this option to the client in the mistaken view that it will be too difficult for the client to watch. Contrary to this view, many clients will grieve more easily and accept more quickly the loss of their pet if they have had the opportunity to say good-bye in this most personal way (Fig. 28–1). The chance to hold their pet and let it know that it is loved dearly while sharing its last moments is sometimes an important first step in the grief process. However, with the benefits to the client can come problems for the veterinarian and his staff. The veterinary team must realize that having the client present can increase their own stress level associated with euthanasia, and every attempt should be made to understand and minimize its effects (see The Stress of Euthanasia in this chapter).

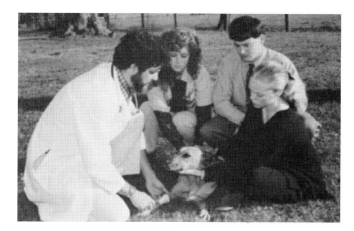

Figure 28–1. Being present during the euthanasia of the companion animal helps clients to say good-bye and complete the responsibilities of pet ownership. At times, clients will want to have euthanasia performed in a "special place," making the event more personal and meaningful.

interruptions are unlikely, the waiting room is empty, and the potential for embarrassment by public exposure is minimized. Early mornings, evenings, or during the lunch hour may be suitable. It is best to schedule at least 30 minutes. The most important aspect of the euthanasia to consider is communication. The unexpected should be avoided at all costs, and before the procedure, the client should be given a detailed explanation of exactly what is about to happen to the pet and what he is about to see. Then the client should be talked through each step of the procedure. The euthanasia should proceed at a pace with which the client feels comfortable. Occasionally pets will urinate, defecate, vocalize, twitch, or gasp after they have become unconscious. Although these reflex acts can be minimized, they will still occasionally occur and will have a far less negative effect if they are expected and if the client is told that they are not a reflection of pain or suffering.

> **TECHNICIAN NOTE**
>
> Communication is critical to a smooth euthanasia when owners are present.

Deciding where the euthanasia is to take place can be important. Using a hospital space that is less sterile than the typical stainless steel hospital examination room is preferred. If the examination room is to be used, at least a blanket should be placed over the table and there should be a chair where the client can sit down. Some clients will request that the euthanasia be performed at home or at some special place. Many veterinarians will honor these requests or use the services of a house call practice for this need. Sometimes just being outside the "normal" environment of the veterinarian facility is a fair and acceptable compromise. A blanket on the floor, the lawn beside the clinic, and even the back seat of the family car might serve this purpose. One important consideration for the veterinarian in choosing the place is that many clients will feel uncomfortable coming back into the room where a pet previously under-

> **TECHNICIAN NOTE**
>
> Many clients will go through the grief process more easily if they are present at the euthanasia.

When the client or family members are to be present, euthanasia should be scheduled for a time of the day when

went euthanasia. Indeed, many clients switch veterinarians because of a lack of sensitivity to this fact by the veterinary staff. To minimize this potential conflict in the future, it is best to choose a space that will not be routinely used for other client-related activities.

Clients who choose not to be present during euthanasia may still wish to see the body of the animal after it is dead. Seeing the animal dead conveys finality and also allows the client the opportunity to say good-bye. Many clients have a difficult time proceeding through the grief process if they have not been given this chance.

> **TECHNICIAN NOTE**
>
> Clients who choose not be present for a euthanasia often still wish to see the body afterward.

Make arrangements in advance concerning how payment for services is to occur. Discuss with the client whether payment is going to be made in advance, at the time of services, or is to be billed later. This can be an uncomfortable subject to broach after euthanasia has occurred.

AT THE END

All of the preparations having been made, the euthanasia should be performed with skill and concern. Each member of the veterinary team should be well trained, know his responsibilities, and be available. The key, as already mentioned, is to expect and plan for the unexpected. Although many methods of euthanasia are deemed acceptable by the AVMA panel on euthanasia, only those that are aesthetically acceptable should be used when the client is going to be present.

> **TECHNICIAN NOTE**
>
> Expect and plan for the unexpected.

If the examination room is to be used, the table should be covered with a cloth or blanket. Some owners will want to bring a favorite blanket for the pet to spend its last few moments on. It is important that they understand that it is possible, indeed likely, that the blanket will be soiled by feces or urine when euthanasia occurs. If the pet is likely to be aggressive or extremely apprehensive, tranquilizing it ahead of time should be considered. If the client is to be present, the animal should be taken away briefly so that a peripheral vein can be catheterized for smooth delivery of the euthanasia solution. It is advisable to put the catheter into a vein in a back leg; this will allow the client to hold the animal and pet its head without being in the way of the veterinarian while the injections are being given. Once the catheter has been placed, the client should be given the opportunity to be alone with their pet for a few moments.

Before administering the euthanasia solution, a saline solution should be injected into the catheter to ensure its patency.

Next, the patient should be anesthetized with an ultrashort-acting barbiturate. This will decrease the incidence of excitement after the euthanasia solution is injected. Once the animal is anesthetized, the euthanasia solution can be injected. Sodium pentobarbital is the most commonly used euthanasia solution. It is a member of the barbiturate family of drugs that depress the entire central nervous system.* When large doses of this drug are administered, as for euthanasia, unconsciousness occurs first, and then breathing stops due to depression of the respiratory center. This is followed by cardiac arrest. The pentobarbital dose, concentration, and rate of administration determine the speed of action. When the drug is administered intravenously, animals die swiftly and quietly. Although intravenous administration is preferred, the drug is also effective when injected intrahepatically and, to a lesser extent, into the peritoneal cavity. Death following intraperitoneal injection may take as long as 15 minutes, however, because of relatively slow absorption. Pentobarbital for euthanasia is available alone or in combination with other drugs. The concentration of pentobarbital in most euthanasia solutions is approximately 20% by weight. The recommended dose is 2 ml for the first 4.5 kg of body weight and 1 ml for each additional 4.5 kg of body weight. Sodium pentobarbital should be administered as rapidly as possible to provide the quietest and swiftest form of euthanasia. The veterinary team should be completely familiar with the use of the euthanasia solution chosen and the possible reactions that might be seen.

As the cerebral cortex is affected by general anesthetic, predominant emotions may take over and the animal may show fear behavior, which is usually characterized by struggling and vocalization. Experimental studies indicate that the animal is not conscious of these feelings at the time. People who have undergone the "excitement" phase during general anesthesia do not remember that it took place. Although trained individuals may understand this "excitement phase" from the clinical standpoint, it is difficult for the owner to understand that struggling and vocalization are not due to pain or discomfort. Thus, the owner's perception is that the animal is not experiencing a peaceful death. Clients who choose to be present should be warned that this phase may occur. The use of an ultrashort-acting barbiturate first will minimize the "excitement" phase.

THE END AS A BEGINNING. . . . AFTER THE END

A gentle touch,
barely audible she purrs,
good-bye, oh good-bye,
a final glimpse of life drifting away,
a lifeless stare;
. . . and then, I am alone.
                                   J. TABOADA

Many veterinary professionals are good at the technical aspects of euthanasia but fall short in supplying what the client needs

---

*Note that all barbiturates are strictly controlled by federal regulations, and accurate accounting of the use of these agents is required. The Drug Enforcement Agency (DEA) of the U.S. Department of Justice is responsible for enforcement of laws governing the user of barbiturates. Sodium pentobarbital is a Schedule II controlled substance and can be obtained only by a licensed medical practitioner, such as a physician, dentist, veterinarian, or approved institution. In addition to the DEA paperwork involved for procuring barbiturates like sodium pentobarbital, careful handling of the drug is necessary after the drug is on the hospital premises. Thorough record keeping is required by law.

after euthanasia has been performed. The animal's death is often only the beginning of a long and difficult odyssey that the client is about to face. Some clients will feel a great sense of relief immediately after the pet's death, but most will soon feel empty, numb, or alone. They may question whether they did the right thing. We can help them by again stressing that the pet's death was painless, assuring them that they did the right thing, and focusing on some of the positive things that the pet brought to their life. At the time of euthanasia, it is important that an environment be fostered that says, "It's all right to cry, it's all right to be emotional, it's all right to begin to grieve." Few of us have the gift of being able to say the right thing at the right time, so sometimes consolation can best be offered in a touch or an embrace. A touch on the arm or a simple embrace will often express best what the client needs to hear: "We care and you are not alone."

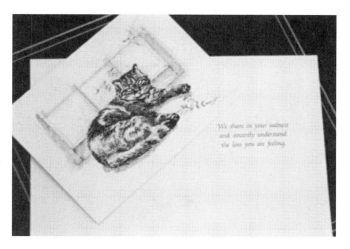

Figure 28-2. After a pet has died, a condolence card or letter from the veterinary practice is an appropriate symbol of support. Many clients will return to a practice that shows this type of caring gesture when they eventually invest in a new relationship with another pet.

> **TECHNICIAN NOTE**
>
> The pet's death is often only the beginning of a long and difficult odyssey.

Many clients, whether present for the euthanasia or not, need assurance that the animal is dead. Clients will feel more assured by the veterinarian who takes the time to listen to the animal's thorax with a stethoscope and shines a pen light into the animal's eyes before pronouncing the patient is dead. For those who choose not to be present, allowing them to view the animal's body can alleviate some of this fear. Before bringing the body to the client, it should be made as presentable as possible. It must always be treated with dignity and respect. Clean any blood from the fur, remove any catheters or bandages, place the tongue in the mouth, and close the eyes. Placing a drop of cyanoacrylate glue* in each eye will keep the eyelids closed. If time permits, bathe and brush the animal before laying it on a clean paper, blanket, or towel in a sturdy box. This will help to make the viewing as pleasant an experience as possible. If the animal's body is sealed in a box (commercially made boxes for home burial are available), let the client know how the body is wrapped and whether any signs of trauma or surgery are present. Even the client who assures the veterinarian that he will not open the box before burial or cremation often changes his mind after leaving the office.

> **TECHNICIAN NOTE**
>
> Always treat the pet's body with dignity and respect.

Having the client bring someone who will be able to drive him home will help him feel less alone and will also ensure a safe trip. It is nice to call clients after they have arrived home to check on them. Attempts should be made to call all clients who have lost a pet to answer any questions and to show

concern. The veterinarian or a staff member may call. The show of concern is always appreciated, helps the client who is having difficulty in dealing with grief, and assures the client that a relationship with the clinic fostered in life has not been ended by the death of their pet. Most clients will eventually choose to get another pet. A sympathy card or handwritten note is usually appreciated. Many beautiful sympathy cards designed for veterinary use are available (Fig. 28–2).

One of the biggest concerns of clients who have just lost a pet is disposition of the body. When possible, all arrangements should be made in advance. The veterinary staff should be prepared with information to assist the client in making these arrangements. Know the laws concerning burial in the practice area. Make available names and telephone numbers of places that offer cremation and pet cemetery burial. If the client chooses to have the veterinarian handle the remains, it is best not to lie to the client concerning the disposal of the animal's body.

> **TECHNICIAN NOTE**
>
> Memorializing the pet can be an important part of grieving for many clients.

Memorializing the pet is a step that many clients find comforting. It can be an important part of grieving for many clients. Offering the client a lock of hair and returning collars or leashes may facilitate these wishes. Having a memorial service, planting a special plant in memory of the pet, framing a photograph, keeping a lock of hair, writing a poem or special letter, offering a memorial scholarship at a veterinary school, or making a donation to organizations such as the American Veterinary Medical Association or a veterinary school foundation are actions that clients may use to memorialize their pet (Fig. 28–3).

---

*Krazy Glue, B. Jadow & Sons, Inc., New York, NY 10010.

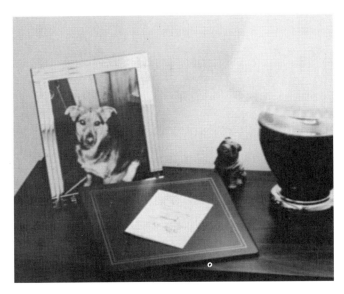

Figure 28-3. Memorializing a pet who has died can be an important part of grieving. A framed photo and a scrapbook are two effective ways to memorialize.

THE STRESS OF EUTHANASIA

Euthanasia is stressful not only to the client but also to the veterinarian and veterinary staff. Frequent performance of euthanasia is a primary cause of burnout within small animal practice (Table 28–1). It is at times even more stressful to the technical staff than it is to the veterinarian because they usually have little control over the situation. Euthanasias that go smoothly as well as "difficult" euthanasias will create stress. "Difficult" or inherently stressful euthanasias include euthanasia in which technical problems arise, instances in which the animal reacts badly to the injections in the presence of the client, and the euthanasia of one's own pet, healthy animals, young animals, and animals for whom one has put a great deal of time and medical effort into fighting their disease. Euthanasia with the client present usually creates more stress on the veterinary staff than when the procedure is performed in the absence of the owner.

Each individual will have to decide for himself in what type of euthanasia he is able to participate and what his tolerance is for euthanasia. A technician may not be able to work effectively in a practice in which the veterinarian's views on euthanasia

• Table 28–1 •

SIGNS AND SYMPTOMS OF BURNOUT	
PHYSICAL SYMPTOMS	**PSYCHOLOGICAL/ BEHAVIORAL SYMPTOMS**
Ulcers	Withdrawal
Gastroenteritis	Overeating
Cardiac arrhythmia	Constant fatigue
Heartburn	Increased alcohol intake
Backache	Agitation
Nausea	Distraction
Skin disorders	Aggressive behavior
	Insomnia

are vastly different from this own. Stress can become intense if these differences are not discussed and reconciled. Veterinarians differ markedly in their views on euthanasia. A survey of British veterinarians revealed that 74% would perform euthanasia on a healthy animal if the owner requested it. A similar survey in Japan reveal that 63% would not. There is room within the veterinary profession for this divergence of views; indeed, the diversity of opinions is one of the profession's strengths.

 TECHNICIAN NOTE

Euthanasia is stressful to both the owner and the veterinary staff.

One of the most important mechanisms of coping with the stress brought on by euthanasia is discussion with colleagues. Having sessions for the hospital staff in which people can openly express their feelings is a good outlet for emotions that, if unexpressed, can cause further stress and lead to burnout. This type of communication allows members of the veterinary team to understand their colleagues' feelings and tolerances for different situations. Members of the team may need to temporarily pass responsibility for euthanasia to their colleagues when they have reached the limit of their tolerance. Other mechanisms of managing stress include taking time off, making time for self, adopting recreational habits, helping clients deal with their grief, and finding strength in relationships formed with colleagues that experience the same stresses. Dark humor is often used to relieve stress. Such humor reduces tension by acknowledging death as part of the setting, but also minimizing, for the moment, its tragedy and finality. In animal shelters or practices in which large numbers of euthanasias are performed, veterinary staff often cope by shifting moral responsibility for killing animals away from themselves to the owners. Care must be taken not to develop an attitude that will be detrimental to the client-veterinarian relationship. (Additional information concerning stress management may be found in Chapter 33.)

TECHNICIAN NOTE

Open discussion of issues surrounding euthanasia can help a hospital's staff deal with the stress.

EUTHANASIA OF LARGE ANIMALS

Euthanasia of large domestic animals presents specific hazards and problems not encountered in companion small animals. Safety must be a major consideration. The jugular vein should be used for injection whenever possible because this will place the person injecting the euthanasia solution in the safest position. On rare occasions, the jugular veins may be thrombosed from disease, and the cephalic vein must be used. However, this puts the individual under the animal's forequarters and in a dangerous position.

Euthanasia-strength pentobarbital can be administered with a large-gauge needle (16 to 14 gauge). The volume of solution is large, and even with a large-gauge needle, the time it takes to inject the solution is relatively long. The animal may go through the same "excitement" phase as that experienced by small animals, and it may come crashing to the ground on becoming unconscious. Generally, large-animal euthanasia should be performed in an area with vehicle access to allow removal of the body. In some instances, the client may wish to bury a large animal. It should be remembered that all of the same emotional concerns encountered in small-animal euthanasia pertain to large animals when a bond has formed between the owner and the animal.

CONCLUSION

Euthanasia is a skill that, like any other skill, must be well thought out and practiced. The entire veterinary team should be involved in a well-coordinated and professional manner. Euthanasia, if performed poorly, can be a disastrous experience for both the client and the veterinary practice. If performed with practiced care and gentle concern, it can be remembered positively for a long time.

Recommended Readings

Arluke A: Coping with euthanasia: A case study of shelter culture. J Am Vet Med Assoc 198:1176–1180, 1991.

AVMA Council on Research: Council Report: Report of the AVMA panel on euthanasia. J Am Vet Med Assoc 188:253–268, 1986.

Fogle B and Abrahamson D: Pet loss: Attitudes and feelings of practicing veterinarians. Anthrozoos 3:143–150, 1990.

Grier RL and Schaffer CB: Evaluation of intraperitoneal and intrahepatic administration of a euthanasia agent in animal shelter cats. J Am Vet Med Assoc 197:1611–1615, 1990.

Hart LA, Hart BL, and Mader B: Humane euthanasia and companion animal death: Caring for the animal, the client, and the veterinarian. J Am Vet Med Assoc 197:1292–1299, 1990.

Kay WJ: Euthanasia. Trends 1 (5):52–54, 1985.

Kogure N and Yamazaki K: Attitudes to animal euthanasia in Japan: A brief review of cultural influences. Anthrozoos 3:151–154, 1990.

Peters TG: Commander. JAMA 260:1460, 1988.

Randolph JW: Learning from your own pet's euthanasia. J Am Vet Med Assoc 205:544–545, 1994.

Tannenbaum J: Veterinary Ethics. Baltimore, Williams & Wilkins Co. 1989, pp 208–236.

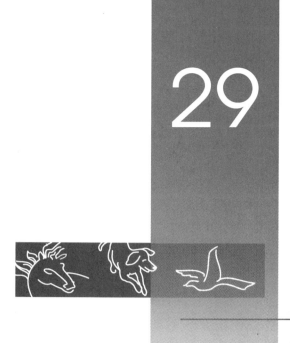

29 Client Bereavement and the Grief Process

*Joseph Taboada • Stephanie W. Johnson •
Sandra S. Brackenridge*

Domestic animals have lived in association with humans for thousands of years. The dog was probably the first animal to be domesticated, a process that probably began at least 15,000 years ago. The domestication of the cat may have begun as early as 7000 BC. Initially these animals were tools used for hunting, hauling, and protection, but over time they have assumed a variety of other roles, not the least of which is companionship.

Today, with more than 58 million families owning one or more companion animals,* pets are considered part of the "extended family network." Surveys and clinical experience indicate that many people consider their pets to be like children, partners, or best friends. Family structures have evolved from traditional nuclear families to single-parent, step-parent, never-married, and widowed elderly families. Due to changing family structure and an increasing number of people who live alone, companion animals have taken on larger roles in people's support systems. With these changes have come added expectations of veterinary health care professionals. Members of the veterinary medical profession must realize that they are not treating just dogs, cats, birds, rabbits, or horses but important members of their clients' family and an important part of their clients' support system (Fig. 29–1).

THE HUMAN–COMPANION ANIMAL BOND

During the twentieth century, society has evolved at a remarkable rate. As a result of the industrial revolution and technological advances, modern society is largely urban rather than rural;

thus the need for companion animals as hunters and herders has decreased. Millions of Americans restrict themselves and their animals to urban life styles. Animals live indoors in apartments or houses with their owners, increasing familiarity, dependency, and bonding.

TECHNICIAN NOTE

Many people consider their pets to be like children.

Society is also more mobile than ever before. It is not unusual for people to change locales and residences several times within a 10-year period. Additionally, the family itself is radically different from the nuclear family of the past. No longer do most Americans live within a short distance of their extended families, and the nuclear family is smaller, consisting of an average of less than two children per family. More than half of American couples divorce, and the single-parent family is becoming common. Because 64% of U.S. women work outside the home, many school-age children return home to be greeted not by their mother but by the family pet. Companion animals provide both parents and children with stability, constancy, and security in a twentieth century littered with losses and personal adjustments.

An increasing number of adults live alone and couples opt to remain childless. Many of these people fill the void with pets, who provide a unique outlet for their owners' needs to nurture and be loved. As health and medical care improves, the

*1996 APPMA National Pet Owners Survey.

723

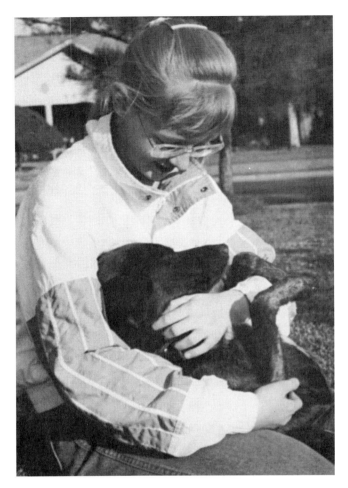

Figure 29-1. Pets have become important members of the "extended family network." They provide tactile contact that can be important for young and old alike.

number of people in the age group above 60 has increased—nearing 25% of the population. Pets fulfill many needs for the elderly, including needs for interaction, exercise, companionship, protection, and motivation to remain active and independent.

Recently, special populations have benefited from contact with animals. As society has realized the special talents of pets, we have found new utilitarian functions for them. Dogs are used with success to assist the blind, hearing impaired, and physically challenged. These specially trained animals provide their owners with independence, companionship, social lubrication, protection, and love. Both cats and dogs have been used successfully in animal-assisted therapy programs for people with all types of physical and mental disabilities. Animals facilitate interaction with people who may be reluctant to interact, and their presence reduces anxiety, lowers blood pressure, and decreases heart rate. Results of some studies indicate that animals may alleviate and/or prevent depression. Survival rates for cardiac patients who are pet owners are higher than for those who do not own pets. In fact, pet ownership is considered an important predictor of survival for patients with coronary artery disease.

In short, the relationships between people and animals

have become physically closer, and the role of animals in the daily lives of their owners has become more emotional and less utilitarian as society has changed. Of the more than 58 million families owning at least one pet, 87% describe their pets as "family members" and cite companionship, love, and friendship as the most important derivatives of the relationship.

TECHNICIAN NOTE

Animals facilitate interaction, reduce anxiety, lower blood pressure, and reduce stress.

The Attachment Between Animals and Humans

The attachment between animals and people is based on such factors as the frequency of contact, pleasant emotional states produced during these contacts, and pleasing behaviors, facial expressions, and body postures displayed during interactions. Pets can generate a sense of well-being and of being wanted, needed, and unconditionally loved and can provide warm, soft, tactile contact (see Fig. 29–1). They can also help people to feel happy by greeting them in familiar and endearing ways.

Strong attachments can form between owners and any type of animal but are probably recognized most commonly in veterinary practice with dogs, cats, and horses. The degree of attachment varies greatly from the utilitarian attachment between a rancher and his or her cattle to the parent/child–type bonding that occurs between some people and their dog or cat. During the nineties the cat has supplanted the dog (58 million) as the most popular pet in the United States, with more than 66 million being owned.* It has recently been estimated that about 50% of these cat owners classify their attachment to their pet as "strong." Of these "strong attachment" owners, about half see their cat(s) as reflections of themselves or of their tastes that are dependent on the owner for love, affection, and care. The other half of the "strong attachment" owners report a reliance on their cat(s) as an emotional crutch, supplying unconditional love and affection and sometimes acting as a substitute for family, friends, or children.

As pets are used to meet many of the changing psychosocial needs of modern society, the intensity of attachment has increased. When pet loss occurs, intensity and duration of attachment are determinants of the significance of the loss and intensity of grief that follows. Attachment is more intense when the animal has functioned in many roles for the owner. The owner of an assistance dog may therefore suffer more intense bereavement than the owner of a dog used only for herding or hunting. Owners who have experienced previous significant losses, adjustments, or traumas and have been comforted by their pet's presence may also exhibit strong attachment and thus intense bereavement.

Benefits of Attachment

As reminders of both pleasant and traumatic events in people's lives, pets can take on symbolic meaning. If a pet is associated

*1996 APPMA National Pet Owners Survey.

with a particular friend, relative, or stage in life, the attachment to the pet can take on added significance. If the pet represents a tangible link to a person or relationship that is now gone due to death, divorce, or other loss, the pet's death may stimulate recurring grief for the lost loved one as well as for the animal itself. Even when the pet is simply another family member, grief can be intense. Grief is also very individual, and each family member may grieve in his or her own way.

TECHNICIAN NOTE

If a pet is associated with an important person or significant life stage or event, it can take on added significance.

Casey, an 8-year-old male Doberman, is brought into the clinic for lethargy and anorexia. After a work-up he is diagnosed as having Doberman cardiomyopathy. Even with appropriate treatment, the prognosis for a long lifetime is poor.

Casey is owned by a 72-year-old widow named Emily who lost her husband to cancer 5 years earlier. During her husband's fight against the disease, Casey was his constant companion. Emily can still vividly remember how Casey, as a young puppy, used to make her husband laugh by chewing on her shoes while always leaving her husband's alone.

Casey was brought to the veterinarian for what was perceived to be a minor problem, but a severe, life-threatening disease was diagnosed. Emily is likely to feel numb initially. The diagnosis is likely to be hard to accept. An important part of Emily's attachment to Casey comes from her relationship with her late husband. Casey represents a tangible link between Emily's life now and the many memories of her life with her husband. Not only is Casey's death going to be hard because of the loss of a faithful companion/family member, but it is also going to bring back many of the emotions that were associated with the death of her husband.

PET LOSS AND VETERINARY MEDICINE

Veterinarians and veterinary technicians are confronted daily with complex issues of attachment, loss, and grief in the course of their patients' illness and death. The diagnosis of life-threatening or terminal disease can be a difficult time for both the client and the veterinary professional (Fig. 29–2). Considering all the emotional and utilitarian aspects of the human–companion animal relationship in modern society, it is not surprising that the breaking of the bond due to the death of the pet is a significant event in the lives of many pet owners. The loss of the pet for many owners is made even more intense and personal in that the pet is often grieved by no one other than themselves. Daily routines are filled with reminders of activities once performed for or with the pet. The loss of a pet often means that a unique, irreplaceable member of the family is gone.

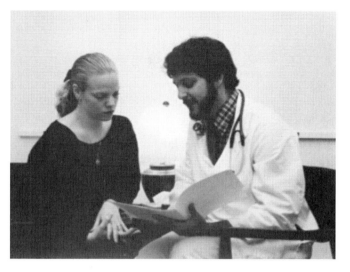
Figure 29–2. The diagnosis of a disease can be a difficult time for both clients and veterinary professionals.

TECHNICIAN NOTE

Veterinary technicians are confronted daily with complex issues of attachment, loss, and grief.

A person's support system is made up of people (and pets) that interact with one another on a day-to-day basis, providing support, comfort, and social interaction. Support systems are especially important during times of loss. Unfortunately, most people who make up these support systems do not understand the full extent of attachment between a pet owner and pet. This lack of understanding can present serious problems for the owner facing the odyssey of grief after the death of a pet.

Because of the general lack of social support from standard support systems for clients who have experienced pet loss and because of the caregiving role filled by veterinarians and veterinary technicians, pet owners often turn to veterinary professionals as sources of support, comfort, and understanding at and around the time of their pet's death. Veterinary professionals usually have a good understanding of attachment. Additionally, veterinary professionals are often looked on as an important part of the pet's life.

TECHNICIAN NOTE

People tend to turn to the veterinary staff during grief over a pet.

The tendency for people to turn to the veterinary staff during the period of grieving the death of a pet places veterinary professionals in an awkward position, however. It demands that they have knowledge that is typically outside the boundaries of traditional veterinary medicine and requires that they find a comfort level in talking about death and the grief process. This is why the areas of attachment, animal behavior, human bereavement, and grief counseling are becoming increasingly relevant to veterinary medicine.

In the sections of the chapter that follow, we describe the normal grief responses to pet loss and offer veterinary technicians and other veterinary professionals a framework from which they can develop a level of comfort with grief and support of the grieving pet owner. The goal is not to transform veterinary professionals into therapists but to give them an understanding of grief and the grief process that will be useful in the day-to-day practice of veterinary client relations. It is best to remember that in most cases, grief responses are normal and healthy and require little or no intervention beyond validation and compassion.

WHEN THE BOND IS BROKEN

Our society has been described as "death denying" because many people are uncomfortable talking about death. We know little about the experience of death, and we fear the unknown, yet veterinarians and their staff must frequently discuss death, participate in causing it, witness it, and deal with the emotions triggered by these experiences.

Although people in the midst of grief have a need and a right to understand what is happening to them, there are few places they can go to get helpful, supportive information about grief. This is particularly true when the loss they are grieving is that of a beloved pet. Like most of society, veterinarians and veterinary technicians rarely have formal training in this area.

• Table 29–1 •

THE STAGES OF GRIEF: HOW VETERINARY PROFESSIONALS CAN HELP
DENIAL
What the client needs most is time, support, understanding, and permission to grieve.
BEFORE DEATH
• Arrange to communicate with the client in person, if possible, where you both can sit down to talk without interruption or distraction. Recognize denial as a normal part of grief.
• Communicate clearly, and reiterate patiently. Phrase statements in words that are concrete and simple for the layperson. Avoid using medical jargon and lapsing into complicated medical explanations.
• Listen actively: Maintain eye contact, use attentive body language, and paraphrase or clarify the client's statements as you respond to him. Give him permission to express his feelings.
• Give the client time to think about and to grasp the reality of information that has been given. Some clients need only a slight pause in the conversation or a few minutes alone. Other clients may need more time to themselves before they comprehend the news of severe illness or actual death.
• Refrain from judging the client as "stupid" or "out of it."
• Remain nonjudgmental and unhurried toward the client, and state that you are available to talk about specifics or about his feelings whenever he's ready.
• NEVER attempt to force the client to "come to his senses" or to move out of denial. He will comprehend at his own pace.
AFTER DEATH
• Encourage the client to view the body, say good-bye.
• Reveal a bit of personal experience (self-disclosure) that relates to the situation. (Self-disclosure allows clients to feel comfortable and not alone in what they are feeling and gives them permission to grieve.)*
• Give permission to grieve.
BARGAINING
• Understand that bargaining is an attempt to control or reverse a dire situation. The client feels irrationally compelled to bargain during the grief process and does not mean to doubt the professionals involved.
• When the patient is terminally ill, do not become defensive or threatened when clients ask for other opinions or consider alternative treatments. Giving information and readings and referral for second opinion will ameliorate bargaining attempts and facilitate commitment to treatment.
• After the death, be sympathetic and educative about the stage of bargaining when clients confide their feelings and bargaining behaviors, such as prayers and dreams (or daydreams) of the pet still alive. Reassure them that the emotional basis for their behaviors and feelings is normal even though it may seem irrational.
• When clients inquire as to when to "replace" their pet, educating them about the role bargaining plays in shopping for a new pet can alleviate future disappointment. State that their dead pet was unique and cannot be replaced, but encourage them to obtain a new pet whenever all members of the family feel ready. Help them to find the type of animal they are looking for while gently steering toward one that is slightly dissimilar to the dead pet. Encourage them to choose a different breed, color or gender, and a new name should be chosen.
ANGER
• Listen actively and let the client know that you understand.
• Arrange for communication in a private room with no distractions. Sit at eye level, and use attentive body language. Take notes if the client is complaining or criticizing.
• Give the client permission to ventilate his feelings. Listen actively using attentive body language, maintaining eye contact, nodding and responses that paraphrase, clarify and indicate your understanding of the client's feelings. (Example: "I can see that you're very angry . . ." or "You feel that diagnosis could have been made sooner. . . .")
• If the client is directly angry at the veterinarian, technician(s), or clinic staff, take a mental step backward, pause with either a deep breath or by counting to 10.
• DO NOT BECOME DEFENSIVE OR RESPOND IN LIKE MANNER to the client.
• Relieve guilt by assuring the client that he did the right thing.
• Educate the client about the grief process and about the role of anger and guilt. Let him know that as he is able to let go of his anger/guilt, he will move toward resolution of his grief.

• Table 29–1 •

THE STAGES OF GRIEF: HOW VETERINARY PROFESSIONALS CAN HELP *(Continued)*
DEPRESSION
• Encourage depressed clients to talk about their feelings in regard to their pet. Follow up clients whose pets have died with a telephone call in a few days and then 2 weeks afterward. • Listen actively. • Attend to the client by positioning yourself at eye level, offering tissues and/or a drink of water, and leaning slightly toward him. A nonthreatening yet compassionate touch on the forearm or on the shoulder communicates empathy and understanding. • Offer a place to sit, a place to be out of the "public eye." • Tell the client that it is all right, and even good, for him to cry. Listen supportively and actively, and touch the client gently on the shoulder or forearm. Some clients are known well enough to embrace, and this can be helpful as well. • Validate the feelings of sadness by letting the client know that he is normal. • Offer to call a family member or friend. • Be a friend. • Encourage and suggest means by which clients can memorialize their pet. Making scrapbooks, planting a tree, writing a letter to the pet or writing the pet's life story all are cathartic activities that alleviate depression due to grief. • If a client expresses continued depression several weeks following the death of his pet, if his support system is poor or if a client expresses a personal wish to die, referral to a compassionate professional counselor is necessary. Although referral may feel awkward, many clients appreciate the technician who states, "Grief due to pet loss is normal, but sometimes there can be no one to talk to, or the grief can be overwhelming. I know of a person who understands what you're going through. Would you like her (his) telephone number, or may I have her (him) call you?" Today, several schools of veterinary medicine employ counselors experienced in pet loss. Many communities have established support groups, and private counselors increasingly view pet loss as significant bereavement.†
RESOLUTION
• Acceptance is achieved once the above four stages have fallen into the background of the client's life. At this point, the bereaved can channel emotional energy into a new relationship. The veterinary professional can help clients reach the resolution stage by offering insight into the grief process through his or her actions and by offering suggestions of reading material or seminars on the grief process.

*When using self-disclosure, take care not to monopolize the time with your own experiences. A short comment that lets the client know that your own experiences parallel and thus validate their emotions is sufficient.
†For a complete list of referral counselors or for a referral, write the Delta Society (see Table 29–3).

Few curricula offer more than a cursory introduction to the concepts of death, grief, and bereavement. On-the-job training is almost always inadequate because few veterinary professionals, especially technicians, have the extent of client follow-up needed to see and understand the full spectrum of effects that grief has on owners. Despite this fact, veterinary professionals are still often the people clients instinctively turn to for support.

Making the job more difficult is the fact that grief and bereavement are emotional and often irrational areas of human interaction. The bereaved may, at times, seem out of control or out of touch with reality. When this happens, those around the griever, including the veterinary professional, may feel uncomfortable; few of us are taught how to support or to deal with people who are irrational or emotional. Compassion is an important sensitivity to draw on when interacting with clients experiencing grief.

Grief is the companion to death. It is the mental anguish experienced by any human being confronted with the loss of an object of attachment. Grief may ensue as an effect of any loss; the loss may be through death, divorce, loss of a job, or even moving or having friends move away. It can be intensely emotional and can affect mind, body, and spirit. Also, grief is a major stressor, able to produce any of the symptoms of stress listed in Chapter 28. When confronted with grief, the bereaved individual goes through a grief process. The term *grief process* implies that there is an intended end or result to be produced through grieving. Thus, the grief process is the means of letting go of the object of attachment to feel better, reinvest, emotionally grow, and attach again.

The veterinary staff is in a unique position to assist clients going through the process of grief. By way of their unique role in the life of the owner and pet, they may be the only people who knew the pet and understood the bond that had developed between owner and pet. Additionally, the veterinarian and the owner may have interacted uniquely in choosing the time of the pet's death (as occurs when euthanasia is performed). To assist clients during the difficult bereavement period, it is helpful to understand the normal grief process and the manifestations of it as applied to pet loss.

Pet Loss and the Grief Process

The death of a pet is all too often regarded as a trivial loss by society, perhaps due in part to the mistaken belief that pets can be easily replaced. There are no socially sanctioned rituals like funerals or memorial services to help grieving pet owners gain support once the bonds between them and their companion animals have been broken. Furthermore, people are rarely granted time off from their jobs to care for sick animals or to make arrangements for them after their deaths. Society also does not allow adequate time for mourning the death of a pet. Most people feel pressured to be "back to normal" within a few days of their pet's death to avoid being labeled as neurotic, hysterical, or overly attached. However, crying, taking time away from work, and wanting to memorialize a pet are healthy responses to the death of a pet. They should not be discouraged, nor should they be judged.

One of the most effective ways for veterinary professionals to assist grieving clients is to educate and reassure them that their feelings and behaviors are normal parts of the grief process. Other ways that veterinary professionals can help are listed in Table 29–1.

TECHNICIAN NOTE

Veterinary professionals can assist clients by normalizing their feelings.

The Normal Grief Process

As stated earlier, the word *process* implies movement toward some end or result. In regard to grief, this movement is accomplished by passing through what have been termed stages, phases, or tasks. The basic emotional process in pet loss is the same as in human loss. However, veterinary professionals who assist clients are aware of some differences and particulars.

Several models of the grief process can be modified to describe the emotional process that occurs during pet loss. Some important ones are exemplified in Table 29–2. For our purposes, we will use the classic model supplied by Elisabeth Kübler-Ross (1969) and extrapolate for the situations peculiar to pet loss.

Dr. Kübler-Ross was one of the first to work extensively with the dying and their families during the late 1960s. She described the grief process as consisting of five "stages": denial, bargaining, anger, depression, and resolution. She used the stages to describe the passage through grief, but it is helpful to remember that these stages are not a linear odyssey. Although people may travel through the grief process in a straight line, they more often fluctuate between stages, bounce back and forth, and feel the entire gamut of grief within minutes, days, or months.

TECHNICIAN NOTE

The grief process consists of five "stages": denial, bargaining, anger, depression, and resolution.

Stage 1: Denial

Denial is a normal defense mechanism that buffers a human being from some unbearable news or reality. It is important to recognize the word "normal" here, as many individuals experiencing denial at the time a poor prognosis is given or during bereavement will seem to all observers to be out of touch with reality. The veterinary staff may wonder whether the client has even heard the veterinarian stating the seriousness

of an animal's illness. A client in denial may listen attentively to a diagnosis of cancer with a poor prognosis but ask only if the toenails can be clipped or if their current flea shampoo is correct. A client informed of the death of his or her pet while it was hospitalized may chatter on about activities for the weekend. A simple form of denial is exemplified by the client who states repeatedly, "It can't be. I don't believe it."

It is tempting when presented with a client experiencing denial to insist that he or she recognize the seriousness of the situation. Many veterinarians and veterinary technicians worry that the client does not comprehend or has not heard correctly. There is no harm in repeating oneself to a client in denial (Fig. 29–3). In fact, restating diagnoses, prognoses, treatment plans, and particulars is advisable. However, clients in denial will accept the unbearable reality of the situation only when they are ready internally; attempts to push them may backfire, resulting in frustration. Usually, a client will begin to ask appropriate questions about the time he or she arrives home and may telephone the veterinary office. Some may even seem to return to reality before your eyes while those toenails are being attended to. The veterinary professional must feel assured that the client has been told the basic information that needs to be given. Remember, however, that it may not have been fully understood; therefore, always leave the door open for further communication.

Although denial reappears later during the grief process, at that time it is usually of little significance to the veterinary staff. Later-stage denial may be manifested as clients reporting during a telephone call or visit that they were sure they had seen their pet that morning or they had absent-mindedly purchased pet food several weeks or months after their pet's death. Denial is reflected by the client's eyes and demeanor and by incongruous questions. The veterinary staff should not feel responsibility to "break through" a client's denial. The client will move out of denial, accepting the reality of the situation, when he or she is ready. The veterinary staff's recognition of the client's denial can prevent impatience and frustration during the veterinary contact.

> Soft Paw, a 15-year-old female domestic shorthair cat, is brought into the clinic for vomiting and anorexia that the owner thinks is due to the ingestion of chicken bones. Physical examination reveals Soft Paw to be thin and pale. Further evaluation reveals that Soft Paw is severely anemic due to renal failure. The prognosis is poor.
>
> Soft Paw is owned by a 20-year-old college student named Ashley who found the cat as a

• Table 29–2 •

KÜBLER-ROSS	WORDEN		ROSENBERG	DERSHEIMER
POPULAR MODELS OF THE GRIEF PROCESS				
Stages	**Tasks**		**Stages**	**Phases**
Denial	I. To accept the reality of the loss		Denial	Shock
Bargaining	II. To experience the pain of grief		Anger/guilt	Acute grief
Anger	III. To adjust to an environment in which the deceased is missing		Grief	Straightening up the mess
Depression	IV. To withdraw emotional energy and reinvest it in another		Acceptance	Reinvesting and reengaging in life
Acceptance	relationship			

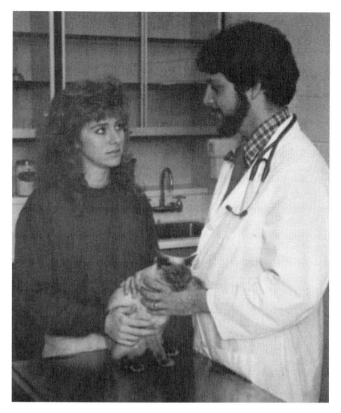

Figure 29-3. Even when dealing with attentive clients, veterinary professionals may be required to repeat themselves several times while clients decide on a course of treatment for their pet.

kitten. Ashley has owned Soft Paw since she was 5 years old. When told that Soft Paw's problems were not caused by chicken bones but were due to end-stage renal failure, Ashley at first did not seem to hear what the doctor had said. A blank stare washed over her face, and for a moment she appeared to be daydreaming. The doctor continued by explaining that there were some treatments that may prolong Soft Paw's life, but they should be considered palliative and not potentially curative. After hearing the doctor's assessment, Ashley smiled, picked up her cat, and turned to leave. "Thank you for your time today," she said as she turned to leave. "I'll try not to let her get into the chicken bones in the future. Oh, by the way, can you trim Soft Paw's front claws? They are getting kind of long."

Ashley came to the veterinarian's office for what she perceived to be a problem brought on by Soft Paw's dietary indiscretion. Ashley had probably not seen her cat eat chicken bones but was grasping for an explanation for why Soft Paw was vomiting, losing weight, and acting lethargic. In all probability, Ashley had been denying that Soft Paw was sick for some time even before making the appointment with the doctor. When the doctor told Ashley the diagnosis, her initial reaction appeared to be that of shock. Ashley's shock—seeming not to hear the results of the evaluation and asking the doctor to perform

something seemingly inappropriate like a nail trim—is part of denial, the first stage of grief.

When a client like the one presented above is encountered, the veterinary professional must realize that the response is a normal part of the grief process. The conversation up to that point may or may not have been heard, but it certainly has not yet been clearly comprehended. The client will be able to acknowledge the seriousness of the situation only when he or she is ready internally. The veterinary professional should repeat things and not become frustrated or impatient. Clip the nails and call the client at home later for further discussions. At that time the client may be ready to acknowledge the reality of the bad disease, and meaningful discussions concerning treatment options can then occur.

TECHNICIAN NOTE

During denial the veterinary professional should repeat things without becoming frustrated or impatient.

Stage 2: Bargaining

Once the reality of death or impending death is realized, the client may show various impotent attempts to control or to reverse the reality. The client is grappling with the stage of the grief process that Dr. Kübler-Ross called *bargaining*. During this stage, the client maneuvers personally and privately, possibly praying and negotiating with God for miracles. The client might add various herbs and old family remedies to food. Children behave like little angels, hoping to be rewarded with a reversal of bad news. The veterinary staff may be subject to various inquiries by the client at this stage, such as, "Have you ever heard of avocado in the food? I read that it may reverse cancer." It is while bargaining that a pet owner may also request permission to obtain a second (and sometimes third, fourth, or fifth) opinion. Bargaining during terminal illness rarely results in harm to the patient, and veterinary staff should reassure themselves of their clients' normality. Be compassionate and when possible answer their questions. Help clients to understand that this stage of grief is normal.

Bargaining after death has occurred may go on without the knowledge of the veterinary professionals involved. Seeking to "replace" the lost animal without grieving at all is a form of bargaining. Many pet owners seek a new pet too soon, and they purchase the same species, the same color, and name them the same or a similar name. Leaving dishes or the dead pet's belongings down for an obviously unusual length of time is another subtle form of bargaining. Through bargaining, the client is unconsciously attempting to control or subvert the grief process.

TECHNICIAN NOTE

Once reality is realized, clients attempt to reverse or control the inevitable through bargaining.

It is important to recognize bargaining as part of the normal grief process. The veterinary professionals who understand the stages of bargaining and denial will avoid frustration in their attempts to provide quality patient care and client service.

> Three days after the euthanasia of his Doberman "Saber," Ron came into the clinic to pay his bill. After reviewing the bill, he asked to speak to the veterinarian, who was busy at the time. Maggie, the technician, led Ron to an examination room and then inquired as to how he had been doing. Ron told her that he had not been sleeping well because of dreams of Saber. He stated that the dreams were pleasant, but he would awaken hoping that Saber's death had been a nightmare. He said, "Sometimes I'll keep my eyes closed for an extra 10 seconds and pray that she's come back, somehow, healthy and happy. But of course, it never works." In addition, he said, "I want to see Dr. Roberts today because I can't stop thinking about Saber's treatment. I know Dr. Roberts is the best vet around, and I'm grateful to him for being so kind to me and Saber. But I feel like maybe something more could have been done."
>
> Ron met with Dr. Roberts for only a few minutes. During this time, Maggie was asked to bring tissues to the room. As Maggie handed him a tissue, Ron said tearfully, "I looked at the whole record. Even while I was doing it, I realized that no information could bring Saber back to life. For some reason, I had to look anyway. Now, maybe, I can let her go."

Although Ron understands that Saber died, he feels compelled to try to control the situation. Childlike and irrational behaviors such as his closing his eyes and wishing or praying that Saber was alive are manifestations of the bargaining stage of grief. Ron's request to view the record might have been viewed by the veterinarian and the technician as challenging or accusatory, yet Ron was not looking for information that could be damaging; rather, he was hoping again to somehow reverse the illness and death of Saber. Bargaining can be frustrating for veterinary professionals unless they understand and assist the client in working through these irrational attempts to "bring their beloved pet back."

Stage 3: Anger

During the grief process, clients may move in and out of the stage called *anger*. Clients coping with this stage may exhibit anger in a wide variety of direct or indirect manners. The anger may be specific or nonspecific in the way that it is directed. Anger may also be exhibited in the form of guilt, which can be defined as anger turned inward.

Anger is a particularly difficult emotion to deal with when a client directs it toward the veterinary professional. Whether or not the client is justified in his stated cause for anger, staff members must use tolerance and patience to avoid responding defensively. Bereaved clients may complain that the illness that resulted in death should have been discovered sooner, should have been treated differently, or should not have been allowed to happen. They may complain that their pet died while hospitalized due to neglect or inappropriate treatment rather than to the tumor revealed by necropsy.

Anger may be apparent in the form of guilt. Clients feeling guilt use language with an abundance of "I should've" statements. They often seek the listening ear of the veterinary professional to ask questions pertinent to absolution from guilt. They may ask whether the food they fed their pet could have contributed to the illness or death. They often ask whether it was the pesticide in their home or in the shampoo that caused a tumor or cardiac arrest. Clients may believe they allowed their pet to be too active or too fat; others may believe they caused the kidney failure in their cat by feeding insufficient diet. These clients can direct anger at themselves, but frequently they cannot find a specific crime that they committed. When possible, the veterinary professional can assist the clients by assuaging their guilt. Reassuring the clients that, in your opinion, they did everything possible for their pet, that they did only what they thought would benefit their pet, and that they made the right decisions for their pet will relieve much of the clients' guilt or anger and assist them in moving through the grief process.

✎ TECHNICIAN NOTE

Veterinary professionals can help by reassuring clients that they did everything possible and made the right decisions.

The client showing indirect and nonspecific anger is not as threatening to the veterinary professional as those who direct their anger specifically toward the veterinarian or veterinary technician. The client who is feeling this type of anger may be gruff or rude and generally hard to get along with. Stating that he is angry, he may be at a loss to express with whom or what he is angry. This type of anger is common in American society. These clients yell at the cashiers, waitresses, and telephone operators, and they drive their cars with aggressiveness and anger. Giving the angry client an opportunity to express his feelings (ventilation) is an effective way for the veterinary professional to help. At times, all that is needed is for the sensitive veterinary professional to explain that, considering the client's loss, anger is a normal feeling. This explanation gives the client permission to grieve effectively.

Indirect and specific anger in a client is most often exhibited by reluctance to pay the bill. On receiving an inquiry by telephone, the client implies that nonpayment is due to anger at treatment by the veterinarian or technician, the pet was neglected, the illness was mistreated, or he (the client) was treated insensitively. Bereavement support can alleviate this client's anger. Listen attentively, state your apologies, if any, and follow up with this client. No admission of mistakes need be made, but the client needs to feel significant and understood.

Although all of the types of anger may be exhibited by one client, it is guilt that may be hardest for the client to relinquish. Yet, direct and specific anger, when justified (or perceived to be justified), is difficult to work through, as well. In continuing to feel guilt and anger, the client avoids letting go of the beloved pet, and the grief process is stymied. Once the client is able to relinquish the guilt or anger, the grief process can continue.

The veterinary professional can assist the client with all

types of exhibited anger by taking a mental step back and a deep breath, committing to a nondefensive attitude, and simply listening. Take notes if possible and reassure the client of follow-up if his anger is directed at veterinary staff. Assuage any guilt if the opportunity arises, and allow the client to ventilate. A few minutes on the telephone or in person may salvage a client relationship and go a long way in assisting the client through the grief process.

> Honey, a 12-year-old male poodle, is presented for a second opinion. He has been having seizures for almost a year. They have been occurring more frequently and have been increasing in severity over the past few months. Another veterinarian has told the owner that the diagnosis is epilepsy and that there is nothing further that can be done.
>
> Not wanting to accept that Honey's seizures cannot be controlled, Charles, a 40-year-old businessman, takes Honey to another veterinarian for a second opinion. The second veterinarian diagnoses the problem as a brain tumor and offers referral to a veterinary school for surgery. While Charles is considering his options, Honey has a severe seizure and dies. Charles calls the second veterinarian to let him know of Honey's death. He refuses to wait for the veterinarian to come to the telephone, is rude to the receptionist, and hangs up abruptly. Two days later, he calls to apologize and expresses feelings of guilt for not bringing Honey to the second veterinarian sooner. He also informs the second veterinarian that he has stopped payment on his check to the first veterinarian. A week later, the second veterinarian is contacted by Charles' lawyer inquiring as to his willingness to testify should Charles elect litigation against the first veterinarian for malpractice.

Charles is showing signs of anger. Anger should be recognized as a stage of grief. It can be directed in many ways. In this case, Charles' initial anger is nonspecific and indirect, being manifested as rude behavior on the telephone. The person taking the telephone call and absorbing the brunt of this initial anger should realize that the anger is not personal and is not necessarily directed at him. He should not react defensively but should listen politely and let the client know that he empathizes and understands. Charles later calls to apologize for his behavior and at that time reveals his feelings of guilt at not making up his mind concerning referral sooner and for continuing to take Honey to the first veterinarian for almost a year. Assuring Charles that the short time over which he was thinking over his options had not made a difference may help relieve some of the guilt. Also assuring Charles that the first veterinarian could not have known of the tumor based on the initial signs and that the same course of events was likely even if he had sought a second opinion sooner may also alleviate guilt and prevent further questioning of the initial veterinarian's diagnosis. By stopping payment to the first veterinarian, Charles is showing indirect and specific anger. Later, the anger is directed specifically at the first veterinarian when Charles seeks the advice of a lawyer concerning the professional conduct of the first

veterinarian. Communication among the first veterinarian, the second veterinarian, and Charles will probably be necessary for Charles to work through the anger stage of grief.

Stage 4: Depression

The stage of the grief process that is termed depression has also been called *grief*. Clients experiencing depression describe their mood as complete, overwhelming sadness, a feeling of "lead in their boots" accompanied by bouts of uncontrollable crying. Intense grief can result in depression, which prohibits a client from functioning normally. Appetite is changed, energy level is lowered, the client withdraws from others, and sometimes the client is unable to go to work. More subtle symptoms of depression include irritability, sleep irregularity, restlessness, and inability to concentrate.

TECHNICIAN NOTE

Depression has been described as complete, overwhelming sadness.

The veterinary professional has occasion to recognize depression due to pet loss when follow-up contacts are made with the client. Depression, when severe, usually sets in some time after the loss. Clients with poor social support systems, elderly clients, and clients with intense and/or symbolic attachment to the pet may experience worrisome depression. When contacts are made several days or weeks after bereavement and it is suspected that a client is depressed, referral can be made to a counselor or hotline specializing in pet loss (Table 29–3). Although referral sometimes feels awkward, it might be gently phrased as, "I know a person experienced in counseling people who have lost their pets." Again, reassurance that grief is normal is of benefit.

TECHNICIAN NOTE

If severe depression is suspected, referral can be made to a counselor or hotline.

Most clients experience the feeling of being overwhelmed by their emotions because of grief. They state the feeling of being out of control in their emotions. They may also state surprise and worry that they are reacting with such intensity to the death of an animal. They may be embarrassed. It comforts clients when veterinary professionals confide that most pet owners feel and act similarly on the loss of the pet. Assuring them of your knowledge of their pet's importance as well as your respect for their grief is valuable to them.

Grief must be worked through, not bottled up; thus, it is a process requiring some emotional catharsis. Many clients cry, and some are uninhibited about expressing anger and sadness. They may loudly complain, and they may sob unabashedly. Becoming comfortable with one's own emotions facilitates comfort with others' emotions. It is human and necessary to feel empathy for grieving clients, but it can also be uncomfortable

• Table 29–3 •

PLACES TO CONTACT FOR HELP OR REFERRAL SOURCES FOR CLIENTS NEEDING HELP WITH GRIEF

The Delta Society
ATTN: Librarian
289 Perimeter Road East
Renton, WA 98055-1329
Telephone: (206) 226-7357
(Can be contacted for a list of referral sources in your area)

Veterinary Grief Counseling Hotlines
Companion Animal Association of Arizona, Inc.
Pet Grief Support Service
P.O. Box 5006
Scottsdale, AZ 85006
Telephone: (602) 995-5885

Pet Loss Support Hotline
Center for Animals in Society
School of Veterinary Medicine
University of California-Davis
Davis, CA 95616
Telephone: (916) 752-4200
(Staffed by University of California-Davis veterinary students; weekdays, 6:30 P.M. to 9:30 P.M. PT)

The Chicago Veterinary Medical Association Pet Loss Support Hotline
Telephone: (708) 603-3994
(Staffed by Chicago VMA veterinarians and staff. Voice mail will be returned daily between 6 P.M. and 9 P.M. ET; long distance calls will be returned collect)

Pet Loss Support Hotline
College of Veterinary Medicine
Cornell University
Ithaca, NY 14853
Telephone: (607) 253-3932
(Staffed by Cornell University veterinary students; voice mail messages will be returned within 24 hours)

College of Veterinary Medicine
University of Florida
Gainesville, FL 32610
Telephone: (904) 392-4700; then dial 1 and 4080
(Staffed by University of Florida veterinary students; weekdays, 7 P.M. to 9 P.M. ET)

Pet Loss Support Hotline
College of Veterinary Medicine
Michigan State University, G100
East Lansing, MI 48824
Telephone: (517) 432-2696
(Staffed by Michigan State University veterinary students; Tuesday to Thursday, 6:30 P.M. to 9:30 P.M. ET)

Virginia-Maryland Regional College of Veterinary Medicine
Virginia Tech
Blacksburg, VA 24061
Telephone: (540) 231-8038
(Staffed by Virginia-Maryland Regional College of Veterinary Medicine; Tuesday and Thursday, 6 P.M. to 9 P.M. ET)

College of Veterinary Medicine
The Ohio State University
Columbus, OH 43210
Telephone: (614) 292-1823
(Staffed by The Ohio State University veterinary students; Monday, Wednesday, and Friday, 6:30 P.M. to 9:30 P.M. ET)

School of Veterinary Medicine
Tufts University
N. Grafton, MA 01536
Telephone: (508) 839-7966
(Staffed by Tufts University veterinary students: Tuesday and Thursday 6 P.M. to 9 P.M. ET; voice mail messages will be returned collect daily)

Veterinary Schools and Colleges with Grief Counseling Programs
University of California
School of Veterinary Medicine
Center for Animals in Society
Davis, CA 95616
Telephone: (916) 752-4200

Colorado State University, Veterinary Teaching Hospital
CHANGES: The Support for People and Pets Program
300 West Drake Rd.
Fort Collins, CO 80523
Telephone: (970) 491-1242

Louisiana State University
School of Veterinary Medicine
The Best Friend Gone Project
Baton Rouge, LA 70809
Telephone: (504) 346-5710

University of Pennsylvania
School of Veterinary Medicine
3800 Spruce St.
Philadelphia, PA 19104-6044
Telephone: (215) 898-5438

Tufts University School of Veterinary Medicine
Center for Animals and Public Policy
200 Westboro Rd.
North Grafton, MA 01536
Telephone: (508) 839-7991

Washington State University, College of Veterinary Medicine
People-Pet Partnership
Pullman, WA 99164-7010
Telephone: (509) 335-4569

University of Wisconsin, School of Veterinary Medicine
Pet Loss Support Group
2015 Linden Dr.
Madison, WI 53706
Telephone: (608) 836-7297

and painful. Separating your own feelings from theirs will allow you to transform empathy into sympathetic gestures that help the client.

> Mary Jo, a 64-year-old widow, brings her 3-year-old dog for examination. She states that the young dog, a mixed breed named Boo, is lethargic and just does not seem to be ``getting over'' the death of her golden retriever, Lucky. As she talks with the technician, she states that even though Lucky died a month ago, Boo is depressed all the time. The veterinarian examines Boo and determines that the dog is in perfect health. Also, Boo wags his tail, strains at the leash, licks the veterinarian and technician, and appears happy and energetic.
>
> The technician, left alone with Mary Jo for a few minutes, inquires as to how she is feeling in regard to the death of Lucky. Mary Jo begins to cry softly and says, ``I just can't stop crying. I miss him so much. I've lost 10 pounds, and I just don't feel like doing anything. Sometimes I stay in bed most of the day. I know my friends and my children think I should be over it, and I don't talk with them about it anymore. I feel silly to be still grieving over an animal. I think I dealt with my husband's death better than this.''
>
> The technician lets Mary Jo talk about Lucky for many more minutes. Some of the time Mary Jo cries, but much of the time she tells amusing stories and both individuals laugh.
>
> Finally, when Mary Jo breaks down into tears again, the technician puts her hand on Mary Jo's shoulder and says, ``I understand now why you're still grieving. Lucky was so special to you, and it might take you a while to grieve. Support and someone to talk to can help. May I provide you with a telephone number of an understanding counselor?''
>
> Three weeks had passed when Mary Jo telephoned the technician. With a new lift in her voice, she reported that both she and Boo were doing much better. After talking with a counselor, she found a way to memorialize Lucky, and she cries less each week. ``I called because I'm ready to look for a playmate for Boo, and, of course, a new friend for me. Do you know of anyone with puppies?''

Without the contact due to Mary Jo's visit for her other pet Boo, her depression may have gone unnoticed by the veterinary professionals. Many times clients suffer through the stage of depression feeling very much alone and as if they have nowhere to turn for help. Depression may occur on and off during the entire grief process (as in the client who sobs uncontrollably just after a pet has died) or depression may become more serious later on in the grief process. At that time, support for the bereaved may no longer be available within their circle of friends and family. It is important to follow up on clients who have poor support systems or who are unusually attached to

their animals. Referral to professionals can be of great assistance in helping these clients resolve the grief process.

TECHNICIAN NOTE

Follow-up is important for those clients with poor support systems or unusual attachments.

Stage 5: Resolution or Acceptance

The stage of *resolution or acceptance* is the feeling that everything is okay, normal functioning is restored, and emotional energy is reinvested. The dead pet has been "let go of" emotionally. This does not mean that the pet is forgotten but that it has been assigned to a special place in the bereaved individual's heart. New attachments can be made without regret and hesitation. Resolution may come easily for some and may be difficult for others. In general, children reach the stage of acceptance and resolution more quickly and more easily than do adults. (For more information on how to help children when a pet dies, see Table 29–4.) As stated previously, the grief process is not linear, and bits of this stage occur with more and more frequency and with longer durations throughout the grief process. Eventually, the client who successfully resolves the grief process feels little, if any, of the first four stages.

There are many factors that may complicate the grief process (Table 29–5). These complicating factors may lengthen the time it takes to reach resolution or, in severe cases, may arrest progress through the grief process without allowing the individual to reach a resolution. Situations in which the grief process is complicated may not affect some individuals' ability to progress but may drastically affect that of others. Few veterinary professionals are equipped to give the special kind of help that these complicated situations may require, but most have empathy and the ability to listen for signs that indicate someone may need help. Early recognition of factors that may complicate the grief process can be helpful when a person appears not to be progressing well through the process. Early recognition may also be important for timely referral in situations in which further assistance is required. Keeping on hand a list of professional alternatives for referral to someone who can give the help that is needed is advised (see Table 29–3 for a short list of potential sources of help).

The question is often raised whether clients should "replace" an animal before they reach resolution of the grief process. The process itself is highly variable in length. It can be as short as a few weeks to as long as many years. Most pet owners are able to reinvest and reattach to a new pet at any time but only after they become aware that replacement of their unique loved one is impossible. If companionship, tactile closeness, and friendship are desired while grieving, it can be obtained through a new pet. Cautioning and encouraging clients to choose animals somewhat dissimilar to their dead pet can be helpful. Having a new pet forced on the grieving individual who is not ready to reinvest in a new relationship will only end up furthering heartache in the bereaved and causing unhappiness in the new pet.

GRIEF AND THE VETERINARY PROFESSIONAL

Those in the veterinary profession deal with client grief on an almost daily basis. Rarely do they think about their own, how-

• Table 29–4 •

HOW TO HELP CHILDREN WHEN A PET DIES

When children's companion animals die, many parents follow their instincts to protect them from pain and grief. Some parents make decisions regarding the pet without discussing them with their children. Some may even lie to their children about the actual circumstances of the pet's "disappearance," preferring to tell them that a beloved pet ran away or was stolen rather than died. These tactics are not used maliciously by parents. They develop from a desire to spare children feelings of pain and from a belief that they, as parents, are inadequately prepared to discuss loss, death, and grief with their children.

Children, however, are tuned into their parents' emotions and, almost without exception, know that *something* is going on in the family. They don't know what that *something* is, but they do know

that it upsets mom and dad. Consequently, children may feel anxious, confused, left out, and even guilty because, without honest explanations of a family crisis, children often feel that they are somehow responsible for the tension level in the home. At later ages, children may also feel betrayed by the parents they trusted when they discover the "truth" about their childhood pet's "disappearance."

The knowledge, skills, and tools for dealing with loss and grief that are developed in childhood are the same ones used in adolescence and adulthood. It is of utmost importance, then, that children be given honest support and information about loss and death so their grief-coping strategies will be healthy, rather than unhealthy, ones.

HOW TECHNICIANS CAN HELP

Parents will often turn to veterinary professionals for assistance in telling their children about the death of a pet. Having books available for them to read and having information yourself to share can help ease an otherwise traumatic situation. Here are some suggestions:

- Always encourage parents to be honest with their children throughout a companion animal's illness, treatment, and death. Never agree to participate in a lie that the parents may want to tell their children to protect them. In the long run, lies create more problems for everyone involved and can be more damaging to children than the pet's death itself.
- Children under the age of 8 do not really understand that death is final. They may believe that a dead pet can return or that they will need food in their grave with them. Young children are also egocentric and believe quite strictly in the law of cause and effect. Thus, they may develop the idea that they did something to cause the pet's death. Therefore, they must be reassured repeatedly that the pet died because it had a disease or an accident or was very old.
- Straightforward explanations and concrete words like dead and died should be used when talking to children about death. Young children do not understand euphemisms and can become upset when they hear terms like "put to sleep." Since they go to sleep every night, and do not want to die like their pet did, attempts at "softening the blow" can actually make the situation more difficult and frightening for children.
- Children need to be held, reassured, and allowed to ask questions. Open communication about death is the desired atmosphere for keeping death anxiety manageable. Pets' names should be used in conversation whenever possible and memories of them should be shared by the whole family. Older children should be included in the euthanasia process, the memorial ceremonies, and the good-bye rituals to whatever extent they wish to be and should be encouraged to demonstrate their sensitivity and compassion.
- It is always helpful to contact children's teachers, care providers,

relatives, and other significant adults so they can help acknowledge the loss and grief process. Adults may observe children playing "funeral" or overhear them talking to friends about a pet's death. While these activities may seem alarming and even morbid to adults, they are normal, healthy responses for children. Children deal with issues through play and experimentation. Unless they are in physical danger, their activities do not, in most cases, require interference.

- For adult information about helping children deal with pet loss, consult the following books:

  Balk DE: Children and the Death of a Pet. Manhattan, KS, Cooperative Extension Service, Kansas State University, 1990.
  Jewett CL: Helping Children Cope with Separation and Loss. Boston, Harvard Common Press, 1982.
  Nieburg HA and Fischer A: Pet Loss: A Thoughtful Guide for Adults and Children. New York, Harper and Row, 1982.
  Quackenbush J and Graveline D: When Your Pet Dies: How to Cope with Your Feelings. New York, Simon and Schuster, 1985.
  Shirl-Potter JW and Koss GJ: Death of a Pet; Answers to Questions for Children and Animal Lovers of All Ages. Stanford, Guideline Publications, 1991.
  Stein S: About Dying: An Open Family Book for Adults and Children. New York, Walker and Co., 1974.

- Children's books that may be helpful in explaining the loss of a pet to children:

  Brackenridge SS: Because of Flowers and Dancers. Santa Barbara, CA, Veterinary Practice Publishing, 1994.
  Morehead D: A Special Place for Charlie. Broomfield, CO, Partners in Publishing LLC, 1996.
  Rylant C: Dog Heaven. New York, The Blue Sky Press, 1995.
  Viorst J: The Tenth Good Thing About Barney. New York, Aladdin Books, 1971.

• Table 29–5 •

FACTORS THAT MAY COMPLICATE THE GRIEF PROCESS
Multiple losses occurring within a related time frame
Loss of a pet that was associated with a special person or event
Loss of a pet on a day that is important, such as a birthday or holiday
Loss of a pet due to factors that may have been preventable
Feelings of guilt about the death of a pet
An inability to afford expensive care that was offered
Loss of a pet due to an illness or situation that previously caused the loss of another pet
Sudden illness or trauma resulting in loss
Witnessing the violent or unnecessary death of a pet
Disappearance of a pet
Lack of explanation as to why their pet died
Situations in which the person experiencing loss has little or no support
Insensitive comments from others who may not understand the bond between the owner and his or her pet
Getting incorrect or bad information concerning the loss of their pet and/or the grieving process
No previous experience with grief
Not being present at the time the pet dies or not having the opportunity to view the body
Not being able to say good-bye

ever. The veterinary professional must realize the grief process that the client is struggling with is not taking place in an emotional vacuum. It is real and touches not only the bereaved but also those around the client, including the veterinary professional. It is common for veterinarians and veterinary technicians to cry with clients, to feel a lump in their throat, and to feel guilty or depressed or experience a sense of failure. The fact that veterinary professionals may go through a grief process each time a patient is lost must be recognized and accepted. Time should be spent thinking about these feelings and responses. Validation of the process within the profession, by way of staff meetings, discussions, and support sessions, can be important in recognizing and dealing with the stresses of "professional grief." Left unacknowledged, the grief process encountered by veterinary professionals can become destructive and lead to burnout. (More information concerning grief and the stresses that it causes can be found in Chapter 33.)

TECHNICIAN NOTE

Left unacknowledged, the grief process encountered by veterinary professionals can become destructive.

Missy, a 10-year-old female mixed-breed dog, had been treated for diabetes and hyperadrenocorticism for approximately 2 years. She recently developed pulmonary thromboemboli and became severely dyspneic. She also developed disseminated intravascular coagulation (DIC). Missy's owners, two sisters going to college together, elect euthanasia rather than see her suffer any further. Both sisters want to be present for the euthanasia. They hold Missy and

say good-bye as the veterinarian and veterinary technician compassionately perform the euthanasia. As the euthanasia solution is being injected, Missy weakly wags her tail. The girls spend about 30 minutes with Missy's body after her death. They alternately cry, hold hands, and tell the veterinarian and veterinary technician remembered stories of a young, healthy Missy playing with the children on their hometown street.

Two days after the euthanasia, the veterinary technician who spent those last few moments with Missy and her owners calls to see how the girls are doing. The technician finds out that they still find themselves crying at times but are doing better. The girls express concern over whether they did the right thing in electing euthanasia. After assuring them that their decision was indeed the best thing for both Missy and themselves, the technician asks if they have done anything special to remember Missy. After a short pause, the youngest sister says that they would like to plant a tree in remembrance of Missy. They have even picked a special place in front of the clinic where Missy spent her last few days. A week later, a small tree is planted on the clinic lawn during a short ceremony in which Missy is remembered. The two sisters, their mother, the veterinarian, and the veterinary technician attend. Afterward, the veterinary technician cries with the sisters. All three feel the sadness of the loss but can smile in shared memories.

Two months after Missy's death, the girls show up at the clinic with proud smiles on their faces and a new puppy in their arms. Archie is a beautiful little schnauzer puppy that they adopted from the local humane society. ``He is a ball of fire,'' laughs the older sister. ``You should have seen what Archie did to his favorite stuffed doll yesterday!'' Both the veterinarian and veterinary technician smile.

The girls are doing well. They have grieved for their lost pet—a process made easier by the compassion and concern shown by the veterinary staff. In being present during the euthanasia, they had a very special opportunity to say good-bye, and by memorializing Missy with a ceremony and by planting a tree, the girls were not only able to remember Missy in a special way but also able to share it with people at the veterinary office who had become part of Missy's (and therefore their) extended family. Through the process of grieving, the girls, and indeed the veterinary staff in this instance, experienced a degree of personal growth. The resolution is symbolized by the channeling of emotional energy into a new relationship with Archie. Missy is not forgotten!

CONCLUSION

Grief and the grief process are difficult to deal with, especially in a society that denies death as much as ours. Despite this difficulty, veterinary professionals are asked to deal with it on a daily basis. Veterinary professionals are rarely trained in the area of bereavement and the grief process, yet despite this shortcoming they are still often the best qualified individuals when it comes to helping clients who have recently lost a beloved pet. Understanding what the client is going through by understanding the basics of the grief process will help the veterinary professional to empathize, maintain a balanced perspective, and be compassionate. The veterinary technician can play a vital role in helping bereaved clients by being available; listening; assuring the client that his feelings, emotions, and struggles are normal; and offering referral when the client thinks he needs more help than his available support group is able to provide. This form of client help will strengthen the bond that develops between the client and the veterinary staff and will result in positive growth and added fulfillment for both the client and the veterinary professional.

The Feeling

. . . alone; the haunting thought of my old friend;
Alone; walking among those who could not possibly understand;
Alone; an unused bowl, an empty collar, a silent toy;
. . . the feeling is so strong;

How could I have let them do it?
What if there was something else that could have been done?
Sometimes I just want to yell;
Sometimes I just want to cry;
Sometimes I just want to die;

. . . the feeling is still so very strong;

I know that it was for the best;
My old friend was so sick, so frail;
We cried together on that day;

. . . the feeling was so strong;

I visited his grave today;
I could almost feel his kneading paws and hear his deep harsh purr;

Today I smiled . . . the feeling is so strong.

J. Taboada

Recommended Reading

Anderson M: Coping with Sorrow on the Loss of Your Pet. 2nd ed. Los Angeles, Peregrine Press, 1994.

Brackenridge SS and Elkins AD: Euthanasia and patient death: Stressors in veterinary practice. Vet Pract Staff 4:1, 8–10, 1992.

Cain AO: A study of pets in the family system. *In* Katcher AH and Beck AM (editors): New Perspectives on Our Lives with Companion Animals. Philadelphia, University of Pennsylvania Press, 1983.

Church JA: Joy in a Wooly Coat. Tiburon, CA, H. J. Kramer, Inc., 1987.

Cohen SP and Fudin CE (editors): Animal illness and human emotions. Prob Vet Med 3(1):1–121, 1991.

Cusack O: Pets and Mental Health. New York, Haworth Press, 1988.

Dershimer RA: Counseling the Bereaved. New York, Pergamon Press, 1990.

Fogle B and Abrahamson D: Pet loss: A survey of the attitudes and feelings of practicing veterinarians. Anthrozoos 3:143–150, 1990.

Frey WH: Crying: The Mystery of Tears. Minneapolis, Winston Press, Inc., 1985.

Haig RA: The Anatomy of Grief: Biopsychosocial and Therapeutic Perspectives. Springfield, IL, Charles C Thomas, 1990.

Harris JM: Nonconventional human/companion animal bonds. *In* Kay WJ, Nieburg HA, Kukscher AH (editors): Pet Loss and Human Bereavement. Ames, IA, Iowa State University Press, 1984, pp 31–36.

Katcher A: Interactions between people and their pets: form and function. *In* Fogle B (editor): Interrelations Between People and Pets. Springfield, IL, Charles C Thomas, 1981.

Kay WJ, Cohen SP, and Nieburg HA (editors): Euthanasia of the Companion Animal: The Impact on Pet Owners, Veterinarians, and Society. Baltimore, The Charles Press, 1988.

Kübler-Ross E: On Death and Dying. New York, Macmillan Publishing Co., 1969.

Lagoni L, Butler C, and Hetts S: The Human Animal Bond and Grief. Philadelphia, W. B. Saunders, 1994.

Lawrence EA: Love for animals and the veterinary profession. *J Am Vet Med Assoc* 205:970–922, 1994.

Messent PR: Social facilitation of contact with other people by pet dogs. *In* Katcher AH and Beck AM (editors): New Perspectives on Our Lives with Companion Animals. Philadelphia, University of Pennsylvania Press, 1983.

Nieburg HA and Fischer A: Pet Loss: A Thoughtful Guide for Adults and Children. New York, Harper and Row, 1982.

Quackenbush JE and Glickman L: Helping people adjust to the death of a pet. Health Soc Work 9:42–48, 1984.

Quackenbush JE and Graveline D: When Your Pet Dies: How to Cope With Your Feelings. New York, Simon and Schuster, 1985.

Rosenberg MA: Clinical aspects of grief associated with loss of a pet: A veterinarian's view. *In* Kay WJ, Neiburg HA, Kukscher AH (editors): Pet Loss and Human Bereavement. Ames, IA, Iowa State University Press, 1984, pp 119–125.

Veevers JE: The social meanings of pets: Alternative roles for companion animals. *In* Sussman MB (editor): Pets and the Family. Marriage and Family Review 8(3/4):11–30, 1985.

Voith VL: Attachment of people to companion animals. Vet Clin North Am Small Anim Pract 15:289–296, 1985.

Walshaw SO: Role of the animal health technician in consoling bereaved clients. *In* Kay WJ, Nieburg HA, Kukscher AH (editors): Pet Loss and Human Bereavement. Ames, IA, Iowa State University Press, 1984, pp 126–134.

Wilbur RH: Pets, pet ownership, and animal control: Social and psychological attitudes. Proceedings of the National Conference on Dog and Cat Control, Chicago, American Veterinary Medicine Association, 1976.

Worden JW: Bereavement. Semin Oncol 12(4):472–475, 1985.

Worden JW: Grief Counseling and Grief Therapy: A Handbook for the Mental Health Practitioner. 2nd ed. New York, Springer Publishing Company, 1991.

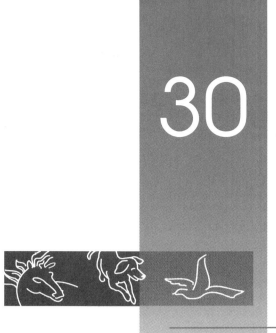

30 Basic Necropsy Procedures

Doo-Youn Cho • Terry R. Spraker

INTRODUCTION

Necropsy (Greek word for *viewing death*) is the postmortem examination of a dead animal. The word *autopsy* (the Greek word for *viewing self*) should not be used in veterinary medicine because of its reference to humans. The necropsy is an important part of the veterinary medical practice for many reasons, the major reasons being to (1) determine the cause of death of the animal, (2) determine the nature and course of the disease and/or pathological process, and (3) assess the accuracy of the clinical diagnosis and the effectiveness or success of the treatment. Necropsy may also need to be performed for medicolegal reasons. In these situations, however, it may be better to submit the animal to a qualified veterinary pathologist. This is important, especially if a particular case were to be challenged in court.

Because the postmortem examination involves dissection of the body and organs and recognition of pathological changes in the tissues, systematic dissection techniques and a knowledge of anatomy are required. During necropsy, proper tissue samples are collected and submitted to the appropriate laboratories for further evaluation.

Knowledge gained through necropsy will aid and enhance the quality of the practice of veterinary medicine in the future.

> **TECHNICIAN NOTE**
>
> Knowledge gained through necropsy will aid and enhance the quality of the practice of veterinary medicine in the future.

PERFORMING THE NECROPSY

Records

The necropsy record is commonly overlooked or poorly completed by veterinarians. The most common excuse is "not enough time." If one is going to take time to do a necropsy, one should "take time" to write down the findings. The necropsy record is important for future reference, especially in medicolegal problems. Pathology or necropsy records should contain at least five items: (1) signalment, (2) anamnesis (history), (3) gross necropsy findings, (4) tentative diagnosis, and (5) tissues submitted to the laboratory.

The signalment should contain the owner's name, address, and telephone number and the animal's species, age, sex, and name. The signalment should also include the animal's clinical case number, date of death, postmortem interval (hours since death), date of necropsy, and necropsy number.

The anamnesis should contain a brief medical history, including clinical signs, duration of illness, and treatments. If the veterinarian is referring the animal to a pathologist and has a special dignostic request (e.g., removal of the spinal cord), this request may be stated in the anamnesis.

The next portion of the necropsy report should contain a brief gross description *(not interpretation)* of organs and lesions. The gross description should contain comments on size, shape, color, consistency, texture, and odor of all organs and a detailed description of all lesions. The last statement of the gross description should list the organs or tissues that were clinically suspected to be involved but are found to have no gross abnormalities.

After the gross description, a tentative diagnosis is made. The interpretation and discussion of lesions and the cause of death of the animal are stated here. The interpretation of lesions should *not* be included in the description of the gross findings.

Finally, a short note should be added if tissues are submitted to a laboratory for microbiological, toxicological, parasitological, or histopathological studies. If tissues are being sent to the laboratory, one copy of the necropsy report with a cover letter explaining specific requests should be mailed with the tissues. Another copy of the necropsy report should be placed with the medical record of that particular animal. (Additional information concerning the medical record can be found in Chapter 4.)

Fixatives

If the veterinarian requests histopathological studies on tissues from the case, the tissues must be properly preserved. *Fixatives* are chemicals that preserve the natural architecture of tissues by causing alteration of proteins, lipids, and carbohydrates and thus prevent *autolysis* (self-destruction). For histopathological studies to be of value, tissues must be taken as soon as possible after death and must be properly fixed. If an animal has been dead for longer than 24 hours or has been exposed to the sun for several hours, autolysis of the tissues will prevent meaningful histopathological studies. The size of tissue to be fixed in the fixative is also important. Tissues should not be more than 0.5 cm thick. The only exception is when fixing brain (which should be hemisected and placed in formalin), eye, and lung tissue.

TECHNICIAN NOTE

If an animal has been dead for more than 24 hours or has been exposed to the sun for several hours, autolysis of the tissues will prevent meaningful histopathological studies.

The most practical fixative for the practicing veterinarian is 10% neutral buffered formalin (formalin can be used for all tissues). Formalin is actually a 3.7% formaldehyde solution and is acidic. The solution has to be buffered to pH 7 or it will cause acid digestion of tissues. Formalin can be easily made and, in tightly closed containers, has a shelf life of a minimum of 6 to 8 months. All solid tissues should be 0.5 cm or less in thickness when placed in the formalin. The total volume of formalin to solid tissues should be approximately 10:1. The 10:1 ratio will allow proper fixation of tissues. If too much tissue is placed in the formalin, the tissues will tie up all of the fixative, leaving some of the tissue unfixed. This unfixed tissue will then undergo autolysis.

Other fixatives of which the veterinary technician should be aware are *Zenker's* and *Bouin's fixatives*. Zenker's is an excellent fixative for eyes, but to benefit from this rapid fixative the eyes should be placed in it within 10 to 15 minutes after death; otherwise formalin is as effective. Bouin's is the preferred fixative for reproductive organ tissues. Neither Zenker's nor Bouin's is recommended for use in private practice because of the involved fixation procedures and cumbersome disposal requirements of the chemicals involved. All fixatives must be clearly labeled, and the proper precautions must be taken to

• Table 30–1 •

FORMULATION FOR FORMALIN, ZENKER'S, AND BOUIN'S SOLUTIONS	
BUFFERED NEUTRAL FORMALIN SOLUTION	
37–40% formalin	100.0 ml
Distilled water	900.0 ml
Sodium phosphate monobasic	4.0 g
Sodium phosphate dibasic (anhydrous)	6.5 g
ZENKER'S SOLUTION*	
Distilled water	1000.0 ml
Mercuric chloride	50.0 g
Potassium dichromate	25.0 g
Sodium sulfate	10.0 g
BOUIN'S SOLUTION	
Picric acid, saturated aqueous solution	750.0 ml
37–40% formalin	250.0 ml
Glacial acetic acid	50.0 ml

*Add 5 ml of glacial acetic acid to 95 ml of Zenker's solution before use. The solution does not keep well after the addition of the acetic acid.

avoid direct contact with these chemicals. See Table 30–1 for formulation of the fixatives.

Equipment

The equipment used for necropsies includes three major categories: (1) protective clothing, (2) instruments and tools, and (3) fixatives. Protective clothing should be worn during every necropsy and includes coveralls or aprons, rubber gloves, and boots. Some infectious diseases are transmissible from animals to humans (zoonotic diseases). When performing a necropsy on animals suspected of a zoonotic disease, including birds (especially psittacines), a mask should be worn in addition to the routine protective clothing and gloves.

TECHNICIAN NOTE

When performing a necropsy on animals suspected of a zoonotic disease, including birds (especially psittacines), a mask should be worn in addition to the routine protective clothing and gloves.

The instruments needed to do a necropsy for both large and small animals include knives, scalpels, scissors, forceps, and saws of various sizes and shapes (Fig. 30–1). Knives should be kept sharp. Dull knives tend to tear and compress tissue and cause compression artifacts on histopathological study. The prosector also has to apply more pressure for cutting, and one is more apt to cut oneself when using a dull knife. Cleavers or saws can be used for removing the brain or spinal cord. Pruning shears intended for cutting branches from trees are useful for cutting ribs of large and small animals. Necropsies should be done in areas that are easily cleaned and disinfected and *not* in surgery or treatment rooms.

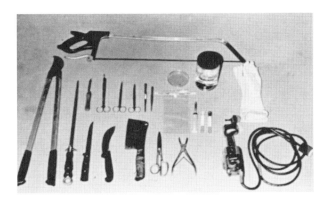

Figure 30-1. Instruments and equipment commonly used during a necropsy include saws, knives, scalpels, forceps, formalin, and gloves.

A covered instrument tray filled with disinfectant, containing scissors, forceps, and scalpels, should be kept near the necropsy table for collection of sterile samples for microbiology (see Chapter 8). Properly labeled fixatives and collection bottles should also be available for tissue samples.

General Procedure

An important point to remember about a necropsy is that autolysis begins immediately after the animal dies; therefore, necropsy should be done immediately after the death of the animal. If it cannot be done immediately, the carcass should be refrigerated. The carcass should not be frozen if a meaningful histopathological evaluation is desired. Freezing disrupts cells by crystallization and melting of intracellular water. In general, the longer you wait to do a necropsy following the death of an animal, the less information the necropsy will provide. Before the necropsy is started, the signalment and anamnesis should be reviewed.

TECHNICIAN NOTE

In general, the longer you wait to do a necropsy following the death of an animal, the less information the necropsy will provide.

There are various techniques for doing a necropsy. The veterinary technician should develop a standard technique that allows examination of all organs and meets the requirements of the veterinarian. The prosector should have a knowledge of anatomy, including normal size, shape, color, consistency, texture, and odor of all major organs. At first, the veterinary technician should follow a step-by-step outline of a necropsy. As the technician gains experience, some alteration in the basic outline may become necessary to check for specific lesions.

Necropsy Technique for the Cow

The animal that most commonly undergoes necropsy by veterinarians is the cow. The reason is the "herd health approach" to bovine medicine. If a farmer has several sick calves, several

morbid calves will often be presented for necropsy so a definite etiological diagnosis can be determined. After necropsy, the veterinarian will usually be able to provide information on prevention of the disease and specific treatments for the other sick calves.

TECHNICIAN NOTE

The animal that most commonly undergoes necropsy by veterinarians is the cow.

Position

Most ruminants (cattle, goats, sheep) are positioned with the left side down because the rumen is on the left side and if the animal is examined from the right side, the internal organs are more easily visualized. Before the animal is opened, all external surfaces should be examined carefully with special attention to eyes, ears, nose, feet, anus, and hocks. For example, a calf with staining of the hocks and tail region with feces suggests scours. This would provide additional insight into the problem and may suggest tissues that need to be taken for histopathological and microbiological studies before opening the carcass. After the external examination, the right forelimb and hindlimb are reflected dorsally until they lie flat on the floor (Fig. 30–2). Reflection of the limbs may be accomplished by raising the leg and cutting the axillary muscles of the forelimb and by cutting the muscles, joint capsule, and round ligament of the coxofemoral (hip) joint of the hindlimb. As the limbs are reflected, the brachial plexus of the forelimb and the sciatic nerve of the hindlimb are examined. After reflection of limbs, the skin is incised from the chin to the anus along the ventral midline, circumventing the umbilicus, adult female mammary glands, and external genitalia. The skin on the right side is reflected to the dorsal midline throughout the entire length of the body (Fig. 30–3). The exposed right side of the animal, muscles, and external lymph nodes should be checked. If the animal is an adult female, the mammary glands, including the mammary lymph nodes, are removed from the carcass and examined.

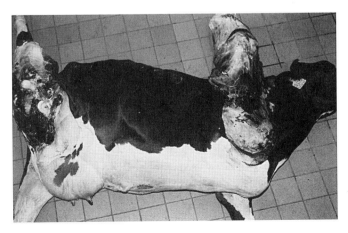

Figure 30-2. The left forelimb and hindlimb have been reflected in this cow.

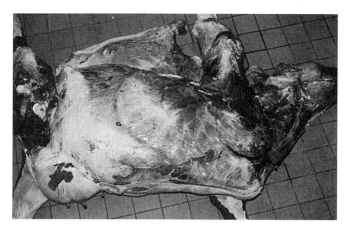

Figure 30-3. The left side limbs and skin have been reflected in this cow.

Exposure of Abdominal and Thoracic Cavities

The abdominal cavity is opened by making an incision through the abdominal wall, starting behind the ribs down to the sternum and then posteriorly along the ventral aspects of the vertebrae (dorsal flank region) down to the pelvic rim. This creates a large abdominal wall flap. This flap is reflected downward. Opening the carcass in this manner allows replacement of the viscera back into the carcass and reattachment of the abdominal wall flap to the vertebrae. This technique will allow easier removal of the carcass from the rancher's pasture.

Once the viscera are exposed (Fig. 30–4), they should be examined for size, position, adhesions, and so forth. The prosector should run his or her hand between the reticulum and the diaphragm in adult cattle to check for adhesions (hardware disease). Next, the diaphragm may be punctured with a knife, and the prosector should listen for the inflow of air into the thoracic cavity. An animal with pneumonia or *pneumothorax* (air in the thoracic cavity) will have a reduced amount of negative pressure within the thoracic cavity. This will result in reduced sounds of inflowing air. Next, the entire right side of the diaphragm is cut along its costal arch to allow observation of the thoracic cavity. Now, using the pruning shears, the dorsal ends of the ribs are cut along the angle of the ribs starting from the thirteenth rib, and then the sternocostal junctions are cut, allowing the rib cage to be removed (Fig. 30–5).

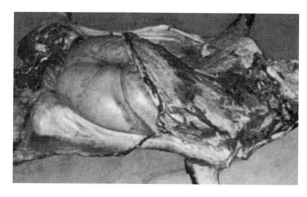

Figure 30-4. Skin reflected, abdominal flap removed, and viscera exposed in a cow.

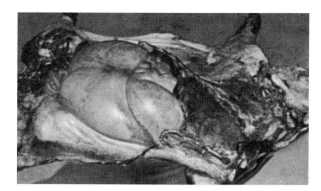

Figure 30-5. Skin reflected and abdominal flap and rib cage removed to expose viscera, lungs, and heart in a cow.

The thoracic and abdominal cavities are now exposed, and all organs are inspected in situ for displacement, size, shape, and color. If organs are noted to be abnormal and cultures are desired, now is the best time to take the samples, before tissues are handled and further contaminated. For example, if a pneumonic lung is observed, the culture should be taken before removal from the thoracic cavity. All microbiological specimens should be taken with sterile instruments and placed in sterile containers (see Chapter 8).

Removal of Primary Organs

The viscera are now removed from the abdominal cavity. First, take four pieces of string and double ligate the terminal rectum and proximal duodenum. After transecting the rectum and duodenum between the double ligatures, begin to pull out the small intestine. Remove the mesentery and cut the attachments to the liver. Next, remove the liver and set it aside. Remove the rumen by pulling it ventrally and cutting its dorsal attachments. Another double ligature is placed around the esophagus as it enters the rumen, thus preventing spillage of rumen contents into the thoracic cavity when transected. The spleen will be attached to the dorsal left side of the rumen and will be removed with the rumen. The urinary and reproductive systems and adrenal glands remain in the abdominal cavity. These systems are removed en masse and are set aside for further examination. The *pluck* (includes tongue, esophagus, thyroid glands, trachea, lungs, thymus, and heart) is removed en masse and set aside. This is done by incising the medial side of both mandibles close to the bone; this will free the tongue. Next, pull the tongue downward to the hyoid bones, cutting through the large prominent keratoepihyoid joints of the hyoid bones. The teeth and hard and soft palates should now be examined. Continue to pull the tongue and trachea posteriorly and cut the tissue between the aorta and the ventral aspects of the vertebrae. Continue the cut between the mediastinum and pericardial sac to the sternum, transecting the aorta, vena cava, and esophagus at the level of the diaphragm.

 TECHNICIAN NOTE

The *pluck* includes the tongue, esophagus, thyroid glands, trachea, lungs, thymus, and heart.

Head

The head is removed by extending the head and transecting the ventral neck muscles down to the level of the atlanto-occipital joint. If cerebral spinal fluid is needed, insert a needle attached to a syringe into the subdural space of the spinal cord and collect the sample. Often, 10 to 12 ml of clear cerebrospinal fluid may be obtained in this way. Next, cut the ventral ligaments of the atlanto-occipital joint, transect the spinal cord, and cut the dorsal ligaments of the joint and the dorsal neck muscles. The oral cavity and teeth should be examined at this time. Place the head aside.

Musculoskeletal System

The muscles of the hindlegs and the forelegs are incised several times and carefully evaluated for muscular lesions. At this time, the prescapular lymph nodes (just anterior to the midscapular region), prefemoral lymph nodes (just anterior and dorsal to the stifle joints), and popliteal lymph nodes (under the ventral aspects of the semitendinous and semimembranous muscles and adjacent to the sciatic nerve and femoral artery) are checked. Stifle and hock joints should be opened in both hindlimbs and at least the carpal joints of the forelimbs should be opened. If joint lesions are found, all joints should be opened. If a culture of joint fluid is needed, open the joint by first cutting the skin over the joint with a clean knife (Fig. 30–6) and then using a sterile scalpel to cut the joint capsule. Open the joint and swab the inside, being careful not to touch the cut edges of the joint capsule (Fig. 30–7).

The internal organs are now examined carefully. The order in which they are examined is a matter of personal preference. For the sake of organization, the techniques used to examine organ systems will be described in the following order: head; lungs, trachea, and thyroid glands; thymus and heart; great vessels and esophagus; liver and gallbladder; spleen; kidneys, adrenal glands, and bladder; genital organs, small and large

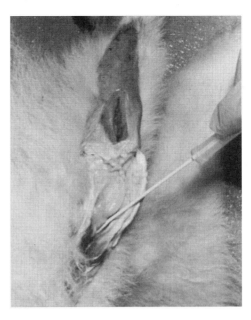

Figure 30–7. The stifle joint is opened, and a culture is taken.

intestines; and pancreas, mesenteric lymph nodes, and forestomachs.

Eyes

The skin over the cranium and around the eyes is removed, leaving the skin around the nose. The skin is left around the nose to enable the prosector to hold the head with more stability. The eyes are removed by grasping the skin that is left around the eyes or the conjunctiva with a pair of forceps and then cutting the loose tissue around the eye with a sharp pair of scissors. The ocular muscles, vessels, and optic nerve are cut, and the entire eyeball is removed. For best fixation, remove all of the loose tissue and muscles from the eyeball. If there are lesions in the eyes or if the animal was known to be blind, the eyes should be removed first. If the animal died by euthanasia, the eyes should be removed within 3 to 5 minutes after euthanasia and placed in Zenker's solution. If the postmortem interval is beyond 20 to 30 minutes, the eyes can be fixed in formalin. If the animal has cataracts, the best fixative is formalin, regardless of the postmortem interval.

 TECHNICIAN NOTE

The eyes should be removed within 3 to 5 minutes after euthanasia and placed in Zenker's solution.

Brain

The brain is removed by cutting away all of the major muscle masses covering the lateral aspect of the cranium (Fig. 30–8). Using a cleaver or saw, two parallel cuts are made, starting at the upper lateral edge of the foramen magnum and progressing anterior to the cranial aspects of the eye sockets. The anterior portions of this cut should be connected. As these two parallel

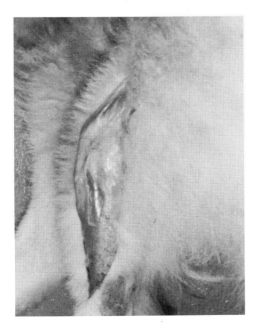

Figure 30–6. Skin is cut, exposing the stifle joint for a joint culture.

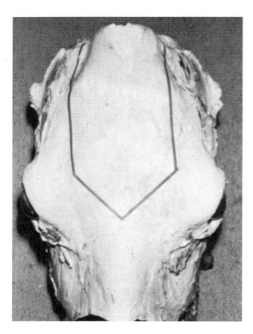

Figure 30-8. Skin reflected from the skull of a cow. The line indicates the location of the skull cut.

cuts are connected, the frontal sinuses will be entered. These structures should be inspected before cutting the bony covering of the brain. After the bony cap is removed (sometimes prying the bony cap with a screwdriver or the tip of the cleaver is helpful), the dura should be cut. Sometimes (especially in young animals), one has to cut the dura as the bony cap is being removed (Fig. 30–9). Make sure that you cut the tentorium cerebelli (the thick portion of dura between the cerebrum and the cerebellum) before removing the brain. If the tentorium cerebelli is not cut, the brain cannot be removed intact and will be divided between the cerebrum and the cerebellum. Now

that the dura and tentorium cerebelli have been incised and removed, grasp the head by the nose and hold it upright. Tap the head lightly on the chopping block to loosen the brain. If brain cultures are desired, they should be taken before removing the brain from the skull. Cultures should include the subdural space, especially around the optic chiasma. Tilt the head backward to allow the brain to roll out of the cranial vault. The optic and remaining cranial nerves must be severed to allow removal of the brain from the skull. Care must be taken not to let the brain drop on the table or on the floor. If histopathological study only is to be done, the whole brain is placed in 3 to 4 liters of formalin. The brain. may be hemisected by cutting along the longitudinal fissure; one half is placed in formalin and the other half is submitted for toxicological, virological, and bacteriological studies. The pituitary gland, gasserian ganglion (fifth cranial nerve), and cerebral retes should be removed and placed in formalin. These structures are removed by making a cut posterior to the optic chiasma lateral to the left and right gasserian ganglion and posterior to the pituitary gland. With a pair of forceps, grasp the dura covering the gasserian ganglion and pull upward, using a scalpel to cut the tissue away from the nerve and the anterior aspect of the fifth cranial nerve as it enters the foramen on both sides. Then peel out the square of tissue that contains the pituitary gland in the center surrounded by the cerebral retes and the gasserian ganglion.

Pluck

The pluck (tongue, esophagus, trachea, thyroid glands, parathyroid glands, thymus, heart, great vessels, and lungs) is examined next (Fig. 30–10). First, locate the thymus gland. In young animals, the thymus is large and located anterior to the heart under the left apical lobe of the lungs. In ruminants (cattle, goats, and sheep), a large portion of the thymus is located on the ventral aspect of the trachea and can extend to the thyroid glands. The tongue is incised at 1-cm intervals and is inspected. The thyroid and parathyroid glands located just posterior to the larynx should be checked. The esophagus is opened and inspected from the oral cavity to the rumen. The trachea is opened along its dorsal aspects down to the bifurcation. The lungs and pleura are inspected. The lungs are examined by palpation. The lungs should be light pink, soft, and spongy, and the pleura should be shiny and smooth. Red, rubbery lungs

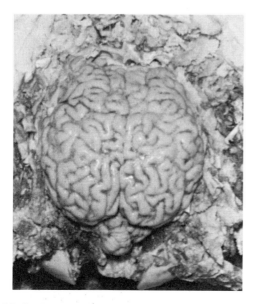

Figure 30-9. Bony cap of the skull and dura removed from a cow to expose the brain.

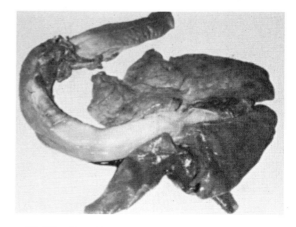

Figure 30-10. The pluck includes the tongue, esophagus, trachea, thyroid glands, thymus, heart, and lungs.

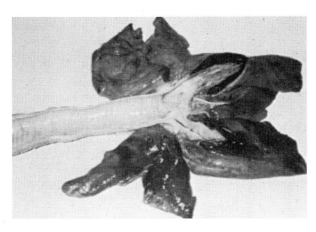

Figure 30-11. Lungs with trachea and main stem bronchi opened for inspection.

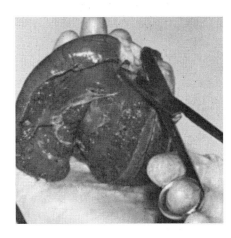

Figure 30-13. After opening of the right ventricle, the pulmonary artery is opened.

usually are edematous and congested. Firm, dark red lungs are usually pneumonic. In bovines, the pleura covering the dorsal aspects of the diaphragmatic lobes is normally thick and opaque. Remove both lungs from the heart and dissect out the aorta. Using scissors, open the trachea, main stem bronchi, and the smaller air passages of the lung (Fig. 30–11). Locate the thick-walled artery and, using scissors, open this vessel and check for emboli. Locate the large, thin-walled pulmonary veins and cut along these vessels, checking for thrombi. If histopathological studies are desired on the lungs, use a pair of forceps to grasp a small portion of lung tissue and, using a sharp scalpel, remove a small wedge of lung parenchyma. Do not squeeze lung tissue to be examined histopathologically, since this causes extensive artifacts.

TECHNICIAN NOTE

Do not squeeze lung tissue to be examined histopathologically, since this causes extensive artifacts.

Heart

If you are right-handed, hold the heart in the left hand so the right ventricle is on your left. The fat encircling the coronary vessels should be checked. An animal that has had a chronic disease or has been in a malnourished condition will have serous atrophy of fat around the coronary vessels instead of white opaque fat. The heart is opened in the same sequence as the flow of blood. The right atrium is opened and inspected. The atrioventricular valves are checked. The right ventricle is opened by starting in the opened right atrium (Fig. 30–12), cutting along the interventricular septum to the tip of the ventricle and then upward and into the pulmonary artery outflow tract (Fig. 30–13). The atrioventricular valves can be more closely inspected now. One should look into the pulmonary artery to check for stenosis (narrowing of the lumen) or other lesions before cutting through it. Now cut through the semilunar valves and up the pulmonary artery. The left atrium is now opened, and the left atrioventricular valves are inspected. The left ventricle is opened by making a straight incision from the atrioventricular valve down to the tip of the heart. The aorta is opened by inserting scissors under the medial cusp of the left atrioventricular valve (Fig. 30–14). As you are opening the aorta, turn the scissors slightly to the right or clockwise; this is done

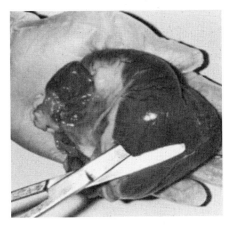

Figure 30-12. The right atria and ventricle are opened first during examination of the heart.

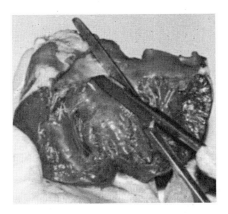

Figure 30-14. The aorta is opened by inserting scissors under the medial cusp of the left atrioventricular valves and cutting upward.

to avoid cutting through the orifice of the ductus arteriosus. The semilunar valves of the aorta should be examined. The atrial septum should be checked for an open foramen ovale, and the ventricular septum should be checked for septal defects. Among the more common heart defects in cattle are high ventricular septal defects. Check the orifices of the left and right coronary arteries (just under the semilunar valves of the aorta). Now make multiple cuts in the myocardium, checking for small foci of degeneration or necrosis. If no lesions are found in the heart, and a section is desired for histopathological study, a small section of the left papillary myocardium is the best place to sample.

Liver and Gallbladder

The liver is examined by first inspecting the capsule and external surfaces. The gallbladder is opened, and its mucosal surface is examined. Remember, an animal that has not eaten for several days before death will have a distended gallbladder filled with thick green bile. To check for a swollen liver, make one deep cut into the parenchyma and wait 10 to 15 seconds; then try to appose the tissue back together. If the liver is swollen, the cut edges below the capsule will bulge, and the cut edges will not match, whereas if cellular swelling is not present, the cut edges will match. The texture of the liver is evaluated by making two deep cuts into the liver parenchyma approximately 0.5 cm in thickness. Using the thumb and forefinger, squeeze the tissue between your fingers. A liver from an animal with chronic heart failure (as with high mountain disease) will be firm. However, the texture of a liver from a cow with ketosis (fatty liver) will be soft and greasy. The portal and hepatic veins should be opened and checked for thrombosis. Next, with the liver lying flat on a table, make multiple incisions into the parenchyma approximately 1 cm in thickness. This opens the organ, exposing internal lesions. If histopathological studies are desired, a small wedge of liver tissue, including the capsule, should be placed in formalin.

 TECHNICIAN NOTE

An animal that has not eaten for several days before death will have a distended gallbladder filled with thick green bile.

Spleen

The spleen should be examined next. The technique for inspecting the spleen is similar to that for inspecting the liver—that is, multiple cuts are made throughout the organ, thus exposing the internal parenchyma. A small wedge of spleen should be taken for histopathological study.

Adrenal Glands

The adrenal glands should still be attached to the anterior pole of the kidneys. The size and shape of the adrenal glands should be noted, and multiple incisions should be made through each organ. Hemorrhagic adrenal glands are often found in calves that have died of acute endotoxemia and scours. Animals that have undergone extensive chronic stress usually have bilateral enlargement of the adrenal glands.

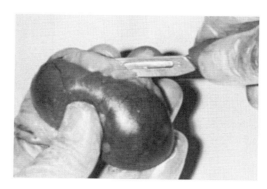

Figure 30-15. The kidney is incised longitudinally down to the renal pelvis.

Kidneys

Examine the external surface of both kidneys. Open the kidney longitudinally (Fig. 30–15), extending the incision to the level of the renal pelvis (Fig. 30–16). Inspect the parenchyma. To check for swelling, fold the kidney back together. The cut surfaces should match. If the cut surfaces do not match but bulge instead, this indicates that the organ is swollen. A small wedge of kidney including capsule, cortex, medulla, and pelvis is taken for histopathological study. Next, the capsule is peeled from both kidneys, and the organ is sectioned in multiple areas. The parenchyma can then be examined thoroughly. With a small pair of scissors, open both ureters. Open the urinary bladder and examine the mucosal surface. Extend the incision through the trigone of the bladder down through the urethra.

Reproductive Tract

In the male, both testicles should be opened and multiple incisions made in both organs so that the inner parenchyma can be examined. The penis and prepuce should be examined and the urethra opened to the glans penis. In females, the vagina and uterus should be opened. Both ovaries should be incised multiple times to inspect the inner parenchyma. The vulva should be checked for lesions also.

Alimentary System

Examination of the alimentary tract is performed as the last major procedure of necropsy to prevent fecal contamination of

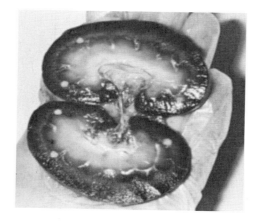

Figure 30-16. A kidney opened and ready for inspection.

tissues and instruments. The alimentary tract is removed from the abdominal cavity in two parts. One part contains the small and large intestines, and the other the rumen, reticulum, omasum, and abomasum. The small and large intestinal tracts are usually examined first. The intestine is removed from its mesenteric attachment and is laid out on the floor. While this is being done, the mesenteric lymph nodes are examined. Next, the intestine is opened. This is best done with a pair of enterotome scissors (scissors made for opening the intestine) over a garbage can. As the prosector opens the intestine, lesions such as ulcers, parasites, necrosis of Peyer's patches, and so on should be noted.

The rumen, reticulum, omasum, and abomasum are opened along the greater curvature of each compartment. The luminal contents are examined for parasites, toxic plants, and foreign bodies as well as for composition and consistency. The mucosal surfaces are checked carefully for lesions such as ulcers and parasites.

Spinal Cord

The spinal cord is the most commonly overlooked system because of the difficulty in removing it. The easiest method to remove the spinal cord on a bovine is to first remove all of the muscles on the right side of the spinal column from the neck to the pelvis. Next, using a large cleaver, cut away the lateral aspects of the cervical, thoracic, and lumbar vertebrae. Be careful as you near the spinal cord not to crush the cord with the cleaver. The entire cord can be exposed with the use of the cleaver. Using a pair of forceps, grasp the dura over the anterior aspect of the spinal cord and pull upward. Use a scalpel or pair of scissors, or both, to cut the left spinal cord nerves and gently pull the spinal cord upward.

Necropsy Technique for the Horse

The basic technique for doing a necropsy on a horse is similar to that for a cow; only the variations will be covered in this section. The prosector should refer to necropsy technique for the cow for a more detailed description of the examination of individual organs. If the horse is undergoing necropsy for insurance purposes, photographs of the entire horse should be taken for proof of identification. The inner lips and ears should be checked for tattoos. In gross necropsy reports of such cases, all identifying marks, such as white socks on specific feet, stars, and tattoo numbers, should be included.

> #### TECHNICIAN NOTE
> Horses should be placed with the right side down (just the opposite of cattle).

Horses should be placed with the right side down (just the opposite of cattle). This allows the best exposure of the spleen, stomach, and large colon. The external parts (especially all orifices) should be examined first. If sections of skin are needed, they should be collected. The animal is opened, as is the cow, by reflecting the limbs and then the skin on the left side of the body. The abdominal wall and rib cage are removed

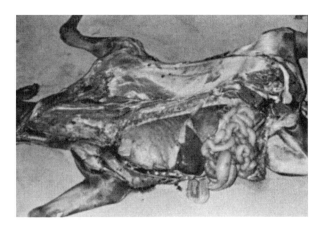

Figure 30-17. Skin reflected, abdominal wall and rib cage removed, and left limbs reflected to expose the thoracic cavity and viscera of a foal.

(Fig. 30–17). The best time to examine proper locations of internal organs and displacement or torsions is immediately after exposure of the internal organs. Any specific cultures that are needed for microbiological procedures should be taken at this time to help prevent contamination.

It is usually easier to remove first the abdominal organs and then the thoracic organs. After opening the abdominal cavity and exposing the abdominal viscera, check the intestines for torsions or displacements. Discoloration of the wall and disorganization of the arrangement of organs are usually the first clue of displacement. Sometimes, the large bowel is so filled with gas that the organs immediately bulge out of the abdominal cavity. When this happens, several small holes may be punctured in the wall of the large colon to deflate the distended bowel. After visual inspection for the location of organs within the abdominal cavity, the bowel and mesenteric attachments should be palpated in search of twists or torsions.

Next, the abdominal organs are removed in a systematic fashion. First, grasp the pelvic flexure on the left side located just anterior to the pelvic inlet. Pull the pelvic flexure outward, thus removing the entire large colon. Place the large colon at right angles to the body. This allows a good view of this organ. Vessels of the large colon can be examined now. The spleen is removed and examined. The left adrenal gland and kidneys are now removed and examined. The abdominal aorta is exposed and opened in its entirely. One should also dissect the anterior celiac and mesenteric arteries to check for verminous arteritis resulting from *Strongylus vulgaris*.

Next, the terminal ends of both esophagus and rectum are located, doubly ligated, and transected. The entire gastrointestinal (GI) tract is removed from the abdominal cavity by pulling and cutting the attachments to the liver and body wall. The ileum may be located just as it enters into the cecum. The ileum has a much thicker wall than the remaining small intestine. The small intestine is now traced proximally to the duodenum and stripped from its mesenteric attachments. The liver can be removed and examined. The right adrenal gland and kidney are removed and examined. The urinary bladder and genital organs are removed and examined.

Removal of the pluck is more difficult in the horse because of the long, narrow mandible. Removal of the tongue and pharynx is facilitated by separating the left and right mandible by cutting the mandibular symphysis with a cleaver or saw. The teeth and the hard and soft palates are examined. The tongue, pharynx, and trachea are then pulled caudally, and the heart and lungs are removed as in the cow. The thyroid glands are checked at this time. It is difficult to remove the heart with the intact pericardial sac. Thus, if excessive pericardial fluids or specific lesions within the pericardial sac are noted, the prosector should open the pericardial sac while the heart is still in the thoracic cavity. Otherwise, when the heart is pulled out with the lungs, the pericardial sac will tear, and the fluid within the sac will be lost.

The inner surfaces of the thoracic and abdominal cavities can now be examined for puncture wounds, such as bullet holes.

Large incisions should be made in all major muscle masses to search for lesions deep in muscles. Keep in mind that intramuscular injections (especially antibiotics) can cause massive areas of necrosis. All joints should be opened and examined. Removal of the head and brain is similar to their removal in the cow. Because the pituitary gland is much larger than in the cow and most of the organ is not covered by dura, it is slightly more difficult to remove the pituitary gland and gasserian ganglion. However, it can be removed with the same technique described for cattle, but additional care should be taken.

The animal's individual organs—that is, heart, lungs, brain, liver, kidney, endocrine glands, and lymphohemopoietic and reproductive organs—are evaluated as described for cattle. The only major difference is the examination of the digestive system. The stomach should be opened above its greater curvature. Common lesions in the stomach are small ulcers due to stomach bots (*Gasterophilus*) and small abscesses just below the margo plicatus caused by *Habronema* spp. The small intestine, small colon, large colon, and cecum should be opened and their mucosal surfaces examined. It is common to see multiple, small 1- to 3-mm lymphoid nodules within the mucosa of the large bowel in horses with moderate to heavy parasite loads.

Necropsy Technique for Small Animals

Most of the necropsy procedures for small animals are similar to the procedure for the cow, except for positioning and the initial removal of organs. The necropsy technique used on the dog will be described; this same technique can be used for other monogastrics, such as cats, ferrets, pigs, and rodents.

The initial step is to examine the skin thoroughly on both sides and especially around the head, neck, ears, paws, and perineum, checking for lesions such as lacerations or swelling (abscesses or tumors). The mouth and teeth should be examined next. If ocular lesions are suspected, the eyes should be

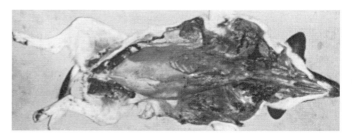

Figure 30-19. The skin is now reflected down to the back of the dog, exposing the chest and abdominal wall.

removed first. If the animal died by euthanasia, the eyes should be fixed in Zenker's solution. If the dog has cataracts, the fixative of choice is formalin, regardless of whether the dog died by euthanasia.

Position and Initial Exposure

The animal is now placed on its back, and an incision is made through the axillary region and muscular attachments of the scapula bilaterally. Another incision is made in each groin area through the muscles of the hindlimbs, transecting the coxofemoral joint capsule and round ligament of each hip. All four legs should now be lying flat on the table, thus stabilizing the carcass. An incision is then made from chin to anus (Fig. 30–18). The skin is reflected on both sides of the animal nearly to the back (Fig. 30–19). Another technique commonly used on small animals is to first make the incision from chin to anus (Fig. 30–20) and then reflect the skin, cut the muscular attachments to the scapula and disarticulate the hip joints, in that sequence (Fig. 30–21). Peripheral lymph nodes should now be examined, especially the prefemoral, prescapular, and popliteal nodes.

The abdominal cavity is opened by starting an incision at the pubis, incising along the lateral abdominal wall, and ending in the center of the last rib. When this incision is made on both sides, and this flap of abdominal muscle is reflected cranially, one can visualize the size, shape, and location of most of the abdominal organs (Fig. 30–22). A small stab incision is made in the diaphragm on both sides to check for negative pressure. Dogs that have been hit by cars commonly have fractured ribs and pneumothorax. With the pruning shears (or scissors, depending on the size of the animal), the ribs are cut in the midregion starting with the last rib and progressing to the first rib. The ribs and sternum are removed. The entire abdominal cavity and thoracic cavity are now open (Fig. 30–23). This complete exposure allows close examination of the organs

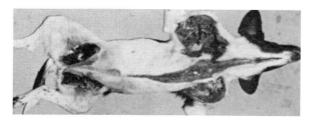

Figure 30-18. All four limbs have been cut and laid flat on the table. An incision is made from the chin to the anus of a dog.

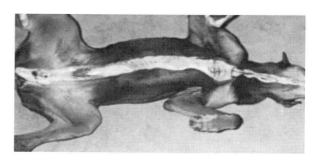

Figure 30-20. Dog with primary skin incision from chin to anus.

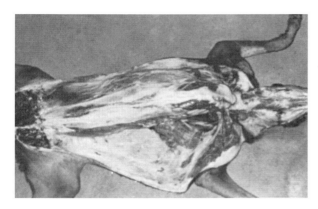

Figure 30-21. Skin and limbs reflected, of a dog. The abdominal chest wall is thus exposed.

without moving them (checking for displacement, tumors, and so forth) and also allows collection of microbiological samples.

Internal Organs

The sequence for removal of internal organs varies with the pathologist and the observation of various lesions during the initial inspection. For the sake of organization, the sequence that follows will be used. Double ligate the terminal rectum if the animal had diarrhea; otherwise, transect the rectum without ligation. Hold the rectum with one hand and begin to pull it out of the abdominal cavity. With scissors, cut the mesenteric attachments of the intestine. While removing the intestines from the abdominal cavity, inspect the mesenteric lymph nodes. As the duodenum is approached, the pancreas will be found. Inspect this organ carefully; pancreatitis is a common disease in dogs. Continue to remove the small intestine, including the stomach. Double ligate the esophagus just behind the diaphragm and anterior to the stomach. Cut between the ligatures. The digestive system from the stomach to the anus can be removed and set aside for further examination. The liver and spleen are removed and set aside. The pelvis is cut so that the kidneys, adrenal glands, ureters, bladder, and female genital organs can be removed en masse. With males, the genital organs usually remain attached to the carcass.

The pluck (tongue, trachea, thyroid, parathyroid glands, esophagus, lungs, and heart) is removed as described for the bovine. As the tongue is removed, tonsils and teeth should be carefully examined. The head is removed as described for the cow.

All muscles should be examined carefully by making incisions deep into the muscle masses. All joints should be opened

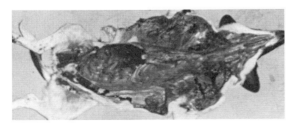

Figure 30-22. Skin and limbs reflected and abdominal wall removed to expose the abdominal cavity of a dog.

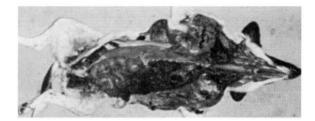

Figure 30-23. Skin and limbs reflected with abdominal and chest wall removed to expose the thoracic and abdominal organs of a dog.

and examined. The stifle joints and both anterior cruciate ligaments should be given special attention in the dog (especially in the smaller breeds, such as the poodle).

Head

The head is examined in a manner similar to that used for the cow. The skin and muscles covering the skull are removed; this exposes the salivary glands and parotid lymph nodes. These organs should be examined and several deep incisions made in order to check the inner parenchyma for cysts and tumors. The brain is removed by means of a small cleaver or stryker saw. In small dogs, a pair of bone rongeurs may be used to easily remove the brain. The pituitary gland and gasserian ganglion are removed as described for the the horse. Remember that the gasserian ganglion is an important tissue to examine histopathologically for the presence of rabies. For rabies diagnosis, the veterinarian should submit either the entire head or one half of the brain frozen and one half of the brain in formalin to a local diagnostic laboratory. The frontal sinuses should be opened and examined, especially in pigs, to check for atrophic rhinitis.

 TECHNICIAN NOTE

For rabies diagnosis, the veterinarian should submit either the entire head or one half of the brain frozen and one half of the brain in formalin to a local diagnostic laboratory.

Pluck

The lungs, trachea, esophagus, parathyroid, thyroid, and thymus should be examined as described for cattle. In dogs, the parathyroid glands are more prominent and should be checked, especially in older dogs with chronic renal problems.

Heart

The heart, great vessels, and valves should be examined. The right and left atrioventricular valves should be carefully checked because of the common problem of degenerative lesions (valvular endocarditis) within the valve leaflets in older dogs. Occasionally, a chorda tendineae cordis is ruptured, and this must be checked before the ventricle is opened. The method to check a ruptured chorda tendineae cordis is to open the atrium only. Then the clotted blood is washed from the ventricle, and the ventricle is filled with water. Using the hands, the ventricle is compressed from the bottom upward. If the chordae tendineae cordis are ruptured, they will flow up and be visualized. This method also helps to evaluate competence of the valves, especially in cases with valvular endocarditis. The heart should now be open as described for cattle. The heart should be incised in 0.5- to 0.75-cm-thick pieces to examine the inner myocardium. Occasionally, dogs with diabetes will have atherosclerosis of coronary vessels, which may result in myocardial infarction.

Urogenital and Digestive Tract

The kidney, bladder, urethra, adrenal glands, and genital organs should be examined as described for cattle. In male dogs, the prostate gland (posterior to the trigone of the bladder as it enters the pelvic canal) should be carefully checked for neoplasia, hyperplasia, or infection. The digestive system is best examined by opening the stomach along its greater curvature, continuing through the pylorus and the intestinal tract along the mesenteric border to the anus. If there is suspicion that the dog has been poisoned, the stomach contents should be saved for analysis. The external surface of the pancreas is examined; then, multiple slices are made to inspect the inner parenchyma of the organ.

Cosmetic Necropsy

A procedure that is commonly requested for pet animals is a *cosmetic* necropsy. A cosmetic necropsy should be discouraged, because it precludes a thorough examination and may result in lesions being missed. A cosmetic necropsy is a postmortem examination done through a small abdominal incision similar to that made for a routine laparotomy. The animal is placed on its back, and a 10- to 12.5-cm incision (depending on the size of the animal) is made through the skin and linea alba of the abdominal wall. All of the abdominal organs are removed through this incision. Next, the hand is inserted into the empty abdominal cavity, the diaphragm is cut, and the heart and lungs are removed. The organs are now examined as described previously. The empty abdominal cavity is stuffed with paper to give the dog a "full appearance," and the abdominal incision is sutured.

> **TECHNICIAN NOTE**
>
> A cosmetic necropsy should be discouraged because it precludes a thorough examination and may result in lesions being missed.

The brain can be removed during a cosmetic necropsy. Wet the hair of the skull, part the hair, and make the skin incision from behind the eyes to the external occipital protuberance. Peel the skin laterally in both directions, separate the muscles of the jaw from the skull and, using a Stryker saw, remove the skull cap. With practice, the intact brain can be removed in this manner. The skull cap is now replaced; sometimes it helps if two small holes are made in the skull cap (one on each side), and an opposite hole is made in the lower portion of the skull. Using a small piece of wire or string, the skull cap can be secured. The skin is sutured, and the hair is flattened. If the eyes have to be removed during a cosmetic

necropsy, the eyelids should be sutured using a subcuticular suture pattern so that the suture is not observed.

The spinal cord can be removed during a cosmetic necropsy, but it is difficult and time consuming. The procedure is similar to removal of the brain. The dog is placed in ventral recumbency, and the hair over the back is moistened and then parted. An incision is made from the first cervical vertebra distad to the base of the tail. The skin is reflected 5 to 7.5 cm on each side of the incision down the carcass. The muscles of the spinal column are dissected from the bone. Using bone rongeurs or a Stryker saw, the dorsal wall, including the dorsal processes, is removed. The cord with the dorsal root ganglia can be removed. The muscles are put back in place, and the entire incision is sutured.

Necropsy Technique for Birds

Avian medicine (including caged-bird medicine and raptor rehabilitation) in the veterinary profession has greatly increased in the past 10 years. Veterinarians and veterinary technicians should be acquainted with a necropsy technique for birds. Remember that psittacine birds may have psittacosis (an important zoonotic disease of humans), and if this disease is suspected, the bird should not undergo necropsy by the veterinarian but should be mailed or hand-carried to the nearest state health department or state diagnostic laboratory.

> **TECHNICIAN NOTE**
>
> If psittacosis is suspected, the bird should be mailed or hand-carried to the nearest state health department or state diagnostic laboratory for necropsy.

The history should be carefully reviewed as with any necropsy. All psittacine birds should be dipped in a bucket of soapy water before necropsy. This is done for several reasons: one reason is that it wets the feathers and helps to prevent aerosolization of organisms that have dried on the feathers, especially *Chlamydia* (psittacosis). The external surfaces of the bird are examined with particular attention to the body orifices. The wings and legs are palpated to check for fractures.

Small birds may be placed on cardboard, and pins may be used to hold the wings open. The bird is placed on its back, and a line is made from the lower beak down over the keel to the cloaca by parting the wet feathers. An incision is made through the skin from the beak to the cloaca along this line. The skin is reflected on both sides, and the legs are disarticulated from the coxofemoral joints (Fig. 30–24). This provides good visualization of the pectoral muscles and abdominal wall. One blade of the scissors is inserted through the bird's mouth and into the pharynx. A cut is made down through the cervical esophagus and crop, thus exposing the upper digestive system. The abdominal wall is grasped with a pair of forceps, and a flap of abdominal wall is removed from the posterior tip of the keel to the cloaca. This exposure opens the abdominal cavity and abdominal air sacs. The sternum and pectoral muscles are removed by cutting through the ribs and coracoid bones with a heavy pair of scissors or poultry shears. As the sternum is removed, the thoracic air sacs, pericardium, heart, lungs, liver,

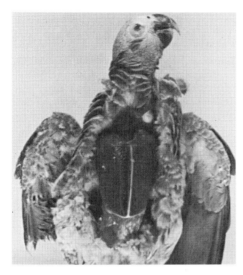

Figure 30-24. Skin is reflected from this African gray parrot to expose the chest muscles and abdominal wall.

thyroid, and parathyroid glands can be easily examined (Fig. 30–25). The heart is removed and examined first. The liver should be removed and examined. The spleen is best found by rotating the ventriculus outward and counterclockwise. The spleen is located at the junction of the proventriculus and ventriculus. The esophagus is grasped with forceps and is transected anterior to the proventriculus. The esophagus may be removed by pulling posteriorly. This results in removing the entire digestive system from esophagus to cloaca. Incise the skin around the external cloacal opening and set the digestive system en masse to the side. If histopathological study is desired on the lungs, kidneys, adrenal glands, and gonads of small birds, it is easier to leave these organs attached within the cavity of the bird. Place this mass of tissue in formalin intact. In larger birds, the lung should be removed. The kidneys, adrenal glands, and gonads are then removed en masse. The gonads are located on the anterior pole of the kidneys, and the adrenal

glands are just under the gonads. Remember that only the left ovary is present in birds. The brain is removed in a manner similar to that described for other animals, except that scissors only are needed to cut through the thin calvarium. The spinal cord is rarely examined in birds because of the difficulty of its removal. The easiest way to examine the spinal cord is to place the whole spinal column in formalin and let the cord fix; then, using bone rongeurs, cut the dorsal wall of the vertebral column and remove the fixed cord. This prevents destruction of the small, soft, unfixed spinal cord. All joints should be opened and slices made in muscle masses (pectoral, leg, and thigh muscles) to check for lesions. All internal organs are examined essentially as described for other animals.

COLLECTION OF SPECIMENS DURING A NECROPSY

Proper collection and identification of specimens during necropsy is a must; otherwise false laboratory results may follow. Some of this information has been covered in previous chapters, so only highlights are discussed here.

Clinical Pathology

Blood deteriorates rapidly after death, especially in large animals. One of the few tests that is somewhat accurate is the use of serum in serological tests for bacterial or viral diseases. This is probably good for the first 4 to 5 hours after death. The best place to obtain serum in an animal that has been dead for several hours is the atrium of the heart or the posterior vena cava. Urine is somewhat stable and can be collected from the bladder with a needle and syringe. If poisoning by ethylene glycol is suspected, urine should be collected from the dog or cat and submitted for analysis. Two common tests done on urine in large animals are ketone bodies (dairy cattle with ketosis) and glucose (lambs with *Clostridium perfringens* type D enterotoxemia). As with diabetes mellitus, a dog that has glucosuria will have a positive glucose test for several hours after death. Remember, however, that bacteria are in the bladder, and they will utilize glucose fairly rapidly.

> **TECHNICIAN NOTE**
>
> The best place to obtain serum in an animal that has been dead for several hours is the atrium of the heart or the posterior vena cava.

Body fluids and cerebrospinal fluid are stable 4 to 5 hours after death if the animal is cooled. These fluids can be collected with a needle and syringe and placed in either a clot tube or an EDTA (ethylene diamine tetra-acetic acid) tube. Joint fluids are stable after death because they usually cool rapidly due to their peripheral location. If one is checking joint fluid for cellular components, the fluid will be representative of the live state for 3 to 4 hours postmortem. However, joint fluid enzymes deteriorate rapidly, and after death they lose their value. Occasionally, impression smears are made during a necropsy to diagnose infections or tumors. Impression smears are made by first blotting the tissue so that most superficial blood is re-

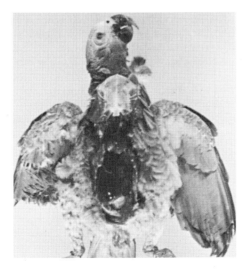

Figure 30-25. The chest and abdominal wall have been removed to expose the lungs, heart, air sacs, and viscera.

moved. Touch impressions on a clean glass slide are then made. (For further discussion of collection and handling of specimens for clinical pathological studies, see Chapter 5.)

> **TECHNICIAN NOTE**
>
> Body fluids and cerebrospinal fluid are stable 4 to 5 hours after death if the animal is cooled.

Toxicology

Collection of specimens for toxicological analysis is common in both small and large animals. The two most common types of poisoning in small animals are ethylene glycol (car antifreeze) and strychnine. Stomach contents and urine should be collected when ethylene glycol is suspected. Stomach contents only should be collected when strychnine is suspected. If heavy metals are expected (i.e., arsenic, lead or mercury), 20 to 30 g of kidney and liver should be collected. Nitrate toxicity is common in cattle; however, analysis of tissues cannot be used. Thus, if nitrate toxicity is suspected, the animal's feed and water must be analyzed. If nitrate poisoning is suspected in an aborted bovine fetus, ocular fluid (aqueous humor) should be collected in a syringe and then placed in a glass tube and submitted to a laboratory for nitrate levels. Further discussion of various toxins is not within the scope of this book; consultation of a general toxicological textbook is recommended.

Microbiology

The most common samples taken during a necropsy are for microbiological culture. Remember that within 5 to 10 minutes after death (and even before death with many debilitating diseases), motile intestinal bacteria may invade the blood and can seed many organs. Bacterial and viral cultures are best taken just after the carcass is opened to minimize contamination. Viral cultures must be taken within 20 to 30 minutes after death; otherwise, the pH change in the tissue inactivates most viruses. A few exceptions do occur, such as contagious ecthyma (sore mouth of sheep) and rabies. Bacterial samples are usually diagnostic for the first 8 to 15 hours after death, depending on how rapidly the animal cooled after death, the specific bacterial organism, or both. When an enteritis is observed and a culture is desired, using sterile instruments, first remove one large mesenteric lymph node and place it in a sterile Whirl-Pak (Fisher Scientific, Englewood, CO). Then, tie off a loop of small intestine (approximately 2.5 cm in length) with string and place it in a sterile Whirl-Pak. If you suspect an infection in a solid organ (e.g., hepatitis or pneumonia), remove a wedge of tissue (approximately 2.5 to 5 cm thick) using sterile instruments and place the tissue in a sterile Whirl-Pak. When an infection of the brain is suspected, two types of cultures should be taken. The first is a swab of the subdural space. This swab is taken under the brain just after the skull cap has been removed, and the head is turned over and tapped so the brain will fall forward before the optic nerve cord and other cranial nerves are cut. The second type of culture is obtained by submission of one half of the entire fresh brain to the laboratory in a sterile Whirl-Pak.

> **TECHNICIAN NOTE**
>
> Bacterial and viral cultures are best taken just after the carcass is opened to minimize contamination.

Joints should be opened carefully; otherwise they are easily contaminated. A method to culture joints is to wash the skin with alcohol and make an incision through the skin over the joint with a sterile scalpel (see Fig. 23–6). Then, using another sterile scalpel, incise through the joint capsule and open the joint to its maximum. Do not touch the cut joint capsule, but swab the far end of the joint space (see Fig. 30–7). All swabs should be placed in either aerobic or anaerobic transport media in an effort to preserve the organisms during transport to the laboratory.

When an animal has died of bacteremia (bacteria in the bloodstream), three culture sites are important: (1) heart blood, (2) spleen, and (3) blood from a lower leg vein. Usually, heart blood is the first to be contaminated by intestinal organisms, followed by the spleen. Many times, even though heart blood and spleen are contaminated, a pure culture of an organism (e.g., *Pasteurella*) can be isolated from blood of the lower leg. The reasons for this are that the blood in the lower extremities cools rapidly and the lower extremities are farther from motile intestinal flora.

Samples obtained for fungal culture are taken in the same manner as described for bacterial samples.

Samples for virus isolation are obtained in the same manner as described for bacteriological cultures except that they must be taken within 10 to 15 minutes after death. The samples should be cooled and immediately taken to the laboratory. If the samples cannot be taken to the laboratory within 30 minutes, the tissues should be frozen. Most viruses are not stable or do not maintain viability if frozen in a refrigerator freezer; thus these samples should be packed on dry ice and taken to the laboratory as quickly as possible.

Samples for fluorescent antibody tests should be collected with clean scissors and forceps. Small pieces of tissue, approximately 0.5 cm², are adequate. For example, if one suspects infectious bovine rhinotracheitis (IBR) in a bovine fetus, several small pieces of liver and lung should be submitted to a laboratory for fluorescent antibody testing for IBR. These samples should be kept cool during transportation to the laboratory. If the transportation time to the laboratory is greater than 24 hours, the tissue should be transported frozen.

A test commonly being used in the laboratory is the electron microscopic scan. This test involves concentrating viral particles from intestinal contents and then identifying viruses with the use of the electron microscope. The technique is especially useful in calves and pigs with scours and with parvovirus enteritis in dogs and cats. A satisfactory sample would be 5 to 10 ml of the lower small intestine contents (in a syringe) for parvovirus in dogs and cats. The sample from pigs and calves is best taken from a mixture of the lower small intestine, rectum, and spiral colon because the viruses seem to be concentrated in these locations, even though virus replication occurs in the upper and middle small intestine. (For further detailed discussion of the collection and handling of specimens for microbiological cultures and tests, see Chapter 8.)

The procedures for collection of specimens for parasitology at the time of necropsy are fairly straightforward. A 4- to 5-g sample of feces from the terminal rectum is best for routine fecal flotation. This will be adequate for cestodes, trematodes, nematodes and *Coccidia* ova or larvae. If parasites are found intact (e.g., lungworms in cattle, liver flukes in sheep or intestinal nematodes in dogs), the easiest method to preserve these specimens is 10% buffered formalin. If the parasites are still alive, it is best to cool them in saline before placing them in formalin. (For further detailed discussion of collection and handling of specimens for parasitology, see Chapter 6.)

SHIPMENT OF TISSUE

Microbiological Samples

All microbiological samples should be tightly packed in transport media or sterile Whirl-Paks. Specimens should be chilled and placed in small styrofoam containers. Two or three ice packs should be included in the container. If transportation time is greater than 24 hours, the samples should be frozen and packed with dry ice (there are a few exceptions; see Chapter 8). Most samples are shipped via mail or other commercial delivery services.

Toxicological and Parasitological Samples

Specimens shipped for most toxicological tests should be frozen and placed in styrofoam containers containing frozen ice packs. Specimens should be double packaged, and the tops of the styrofoam containers should be well sealed. Parasitological samples should be kept cool, and parasites should be preserved in formalin. These samples can then be packaged in styrofoam containers and shipped. The most common means of transporting samples are by the U.S. Postal Service or other commercial delivery services.

Clinical Pathology Samples

Transportation of clinical pathology specimens to the laboratory should be done as quickly as possible. Several private laboratories have a carrier service to pick up samples and deliver them to the airport and then transport them to the laboratory by air. These laboratories usually have special shipping instructions that should be consulted. Otherwise, clinical pathology samples should be cooled, packaged in a styrofoam container, and shipped to the laboratory as soon as possible. Serum should be transported frozen and on dry ice. (For further discussion of collection and handling of specimens for clinical pathological studies, see Chapter 5.)

Histopathology Samples

Samples for histopathological study should be placed in small, well-sealed glass or plastic containers containing formalin. The tops of the containers should be taped to ensure that shaking or vibrations that occur during transportation do not loosen the lids and allow formalin to leak. If multiple tissues are to be sent via mail or bus, tissues should first be allowed to fix properly in the proper volume of formalin (10:1, formalin to volume of tissue); then the tissues can be placed in a smaller jar filled with formalin and shipped to a diagnostic laboratory. This procedure reduces the weight of the package to be shipped. For example, if an expensive insured stallion has undergone necropsy, the tissues collected may fill two 4-liter jars of formalin (remember the 10:1 formalin to tissue ratio). Formalin weighs approximately 4 kg per 4 liters. This would result in more than 8 kg of substance. The best way to reduce the weight is to allow the tissues to fix for 3 to 4 days, and then place all the tissue in a 1-liter jar and cover the tissue with formalin. This will adequately keep the tissues during transportation.

Recommended Reading

Andrews JJ (editor): Necropsy techniques. Vet Clin North Am Food Animal Practice, Vol 2/No 1, 1986.

Strafuss AC: Necropsy: Procedures and Basic Diagnostic Methods for Practicing Veterinarians. Springfield, IL, Charles C Thomas, 1988.

Van Kruiningen HJ: Veterinary autopsy procedure. Vet Clin North Am 1:163–189, 1971.

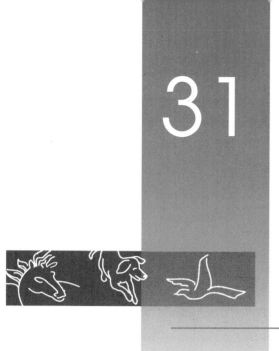

31 Veterinary Practice Management

Roger L. Lukens • *Dennis M. McCurnin*

INTRODUCTION

Each veterinary practice is a business that offers medical care to animals with their owners' consent. Only willing owners consent to pay a fee for professional services provided by the veterinary team. The total cost of providing these services is paid by the clients of the practice. Therefore, marketing efforts must effectively attract (and retain) sufficient clients to each practice or it will go bankrupt! No professional veterinary business will survive long if it is not profitable.

The highest quality of care possible for the animals must be offered to their owners in a cost-effective (not cost-cutting) manner; this is extremely important to both animal and owner. A high-quality practice requires keeping up with the latest medical knowledge and technologies. It also requires the most effective and caring communication possible with owners by the entire veterinary team. Communication is absolutely necessary to inform, educate, and obtain owner compliance with the veterinarian's recommendations for treatment plans to benefit the animal.

The profitability of the practice and the care of the client's animal are at risk if the veterinary team fails to deliver quality medical care for the animal coupled with caring effective communication with the owner. The services of the veterinary team are not successful unless (1) the patient is helped and the client understands the service, (2) the client is pleased with the caring attitude of the team, (3) the client tells others of their enthusiasm for that practice, and (4) the client wants to return for future veterinary care of his or her pets. Veterinary technicians are very important to the success of the veterinary team in accomplishing these goals.

Effective management of the veterinary practice as a business is also necessary because of increased competition, grow-ing malpractice threats, new technology, shifting client expectations, and continuing inflation of medical equipment, supplies, and personnel costs. All these risks and challenges must be well managed to enhance both productivity and quality of patient care. It has been said, "What is good business may be bad medicine, and what is good medicine may be bad business." Veterinary practice represents the *art* of balancing both business and medicine to meet the needs of patients, clients, and the veterinary team.

ROLE OF VETERINARY TECHNICIAN IN MANAGEMENT

Technicians have an ever-increasing role in practice management. In most practice situations, the technician will usually be involved in management of the patient, client, equipment, and inventory. They may also be involved in staff, facility, and business management. To develop management skills, one must be willing to assume increasing levels of responsibility. As the practice changes in staffing, number of cases, facility, type of clients, new technologies, and so forth, the veterinary technician must adapt his or her management skills to these changes.

The role of the veterinary technician in management will vary depending on the type of practice and the previous experiences of the technician and veterinarian. The technician who can (1) conceptualize the vision and goals set by the veterinarian for the practice, (2) efficiently organize each area in which they are given responsibility, (3) become a productive team player and a good communicator, and (4) develop the ability to solve problems constructively to enhance both patient care and the veterinary team will usually be given a greater role in practice management.

To be effective, the veterinarian-owner must act as overall hospital chief executive officer and delegate appropriate areas of responsibility to the veterinary technician as well as to other members of the team. Effective delegation of responsibility to the technician must include technical procedures of medicine and surgery. Ideally, veterinarians diagnose, prescribe, and perform surgery, and technicians perform venipunctures, laboratory tests, and treatments; expose and develop radiographs; and anesthetize, prepare, and manage recovery of surgical patients. The veterinary technician should delegate most non–income-producing tasks to aides, assistants, and/or animal caretakers. Clinic aides restrain, move, feed, and exercise the animals and assist both technicians and veterinarians when needed. The receptionists handle scheduling, receiving, discharging, billing, and related front office duties. There should be a direct relationship between the salary level paid and the income produced (productivity) for each veterinary technician and veterinarian if effective delegation is occurring.

 TECHNICIAN NOTE

The veterinary technician should delegate most non–income-producing tasks to assistants or aides.

Practice management skills are necessary in all types of practice. To be effective in practice management, the veterinarian and technician must each be an effective people manager. This requires both excellent communication skills and a policy and procedures manual for the practice team. The veterinarian and technician must work together with the rest of the staff as both a *management team* and a *medical team*. Unfortunately, most colleges provide little training in hospital or people management for either technicians or veterinarians because it takes students so much time and effort to gain the medical expertise, technical skills, and confidence necessary to succeed medically. However, there are many new resources available to meet this need for management training after graduation, including continuing education short courses, books, journals, and consultants.

VETERINARY PRACTICE MANAGEMENT AREAS

Veterinary technician students are naturally interested in managing the nursing care of patients. They realize the necessity of effective client communication to benefit the patient and begin to understand the business side of medicine only after gaining significant experience in a veterinary practice. Managing equipment, facility, staff, and marketing are not of much interest until one has experienced problems or limitations in these areas that have a negative impact on patient care (or technician salary).

Each of these areas (Table 31–1) must be coordinated with the other areas to achieve an effective working unit that can meet the veterinary team's goals for the operation (strategic plan). A successfully managed practice enjoys success and accomplishment with people, both internally and externally. Failure to properly manage patients, people, and the business leads to a reduction in the quality of service rendered, staff

• Table 31–1 •

MANAGEMENT AREAS	
Management areas include:	Marketing
Facility design	Building
Patient care	Equipment
Client communications	Medical records
Human resources	Inventory control
Finance	Computerization

dissatisfaction, a disorganized practice, dissatisfied clients, and a deteriorating business.

Veterinary Facility Design

Numerous terms are applied to veterinary facilities. The American Veterinary Medical Association (AVMA) has developed guidelines (Table 31–2) for consistency in naming veterinary facilities to avoid confusion by the general public. In addition, many state practice acts and regulations not only have been updated to specify standards of practice and professional competency for both veterinarians and technicians but also have adopted facility and equipment requirements and hired inspectors to ensure that these standards are being met. The American Animal Hospital Association (AAHA) has extensive standards of excellence that cover most of the management areas listed in Table 31–2 that must be met to have the hospital accredited by AAHA.

Location is the primary factor (other than referrals from satisfied clients) in attracting new clients. Location will often dictate slow or rapid practice growth. Location provides visibility for potential clients and allows existing clients to easily find the practice. Prime locations within shopping centers and on

• Table 31–2 •

VETERINARY FACILITY NOMENCLATURE

Office—Room where limited or consultative type of practice is conducted

Mobile facility—A vehicle for making house or farm calls *or* a vehicle equipped with special medical and/or surgical facilities; both must have a permanent base of operations (published address and telephone number)

Clinic—Outpatient practice facility *not* offering overnight patient confinement

Hospital—Inpatient practice facility offering overnight hospitalization of patients

Emergency facility—Emergency practice facility that focuses primarily on treating and monitoring emergencies with veterinarian and staff who are always available (during specified hours of operation) and equipped to provide timely and appropriate level of emergency care

On-call emergency service—Veterinarians and staff are not on premises all the time but are available via on-call basis to handle emergency calls

Referral center—Staffed with board-certified specialist veterinarians who receive referrals from the primary care practitioners of the above facilities; sometimes called secondary care facility

Animal medical center—A large facility (veterinary teaching hospitals and large corporate practices) offering consultative, clinical, and hospital services to referred clients and their local veterinarian; also performs significant research on animal health problems and conducts advanced professional education programs; sometimes called tertiary care facility

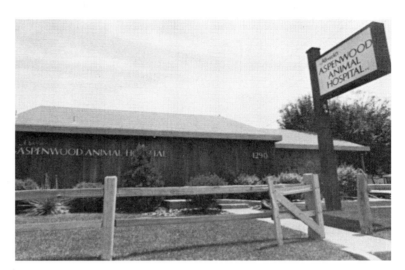

Figure 31-1. Hospital signs should be professional and clearly visible from the street.

main streets are expensive during the initial investment period but will repay the investment by increasing practice growth. Location of the facility must therefore be considered by veterinary technicians when selecting a practice for employment.

Furthermore, the *practice sign* must be evaluated for visibility and professional appearance. The optimum would be a well-placed, neat, professional sign that allows the client clear visibility and direction (Fig. 31–1). The sign becomes even more important during an emergency. Some form of lighting will allow clients to identify the building after dark and more easily identify the building entrance.

Attention must be given to the *parking lot area.* Litter must be picked up, and plants and grass must be tended. The parking lot entrance and exit should be clearly marked by signs (Fig. 31–2). Parking spaces should be outlined by parking stripes. The parking area should be reserved for clients only, with employee parking behind the building or in a remote area away from the building entrance.

The *entrance* to the veterinary facility should be in full view and well marked to allow easy access by the new client. If more than one entrance is available (i.e., small animal and large animal or canine and feline), each entrance should be marked. To prevent client congestion, entrance and exit should be separate. Practice employees should not use the public entrance of the building. Furthermore, routine deliveries and

service activities should enter and exit the building away from client contact when possible.

Professional activities within a hospital can be grouped into four areas: (1) *outpatient*, (2) *inpatient*, (3) *surgical*, and (4) *support*. Depending on the practice size and type, the veterinarian, technician, or both may work in all four areas or focus in one or more areas.

> **TECHNICIAN NOTE**
>
> The four professional areas of activity within a hospital are outpatient, inpatient, surgical, and support service.

Outpatient Area

The first area to be discussed is the outpatient area. This area is composed of the *reception area, examination rooms, laboratory, pharmacy,* and *public restrooms.* Most commonly, clients will only have access to this area of the hospital. Special attention must be paid to maintain the outpatient area in a clean, organized, quiet, and odor-free condition. Because the client's first contact is with the outpatient area, lasting impressions are made, which may raise or lower the overall client confidence level. A disorganized, dirty, smelly, noisy area will be remembered just that way. Veterinarians and technicians must be well groomed, clean, and professionally attired. A professional appearance is mandatory for a professional image. All personnel in the outpatient area should refrain from smoking, eating, and drinking when clients are present.

The *reception area* should always be considered by all hospital employees as a reception or client greeting area and not as a "waiting" room. The reception area should be comfortable and project a feeling of warmth, not a sterile feeling. Plants will help to create this warm feeling, but they must be well cared for. Dead or dying plants in the reception area will not send a positive message to the client. Warm colors will also help to brighten the area. Reading material, if present, should be complete and not torn up or half missing. A well-maintained fish aquarium and attractive wall hangings or paintings will relax the guests (Fig. 31–3).

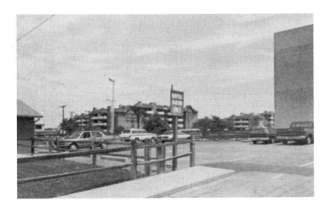

Figure 31-2. Client parking lot should be clearly designated and clean.

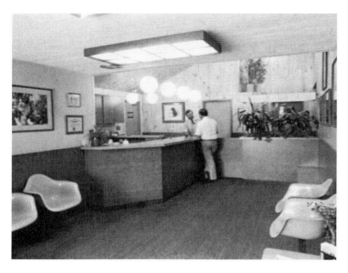

Figure 31-3. Reception area should give a warm, comfortable feeling to clients and staff.

The client should spend only a short period of time in the reception room before being escorted to one of the *examination rooms*. As a general rule, two examination rooms should be available in the outpatient area for each veterinarian. The examination areas should be decorated in warm tones, as is the reception area. Medications, examination equipment, records, and so forth should be secured or out of sight so that neither clients nor their children will be tempted. It is extremely important that the examination room be clean and in excellent repair as the client will spend the greatest amount of time there (Fig. 31–4). Soiled floor or wall covering, dirty sink, and marred door will be noticed and remembered by the client.

The *laboratory* and *pharmacy* should be organized and clean. Clients will only occasionally visit these areas and should always be accompanied by a hospital employee. In some practices, the laboratory and pharmacy will be combined for more efficient use of floor space (Fig. 31–5). The *public restrooms*

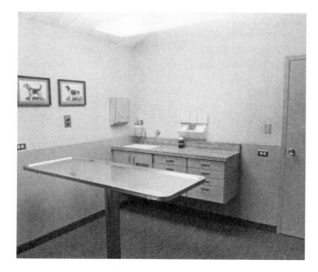

Figure 31-4. Examination rooms should be warmly decorated, clean, and in excellent condition.

should be cleaned and inspected regularly and should be conveniently located for client use.

Inpatient Area

The second work area is the inpatient area, consisting of a *treatment area, patient wards or stalls*, an *isolation area*, an *exercise area*, an area in which *necropsy* is performed, a *kitchen*, and a *bathing* and *grooming* area. The client has much less contact with this area than with the outpatient area, but constant attention must be given to maintain a clean, odor-free environment to prevent nosocomial infections of patients (Table 31–3).

Kennels, runs, and stalls must be cleaned several times during the day. Hospitalized patients must have closer attention than animals who are just boarding. Sick animals often cannot control urination and defecation; therefore, more frequent attention to these areas will usually be required. Some pets are not used to eliminating indoors and will be reluctant to urinate and defecate unless they are in an exercise run. To maintain a quiet environment in public areas of the hospital, patient wards must be well insulated to reduce noise.

If large animals are hospitalized, adequate holding stalls will be necessary, with regular attention given to cleaning the stall and grooming and exercising the patient. When exercising either a large animal or a small animal patient, absolute security must be maintained at all times. Fenced areas should always be used to ensure that in the event of escape, the animal will still be contained (Fig. 31–6). The veterinarian, hospital, or both assume all liability for an animal entrusted to them. Few experiences will match the helpless feeling of watching an escaped dog, cat, horse, cow, and so forth run off into the distance (especially if close to a busy street or highway).

Because of the security problem, the ward or stall area of the hospital should be adjacent to the *exercise area*, with an escape-proof fence or walls connecting the two. Exercise areas for small animals ideally should be located within a well-insulated area of the hospital in which the temperature and humidity can be maintained at a constant level. Most city zoning laws will allow a small animal hospital to be located in proximity to residential areas because modern construction techniques use totally enclosed, attractive, and well-insulated designs.

TECHNICIAN NOTE

Animal security within the hospital must always be a high priority. Animals that escape are the legal responsibility of the hospital.

Large animal hospitals or hospitals caring for both large and small animals will usually be required to locate in a less developed area of a city to allow exercise areas and odors to be properly addressed. Fewer veterinary hospitals now board either large or small animals on a regular basis. When boarding is offered, it should be explained to the client as "veterinary-supervised boarding." The recent trend has been away from construction of large boarding facilities as part of an animal hospital. Because of both the cost of construction and the cost of hospitalization, most veterinary practices work on an outpatient basis whenever possible. Construction and labor

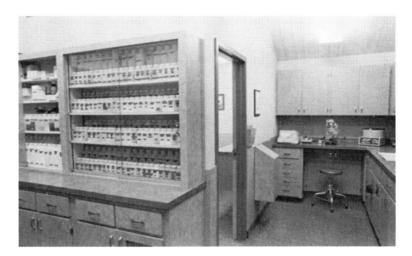

Figure 31–5. Combination pharmacy and clinical laboratory.

costs have made long-term hospitalization a financial burden to both client and veterinarian.

In certain instances, animals with infectious diseases must be hospitalized. Adequate *isolation facilities* must be available before a patient with an infectious disease is admitted. The isolation area should have only one entrance and exit, with proper disinfectant and clothing protection available. The air handling system for the isolation area must be separate from the remainder of the building. In the event that adequate isolation facilities are not available on the premises, the case should be referred to a veterinarian who has the proper facility. All treatments and handling of the infectious patient should be done by one or two persons only. The patient should be treated within the isolation facility and should not be taken to the main treatment room unless absolutely necessary. Special precautions are imperative to prevent nosocomial infections (see Table 31–3).

The *treatment area* should be the central hub of the hospital (Fig. 31–7). Patients from both the wards (inpatients) and examination rooms (outpatients) will be presented to this area for diagnostic procedures, medication administration, and recheck procedures (cast, bandage, or splint changes or removal).

Certified veterinary technicians are increasingly performing the medical treatments and other nursing procedures prescribed while the veterinarian is in surgery or seeing outpatients. One of the technical staff should have the primary responsibility for organization and cleanliness of the treatment area.

On occasion, clients will accompany the patient to the treatment area to assist with a bandage change or other minor procedure. The area, therefore, must be presentable at all times. In addition to the routine treatment functions carried out in the treatment room, many hospitals also use this room for preparation of the surgical patient. In the smaller practice, the treatment room may also contain x-ray facilities, laboratory equipment, or both. Because of the high traffic volume in the treatment area, hair and other debris will build up rapidly and should be removed with a vacuum cleaner on a regular basis to prevent nosocomial infections.

The *kitchen* in a small animal hospital should be an area in which food is stored and prepared. Usually, both canned and dry foods are available, and it should be stored in dry, rodent-proof containers. An automatic dishwasher is of great value if any quantity of dirty pans must be cleaned on a daily basis. It will also sanitize the pans with very hot water and remove soap and disinfectant residues. Hot and cold running

• Table 31–3 •

NOSOCOMIAL INFECTIONS

Definition—New infections acquired by patients in the veterinary facility
Examples of nosocomial infection sources:
  Staff—Unwashed hands; contaminated equipment, including dirty needles, clothing, and boots; inadequate cleaning and disinfecting protocols; breaks in aseptic technique
  Other patients—Direct contact, airborne droplets, hair, excrement, blood
  Environment—Cages, feed or water pans, dust, bedding
Staff prevention: Always wash hands between every patient
                 Always wear clean clothing and boots
                 Always follow established cleaning, disinfecting, sterilizing, and aseptic protocols
                 Train all staff in preventative protocols
Note: Recent studies indicate that human hospital workers wash their hands less than one-half of the time before touching human patients: one factor in the recent increase of nosocomial infections in human patients!

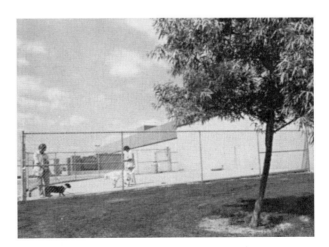

Figure 31–6. For security, fenced enclosures should always be used for outside exercise.

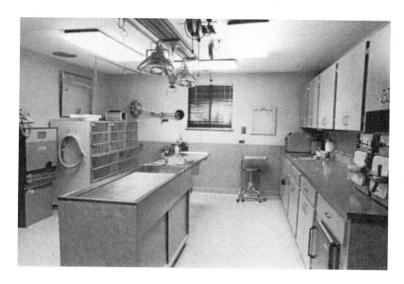

Figure 31-7. Centralized treatment area accommodates both outpatient and inpatient treatment.

water, a sink, countertop space, and a refrigerator should be available in the kitchen (Fig. 31–8).

In the large animal hospital, the *feed room* will usually contain several grain mixtures and ration supplements. All materials must be stored in dry, rodent-proof containers. Grass hay, alfalfa, and bedding straw should be stored in a dry area protected from the weather to prevent mold and mildew. Moldy hay or alfalfa should never be fed to an animal because of possible toxicity.

The *bathing-grooming area* in the small animal hospital will usually consist of a raised bathroom tub (elevated about 60 to 90 cm [Fig. 31–9]), a combing table, and a dryer cage. It is critically important that all patients dismissed from the hospital be clean and dry. Grooming services within the hospital are sometimes discouraged, but attention to daily grooming of all patients by all employees is necessary. Attention to grooming is also important in the large animal patient (especially the horse) and is usually done in the stall on a daily basis.

The final area to be discussed within the inpatient work area of the hospital is the *necropsy area*. The veterinary technician is able to perform a prosection (initial dissection) for the veterinarian to quickly inspect all organs for lesions and decide what specimens should be collected. The technician will collect, prepare, and ship the designated specimens to a diagnostic laboratory (see Chapter 30). The necropsy area should be located in an isolated place in the building and be well lighted and well ventilated. Hot and cold running water and a drain should also be present. Necropsy tables or racks may be used for small animals, whereas the necropsy floor is usually used for large animals. Gloves, boots, and aprons should be available in addition to specific necropsy instruments and specimen bottles. The availability of a 35-mm camera or videocamera is helpful to record specific lesions.

In conclusion, the hospital inpatient area is the most labor-intensive section because of patient contact. Most hospitals expend the greatest amount of effort in maintaining this area. Most employees spend their greatest amount of time in this area performing direct animal care, diagnostic procedures, and nursing treatments. The outcome of most cases will be determined here.

Surgical Area

The third work area in the hospital is the *surgical area*, which consists of the *preparation room, operating rooms, radiology*

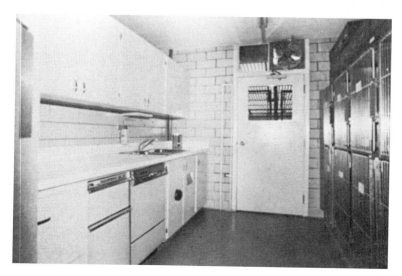

Figure 31-8. Hospital kitchen should contain diet materials, dishwasher, counterspace, and refrigerator.

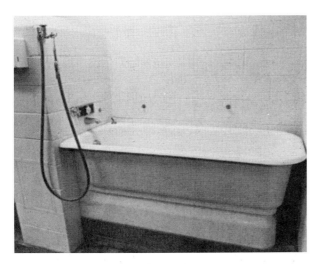

Figure 31-9. Bathing tub elevated 80 cm from floor to aid in controlling animal during bath.

section, and *recovery room*. All four areas in the surgical section must be in proximity to one another. Frequently, the surgeon may need to obtain a postoperative radiograph of a fracture reduction to determine bone alignment or implant placement. When neurosurgery is to be performed, the surgeon may request a myelogram just before surgery; this requires that the patient be moved from the preparation room to the radiology section, back to the preparation room, and then into surgery.

As stated earlier, the *preparation room* may also be the treatment room. All presurgical preparation of the patient, surgeon and technician should take place outside the operating room. Instrument preparation and sterilization usually will be completed in the preparation room. Clipping and scrubbing the patient and hand scrubbing of the surgeon and technician should be done before entering the operating room. Again, a vacuum cleaner should be available in the preparation room to remove all loose hair from patient, table, and floor.

The *operating room* itself should be a "dead end" room with only one entrance-exit (Fig. 31–10). No one should enter the operating room without proper clothing, shoes, cap, and mask. The operating room should be used only for surgical

procedures and must not double as a treatment or examination room. Storage cabinets should be kept to a minimum and should contain only items that are used in surgery. Items used elsewhere in the hospital should not be stored in the operating room. Countertops should be kept to a minimum because flat surfaces collect dust and must be wiped down daily. Some flat surface is desirable to allow opening of packs and layout of instruments.

TECHNICIAN NOTE

The operating room (OR) must be used only for surgery and cannot be used as an examination or treatment room.

Wall-mounted radiographic viewers should be present to allow several views of a body part to be observed at once. Surgery lights, oxygen outlets, and patient monitors should be ceiling- or wall-mounted when possible. Floors, walls, and ceiling should be washable, smooth and seam free to allow complete and easy cleaning. Cleaning under the surgery table base as well as the floor and flat surfaces should be performed daily. The air handling system for the operating room should be separate and should create a slightly positive pressure to prevent dust and other debris from entering the room from other rooms when the door is opened.

All cleaning materials and utensils used in the operating room should be restricted to use in this room. Mops and sponges that are used elsewhere in the building and are then used in the operating room will bring additional contamination into the room. The cleanliness of the operating room is everyone's concern to prevent nosocomial infection of the surgical site.

The *radiology area* should be located near the operating room, the preparation room, and the treatment area (for diagnostic workups). The radiology section should not be visited by clients during film exposure because of potential radiation. Protective aprons, gloves, and film exposure badges should always be worn by all personnel in radiology. The technician will usually be responsible for equipment maintenance, expo-

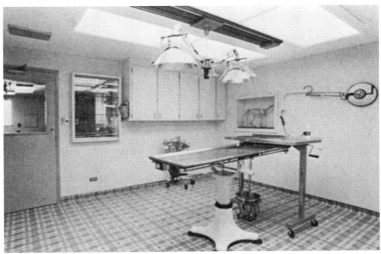

Figure 31-10. Surgical room with one door for both entrance and exit, ceiling-mounted lights, and minimal countertops.

sure, developing, and filing radiographs. In most surgical orthopedic cases, the radiology area will be visited after surgery to evaluate bone alignment or metal implant placement, or both, before placing the patient in the recovery room.

The *surgical recovery area* should be monitored at all times by a technician until the endotracheal tube has been removed. The recovery area may be in a room adjacent to the treatment room or behind a glass partition in the treatment room, or the recovery process may occur on a blanket on the treatment room floor. Wherever surgical recovery occurs, the patient should be closely monitored by the technical staff. *Under no circumstances* should any patient recovering from anesthesia be left unattended in the ward, stall, or elsewhere with an endotracheal tube in place.

In review, the surgical work area is a very technical and equipment-oriented area. Clients will not be permitted in this area except in unusual circumstances. The skill level of technical support in this area is very high, requiring familiarization with anesthesia, induction and administration emergency procedures, radiology, surgical assisting, medical-surgical nursing, fiberoptic equipment, sterile technique, sterilization, monitoring equipment hook-up, electrosurgical equipment, necropsy techniques, and so forth.

Support Area

The fourth work area of the hospital is the hospital support area. This area contains, somewhat by default, some of the "leftovers," but it also contains the planning and management areas of the hospital. The support area contains the *professional offices, business management office, library, employee lounge,* and *storage-inventory* areas.

TECHNICIAN NOTE

The support area of the hospital contains the professional offices, business management office, library, employee lounge, and storage areas.

In smaller practices, the *professional office, business management office,* and *library* will be in one room. In some multiperson practices, each veterinarian may have an office or desk area in addition to the hospital manager's office. Larger practices may also have a library and conference room combination in which weekly staff meetings and conferences can be held.

The role of the hospital manager will vary according to practice size and management philosophy, but his or her office will usually be in proximity to the admissions-discharge functions of the hospital. Credit policy, accounts receivable, inventory control, purchasing, receiving orders, accounts payable, computer information management, management reports, personnel activities, and so forth will usually be handled by the hospital manager. In many practices, these functions are divided among the technical staff, and the veterinarian or veterinarians will assume the overall management role. For most veterinary technicians, some management skills will be required for advancement. Hospital management is now developing into a

specialty area of veterinary medicine for nonveterinarians (Table 31–4).

The *professional office* of the veterinarian functions as a client consultation area, a medical management area for discussing new products with salespeople, and a professional management area for writing medical records, contacting clients, and discussing difficult or interesting cases with other veterinarians or staff (Fig. 31–11). Many office hours are spent by the practicing veterinarian in studying and reading textbooks, journals, reference materials, and computer information. Veterinary technicians must also keep up with the latest advances in nursing, imaging, and laboratory procedures.

The last portion of the support area is *storage*. From the management viewpoint, hospital storage space is the most expensive floor space in the building because this space produces the least income. Therefore, the storage areas must be given close attention so that this valuable space will function as efficiently as possible. Supplies and equipment that are no longer used or usable should be removed to make room for the essential items. Inventory control (not overstocking or understocking) and space organization will ensure maximum utilization. Items that can be hung on the wall or ceiling should be removed from the floor. Metal or wooden shelving will organize space for bulk drugs, food, and cleaning supplies. Flammable or toxic materials should be safely marked and stored away from foods or drugs.

In summary, the four major hospital work areas (outpa-

• Table 31–4 •

SOCIETIES WITH OR DEVELOPING SPECIALTY CERTIFICATION PROGRAMS
Veterinary Emergency and Critical Care Society (VECCS) Academy of Veterinary Emergency and Critical Care Technicians (AVECCT) 16729 San Pedro San Antonio, TX 78232 AVECCT members can be certified as veterinary technician specialists-emergency and critical care *and will use* VTS (Emergency/Critical Care) after their name and state certification (i.e., Jane Doe, RVT, VTS (Emergency/Critical Care).
American Society of Veterinary Dental Technicians (ASVDT) P.O. Box 1636 Venice, FL 34284-1636
Veterinary Technicians Anesthetist Society (VTAS) Academy of Veterinary Technician Nurse-Anesthetists (AVTNA)—proposed c/o Charles Hoffman Scott-Ritchey Research Center Auburn University College of Veterinary Medicine Auburn, AL 36849
Veterinary Hospital Managers Association, Inc. (VHMA) 48 Howard Street Albany, NY 12207 To be certified, a VHMA member must be actively employed as a veterinary practice manager (not necessarily a technician or DVM), achieve 18 college credit hours in business management, pass VHMA written and oral exams, and participate in 6 days of management continuing education every 2 years. The designation of certified veterinary practice manager (CVPM) is conveyed to successful applicants (i.e., Jane Doe, CVPM; if a registered technician, Jane Doe, RVT, CVPM).

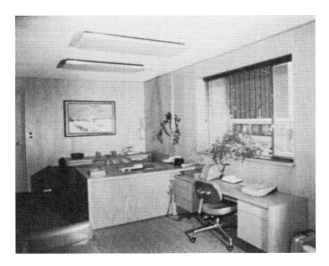

Figure 31-11. Professional private office to be used for consultations, study, and maintenance of medical records.

tient, inpatient, surgery, and support) are somewhat separate in function but are related in patient care and support. The smaller the practice, the less distinct will be the above areas. Furthermore, the smaller the practice, the fewer is the technical staff and assistants, resulting in less opportunity for the veterinary technician to focus on one work area. This is not to imply that the smaller practice is less desirable. Sometimes, to the contrary, the smaller practice can provide more personal satisfaction because of closer contact with the entire operation and a diversification of job roles. Each technician and veterinarian needs to choose the type of practice with staffing patterns that provide the greatest personal and professional satisfaction.

The four work areas that have been discussed are important from both client-patient and hospital organization viewpoints. The client wants personalized and professional service that is efficient, thorough, and cost effective. If each employee fully understands and enjoys his or her work area, the client and patient will usually experience satisfaction. However, the veterinary team must be efficient at handling the required number of patients to provide the cash flow required to stay in business. The traffic flow (i.e., the movement of the client-patient from admission to dismissal) becomes very important to accommodate the required number of clients each day.

Client Traffic Flow Patterns

The client first enters the reception area, and the admission process begins. The receptionist initiates the proper business and medical records for each case. The client is escorted into one of the examination rooms. A preliminary history and examination (including temperature, pulse, and respiration [TPR]) may be taken by the technician before the veterinarian arrives. After examination and consultation with the veterinarian, either the client will leave the animal (hospitalization for further diagnostic tests, treatment, surgery, or observation) or the patient is treated and, if necessary, medication is dispensed before the patient returns to the receptionist for dismissal. In the event that the patient is dismissed (outpatient), the client settles the account and is scheduled to return for a reexamination or to call with a follow-up report. During the routine outpatient visit,

the client usually only contacts the outpatient work area. The client traffic pattern for an outpatient visit is reception → admission → examination → (pharmacy) (laboratory) → dismissal.

If the patient is hospitalized, the client may have some contact with the inpatient area in addition to the outpatient area. A typical client traffic pattern in the hospitalized case would be reception → admission → examination → treatment area or surgical area → admission (discussion of dismissal and payment-credit policy). The client would leave the hospital and return to the reception area on the day of dismissal.

On dismissal of hospitalized cases, the client enters the reception area and usually receives patient information from the receptionist or technician. The client then proceeds to the examination room for a brief consultation with the veterinarian followed by home care instructions and demonstrations from the technician. To reduce confusion at dismissal, it is advisable for the client to return to the dismissal area and settle the account prior to presenting the patient. Once the patient has been returned to the client, communication may be difficult during the reunion process.

In addition to the routine inpatient and outpatient client traffic pattern, a third type of contact exists when the client visits a hospitalized patient. In this event, the client usually makes an appointment with the receptionist to visit the animal at a specific time that is convenient to both the client and the hospital operation. When the client arrives, he or she will proceed directly to the examination or treatment room. Visiting patients in the ward is usually discouraged because other patients are disturbed. During the visit with the animal, a technician (or veterinarian) should be present to answer questions concerning care and progress made by the patient. The client should always visit with the veterinarian at some point—in the examination room or the treatment room or in the veterinarian's private office.

Client visits are often beneficial for both patient and client. The mental attitudes of client and patient can be strengthened, and communication can be improved between veterinarian and client. Client visits should be encouraged rather than discouraged.

Client Management

The most important person in any practice is the client. The practice of veterinary medicine is truly a *people business*. Everyone in the practice must enjoy working with and problem solving for the people served by the practice. Veterinarians and technicians who do not like working with people and their animal problems should not be employed in practice. Many other professional careers are now available to individuals who desire less public contact.

 TECHNICIAN NOTE

The most important person in any practice is the client!

Value of the Client

The availability of veterinary service in the United States appears to be at an all-time high. New schools of veterinary medicine and expanded enrollment at existing schools have resulted in this increased availability of graduate veterinarians. The net result of the increasing supply of veterinary practitioners is increased competition for clients among established and new practices. The practices that will financially survive must offer expanded services that are competitive and cost effective by using both technicians and assistants effectively to leverage veterinarians' productivity.

How valuable is the client? The practice will collapse unless old clients are retained and new clients are continually entering the practice. Clients are the "lifeblood" of the practice. Everyone in the practice works for the client. Some practices would like to think that they control their clients, but client loyalty is seldom mandated. Loyalty is won with hard work and dedicated service to each client. The only unique product that a veterinary practice has to offer is service. If everyone in the practice understands that his primary role is to provide the finest quality medical care possible to the patient with the end result being a pleased and informed client, the practice will grow. If the staff attitude becomes one of negative feelings toward clients (i.e., not another one of these!), the practice will dwindle. Our facilities, equipment and techniques may be the finest available, but they will remain unused until clients willingly authorize or request our services.

Client Selection of a Veterinarian

How does a client select a veterinarian? Most clients with small animals will select a veterinarian because the practice location is convenient. Following closely after practice location, recommendations from friends is ranked next. Once a practice is selected, the individual veterinarian will be evaluated in the following areas: (1) personality, (2) gentleness in handling the animal, (3) communication, and (4) professional knowledge. In the selection process it becomes readily apparent that practice location, facility appearance and recommendations from satisfied clients are extremely important to practice growth. Once the client enters the hospital, the ability of the veterinarian and staff to project a *concerned, caring personality*, the expertise used in carefully handling the animal, and the clarity of the communication are the most important determining factors. It is interesting to note that professional knowledge falls to the bottom of the list. The general public has a limited informational basis by which to judge the professional knowledge of a physician, dentist, attorney, or veterinarian.

> **TECHNICIAN NOTE**
>
> Practice location and personal referrals are the two most common methods by which new clients find the veterinarian.

When does the veterinary technician have an impact on the client selection process? Clients always view the hospital staff as an *extension* of the veterinarian. Therefore, your personality, patient-handling techniques, and caring communication skills become critically important in this whole process.

Clients with large animals usually select a veterinarian based on recommendations from others. Once the veterinarian arrives at the farm or ranch, the selection process is the same

as the one used by small animal owners, with the addition of economic return. In food animal practice, the veterinarian must become an economic asset to the overall operation, or the client cannot afford veterinary services. Pet animal practice (i.e., small animal and horse) has some economic limits, but the sentimental and emotional attachment (human-animal bond) of the client to the pet is relied on to extend that economic limit, which the food animal client may not do.

Evaluation of the Client

Your attitude toward yourself will reflect how you handle clients. If you are excited, happy, and positive about yourself and what you are doing, this will dominate your client relations. One of the most infectious conditions we can have is *enthusiasm*. Enthusiastic people turn other people on! Enthusiasm is caught, not taught. The client must be handled effectively so that we do not cause a positive client to become negative. Conversely, we want to deal with a negative client exposing them to a friendly and positive environment, identifying their needs, and trying to help them.

Generally, after you work with a client for a short period of time, you get enough feedback to make some judgments about the client's expectations. These expectations are in the form of client-pet relationships, client-hospital relationships, and one-on-one personal relationships. Do not make the mistake of judging clients by their outward appearances only. Clients who appear to have nothing materially may value their animal highly and have resources to support veterinary care. In contrast, clients who drive up in a luxury car and have expensive clothes may not have the animal's best interests in mind and may be financially overextended. You cannot judge a book by its cover, and you cannot judge people by their appearance.

> **TECHNICIAN NOTE**
>
> Do not judge the client's ability to pay by his or her appearance.

In most instances you and your veterinarian will have to discuss pet values with the client and give the client the opportunity to express himself or herself. One of the most important roles in client communication is to establish the value of the animal in that client-pet relationship. Some clients will be difficult to really figure out, and you may never feel as if you understand their intent or interest level.

Client Communication

Sharpened interpersonal communication skills can serve to develop and expand veterinary service markets. Improved communication between client and veterinarian, client and technician and technician and veterinarian results in more personalized professional care. Reduction in spendable income may reduce demand for elective procedures, but this can be offset by providing a more comprehensive preventative medicine program through improved communication skills. Clients are unable to make service selections until they fully understand all options. It has been said: "I don't care how much you know until I know how much you care!"

• Table 31–5 •

SIX Cs OF PROFESSIONAL CLIENT RELATIONS	
Caring	Competence
Courtesy	Communicator
Compassion	Concern

Common courtesy and genuine concern affect all professions and businesses. The world as a whole is becoming more depersonalized and people do not count as individuals; they are a means to an end (i.e., making a profit). When a veterinary practice loses sight of the individual pet or client, or both, the personal service feeling is lost to both parties. Courtesy is acknowledging the clients as soon as they enter the reception room, carefully explaining why an appointment is helpful, calling clients by name, asking about the clients' families—in short, treating clients as the important guests they are in your hospital.

Courtesy also extends to telephone manners. All calls should be answered by the third ring; the caller should be greeted by "Good morning, this is ABC Animal Hospital, Kathy speaking, how may I help you?" The caller immediately knows that he has reached the correct hospital and that Kathy is there to help him. Telephone courtesy is just as important as personal courtesy because most clients have their first contact with the hospital by telephone.

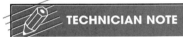

TECHNICIAN NOTE

All telephone calls should be answered by the third ring, although callers prefer the telephone to be answered on the first ring.

If the veterinary staff of a hospital treat each caller and each client with common courtesy, the feeling that the client will receive is genuine concern. A lack of concern for people and their pets' problems is a common complaint received by veterinary hospitals. If you treat each client as you would like to be treated when you are selecting or securing service, the result will be happy clients who experience courtesy and concern (Table 31–5).

Closely accompanying the issue of courtesy and concern is effective communication. The majority of complaints against veterinarians are the result of improper or misunderstood communication between veterinarian or practice personnel and client. To communicate completely, we must have concern for *both* animal and client. Additionally, we must learn to *listen* to the client and then communicate a caring attitude as well as information that is understandable and effective. Most people *hear* other people talking, but few people have developed the ability to listen effectively. The successful veterinary team must develop this ability.

To ensure effective communication consider these four areas: (1) Use terminology that the client will understand; scientific terms can be confusing to the client. (2) Do not rush through the information just because you are hurried or because it appears to be "common knowledge" to you, or the client will feel "brushed off." (3) Do not assume a superior manner or tone to the extent that the client feels "put down." (4) Use effective communication techniques for obtaining a history (see Table 31–6).

In short, show concern and attempt to treat each client with honesty and as a very special person. If the communication is open, honest and caring, it will be effective and most problems can be prevented. One of the most common reasons for veterinarians to refer clients to other veterinarians is not for medical or surgical considerations but because of the inability to cope with the client or situation. This usually results from the lack of inappropriate communication skills.

• Table 31–6 •

COMMUNICATION TECHNIQUES FOR INTERVIEWING CLIENT		
Open-ended (or Probing) Questions	*vs.*	***Leading (Yes/No) Questions***
Who?		Did?
How?		Was it?
What?		
When?		
Where?		
Answers will be detailed descriptions.		Answers will be yes or no even if client is not sure!

One-Word Acknowledgment
Use one word (e.g., oh, okay, yes) with eye contact and voice inflection that imply you understand and want him or her to continue talking. This can be done with eye contact, nonverbal signs of active listening, and verbal silence with some clients.

Accent Questions
Restate one or two words used by the client in a questioning tone, which serves to request the client to elaborate on the description of events or signs.

Paraphrasing
Restate client statements (in your own words) to check with the client whether you understand what the client is trying to say before going on in the interview. Use periodically in each segment of the interview to give the client an opportunity to clarify or confirm your understanding.

Summarizing
Restate main points at the end (or at end of major segments) to emphasize key points and inform the client about what is going to happen next.

Only about 40% of all communication is verbal. Sight, touch, smell, sounds, and body language are all important factors. What the client sees on entering the parking lot or reception room, what is heard once in the building, what odors and sounds are perceived, and what body language is used (e.g., nod of the head, raised eyebrows, smile) are taken in by the client to form a total picture (positive or negative) of the practice.

TECHNICIAN NOTE

About 40% of all communication is verbal; 60% is body language and environmental factors.

Listening is an extremely important communications skill. The skill of listening must be practiced on a regular basis to become effective. Many people would rather talk than listen. Often, the client will assist in the diagnosis by providing important clues in the history if only we will listen. Active listening involves listening to clients and then verbally rephrasing their messages back to them for verification. This technique ensures that the client was heard correctly and the technician or veterinarian received the entire message.

Listening requires understanding of both the *music* and the *words*. The correct words must be sent and received. In addition, the nonverbal music (facial expressions, hand gestures, body stance, and so forth) must also be observed and understood to allow complete communication.

Client Expectations

Most clients expect the following five things during a consultation with a veterinarian: (1) examination of the animal, (2) diagnosis (cause if possible), (3) prognosis (predicted outcome), (4) treatment plan, and (5) fee estimate. Communication of prognosis, treatment plan, and fee estimate is difficult for many veterinarians. Clients feel unprepared to make judgments without this information and often complain if complications occur. Malpractice (professional negligence) concerns can be virtually eliminated if these areas are effectively handled with the client. Again, the veterinary technician should be part of the communication team in these areas. Clear, effective communication is a team effort.

Common Complaints from Clients

When dealing with a cross section of the public, as most practices do, complete satisfaction for all clients can never be obtained. However, when clients do have complaints, careful attention must be given. To reduce the number of complaints from clients, several potential problem areas will be addressed. The more common areas of client complaints you will have to deal with are fees, courtesy-concern, communication, appointment schedule, sanitation and quality of care.

Every client deserves a complete explanation and breakdown of all anticipated costs of each service to be performed. Whenever communication fails to become complete, client complaints will result. One of the most sensitive issues practitioners deal with is financial estimates. Quoted fees must be written down and honored unless revised with full consent of the owner. The most common client complaint will concern

fees. The use of a fee-estimate sheet and up-front, open communication will eliminate most fee complaints.

The use of appointments has been found by most practitioners to be helpful to both client and veterinarian if properly used. Practices that have an appointment system but always seem to have people waiting have a management problem. Clients do not like to wait any more than you do when you have an appointment. Society is geared to drive-in service, fast food, instant automatic banking, cellular communications, one-stop shopping, microwave cooking, and so forth; no one expects or likes to wait.

Appointment schedules on occasion will be disrupted by an emergency. When clients consistently have to wait, more veterinarians may be needed, office visits may need to be shortened or additional appointment hours may need to be scheduled, to reduce the backlog. When appointments are going to be delayed, common courtesy dictates that an explanation be given and a specific appointment time stated as soon as the client arrives. The client always should be given the option of rescheduling the appointment to a more convenient time or leaving the pet and returning to pick it up later in the day. When time permits, scheduled clients should be called by the receptionist and rescheduled before they leave home to ease an overburdened schedule caused by an unexpected emergency.

Hospital cleanliness is important to the client, and the lack of it can result in complaints. If the veterinary hospital is to be considered a medical facility, odors and sanitation must be rigidly monitored by all personnel. The reception room, examination rooms, and public bathrooms must be inspected and cleaned regularly. Whenever a pet soils an area, it must be cleaned quickly and thoroughly. Deodorizers may be of benefit to help clear the air but should not be used to "cover up" a sanitation problem. The hospital wards should be cleaned frequently to avoid odor build-up. The ventilation system should be capable of exhausting all air in the building within 15 to 20 minutes. In addition to exhaust fans in the wards, fans are useful in the examination rooms and laboratory areas.

The last common client complaint area centers on the quality of care offered to the patient and the client. Often, animal owners are hesitant to accept one veterinarian's opinion. As in human medicine, seeking multiple opinions on a case has become routine. Specialists have become more commonplace in veterinary practice, and veterinary clients are requesting second and third opinions. Multiple opinions have been good for both the patient and the client, but they require veterinarians to be thorough and up to date with their information and techniques.

Veterinary clients are no different from any other segment of the population; our clients just happen to own animals. Most of the negative confrontations with clients arise from a lack of common courtesy or from communication failures. Being aware of common pitfalls will allow us to concentrate more effort on those areas, thereby reducing complaints.

The Difficult Client

Some clients remain difficult to deal with regardless of the best efforts of everyone in the practice. Some of these difficult people actually enjoy being difficult. The attitude of the difficult client toward the technical and reception staff may be different from the attitude toward the veterinarian. A very difficult, demanding person can suddenly become quite reasonable when the veterinarian enters the room. When this happens, do not feel that you have failed but rather work a little harder to understand and win the client's trust.

In dealing with someone who is politely complaining, listen to understand their perceptions and feelings and attempt to convey that you understand the problem (you will appear to be agreeing; this will help reduce the level of the confrontation). A good example would be the common complaint that fees are too high, which can be answered by, "Yes, fees are high. Everything is too high these days!"

In situations in which the client appears to be unreasonable about the complaint, establish the specific problem (i.e., fees, unsatisfactory treatment result, poor communication) and then indicate to the client that you would like for him or her to speak to the veterinarian. Once the unreasonable client has been identified, escort the client out of the reception room and into an examination room away from other clients; then, have the veterinarian handle the problem as quickly as possible.

The most difficult people to reason with are people who have been drinking or are on drugs. Be careful how you handle these people because they could become violent and uncontrollable. In situations in which drugs or alcohol has been consumed to excess, law enforcement officials should be contacted to handle the situation.

Never argue with a dissatisfied client. The client is always right, even when wrong. If a client leaves angry, 10 other people are told how terrible you, your veterinarian, and your hospital are. When the client leaves the practice as an enthusiastic client, he will only tell three other people. We cannot have clients leaving angry. Sometimes we must all "eat a little crow" to keep the client's good will. In the long run, this will benefit all concerned.

TECHNICIAN NOTE

Never argue with a dissatisfied client.

Patient Management

Patient management and client management go hand in hand. Both should be handled together, but for the sake of this discussion we have separated them.

Patient management can best be described by outlining the typical case as it moves through the hospital. The first contact is with the receptionist. The receptionist should move the patient and client as quickly as possible into an examination room. A patient presented as an emergency should receive priority. An emergency case is always any case that the *owner* feels is an emergency. Most of these cases are not emergencies, but each should be managed as if it were to ensure client satisfaction with quality of service.

In many practices, the patient will be escorted into the examination room by a veterinary technician. The technician will continue to develop the medical record by obtaining the temperature, pulse, respiration, and weight of the patient. Additional informational questions and a brief physical examination may also be helpful to the veterinarian (see Table 31–6).

Once the veterinarian enters the examination room, the patient and owner should be introduced to the veterinarian by

the technician. Name tags should be worn by all personnel to help the clients remember whom they have met. A veterinary assistant should assist the veterinarian in the physical examination by restraining the patient as necessary. If blood, urine, or skin specimens are needed, the technician should usually take the patient to the treatment room and conduct these procedures away from the client with the help of an assistant. Once a diagnosis has been made by the veterinarian, the patient will either be treated and released or will be hospitalized.

If the patient is to be treated and released, the technician will often give the treatment and will prepare prescriptions as needed. The technician will explain (or demonstrate) how to administer home medications or treatments and will then escort the client to the receptionist for dismissal and fee payment.

When the patient is to be hospitalized, the technician will escort the patient to the ward and ensure that the necessary items are present to make the patient comfortable. The veterinarian will establish each treatment regimen and evaluate its success. During hospitalization, the technician will maintain and manage most of the routine treatments, therapy, laboratory tests, and medical records while delegating exercise, feeding, and grooming to assistants or animal caretakers. Often the daily phone contact with the client will be through the technician. A blackboard or bulletin board in the treatment room can be used to remind personnel of the diagnostic, treatment, and surgery schedules for hospitalized patients. All patients should be evaluated several times daily, and these evaluations should be documented with appropriate records. Walking through ward rounds can be very helpful to all personnel to keep everyone updated on each case.

The dismissal of a hospitalized patient is similar to that of the outpatient except that dispensed medications and patient clean-up must be completed before the owner's arrival. When dismissing a hospitalized patient, the following points should be considered: (1) an itemized fee statement should be ready at the time the owner is called to pick up the animal, (2) all medications should be prepared in child-proof containers with proper labels, (3) the veterinarian should be available for consultation with the client, (4) the technician should be available to demonstrate treatment and home care techniques with hand-out instructions for home reference, (5) fee collection should take place, (6) the next appointment or recheck should be scheduled, and (7) the patient should be presented dry, clean, and odor free. Some conditions dictate that the patient be presented before fee collection and the scheduling of the next appointment. When this occurs, someone should be available to hold or control the animal until the client has completed the dismissal process.

The technician can be extremely valuable during the dismissal process by explaining to the client what to do if specific possible events occur (through reenforcement of directions given by the veterinarian). Clients will often ask technicians questions that they forgot or were afraid to ask the veterinarian.

Most clients will judge the total care an animal has received by the condition and appearance of the animal at dismissal. The patient should always be as clean or cleaner than when admitted. If an animal soils itself just before dismissal, always clean or bathe the animal before sending it home even if the client has to wait a few minutes longer. The client should be informed that the animal has accidentally soiled itself, and you are cleaning it up; "We certainly do not want him to leave dirty." When dismissing surgical patients, in addition to the animal itself being clean, the surgical incision, bandages, splint, or cast must be clean and dry. The surgery technique will be judged by the neatness of hair removal at the surgical site and the appearance of the incision.

TECHNICIAN NOTE

Never send home a patient that has soiled itself.

Personnel Management

Personnel in a practice may be managed directly by the veterinarian or, if the practice is large enough, one of the staff may become the manager. This person will often control the business, personnel, and building functions. Regardless of the size of the practice and how it is managed, each position within the practice should have a back-up person who is cross-trained in that area to take over when sickness, vacation, and emergencies arise. Without a cross-training plan, the practice may become crippled when one person is gone. This is especially true in the smaller practice.

In most practices, the staff duties can be divided into the following job areas: (1) *reception*, (2) *examination room or front office duties*, (3) *in-patient* or *back office duties*, and (4) *building, kennel, and barn maintenance*.

The receptionist is a key position in any hospital operation. She is the first and last to speak to the client. The "life blood" of the practice (clients) must filter through the receptionist via the telephone or one-on-one contact in the reception room. She or he must be a friendly and caring person. The entire mood of the practice and, to a great extent, the attitude of the client will be determined by the communication skills used by the receptionist. For example, the receptionist should screen patients and schedule undiagnosed medical problems or cases requiring radiography earlier in the day so that the client will have a diagnosis before the day's end. The receptionist greets clients, starts the medical record by obtaining some history, answers questions by telephone, makes appointments, handles the records for patient dismissal, answers general medical questions, quotes certain fees, maintains a schedule of all veterinarians, handles money and bank deposits, and manages accounts receivable and other duties as assigned. In short, the receptionist in most practices is a superperson.

A veterinary technician is usually assigned to *examination room or front office* duties. In some practices, the receptionist duties and front office duties will be performed by one person. The role of this individual may include back-up or fill-in for the receptionist in addition to assisting in the examination rooms, obtaining medical histories, filling prescriptions, restraining patients, administering medications, demonstrating treatment techniques to clients, obtaining blood samples, performing laboratory work, escorting patients to the wards, dismissing patients, maintaining the examination, laboratory and pharmacy areas in a clean and orderly manner, and other duties that are necessary for smooth patient flow in the public areas of the hospital. Efficiency is enhanced with multiple examination rooms and an assistant or orderly assigned to assist both technician and veterinarian. Every patient must be examined by a veterinarian to ensure that existing problems are not overlooked (e.g., her-

nias, retained testicles, external parasites). Patients should not be admitted unless a veterinarian has had contact with the patient and client to establish a legal client-patient-veterinarian relationship.

The duties in the *in-patient area (back office)* are more isolated, and there is usually less client contact. Most of these duties are performed by a team of technicians and assistants. These duties include administering or monitoring anesthesia, or both, preparing patients for surgery, monitoring postsurgical patients, surgical assisting, collecting laboratory samples, performing dental cleanings, administering and monitoring treatments, exposing and developing radiographs, performing laboratory work, maintaining medical records, maintaining surgical and anesthesia logs, providing direct medical and surgical nursing care and maintaining the surgery, treatment and radiology areas. *Maintaining building, barn, and wards* in a clean and orderly manner and other duties that are necessary for hospitalized patients to be well cared for are usually delegated to assistants and caretakers and supervised by a veterinary technician. Large practices usually employ animal caregivers to clean, bed, and feed patients, allowing the veterinary technician to perform additional technical support functions.

The role of the technician is determined by the staffing and delegation patterns as well as the size and type of practice. Large private and institutional practices have the case load to allow the technical staff to become very skilled in one area. Examples of these areas would be surgery, intensive care, anesthesiology, cardiology, internal medicine, radiology, clinical pathology, and office management. Specialty societies and certifications for veterinary technicians are now available in critical care, dentistry, anesthesia, and management (see Table 31–4). If the scope of the practice allows, the technician may choose to deal with only small animals or large animals in these areas.

A veterinary technician must be able to work in all areas of the hospital. The most common form of technical support in veterinary practice involves the utilization of the generalist type of veterinary technician. For a technician to function effectively as a generalist, a broad base of information and techniques must be mastered and maintained with cross-training in all technical areas. Being a high-quality generalist is not an easy task.

Veterinary Technician Specialties

Emerging veterinary technician specialties is a new development of the mid-90s in the profession. The use of the word *specialist* is reserved to those who pass an advanced examination (the same is true of veterinary specialties) administered by each respective group (see Table 31–4). It is misleading to the public to call anyone a specialist (even though one's knowledge and expertise may be advanced) until they are credentialed by a specialty organization that meets national standards. The North American Veterinary Technician Association is recognized by the AVMA as the accrediting body for veterinary technician specialties.

It is important to note each of these specialties have a society (an organization of individuals interested in a particular area of veterinary technology) that is open to any interested veterinary technician. The society serves to provide advanced educational materials to its members, some who are studying for specialty certification, some who are certified, and some who are interested in learning the specialty information without sitting for the examinations. Some societies are broader in scope like the Veterinary Hospital Managers Association, Inc., which is open to anyone (including nontechnicians) involved in veterinary practice management. Those who are certified become members of the respective academy.

Job Descriptions

Regardless of the job role in the hospital setting, all personnel should have a detailed job description. A job description will allow both employee and management to maintain a clear understanding of areas of responsibility. Job descriptions are useful when hiring new employees or replacing employees.

Through the use of the job descriptions (expectations) and periodic performance evaluations, employees can be rewarded according to their performance, poor workers can be guided and encouraged to improve, and chronically poor workers can be discharged. One of the most common mistakes in personnel management is to put off regular employee evaluations. Personnel problems resulting from poor work performance do not just go away, they only become worse. Therefore, a job evaluation system that is applied equally to all employees needs to be maintained. Employees cannot improve performance unless they are given an opportunity to identify shortcomings. If improvement is not observed within a reasonable period of time, both practice and employee will probably be better off through employee dismissal.

Hiring Procedures

When hiring a new employee, it is important that all employees have input into the decision if teamwork is to be expected. This is a very important decision. The cost of selection, training, and adaptation can equal 1 year's salary. A bad choice means disruption, turnover, and a loss of thousands of dollars to the practice.

A simple method of candidate evaluation that will satisfy most employees is to have two or three employees interview each candidate first and then make recommendations to the veterinarian. The screening committee should establish specific questions to ask each candidate using the job description prepared for that specific job. The recommendations made to the veterinarian should include suitability, personality, professionalism, knowledge, experience, dress, and other interview assessments. The veterinarian should have the final word on hiring and firing unless a practice manager has been hired for personnel management.

The major steps in the hiring process are to (1) analyze personnel requirements, (2) develop a specific job description, (3) develop a set of interview questions, (4) announce and advertise the position, (5) review the applications and resumes, (6) rank the candidates for interview, (7) check references, (8) interview the top-ranked two to four candidates, (9) make a final selection, (10) offer the job to the best candidate, and (11) establish a starting date.

The analysis of personnel requirements will be done by the veterinarian or office manager based on the needs of the practice or business. Once the general need for the position(s) has been established (or replacement approved), a detailed job description must be prepared or the previous job description updated. The job description is usually developed on one page and consists of four or five job functions outlined in one or two sentences each. Each job function is then assigned a percentage

of time. Once the job description is developed or updated, it can be used to write the advertisement to search for a specific individual. To prepare for the interview, a set of interview questions needs to be developed.

Some interview questions are unlawful or discriminatory and should not be asked (such as questions on race, religion, national origin, sex, handicaps, marital status, and so forth). Questions should always be open ended (see Table 31–6) and allow the candidates to express themselves. The following requests and questions could be considered when preparing interview questions: (1) Please review your previous position. (2) Describe your best boss. (3) Describe your worst boss. (4) What did you like best about your last position? (5) What did you like least about your last position? (6) What specific skills and abilities do you have that apply to this particular position? (7) What are your short-range and long-term employment goals? (8) What accomplishments made you most proud? (9) What type of working relationships do you want to cultivate? (10) How do you feel about constructive criticism and formal evaluation? (11) How do you feel about being on call several times per month? (12) Do you have any questions you would like to ask?

During the interview, the evaluator should ask each candidate the same questions so the responses can be compared. The interview period is the time to evaluate motivation, personal appearance, and personal hygiene. The job description, salary, and benefits should be reviewed. Each interviewer or interview team should limit their part of the interview to 30 minutes.

After the interview, personal references should be checked and past supervisors contacted. When all the above material has been collected and weighted, the individual who is the best person (and match) for the position should be offered the job.

When the final selection has been made, the most common initial contact will be by telephone. During the telephone call, the job description should be reviewed, salary and benefits discussed, and starting date established. When the above steps are followed, the best candidate should be more easily identified and successfully hired.

A potential problem in personnel management is internal communication. To avoid internal disputes, weekly (or monthly) staff meetings should be held to detail all employees on various aspects of hospital operation. Often, notes on a blackboard just do not do the job! These meeting can also be used to develop teamwork via group problem-solving techniques.

 TECHNICIAN NOTE

Practice staff meetings should be held at least once per month to ensure open communications.

Delegation Principles

Personnel costs may be reduced by hiring the correct personnel for the job and delegating properly. Too many practices are still trying to hire a new veterinarian to perform veterinary technician duties. Many also hire veterinary technicians to perform non–income-producing duties of assistants and caretakers. Consequently, the practice spends more money than necessary on personnel and frustrates a new veterinarian or technician in the process as well as limiting income produced.

Both veterinarians and veterinary technicians should be paid according to gross income produced; therefore, aides and assistants hired at near-minimum wage levels should be relied on as much as possible to perform most non–income-producing tasks, like restraint, cleaning, and animal husbandry. Veterinarians should focus on making diagnoses, prescribing treatments, and performing surgery while delegating billable treatments, anesthesia, dental prophies, imaging, and laboratory procedures to certified veterinary technicians.

Personnel management is important because the greatest percentage of overhead is in personnel. All personnel must work as a team. Working *with* someone is always better than working *for* someone. All practice employees (including veterinarians) must be as productive as possible to provide a profitable and pleasant working environment. Veterinarians and technicians are usually not professionally trained to be managers. Both must work together to have a successfully managed practice, which will result in career satisfaction, not just a job.

Business Management

Professionals as a whole would like to abstain from the business side of practice and concentrate exclusively on professional (medical) activities. In reality, without the business side of any profession, there would be few opportunities to practice that profession. The business management aspects of practice can become as challenging as patient management. Available time, lack of interest, and/or minimal experience are the limiting factors.

Clinical signs of poor business management are lax credit policies, increasing accounts receivable (total dollars clients owe), reduced operating capital, lowered gross income, lowered net income, increasing personnel costs, increasing overhead, reduced client numbers, and reduced average transaction fee per patient. Tests used to confirm your diagnosis of poor business management include complete review of monthly business information to establish trends, comparison of this month's data to the same month 1 year ago, review of fee schedule, review of credit policy and review and comparison of inventory levels, and turnover rates.

Prognosis is generally good once the diagnosis of poor business management has been supported by a review of the diagnostic tests. Treatment will usually need to continue for the life of the practice. Some recommended treatments for the poor business management syndrome follow: Establish a firm and written credit policy with few exceptions. Make use of a written fee estimate sheet to itemize all patient charges. Prior to admission, have the owner sign and retain one copy. The credit policy should be clearly stated on the fee estimate sheet (see Chapter 4 for example of fee estimate form). Make use of appointment systems to schedule clients for the most efficient use of time.

The practice fee schedule should be reviewed and updated at least every 3 to 6 months, and a current printed fee schedule should be available near each telephone. Daily work schedules should be planned each morning to divide the work into work blocks. Some days, noon hours will not be able to be taken when the surgery schedule is heavy or unexpected emergencies arise. Accounts receivable need to be monitored monthly, with appropriate follow-up telephone calls and letters to stimulate payment in a timely manner.

Accounts payable should be handled in a way to allow discounts for prompt payment. Accounts that do not provide discounts should be paid near the due date to conserve working capital. No account should be allowed to be past due. A poor credit image is difficult to remove.

Close attention to inventory levels of surgical supplies, pharmaceuticals, cleaning supplies, x-ray film, and so form will ensure that an adequate stock is maintained without oversupply (Table 31–7). Inventory (second largest expense area) should turn over approximately every 45 to 60 days. Beware of the "deal" that gives you a year's supply of an item, because that item also ties up capital for a year. Some inventory items will turn over 12 to 20 times per year (e.g., pet food) and will be sold before the supplier is paid.

One tool for analyzing and correcting poor business management is the minicomputer. The office minicomputer can provide on-line storage and have information readily available at the push of a button. The minicomputer can provide income analysis, accounts receivable information, vaccination reminders, accounts payable information, inventory control, client information analysis, patient diagnosis analysis, and so forth. Computerization is becoming increasingly cost-effective, and well-designed programs are now available through several vendors. Additional information about computers in veterinary medicine is found in Chapter 35.

If these treatments are properly applied, the outcome from "the poor business management syndrome" should be complete recovery. The result of improved management is a sound and stable veterinary practice that pays dividends to clients, patients and employees.

Professional Marketing

Some professionals feel uncomfortable with the idea of marketing because the scope of activity has been poorly understood.

• Table 31–7 •

INVENTORY MANAGEMENT FORMULAS

$$\text{Turnover rate* of an item} = \frac{\text{Yearly inventory expense for item}}{\text{Average cost of item on hand at any one time}}$$

$$\text{Average cost of inventory on hand at one time} = \frac{\text{Inventory at midyear} + \text{Inventory at year's end}}{2}$$

*Pareto's law, or the 80/20 rule, states that 20% of the items account for 80% of the annual inventory expenses; this suggests that the above formulas should be used to evaluate and adjust the turnover rate of the biggest expense items to attain the "ideal turnover rate."

Adapted from Lukens & Landon's Effective Inventory Control. West Chester, PA, Smith Kline Beecham (Pfizer), 1993.

Often, the connotation of marketing is advertising. However, advertising is only a portion of the total marketing picture. Professional marketing has numerous definitions, but the one that will be used here is "the communication of professional services and goods offered to existing and potential clients." The veterinary technician will continue to be a necessary communicator of professional services and goods offered by the practice.

What Is Professional Marketing?

Professional marketing consists of all activities that increase awareness of professional services and goods. Marketing occurs through effective client relations; appearance of the hospital, clinic, or ambulatory vehicle; listening to owner's opinions; convenient practice location; a polite support staff; offering full-service care; sending client service reminders; being neat and clean; using business cards; sending client educational newsletters; providing nutritional counseling and dietary management; providing emergency service; offering pet and livestock supplies; giving career talks at high schools; leading 4-H, FFA, or scouting groups; attending dog/cat/horse shows; having producer or client educational nights; being involved in a community service club; advertising in the yellow pages of the telephone book; providing handout material to clients; having an attractive and well-located building sign; sending thank-you and sympathy cards to appropriate clients; appearing as a guest on radio or television shows; writing a newspaper animal column; using attractive letterhead stationery; becoming active in professional associations; group advertising in the newspaper about the annual rabies vaccination clinic; and so forth.

Animals are totally dependent on owner awareness of health care needs. Professional marketing should be designed to help more animals by informing and serving more clients. If successful, it will result in increased practice income through increasing client numbers of and/or amount of each client transaction. It requires balancing improved animal health and public health with the needs and goals of the practice.

Professional marketing has now become a part of practice and should be used with the same skill and currentness as medical, diagnostic or surgical procedures. Continuing education in the areas of marketing and practice management are as necessary as any other veterinary medical discipline. The question is no longer, "Should we market," but "How should we market?"

The profession needs to continue to be acutely aware of professional ethics and maintain the highest degree of professionalism. Professional marketing is not opposed to that position and philosophy when properly applied. The first step must be to accept marketing as a useful practice tool. The next step is to gain understanding in techniques available and then apply those techniques to the practice and the profession.

The Business of Veterinary Medicine

One of the most critical questions a veterinarian should ask is "What business am I in?" To be able to conduct a successful professional business, one must be clear about specific business objectives. Some practitioners believe as long as high-quality medical and surgical skill is delivered, the client will continue to use their service based on the quality of service alone. Fortunately, clients today are usually well-informed consumers and are looking for both quality *and* value. The average client

lacks the professional background to accurately judge the quality of medical or surgical services performed. However, they do have the ability to judge the quality of care *they* received personally and the value of the service received. The client's perceived value of services is the reality of the practice's quality.

Veterinary medicine is in the *people service* business. The profession cares for animals but provides professional services to their owners. If one understands that she or he is in the people service business, a completely different orientation will take place. When clients call on the telephone, for example, they are not interrupting the veterinarian's or technician's time in the examination room or surgery room; they are the reason for the existence of the examination room and surgery room. Veterinary practices do provide high-quality professional service to animals but only after the agreement and support of the owner/client.

✎ TECHNICIAN NOTE

Client phone calls are not an interruption because clients are the reason for the existence of the practice.

The professional success of most veterinarians and technicians is the result of *interpersonal skills* rather than strictly clinical skills. The ability to relate to people and their problems will allow the practice the opportunity to provide high-quality veterinary medicine (Fig. 31–12).

Once the practice is viewed as a people service business, marketing of those services becomes possible. The product to be marketed is *high-quality, people-oriented professional veterinary medical service.*

Marketing techniques must benefit the profession as a whole to achieve maximum success. The overall program must promote the *benefits* of veterinary services rather than the specific service.

If one were to compare a program of the benefits of immunization with one that sold a vaccination, the long-term effects are evident. A program that details the benefits of immu-

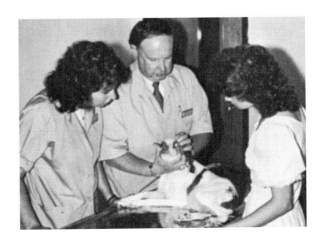

Figure 31-12. Technician, veterinarian, and client communicating as a team about patient care.

nization can build in a physical examination, dental care, nutritional management, and so forth on an annual basis. The approach of selling a vaccination is just that—promoting a vaccine.

The program of promoting the benefits of a high-quality, people-oriented professional veterinary medical service must be the end goal.

Practice Marketing

Practice marketing cannot become a "bag of tricks" to be pulled out as a last resort when all else fails. Marketing must become a practice and professional philosophy that is driven by client needs. The profession must understand the veterinary needs of the client. A compromise must be reached between what we think the client needs and what the client feels is needed for his or her animal.

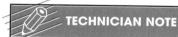

TECHNICIAN NOTE

Marketing must become a practice and professional philosophy driven by client needs.

The first step in a marketing plan, then, is to determine client needs. One must listen closely to services being asked for by each client. Determine what service trends are going on within the practice in response to economic growth of the community. As an example, both spouses usually work today. This results in some people being unable to seek veterinary care during the traditional 8 A.M. to 5 P.M. time period. The typical client also has less free time to devote to shopping around at several stores for items when all items could be purchased at one convenient location. By listening to clients and observing service needs, the practitioner may opt to extend the practice hours two evenings per week and open later in the mornings on those days. The practice may also expand services to include veterinary supervised boarding and offer selected non-professional supplies like grooming aids.

The practice owner must determine the direction of the marketing plan by listening to client needs and gathering additional facts concerning community trends. The marketing process will then be guided by current facts and psychodemographic information.

Specific Marketing Techniques

Marketing techniques will not overcome the effects of poor client relations within a practice. Unless effective client communication and client orientation are practiced on a client-by-client basis, marketing will be unsuccessful.

Professional marketing can be divided into *internal* and *external* marketing. Internal marketing techniques are the day-to-day activities that occur within each practice, whereas external marketing involves techniques used outside the practice. The purpose of both internal and external techniques is to enlarge the number and size of client transactions.

Internal Marketing

Internal marketing is aimed primarily at the existing client base. These techniques are attempting to educate and inform current

clients about various veterinary services and service programs. They also should generate client enthusiasm for the practice. The following methods are meant to serve as an idea base and not as a complete listing of techniques.

Client Relations. The most important technique to use in any marketing program is personalized, sincere client care. Most clients require as much attention and care as the patient. Clients today want both high technology and high touch. Personalized service that places emphasis on each individual client will allow the opportunity for excellent communication to be established. Both veterinarian and technician must be skilled communicators as well as technically skilled professionals.

Practice Appearance. The visual appearance of the clinic, hospital or ambulatory vehicle is the first outward signal to the client concerning the potential quality of service. One must consider the appearance of the building (repair, paint, cleanliness) and the grounds (Fig. 31–13). Plantings and grass must be neat and trimmed and the parking lot clean and well signed for parking. The interior of the building must also be clean, well cared for, and odor free. Silent marketing messages are sent to clients through the appearance of the facility.

A practice facility does not have to be new or have the latest equipment to project a positive image. The older facility that has been given proper care and maintenance will exhibit a strong marketing message of "we care" to people passing by each day.

Support Staff Utilization. Most of the internal marketing carried on within a practice will be through the veterinary team members. Support staff activities will augment the efforts of the veterinarian in client relations and personal appearance. Primarily, veterinary technicians and receptionists will be responsible for recommending services or goods and following up on hospital programs that require appointments or individual client contact. These team members are regarded as an extension of the veterinarian and must have a professional approach to client management.

Technical staff will usually deliver the majority of client education with the assistance of receptionists. Handout materials, visual aids and video presentations will help the staff in their educational efforts. The staff will need detailed information concerning the various preventative health programs from the veterinarian. To be able to promote the product, everyone needs to be clear about the product. Therefore, the veterinarian

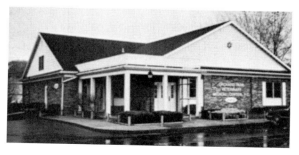

Figure 31–13. Exterior appearance of the hospital should provide a positive image.

and the support staff must work together as a service team, all delivering the same high-quality service.

Professional sales point displays can add another level of service for clients. These displays need continuous monitoring by support staff to provide "on the spot" professional information. Areas in which support staff should have in-depth knowledge include nutrition, parasite control (internal and external), grooming aids, dental care, immunization programs, obedience training, and rearing orphan animals. In addition, support staff must be on the constant lookout for new clients and additional services. Staff members who are active in dog clubs have continual access to new potential clients. New clients may not be aware of services offered, and so all staff members must be willing to provide program information at any time. When certain key support staff members are given a small percentage of income from all new services and new clients they provide the practice as an incentive, a new wave of enthusiasm may develop in everyone.

Full-Service Care. Listening to client needs will verify that clients want full-service care when possible. People are exposed to 1-hour photo processing, 1-hour eyeglasses, 7-Eleven, fast food restaurants, K-Mart, Wal-Mart, drive-through banking, and so forth. Convenient, fast, economical, one-stop shopping is the rule for single-parent families and families in which both husband and wife work. People are now asking for this same type of convenient service in their veterinary care. In small animal practice, full-service care would include prepurchase counseling concerning pets, human-animal bond and behavioral problem counseling, pediatric care, preventive medicine, nutritional counseling, nutritional management, veterinary supervised boarding, geriatric care, dentistry, bereavement counseling, cremation service, and full routine veterinary care. The service would extend from birth to death.

In a full-service practice, various programs can be packaged for marketing. The goal of marketing is to sell a *program,* not an individual service. The emphasis of a quality practice is to provide preventative health care, not just disease treatment. A small animal practice might have a complete health maintenance (wellness) program for new puppies as well as puppy training classes. This program carries into adulthood and on into the geriatric period. The wellness program could include annual physicals, nutritional counseling, dental care, immunizations, and so forth. Nutritional counseling would include pediatric, adult, and geriatric care as the patient matures. As clients continue their regular contact with the practice to purchase foods, the practice has a regular opportunity to market other health preventative care services.

Client Reminders. One of the more successful early attempts at practice marketing was through the use of a vaccination reminder system for small animals. During the early discussions on the use of a recall system, many practitioners felt it was unprofessional to send a reminder card to clients because it was advertising. No one was considering the service provided to the client and animal. Most veterinarians thought only of how it would appear to other veterinarians.

Charles, Charles and Associates discovered that sending vaccination reminders was more important to clients than having boarding facilities or an attractive building. Clients want to be reminded when specific services are to be done. However, clients prefer to receive reminders by mail rather than by telephone.

> **TECHNICIAN NOTE**
>
> Clients now expect the practice to send annual vaccination reminders.

A reminder system is a major marketing feature of most practice management computer software packages. A system that has the capacity to generate only one reminder is not nearly as valuable as a system that will produce a second and third level of accountability. Using a system that will allow a second or third notice to be sent will greatly increase the service return rate.

Most practices now accept the use of a reminder system as a valuable marketing tool for routine immunizations. The reminder system must now be expanded to include other routine services for the clients. Additional use in the small animal practice could be in the areas of dental hygiene (routine cleaning), annual physical examination, geriatric care, hip-dysplasia evaluations, heartworm evaluation, and so forth. The suggestion of an annual physical examination may appear on the surface to be a poor recommendation in light of physicians now recommending fewer annual physicals. However, considering that the dog and cat age seven to nine times as rapidly as humans and that the diligent veterinarian and technician are able to find a potential problem on almost every physical examination, many clients will take advantage of the service when offered. When performing the examination, the veterinarian and technician must explain and demonstrate the findings to the client (i.e., potential problem with ears, eyes, teeth, anal sac, hair coat, obesity, and so forth) (Fig. 31–14).

Small animal geriatric care is another relatively untapped market area. When patients reach a specific age (i.e., 7 to 8

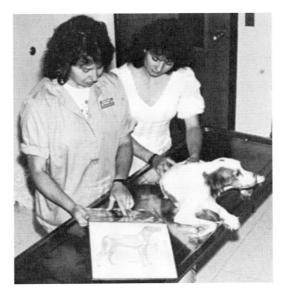

Figure 31-14. Technician explaining diagnosis to client using visual aid.

years of age), a reminder letter could be sent to the client providing information on specific conditions to be monitored. The letter could approach the client by "Congratulations, Blacky has just become a senior canine citizen. When dogs reach about eight years of age, the care necessary to prevent and monitor disease changes. We would like to provide the following information to allow Blacky to enjoy his new senior status: . . . " This letter could be developed on the word processor and recalled by the computer at a specific age.

Another area in which a reminder system could be used is to recall young animals that have been previously vaccinated but not yet neutered. The recall of un-neutered animals is an opportunity to market ovariohysterectomy and castration services. This reminder may attract some of the clients who would otherwise go to a low-cost spay and neuter clinic. A personalized word processor letter could detail the specific features of the service, which is not possible from the spay and neuter clinics.

The use of a recall system allows the market to be segmented (targeted). An example of market segmentation would be to send all feline owners a reminder about leukemia vaccination.

Personal Appearance. The personal appearance and hygiene of each staff member are a reflection of the quality of the practice. Clients quickly relate personal appearance to the sanitation and level of quality of the practice. If someone does not care enough to change a dirty smock, or dirty coveralls or boots, why should they care enough to provide the highest-quality service? Not only should hand washing occur between every patient, it should be practiced in front of the client. Personal appearance marketing works just as building appearance—an outward signal of internal activity (Fig. 31–15). A professional image is perceived by the client when all hospital members have a professional appearance.

TECHNICIAN NOTE

Personal appearance is a direct reflection of practice quality.

Handout Materials. Marketing with handout materials has been used for a number of years. The quantity and quality of commercially available handouts are continually increasing. Most commercial companies realize the value of client-oriented professional literature. These pieces should be carefully reviewed by the practice so only acceptable material is made available to clients. Once the material has been reviewed and useful pieces selected, all staff members must be made familiar with how and when they should be used. A professional rubber stamp can be purchased with the practice name, location, and telephone number on it and used to personalize all handout materials. Handout material must be handed directly to the client by the veterinarian or technician to be most effective (Fig. 31–16). Handout materials displayed in the reception room for clients to pick up are often not well utilized. Clients will pick up material from a display rack and take it home, but few will ever read it.

In addition to commercial handouts, materials may be purchased from organized veterinary medicine. The American Vet-

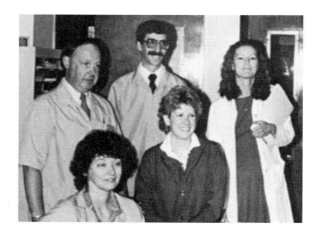

Figure 31–15. A professional appearance is a marketing tool.

erinary Medical Association, American Association of Equine Practitioners, and American Animal Hospital Association, among others, have useful client handout materials.

Practices may also produce their own informational material. Quality handouts on whelping, ovariohysterectomy, cystic calculi, colic, mastitis, and so forth can be easily prepared on the word processor. Discharge instruction handouts are very effective because clients often forget verbal explanations and instructions. Practice information brochures can also be produced to more fully explain practice hours, services, equipment, facilities, and staff function (Fig. 31–17). Other forms of handout materials used on a regular basis are business cards and letterhead stationery. These have become so commonplace they are also forgotten; however, they are effective forms of marketing. Business cards should be made available to clients from *both* veterinarians and key support staff, especially veterinary technicians.

Sympathy and Thank-You Communications. A very personal marketing approach is to appropriately use sympathy and thank-you types of communication (Fig. 31–18). One may choose to use commercially prepared cards or develop a letter format on the word processor that can be personalized. Regard-

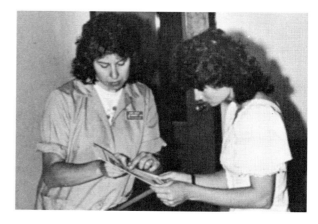

Figure 31–16. Technician explaining and providing a handout to client.

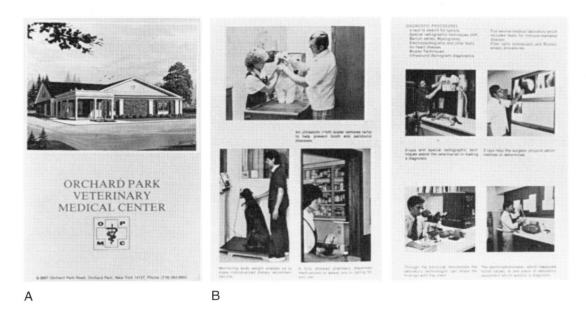

A   B

Figure 31-17. Practice information pamphlet: cover (A) and inner page (B) examples. (Courtesy of Orchard Park Veterinary Medical Center, Orchard Park, NY.)

less of the format used, the use of personal messages to specific clients for specific purposes has an everlasting positive effect.

In the case of a newly referred client by a current client, a note or card to both the referring client (thanking them for the referral) and the new client (welcoming them to the practice) is appropriate. The sympathy card or personal note is helpful to demonstrate open concern for the feelings of the client during his or her emotional loss. The expression helps the client deal with the loss and allows the client to understand the "I care" attitude of the practice for both the client and pet.

Newsletters. Charles, Charles and Associates reported the use of newsletters is related to increased number of clinic visits by dog owners. The use of newsletters will increase client activity through improved understanding and education about veterinary services. Educational goals for newsletters should be to inform animal owners of signs of illness, to make seasonal animal health care recommendations (i.e., heat stroke in summer), to review health care programs, and to introduce key

staff members. Many clients do not understand how to tell whether an animal is ill or in serious condition. This lack of knowledge is especially true for cat and horse owners.

The horse is difficult for the average client to evaluate when the animal is experiencing abdominal pain from colic. Unless the owner is familiar with the specific signs of abdominal pain, the animal's condition may become critical before attention is sought. It is also difficult to tell when a cat is ill. Normally, cats sleep a lot, cover their feces and urine, and tend to be loners. It becomes difficult to really know when they are ill unless the owner understands normal cat behavior traits.

Newsletters will allow the client to be exposed to specific pieces of information that will help the owner to know when to call a veterinarian for help. Total health care plans can also be explained to allow the owner to be aware of full-service health care that extends beyond vaccinations. The newsletter should help market the benefits of healthy animals.

Newsletters can be sent to specific segments of clients in the practice computer base; however, they can also be provided through a hand-generated list or passed out to each client as they enter the practice. Most veterinarians do not have the experience or time to compose a complete newsletter three or four times per year. The practice managers, veterinary technicians, and/or receptionists may develop articles for a practice newsletter, or consideration can be given to purchasing a professionally edited newsletter service.

Each newsletter should be personalized by the practice to allow the reader easy access to the practice's location and telephone number. Another advantage newsletters have in overall marketing is the ability to reach the nonuser. If the client receiving the newsletter passes it on to a nonclient friend, the nonclient has an opportunity to be exposed to various veterinary services offered by the practice.

Special Services. Practices can either expand existing services or add new services to increase their market share. In a small animal practice, market expansion might be in the areas of

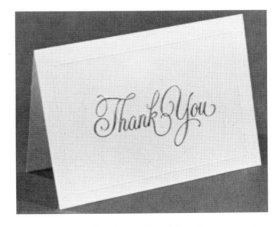

Figure 31-18. Example of thank-you card.

birds and exotic service, bereavement counseling, prepurchase evaluation of pets to determine suitability for family, behavior counseling, nutritional counseling (i.e., puppy, adult, senior), dental care (i.e., endodontics, periodontics, orthodontics), geriatric care, cremation service, emergency care, and intensive care unit. Because most small animal clinics cater to dogs, many cat owners do not feel welcome or comfortable in an environment of dog pictures on the walls and barking dogs in the reception area. Practices that want to increase feline clients might be well rewarded by considering the needs of cats and cat owners when remodeling. Having a separate reception area for cats and keeping cats in a separate ward should be a starting point. Our own attitudes about feline care may be the primary reason for serving only 70% of the cat owners with professional veterinary care.

Sales Point Displays. When displays are being considered as an internal marketing technique, several important points must be contemplated if they are to be maximally successful. First, the practice must define the clients' needs. The specific products must be carefully selected and priced. An appropriate location(s) must be established in the clinic or hospital that may be monitored at *all* times by the technical staff (Fig. 31–19). The products must be attractively arranged and kept neat and clean. Prices must be clearly marked on all products.

The most important difference between a hospital or clinic display and a retail store display is the *professional* advice that goes along with each item sold. Professional counseling is not available at the feed store, grocery store, department store, or mail order outlets. The technical staff will play a key role in product information for the client.

Professional displays may be limited product lines confined to an examination room, a specific area of the reception room, or a special room adjacent to the reception room.

Animal Care Talks. Veterinary technicians and veterinarians can both become involved in providing veterinary medical care talks to grade school and high school students as well as to adult clients. The most effective and unique visual aid is a live animal. These presentations can provide information on routine animal health care, first aid activities, signs to look for when an animal is ill, and general information on educational requirements of veterinarians and technicians. These presentations also help to change the established "norms" about animal care.

When a presentation has become polished, service clubs

in the community make excellent audiences. Talks to service clubs are helpful to enhance awareness of quality medical care provided by the individual practice and the profession. A slide or video presentation that features both veterinarian and technician in their "team" roles is very effective.

The veterinary technician could present information on care of the new puppy or kitten, information on exotic pets and birds, first aid, feeding the pet, whelping and queening, hip dysplasia, parasite control, pet obedience training, and pet selection. Client education programs should be given on a regular basis and offered at convenient times. Attendees should be provided with handout material to take home for future reference.

TECHNICIAN NOTE

Technicians can present client education programs to expand professional services for preventive medicine.

When the education program is held at the practice, a complete tour of the facilities should be planned. Clients are interested in seeing hospital equipment and understanding more about hospital care. An annual hospital open house is an excellent image builder to clients. Having a "behind the scenes" tour is something most clients have not had an opportunity to experience. Many will be "amazed" to see x-ray, anesthesia, surgery, and laboratory equipment "just like in a human hospital." Children are especially impressed with "show and tell" demonstrations using live animals.

By providing client education opportunities, the client becomes more bonded to the practice. When veterinary problems arise, the client is more apt to contact the practice who has provided the inside look and veterinary medical information.

External Marketing

Most external marketing activities are aimed at expanding current client activity and identifying new nonclient activity. External marketing can be carried out by an individual practice, group practice, organized veterinary medicine, and commercial companies.

Some types of external marketing are currently being utilized in many practices. The use of newsletters (direct mail to nonclients), telephone yellow page listings, building signs, client education nights, community service activities, and AVMA's National Pet Week materials expands the image of the practice to clients and nonclients. When a practice wants to penetrate into the nonclient base, one must make use of advertising.

Professional Advertising. Professional advertising includes hospital signs, telephone book listings, practice newsletters, vaccination reminders, professional business cards, and so forth. However, the focus on advertising in this discussion will center on the more "hard-core" forms of advertising: yellow pages of the telephone book, newspapers, magazines, radio, direct mail, and television.

Attitudes concerning advertising differ between the professional and the consumer. A great majority of professionals (physicians, dentists, attorneys, veterinarians) are against adver-

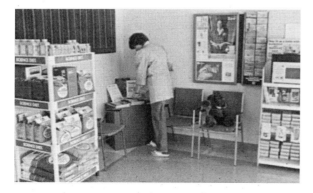

Figure 31-19. Professional display in reception area being monitored by a staff member.

tising for a variety of reasons: it seems to be unprofessional and unethical, and lowers status, credibility, and sense of dignity. Just as professionals feel strongly negative toward advertising, consumers feel strongly positive. Consumers generally feel advertising by a professional would not compromise that professional's credibility, status, image, or dignity as long as it is honest and not misleading. In fact, most consumers believe advertising by professionals would help them make a more intelligent choice.

Telephone Yellow Pages. When a yellow page advertisement is deemed appropriate for external marketing purposes, several guidelines should be followed. First, the advertisement should not be larger than one-fourth page; advertisements larger than one-fourth page are perceived as being more unprofessional by the consumer. Second, the advertisement should be set in one color (preferably black). The use of multiple colors (such as red and green) is again perceived by the consumer as being less professional.

Newspapers. Newspaper advertising, like telephone yellow page advertising, is useful for initial impact when opening or expanding a practice. Many professionals will have a newspaper listing when opening a new practice, when relocating an existing practice or when adding new associates to an existing practice. The continual use of newspaper advertising by veterinarians has been largely prohibited by cost.

Probably the best form of newspaper advertising for veterinarians is the "animal care information" format. Weekly animal care information columns are a public service, and newspapers are always seeking educational material. "Pet columns" have become popular reading as the public begins to acknowledge and understand the human-animal bond. To address the need for weekly newspaper columns, several private column services have sprung up that will provide the practitioner with 52 professionally written stories on animal care each year. This service can be purchased by individual veterinarians or through associations.

Radio and Television. Veterinary associations can obtain air time essentially free by participating in talk shows. The subject of animals, animal care, and animal behavior is a fascinating subject to most listening and viewing audiences. A number of the larger radio and television markets have regularly scheduled talk shows (some hosted by veterinarians) that have a question-and-answer format devoted to animal care. The talk show format is an excellent opportunity for associations that have articulate and knowledgeable veterinarians and technicians to sell veterinary medicine for the profession as a whole.

The bottom line for all individual practices and most smaller group practices is advertising is too expensive to be carried out on a regular basis. The only medium that has consistently been used to attract nonclients is the telephone yellow pages. Other forms of advertising (i.e., television, newspaper, magazines, radio) must be supported by organized veterinary medicine and commercial companies. Increased interest in promoting veterinarians and veterinary practice has come from commercial companies on the realization that individual practice expansion results in commercial expansion.

Community Activities. Veterinary practices that are engaged in community activities have a much wider client contact base.

Veterinarians and technicians can both become involved in community service through Girl Scouts, Boy Scouts, 4-H Veterinary Science Leader, school board, humane society, country club, Rotary, Lions, and church activities. Potential client contacts are made in the course of "being involved." In addition, one becomes more knowledgeable about the species, breed, and show circuit problems when participating in animal breed clubs.

One should not join a community activity only to make client contacts. Practice is too time consuming for both veterinarian and technician to become involved in too many activities or activities that are not personally rewarding. However, these activities are an important marketing tool in addition to being necessary for supporting the community.

Graduate Technician Self-Marketing

Veterinary technicians must learn to choose employment in practices in which veterinarians will delegate sufficient billable technical tasks to allow the technician to generate income. This must be sufficient to provide adequate leveraging of the veterinarian's productivity to provide a professional salary sufficient for the technician to stay in the veterinary technology profession. The IAMS publication "How to Market Yourself—A Veterinary Technician Placement Program" is an excellent resource to plan this critical choice.

TECHNICIAN NOTE

Leveraging of the veterinarian's productivity through delegation of billable tasks will provide adequate salary for the technician.

The second phase of technician marketing occurs after the initial adjustment period of employment. Once a technician is a productive and trusted part of the veterinary team, strategies must be undertaken to improve and enhance the technician's productive role on the veterinary team. "I can do that" spoken at appropriate times is one of many ways to encourage greater delegation. Keeping a log of technical duties performed by the veterinarian and preparing a written summary with an analysis of potential time (and money) saved can also be effective. The same process can be applied to tasks that could be more economically done by a minimum wage assistant.

Obviously, there must be some role delineation between the technician and assistants and between veterinarians and technicians while the most productive teamwork possible is maintained. In general, tasks should be delegated to the lowest paid person who can perform them correctly, especially when other income-producing tasks are waiting. However, no one should avoid their fair share of unpleasant tasks at the cost of destroying a cohesive team!

Building Maintenance

The largest capital investments of a veterinary hospital practice are the building, land, and equipment. Clients often evaluate the level of animal care by the appearance of the building and grounds. Maintenance of building and grounds through paint-

• Table 31–8 •

ELECTRICAL EQUIPMENT SAFETY RULES

The patient

- Avoid touching the animal and any conductive metal surface of an electrical instrument at the same time.
- Be sure all electrical equipment in the vicinity of or attached to the animal is effectively grounded with three-wire power cords and do not allow any equipment with two-prong plugs in the animal's vicinity.
- When two or more electrical instruments are used near a patient, connect them to the same wall outlet. Also, remove all unnecessary electrical equipment from the animal's environment.
- Always plug electrical equipment into the wall outlet with the equipment power switch off.

Power cords

- Avoid using extension cords with any patient instrumentation, and never use a two-prong to three-prong cheater adapter on two-wire outlets.
- Keep electrical cords out of well-traveled pathways and do not step on or roll equipment over electrical cables.
- Plug and unplug the power cord of the equipment by holding onto the plug firmly and straight.
- Before power cords and their connectors are used, carefully check for intermittent or loose connections, frayed wires, cracked connectors, and overall quality.

Appliances

- Check all electrical appliances (especially motorized devices) periodically for current leakage and ground wire continuity.
- If performance of an instrument is unsatisfactory or a tingling sensation is felt from it, remove it from use and have it checked.
- Keep fluids, chemicals, spillable products, and heat away from electrical equipment and cables.

General

- Know the location of circuit breakers for each wall outlet serving clinical areas.
- Remember, body moisture or perspiration lowers electrical resistance and permits greater current to flow.
- Use common sense when working with electrical equipment.
- Remember that the patient is in the electrical environment and could become part of an unsuspected circuit.

Adapted from Swift C and Carithers R: Electrical safety for the veterinarian: Macroshock hazards. JAVMA 172:903–910, 1978.

ing and repair of the interior and exterior of the building along with meticulous care of the lawn, shrubs, trees, and flowers translates into a caring feeling to the client.

General maintenance within the building is an ongoing responsibility. Floors, flat surfaces, walls, cages, runs, and stalls must be kept sparkling clean and odor free. To reach this goal, *everyone* in the practice must assume some of the responsibility. No one should hunt for someone else to clean up a fresh urine or fecal deposit; it is quicker and easier to clean it up by yourself.

Equipment maintenance and cleaning should be an ongoing activity as well. Each major piece of equipment should be assigned to a specific member of the hospital team. Certain items should have a specific recorded maintenance schedule to ensure proper servicing (e.g., anesthetic machines, x-ray developer solutions, autoclave, microscope, clinical pathology laboratory instruments, computer terminals, central vacuum system). A file of warranties and instruction manuals must be used to develop the schedule of required maintenance. Other items need to be cleaned or serviced, or both, after each use, such as electric clippers, surgical instruments, endoscopes, otoscope,

ophthalmoscope, Bard-Parker instrument tray, and gas levels of oxygen tanks.

If each equipment item has an assigned responsible maintenance person, all equipment will last longer and always be ready when needed. Nonmedical equipment, such as typewriters, calculators, air conditioning and heating units, lawn mowers, and hospital vehicles, must also be assigned to those responsible for their use.

A veterinary technician, animal handler, or veterinarian should be aware of some easy-to-follow rules to minimize macroshock hazards (Table 31–8). Too often people become careless when working around electricity, from either habit or being in a hurry. Taking the time for a refresher session in electrical safety and/or checking equipment to ensure it is in proper working order (including nonfrayed cords) can prevent tragic accidents.

In conclusion, practices that will flourish in the twenty-first century will be those that integrate well-trained technicians with responsible client communication, deliver high-quality medicine and surgery, maintain good client-patient and personnel-business management, practice in attractive facilities aided by a good location, and practice preventative maintenance on the facility, equipment, and grounds. These flourishing practices will be exciting and rewarding for clients, patients, and staff.

Recommended Reading

Finch L: Telephone Courtesy and Client Service. Schaumburg, IL, AVMA, 1991.

Gerson RF: Beyond Customer Service: Keeping Clients for Life. Schaumburg, IL, AVMA, 1993.

Haberer JB and Webb MW: Teamwork: 50 Ways to Make It Work in Your Practice. Schaumburg, IL, AVMA, 1996.

Lukens RL and Landon RM: Effective Inventory Control. West Chester, PA, Smith Kline Beecham (Pfizer), 1993.

McCarthy JB: Basic Guide to Veterinary Hospital Management. 2nd ed. Lakewood, CO, American Animal Hospital Association, 1995.

McCurnin DM (editor): Veterinary Practice Management. Philadelphia, J.B. Lippincott Co., 1988.

Pettit TH: Hospital Administration for Veterinary Staff. Goleta, CA, American Veterinary Publications, 1994.

Scott D: Client Satisfaction: The Other Half of Your Job. Schaumburg, IL, AVMA, 1991.

Wise JK: The Veterinary Service Market for Companion Animals 1992. Schaumburg, IL, AVMA, 1992.

Manuals and Directories

AAHA Hospital Standards and Accreditation Manual. Denver, CO, American Animal Hospital Association, 1995.

1997 AVMA Membership Directory and Resource Manual. 44th ed. Schaumburg, IL, AVMA.

How to Market Yourself: A Veterinary Technician Placement Program. Dayton, OH, The IAMS Company, 1995.

Waltham Veterinary Hospital Manual (for Veterinary Technicians). Vernon, CA, Waltham, 1993.

Journals

DVM, The Newsmagazine of Veterinary Medicine. Cleveland, OH, Advanstar Communications, monthly.

Trends. Denver, CO, American Animal Hospital Association, monthly.

Veterinary Economics. Lenexa, KS, Veterinary Medicine Publishing Group, monthly.

Veterinary Practice Staff. Los Angeles, Veterinary Practice Publishing Co., bimonthly.

Veterinary Product News. Mission Viejo, CA, monthly.

Veterinary Technician. Trenton, NJ, Veterinary Learning Systems, monthly.

Management Short Courses

Veterinary Management Development School, Denver, CO, contact AAHA for details.

Veterinary Management Institute at Purdue University, contact AAHA for details.

32 Personal Leadership*

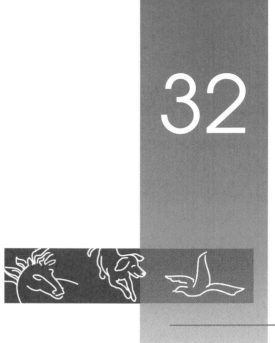

Ray L. Russell

INTRODUCTION

Study and application of the principles in this chapter will help you develop the skills of *personal leadership* (PL) (Russell, 1996A). The most important business in life is the business of leading yourself to be all you can possibly be through the process of PL.

In a time of rapidly changing technology, when there is so much new information to learn, it is easy to overlook the importance of continuing to learn some of the so-called soft skills, such as communication, leadership, and interpersonal relations. For a veterinary practice to reach its potential, it is important to maintain a balance between critical technical skills and leadership skills. If you are willing to pay the price to develop PL skills, you will become an even better technician and a greater asset to your practice.

The importance of learning these skills is pointed out in a poll taken by the American Management Association that revealed two of three workers in America believe their supervisors are incompetent. This is a shocking indictment of the failure of management to learn and practice PL.

> **TECHNICIAN NOTE**
>
> Two out of three workers believe their leaders are incompetent.
> —American Management Association poll

There will always be a demand for position or public leadership; however, our changing world will necessitate greater emphasis on PL than on organizational leadership.

*© Ray L. Russell 1996. All rights reserved.

> **TECHNICIAN NOTE**
>
> A major shift is occurring today from organizational to personal leadership.

Our quest should be to find better methods of leading, managing, learning, teaching, motivating, and interacting with others. Acquiring new competencies will be necessary to effectively compete and adapt to the challenges of society, which are different than anything we have previously experienced.

Competent technicians and front office staff are absolutely essential to the operation of a successful practice. In managing my clinical practice, I often said, "I would rather replace a veterinarian than a technician or receptionist." I have had many outstanding technicians; however, one technician who was also a behavioral consultant opened up a new dimension in our practice with her knowledge of animal behavior. Kay Bickford added to her value as a technician because she had answers and training techniques for clients with pet behavioral problems.

Kay's interest and knowledge of animal behavior started when she was a young child. She trained her dogs to do unusual things; her German shepherd rode bareback with her on her horse. Kay said, "My best friends were my dogs." She developed a reputation in show circles by training and showing her golden retrievers. Her proficiency in working with canine behavior is attested to by the fact that she trained five of the number 1 obedience dogs in the country.

Kay's advice to new veterinary technicians is as follows:

1. Love animals; be firm with them so they will not make a mistake that could harm them.

2. Go through the best technician program available and become certified.
3. Talk to veterinarians and find out what they want in a technician.
4. Get all the experience you can by doing the dirtiest jobs and working your way up. Do not worry about the pay. If you are good, the pay will follow.
5. Treat people like they are long-lost relatives.
6. Enjoy what you do.

Kay is an outstanding example of a personal leader who has led herself to master skills that have complemented her technical training. Her willingness to learn, be unique, and deliver quality service as a technician and behavioral consultant landed her a popular radio talk show on pet behavior that has aired the past 5 years on KFYI in Phoenix, AZ.

OTHER ROLES

Your role as a veterinary technician may often expand beyond the work you do as a technician into the management of the practice. In this role, you need to be sure the practice is in compliance with OSHA controlled substances and environmental standards. In addition, many technicians need to learn how to do the following:

- Order drugs and supplies
- Hire staff, negotiate contracts, and review performance
- Operate computers, faxes, and other business equipment
- Supervise, train, and provide leadership to the practice staff
- Handle payables, receivables, and deposits, and balance the checkbook

If some of these roles are new to you, you may have to lead yourself to obtain the information and training to learn these skills in addition to keeping current with the advances in technology. Life-long learning is essential to contributing to a successful practice as well as having the quality of life you deserve.

WHAT IS LEADERSHIP?

Everyone has his or her own definition of *leadership,* and most use the word without a clear understanding of what it really means. This is understandable because there are more than 350 definitions according to leadership authorities.

My favorite definition of a *leader* is someone who knows where they are going and can convince others to go with them.

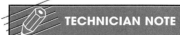

TECHNICIAN NOTE

Leaders know where they are going and can convince others to go with them.

President Harry Truman said, "Leadership is the ability to get other people to do what they don't want to do and like it!"

The management and leadership guru Peter Drucker taught, "The essence of leadership is performance. The ultimate task of leadership is to create human energies and human vision. Lifting vision, raising performance, and building personality is the very essence of leadership."

Regardless of the definition, one thing is certain—there is a huge leadership gap in the world at a time when leadership is needed the most.

BOTTOM-UP PERSONAL LEADERSHIP

Recently, I spent the night at the Madison Concourse Hotel while speaking at the University of Wisconsin. At the conclusion of my meeting, a student who was employed at the hotel drove me to the airport. In our conversation about his work at the hotel, he said, "I think I could do a better job of managing than the manager of the hotel. Eight of our student employees are turned off by how they are treated by management—their attitude is terrible and morale is low."

This student decided this was the wrong attitude to have, so he arranged a meeting with his department and they all agreed to put the customer first. They decided to do everything in their power to help each hotel guest feel glad he or she stayed at the hotel.

Instead of being a "hostile takeover" by the employees, it became an employee "make-over." Their department completely changed, and it is now the very best and most motivated department in the hotel. He told me, "Everyone works harder and we enjoy our work so much more—we take pride in giving our very best to every customer."

The employee responsible for this turnaround acted on his own without any direction or authority from management. His personal action changed the attitude of every employee on the busing staff and energized the department. His motivation and attitude of quality customer service had a positive impact on all the other employees. This demonstrates the power of one person who exercises PL.

Bottom-up PL was very effective in changing attitudes and creating positive results for the entire organization. Top-down leadership may not have been nearly as effective.

In your role as a veterinary technician, your own PL can have a positive influence on the entire practice. Let's discover how you can build these skills so in addition to your technical skills you can have a major impact on the staff and clients in your practice.

A NEW LEADERSHIP MODEL

PL is a new leadership model that radiates life, spirit, and energy to all who come within the leader's energy field. It enables and empowers individuals to visualize and achieve the pictures they paint.

How can PL be defined?

TECHNICIAN NOTE

Personal leadership is the ability to create a vision, develop a strategy, and generate the energy and empowerment necessary to accomplish personal objectives.

Study Figure 32–1 and observe the visual relationships of the five elements of PL. As you study the model, you will see an interrelationship among the parts. The two-way arrows illustrate a dynamic synergism in leadership. If any part of the model is neglected or eliminated, the energy and empowerment components are weakened.

The PL model is very direct and straightforward. Learn to do these five things well and you will be on your way to being a successful personal leader.

Five Principles of Personal Leadership

1. Paint a picture.
2. Develop a personal strategy.
3. Energize self.
4. Personal empowerment.
5. Set an example.

These five principles will make you a proactive PL when you understand and apply it to your life. As you read about each of these principles, ask yourself the following questions:

1. Do I have a clear picture in my mind of what I want to achieve for the rest of my life?
2. Have I written a strategy for accomplishing my vision?
3. How much energy am I willing to put into accomplishing my strategy?
4. Do I have the personal empowerment to make my vision come true?
5. Am I setting a quality example for my family, friends, and coworkers?

Painting a Picture

Pictures are worth a thousand words. Some people have the natural ability to visualize and dream, whereas others have to work at developing this skill. Seeing clear, living pictures painted in color inside your mind is an important quality to develop. These pictures may or may not be your own ideas. Leaders can visualize what the finished product will look like and have the ability to see things as they will be in the future. *Vision* is a constant source of internal drive and motivation; it keeps you focused on your purpose in life.

> ✏ **TECHNICIAN NOTE**
>
> Successful people have developed the habit of doing what failures don't like to do. They don't like to do them either, but their dislike is subordinated to their strength of purpose.
> —E.N. Gray

Power of Purpose

When you have purpose in your life and work, you generate an energy that propels you forward to achieve your objectives. My *purpose statement* was about 50 words long when I first wrote it. Each year, I have refined and shortened it. After years of experimenting and refining my statement, I have arrived at an eight-word purpose statement: Raise people and organizations to their highest value.

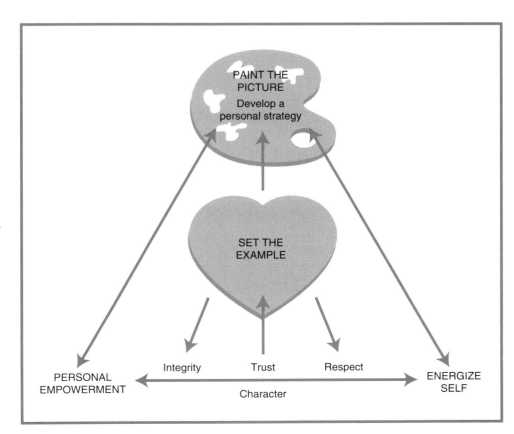

Figure 32-1. Personal leadership model.

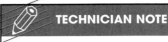

Raise people and organizations to their highest value.

—Ray Russell

Purpose is often referred to in business as a *vision* or *mission statement*. Technically, there is a difference between vision and mission; however, for our purposes, I use painting a picture, mission, or purpose interchangeably.

Unless you have clearly identified your mission, you are likely to wander—not focusing on what is most important. Many business owners struggle and even go bankrupt because they have lost sight of the mission. If businesses fail, it is reasonable that each of us also may wander and lose focus if we have not clearly identified our own purpose or mission. Consider the following mission or purpose statements:

- Quality without compromise . . . because we care (James S. Reid, VMD, Vienna, VA)
- Serve others each day by some small act of service (Loe Pierce, Sandy, UT)
- Because we care . . . we treat them like family (Terry Sippel, DVM, Wichita, KS)

Gita the philosopher, said, "You are what you believe in . . . and [you will] become what you believe you can become." Developing and living your *purpose* will *energize* and *empower* your life.

I have met several people who have achieved extraordinary results in their lives. When I asked them how they were able to accomplish seemingly impossible projects, they frequently told me it was constantly before them in their mind's eye.

The ability to clearly see and paint vivid pictures of how things will appear when they are finished is an important talent for people to develop. Two people who exemplify what can be accomplished when they painted a picture in their mind are Dr. Otto Shill and his wife, Betty.

I first heard of Otto from my mother-in-law, who taught him in the seventh grade. She said he was not interested in school and was an unmotivated learner. She wondered what would ever become of this boy who grew up on a small dairy farm.

Otto enrolled in college with aspirations of becoming a veterinarian. He was accepted into the College of Veterinary Medicine at Kansas State University and 4 years later graduated second in his class.

Betty's parents were divorced when she was 16 months old. Her mother died when she was 8, so she lived with various relatives during her childhood. She became a registered nurse and worked for 1 year as a school nurse and then returned to college for further study.

Otto and Betty were married during Otto's first year in veterinary college. She worked for a pediatrician to support them while he finished school. Before Otto graduated, Betty contracted poliomyelitis and was hospitalized for 4 months; for 1 of those months she lived in an iron lung. After the acute illness, she began the long process of rehabilitation to overcome the extensive paralysis.

On graduation, Otto became an associate in a veterinary practice in El Paso, TX, while awaiting his call into the Air Force. During this time, he was exposed to rabies and had to take the Pasteur treatment. He reacted to the treatment, developed transverse myelitis, and for 3 weeks was unable to move from the waist down. He was told if he ever had to take the treatment again, he would die.

Otto recovered to the point where he was able to enter the Air Force and spend the next 5 years doing public health and radiation research. He resigned from the Air Force to return to medical school. At graduation, he received the Wintrobe Award as the outstanding student of his class. After his internship, he moved to Houston, where he completed a 4-year residency in otolaryngology at Baylor University College of Medicine.

Otto and Betty have five children—three by birth and two by adoption. Betty miraculously was able to raise her three sons and two daughters, even though some observers may have wondered how she could manage with her physical impairment and paralysis. The Shills' experiences have given them a deep appreciation for life. They also know the heartache of losing a 25-year-old son to death.

If you feel you are not able to lead your life through education, finding the right practice, or take care of your family (even if you are a single parent), just observe the determination and power of painting a picture in your mind by following the examples of Dr. Otto and Betty Shill.

Develop a Strategy

The Small Business Administration reports lack of planning as one of the principal reasons businesses fail. Consequently, one of the primary reasons people do not achieve as much as they could is because they fail to make personal plans. When a person fails to plan, they are operating by *chance* instead of by *choice*.

If you fail to plan, you are operating by *chance* instead of by *choice*.

Pictures painted in the mind's eye will become reality when clear and vivid personal strategies are developed and acted on.

In 1980, several veterinary technicians saw the need for greater self-directed learning and advancement of their profession. The PL of these technicians resulted in the organization of the North American Veterinary Technicians Association (NAVTA) at a meeting in East Lansing, MI, in 1981.

NAVTA has had a positive influence on uniting members of the technician profession, encouraging self-directed learning, and advancing careers through knowledge gain.

Patrick Navarre, Executive Director of NAVTA, has this advice for students in high school who have an interest in pursuing a career in veterinary technology: "Get a solid foundation to build your career on by becoming proficient in English, math, and science. It is also important to learn all you can about communication and interpersonal skills."

While serving as a member of the American Animal Hospital Association (AAHA) Board of Directors, I learned an important lesson about the power of a written strategy. The board had a strong desire to move the national headquarters to a city more centrally located and near a major airport. It was interesting to observe the excitement among the board members; however, after a period of time, the energy died. The headquarters were never moved because the board failed to develop a written moving strategy.

As fate would have it, several years later I became the executive director of AAHA. I moved my family from sunny Arizona to Indiana so we could live close to the association headquarters. After my first year, it became apparent that we were limiting our growth by remaining in this location.

Even though the board had wanted to move several years previously, it had given up hope because of the expense and difficulty involved in moving the computer system. Interest was revived when a clear, written moving strategy was presented to the board, which they quickly approved. As the strategy was implemented, Denver, CO, was selected over eight other cities.

Following this written strategy made the move easier than expected. The move and eventual construction of a new headquarters injected a new enthusiasm into the membership. The many dedicated volunteers, staff, and members have earned AAHA the reputation of being one of the finest nonprofit associations in North America. Many people and organizations never reach their potential because they do not take the time to develop a *written strategy*, which has the power to turn dreams into reality.

Energize Self

Many of us have developed habits that rob us of natural energy. To stay energized, avoid the following *enemies of energy*, or *energy drains*.

The Common Enemies of Energy Are:

- Low self-esteem
- Inaction
- Worry
- Fear
- Criticism
- Anger
- Negative thinking
- Jealousy
- Dictatorial leadership style
- Poor physical and mental conditioning

Avoid these energy robbers like the plague. They are contagious and extremely destructive to high energy.

In addition to avoiding things that drain your energy, there are numerous ways to *build energy*.

To Develop Greater Personal Energy:

- Take charge of your life, and "just do it."
- Keep in top physical and mental condition.
- Learn something new every day.
- Communicate effectively.
- Act enthusiastically.
- Associate with high-energy people.
- Lose yourself in serving others.
- Build up other people.
- Set a powerful example.
- Listen; give others your full attention.

- Express sincere interest and concern for others.
- Look on the bright side of life.
- Relax; take time for recreation *(re-creation)*.
- Build your self-confidence, commitment, and control.
- Develop a "light touch"; have a playful attitude.

Life is energy! Death is when all the energy leaves the body. Energy is the fuel of PL. If you should lose your zest for living, you may die when you are 20, even though you may not be buried until you are 80.

 TECHNICIAN NOTE

Life is exciting and interesting to interesting and exciting people. It is only dull and boring to dull and boring people.

The quality of your life will largely depend on the degree to which you keep your life active and involved.

The First Seeing Eye Dog

One of the most energized persons I have ever known was Dr. Mark L. Morris, who is well known in the veterinary profession because of his contribution to nutrition and organized veterinary medicine.

Mark once told me about his experience in researching and developing Science Diet Prescription Diet k/d in the clinical laboratory and in his kitchen at his Raritan Hospital for Animals. One of his clients was a blind man, Morris Frank, whose dog, Buddy, was the first seeing eye dog. Buddy had kidney failure, and Mark and his wife, Louise, were preparing food for Buddy in the hospital kitchen. Mr. Frank persuaded Mark to put the k/d in a can so he could take this special diet on the road to feed Buddy while he was traveling around the country raising money for the Seeing Eye Foundation during its formative stage.

When I learned that Mark had died at the age of 93, I reflected on the dynamic role this visionary personal leader had played in pioneering small animal practice, nutritional knowledge, organized veterinary medicine, and companion animal research. I thought of all the pets throughout the world that have benefited from his research and innovative contributions to animal nutrition.

Before Louise died, she best described her husband as he was approaching his 80s; she said, "Mark is still vigorous, coming up with a fresh idea every few days to improve the profession or the country."

Dr. Morris is an example of one of the most energized, empowering, and unique personal leaders I have known.

Personal Empowerment

Empowerment has been a much overused "buzzword" in recent years. Some authorities say you cannot empower a person, just like you cannot motivate them. Motivation is internal; it is something you do to yourself.

Anything that causes an increase in performance or improves your ability to lead yourself to accomplish your purpose is empowerment. You are empowered if you have the ability to get things done and can achieve your objectives.

The word *power* comes from the Latin word *potere*, which means "able." *Roget's II New Thesaurus* defines *power* as "the capacity to exert an influence or force."

Think of empowerment in terms of having personal power or the ability to act and take ownership for your actions. When you fail to act, you lose personal empowerment.

H.B. Karp wrote, "Power is strictly an interpersonal phenomenon and is measured in terms of obtained objectives. . . . You cannot empower or dis-empower anyone else and nobody else can do this for or to you either. . . . Power resides with the individual, authority resides with the organization."

A very successful businessperson who exemplifies this is Dan McCormick. His burning desire, consistency, and work ethics have carried him to the top of his businesses. I asked him what his secret was in earning $1.5 million in his first four years in business. He said, "Life is a marathon—not a 100-meter dash." His formula is:

1. Do not let other people steal your dreams.
2. Be teachable; read motivational books and listen to tapes.
3. Find a mentor you respect and model their behavior.
4. Be consistent.
5. Develop a burning desire.
6. Paint clear vivid pictures in your mind of what you want to achieve.

Rudy Lavik, a university professor, took control of his life by running several miles each day. He continued to run nearly every day well into his 80s. Rudy said, "We are soft—we need to run an extra mile each day and read an extra book each week."

> **TECHNICIAN NOTE**
>
> We need to run an extra mile each day and read an extra book each week.
> —Rudy Lavik

The personal discipline exemplified by Rudy is an essential characteristic for PL to develop. Discipline builds character and will help you become a great technician.

There is a big difference in being interested in something and in being committed. When you are interested, you will do it when it is convenient. When you are committed, you will do it no matter what it takes. You will find a way to accomplish your objective with no excuses.

The two essential empowering skills technicians must learn are *people skills* and *performance skills*. You may be a very competent technician, but until you develop these skills, you will not be as effective as you could be.

Interpersonal Skills

Business and professional people are learning to understand the vital importance of developing interpersonal skills. Recent research reveals that 70% of all litigation with physicians is the result of poor attitude, relationships, or communication skills. More than 200 practice owners told me that it was difficult to find employees who have the ability to communicate with and relate to clients (Russell, 1994).

If your role as a technician also requires you to supervise other staff members, you should recognize that many managers have tried to manage people like inventory, which will not work. You manage things and lead people. Both management and leadership are necessary to a successful practice, but most people do not possess both skills.

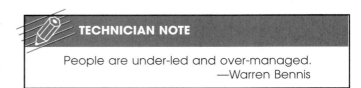

> **TECHNICIAN NOTE**
>
> People are under-led and over-managed.
> —Warren Bennis

Trust and respect form the foundation on which all human relationships are built. You can respect a person without agreeing with him or her. The secret is to learn to disagree agreeably. Relationships grow stronger when every encounter is a win-win situation. Even when it is necessary to discipline or terminate employees, you can preserve the person's dignity by treating him or her with respect.

Research demonstrates that the more you understand about other people and yourself, the more effective you will be in working relationships. Sensitivity to these differences will strengthen your relationships.

As you observe others, try to recognize their primary behavioral style. With practice, you can read other people and predict their style by the way they walk, talk, sit, and gesture. Other clues regarding their style may be discovered by the appearance of their desk, yard, and cars.

People are quite predictable in their behavior, so the ability to read people will assist you to more effectively interact with others. As you focus on the other person, your own interpersonal relationships will usually improve.

Let me reemphasize that it does not matter what style you are. There is no need to change your style, unless a certain behavior is affecting the success of your work, marriage, or relationships. You can learn to blend your style when this would improve your job or relationships with others.

For several years, I have used computerized behavioral reports (Managing for Success, 1991) as a tool to build strong practices and businesses. These reports are simple and accurate. They are useful in helping staff members understand themselves, their clients, and other staff members. After completing a 24-question instrument, the computer will print a 14- to 20-page report about your unique behavior, with startling accuracy. This report is used by many executives, supervisors, and other business and professional leaders.

These computerized reports are a valuable tool in helping students, technicians, and practitioners develop skills in leadership, team building, client service, staff supervision, and mentoring. This technology combined with training has produced significant improvements in productivity and helping people work together. It is the operations manual for working with people.

The computer report will describe your:

- General characteristics
- Value to the organization
- Checklist for communication
- Cautions on communication
- Ideal environment

- Perceptions
- Natural and adapted style
- Motivated style
- Keys to motivating
- Keys to managing
- Areas for improvement
- Action plan

I have observed significant improvements in productivity, service/quality, teamwork, and profitability as a direct result of the use of these reports (Russell, 1996B). It is a particularly effective tool for improving communication within organizations.

Developing Rapport

We tend to be attracted to people who are similar to us. This attraction or relationship is referred to as being in rapport with others. *Rapport* is defined as a harmonious, empathetic, or sympathetic relation with mutual trust to another person.

Rapport is essential for successful communication; it is the glue that holds together relationships. Exceptional client service depends on developing and maintaining harmonious relationships.

Many business and professional owners have said their greatest need is to find employees who can relate to their customers. It is relatively easy to find people who have good technical skills but more difficult to locate employees who can relate to and communicate effectively with clients.

A technology known as neurolinguistic programming, or NLP, was developed by Dr. John Grinder and Richard Bandler. Dr. Michael Brooks, an industrial psychologist, presents this technology in his books *Instant Rapport* (Brooks, 1989) and *The Power of Business Rapport* (Brooks, 1990). He describes how people experience the world through one of three senses: *sight, sound,* or *feelings.*

If you can diagnose whether your clients or associates are visual, auditory, or kinesthetic, you have a better chance of establishing rapport with them. Until rapport is established, there will be no openness and trust, which are needed to communicate and relate effectively.

Observe clients closely, and become sincerely interested in them. Listen carefully, noticing their voice, rate of speech, and tone. Pay attention to their eyes and position of their pupils. Match and mirror their rate and tone of speech and body language. This will assist you in quickly developing rapport.

Communication

Most people are completely unaware of their communication habits. They may say one thing yet convey a different message because of their nonverbal language. If this happens to you, analyze your speaking and listening habits.

The ability to clearly communicate your message through written and spoken language is important for leading yourself to accomplishing your objectives.

When you communicate, do you speak rapidly? Slowly? Talk too much? Or not enough? Is your verbal message saying one thing and body language something else? Do you have credibility? Are people influenced by your message?

Most people think they are good communicators; however, after a review, they frequently find weaknesses that can be corrected with identification and coaching.

Listening Is Essential to Effective Communication

The inability to communicate effectively with others is often the reason for a breakdown in relationships. After working with many different organizations over the years, it has been my observation that the majority of problems originate because of a failure to communicate. Much of this problem is specifically related to our listening skills.

Even when people think they listen, they commonly retain less than 25% of what they hear. The ability to be a good listener is one of the rarest yet most important of the interpersonal skills. You really feel important when a person listens to you, really listens, with his or her ears and heart.

There are many reasons why people do not listen. Frequently, they are busy talking or preoccupied with what they will say next. Being aware of your listening barriers will improve your ability to listen.

Here are some tips for becoming a better listener:

- Have a desire to listen.
- Maintain eye contact and concentrate on the other person.
- Listen with your heart, ears, and eyes.
- Take notes.
- Build rapport by pacing the speaker (match and mirror gestures, voice patterns, and expressions).
- Tell someone else what you have learned.
- Do not jump to conclusions.
- Control distractions.
- Expect to be a good listener.

Be aware of what kind of listener you are. Work at it, and you will build stronger relationships. Other people will like you more, and you will have a greater capacity to contribute to the practice.

Make Others Feel Important

One of the most effective listeners I have known is Dr. Jacob Mosier, former president of the AVMA and former head of clinics at Kansas State University. He seldom talks about himself. His eyes are focused on you while he asks questions to draw out your comments. His complete attention and interest make you feel very important! If you can emulate his example in speaking to clients and other staff members, you will greatly increase your effectiveness.

Develop a Light Touch

Life would be a lot happier and more interesting if there were more people with a sense of humor. I was recently in a practice in which a technician was a great example of a person with a light touch. This technician intently listens to clients with her heart and eyes. Her keen sense of humor erases any communication barriers and instantly draws people to her. She makes a client feel important because of her sincere interest and sense of humor.

Practical Ideas to Build Rapport and Develop Relationships

Try the following simple practical suggestions, and you will be amazed at how your interpersonal relations with clients will improve.

- Greet clients with a warm salutation.
- Look them in the eye, smile, and call them by name.
- Develop rapport.
- Become genuinely interested; find out about them.
- Ask more questions, talk less, and listen more.
- Welcome criticism, and avoid being defensive.
- Make every person you meet feel important.

There is a saying in business, "If you don't succeed with people—you don't succeed in business." Interactive skills are synonymous with being a successful technician.

Set the Example

At the center of the leadership model is the heart of a leader. This represents the role model that is the most important part of leadership.

Your character is the building block of PL because you must be able to look yourself in the mirror with respect; otherwise, your energy and confidence are diminished. You must know what John Gray meant when he said, "Success lies in doing not what others consider to be great, but what you consider to be right."

> **TECHNICIAN NOTE**
>
> Success lies in doing not what others consider to be great, but what you consider to be right.
> —John Gray

The heart of PL is example. Values, character, trust, respect, and integrity are the core of your example. It has been said that "the way one wins shows much of their character, and the way they lose shows all of it."

Dr. Albert Schweitzer, the French theologian and jungle physician, said, "Example is not the main thing in influencing others. It is the only thing." He taught, "There are only three ways to teach. . . one is by example, two is by example, and three is by example!"

Dr. Hugh Nibley said, ". . . leadership is an escape from mediocrity . . . the leader being simply the one who sets the highest example."

It is important to feel good about yourself and recognize your worth. The feeling that you are a person of value is closely related to your development as a personal leader. Your ability to set a good example is also closely linked to your self-esteem.

The Journey of Jim and Naomi Rhode

A good example of two inspirational role models is provided by Jim and Naomi Rhode. They developed one of the most successful medical marketing companies in the world; they develop, design, manufacture, and distribute products to help health care professionals communicate with their patients and clients.

They supply more than 14,000 products to customers in North America, Europe, Australia, and Japan; these products range from consumable and disposable infection-control products to "soft paws" for the veterinary profession, which keep cats from scratching the furniture.

Naomi Rhode, CSP, CPAE, and a graduate of the University of Minnesota, is a motivational speaker who is in great demand. She was elected president of the National Speakers Association and has served in numerous other leadership positions.

Despite their busy schedules, Jim and Naomi have been able to maintain a balance in their business, family, and church. I asked them, "What has been your greatest internal motivation for accomplishing so much?" They answered, "Our involvement and love for the spiritual part of life are what light the fire within us." Naomi added, "Our family, faith in God, and dedication to living life abundantly are most important to us. Through the years, we have come to know the value of little things. Our lives have been happy and fulfilled as we have been able to serve others."

> **TECHNICIAN NOTE**
>
> Our energy comes from the love of the spiritual part of life.
> —Naomi Rhode

BE A LIFE-LONG LEARNER

Knowledge is power! Keeping current requires the processing of a huge amount of information. Jeanne Bosson, a technician at the Brown Road Animal Hospital, says, "Take every seminar you can; study during your free time." Vicky Kasel from the Gilbert Veterinary Clinic echoes this advice. She said, "After 30 years' experience as a veterinary technician, the most important thing I can say is don't become stagnant; keep learning." Unless a person is truly motivated to life-long learning, he or she will fall hopelessly behind.

B.F. Skinner writes, "Education is what survives when what has been learned has been forgotten."

> **TECHNICIAN NOTE**
>
> Education is what survives when what has been learned has been forgotten.
> —B.F. Skinner

Formal education is a place to start, but it will not fulfill all your learning requirements throughout life. Workshops, seminars, training sessions, coaching, videos, audiocassettes, interactive computer programs, and visits to other practices are other excellent sources of new information. Also, there is no substitute for reading and studying books and periodicals.

If you have a desire to get a formal education but feel you cannot afford it, consider Dr. Gabor Vajda. Looking back on his childhood, he remembers the bombings, deaths, and destruction in his neighborhood in Bolatonszemes, Hungary; his family lived on a small farm in this village of about 1000 people during the dark days of World War II. His father was away fighting in the war, and the Vajda family had to fend for themselves, surviving on only the crops they could grow.

When conditions improved after the war, Vajda accompanied a German country veterinarian on his farm calls to neighboring farms. His love for animals grew and his boyhood dream of preventing suffering and diseases among animals became dominant in his mind.

He prepared to become a veterinarian and was studying veterinary science at the University of Budapest when the Communists again took over the country in the Hungarian Revolution. Gabor protested the presence of tanks and destruction of thousands of lives. His family's farm and business were taken over by the Communists, and Gabor and his younger brother fled the country. They were successful in getting to Salzburg, where they obtained sponsorship to immigrate to America. Gabor spent 3 months learning to speak English and was accepted into the Iowa State University College of Veterinary Medicine. Four years later, he graduated with a doctoral degree in veterinary medicine. He paid his way through school by milking cows, making doughnuts, caring for a research colony of beagles, and working as a janitor.

Gabor obtained his first position with Dr. Bella Marriassy, who had also escaped from Hungary after the war. Through hard work and sacrifice, he eventually was able to lease his own small animal clinic. In the next few years, he worked 7 days a week, concentrating on delivering quality medicine and exceptional client service. His efforts earned him the respect of his clients and colleagues, as attested to by being selected Arizona's Veterinarian of the Year and later being elected the national president of the American Animal Hospital Association.

How was Gabor able to overcome the obstacles that hold back most people? He told me that he was able to achieve his dream despite a lack of money and family support because he had confidence that he could achieve his goals. He said, "I have never known failure—I believed I could accomplish anything through hard work and by giving other people their money's worth."

> **✎ TECHNICIAN NOTE**
>
> I have never known failure—I believed I could accomplish anything through hard work and by giving other people their money's worth.
> —Gabor Vajda

The advice Dr. Vajda would give to others who would like to be a stronger personal leader is to:

- Love people; put people first.
- Always be sincere, appreciative, and grateful.
- Treat others with respect.
- Be willing to work as hard as necessary to achieve your goals.
- Be honest and open, and count your blessings.

Dr. Vajda lives by the philosophy of Bernard Shaw, which (paraphrased) is, "Life is like a burning torch; live it to its fullest and pass the torch along to others."

OVERCOMING OBSTACLES

It is easy to look at other people with envy, not realizing the obstacles they have had to overcome to achieve success.

A good example is Emmett Smith. He was diagnosed with a fatal brain tumor and given no hope of living. A decision was made to have experimental surgery that had been performed only four times. Two of the patients had died on the operating table, and the other two were vegetables for the rest of their lives.

After Emmett's surgery, he was partially paralyzed and confined to a wheelchair. His inner balance system had been destroyed. To complicate matters, infection set in, and he again was given no hope of survival. However, after 14 days of a temperature of 104°F, he miraculously began to respond and slowly recovered.

Most people would have resigned themselves to remain in the wheelchair for the remainder of their lives, but not Emmett! He challenged himself to not only walk again but also run 20 miles just 1 year from the day of his operation. As impossible as it seemed, Emmett had the faith and determination needed to lead himself to accomplish this goal.

Emmett literally forced himself to get out of the wheelchair and start walking. He struggled because he could not maintain his balance and would fall. He eventually conquered this problem and threw away his canes. Soon he was able to jog slowly. At exactly 1 year after his surgery—through sheer determination, practice, and persistence—he accomplished his goal of running 20 miles. Emmett believes, "It is how you handle the difficulties in your life that determines your success." Experience taught him that true happiness is achieving victory over self.

> **✎ TECHNICIAN NOTE**
>
> It is how you handle the difficulties in your life that determines your success. True happiness is victory over self.
> —Emmett Smith

Emmett demonstrated that the human spirit cannot be held down if there is a will to fight back and succeed. In his speeches, he challenges others to find success and happiness in life by doing the following:

1. Meeting trouble as a friend
2. Realizing that all great human endeavor results from doing common things in an uncommon way
3. Taking chances; the fear of failure holds back people
4. Daring to meet luck half-way
5. Daring to be honest
6. Setting an example; being a role model

Regardless of your circumstances, problems, or challenges, you can achieve your personal objectives if you believe in your goal and are committed to overcome all obstacles to achieve your goal.

ALL THINGS ARE POSSIBLE

Ryan Zinn, the son of a Tiffin, OH, veterinarian, is a 100- and 200-meter sprinter. He was voted the most valuable member on his Sycamore Mohawk High School Track Team and elected captain of the 4 × 100 relay team, which set a new school record.

You may wonder, what is so unusual about this? The remarkable thing is that he accomplished this with someone else's heart. Yes, Ryan is proud of the fact that he is alive today and just graduated with a degree in mechanical engineering from The Ohio State University. He has the heart of a 21-year-old college ROTC and honor student, which was transplanted into his chest cavity when Ryan was only 15 years old.

Ryan is not only an unusual athlete but also a scholar and leader. He graduated as valedictorian of his high school and had a 3.1 grade point average in the very competitive College of Engineering at The Ohio State University.

I wondered how Ryan was able to keep going, without slowing down, in the face of death. Ryan said, "I focused on what I could do—not on what I couldn't do."

TECHNICIAN NOTE

I focused on what I could do—not on what I couldn't do.

—Ryan Zinn

How was Ryan so successful in recovering from this life-threatening event? He has been successful in leading himself through his stroke and transplant surgery by learning to do the following:

1. Follow and learn from the example and values of parents
2. Be goal oriented
3. Manage time effectively
4. Relate well with other people
5. Never give up
6. Recognize that no matter how tough it may seem, it always gets better

THE PRECIOUS FAMILY-PET BOND

Dr. Martin Becker from Twin Falls, ID, has dedicated his life to promoting "the celebration and protection of the family-pet bond" on a global basis.

A highly motivated and skilled communicator, Martin's goal is to educate and enlighten the practice staff on everything they need to delight clients and nurture and protect animals. He believes, "To be a successful technician, you should treat every animal as if [his or her] owner was watching."

His parents taught him the following ideas to help him craft emotional wealth and financial success:

1. The harder you work, the luckier you'll get.
2. Don't look for opportunities. Create them!
3. If you want your ship to come in, you've got to send some out.
4. R.O.A.: Be responsible for (your) own actions.

"Every day when I leave my house, I pause to look at our family mission statement, which is at eye level on the door: Remember yesterday; live for today; plan for tomorrow; no regrets!"

TECHNICIAN NOTE

Remember yesterday
Live for today
Plan for tomorrow
No regrets!

This is good advice for technicians or any personal leader who wants a better quality of life. If you want to accelerate your personal growth, follow Martin's example and do not wait for success to fall into your lap. Make your own mark on society by having a purpose, developing a strategy, taking action, evaluating your progress, and living a life of self-improvement. Dr. Becker truly believes, "You won't get to the top of the mountain by falling there!"

APPLICATION OF PERSONAL LEADERSHIP

PL will lift vision to higher sights, raise performance to higher standards, and build personality beyond its normal limitations. If you will faithfully follow the PL formula and apply these five principles, you will be amazed at the results you can achieve in practice as well as in your personal life. Do not be discouraged if you sometimes fail. Just remember, no one succeeds 100% of the time. Keep in mind that losing is the first step to winning. Failing should not be thought of as a failure, but as a valuable learning experience.

TECHNICIAN NOTE

Losing is the first step to winning.

The ups and downs in life make you committed to improvement and energized to accomplish tough projects. Recall a time you were discouraged and a time when you were successful. Success energizes you to try harder.

TECHNICIAN NOTE

Knowing is not enough, we must apply; willing is not enough; we must do.

—Goethe

Why do you think there are so many half-read books, uncleaned garages, and diets and exercise programs that have been started and stopped? We have failed to lead ourselves to accomplish our objectives. It could result from not having a specific plan to achieve our objective, a weak commitment, or failure to follow the five principles of PL.

My challenge to you is to read and reread this chapter and then apply this information after you have made a commitment to lead yourself to be all you can be. Reading this chapter will be beneficial, but real power will not come from reading but from the application of PL.

Suggested Reading

Brooks M: The Power of Business Rapport. New York, HarperCollins, 1990.

Laborde GZ: Influencing With Integrity. Palo Alto, CA, Syntony, 1983.

Russell RL: The Miracle of Personal Leadership. Dubuque, IA, Kendall/Hunt, 1996.

Russell PL: "People: The Keys to Profitability." Semin Vet Med Surg 11: 1996.

References

Brooks M: Instant Rapport. New York, Warner Books, 1989.

Brooks M: The Power of Business Rapport. New York, HarperCollins, 1990.

Managing for Success Software: Employee Manager Version. Scottsdale, AZ, TTI Software, Ltd., 1991.

Russell RL: Preparing veterinary students with the interactive skills to effectively work with clients and staff. J Vet Med Educ 21:40, 1994.

Russell RL: The Miracle of Personal Leadership. Debuque, IA, Kendall/Hunt, 1996A.

Russell RL: "People: The Keys to Profitability." Semin Vet Med Surg (Small Animal) 11: 1996B.

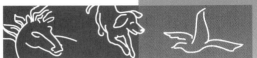

33 Stress and Its Management

Sandra S. Brackenridge

During the past two decades, information from the medical community regarding stress and its deleterious effect on human beings has been abundant. According to current research, stress is responsible for physical illness, mental illness, and even death more often than any other factor. Furthermore, stressful living has become accepted, even considered unavoidable, in our technologically modern, fast-paced society. In choosing to work in veterinary medicine, especially if responsibilities entail direct service to clients, one chooses a work environment with a high potential for daily stress. However, stress can be managed, controlled, and sometimes alleviated through personal and professional awareness, understanding, monitoring, and revision of lifestyle. This chapter provides a basic understanding of stress, identification of some of the stressors in life and those specific to veterinary medicine, suggestions for management and coping, and awareness of burnout signals.

TECHNICIAN NOTE

In choosing to work in veterinary medicine, one chooses a work environment with a high potential for daily stress.

A DEFINITION OF STRESS

Stress can be defined as the state produced when the body responds to any demand for adaptation or adjustment. The infinite demands that produce this response state are called *stressors.* These stressors may be external (e.g., time schedules and workload), environmental (e.g., heat, cold, noise), or inter-

nal (e.g., emotions and sensitivities). The nature of stress is nonspecific in that certain biochemical reactions are common with exposure to all types of stressors. However, stress is not always negative. Stress responses can be pleasurable and even beneficial in certain situations.

GOOD STRESS/BAD STRESS

Stressors can mobilize a person into being energized in order to meet specific challenges and take action. As action is taken, the body's stress management system functions in exactly the way it was intended, and with "good" stress, the person experiences a feeling of satisfaction, relief, or exhilaration. Stressors can also be excessive in number or intensity, prolonged, and unavoidable. When a person experiences stressors of this nature, the stress reaction of the body works overtime. The body mobilizes, attempts to adjust to an ongoing drain of energy, and eventually becomes overwhelmed and exhausted. Three factors determine whether stress is negative or positive: *choice, control,* and *consequences.*

TECHNICIAN NOTE

Stress may be negative or positive depending on choice, control, and consequences.

Choice

When a person responds to a stressor that is perceived as self-chosen, the response itself is viewed more positively. Generally speaking, if individuals are attracted to veterinary medicine, pursue training, and obtain their desired employment, they will be more likely to perceive stressors encountered at work without excessive negativity or resentment. However, if employment in veterinary medicine is perceived as necessary simply to make ends meet financially, or if the person feels his or her true career choice is an impossibility, stressors common to veterinary medicine may be less tolerable. For example, an aggressive animal may be perceived as a challenging stimulation by one who has chosen this career, whereas the same animal would be perceived as a burden or an obstacle by one who truly wishes to be in a different position of employment.

Control

Good or bad stress is also determined by whether the stressor is perceived as within the person's control. In veterinary practice, clients control the schedule, patients provide emergencies and unpredictability, and employers control much of the working environment. When staff are consulted as to scheduling and offered control over certain areas of the working environment, the stressful effect of these factors can be minimized. Again, an aggressive animal provides a good example. Such a situation can seem intolerable when the client insists on being present during treatment, and the employer refuses to muzzle the animal. However, when the client responds in the desired way, and when the employer considers others' opinions, the staff feel that the treatment of the animal and the aggression is within their control. Although the aggressive animal continues to be a stressor during the working day, perceived control of the stressor alleviates much of its negative impact.

Consequences

Stressors are more likely to be perceived as positive stimulation when consequences can be anticipated. In veterinary medicine, the death of a patient is always a source of stress. However, when the animal is properly diagnosed and death is expected or euthanasia is performed, stress in the situation is manageable. On the other hand, when an apparently healthy animal unexpectedly dies during surgery, treatment, or boarding, resulting stress can feel acutely negative and overwhelming. Because the stressor could not have been anticipated, the stress response has become "bad" stress.

Therefore, each stressful situation provides an opportunity for choice, a feeling of control, and anticipation of consequences. Table 33–1 provides further examples of good and bad stress within veterinary medicine. Because stress is unavoidable, knowledge of these three factors can help one to transform adverse stressors into tolerable stressors.

STRESS AND THE BODY

Stress, whether good or bad, is a response of the body. An understanding of how and where stress originates within the body, its pathway, and the physical toll it can extract is necessary to manage stress and maintain good health.

Flight or Fight

We are equipped, as are all mammals, with a physical system to assist us in handling threatening situations. This system has

• Table 33–1 •

	GOOD STRESS	BAD STRESS
EXAMPLES OF GOOD AND BAD STRESS		
Personal	You exert yourself and win a game of tennis.	Your car breaks down and you must walk 3 miles for help.
Professional	You are asked to speak at the next professional conference.	A co-worker fails to show up for work, and you must work doubly hard.
Personal	You throw a party for 150 people.	Your house is burglarized.
Professional	You perform euthanasia on an elderly animal, and the family thanks you.	A young animal unexpectedly dies while boarding.
Personal	You re-enter higher education.	Your spouse is laid off.
Professional	The practice expands, you work harder, but your income increases.	A type A co-worker constantly competes with you.

been necessary for our survival as a species. Historically, this physical system enabled us to flee or to fight when externally threatened. In the primitive state, our enemies included wild animals, other primitive peoples, and natural occurrences. Today, this physical system shifts into gear when anything or anyone is perceived as threatening, externally or internally. In fact, perceived threat is chronic. We drive defensively and cope with pollution of all sorts, and crime has become a realistic cause for concern. Internally, we fear bad news, losses, rejection, and failure; we are threatened by financial crises, inconsideration by others, illness, and aging. The list of internal stressors is unique to every person, depending on background, temperament, and aspirations. The stress response is nonspecific and is mobilized when one is faced with any of these threats, perceived or real.

The Pathway of Stress

Dr. Hans Selye, who is often called the father of stress research, termed the body's response to stress the general adaptation syndrome (GAS). On a person's exposure to any threat or stressor, the first phase of GAS, the alarm reaction, is elicited. After this phase, the person enters a stage of adaptation or resistance. If the stressor continues to threaten, the person enters a third phase, which Dr. Selye called the stage of exhaustion. Unless interrupted, and if the stressor is severe enough and present long enough, the third stage results in physical illness, burnout, or even death.

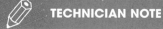

TECHNICIAN NOTE

The general adaptation syndrome (GAS) is the body's response to stress.

During the alarm phase, the body's physical system designed for fight or flight is mobilized. The human body is "supercharged" for action with all muscles and organs in a state of readiness. Many changes are happening internally. The real or perceived stressor signals the hypothalamus to produce hormones such as endorphins. These hormones stimulate the autonomic nervous system as well as the pituitary gland. The autonomic nervous system affects the digestive system and other vital organs. The stimulation of the pituitary gland increases blood flow, discharging more hormones into the blood stream. This action stimulates the adrenal glands, which affect breathing, cortisone production, muscle tension, perspiration, and blood sugar levels. Figure 33–1 charts the pathway of the stress response through the body.

The stimulation of the adrenal glands is responsible for many stress-related illnesses. Increased epinephrine production causes increased respiration and heart rate. Rapid breathing causes the injection of additional oxygen into the bloodstream, which alters the amount of carbon monoxide in the bloodstream and causes dry mouth, irritated nasal passages, and chest contractions. A prolonged increase in heart rate can cause hypertension, leading to cardiovascular problems. The pituitary and adrenal glands influence cortisone levels, which are responsible for the body's immune responsiveness. Prolonged muscular tension, caused by the adrenal glands and by stimulation of the autonomic nervous system, results in various aches and pains, as well as digestive disorders. Stress-induced digestive disorders are exacerbated by the fluctuation in blood sugar levels, resulting in poor eating habits, ulcers, nausea, or constipation. Prolonged stress can result in ongoing endocrine disorders. Table 33–2 shows the various physical disorders that can be considered stress-related disorders.

All of the mentioned physical changes originally occur during the alarm phase of GAS. However, when the stressor or stressors continue, the adaptation phase ensues, in which the body attempts to adjust to its new level of activity. When

• Table 33–2 •

PHYSICAL PROBLEMS TRIGGERED BY STRESS	
Insomnia	Chest pains
Headaches	Hypertension
Allergies	Heart attacks
Temporomandibular joint (TMJ) disorder	Sexual dysfunction
	Chronic fatigue
Nausea	Depression
Indigestion	Dizziness
Heartburn	Anxiety
Backaches	Alcoholism
Ulcers	Muscle aches
Colitis	Dry mouth
Problems swallowing	Facial tics
Hyperventilation	Erratic breathing
Asthma	Upper respiratory illnesses
Rheumatoid arthritis	Nosebleeds
Dermatitis	Perspiration

exposure to the stressor continues, any level of adaptation that the body has acquired may be lost, depending on factors unique to each person. Exhaustion may appear physically, or it may be demonstrated psychologically. Burnout can be defined as psychological, and sometimes physical, exhaustion prompted by prolonged subjection to a stressor without adaptation or interruption.

Although all human beings will respond to stressors through activation of the above described physical syndrome, not all will proceed through all three phases of GAS. Whether a person can adapt to stress, what stressors are felt most acutely, and which physical or psychological manifestations of stress will appear depend on various factors, including personality.

PERSONALITY FACTORS

Certain personality variables predispose individuals to susceptibility to stress or to resistance to stress. These variables may be inherent in the personality, or they may be learned behaviors and attitudes. Science has not yet determined how much of the personality is genetic and how much is learned, but personalities can be grouped into types. Personality type is a reliable indicator of predisposition to stress-related disorders.

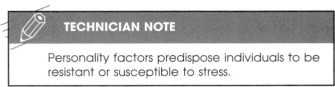

TECHNICIAN NOTE

Personality factors predispose individuals to be resistant or susceptible to stress.

The Stress-Prone Individual

The term *type A personality* was first used by Dr. Meyer Friedman and Dr. Ray Rosenman in their book *Type A Behavior and Your Heart*. In one study, it was concluded that type A personalities were three times as likely to have coronary artery disease, and personality type was found to be the most reliable predictor of heart attack. People are type A if they are competitive, impatient, perfectionistic, often angry, suffering from "hurry sickness," and insecure.

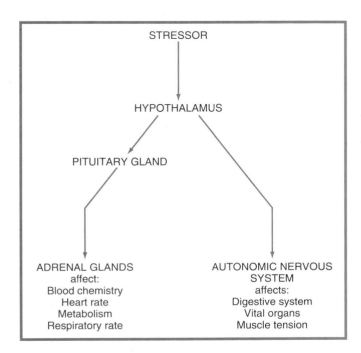

STRESSOR
↓
HYPOTHALAMUS
↓
PITUITARY GLAND

ADRENAL GLANDS
affect:
Blood chemistry
Heart rate
Metabolism
Respiratory rate

AUTONOMIC NERVOUS SYSTEM
affects:
Digestive system
Vital organs
Muscle tension

Figure 33–1. Pathway of the stress response through the body.

TECHNICIAN NOTE

Type A people are susceptible to coronary artery disease.

Overt and covert feelings of competition with others represent a characteristic of type A personalities. These feelings may be motivated by an ambition to win or succeed, or they may stem from a fear of defeat or failure. Specific areas for competition may be chosen, such as within the workplace, or the type A person may compete in every activity, even in driving, recreation, and social groups.

Type A personalities are impatient, and they find it trying to stand in line or to wait. They would rather be late to appointments than be left waiting; thus, type A personalities can be chronically late. They are impatient with receptionists, waiters and waitresses, car repairmen, and, frankly, almost anyone on whom they depend for service. They are also impatient with employers and sometimes with their families. This behavior may be motivated by the need to be in control of situations, or it may be motivated by the desire to avoid anxiety-provoking thinking time.

Perfectionism is a characteristic included in identification of many personality types, and it is also a sign of type A personality. The need for approval and the desire to avoid criticism are paramount in their minds. Combined with their competitive behavior, perfectionism accounts for the priority type As seem to place on performance. They have difficulty delegating and appear critical of others to whom they do delegate. Type As wage a true inner struggle between the need to share responsibility and fear that delegation will backfire on them.

Hostile and *aggressive* are terms often used by co-workers to describe a type A personality. Because the type A personality is competitive and impatient, he or she will expect the same from others. They then defend themselves against what they perceive as other people's aggression and hostility. As a self-fulfilling prophecy, they often find themselves working with others who are also type A. Their sense of humor is often directed toward others' inferiority, and they have difficulty believing that anyone likes them for themselves rather than for their performance. As a result, type As can be difficult as employers and as fellow employees. Ironically, they usually obtain rave reviews from their own supervisors or mentors.

The type A individual suffers from what Friedman called "hurry sickness," or polyphasic behavior. This is the easiest behavior to identify, as type As constantly seem to juggle more than one activity at a time. They talk on the telephone at the same time that they write in charts and eat lunch. Type A secretaries are able to simultaneously answer the telephone, file charts, and schedule appointments. A type A technician might be found attending to a patient, setting up for surgery, and taking a telephone call from a client at the same time. Type A personalities impose too many deadlines on themselves. In short, they deprive themselves of opportunities to relax, while thinking that efficiency is another word for speediness in all activities.

Often, type A individuals appear judgmental of others; however, they are usually most judgmental about themselves.

They have high standards and high expectations for themselves and for others. This behavior stems from insecurity about their own worth, and they are constantly trying to prove their worth through performance, production, and status. Type As are often truly compassionate individuals, empathic to the pain and sensitivities of others.

Although type A behaviors place these individuals at risk in regard to stress, many of the same behaviors are responsible for the success that type As experience in their chosen field. In veterinary medicine, as in many other professions, there is a higher proportion of type A individuals at the top of the profession. Veterinarians often exemplify type A behavior, and thus technicians frequently work for type A individuals. Because of the fact that type As often approve of behavior similar to their own, these same veterinarians enjoy employing type A technicians as well.

An alternative to the type A personality is termed the *type B personality*. To determine whether you are a type A or type B personality, answer and score the questionnaire provided in Table 33–3. No one is a perfect type A or type B, but the more that type B fits one's personality, the lower the incidence of stress-related illness.

The Stress-Hardy Individual

Research has focused on personality types who are stress prone as well as on the characteristics of individuals who are more resistant to stress. Friedman and Rosenman described type B individuals who are more resistant to stress-related illness. Other studies use the term *hardiness* to stress and outline certain components of the personality that appear to protect against stress.

• Table 33–3 •

TYPE A OR TYPE B?		
	TYPE A	**TYPE B**
1. I become impatient when events move slowly.	____ Often	____ Rarely
2. I bring work home from the job.	____ Often	____ Rarely
3. I set deadlines and schedules for myself.	____ Often	____ Rarely
4. I feel guilty when I relax and "do nothing."	____ Often	____ Rarely
5. I speak, eat, and move at a quick pace.	____ Often	____ Rarely
6. I am achievement oriented.	____ Very	____ Slightly
7. I have a strong need for success.	____ Yes	____ No
8. I hurry through or do not finish sentences.	____ Often	____ Rarely
9. I try to do two or more things at once.	____ Often	____ Rarely
10. I like to count my achievements and possessions.	____ Yes	____ No
11. I have angry or hostile feelings toward competitive people.	____ Often	____ Rarely
12. I am generally observant of my surroundings.	____ Yes	____ No

TECHNICIAN NOTE

Type B people are more resistant to stress.

Type B individuals have realistic expectations and are not worried about failure. They have an appreciable acceptance of themselves, which is not based on status or production. Type Bs have a good sense of security and self-esteem, and they are comfortable delegating responsibilities to others without fear of backfire. Deadlines are based on an appraisal of what the type B can do, not on a misperception of what others believe they should do. Type B individuals enjoy time off for recreation and quiet time. Type Bs can be as ambitious and successful as type As, sometimes more so. In fact, because they do not suffer from the same sense of urgency as type A personalities, type Bs can avoid mistakes and therefore be more efficient. They have good relationships in their world because they are not hostile, guarded, or judgmental.

Other qualities of personality that help individuals in their resistance to stress have been identified and grouped under the term *stress hardy*. These individuals have in common three notable attitudes toward living that appear to make a difference in their response to stress:

1. *Control.* Hardy individuals approach experiences with the attitude and belief that they are in control of their own life, responses, and destiny. They believe that they can influence events and do not have a "victim" attitude. They take responsibility for what happens to them and for the situations in which they are placed.
2. *Commitment.* Hardiness also indicates an attitude of curiosity and involvement in situations that are faced. They do not withdraw from situations; instead, they attempt to understand the people and activities in their life.
3. *Challenge.* The belief that change and adjustment is exciting and conducive to personal growth is important to hardy individuals. They see life as an opportunity to learn and develop as people, and experiences of all kinds help them to do so.

Hardy individuals ride out stress or cope with it better. In addition, they are often people who have deeply spiritual connections. This spirituality is not necessarily dependent on affiliation with any religious institution, yet it is important to hardy individuals in their private moments, their belief systems, and their approach to life.

Thus, personality can be an advantage or disadvantage in regard to stress management. Certain qualities of behavior and of attitude may buffer a person against stress, and awareness of these personal risk factors is the first step in managing stress. Identifying specific stressors is the next step.

IDENTIFYING STRESSORS

A veterinary technician's stressor load includes general stressors and those that are unique to veterinary medicine. There are life event stressors, environmental stressors, personal stressors, client stressors, and career stressors common to many technicians.

TECHNICIAN NOTE

Technicians are often subjected to stress from the environment, workplace, clients, and personal issues.

Life Event Stressors

Many events encountered within a lifetime are stressful, regardless of the perception of the event as positive or negative. Thomas Holmes and Richard Rahe created a scale that allows us to measure the impact of 43 life events. This scale is presented in Table 33–4. An individual who accrues more than 300

• Table 33–4 •

THE SOCIAL READJUSTMENT RATING SCALE	
LIFE EVENT	**NUMBER OF LIFE CHANGE UNITS**
Death of a spouse	100
Divorce	73
Marital separation	65
Jail term	63
Death of close family member	63
Personal injury or illness	53
Marriage	50
Fired at work	47
Marital reconciliation	45
Retirement	45
Change in family member's health	44
Pregnancy	40
Sex difficulties	39
Gain of new family member	39
Business readjustment	39
Change in financial state	38
Death of close friend	37
Change to different line of work	36
Change in number of arguments with spouse	35
Mortgage of $100,000	31
Foreclosure of mortgage or loan	30
Change in work responsibilities	29
Son or daughter leaving home	29
Trouble with in-laws	29
Outstanding personal achievement	28
Spouse begins or stops work	26
Begin or end school	26
Change in living conditions	25
Revision of personal habits	24
Trouble with boss	23
Change in work hours or conditions	20
Change in residence	20
Change in schools	20
Change in recreation	19
Change in church activities	19
Change in social activities	18
Mortgage or loan less than $100,000	17
Change in sleeping habits	16
Change in number of family get-togethers	15
Change in eating habits	15
Vacation	13
Christmas	12
Minor violations of the law	11

Modified from Holmes TH and Rahe R: The Social Readjustment Rating Scale. J Psychosom Res 11:213–218, 1967; with permission.

life change units within a year is at risk for stress-related illness. If the total is 150 to 299, the risk is reduced by 30%. Only a slight risk is posed if the total is under 150 life change units. The scale is only an indicator, however, and some people are simply more susceptible to stress than others. Total stressor load must be analyzed to determine true risk for stress-related illness and the need to alleviate stress load.

Environmental Stressors

General environmental stressors include climate and weather, pollution, where one lives and works, crime, traffic, and so forth. Other environmental stressors include the people with whom time is spent; for example, a mother-in-law who has come for a month-long visit may be a stressor for some individuals. Government concerns, such as the threat of war or IRS auditing, may be an environmental stressor. Many environmental stressors can affect individuals in their personal and professional lives. Identification of general environmental stressors can help in determining stressor load and need for revision of lifestyle.

Veterinary environmental stressors, which are more pertinent for the purposes of this chapter, may also be numerous and greatly affect an individual's stress level. Environments will differ for those who work in a small animal clinic and for those who work in large animal or mixed animal practices.

Environmental stressors in a veterinary practice may include noise level, space limitations, equipment and supply factors, orderliness, record-keeping factors, scheduling demands, geographical area, co-workers, and population served. Noise in a clinic is often constant, due to vocalization of animals, telephone ringing, and conversation. Most people who work in a clinic accustom themselves to the noise level and are able to tune it out. However, if the stimulation becomes irritating, more frequent breaks may be required to combat this stressor.

Space limitations are also a stressor in most veterinary practices. Clientele and staff frequently become larger in number before the addition of space is discussed or affordable. Crowding is stressful for humans, and each person in a practice needs his or her own personal space, even if it is just a locker or desktop. Attention should also be paid to arrangement, design, colors, lighting, temperature, and flow of traffic, all of which has been shown to affect stress levels. Clinic arrangement should make work easier and not more difficult. Equipment and supplies should be available and accessible to avoid unnecessary stress, and this is true in all practices, whether stationary or mobile. Inadequate equipment is a stressor and should be discarded. Maintain equipment regularly to avoid the stress of breakdowns and burdensome catch-up maintenance. Orderliness in storage is important, as is storage near the working area. Orderliness and efficiency are necessary to avoid stress in record-keeping. Computers have become a huge asset in record-keeping, but training must be thorough and provided to all staff so that software is an asset, not an additional stressor. Most software companies offer support in sales contracts and should be required to provide training. In addition, forms should be customized, whether on computer or manually, to the needs of the practice, assisting in speed, accuracy, and efficiency without stress.

Scheduling can be one of the most formidable veterinary environmental stressors. Despite best efforts, schedules frequently go awry due to emergencies, a verbose client, or unexpected lengthy surgery or treatment. In a small animal clinic, scheduling is frequently interrupted by an emergency, such as an animal hit by a car or a resident case in cardiac arrest. In an equine practice, a case of colic can disrupt scheduling for several days. All staff must work together to ensure that scheduling is as stress free as possible, allowing breaks while allowing a good level of productivity. Type A employers may need to be approached as to the problem of overscheduling if necessary. Walk-ins or emergencies on a slower day may be manageable, but the same case during a busy day may be stress producing. Encourage the development of policy regarding walk-ins and emergencies, making certain that all opinions are heard.

Geographical location is important, especially in large animal or mixed practices. Traffic, distance, and travel time to and from appointments may require special flexibility in scheduling. Emergencies and the unexpected occur frequently and can be stressful if one is compulsively attached to schedule. The stressors of population served and co-workers will be discussed later under Career Stressors.

Personal Stressors

Each person brings to employment certain qualities that make them either resistant to the stressors in veterinary medicine or sensitive to those stressors. Amount of experience is a factor in that all initial employment in a chosen field is stressful. Moreover, each person's temperament is unique and may or may not be suited to the various duties of being a veterinary technician. Some people are naturally more sensitive to stimulation and environmental stressors. Some people are more comfortable with animals than with clients, finding professional contact with clients stressful. Yet in most practices, technicians will be expected to deal with both animals and people. Flexibility is a quality of temperament necessary to manage stress in veterinary medicine. Each person also brings the baggage of individual personal problems and backgrounds. These make the person vulnerable to certain types of people, certain situations, and certain animals that are reminders of similar personal experiences. Furthermore, the coping with various stressors in one's personal life (e.g., relationships, family) makes one more vulnerable to stressors within the workplace.

Self-confidence and self-esteem are important in the workplace and in all areas of life. Without those two qualities, almost every situation is stressful. With successful experience and acceptance and support by co-workers and employers, both qualities will develop to their fullest positive extent in a healthy person. If an individual struggles constantly with confidence and self-esteem, counseling can help in management of stress and avoidance of further deterioration in these areas.

Some professionals believe that people who work with animals are empathic by nature. After all, they learn to recognize pain and contentment in patients who cannot use words. Empathy can be defined as the vicarious experience of another person's emotions. Furthermore, empathy has been said to be the foundation of compassion. Yet, empathy may be stressful in a veterinary environment, where patients are often in pain and treated without benefit of the talent to inform or to object. Empathy also is stressful in situations of patient death and euthanasia when the experience of another person's grief is painful. It cannot be avoided, but it can be useful in every work situation. Technicians must learn to distinguish between their own empathy and another person's emotions to manage stress.

Client Stressors

All clients may be stressors for one who would rather spend time with animals than with humans. However, there are certain types of clients who are always stress producing. The elderly client, angry client, independent client, and grieving client are mentioned most often as the most difficult to deal with and, therefore, most stressful.

TECHNICIAN NOTE

The angry and demanding client always produces stress for the technician.

The *elderly client* is often attached to a pet. In fact, the animal can even be important to the quality of life of an elderly person who is widowed and living alone. Because of the health problems of the elderly, their decreasing mobility, their ever-fluctuating memory, and sometimes their loneliness, more time can be expended with these clients than with all others combined. Instructions are given and are not always understood, or they must be repeated several times. When in the clinic, the elderly would like to talk not only about the animal being treated but also about all of the animals they have owned, and even their children's animals. When an animal desperately needs conscientious treatment, treatment is not always followed by the elderly client, who cannot bear to leave the animal for treatment at the clinic. One can manage the stress of elderly clients by scheduling them for slower times of the day, allowing time to talk, returning their telephone calls when extra time can be allotted, and talking to their loved ones when painful decisions must be made. When an elderly person is your client, take a mental step backward, take a deep breath, and be patient.

The *angry client* can disrupt a perfectly good day. If the technician's confidence is not functioning well, the angry client can quickly find and mangle all of his or her sensitivities. No matter what the provocation, the angry client feels that he (or his animal) has been neglected, abused, or taken advantage of in some way. Assuming a defensive position is counterproductive with angry clients. Listening to their complaints, even making notes, reporting what they have said, and following up with them and their complaints can salvage positive feelings. Even when an angry client's accusations are correct, listening is the best response. Making excuses or defending actions will not alleviate the anger. These clients need the feeling that they, and their animals, are cared for, paid attention to, and important. Contact with angry clients, even when remediation has been successful, produces stress, and support from other staff members is essential to relieve stress.

The *independent client* is the client who consults a veterinarian but continues to treat his animal in his own predetermined fashion. Such clients hear only what they decide makes sense in regard to instructions. They may have attempted every old-fashioned remedy before the animal is seen for treatment. They may be uneducated clients, or they may be clients who have obtained higher education, even within another area of medicine. In short, they act as if they know more than the professionals do about treating the animal. These clients unwittingly provoke anger and frustration among the veterinary team. To resist stress in dealing with independent clients, hear them out and tell them that you agree with some of their points. Explain, in terms that they can understand, your opinion as to diagnosis, justification for the diagnosis, and treatment. Treat them importantly, and make them feel as though they are a part of the treatment team, and as though their opinions are carefully considered.

The *grieving client* is a stressor due to the emotionality of the situation. As mentioned, empathic response is helpful to clients yet stressful for the veterinary professional. Death of a patient is always stressful in veterinary practice. Not only do technicians frequently witness death and participate in causing death, but they face the grief of clients, and sometimes they must even deal with their own grief for the patient. Management of this stressor involves several activities. First, technicians must separate their own feelings of grief (and/or failure and guilt) from the client's feelings. Second, they must deal with their own philosophy and feelings about death, including their feelings about their own and their loved ones' deaths. Third, technicians can become more comfortable with functioning during times of client bereavement. Literature and seminars are available that allow veterinary professionals to learn how to deal with bereavement. The chapter on bereavement in this textbook gives assistance in this situation. An understanding of the stages of grief and what the technician may do to help clients during each stage is necessary to make the technician more comfortable in dealing with bereavement. Grief is an emotional process that cannot be avoided and must be experienced. Nothing can transform the bad news into good news, but certain behaviors can allow an individual to confidently support others through bereavement.

Career Stressors

In choosing a career as a veterinary technician, individuals open themselves to various stressors. Veterinary technicians frequently must cope with long hours and demanding work responsibilities in return for minimal financial compensation. As in many careers, they must also cope with stressors provided by participating in a medical team.

Daily vulnerability to stress is much more justifiable when monetary compensation is on a par with the level of risk. Unfortunately, the salaries of veterinary technicians (and many veterinarians) do not reflect the long hours and demands of their careers. Technicians must at some point decide whether they can cope with this reality on a long-term basis. Only a conscious decision to accept a financial ceiling to remain in this rewarding career can prevent resentment due to terms of financial compensation.

Finances in the 1990s are a stressor for most Americans. Budgets, consumer counseling services, and cutting back on credit can help. Veterinary technicians must accustom themselves to this stressor as ongoing, and they must use management techniques to cope.

The long hours of sometimes intense physical work to which veterinary technicians expose themselves is another stressor. Fatigue is an enemy that must be guarded against if one is to successfully manage stress. Becoming overtired, missing breaks, and working too many hours per week should be infrequent occurrences if longevity on the job and good health are desirable.

Work responsibilities for most veterinary technicians are demanding and stressful. Often, the veterinary technician spends more time caring for the animals and the clients than does the veterinarian. High-pressure cases, full schedules, emergencies, demanding clients, and monotonous tasks are stressors that can take their toll.

Finally, working as part of a medical team has advantages and disadvantages. When relationships within a medical team are amicable, compatible, and supportive, benefits in terms of stressor tolerance can be notable for each person. However, when there is even one conflictual relationship within the team, all members are vulnerable to the stress of this conflict. Communication, fairness, and trust within the team are necessary to meet the demands of the career. All team members should work conscientiously to ensure that the team functions as a buffer against stress rather than having the opposite effect.

Evaluation

After identifying all stressors in an individual's life, the total stressor load should be analyzed. Which stressors can be alleviated? Which ones can be prevented? In the workplace, team effort is usually required to alleviate many of the stressors mentioned in this chapter. If other people must be involved in lowering the stressor load, are they willing to cooperate to do so? Now, take a look at how much of the stress is ongoing and unavoidable. The following section discusses techniques for coping with stress and building stressor resistance.

COPING WITH STRESS

Resistance to stress can be developed by instituting new habits within the lifestyle, increasing mental health and awareness, developing support systems, and performing relaxation activities that are known to miraculously protect against stress within the body and psyche. Some of these techniques may require more extensive explanation than this chapter can provide, and the reader is encouraged to consult Recommended Reading for more information. Table 33–5 outlines some common solutions for stressors found in the environment, career, and personal life.

TECHNICIAN NOTE

A slightly altered lifestyle along with certain mental and physical requirements can combat the effects of stress.

Stress Resistor Habits

Individuals can become more resistant to stress if they incorporate specific healthy habits into their daily lives. Attention to certain mental and physical requirements and the institution of a slightly altered lifestyle can combat the effects of stress. Aspects of nutrition, sleep, exercise, and mental recreation are relevant in the management of stress.

Nutrition is important in coping with stress. Regular healthy eating habits are the best protection against stress.

• Table 33–5 •

STRESSOR TYPE	STRESSOR	SOLUTION
ALLEVIATION OF STRESS		
Environment	Noise	More frequent breaks
	Space	Redesign of clinic
	Equipment	Maintenance, discard faulty equipment
	Orderliness	Organization with routine staff maintenance
	Records	Customization of forms, computerization with consultation and training
Career	Scheduling	Team scheduling with attention to breaks, avoid overscheduling
	Geography	Avoid compulsivity in scheduling, make schedules flexible, maintenance of transportation, communication links
	Co-worker conflicts	Team meetings, mediation
	Client population	Training of staff in communication
	Finances	Budgetary counseling
	Long hours	Vacations, shift work
Personal	Personal/home/family	Counseling, peer support

However, during more stressful periods or if one is living a highly stressful daily life, the body's requirements are somewhat altered. Protein is important in counteracting the impact of stress on the body, and attention should be paid to the consumption of adequate protein while under stress. Vitamin C is helpful in combating the lowered immune response that stress produces and in avoiding stress-related illness. Vitamin D, calcium, iron, and the B-complex vitamins are thought to be important in reducing the impact of stress on the body and the psyche as well, especially in women. Because the amount of sugar within the bloodstream is altered during the body's response to stress, many people have a tendency to overeat or to eat too many sugars, fats, and carbohydrates during stressful periods. This tendency should be avoided because it is directly counterproductive in alleviating stress. Finally, good nutrition includes moderation in negative habits such as the use of alcohol, caffeine, tobacco, and sodium.

Sleep is often neglected by veterinary professionals. More and more information from researchers is becoming available involving sleep, our need for it, and the type and duration of sleep we need. Every person has a unique set of requirements for duration of sleep, and one must examine this habit over a period of time to determine how much sleep makes him or her feel best, work best, and enjoy rising in the morning. An optimal amount of nightly sleep is important in coping with stress, as is the type of sleep. The phase of sleeping called rapid eye movement (REM) sleep is when dreams occur. This phase does not occur normally in those who use drugs or alcohol or in those who are constantly tired and sleep deprived. In addition, it is known that this phase is abnormal in many people with mental illness. Good sleep habits particular to each individual provide the rest that both the body and mind need to be strong in response to stress.

Exercise is one of the best antidotes to stress. Its benefits include release from tension, restoration of normal chemical balance, resistance to the physiological reaction to stress and resultant cardiovascular diseases, and relief from depression. To achieve these benefits, an exercise program should be convenient and inexpensive, be rhythmic and part of a daily routine, and require some exertion and concentration. Because aerobic exercises can be performed free, indoors or outdoors; are rhythmic; and require focus, they are well suited for incorporation into a program of stress management.

Mental recreation describes the activity of pleasantly refocusing the mind away from stress-producing thoughts. So many stressors involve mental and emotional components that no coping program is effective unless there is attention to strengthening and relaxing the mind. Humor is important because laughter produces endorphins and combats illness. It is helpful if habits are developed so that some time is spent amusing ourselves, even laughing, each day. Television is sometimes, but not always, helpful. Other sources of humor include various forms of literature and art. The best source of humor is oneself, and learning to laugh at oneself is an irreplaceable gift.

Various other forms of mental recreation exist. Music, reading, and conversation are pleasing and interrupt the stress response. Hobbies that are enjoyable and require concentration are also effective. Contact with animals, coincidentally, has been found to lower blood pressure, respiration rate, and pulse rate. Animals are certainly available to veterinary technicians, but some time each day could be spent enjoying them rather than working on them. Spirituality and prayer are also effective in refocusing mental activity. Some form of mental recreation should be built into the weekly routine for each individual.

Mental Health and Awareness

Mental health is the best predictor of physical health. When an individual's stressor load includes a higher proportion of personal stressors from their present and past personal backgrounds, a more concentrated effort toward mental health may be recommended. Fears of rejection, inadequacy, or abandonment and problems with self-esteem, relationships, depression, or anger may render a person more vulnerable to stress.

Awareness, not only of one's own state of mental health but also of what personal stressors are and how one reacts to stressors, can make management of stress more effective. Which parts of the body are the first to react or are more sensitive to stress? How does the person respond to stress emotionally? Behaviorally, where and with whom is stress released, and are those behaviors inappropriate or hurtful to others? Individuals may need professional help to answer these questions and to change their external and internal lives. Counselors can be of help in this area. In choosing a counselor, make sure that the professional is licensed in your state. Interview the counselor and ascertain that his or her style and philosophy are compatible with those of the person to be treated. Finally, choose a counselor who appears knowledgeable about stress and the medical field and who is goal oriented.

Support

One of the more essential coping techniques concerns human relationships. Friendships, support, and ventilation of feelings are vital for human mental health in general but are also necessary for stress resistance. Veterinary technicians may need to work at developing healthy support networks at work and outside of work. Spouses cannot be the only resource for support because the system then becomes out of balance and the marriage begins to take pressure. Staff meetings and socials can help to develop rapport between co-workers. Employers should be required to offer support to their employees in many ways. Association meetings and conferences are another way to develop professional friendships and widen support networks. As mentioned, the veterinary medical profession, at all levels, is stressful, and the stressors within employment are common to many individuals. The feeling of commonality with others, even in stress, can be helpful in managing stress. Creative solutions for common stressors can be shared within office relationships, and some stressors can even be alleviated.

Relaxation Techniques

Dr. Herbert Benson wrote a book in 1975 called *The Relaxation Response*, in which he popularized the response of the body to self-induced relaxation techniques. Meditation, self-hypnosis, and power naps all have the same function in eliciting the relaxation response. The benefits of these techniques are extensive and are listed in Table 33–6. This chapter cannot possibly teach all of these valuable techniques; however, two of them, progressive muscular relaxation and autohypnosis, are described in Tables 33–7 and 33–8.

When All Else Fails: Burnout

Burnout is psychological, and sometimes physical, exhaustion due to prolonged, uninterrupted exposure to a stressor or stressors. Many individuals in the veterinary profession suffer from burnout; veterinarians may burn out within 15 years and veterinary technicians within a shorter period of time. Physical symptoms of burnout include any of the illnesses noted earlier in the chapter, such as ulcers, gastroenteritis, cardiac arrhythmia, and even heartburn, backache, or nausea. Early behavioral symptoms of burnout include withdrawal, overeating, increase in alcoholic intake, constant fatigue, agitation, distraction, aggressive behaviors, facial tics and spasms, and increased spending. Georgia Witkin-Lanoil, Ph.D., wrote about the psychologi-

• Table 33–6 •

BENEFITS OF THE RELAXATION RESPONSE
1. Oxygen consumption is lowered to a degree commonly reached only after 6 or 7 hours of sleep.
2. Heart and respiration rates are decreased.
3. Blood flow and skin temperature increase (circulation eases).
4. Electrical resistance of the skin increases markedly, suggesting decreased anxiety.
5. EEG shows high alpha and occasional theta, beta, and delta waves, suggesting a fluid level of consciousness comprising both wakefulness and deep sleep.
6. Desensitization regarding disturbing thoughts or stimuli
7. Enlivening after relaxation, a fresher view of the world
8. Greater equalization in the workload of cerebral hemispheres
9. Sharpened alertness, improvement in stress-related illnesses, increased productivity
10. Decrease in depression, self-blame, and irritability

• Table 33–7 •

PROGRESSIVE MUSCULAR RELAXATION

1. Frown hard, count to 10, let go. Repeat. Repeat again.
2. Squeeze eyes shut, count to 10, let go. Repeat. Repeat again.
3. Wrinkle nose while counting to 10. Let go. Repeat twice.
4. Press lips together, count to 10. Let go. Repeat twice.
5. Tighten neck, pushing back. Count to 10. Let go. Repeat.
6. Lift left shoulder up, tighten, relax. Again.
7. Lift right shoulder up, tighten, relax. Repeat.
8. Press arms back against imaginary wall. Tighten. Relax. Repeat.
9. Clench fists, count to 10. Let go. Repeat.
10. Slump over, let head fall forward, and up. Repeat.
11. Tighten buttock muscles, count to 10, relax. Repeat.
12. Tighten leg muscles, count to 10. Relax. Repeat.
13. Flex feet, count to 10, relax. Repeat.
14. Repeat whichever spots were tense, at least once.

cal warning signs, which she characterizes as the "Six Ds." They are defensiveness, depression, disorganization, defiance, dependency, and decision-making difficulties.

TECHNICIAN NOTE

When stress becomes overwhelming, burnout occurs.

When burnout has occurred, the professional hates to get up and go to work, has lost passion and enthusiasm for the once-loved career, and feels lost internally. Good counseling

• Table 33–8 •

AUTOHYPNOSIS

1. Put your feet flat on the floor, and support your hands on your lap. Sit up straight but comfortably. Roll your head to loosen your neck.
2. Pick a focal point for your eyes.
3. Breathe in deeply through your nose, out through your mouth, using your abdomen to breathe. Repeat twice.
4. Begin saying the word "relax" silently as you breathe normally and let your eyes close.
5. Repeat the word "relax" in rhythm with your breathing.
6. Let your thoughts come, note them, and let them go. Then return your attention to the word "relax."
7. Just let yourself relax, feel peaceful, and feel safe as you repeat the word "relax." You may stay in this space for 10 minutes. . . .
8. Now take a slow, deep breath, hold it, and breathe out. Begin to open your eyes as you take another breath, breathe out. Stretch, and move about slowly.

may help in reversing the burnout, but many times professionals consider and make a career change. To recover from burnout, one may need counseling and support. Reconnection with the initial enthusiasm is important; once desire to remain in the career has been established, reorganization of lifestyle and business regimen may be necessary.

Yet the individual who is burned out is often the last to know. Loved ones and co-workers may recognize the syndrome much earlier than does the individual in question. As with many emotional problems, when the defense mechanism of denial is in place, the individual will only move to awareness when ready and able to cope. Working (or living) with this individual can be frustrating and difficult. Offer support, gentle confrontation and observations, readings, personal experiences, and, most importantly, LISTEN. Encourage vacations, start an office exercise program, be creative. Suggest counseling only if the relationship is a close one, and if the individual would not be alienated by the suggestion.

SUMMARY

Stress is a fact of life in the 1990s, and it is a problem within the field of veterinary medicine that can cause mental and physical problems and even disrupt this rewarding career. However, it can be prevented, alleviated, and managed to the extent that its ramifications are not severe. The changes made, originally intended for management of stress, can also enrich lives and provide untold secondary rewards.

Recommended Reading

Allison L: Beat Stress! Boca Raton, FL, Globe Communication, 1992.
Benson H: The Relaxation Response. New York, Wm. Morrow and Co., 1975.
Boryshenko J: Mending the Body, Mending the Mind. New York, Bantam Books, 1988.
Brackenridge S and Elkins D: Stressors in veterinary practice. *In* Brackenridge SS and Elkins D: Stress Management for the Veterinary Practice Team. Santa Barbara, CA, Veterinary Practice Publishing, 1996.
Brackenridge S and Elkins AD: A team approach to a successful veterinary practice—with minimal stress. *In* Brackenridge SS and Elkins D: Stress Management for the Veterinary Practice Team. Santa Barbara, CA, Veterinary Practice Publishing, 1996.
Brackenridge S and Elkins AD: The effects of burnout. *In* Brackenridge SS and Elkins D: Stress Management for the Veterinary Practice Team. Santa Barbara, CA, Veterinary Practice Publishing, 1996.
Elkins AD: Burnout: Is it a problem for the veterinary practice team? Vet Practice Staff 2:1, 1990.
Friedman M and Rosenman RH: Type A Behavior and Your Heart. Greenwich, Fawcett Publications, 1974.
George JM, Milone CL, Block MJ, and Hullister WJ: Stress Management for the Dental Team. Philadelphia, Lea & Febiger, 1986.
Hanson P: The Joy of Stress. Kansas City, MO, Andrews and McMeel, 1985.
Selye H: Stress without Distress. Philadelphia, J.B. Lippincott, 1974.
Witkin-Lanoil G: The Male Stress Syndrome. New York, The Berkley Publishing Group, 1988.

34 Professional Development

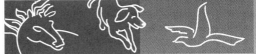

Sheila R. Grosdidier

> *All of our life is but a mass of small habits—practical, emotional, intellectual and spiritual that bear us irresistibly to our destiny.*
>
> WILLIAM JAMES

As individuals, each of us wants to be successful. Of course, when we ask ourselves what the definition of success is, we learn that there are many interpretations. In a career, crisis occurs when success isn't happening. Then, frustration, anger, and disillusionment bring crises to peaks, resulting in lower self-esteem, conflict with coworkers, incompatibility in the workplace, and career dissatisfaction. This is happening at an increasing rate in veterinary technology today. The average veterinary technician remains in practice for an estimated 7 years. The reality is that many of these people, given an opportunity to build strong professional skills, can avert crisis and enjoy additional success in the veterinary profession.

This chapter is about using tools and skills that are critical to securing goals and fulfilling expectations. Although the situation is improving, the important and valuable information provided in this chapter is not usually presented to the student or veterinary technician. If it were, professionally we might enjoy a more satisfying career.

Each of us exists within three different worlds: professional, public, and private. The professional world encompasses our life at work: clients, patients, colleagues, and the like. The public world is made up of friends and family, our interests, and volunteer areas. Our private world revolves around us: who we are, our private thoughts, spirituality, integrity, and character. Although these worlds are tightly interwoven, each contributes to what we are, our foundation, our essence, ourselves. Each day we are participants in each world and it is through the development of professional interpersonal skills,

such as our self-esteem, ability to listen, and manage conflict, that the most dramatic maturation process occurs.

TECHNICIAN NOTE

Each or us exists within three different worlds: professional, public, and private.

BUILDING SELF-ESTEEM

Usually, we do not take time to look within ourselves to understand who we really are and what we want from our lives, let alone our careers. When we do this, however, we learn more about ourselves, and also have a better understanding of others. Accomplishment on a professional level is irrevocably bound to self-esteem. People with low self-esteem seldom accomplish their goals, take risks, or develop strong trust in others. Frequently, they bear the burden of doubt and self-blame.

TECHNICIAN NOTE

Two out of three Americans suffer from low self-esteem.

DESTROYERS OF SELF-ESTEEM

Recognizing the Attitude

I'm-not-good-enough statements
Other people are always right
Always apologizing for everything
If I can't do it perfectly, I won't do it
Not forgiving mistakes
If people knew me, they wouldn't like me
I have no control over who I am
I'm always making mistakes
Blaming others and ourselves
Compared to others, I'm not adequate
I can't change

PAVING THE ROAD TO SUCCESS

High Self-Esteem:
- Presents a positive image
- Increased energy level
- Sustains feeling of self-worth
- Enhances positive attitude
- Increases satisfaction in career
- Affects risk-taking
- Encourages the pleasing of self, instead of others
- Reinforces value of own ideas
- Builds rapport
- Increases confidence and conviction
- Enhances decision-making ability

It is important that the individual see himself or herself in a decidedly positive light.

The economic need for large numbers of people with decent levels of self-esteem is unprecedented and represents a turning point in our evolution.
NATHANIEL BRANDON, *The Six Pillars of Self-Esteem*

Self-esteem is built on understanding and knowing the innate value of success. Ask your friends and family to define self-esteem. Expect to hear many definitions and opinions. Self-esteem is not a solitary entity that you might use, but a multifaceted conglomeration. It is the innate understanding of self-worth, the confidence to think and cope with challenge, a realization of worthiness. And it is right to assert our own needs, pursue our goals, maintain our values, and take pleasure in the achievement of these goals. Sound good? Now where do we go to get it? The ability to secure and enhance personal self-esteem dwells within every human being. However, every individual also maintains thoughts and deeds that destroy self-esteem and confidence, as well. Self-esteem affects all aspects of what you think and how you act.

When the first positive behavior modifying step is taken, the ultimate result is a positive change in self-esteem. Through conscious effort, change is not only possible, it is inevitable. As a building technique, take the time to develop an actionable plan and implement and evaluate its outcome. Choose one of the following concepts on building self-esteem and construct your plan. When you finish, select another, until you've completed all of them. By following the Action Planning worksheet, actionable plans can be realistically outlined. This method of devising and executing strategies for building self-esteem can be used, as well, to achieve any goal.

SELF-KINDNESS

Remember as a child the delight of a small gift, a trip to your favorite park, or meeting with friends to share secrets? As time passes, the feeling of delight may be lost, yet the essential element remains and these pleasant experiences affect self-esteem. Creating an environment where success is rewarded and celebrated is paramount in sustaining self-esteem. In any positive transformation, there must be dividends that mark the milestones of achievement. Personal and inexpensive rewards help erase our desire to punish ourselves and remember only negative experiences. Reward yourself and replace self-defeating negative habits with positive gratifying ones that build confidence.

NEGATIVE SELF-ESTEEM

Identifying the Attitude

Avoiding eye contact
Nervous behaviors
Slow to interact in groups
Poor posture
Second-guessing
Constant need for reassurance
Indecision
Fearfulness
Excessive hesitation/caution
Resentfulness
Anxiety
Frustration
Stuttering/inarticulate speech

 TECHNICIAN NOTE

Personal and inexpensive rewards help erase our desire to punish ourselves and remember only negative experiences.

THE 747 RULE

Have you noticed an interesting fact about jet airplanes? They may attain speeds of over 400 miles per hour, but they don't have a rearview mirror! The plane travels on a steady course toward a goal and doesn't need to be constantly looking back at previous locations. People without confidence often dwell continuously on prior mistakes, sometimes to the point of disability. Mistakes are learning experiences, and once experienced should be discarded. Most mistakes have a short life span and only survive when we continue to breathe life back

ACTION PLANNING

- Construct an action plan that will assist you in meeting your goals.
- Make sure that every step of your plan is SMART.

*S*pecific: Make every step very precise.
Example: ``I will speak with Ms. Jones and ask her to be my mentor and ask her to meet with me for twenty minutes twice a week.'' (Not: ``I will ask Ms. Jones to help me.'')

*M*ethod: Devise how you will make the step occur.
Example: ``I have arranged to get to work twenty minutes early on Tuesday and Thursday.'' (Not: ``Meet twice a week with Ms. Jones.'')

*A*ctionable: Use words that demonstrate action.
Example: ``I have arranged to meet twice a week.'' (Not: ``Check with Ms. Jones sometime.'')

*R*ealistic: Take small but reasonable and achievable steps to build your confidence.
Example: ``I will meet twice weekly for twenty minutes each time.'' (Not: ``I will meet daily for an hour with people who can help me.'')

*T*ime-oriented: Build a time frame so you can see your progress. Stay on schedule.

SAMPLE VISION:	ACTION PLAN WORKSHEET	Write your ultimate goal here. ← What do you want to achieve?	
SMART Steps	Resources Needed to Complete Step (People, materials, etc.)	What Could Prevent This from Getting Done? (What will I do about it?)	Completion Date
1 2 3 4			

into them—time and time again. Let them die a natural death (or maybe euthanasia is indicated in some circumstances!). Learn from mistakes and move on.

SEEING IS BELIEVING

Confidence and improved self-esteem are infectious. One good measurement of determining your progress is to ask yourself, How would a confident person approach this task? Selecting a mentor who exemplifies traits that you admire, such as high self-esteem and self-confidence, can assist you. This person knows the path you are traveling, so why not stop and ask for directions? Make a list of your mentor's attributes that illustrate

self-confidence and self-esteem. How can you implement these concepts?

It is time to reprogram the programmer. Building and sustaining a strong sense of self-esteem takes effort and persistence and a continuous review of the benefits. The elementary process that guides self-esteem is the sum total of repeated

SELF-REWARD GUIDELINES

- Give yourself permission to reward YOU
- Avoid rewards that cause personal damage (bingeing, extravagant spending)
- Reward yourself to diminish unpleasant tasks
- Make rewards a habit
- Choose rewards that are personally meaningful

REWARD YOURSELF

- BUY yourself flowers
- CALL an old friend
- RENT your favorite video
- TAKE a bubble bath
- TAKE a break
- START a new hobby
- TAKE a friend to lunch
- WATCH the sun come up with a loved one
- TAKE an afternoon herbal tea break
- HAVE a massage
- TRY a new cologne
- TAKE up a new sport
- READ a novel
- SET a time to stop working
- SEND a note to yourself about how well you did. Put it on your refrigerator.

OUTER REFLECTIONS OF INNER SELF-CONFIDENCE

Eye contact
Non-defensive posture
Confident tone of voice
Self-motivation
Seldom fidgets excessively
Professional attire in the workplace
Defends own ideas
Assertive
Not easily discouraged
Strong handshake

THE SUPER SEVEN OF SELF-ESTEEM

1. Each day I take time to be nice to myself.
2. I understand that judging others can diminish my self-esteem, so I will stop labeling others as "bad" or "good," etc.
3. I do the best job I can; realistically, that's all I ask of myself.
4. I will not set unreasonable expectations for myself.
5. I am capable of achieving anything I care to dream.
6. I will not dwell on failure while overlooking my success and I will remind myself of my best moments.
7. I will assert my rights and stand up for my decisions.

---

responses to specific behaviors. Take, for example, the programming of a computer. Before it is initiated the hard drive contains no stored information and is waiting for the opportunity to begin accumulating information in memory. As time passes the computer houses (in memory) vast bits of information. Essentially, the human mind operates the same and responds to past experiences. The child who is repeatedly told he or she is stupid responds to the experience by adding "I am stupid" to the memory banks. As a result, the child's hard drive is filled with negative information that will affect every future decision. Acceptance of the negative is easier than asserting the positive. Because nearly 70% of all information transmitted daily to the human mind is negative, positive images become a self-decision and require the human programmer to use a different file to retain information.

TECHNICIAN NOTE

Acceptance of the negative is easier than asserting the positive.

Begin the change by replacing "I can't do that" and "I always mess up" with "Yes, I can" and positive directives that represent strong self-confidence. The Super Seven of Self-Esteem reviews examples of positive self-talk phrases. Write these positive sentences down or create statements for yourself. Read your phrases morning and night, then post them conspicuously, for example, in your car (hopefully not on your windshield), on the bathroom mirror, or in your work area. Repeat those phrases several times during the day. Habits are formed by repetitive performance of given behaviors. Each time you find yourself making a negative comment or thinking negatively, conscientiously replace the thought with a comment from the list. Continue this process for at least 60 days and you will realize that negative, self-destructive statements are being deleted from memory and being replaced with positive responses that boost your hard drive.

JUMP-STARTING THE PLAN

Start now, it isn't necessary to wait until you have developed a fully outlined plan. Review the points in Jump-Starting Your Self-Esteem and start your journey to self-esteem by doing at

least one of these points immediately. *Don't hesitate! Don't equivocate!* See the meaningful impact that will motivate your strategy to fulfill your commitment to succeed.

BUILDING STRONG LISTENING SKILLS

Wisdom is the reward you get for a lifetime of listening when you'd have preferred to talk.

DOUG LARSON

In the high-stress workplace, veterinary health care team members encounter problems that arise from poor communication. The consequences are frustration, anxiety, and a conflict-ridden environment. How can a statement you've made be misunderstood so easily? When was the last time that you've been able to have a true and meaningful exchange of ideas with an associate? The answer to these questions is dependent on your ability to formulate and implement strong listening skills.

JUMP-STARTING YOUR SELF-ESTEEM

SHARE with trusted friends your desire to improve your self-esteem, and be surprised when they tell you how important you are to them.

MAKE a list of 12 important tasks you have accomplished in the last year; include the names of people who have benefited from your accomplishments. Post this list on your bedroom mirror.

TEACH someone a skill that you are good at and feel how pleasant an experience it is to have someone benefit from your ability.

COMPILE a list of what will be different in your life when you have fully developed a strong self-esteem. Be specific. Place these thoughts in an envelope and seal it, not to be opened for 1 year.

BENEFITS OF GOOD LISTENING

Adopting an Attitude
- Increase mutual respect
- Decrease miscommunication
- Demonstrate empathy
- Supply information to help solve problems
- Allow others to test feelings
- Decrease conflict
- Build stronger relationships
- Identify opportunities for resolution

SHARPENING YOUR SKILLS

Listening Techniques
- Use a posture that shows interest (lean in toward the speaker)
- Maintain eye contact
- Show affirmative gestures (nod your head, smile, etc.)
- Find an appropriate environment
- Do not think of responses until the talker has stopped talking
- Do not interrupt
- Use positive body language (good posture, open position to speaker)

> ✎ **TECHNICIAN NOTE**
>
> The average person only listens to about 40% of what is being spoken.

How would you describe a good listener? Most likely, the words "sincere," "compassionate," "patient," "centered," and "intelligent" would be included in your answer. Consider your current listening habits. Are you easily distracted, often forgetting what someone has said? Do you find yourself drifting from the topic being discussed? If any of these phrases sound familiar, you are not alone. The average person only listens to about 40% of what is being spoken, whereas the majority of what is spoken is never secured, retained, or remembered. This can be attributed to the fact that the spoken word is being paced at around 150 words per minute, while listening skills are capable of being comprehended at a much higher rate. This fact explains why we become distracted. Therefore, considering the amount of spoken information and conversation exchanged

daily through daily oral communication, 60% of which is un-evaluated and unprocessed mentally, it is not surprising that miscommunication occurs.

In the workplace, the highest percentage of communication is oral. The total listening process begins with making the distinction between hearing and listening (two terms that are frequently used interchangeably, but which are not interchangeable). Hearing is the physical aspect of capturing sound waves that contact the ear drum. Listening is the conscious psychological process that follows the physical process, which is responsible for assessing and retaining the meaning of the interchange. Listening is an active obligation that seizes and preserves what is being shared by others. The nature of active listening is demonstrated in Sharpening Your Skills.

Before initiating skills that will build powerful listening competence, it is important to understand the elements that prevent or curtail good listening. Review the list of common barriers in Listening Barriers and identify which of those elements affect your listening capabilities. In a conversation, look for instances when a barrier detracts from your ability to listen. Use the acronym IDEAL and disable the barrier. Utilizing the IDEAL process will enable you to eliminate Detractors and Distractions and enhance your listening skills.

Suit the action to the word, the word to the action.
William Shakespeare

There is a certain responsibility that comes with listening. The accomplished listener takes the learned techniques beyond what is just being said and attends to what he or she sees, which is a part of the message. The phrase "Thank you for

---

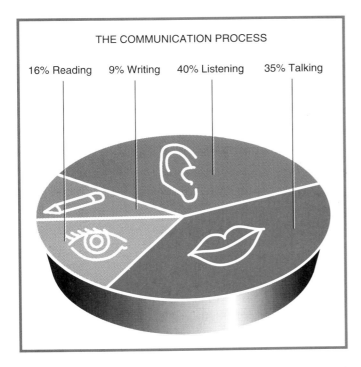

THE COMMUNICATION PROCESS

16% Reading   9% Writing   40% Listening   35% Talking

LISTENING BARRIERS
- Lack of eye contact
- Excessive body motion
- Inattentiveness
- Incompatible environment (noise, too many people)
- Interrupting
- Looking around the room
- Closed body language

coming today" is traditionally seen as a greeting or departing phrase of kindness, yet if spoken with irritation, bitterness, or a glaring look of anger, a whole new connotation is derived. Listening is an instrument that assesses nonverbal clues as well as oral phrases, even when one contradicts the other. Remember the last time that a client said that he or she was satisfied with a service but the person's body language, facial expression, and tone of voice said something different? Use your eyes as a potent listening tool along with your ears.

The active listener is actively in control of the conversation. Active listening skills such as direct eye contact indicate interest and convey focus that will keep the speaker's attention. Active listening skills have a nourishing effect on a speaker by conveying the feeling that he or she is not just being heard but understood. This sophisticated level of listening not only reduces the opportunity for miscommunication but also invites the speaker to share additional information. Initially, it is important to understand what the other person is saying before asking him or her to understand your viewpoint. Think about the last time someone interrupted you when you were talking. As you attempted to convey your thoughts, the person interrupted, possibly adding inappropriate, irrelevant, or unimpor-

tant opinions. What you were going to say was diminished and became less important and the chances that a positive and meaningful exchange would occur were reduced. Always consider that understanding should always precede being understood.

TECHNICIAN NOTE

The active listener is actively in control of the conversation.

Each person has an objective in listening. When building listening skills, it is essential to acknowledge, appraise, and understand. Listen carefully to what the speaker is saying. Also, show the speaker and others in the listening group that you understand what has been said, and, of course, encourage the speaker to continue and complete the message.

The techniques used in developing successful listening skills are deceptively simple, yet their application is frequently discomforting, if not painful. However, learning and using these techniques is worthwhile because of the advantage they bring in establishing a rapport in your workplace. Approach and adopt these techniques as your own. Initially, try to practice one or two of these skills. Then, as your confidence builds, you'll discover that learning the rest of them is easy.

Empathic listening is a valuable asset in veterinary practice because so many painful and tragic experiences occur there. Most clients encounter a variety of emotions surrounding the death of their pet and empathic listening is a nonthreatening and nonjudgmental method of providing a respectful environment. Judgment is an element that clients can rightfully find objectionable and alienating. Perhaps the client says, "I will miss Fluffy immensely. I don't know what I will do without her." An empathic listener would reply, "You are going to miss Fluffy and it is hard to be without her." Note that no judgment, advice, or evaluation has been made, just an exchange that shows caring, understanding, and empathy. Further discussion about bereavement may be found in Chapter 29.

Listening skills are tools that enable strong communication

exchanges to occur in the workplace, with coworkers, employers, and clients. When these skills improve, common pitfalls become more evident. The same strategy that you've employed in building listening skills can be used to enhance and expand oral communication.

Effective interaction with others dramatically improves the ability to triumph in the workplace, to develop strong business relationships, and to diminish conflict. And, perhaps, the advancement of technology that transfers information through impersonal methods such as fax or e-mail substantially emphasizes the necessity for powerful listening skills and cohesive communication. Listening is the foundation of all other communication activities.

EFFECTIVE CONFLICT RESOLUTION

The word "conflict" brings to mind angry words exchanged in a heated moment or, conversely, thoughts or feelings left unexpressed to avoid a confrontation. Conflict is frequently inevitable in veterinary practice. How coworkers respond to uncomfortable situations can ultimately determine the success of their careers. Inability to manage conflict hinders advancement and potentially results in technicians relinquishing jobs. Often, it is the people who work the hardest and love their job the most who become the first casualties. Indeed, conflict is often the primary reason people leave their jobs.

TECHNICIAN NOTE

Inability to manage conflict hinders advancement and potentially results in technicians relinquishing jobs.

There is good news. It is not necessary to run from conflict or to feel trapped in an endless cycle of angry outbursts that fracture business relationships and escalate to unbearable situations. Emotionally electrified circumstances can be faced directly, and confrontation can be managed in a win-win manner. It is possible to reduce tension and effectively resolve conflict by planning and engaging some uncomplicated steps.

CHANGE YOUR PERSPECTIVE

In a conflict situation each participant has a contrasting perception of what occurred in the disagreement. What the listener *believes* the speaker is saying becomes more important than the information the speaker is actually presenting. It is important to remember this—the emotional response of what is occurring overrides and dramatically escalates the situation. An example of this occurs when someone angrily shouts at another person for what the recipient perceives as no apparent reason. The angry person knows that something quite offensive has happened but the other looks on in disbelief over the coworker's sudden outburst. Again, it's not what is said but what is perceived that becomes the issue. Perception becomes reality. Remember this the next time you are listening to a client explain what he or she thought the directions on the medication bottle said. (It is amazing how the mind remembers and interprets what is said. Perception is reality!)

FACING THE FEAR OF CONFLICT

Instilled in many of us at a young age is the fear of conflict and the desire to avoid disagreement. "Don't rock the boat" may have been a common saying heard during your developmental years. The first step in conflict resolution is to embrace the idea that discord need not be negative and can be a positive, if not uplifting, experience with a little skill and technique. A review of some positive benefits of conflict can be found in Facing & Resolving Conflicts. Now is the time to rid yourself of the fear of conflict. Write down all of your fears concerning conflict and confrontation. Now begin reading the list out loud, paying close attention to what your feelings were and how they influenced the conflict situation. After you have taken the time to closely review your list, start ripping the paper into small pieces, and as you discard the pieces into the wastebasket, focus on how you will now replace those "discarded" fears with positive and beneficial efforts.

MISUNDERSTANDING: THE MOST COMMON BEGINNING OF CONFLICT

As we now understand perception, it is essential to begin utilizing techniques that will lessen the occurrence of misunderstanding. One example of a method that works well in a group situation follows. You are participating in a monthly staff meeting at the veterinary clinic and the conversation becomes heated, rising in volume. Finally, no one can hear what anyone else is saying. This is a good opportunity to employ a rephrasing technique that establishes a guideline that alleviates miscommunication. To apply this technique, each person in the group, before speaking, must repeat what the preceding person has said. This fulfills two requirements: The opportunity to address the group is prerequisite by listening to what others are saying and it gives the original speaker an opportunity to correct content and perception. This procedure asks all parties to enhance their listening skills and to understand the different styles that people use to present their thoughts. Although the rephrasing technique may take skill to achieve, it often signifi-

FACING & RESOLVING CONFLICTS
Opportunities
To Strengthen:
- Social and work relationships
- Constructive skills
- Personal development

To Encourage:
- Awareness—that different does not mean ``bad''
- Acceptance of differences
- Alternative ways of thinking and acting

To Increase:
- Self-esteem
- Ability to adapt to diversity

To Decrease:
- Stress

To Learn:
- More about others
- More about ourselves

cantly alleviates misunderstandings and ultimately lessens the potential for conflict.

TAKING STEPS TO MANAGE CURRENT CONFLICT

"If Jane makes one more snide comment, I won't be responsible for my actions. It's ridiculous that she thinks she can get away with everything, and now she is thirty minutes late! I can't take anymore!" says Mary. Chances are that conflict is imminent in Jane's life. Before Mary confronts Jane, it is paramount that she decide upon a plan that will achieve her desired goals and keep the situation from deteriorating into open warfare. A plan will instill a greater opportunity to successfully resolve the situation and obtain the benefits outlined earlier.

The first step is to identify potential roadblocks that prevent conflict resolution. The most common problem is the use of language that will be a barrier to communication. Common phrases often elicit negative behavior from people, especially in emotionally charged situations. Examples of these phrases that can be viewed negatively can be found in Fightin' Words & Phrases. By avoiding these potentially antagonizing phrases, the focus can turn to strengthening intercommunication. Listening skills are of paramount importance in untangling disharmony. *Your ears protect your mouth from your feet.* The focal point in a conversation that is accelerating toward conflict should be understanding what the involved individuals *perceive* as the problem. Note the word *perceive*. What is relevant and obvious may not be what is perceived.

TECHNICIAN NOTE

Listening skills are of paramount importance in untangling disharmony.

Understanding perception is the key to uncovering fundamental issues and building the bridge to resolution and harmony. So, what prevents people from listening to what's being shared? If asked, most people would say that they see themselves as charitable, self-controlled, and patient when they interact with others. Actually, actions are often impulsive, and instead of actively listening, a response is being formulated while the other person is still speaking. The moment the mind engages to consider the response, the person is no longer listening to what is being said. The likelihood that he will miss the essence of what someone wants him to understand is lost. Lessening this tendency can be achieved by utilizing the "three-second rule." The rule is this: before you begin your reply to someone, wait three seconds after they have finished, using that time to formulate your response. This is a useful tool that should be shared with others, as well. It demonstrates listening skills and a desire to fully hear all that is being said. Conflict is often about looking at differences, rather than similarities. The three-second rule can demonstrate that you are searching for those similarities.

Often anger, anxiety, and frustration can decrease our ability to listen to another's comments, which illustrate that we value our own thoughts more than those of others. These barriers can be overcome by thinking of listening as an attitude rather than a skill that can be turned off and on at will. You must be a good listener to be successful and the benefits of good listening are diverse and directly linked to resolving and diminishing conflict.

CREATING A RESOLUTION

Conflict identifies diversity and not everyone shares your view of any particular predicament. The emphasis in resolving a problem should be directed to returning all participants to the workplace where each can function productively and comfortably. To achieve this, conflict should be welcomed as an opportunity to resolve differences.

Take these six steps in managing conflict, remembering that each step must be taken and thoroughly understood before proceeding to the next. Also, acknowledge that someone must step forward and take a leadership role. Disintegration of a plan or failure to resolve a problem is a signal that all steps were not completely accomplished and it is necessary to repeat the process to secure the desirable result.

Step 1: Prepare the Environment

The environment will be the foundation upon which the resolution is based. Yet frequently, the foundation is overlooked. To adequately treat a wound, it is necessary to first appropriately prepare the site in a manner that will reduce infection and lessen the chance of complications. In the arena of conflict resolution, preparation of the site will reduce present misunderstandings and future complications.

It is important that the foundation be competently prepared, the location made acceptable to all participants, and that preliminary well-formulated ideas are outlined. Just as it would not be appropriate to confront a coworker in a group with other associates, it is also inappropriate to ask someone to consider his or her conflict resolution process at 5:10 P.M. on Friday evening. Preparation is integral to effective resolution. Problems are resolved more easily when everyone is comfortable, and aware that the others are valuable participants. This may prove difficult if everyone cannot agree on the real problem (remember that perceptions may vary). The leader must continue to emphasize that everyone benefits from the problem resolution, even those who are not convinced that a problem exists.

Choose a time and a place that lessen the chances for interruptions by orchestrating a quiet environment that allows sufficient time to solve the problem. A 20-minute marathon session may not produce an acceptable outcome. Likewise, extended meetings that allow too much ruminating can be detrimental to the process. Short meetings are less painful, as everyone can see that progress is being made.

FIGHTIN' WORDS & PHRASES

``You made me . . .'' Places blame
``Should . . .'' Places blame
``Never . . .'' an extreme generalization that seldom applies
``Always . . .'' an extreme generalization that seldom applies
``I can't . . .'' Implies an unwillingness to try
``But . . .'' Negates everything said to that point

HOW TO RESOLVE A PROBLEM

Guidelines

- Forge a feeling of collaboration and partnership
- Diminish the feeling of US and THEM—emphasize WE
- Emphasize interest in overall business relationship and productivity
- Be positive
- Review benefit of conflict with group/other persons
- Be realistic
- Outline expectation for meeting
- Be brief—but specific

A location for the encounter is another point to consider. Everyone involved should be content with the location. The locale should diminish distraction and not represent a place where something bad frequently takes place, nor should it represent another participant's turf. Many persons are also placed in a more comfortable mode if refreshments are offered. The location must also have room for everyone to be seated facing one another to encourage interaction.

As an essential element in preparing the foundation, the leader's and speakers' comments should elicit a sense of collaboration. It is important to motivate each participant to begin the resolution process, especially when derogatory or angry comments have been exchanged in the past.

Step 2: What Is the Problem?

We are each the sum of perceptions derived from a lifetime of influence, learning, and experiences. These perceptions influence how we respond to others. Past perceptions mold attitudes and facilitate diversity among human beings. Above all, respect for this diversity must be maintained. Different isn't bad, just different! Without respect, the foundation of the conflict resolution process will crumble. It is time to undertake the operation of understanding each person's perception of the conflict. People involved in a conflict often have dramatically different views and intensity of feelings. Clarification of everyone's views will begin the collaboration process.

TECHNICIAN NOTE

We are each the sum of perceptions derived from a lifetime of influence, learning, and experiences.

Collect everyone's perception about the conflict and organize these thoughts. Identification of priorities is equally beneficial. As conflict rarely occurs overnight, it seldom resolves itself in a day. Be prepared for a lengthy list of perceptions, particularly if more than three people are involved. All issues must be held with respect, although they can vary in how they are organized on the list.

Compile and clarify the components of the conflict on your list before proceeding to the next step. Although individuals may see their entire environment as a battlefield, encourage these persons to remember that this conflict is only one single facet of their overall professional relationship. Just as the fracture of a femur doesn't mean a patient's condition is poor, the presence of problems should not affect overall job performance or overall job satisfaction.

Step 3: Understand All the Pieces

Clarifying the important aspects of the problem should be directed toward identifying and assessing the needs of each individual. Remember that each participant is a sower of the seeds of discontent, which was harvested to produce conflict. For this reason each area of frustration, anger, inappropriate action, and miscommunication must be acknowledged, addressed, and analyzed. After each person becomes aware that his or her input is valued and that each problem has been defined, it's time to move on to step 4.

Step 4: Developing a Plan

The planning phase asks participants initially to focus on the present and future while minimizing experiences from the past. Reaching for answers in the present helps relinquish the negative impact of past occurrences. From past experiences we learn what steps might have been taken earlier to forestall the present problem. Everyone should be reminded that satisfying experiences were enjoyed in the past and that resolution of this conflict should be each participant's reward.

Exploring possibilities and gaining insight from each person initiates a successful resolution plan. In exploring previous steps, an outline of elements for reconciliation exists. It is now time to accurately define the ideas, thoughts, and suggestions that allow the participants to move forward to step 5.

Step 5: Envisioning a Plan

To envision a plan, begin by conceiving the possibilities. List as many options as possible. A list of questions that facilitate choosing options can be found in Identifying Actionable Steps. As the list builds, an actionable plan can be envisioned. Sometimes the list of issues to be resolved may look insurmountable, but keep in mind that only after a problem has been identified can it be resolved. Each issue is a step toward a fulfilling and

IDENTIFYING ACTIONABLE STEPS

"Mind Joggers"

- Ask yourself how a "hot situation" could have been cooled down earlier.
- Draw a mental picture of what a perfect work environment would look like.
- Make a list of all options that could assist you in resolving the problem.
- Brainstorm—Write down everything that would be gained from resolving the problem.

QUALITIES OF ACTIONABLE STEPS

Actionable Steps:
- Show no favoritism
- Respond to at least one need or issue
- Build confidence and trust
- Improve the foundation to sustain a resolution and partnership
- Demonstrate compatibility with everyone's needs
- Encourage everyone's participation
- Result in mutual satisfaction for all participants

---

productive environment. Remember that resolution is a process, not an event, and keep reminding everyone of this fact. Do not rush to a quick solution. Instead, maintain a balanced, steady pace and make sure that all issues have been accurately resolved. Achievable action steps are illustrated in Qualities of Actionable Steps. By following these cues your outlined steps possess the greatest opportunity for success. Actionable steps must be reasonable and have the ability to inspire confidence in the outcome. They demonstrate to those involved that an answer is being placed and measured for accomplishment. Actionable steps must meet the given criteria to substantially enhance the resolution process.

TECHNICIAN NOTE

To envision a plan, begin by conceiving the possibilities.

Step 6: Everyone Wins

When actionable steps are identified, a logical order must be defined and implemented. Part of the process of conflict resolution develops skills and techniques that foster improvements in professional relationships that will enable an enjoyable environment in the workplace.

Agreements for conflict resolution must also be actionable and realistic because they embody the actionable steps previously outlined. These agreements should address the needs and issues established earlier. The mutually beneficial agreement plan replaces typical bargaining techniques because it fulfills the needs of all persons without dwelling on past demands. It emphasizes shared needs and goals.

This process is time-directed, so that everyone maintains the feeling of forward motion and can visualize positive impact. As agreements are formed and implemented, measurable points are indicated against a schedule to demonstrate that results are forthcoming. Seeing and enjoying the fruits of one's labors increases rapport and improves relationships and frequently improves a successful team. A successful team diminishes future conflict by not letting conflict negatively affect its team foundation.

Leadership of this process requires someone to step forward and motivate the participants. The leader is required to be the conscience of the others. It is his or her duty to remind individuals of agreements and to probe for details and information.

TECHNICIAN NOTE

The leader is required to be the conscience of the others.

Even in the most serious conflicts, this six-step process can be accurately applied and advantageous conclusions obtained. A leader's role in resolving conflicts is one of the most useful skills for resolving problems in the workplace. The specific role of the leader and skills of personal leadership may be found in Chapter 32.

CONCLUSION

Conflict is a part of life that should be accepted without negativity, and embraced as an opportunity. The benefits of managing conflict go beyond resolving difficult situations. Possessing resolution skills will also enhance personal self-esteem, strengthen control during negative situations, and provide confidence from the knowledge that conflict need not be feared.

Give us the serenity to accept what cannot be changed, courage to change what should be changed, and wisdom to distinguish the one from the other.

REINHOLD NIEBUHR

Recommended Reading

Adler M: How to Speak, How to Listen. New York, Collier Books, 1983.
Bloomfield HH and Cooper RK: The Power of Five, Emmaus, PA, Rodale, 1995.
Bolton R: People Skills. New York, Touchstone, 1986.
Bourdeaux D: 12 Steps to Personal and Professional Development. Mill Valley CA, Wildflower Press, 1993.
Brandon N: The Six Pillars of Self-Esteem. New York, Bantam Books, 1995.
Butler G and Hope T: Managing Your Mind: The Mental Fitness Guide. New York, Oxford University Press, 1995.
Covey S: The Seven Habits of Highly Effective People. New York, Simon & Schuster, 1989.
Deep S and Sussman L: What to Say to Get What You Want. Reading, MA, Addison-Wesley, 1992.
Deep S and Sussman L: Yes, You Can. Reading, MA, Addison-Wesley, 1996.
Fuller G: The Workplace Survival Guide. Englewood Cliffs, NJ, Prentice Hall, 1996.
Gabor D: Speaking Your Mind in 101 Difficult Situations. New York, Fireside Books, 1994.
Glaser C and Smalley BS: Swim with the Dolphins. New York, Warner Books, 1995.
King L: How to Talk to Anyone, Anytime, Anywhere. New York, Crown, 1994.
Markham U: Creating a Positive Self-Image. Rockport, MA, Element, 1995.
McKay M and Fanning P: Self-Esteem. Oakland, CA, New Harbinger, 1992.
Newman F: Let's Develop. New York, Castillo International, 1994.
Null G: Be Kind to Yourself. New York, Caroll & Graff, 1995.
Scott GC: Resolving Conflict. Oakland, CA, New Harbinger, 1990.
Seligman ME: Learned Optimism. New York, Pocket Books, 1990.
Siress R: Working Woman's Communication Survival Guide. Englewood Cliffs, NJ, Prentice Hall, 1994.
Weeks D: 8 Essential Steps to Conflict Resolution. New York, Putnam, 1992.

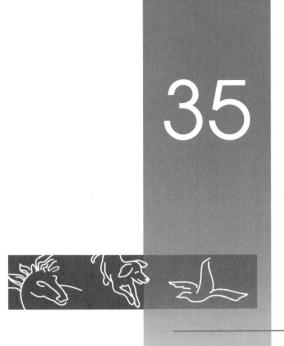

35 Computer Applications in Veterinary Medicine

Richard J. Hidalgo • *Robert A. Holmes*

As with all new and popularized innovations, final applications are often left to the imagination of the user. Computers are the greatest inventions of modern times as they have completely revolutionized many occupations and industries. However, one must ask the inevitable questions: Should computers be used in veterinary medicine? Why should computers be used in the profession? How can these instruments be used to the greatest advantage?

Before answering the question whether computers should be used in the practice of veterinary medicine, one should consider why these devices are used at all. The only logical reasons for using computers in this profession or, for that matter, any other profession or industry, is that the instruments do some aspects of the job that humans are incapable of doing or that the instrument can accomplish certain functions better than humans. For example, it is known that computers are more efficient at handling large volumes of data and repetitive tasks, whereas humans are better suited for decision-making. Although one could argue that veterinarians have practiced successfully for over one hundred years without computers, it would be difficult to deny that computers are capable of doing many chores better, faster, and more conveniently than humans. The ultimate decision to computerize must be based on whether the instruments improve service to the animal-owning public and provide an adequate return on investments of time and money. We are convinced that computers can fulfill both of the above criteria—provided they are utilized efficiently.

Much of the chapter is devoted to describing how computers can be used to the greatest advantage in the practice of veterinary medicine. Its aim is to provide the reader with insights into routine and innovative uses of computers in veterinary medicine. Because of space limitations, the discussion is limited to applications in private practice. However, the same principles can be applied to public, industrial, and academic veterinary medicine.

Before entering into discussions of applications in the profession, a brief introduction to the terminology of computers is warranted. A detailed list of computer terms is provided for the convenience of the reader in the Glossary at the end of the chapter.

COMPUTER HARDWARE

Hardware utilized in computerization of a veterinary medical practice includes any digital or analog device used to develop or process an electronic signal. Hardware includes the central processing unit(s) (CPU) and peripheral devices, such as monitors, printers, plotters, scanners, modems, disk drives, tape drives, and terminals. Simply stated, hardware is the "machinery" over which a computer system runs. Hardware systems come in as many varieties as there are manufacturers. As is the case with other applications, veterinary practice management programs can usually be run on any of a variety of computers. With the steady increase in computing capacity and decrease in cost of computers, the decision regarding which hardware to purchase has become much easier. However, it is emphasized that the type of hardware purchased for a veterinary practice should be dictated primarily by the type of software selected.

One should not even consider computer hardware unless he or she has a firm idea of what the hardware will be expected to do. Some of the decisions that must be made before committing to a particular brand or model of computer include: (1) the number of users that will have simultaneous access to the software, (2) the number and location of the data entry stations, and (3) the sophistication of the software programs (e.g., color screens, interactive diagnostic programs, bar coding). Another prime consideration in the selection of hardware is availability of rapid and reliable service. Rapid service generally equates with a company that guarantees overnight replacement of malfunctioning hardware. Such service is offered by both local and remote companies.

TECHNICIAN NOTE

Before purchasing computer hardware, always assess the tasks to be performed, then select the software that best accomplishes the task, then select the hardware that is best suited to run the software.

COMPUTER SOFTWARE

Software for computerization of a veterinary practice is by far the most important consideration. Software consists of the operating system, the application program, and, with some practice management programs, the networking platform. The operating system is the software platform, which enables the computer to operate the application program. The most commonly used operating system in veterinary practices is DOS (disk operating system). The DOS system is the operating system that was specifically developed for IBM personal computers and is used in all IBM-compatible computers. The DOS platform has the disadvantage of being a single-user, single-application system, meaning that only one person is allowed to use the application program and only one application program can be operated at one time. It has the advantages of being fairly simple to use and of having been in use for many years. Most persons with moderate experience with computers have a working knowledge of DOS.

Another single-application, single-user operating system that is commonly used to run veterinary practice management applications is the Macintosh system. Although less popular than the DOS operating system, the Macintosh system has die-hard proponents who are partial to a graphical-user interface and are adept in use of the mouse. The graphical-user interface provides the user with access to application programs through icons and pull-down menus. A distinct advantage of the later versions of the Macintosh operating system is that networking capabilities are built into the system.

The UNIX operating system (and its XENIX, ULTRIX, System V and AIX versions) is a multitasking, multiuser system. It has the advantages of being capable of executing larger programs and executing programs faster than DOS. In addition, UNIX allows multiple users simultaneous access to the same application. Disadvantages of this operating system are lack of standardization between versions and increased skill and knowledge required to operate and maintain the system.

The networking platform is software that enables: (1) CPUs to communicate with one another and with the server (the main CPU that runs the operating system and networking and application software); (2) dumb terminals to communicate with the CPU, and (3) CPUs to communicate with remote peripherals, such as printers and disk drives. The need for networking

software to run veterinary hospital management systems is usually minimal because of the moderate size of most practices. Even when multitasking systems are used in veterinary practices, terminals are usually connected directly to the CPU. Occasionally in large practices and when two or more practices are linked together, networking systems are employed.

The importance of the application software warrants an indepth discussion which will be presented later. However, the section on application software will be preceded by uses of computers in a veterinary practice. Currently utilized applications are discussed and an attempt is made to predict future uses as technology develops.

USES OF COMPUTERS IN A CLINICAL PRACTICE

It is appropriate to begin this section with the premise that uses of computers in veterinary practices are limited only by the imagination of the software developers and the users. It would also be appropriate to remind the reader that the only justifications for use of computers are that tasks will be performed faster, more efficiently, or more reliably and that there will be a fair return on the investment. With the above statements in mind, computer uses will be examined. Computers in veterinary practices are commonly used for accounting, drug and supply inventory management, medical records management, client communication, hospital management, general practice management, computer-assisted diagnostic programs, and other practice-related programs. Each of these functions has several facets and is discussed individually.

Accounting

Accounting is the most commonly used and probably the most important computer application in veterinary practices. It is the nucleus around which most, if not all, veterinary practice management software was designed. In some instances, this is the only use made of computers in certain practices. In fact, the accounts receivable or the amounts owed to the practice is the only record maintained on the computer. If the sole purpose of a computer system is to maintain only accounts receivable, one could easily create his or her own custom application utilizing one of several commercially available spreadsheets or database programs. Maintaining only accounts receivable records on a computer is not recommended.

TECHNICIAN NOTE

Accounting is the most commonly used and probably the most important computer application.

There are several advantages of utilizing a complete accounting package. Among these advantages are accurate accounting of expenditures, automated client billing, credit management (alerts operator to clients who have more than the allowable balance or who are bad credit risks), business management reports (daily, weekly, monthly, and annual), and maintenance of tax records. The advantage of automated client billing with professional itemized bills and automated addressing is sufficient, at least in our minds, to warrant a comprehensive computerized accounting package.

Scheduling

Scheduling is one of the most valuable features of veterinary practice management software programs and should be utilized to its maximum. Proper use of the scheduling program can balance workloads between days, can fill in appointment gaps with immunizations, heartworm checks, and routine dental maintenance, and can minimize the number of clients who become angry because of long waits in the reception area. The success of the scheduling module of the practice software is dependent not on the veterinarians, but on the receptionist or receptionist-technician. In order to attain maximum efficiency in scheduling, the receptionist must be courteous, forceful, and resourceful and must make on-the-spot decisions that have impact on the whole veterinary team.

Scheduling modules of veterinary practice management programs all work in basically the same fashion, but some are much more efficient and user-friendly. When in the market for veterinary practice management software, seek one with a scheduling module that has the following attributes: effortless shuttling from the scheduling module to all other functions within the practice management program, ability to schedule appointments of variable lengths of time, and ability to graphically display daily and weekly schedules of all providers of veterinary services. Additional features that are desirable in a scheduling program are ability to time multiple simultaneous events and to set multiple alarms and ability to monitor patients' arrival time in the reception area and departure.

Inventory Management

Drug and supply inventory are important functions of veterinary practice management programs that are, without a doubt, best done by computers. Management of drug and supply inventories so that the practice does not run out of an item, does not have to pay high prices for overnight shipment, or does not become overstocked can result in a considerable savings over a 1-year period. The ability to determine with a few keystrokes the amount of any drug or item on hand, its cost and retail value, and the automatic notification when inventory numbers reach predetermined levels is highly desirable. However, the reader is cautioned that a significant initial investment is necessary to establish the inventories and a moderate amount of time and effort is required to maintain inventory accuracy.

In addition to drug inventory, many practice management programs have additional desirable features associated with the pharmacy program, either as part of the overall package or as add-on modules. Features frequently included in the pharmacy package are automatic reordering including customized order forms, a database of drug and supply vendors, automatic prescription label printing, and a drug formulary. An acceptable drug formulary provides drug uses, dosages by species, contraindications, and, in some cases, built-in calculators and programs to calculate specific dosages.

Medical Records

Maintenance of good medical records on every patient is imperative in the practice of quality veterinary medicine and has strong legal implications. The medical record, as used in the context of this discussion, is the chronological record of all physical observations, electronic measurements, imagery, and laboratory data collected on a patient, and all therapy administered. Medical records may be as extensive as problem-oriented medical records (known as POMRs) or as simple as small cryptic notes on observations and therapy. In POMRs, each problem observed in an animal or reported by the client is recorded and "SOAPed." The acronym SOAP is used to describe four steps in dealing with each problem: *s*ubjective observations, *o*bjective data, *a*ssessment, and *p*rocedures performed. Additional information on medical records may be found in Chapter 4.

Medical records on patients must be kept if acceptable veterinary medicine is to be practiced and, from a legal standpoint, a client-patient relationship is to be documented. Whether to keep them in hard copy or electronically is a decision to be made by the owner or administrator of the practice. After this decision is made, a number of decisions on operational procedures must be made and accurately communicated to all members of the practice team. Who is allowed or required to make entries into the medical record? When and where are these entries made? If medical records are maintained electronically, who has access to the information?

Complete and detailed medical records are imperative to the practice of sound, modern veterinary medicine. No matter how good our memories are, it is unlikely that anyone can maintain knowledge of even the common signalments of temperature, pulse, and respiration from day to day. To think that one can mentally maintain the entire medical history of even a few patients is truly foolhardy. Furthermore, consider the scenario of different veterinarians seeing the same patient on different days or on different office visits. There is no better means of communication between veterinarians in the same practice than through good records. This same argument holds true for communication between the veterinarian and the veterinary technician, the referring veterinarian, and the diagnostic laboratory.

> **✎ TECHNICIAN NOTE**
>
> Electronic patient records are legal medical records and must be maintained for a minimum of 4 years (3 years plus the current year).

Maintenance of complete and accurate medical records has profound legal implications. Following a problem that developed involving over-the-counter dispensing of prescription drugs by veterinarians and their staff, it was determined by the court that the simple dispensing of a drug was a violation of state practice acts. It was ruled that veterinarians may dispense prescription drugs *only* to clients when there is a "client/patient/veterinarian relationship." This is usually interpreted as that relationship in which the client's animal was recently physically observed by the prescribing veterinarian. The best proof of such a relationship is an accurate medical record. Aside from proof of the client/patient relationship, medical records are the best evidence that a veterinarian can have in court when accused of malpractice. False malpractice suits, although not anticipated by anyone, are filed even by the best of clients because of some misunderstanding between client and veterinarian or because of financial problems experienced by the client. Electronic medical records are legal and, just as with hard copy records, they must be maintained for a minimum of 4 years (3 years plus the current year).

Practice Management

Practice management, as used in this discussion, involves analyses of all areas of the practice of veterinary medicine with the ultimate goals of improving the efficiency of service, lowering the cost of that service, and improving the income generated by a clinical practice. Computerized systems for operation of clinical practices provide the ultimate tool for true practice management. A majority of the commercially available practice software packages have the ability to automatically analyze the practice and to provide daily, weekly, monthly, and yearly reports. Reports built into the various software packages vary greatly, but most provide analyses of expenses and income. Other analyses that are helpful to the owner or administrator of a veterinary hospital include analyses of time, services, and personnel. Analysis of the average time spent with each appointment should be the basis for scheduling appointments and the cost of an office visit. Analyses of time required for various medical and surgical procedures should also be the basis of charges assessed. Analysis of services provides the administrator with knowledge of income generated by each service of the practice and which service warrants additional personnel or which is overstaffed.

Practice management capabilities of many commercially available software packages include the ability to determine the revenue generated by each of the veterinarians in the practice. Unfortunately, analyses of other members of the veterinary team are not directly possible with most software. However, if one has an accurate analysis of the various services in a veterinary hospital, it is possible to make fairly reliable inferences as to the productivity of personnel in charge of, or associated with, a particular service.

Electronic Mail

Some veterinary practice software includes electronic mail (e-mail). This feature is considered useless in some veterinary practices and essential in others. As a general rule, the larger the practice, the more valued is e-mail. This is particularly true of practices in which personnel work in more than one shift per day or where two or more clinics are under the same administration. E-mail is an excellent means of communication in a practice provided everyone agrees or is required to use the feature.

E-mail has gained importance and popularity in recent times among veterinarians in private practice as a result of access to the Internet and commercial network services. Use of e-mail through the available networks enables veterinarians to communicate with colleagues, veterinary specialists, emergency clinics, diagnostic laboratories, university faculty, drug and pharmaceutical companies, and government regulatory agencies without having to "play telephone tag."

Word Processing

Although word processing is available as a stand-alone software program, most veterinary practice software packages integrate a word-processing program into the overall package. Such an arrangement allows the word-processing program to merge with patient records for the purposes of billing; sending appointment, immunization, dental, and heartworm test reminders; and sending newsletters and special announcements concerning the practice. In addition, word-processing packages are used to communicate with referring veterinarians, regulatory agencies, diagnostic laboratories, and many others.

Next to accounts receivable, the word processor is probably the most important part of the integrated veterinary practice software. The word-processing program is an important key to client communication which, in turn, is the key to a successful practice. One should be cautioned that the word-processing programs integrated into practice management programs are not always the most efficient available. If one is considering purchase of a practice management program with a less-than-ideal word-processing module, one should determine whether the word-processing program of his or her choice will mail-merge with the practice management program.

The word-processing portion of the veterinary practice software is one of the primary means of communication between the practice and the public that it serves. For this reason, when using the word processor to communicate, one must be careful to "put your best foot forward." Stated from another viewpoint, it is important not to portray the clinic or the profession in a negative way. An error in subject-verb agreement or syntax made in a telephone conversation with a client may be quickly forgotten, but a glaring error of tense or spelling in a document makes a lasting impression on most people. Any document, whether a fee statement or a newsletter, that is forwarded from a veterinary clinic should be and *look* professional. The document should be on professional statement forms or letterhead with an appropriate logo. Documents should be free of typographical, grammatical, and spelling errors and should be printed by a letter-quality printer, preferably of the laser variety, on quality bond paper.

Aside from merely being a mode of communication, the word-processing software can be one of the most effective practice-building tools. Consider the effectiveness of a well-timed letter of sympathy to a client who is grieving the loss of a loved pet. The letter need not be original but should be sincere and should reflect the caring nature of the veterinarian and his staff. It is not recommended that the same sympathy letter be sent to all clients or that an original letter be composed for the death of every animal that dies in a clinic. A happy medium is probably the best answer. In other words, one could have the basic letter stored in an electronic file. Comments concerning the specific animal can be added to the letter to make it appropriate for the specific client and pet.

Another practice builder that can be generated with the aid of the word-processing program is a newsletter. Newsletters are means of keeping clients in touch with the veterinary hospital and its staff. Newsletters should be professional in every respect and should provide clients with information that they can use (Fig. 35-1). If the newsletter is perceived as being an advertisement for the veterinary hospital, its effectiveness will be greatly reduced. Clients appreciate helpful topics on feeding and care of their animals, on diseases that occur with regularity in the area, and on changes in the services and procedures of the hospital. With the modern technology available today, word-processing programs should be used to develop the basic newsletter. The newsletter should then be formatted and "pol-

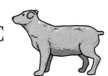

NEWS FROM
BRIARCREST VETERINARY CLINIC
12056 N. Lincoln Street
Baton Rouge, LA 70833

Dr. Robert L. Geaux
Dr. Scott R. Day

Dr. Suzanne Charles
Dr. Joyce A Brown

DR. BROWN JOINS BRIARCREST

Dr. Joyce A. Brown will join Briarcrest Veterinary Clinic as an Associate on January 1, 1998. Dr. Brown received her DVM degree from Texas A & M University in 1992. She was associated with a private practice in Dallas, TX for two years and recently completed a residency in companion animal surgery at the Animal Medical Center in New York, NY. Dr. Brown specialized in orthopedic surgery and has a particular interest in corrective spinal surgery.

As a student, Dr. Brown was active in various student organizations, particularly those involving rehabilitation of wildlife and use of pets in geriatric medicine. Since graduation, she has managed to find time to breed and obedience train Golden Retrievers.

Dr. Brown is married to Mr. Harold L. Brown, a registered pharmacist, and has one daughter, Jill. They will make their home at 10020 N. Meadowbrook Ave., Baton Rouge, LA. Welcome, Dr. Brown, to Briarcrest and Baton Rouge.

HURRICANE JUDY AND YOUR DOG

Hurricane Judy that struck the area on August 25, 1997 had very little direct effect on pets in the Baton Rouge area. However, as a result of the storm and the associated rains, the mosquito population in and around the city has increased greatly. This has increased the probability of heartworm transmission in dogs in the area. If you have not had your dog on heartworm preventive medication, it is recommended that you have the dog tested as soon as possible and that you maintain it on preventive medication. If you have any questions concerning the disease please call the clinic and ask one of the veterinarians.

Please be aware that the state practice act prohibits veterinarians from dispensing prescription drugs for animals without a veterinarian–patient relationship. This has been interpreted that veterinarians cannot dispense heartworm preventive before testing the dog for infestation and that prescriptions cannot be renewed unless the animal is tested annually.

NEW OFFICE HOURS FOR BRIARCREST

In order to better serve our working clients, Briarcrest Veterinary Clinics will be open on Tuesday evenings from 5:00 to 8:00 pm. The new office hours are in addition to the regular hours of the clinic which are 8:00 am to 5:00 pm on Monday through Friday and 8:00 am to 12:00 noon on Saturday.

Figure 35-1. The first page of a newsletter from a veterinary practice to its clients. The newsletter was produced on a modern word processing program and is short, attractive, and informative.

ished up" with desktop publishing software before it is published. The desktop publishing program enables one to incorporate graphics, such as the hospital logo, with columns of text to produce attractive newsletters. The desktop publishing software is not usually part of commercially available veterinary practice software.

TECHNICIAN NOTE

Newsletters should be professional in every respect and should provide useful information for clients. They should not be perceived as overly commercial.

On-Line Services

Network services available to veterinarians and veterinary technicians within the last few years are unprecedented and most exciting. Veterinarians and technicians have access to two networks devoted specifically to veterinary medicine. The network that first became available to veterinarians was the Veterinary Information Network (VIN), a privately owned network carried by America Online network. The most recent veterinary network, the Network of Animal Health (NOAH), was developed by the American Veterinary Medical Association (AVMA) using CompuServe as the carrier. Veterinarians usually access these networks via modems. Both network carriers have local access phone numbers in many cities in the United States and around the world. Access to the veterinary networks can also be achieved via the Internet. Services currently available through the veterinary networks include special interest bulletin boards or messaging services, e-mail; real-time chat capabilities, electronic medical literature retrieval systems, online consultation with specialists, special interest conferences, continuing education, and access to veterinary medical databases. Additional services that the veterinary networks are predicted to provide in the future include interactive continuing education programs with visual images and sound, efficient transmission of medical images (x-ray computed tomography [CT], ultrasound, and magnetic resonance imaging), electronic purchasing from veterinary biological and pharmaceutical companies, and diagnostic programs based on artificial intelligence.

Access to the Internet is becoming increasingly available to veterinarians and veterinary technicians in private practice. Subscribers to the two veterinary networks automatically have access to the Internet. Others obtain Internet access through private local Internet access providers. Interestingly, some of these providers enable veterinarians to access the two veterinary networks via the Internet at rates that are considerably cheaper than long-distance access. This is particularly beneficial to veterinarians who live in areas without CompuServe and America Online local access telephone numbers.

Many World Wide Web (www) sites are accessible through Internet service providers (ISP) and do not require connections to services such as America Online or CompuServe. The most popular Web site in veterinary medicine is Net Vet at http://www.netvet.wustl. The home page for the American Veterinary Medical Association can be reached at http://www.avma.org.

Access to the Internet by the practicing veterinarian and his or her staff is important today and will be increasingly important in the future because, in addition to providing access to information from throughout the world, it provides an electronic link to academic and regulatory veterinary medicine. Internet access provides practicing veterinarians with e-mail access to faculty specialists at veterinary schools throughout the world, to diagnostic laboratories, and to regulatory agencies such as the Food and Drug Administration (FDA), U.S. Department of Agriculture (USDA/Animal and Plant Health Inspection Service [APHIS]), the Drug Enforcement Administration (DEA), the Occupational Safety and Health Administration (OSHA), and state boards. It is predicted that practicing veterinarians and veterinary technicians will have electronic access to approved continuing education programs from veterinary schools and veterinary technician programs in the near future.

Miscellaneous Applications

Veterinary practice software contains many useful features not previously mentioned. These vary with the software packages and include but are not limited to: spreadsheets; database programs; and programs for herd health management, inventory management, tax computations, employee time clock, and vehicle logs. Veterinary practice software is usually not purchased for these programs, but they do constitute significant added value.

PROGRAMS TO COMPLEMENT PRACTICE MANAGEMENT SOFTWARE

Computers in veterinary practices are seldom used exclusively to execute practice management programs. Most persons who are familiar with computers are partial to certain software programs and could not function without them. It is unlikely that any practice management program will have all the features desired by all users. Fortunately, users with unique requirements can execute their favorite programs on the same computer that is used for the practice management program. This section is dedicated to discussion of some programs that can

be used to supplement or even enhance the practice software. The purpose of the section is to suggest useful programs and not to endorse any specific application or program. The reader should not consider this a complete listing of useful utility programs.

Among the most useful software programs are the general utility programs, which assist users in such tasks as recovery of deleted files, recovery of a "crashed" or erased hard disk, optimization of hard disk functions, and routine file management (such as copying, moving, erasing, renaming, and changing of attributes). Most of these programs provide for back-up of hard disk data, either in the regular or condensed modes. A convenient and reliable method of backing up data from the practice management program, whether provided in the program or as a stand-alone utility, is absolutely essential. Without a good daily back-up, a simple power failure or the inadvertent flip of a switch could cost the practice thousands of dollars and the loss of patient and client records.

Another important group of programs for users of practice management programs operating in the DOS platform is antivirus computer software. The software should include detection and destruction modules. The detection antivirus program should be installed to become resident in the random access memory (RAM) when the computer is booted up and should remain there as long as the computer is in operation. The detection module will automatically stop any application program in progress and alert the user when a virus is introduced into the memory. The destruction module will destroy the virus and usually restore files to their original form. Antivirus software is important, particularly if floppy disks are brought from home and other external sources.

If users are to access remote computers and networks, a communications package is needed in addition to a modem. The communications programs facilitate and, in most cases, automate the communication between computers. These programs facilitate communication between CPUs whether they are networked together or linked via telephone lines and modems. Some vendors require users of their practice management software to purchase modems and communication programs. This allows the vendors to service the software and to detect and correct problems remotely.

The professional and technical staff of veterinary hospitals are frequently called upon to make presentations to student groups, civic clubs, and professional organizations. Such presentations are best received when supplemented with quality visual aids, such as text and graphic photographic slides and overhead transparencies. These visual aids can be custom-designed at the clinic with the aid of graphics or presentation programs. If one purchases transparent sheets, attractive images for use on an overhead projector can be generated on any good laser printer. For production of photographic slides, one must usually transport the image either electronically or by disk to specialized photography laboratories.

One type of software program that is utilized by many veterinary practices is desktop publishing. This program is utilized in the preparation of newsletters, announcements, letterhead, attractive statements, and the like. All desktop programs permit importation of text from word-processing programs and graphic images from graphic programs and clip art libraries. With a little practice and imagination, one can prepare documents and brochures that are comparable to professionally designed publications.

TYPES OF COMPUTER CONFIGURATIONS IN A CLINICAL PRACTICE

In determining the type of computer configuration to employ in a veterinary hospital, it is important to first determine the uses for the computer, the flow of traffic within the hospital, and, finally, who will be entrusted to enter data into the system. When these questions have been answered, the software can be selected. Once the decision on the software is firm, it is possible to select and configure the computer hardware.

The most common configuration of computer hardware in veterinary hospitals is the single personal computer operating in the DOS or Windows operating system (Fig. 35–2A). Since this system has one station for data entry, this important task is often entrusted to one employee, usually the receptionist. The receptionist obtains information, usually in written form, from several areas of the hospital, such as the examination room, treatment room, pharmacy, surgery, laboratory, and kennel. This is an efficient arrangement with minimal chance of error. However, it still requires some written exchange before the data are entered into the computer.

Another configuration seen fairly frequently in veterinary practices, particularly those in which several veterinarians are employed, is the multitasking personal computer or workstation with terminals directly attached (Fig. 35–2B). In this system, terminals are located in each of the service areas, such as surgery, treatment rooms, and laboratory. Several persons enter data that feed into the main CPU. With this system, it is important that the staff understand who is responsible for data entry and that those persons are trained properly. The chances for errors with this type of system are greater than the single-tasking, single-user system, but proper training and supervision minimize errors in data entry.

TECHNICIAN NOTE

The most common configuration of computer hardware in veterinary hospitals is the single personal computer operating in DOS or Windows.

A third system, which is equivalent to the multitasking workstation with attached terminals, is that of several personal computers located in service areas that are linked on a network to a network server (Fig. 35–2C). In this system the personal computers are capable of serving as terminals to the network server or they can be used independently as stand-alone computers. The system is often constructed from existing personal computers. The advantages and disadvantages are essentially the same as for the system built around the multitasking personal computer.

A system that is occasionally used in large veterinary practices is a minicomputer to which terminals are attached either directly or via a network. The advantage of this type of network is that the CPU is faster and capable of accommodating more simultaneous users. The disadvantages are initial cost, cost of maintenance contracts, and the need for technical personnel to maintain the system.

FACTORS INVOLVED IN THE SUCCESS OR FAILURE OF THE COMPUTER SYSTEM

Of primary importance in the success of a computer system is the selection of the proper practice management software program. There are at least two dozen practice management software programs commercially available that are designed specifically for veterinarians. Some of these programs are marketed and intended to be used just as they are installed. Others are sold as modules, and veterinarians can purchase only the desired modules. Some vendors, on the other hand, will customize the program to suit a particular need. Before purchase, there should be a clear understanding between the purchaser and the vendor as to whether modifications to the program are permitted and the cost of such modifications.

Most veterinary software programs were designed to accomplish the same basic tasks, but they often do so in different fashions. In addition, the kinds and numbers of utility and special programs included in the packages differ greatly. Therefore, before selection of software, the type of veterinary practice and the long-term goals of the practice should be considered. After matching the software to the type of practice, a number

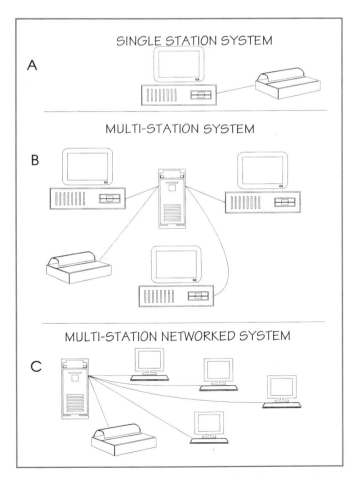

Figure 35–2. Three of the most common hardware configurations used in veterinary practices. A, The single-station system is usually operated by the receptionist. B and C, The multi-station systems allow data entry from several sources. Configuration C is more complex and is used when a practice is particularly large and/or has multiple locations.

of considerations need to be made before the final decision to purchase takes place. There must be a well-understood agreement between the vendor and the purchaser as to whether both hardware and software are provided, type and cost of hardware and software support (maintenance contracts), technical manuals and training provided, frequency and cost of software updates, cost of customized letterhead and labels provided by the vendor, and cost of customizing the software to the practice.

When purchasing software from a vendor, it is important to realize that the software was designed for average veterinarians in average practices. Therefore, it is safe to assume that it is unlikely that any of the available software will contain all of the features that one desires. This then leaves the purchaser with two alternatives: purchase the software and be satisfied with a program that has 85% to 90% of the features desired or purchase the software and pay to have it customized. With this in mind, it is important for the purchaser of practice software to review the programs thoroughly to avoid disappointment later when it is discovered that the software purchased does not have all the desired features.

One of the prime considerations in the selection of practice software is availability and quality of technical support for the software. It is extremely important that the contract to purchase a practice management software package include specifications as to the type and amount of training the vendor will provide for the hospital staff. The contract should also specify the amount of technical support the purchaser is entitled to, the cost per unit of time, and at what time of day the support is available. Response time by the vendor should also be specified. Software support, even for the most experienced users, is necessary because problems, such as file corruption, invariably occur. The time to negotiate these service needs is at the time of purchase, not when a problem develops.

TECHNICIAN NOTE

One of the prime considerations in the selection of practice software is the availability and quality of technical support.

Technical support for computer hardware is as important as that needed for the software. Whether the hardware is purchased separately or with the software as a total package, a service contract should be negotiated prior to the purchase. Response time of the vendor, minimum service fees, and initial warranties should be included in the contract. In addition, specifications for the vendor to provide comparable hardware on loan while nonfunctional instruments are being repaired is highly recommended.

Of all the factors involved in the success or failure of a computerized veterinary practice system, the personnel of the hospital are the most important. The owner of the practice may be a genius with a doctorate in computer science, but if the staff of the hospital are improperly trained or unmotivated, the computerized system is destined for failure. It does not really matter whether the owner, the receptionist, or the kennel help enter charges for an office visit; it is imperative that someone be charged with the responsibility and that he or she discharge

it. Income is lost daily because someone forgets to enter charges for services rendered or drugs dispensed.

In computerized practices, it is important that the management delegate the responsibilities for all aspects of the system. There should be no question as to who has the responsibility to enter charges from the various hospital services, who has authority to grant credit and discounts, who can initiate or delete a record, and, most important, who is responsible for back-up of the system. Once decisions have been made as to the duties of the hospital staff, it is the responsibility of management to provide training in operation of the system.

Computerization of an established practice is highly recommended but is not without a certain degree of trauma to all concerned. First of all, staff are asked to convert to a system that intimidates, if not terrifies, a fair percentage of the general population. Second, the staff are asked to learn a new system that is difficult for some to comprehend. Third, staff are usually asked to work twice as hard during the transition period because they are required to use both old and new systems simultaneously. They are asked to endure all of this on the good faith that their jobs will be made easier by the computer. The transition can be improved if there is some incentive for the hospital staff to take on this added burden.

It must be pointed out that the degree to which the hospital staff's jobs are made easier depends on the investment of the staff in learning the finer points of the software. It is safe to say that the more features of the program that are used, the easier the duties of the hospital staff become. There is truth in the old adage, "the duration of the assigned tasks usually fills the time allowed." Therefore, the greatest advantage of proper use of the practice computer system is the marked increase in efficiency.

A discussion of computer use in veterinary practice would be lacking without a brief discussion of do's and don'ts. The discussion will begin with the don'ts. When a veterinary practice is computerized, there is the risk, or at least it is the perception of some clients, that the business is being "dehumanized." Many people have experienced the frustration of trying to correct an error in billing from a large department store or credit card company. The person one usually speaks to seems to be a lifeless individual who is not ashamed to be subservient to "the computer." These individuals seem reluctant or incapable of making even the most trivial decisions on their own. Veterinary medicine must not become dehumanized. With this in mind, there are a few don'ts to be recommended.

Receptionists should greet clients with eye contact and a warm personal smile. Computer monitors should not be positioned so that they will interfere with the receptionist's view of the clients or vice versa. Receptionists should not hide behind the monitor. It is necessary to view the monitor when entering data on a client's record or when totaling a bill, but questions should not be asked of clients without providing periodic eye contact (Fig. 35–3). Finally, when a client points out an error on the record or the bill, do not blame the error on "the computer." In today's society, where most people have some degree of computer literacy, blaming human mistakes on a computer is no longer acceptable. Furthermore, it tends to aggravate most people.

Now for the do's of computer use in a veterinary practice. For reasons previously mentioned, it is recommended that the veterinary technician take the initiative in learning the practice management system. Given adequate time, this can be accomplished by merely reading the manual(s). However, training

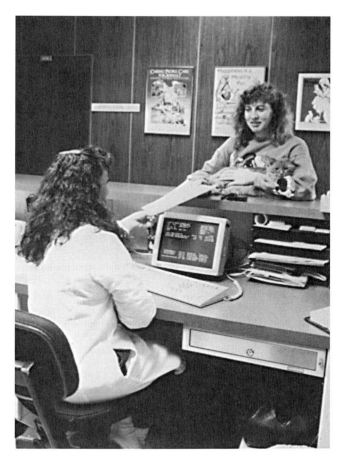

Figure 35–3. The proper placement of the computer and monitor in a reception area. Note that the view between the client and the receptionist is not impaired by the monitor.

provided by the vendor is usually the most cost-effective. Remember that the more one knows about the computer system, the more efficient it will make the user. It is equally important to take the time to learn aspects of the system that are assigned to fellow workers and to train someone else to handle your responsibilities (cross-training). This ensures continuity in the veterinary practice when someone leaves the practice, is sick, or is merely on vacation. Another do that is worthy of mention and emphasis is to maintain the security of the system and the confidentiality of patient records. This entails scrupulous care to maintain the confidentiality of passwords and to ensure that monitors are not positioned in such a manner that clients and other outsiders are able to read patient records. Patient-veterinarian confidentiality is regulated by state law and professional ethics.

BASIC COMPUTER USAGE

The purpose of this section is to acquaint the reader with the basic use of the computer operating system, the structure of hard and floppy disks, and a few of the commands that are essential for the beginning computer user. Since a majority of commercial veterinary practice management software programs were designed to operate in the DOS operating system, this discussion is limited to that system. More and more of the veterinary practice management programs have been adapted to the Windows environment. This graphical environment operates within the DOS operating system. An exception to this statement is Windows95 which serves as a complete operating system. The intuitive nature and simplicity of Windows make a discussion of this environment unnecessary.

When the electrical power of a computer is turned on, the computer boots up and becomes ready to operate. The DOS operating system becomes functional and, in most instances, the practice management software is automatically loaded into the RAM and the proper menus or icons appear. The installer of the software program has placed certain commands in the AUTOEXEC.BAT file, which cause the practice management software to be activated whenever the computer is turned on. This makes it easy for the uninformed user and even the most experienced user, since it saves several steps. But what if something happens to interrupt the software operation and the computer returns to the DOS prompt? What should be done? Two things can be done: the computer switch can be turned off and on again or one can reenter the practice management software using one or two simple commands. The purpose of this section is to acquaint the reader with the operating system and the structure of fixed and floppy disks so that he or she will not be lost when inadvertently switched back to the operating system and will feel comfortable in switching between computer applications.

If the installer of the practice management software program has not added the proper commands, the computer, when turned on, will progress through a series of self-tests and will stop with the DOS prompt (C>) displayed on the screen. To know how to progress from this point, the operator must know the structure of the hard disk (how the files are arranged) or must know how to inquire about the disk organization. The DOS commands to inquire about the disk, to change directories, and to switch from floppy to hard disks are easily remembered. However, it is important to understand the organization of disks before one can utilize these commands effectively.

In order to maintain some order to hard disks, and even floppy disks, files are stored in directories and subdirectories. The concept is simple to comprehend if one considers the directories as file cabinets and the subdirectories as file folders. Since everyone who uses file cabinets and file folders has his or her own "filing system," how is one to know exactly how the files are stored? There are two ways to determine the file arrangement. The first method is to type "DIR" at the prompt and press the "Enter" key. This command will cause the DOS operating system to provide a list of directories and files that are in the main or root directory. Files are listed by name, which consists of eight characters or less, a period, and then an extension consisting of up to three characters (such as config.sys).

Directories, on the other hand, consist of names (usually of software programs) followed by the notation, <DIR>. If one wants a list of only directories, type "DIR *." at the prompt. Another method of determining the directory structure of a hard disk is to type "TREE" at the DOS prompt. This command provides a diagram of the directories and subdirectories on a hard disk. However, the tree command is only available in Version 3.3 and later versions of DOS.

Once one has determined the structure of the hard disk, there is still the task of maneuvering from one directory to another. This can be accomplished with a few easy DOS commands. To return to the main or root directory, simply type

"CD" at the DOS prompt and press Enter. To switch to any of the directories from the root directory, type "CD" followed by the exact name of the directory (such as CD\WPWIN\MACROS). In the same manner, to access a subdirectory, simply type "CD" followed directly by the directory name\subdirectory name (such as CD\WPWIN\MACROS). To determine what files are contained in a directory, simply type "DIR" at the DOS prompt. If the list of files is longer than the screen display, simply type DIR/P to have the list of files presented one screen at a time. Another command that can be used in this situation is "DIR/W." In this case, the files are displayed in the wide format (five columns across the screen) without dates or file sizes.

Another function that should be known but used with extreme caution is the format command. Even if one has a hard disk on the computer, there is frequent need to store files on floppy disks. Reasons for storage of files on floppy disks include freeing up space on the hard disk and making back-up copies of important files to protect against loss should the hard disk crash. Before floppy disks can be used to store files, they must be formatted by the DOS operating system. This simple procedure is initiated by typing "format" followed by "A:" if the disk to be formatted is in the A: drive. The operating system automatically formats the diskette to be compatible with the disk drive. If one is using a high-density drive and wishes to format the disk for use in a double-density drive, simply type "format/F:* A:", where the * specifies the size of the diskette to be formatted (such as 360, 720, 1.2 or 1.44 Mb). Typing "format" without typing the letter of the floppy drive followed by a colon can result in the reformatting of the hard disk. This is a disaster because all data stored on the hard disk are lost.

TECHNICIAN NOTE

Warning: Typing ''FORMAT'' without typing the letter of the floppy drive followed by a colon can result in reformatting of the hard disk with loss of all programs and data files.

Most software programs come with well-written manuals. However, almost without exception, there is new and important information about the application program that is not included in the manual. This information, which is usually contained in text form in the "readme" file, is usually important to the user and should be read. The way to read this material is to either print it out in hard copy or to print it to the screen. To accomplish the former, simply type "copy read.me [or whatever is the exact name of the readme file] prn." To print the file to the screen, type "type read.me [or whatever the exact name of the readme file] more." If one forgets the "more," the entire file will scroll down the screen, and one will only be able to read the last page of the text.

There are several other DOS commands that would be useful to casual computer users. These include commands to make, rename, and delete files and directories. However, the purpose of this discussion is to give users of veterinary practice management software some minimal knowledge of the DOS operating system. For more in-depth reading on the operating system, the reader is referred to the DOS manual, which is usually provided when the computer and operating system are purchased.

IMPLICATIONS FOR THE FUTURE

There are computer software packages available to veterinary practices that offer many new and innovative features. However, these are only hints at what will be available in the near future. With the few exceptions where clinics within a practice are linked by a network, veterinary computer software programs are stand-alone packages. Some have modems that are used primarily by the vendor for technical support. The software of the future will emphasize communication external to the practice. Such communication will be rapid, have worldwide access, and will be transparent to the user (Fig. 35–4). The communication of the future will have graphic and voice capabilities and will offer many conveniences that are unheard of today.

Through the communication packages of the future, veterinary practices will be able to communicate with diagnostic laboratories, regulatory agencies, the AVMA, veterinary schools, consultants, colleagues, and drug and pharmaceutical vendors. In the future, veterinarians will receive reports from diagnostic laboratories via e-mail and will transmit images (x-ray, CT, ultrasound, and magnetic resonance imaging [MRI]) to specialists and will receive timely diagnoses via specialized networks. Practice computer systems of the future will enable veterinary practices to purchase drugs, pharmaceuticals, and supplies directly from the vendors with a few keystrokes and probably with significant discounts.

Veterinary practices of the future will have access to computer-assisted laboratory and clinical diagnostic programs, many of which will be based on artificial intelligence. This will enable veterinarians and veterinary technicians to be more accurate in their diagnoses and will reduce the amount of information that must be memorized. In addition, continuing education will become more accessible to veterinarians and the entire practice team. Individuals, within the confines and comfort of their offices or workstations, will have access to a wide variety of quality continuing education programs that are interactive and feature text, sight, and sound. The practice of veterinary medicine in the future will be made more exciting and productive through the use of computer technology.

PRACTICAL APPLICATIONS OF HOSPITAL COMPUTERIZATION

The 1991 issue of American Animal Hospital Associations (AAHA) magazine *Trends* estimates that from their survey of 35 commercial software vendors in 1988, there were 3300 users of veterinary practice management software. By 1989, the figure had risen to 5300 users, and by 1991, they estimated 9153 users. They also estimated that 80% of the small animal practices in 1991 had some computerization. The June 1995 *Trends* computer issue indicated there were 21 software vendors with over 12,000 installations. The June/July 1997 *Trends* computer issue listed 30 software vendors with more than 19,000 installations (Bohlender, 1997).

Nearly every aspect of veterinary medicine has been computerized—from rabies tag tracking to diagnostic programs. The veterinary hospital team (owner, professional staff, technologist, and receptionist) must determine what tasks are done in

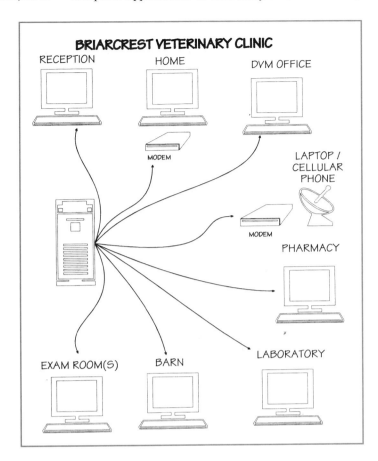

Figure 35-4. Potential input sources for a modern veterinary practice management system. Access to the system from the home allows the veterinarian to make management evaluations and decisions at his or her leisure. Access from the client's premises saves time and effort by permitting direct entry of population data.

practice and then decide which tasks they want done by a computer, which tasks are best done by people, and which tasks are best done by people with the assistance of a computer. Computers are good at storing and processing large volumes of data and doing repetitive tasks, but poor at decision-making and thought processes. People, on the other hand, are relatively inefficient at remembering large volumes of data or doing repetitive tasks, but are better at decision-making—especially with subjective or emotional issues. The computer has no morals; it is brutally cold when it comes time to sending bills regardless of the person's ability to pay, employment status, and so forth. Every practice is faced with certain moral or ethical decisions that the computer is incapable of making. Therefore, in spite of the great strides in computerization, the functions of the daily practice must be tempered with human judgment.

Practice management computer programs are developed and designed to manage information by storing data, assembling facts, and performing calculations. As a part of managing data, the computer provides an excellent means of communicating the information. The term "practice management" is something of a misnomer because the program does not manage the practice; the hospital team manages the practice. The computer system just collects and assembles information in a format that is useful to the various members of the hospital team. In human hospitals, practice management programs are called hospital information systems (HIS), which is a much more descriptive and accurate term.

Since no two practices are alike, the tasks in which the veterinarians, technicians, and receptionists are involved must be itemized and the advantages and disadvantages of computerizing discussed. Only after these items are resolved can the computer software be selected. The benefits may not be readily identified and may be somewhat intangible, and must be balanced against the cost of receiving those benefits. Some of the tasks that should be considered are shown in Table 35–1.

Demographic Data Collection

At the heart of any system, be it paper or computer, is demographic data collection (Fig. 35–5). In essence, there is no option—names and addresses must be collected. Having demographic data computerized has many advantages. Looking up names and addresses is much faster and easier than searching a paper record system. The data are accessible from any computer in the hospital, and even from home through a modem hook-up. One is not limited by the physical restraints of a paper record system. Paper records can be in only one place at a time, whereas electronic data are accessible to any staff member at any terminal or computer.

Traditionally, HIS programs have been developed around client and patient demographics and accounting functions. This has occurred because the demographics are easy to program, and numerous accounting software packages that are already developed are plugged into the system. Therefore, one of the prime uses for HIS has been tracking demographic information and accounting.

• Table 35–1 •

COMPUTER APPLICATIONS IN VETERINARY PRACTICE

Demographic data collection
  Name, address, phone number of the client
  Name, age, sex, species, breed, color of the animal
Scheduling time use
  Client appointments by doctor
  Boarding reservations
  Vacation scheduling
  Conference scheduling
Billing
  Accounts receivable
  Accounts payable
Mass mailings
  Monthly statements
  Newsletters and client information
  Reminders
    Vaccinations, fecal/dental examinations, heartworm tests
    Rechecks and follow-ups
Inventory management
  Drugs; controlled substances
  Supplies
Financial
  Cash drawer reconciliation
  Deposit slips automatically generated
  Payment records—cash, check, credit card receipts
  Payroll calculations
  Profit and loss reports
  Productivity reports—which areas are making or losing money
  Fee code entry to keep track of client's and patient's bill
    status
  Income analysis
  Practice profile and analysis
Medical records
  Patient's history
  Daily progress reports and treatment records
  Laboratory data storage and retrieval
  Surgical procedures
  Diagnostic codes—storage and retrieval
  Physical examination results
  Fee code entry to keep track of treatments done and
    prescriptions
  Certificates and forms:
    Vaccinations, rabies tag number tracking
    Spay/neuter
    Euthanasia
    Release forms—surgery
Communication
  Patient's medical and financial records available to all staff at
    any time
  Security—who can and cannot access certain data
Diagnostic aids
  Diagnostic programs
  Drug formulary
Remote modem communications
  Home to hospital
  Ranch or farm to hospital
  Satellite clinic to hospital
  Meeting or conference to hospital
  Cellular phone to hospital

Scheduling Time Use

Appointment scheduling can be beneficial, but its usefulness will be dictated, to a large degree, by the software vendor. The convenience of using the scheduling function will determine its use. If the receptionist has to work his or her way through several menus to get from one function to another, scheduling or any other function probably will not be used. The receptionist may opt to continue to use a pencil, eraser, and book. Assuming the software is convenient to use, scheduling can have some major advantages. The schedule is visible from any terminal in the hospital or from home or a remote site through a modem connection. The schedule will not only let everyone know what appointments are scheduled, but will tend to keep the whole staff on time (Fig. 35–6). Most of the larger programs will have appointment schedules by provider, so that each individual can have his or her own appointment schedule. Areas in which the scheduling should be considered are:

1. Routine appointments
2. Surgery
3. Boarding
4. Grooming
5. Vacations
6. Conferences
7. Dentistry
8. Geriatric work-ups
9. Radiology
10. Consultations (specialists, colleagues, vendors)

Billing

One of the most desirable features of a computer program is the ability to keep track of billing—not only accounts receivable but also accounts payable. Accounts receivable and payable are features that are at the heart of most software programs and are used as integral sections of all programs. With these data, profit and loss figures can easily be generated. The ability to automatically send statements at the end of each month is one of the major benefits of computerization.

Adding new charges to a patient's record does several things. First, the fee codes become part of the medical record of that patient and give a history of what was done to that patient and the date on which it was done. Second, in hospitalized or complicated cases, the fees entered give a running total of expenses incurred to date and allow estimates to be provided for clients. Third, if there are financial limitations on the treatment regimen, the fee totals keep everyone informed of the status. Finally, the time saved at the end of the month to send statements is greatly reduced. Most software packages let the practice define the dates of the billing cycle, and the computer does the rest.

On the other end of the billing spectrum are those bills for which payment is overdue. When charges are entered into the computer, an internal date timer is set. It keeps track of when charges were made and when payments were made. On a command, the computer will calculate which clients have owed money for specific periods of time. Clients who have an account balance of more than 30 days might be sent a nicely worded reminder. For those who have account balances of over 60 or even 90 days, the reminders might be more stern and pointed. If desired, the system can calculate and add service or interest charges for overdue accounts.

Mass Mailings

Mass mailings will provide service information to clients and generate additional client visits while saving time. Private practices rely heavily on return business to survive; therefore, re-

```
                        BRIARCREST VETERINARY CLINIC

        10/16/97      P A T I E N T   C H E C K - I N   R E P O R T      PAGE 1

                    NAME: KILLER                   IDENT: 2914864 DOG
                 SPECIES: CANINE              OWNED BY: ROBERT A. HOLMES
                   BREED: CHIHUAHUA                    4423 LAKE LARTO CIR.
                   COLOR: BROWN                        BATON ROUGE,  LA.
                BIRTHDAY: 9/22/88  SEX: M
                                                      70816
        RABIES TAG: 153                         TELE: (504)  291-4864
        ANI. NOTES:                          BALANCE:    193.77-
        CL1. NOTES: LINDA T.                    CURR:    193.77- 30DAY    .00
        CL2. NOTES: Linda and Bob               60DAY:      00 90DAY      .00
          REMINDERS  (DUE DATES)              WEIGHTS:
        ** 0/00/00 RABIES  ** 0/00/00 DAPLB  WEIGHTS: 9/22/88 - 7 LB  oz
        ** 0/00/00 DAPLC   ** 0/00/00 CORONA WEIGHTS:         - LB  oz
           9/22/98 HWTEST     9/22/98 FECAL   WEIGHTS:         - LB  oz
        ** 0/00/00 DM      ** 0/00/00 PARVO  WEIGHTS:         - LB  oz


               ** SERVICE/VACCINATIONS DUE IN NEXT 30 DAYS.
               ** SERVICE/VACCINATION PAST DUE.
        ACCESSION # 3993
        REASON FOR VISIT: YEARLY HEALTH MAINTENANCE


         DATE    INVOICE  DESCRIPTION                          PROVIDER


        09/22/97 0001142  ANAL SACCULECTOMY                       DD
                          NYS, NEO, THIO, TRIA, ON.15c            DD
                          DISTEMPER/MEASLES K9                    DD
                          EXAM, FECAL, FLOATATION                 DD
                          H.W.D., KNOTT'S                         DD
```

Figure 35–5. Example of a patient check-in report showing the type of information included. The client demographic data include owner's name; animal's weight, breed, and sex; immunization reminder data; current balance; and current invoice.

minders are a good method of encouraging periodic, routine health care. Traditionally, vaccination; dental, fecal, and heartworm examinations; and routine health examination reminders are used whether or not the practice is computerized. The ability to send client reminders has long been one of the most popular enticements for buying a computer system. Most software programs have a feature that allows linkage of a fee code entry with a trigger to automatically generate a reminder letter or postcard. For instance, when a rabies vaccine is charged to a patient, five steps are immediately done by the computer: (1)

```
                        BRIARCREST VETERINARY CLINIC
        ------------------------------------------------------------------
        10/16/97                PRINT APPOINTMENT FILE BY DATE      PAGE 1
        ------------------------------------------------------------------

        ITEM        #      DATE      TIME      MINS    CLIENT ID   CLIENT NAME        PROVIDER

                    7   10/14/97   08:00A      15      2914864    HOLMES, ROBERT A.      CM
          FOR: DOG                 PURPOSE:  YEARLY  HEALTH MAINTENANCE
                                   NOTE:

                    8   10/14/97   09:00A       1      2919999    HIDALGO, RICHARD J.    CM
          FOR: 2                   PURPOSE:  OVH SURGERY
                                   NOTE:

                    9   10/14/97   10:00A       1      MCCURNIN   MCCURNIN, DENNIS       CM
          FOR: SAM                 PURPOSE:  NEUTER
                                   NOTE:
```

Figure 35–6. Example of a list of appointments by date for one veterinarian in the practice. These lists are printed early in the morning and are helpful to veterinarians and staff in providing optimal service to clients and optimal time utilization.

The vaccination becomes part of the patient's medical record. (2) The inventory quantity of the vaccine is updated. (3) A rabies tag certificate is generated. (4) A reminder card is generated and printed at the proper time. (5) The fee is entered on the client's bill.

Internally, the computer keeps track of when a vaccination was given and then calculates when the next visit needs to be scheduled. This information, which is stored in the computer for automatic reminder generation, is also readily available for display on the computer screen if a client should inquire about a pet's vaccination status.

Other "reminders" can be developed and are usually lumped under a category of "word processing." Reminders or newsletters can be directed to certain types of clients if they are coded properly. For instance, if a new feline leukemia vaccine becomes available, this information can be sent to all feline-owning clients. General information, such as a new staff member, a change in operating hours, or other items of widespread interest can be easily disseminated to all clients or to specific types of client (e.g., all clients who own animals over 10 years of age).

Inventory Management: Drugs and Supplies

This is an application that will take serious consideration before implementing. Much information can be generated from inventory management, but a tremendous amount of time can be spent maintaining the inventory. Therefore, the cost versus benefit must really be evaluated thoroughly. Inventory items used on the patient must be entered into the system in order to generate charges for the client. This is the minimal level of activity needed for inventory management (Fig. 35–7). Quantitative inventory management could turn into an overwhelming job. The computer will subtract an item whenever it is dispensed or used, but a person must be in charge of entering quantities into the computer when shipments arrive. Entering quantities of received inventory items can be a job that is easily put off by piling the receiving reports on a desk and thinking that someone will get back to it later.

In a relatively small practice that does not keep a large inventory, implementing all of the features of inventory management may not be needed. Multisite practices or practices with a large inventory might need to implement all of the features. Just because a feature is in the system does not mean that it has to be used.

If inventory management is an area of concern, bar coding systems might be considered. Each drug or supply is given a bar code number that is linked to the individual drug information. The system then becomes similar to a grocery line checkout. When a drug is dispensed, the bar code wand is run over the bar code label and the quantity of drug is entered. As with the rest of the inventory program, there is a cost-versus-benefit ratio. The bar code system may save some time when dispensing, but someone at an earlier time had to generate the bar code labels and place them on the drugs.

Financial

Cash drawer verification, automatic deposit slips, and payment method itemization are features that are usually most helpful to the reception and accounting staff. During the daily transactions, the computer keeps a record of what charges were paid and by what method—cash (amount tendered and change given), check, or credit card. At the end of the day or at the beginning of the next day, reports and deposit slips are automatically generated so that the day's transactions can be reconciled.

Practice profile and income analysis have often been touted as one of the main reasons to purchase a computer system. These types of reports are generated daily, monthly, yearly, or for any period desired. They are usually tied to the daily fee entries (Fig. 35–8) and give an overall analysis of the activities of a practice. As professional marketing becomes more sophisticated, more data are needed to make management decisions. Can the practice justify additional staff? Will the volume of a certain laboratory procedure justify buying an instrument for that procedure? Are the fees for radiographs at a level to support all costs of the film? Where do clients live? Who has referred clients to the practice? Can the practice afford a salary increase for all staff?

Usually, when statements are done, month-to-date and year-to-date statistics are generated. Which doctor did which procedures? How many of each type of procedure were done? How much income was collected? These data can provide valuable information when making management decisions. If the inventory management portion of the program is maintained, a list of vendors with accounts payable will be generated.

When all charges for a patient are entered into the computer system, monthly billing becomes a relatively painless chore. The ability of various staff members to access a client's bill status can be an important part of the program. One of the main things that both the client and the hospital have in common is the status of charges for a patient. It is easy to let charges get out of hand, especially on a hospitalized case. It is in the best interest of both parties that an accurate record of charges be kept.

Medical Records

The ability to enter medical histories and treatments for a patient is a feature that has evolved with cheaper and more powerful computers. Entering medical data on a patient can be one of the most useful tools in a computer system. Again, most of the larger software companies have a part of the program where data such as the problem list for the patient, the current and past histories, vital signs data, laboratory data, daily progress reports, and diagnosis codes can be entered. Instead of entering all this information on paper, which is useful only to the person who possesses the medical record, the information in the computer is accessible to anyone at a terminal.

One of the features in most larger programs is the ability to attach a status code to hospitalized patients or to patients who are admitted for the day. A set of codes can be devised to aid communication between the veterinarian, technician, and receptionist. Instead of questioning the veterinarian or technician when a client calls with an inquiry, the receptionist can enter the code for that patient and get the answer. For instance, if a patient is ready to go home, the receptionist could access that patient's record and get that information without interrupting the veterinarian or technician. Another response to the code might be that the veterinarian or technician needs to talk to the client about the patient.

Many programs have the ability to create customized data entry templates to enter medical records information. For in-

```
                        BRIARCREST VETERINARY CLINIC
------------------------------------------------------------------------
10/16/97         INVENTORY FILE SHORT LIST SORTED BY  -  DESCRIPTION         PAGE 1
------------------------------------------------------------------------
DRUG NUMBER          DESCRIPTION              VENDOR     UNIT COST  QTY  QOH     PRICE

AMIGLYDE             AMIKACIN 250MG/ML        FORT DODGE    1.8229       0.00     3.65
CLAVAMOX 250MG       AMOX 200/ CLAV 50                       .2149    -282.00      .43
CLAVAMOX 375MG       AMOX 300/CLAV   75                      .3226       0.00      .65
CLAVAMOX 125MG       AMOX 100/ CLAV 25                       .1094       0.00      .22
CLAVAMOX  62 . 5     AMOXI  50/ CLAV 12.5                    .0565     165.00      .11
CLAVAMOX SUSP        AMOXI CLAV SUSP 62.5MG/M               1.4800       0.00     2.96
AMOXITABS 100        AMOXICILLIN 100 MG TABS                 .0409     -80.00      .08
AMOXITABS 200        AMOXICILLIN 200 MG TABS                 .0635     -24.00      .13
AMOX SUSP 250        AMOXICILLIN 250MG/5CC                  2.2000      -1.00     4.40
AMOXITABS 400        AMOXICILLIN 400  MG.                    .1070    -349.00      .21
AMOXITABS 50         AMOXICILLIN 50MG TABS                   .0255     -11.00      .05
AMOXIDROPS           AMOXICILLIN 50MG/ML15CC                 .7000     -13.00     1.40
FUNGIZONE            AMPHOTERICIN  B          SQUIBB       23.9000       0.00    47.80
AMPICILLIN 125       AMPICILLIN 125MG/5CC                   1.6500       0.00     3.30
AMPICILLIN 250       AMPICILLIN 250 MG.                      .0495       0.00      .10
POLYFLEX             AMPICILLIN 25GM.         FORT DODGE   24.7500       0.00    49.50
AMPICILLIN 500       AMPICILLIN 500 MG.                      .0985       0.00      .20
SOD AMP 1GM          AMPICILLIN SODIUM 1 GM                  .4300       0.00      .86
AMP EQUINE           AMPICILLIN SODIUM 3 GM   SK BEECH      2.7300       1.00     5.46
SOD AMP 500MG        AMPICILLIN SODIIUM 500 MG               .5200       0.00     1.04
BACITRACIN           BACITRACIN USP 50 MU     UPJOHN        2.9100       0.00     5.82
GEOCLLIN             CARBENCILLIN 382 MG                    1.3971       0.00     2.79
CEFA - DRI           CEFA - DRI                              .9600       0.00     1.92
CEFA - LAK           CEFA - LAK                              .9400       0.00     1.88
CEFA - TABS 1GM      CEFADROXIL 1 GM.                       1.2330       0.00     2.47
CEFA - TABS 200GM    CEFADROXIL 200 MG                       .2270       0.00      .45
CEFA - TABS 100 GM   CEFADROXIL TABS 100MG                   .1238       0.00      .25
CEFA - TABS  50GM    CEFADROXIL TABS 50MG                    .0737       0.00      .15
CEFA ZOLIN 10GM      CEFAZOLIN 10GM                        20.2800       0.00    40.56
CEFA ZOLIN  1GM      CEFAZOLIN SODIUM 1 GM                  1.9500       0.00     3.90
CLAFORAN 1GM         CEFATAXIME 1GM                        11.0900       0.00    22.18
FORTAZ 1GM           CEFTAZIDIME 1GM          FORTAZ       22.1600       0.00    44.32
FORTAZ 500MG         CEFTAZIDIME 500 MG                     5.5400       0.00    11.08
NAXCEL 4GM           CEFTIOFUR SOD 4 GM       UPJOHN       23.3200       0.00    46.64
NAXCEL 1GM           CEFTIOFUR SODIUM 1 GM    UPJOHN        6.6200       0.00    13.24
CEPHALEXIN 250       CEPHALEXIN 250 MG.                      .1400       0.00      .28
CEPHALEXIN SUS       CEPHALEXIN 250 MG/ML SUSP              5.4400      -3.00    10.88
CEPHALEXIN 500       CEPHALEXIN 500 MG                       .2800       0.00      .56
CHPC   500MG         CHLORAMPHENICOL 500 MG                  .0337       0.00      .07
CHPC   1GM  INJ      CHLORAPHEN SOD SUC 1GM                 1.7500       0.00     3.50
CHPC   250MG         CHLORAMPHENICOL 250 MG.                 .0337       0.00      .07
CHPC   PAL SUSP      CHLORAMPHENICOL 30MG/ML                .2118       0.00      .42
CIPRO 250MG          CIPROFLOXACIN 250 MG.                  1.9962       0.00     3.99
CIPRO 500MG          CIPROFLOXACIN 500MG                    2.1594       0.00     4.32
ANTIROBE SOLN        CLINDAMYCIN 25MG/ML SOL               2.1100       0.00     4.22
ANTIROBE 150MG       CLINDAMYCIN 150MG CAPS                  .3938       0.00      .79
ANTIROBE 25MG        CLINDAMYCIN CAPS 25                     .0653       0.00      .13
ANTIROBE 75MG        CLINDAMYCIN CAPS 75MG.                  .2100       0.00      .42
```

Figure 35-7. Example of a pharmacy inventory list sorted alphabetically by the common name of the drug. The list contains vendor, unit cost, selling price, and quantity on hand for each drug.

stance, a form could be developed that would allow the CBC (complete blood count) results to be recorded, and the program would guide one through the form, item by item, for data input. A template could be developed to record vital signs and enter physical examination data. These data then become part of an individual animal's history. Customized patient forms are an area where the staff must make some real decisions on how much, if any, patient data they want on the computer. Gener-

ally, this feature is a plus because it gives everyone easy access to those data. The legality of computerized medical records versus paper records has always been in question. In general, if adequate back-ups of the hard disk are made and there is a reasonable amount of security in the system, electronic medical records have had equal legal status with paper records. Since laws might vary among states, it would be wise to obtain a legal opinion before starting.

BRIARCREST VETERINARY CLINIC

CLINICIAN _____

HOSPITALIZATION

H7AVLG	HOSPITAL BIRD	8.00
H2HOSC	HOSPITAL CAT	12.00
H9CARN	HOSPITAL - DOG	15.00
H9FER	HOSPITAL FERRET	8.00
H9ICU	HOSPITAL ICU	50.00
H1HOIS	HOSPITAL ISOLATION	18.00
H9PRIM	HOSPITAL PRIMATE	18.00
H9RL	HOSPITAL RABBIT	8.00
H8REP	HOSPITAL REPTILE	8.00
H9ROD	HOSPITAL RODENT	8.00
H9HOO2	OXYGEN CAGE, DAY	20.00
H9PC	PET CARRIER	8.00
H9SD	SPECIAL DIET	0.00
HOTHR		0.00

PLACE CAGE LABEL HERE

EXAMINATIONS

PS9AH	EXAM AFTER HOURS EMERGENCY	60.00
PS9EXI	EXAM, OFFICE VISIT(INITIAL/NEW PROB	25.00
PS9REV	EXAM, REVISIT	18.00
RE9HSA	HEALTH CERTIFICATE	15.00

DIAGNOSTIC PROCEDURES

PS9CAL	CALCULI ANALYSIS, UCD -(M O RX ROO	37.00
PS9CSF	CSF TAP PROC ONLY	20.00
E9ECG	ECG	25.00
PS9BR	ENDOSCOPY	50.00
PS9NW	NASAL WASH	20.00
CP9PPP	PCV / PLASMA PROTEINS	8.00
PS9SS	SCRAPING SKIN	10.00
TH9SAI	SEMEN COLLECTION-AI	30.00
PS9EGS	SWAB EAR GRAM STAIN	8.00
PS9EM	SWAB EAR MITES	8.00
TH9VC	SWAB, VAGINAL CYTOLOGY	8.00
PS9TTW	TRANSTRACHEAL WASH	30.00
PS9ODC	OTHER DIAGNOSTIC CHRG	0.00

VACCINATIONS

RE9LRI	CITY LICENSE, RABIES	6.00
IM1C	CORONAVIRUS	15.00
IM1DM	D-M	25.00
IM1D2B	DA2PL BOOSTER	30.00
IM1DCV	DA2PL-CPV-CV	30.00
IM2FLV	FELV	25.00
IM2FVC	FVR-CP-CHLAMYDIA	25.00
IM2PB	PANLEUK, BOOSTER	25.00
IM1PB	PARVO BOOSTER	15.00
IM9RAB	RABIES	15.00

THERAPEUTIC PROCEDURES

T9ABS	ABSCESS: INCISE/DRAIN	25.00
T9AS	ANAL SAC IRRIGATION/	15.00
T9BP	BANDAGE	0.00
T9BAT	BATH	12.00
PS9BD	BATH/DIP	15.00
T3CA	CAST-APPLICATION	25.00
T9IVC	CATHETER, IV	7.50
OP1CL	CATHETER LACRIMAL DUCT	5.00
T9CUF	CATHETER,URINARY	5.00
T9DW	CLEAN & DEBRIDE WOUND	30.00
T9CPT	CLIP	10.00
SO9LHC	CLOSED REDUCT HIP	50.00
DN9CL	DENTISTRY CLEAN ONLY	30.00
DN9EXT	DENT., TOOTH EXTRACTION	10.00
PS9DIP	DIP ONLY	10.00
TH9DYS	DYSTOCIA MANIPULATION	30.00
T9ENEM	ENEMA	15.00
T9GLF	GASTRIC LAVAGE	15.00
T1HTP	HEARTWORM TREATMENT	200.00
T9HYD	HYDROTHERAPY	15.00
T9EL	LAVAGE, EAR	10.00
T9NT	NAIL TRIM	10.00
T9NOA	NASAL OXYGEN ADM. (SUPPLIES ONLY)	10.00
T1TBCA	TRANSFUSE, BLOOD, CAN	50.00
T2TBFE	TRANSFUSE, BLOOD, FEL	40.00

T2TBFE	TRANSFUSE, BLOOD, FEL	40.00
T1RBCC	TRANSFUSE, PACKED RBC CA	40.00
T2RBCF	TRANSFUSE, PACKED RBC FE	25.00
T1TPPL	TRANSFUSE, PLASMA CANINE	40.00
T9TPFR	TRANSFUSE, PLASMA, FELINE	40.00
T9TRC	TREATMENT ROOM SUPPLIES	0.00
T1URO	UROLITHIASIS, DOG	20.00
T2URO	UROLITHIASIS, TOMCAT	20.00

ANESTHESIA

A1BHI	CAN BARB / HALO (1ST 0.5 HR):	50.00
A1VKH1	CAN VALIUM/ KET./HALO(1ST 0.5 HR):	40.00
A2H1	FEL/FERRET HALO (1ST 0.5 HR):	50.00
A1HADD	CAN & FEL HALO(ADDITIONAL 0.5 HR)	40.00
A1NR	NARCOTIC REVERSAL AGENT (1 ML)	15.00

OTHER IV ANESTHETIC PROTOCOLS:

A1OWO	IV. ANESTHESIA W/O CATHETER	30.00
A1OW	IV ANESTHESIA W/ CATHETER	45.00
A1PO5	POST-OPERATIVE SEDATION	25.00
A1POO	POST-OPERATIVE OXYMORPHONE (1 ML	15.00
A1LOC	LOCAL/EPIDURAL ANESTHESIA	35.00

EUTHANASIA

PS9EUT	EUTHANASIA SA (INCLUDES DRUGS)	15.00

ORTHOPEDIC SURGERY

SS3CVO	AMPUTATION, LEG	500.00
SS3GPD	AMPUTATION, TOE(S)	200.00
SS3CTH	ARTHRODESIS	500.00
SS3IEH	BIOPSY BONE	350.00
SS3NEC	CRUCIATE	600.00
SS3OVP	DEWCLAW, MATURE, PER FOOT	35.00
SS3PL2	FEM HEAD OSTECTOMY	200.00
SS3PA	FRAGMENTED CORONOID	400.00
SS3REC	IM PIN CLOSED	150.00
CP9RK	IM PIN, OPEN	0.00
SS3SPE	INTERTROCHANT OSTEOT	500.00
SS4C2	LIGAMENT REPAIR	200.00
SS3UE	LUX ELBOW, OPEN	150.00
SS3VEN	LUX HIP, OPEN RED	250.00
SS3UH	LUXATION HIP,CLOSED REDUCTION	100.00
SS4CB	LUX HOCK, OPEN REDUCTION	250.00
SS4C1	LUXATION PATELLAR	500.00
SS4CAE	LUXATION SHOULDER, OPEN	300.00
SS4CAS	LUXATION STIFLE	400.00
SS4CT1	MANDIBULAR SYMPH FX	150.00
SS4COM	MENISCECTOMY	150.00
SS4D2H	NONUNION-PLT & GRFT	500.00
SS4DH1	OSTEOCHONDROSIS	400.00
SS4EP	OSTEOTOMY, CORRECT	400.00
SS4EN2	OSTEOTOMY, PELVIC	500.00
SS4IRS	PECTINOTOMY	150.00
SS4LNB	PLATE FIXATION	400.00
SS9OFA	REMOVE ORTHOPEDIC DEVICE,COMPLE	150.00
SS9OFJ	REMOVE ORTHOPEDIC DEVICE,SIMPLE	75.00
SS4OV1	SCREW FIXATION	150.00
SS4PI3	TENDON REPAIR	200.00

Figure 35-8. The front page of a typical fee sheet used in conjunction with a computerized veterinary practice management system. Fee sheets are used by veterinarians and other hospital personnel to communicate with the person or persons responsible for entering charges in the computer. The charges for supplies, drugs, and services are made by entering the short codes.

Communication

A networked hospital computer system encourages the communicating and sharing of hospital information (Fig. 35–9). With the traditional paper system, information is in the hands of the beholder. Essentially, only one person at a time has access to the records. A networked computer system makes information available to those at any computer on the network, either locally or remotely, and to those with proper security clearance.

The veterinarian can enter treatment instructions at one terminal and a technician may read those instructions at another terminal. The receptionist may be at a terminal and look up a patient's discharge status in the computer so that the client can be informed. Patient check-in reports generated when a patient arrives provide a printed history for the patient. The veterinarian, technician, or receptionist can quickly glance at the complete medical history to determine patient needs.

The ability to use the computer system to communicate between staff members will evolve. As members of the team become comfortable with the basic program, they will start to explore new ways to use the system. Most programs allow a great deal of flexibility in the way communications can be approached. Individual electronic mailboxes and message centers can be developed for each staff member.

Diagnostic Aids

Some of the major software companies now are selling diagnostic programs as an option. In most of the programs, a species is selected, signs are entered, and a list of diagnostic possibilities, ranked from the most likely to the least likely, is produced. From that list, a diagnosis may be chosen, or possible diagnoses on the list may jog the doctor's memory and prompt other diagnostic tests. Actually, the programs do not really provide a diagnosis; they just provide a list of possibilities. Many of these programs have been called "memory joggers." True "diagnostic" programs that are highly accurate have yet to be developed. This also is true in human medicine, where there has been a great deal of effort expended. Diagnostic programs undoubtedly will be refined with increased knowledge of medicine and with advanced programming techniques. Are diagnostic programs worth the money? This will be answered only by a complete demonstration of the particular program. Other diagnostic tools, such as electrocardiogram and echocardiogram analyzers, are available as stand-alone machines, but they usually are not integrated into hospital software packages.

Remote Communications

Remote communication is an area that is too often overlooked, possibly because it seems too difficult. High-speed modems, advanced telephone systems, and cellular telephone systems allow broad communication that the hospital team should consider. Remote systems could be used for a multihospital system, communication between the practice and home, remote communication between farm or ranch and the hospital, communication from a meeting to the hospital, or even cellular phone communication to the hospital. All that is required are modems on the sending and receiving ends and the appropriate communication software. This is where good support from the software vendor can be a real asset. What may seem technically beyond the hospital staff should be relatively easy for the software company.

Communication between staff members can be greatly enhanced with remote communication. For instance, the veterinarian could dial in to the hospital computer and receive progress reports on a case. The veterinarian also could leave instructions for certain staff members. Veterinarians occasionally receive phone calls at night from a person who has found a lost dog with their hospital's rabies tag. With remote communication, the veterinarian can dial into the hospital system, look up the rabies tag number, and contact the owner about the lost pet. In the BC (before communication) period, one would have had to make a trip to the hospital to look up rabies tag information.

The Process of Software Evaluation

In the evaluation of a veterinary hospital computer system, not only the veterinarian but also the technician and receptionist should have significant input into the selection process. Computerization is an area where all members of the team must be happy for the system to succeed. This is not a process, for instance, whereby a surgical instrument is evaluated only by the veterinarian because he or she will be the only one using that instrument. In fact, one of the main objectives of installing

Figure 35-9. Example of a printout of a list of hospitalized patients showing client name and identification number, veterinarian in charge of the case, and unpaid balance of the account.

```
                    BRIARCREST VETERINARY CLINIC
-------------------------------------------------------------------------
10/16/97      INVENTORY FILE SHORT LIST SORTED BY - DESCRIPTION    PAGE 1
-------------------------------------------------------------------------
PATIENT      OWNED BY            CLIENT-ID   --DATE--   CASE#   PROV   STATUS

11111111   FLINTSTONE, FRED      FLINT       10/02/97   1144    DD      H
2          HIDALGO, RICHARD J.   2919999     10/16/97   1146    CM      O
33933      HOLMES, ROBERT A.     2914864     10/16/97   1145    CM      H
SAM        MCCURNIN, DENNIS      MCCURNIN    10/16/97   1147    CM      P


***  HOSPITAL FILE CLIENTS - CURRENT BALANCE: $45.39 -
***  HOSPITAL FILE CLIENTS - 30 DAYS BALANCE:  $.00
***  HOSPITAL FILE CLIENTS - 60 DAYS BALANCE:  $.00
***  HOSPITAL FILE CLIENTS - 90 DAYS BALANCE:  $.00


***  HOSPITAL FILE CLIENTS  -  TOTAL BALANCE: $45.39 -
```

a computer system should be to make communication better for everyone—this is not just a tool for the veterinarian.

The first task in deciding to computerize is for the veterinarian, the head technician, and the receptionist to sit down and decide what they want the computer to do for them. Initially, do not even consider what computer to use; consider only the tasks to be done. The next step is to contact several software vendors for a demonstration or to visit exhibits at one of the national or state meetings (such as AVMA, AAHA, Western Veterinary Conference, and so forth). During the demonstration, you will probably be overwhelmed by all of the things these computer systems will do. This is what the vendor wants. One needs a list of requirements prepared to help focus and direct the demonstration. Most of the full-featured programs that have been around for a long time all do pretty much the same things. The things to look for are how they get the jobs done, how easy they are to use, and the staff support and training.

TECHNICIAN NOTE

The first task in deciding to computerize is for the veterinarian, head technician, and receptionist to decide what tasks they want the computer to do.

How does one decide which software vendors to evaluate? Periodically, different veterinary publications will publish a list of current practice management software. Both AAHA's *Trends* and *Veterinary Forum* publications list at least 30 vendors. These articles generally provide a brief synopsis of the state of veterinary practice management computing and then publish a list of vendors and the main features of their programs. These are excellent articles as they usually provide information such as the length of time the company has been in business, number of employees, number of installations, hardware and software platforms, prices, and main features.

There are several items that need to be considered when choosing a software vendor. How long has the company been in business and how many programs have they sold and are in operation? "In the beginning . . ." of the veterinary computer revolution (1970s), some of the hospital systems were programmed by individual practitioners who had an interest in computers and programming. The practitioner used the program in his own practice, and if someone else liked it, the program would be disseminated. Some of them developed into larger systems if there was enough financial backing, but for the most part they were unsuccessful. The competition in the software market is fierce, and the computer cemetery is filled with hundreds of programs and companies. Programs need to be purchased from survivors; they probably have a reliable product and service. Therefore, look for longevity and number of installations.

A vital element to look for is support for both hardware and software. This is a feature that is not given enough attention but is of extreme importance. Most companies concern themselves primarily with software and provide the hardware as a service to the customer. What kind of software support do they provide and during what hours of the day do they provide it? The vendor should know its program inside out; there are often

features or shortcuts that are not documented in the instructions. Even those of us who think we know what we are doing with computers have to rely heavily on software support because the systems are proprietary. Without easily reached, competent support, the system will *never* survive. A monthly support fee will usually provide telephone support and upgrades when new programs are developed. The number of upgrades and the regularity with which upgrades are issued is another indicator of the stability of the program and the company. A progressive company will consistently be improving its product.

Probably the last feature to evaluate is hardware. There is an idiom in the computer world that states that one should always select the software first; there will always be a computer to make it run. Networking and multiuser, multitasking computers have changed greatly since the early 1970s. Computer hardware has become so inexpensive and powerful that it is much less a concern than before. The prices of powerful computers have come down drastically in the last few years and there are wide selections of computers and operating systems that actually work!

Most vendors offer a package system of software and hardware, and in general, it is worth buying the package. Most practice personnel do not have enough knowledge or time to buy and install their own computers and networks. Prices at the local computer store may look slightly better than those of the software vendor, but the local person is probably not knowledgeable about the particular practice management software package to be of real support. The software vendor has tried and developed the software on a particular type of computer on which he or she knows it will work. The vendor probably will not provide hardware support, and possibly not even software support, if you do not comply with their hardware specifications.

The larger software companies usually provide an on-site demonstration by a trained representative; this is highly desirable. This is the time to get a good overview of the software. It also is the time to ask questions. "Can the computer do . . . ?" "How does the computer do . . . ?" It is a good time to let the staff use the system and see how easily it will do the everyday functions. Smaller companies may not have the resources to send a representative but will allow on-site evaluation of the system for some period of time. Evaluation of systems at meetings is an alternative, but usually things are too hectic to be able to really sit down and do a good evaluation.

It is during the demonstration or the evaluation period that a decision should be made regarding what portions of the program are needed. Most programs are built-in modules that can be added to the basic system. A small animal boarding and grooming package would be of no use to an equine practice. An equine trainer list would be of no use to a small animal practice. This is a good way to hold down prices by buying just what the practice can use.

The Decision to Buy—What Happens Next?

After the decision to buy is made, what happens next? Depending on the agreement with the vendor, your delivered computer system will be set up either by you or by the vendor. If a single-user computer system has been purchased and the software is already loaded into the computer, setup will be minimal. It is usually worth the extra expense to have the vendor set up a networked system. Network operating systems are complex and require trained personnel for installation and management. Extensive network maintenance is far beyond the capabilities of most practices.

After installation is complete, the next step is training on the actual system. Most of the large vendors provide on-site training for some period of time, usually 2 to 5 days. During the training period, a reduced appointment schedule is recommended as it becomes too hectic to handle a normal business load and learn the computer system. This is the time when all staff members need to be deeply involved in the new system.

No matter how easy the program is to use and no matter how intelligent the staff, the initial stages of computerization are traumatic. It is amazing, though, how soon things return to "normal." Most programs are well organized and intuitive so that everyday functions become second nature in a matter of days.

A major area of trauma will be working with two systems for a period of time, using both the computer system and the old paper record system. If the practice is new and client records are not extensive, it is better to completely switch to the new computer system and not to use the old paper system. Transferring data from the old paper system to the computer system is extremely time-consuming and labor-intensive.

Glossary

ASCII—American Standard Code for Information Interchange. A standard format for representing characters. This format is used in text files and is useful when files are shared between programs.

AUTOEXEC.BAT file—A file containing disk operating system (DOS) commands written in ASCII text form, which is automatically executed when the computer is turned on or booted.

Batch file—An executable file with DOS commands written in ASCII text, which is used for automating frequently used commands.

BIOS—Basic input/output system. This is part of the read-only memory (ROM) of the central processing unit (CPU), which is installed in the form of a chip and which controls how the CPU interacts with the screen, keyboard, printer, and other peripheral devices.

Bit—Unit of data in binary form; the smallest storage unit for data in a computer.

Byte—A fixed number of bits that represents a character. The most common byte size is eight bits.

CD-ROM—Compact disk read-only memory. A data storage system based on conversion of data from digital to analog and storage of the analog data on optical disks.

CPU—Central processing unit. That part of a computer or computer system responsible for the actual computations.

CRT—Cathode ray tube. This is the electronic tube making up the visual display of the terminal or the computer.

Database—A collection of interrelated data stored together with a minimum of redundancy to serve multiple applications.

DOS—Disk operating system. This is software that controls movement of information in a computer and allows the CPU to use peripheral devices, such as printers, diskette drives, and fixed disk drives.

Driver—A set of commands that are used to run a peripheral device, such as a printer.

EGA—Enhanced graphics adapter. This acronym refers to the ability of a computer to display graphic images in color.

E-mail—Electronic mail. An electronic method of communication between network users.

Extended memory—The random access memory (RAM) of a computer in excess of 1 megabyte.

Expanded memory—The RAM of a computer in excess of 640 kilobytes and less than 1 megabyte.

Facsimile—A device for transmission of graphic files from one location to another. The graphic image is converted to digital signals by the sending device, and the receiving device converts the digital signals to a graphic image. Facsimile machines act as remote copying machines.

File—A collection of one or more records.

Fixed disk—A high-volume magnetic storage device that is usually built into the computer.

Floppy disk—Small, portable, magnetic storage devices for storage of computer programs and data.

Font—A specific typeface, including its point size and weight.

FTP—File transfer protocol. A protocol for remote transfer files from one CPU to another.

Gopher—A program that facilitates access and retrieval of textual (ASCII) information on servers connected to the Internet. Gopher is also referred to as a text browser.

Graphics display—A CRT or monitor that is capable of displaying graphical images.

Hardware—A digital or analog device that is capable of detecting, transmitting, or processing electronic signals.

Home page—A specific hypertext markup language (HTML) program which provides text and graphical information which is retrievable from a World Wide Web server.

HTML—Hypertext markup language. A system for marking up documents which instructs browsers on how to present the document and enables documents (even remote) to be linked by specific tags.

Internet—A worldwide electronic network of interconnected computers operating in Transmission Control Protocol/Internet Protocol (TCP/ICP).

LAN—Local area network. An electronic network permitting communication between the CPUs or CPUs and peripheral devices, such as terminals, printers, and plotters.

Language—A computer language is a particular format in which programs are written, e.g., BASIC, FORTRAN, COBOL, and MUMPS.

MB—Megabyte. One million bytes; refers to amount of memory available or used. To be more specific, it is 1024 kilobytes or 1,048,576 bytes.

Modem—A device that accepts a digital signal and converts it into an analog signal and accepts an analog signal and converts it to a digital signal.

Operating system—Software that enables the computer to run the application software programs.

Optical scanner—A device that converts printed text or graphic images to digital files.

Printer, daisywheel—An impact printer that functions by a device striking a wheel containing the alphabet and the numbers 1 to 10.

Printer, dot matrix—An impact printer that functions by pins striking the inked ribbon to form the letters, numbers and graphical forms. Dot matrix printers have from 9 to 32 pins. The more pins in the print head, the better the quality of print.

Printer, ink jet—A relatively inexpensive, letter-quality printer which operates by fluid ink being forced through nozzles and transferred to the paper by resistive heaters.

Printer, laser—A printer that produces high-resolution images utilizing the same process as photocopy machines.

RAM—Random access memory. Memory that is used to store application programs and data while the program is in use. All data in RAM will be lost when the computer is turned off.

ROM—Read-only memory. That part of a computer memory that contains prewritten instructions. These instructions cannot be erased or rewritten by application programs.

Server—A computer which provides digital programs and information which can be accessed by networked computers and terminals.

Software—Written instructions that enable the computer to conduct desired functions. The software includes the operating system, application programs, utility programs, and other types of programs.

Tape drive—A high-speed storage device that reads from and records data on magnetic tape. This type of storage device is often used for archiving or "backing up" programs and data.

Telnet—Software that enables one to access and manipulate a computer from a remote CPU.

Terminal—An input/output device with a visual display and keyboard that is utilized to send and receive data from the CPU. Terminals are referred to as "dumb" terminals because they are incapable of processing information.

VGA—Video graphics adapter. A board installed in a computer which allows one to view graphical images in color.

WAN—Wide area network. This is usually a network linking two to several LANs.

Web browser—A program that facilitates access and retrieval of graphical data and HTML documents from World Wide Web servers connected to the Internet.

Windows—An operating system with a graphical interface that allows two applications to be active at the same time and the transfer of information between applications.

World Wide Web—A group of computers interconnected via the Internet which provide access to graphical data and HTML documents.

WYSIWYG—"What you see is what you get." This acronym refers to programs that print exactly what is seen on the display screen.

Reference

Bohlender E: Finding the right software for your practice. Trends 8:29–41, 1997.

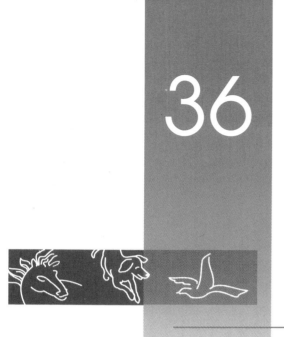

36 Occupational Health and Safety in Veterinary Hospitals*

Diane McKelvey

By the very nature of their work, veterinary technicians are frequently exposed to potential safety hazards, including bite wounds and other animal-related injuries, laboratory accidents, x-ray radiation, waste anesthetic gas, noise, and toxic chemicals. This chapter surveys these and other potential dangers and the means by which injury or disease can be prevented. Zoonotic diseases are covered in Chapter 7.

There are many published surveys of injury and disease in veterinary hospital workers. A study of 773 insurance claims made by injured American veterinarians between 1967 and 1969 (Thigpen and Dorn, 1973) found that most injuries occurred on a farm or ranch. The authors state:

> While in the process of treating, restraining, castrating or examining animals, the veterinarians were bitten, kicked, gored, pawed, knocked down, trampled, run over, and even fallen upon by these animals. While treating resisting farm animals, veterinarians cut themselves, fell, stumbled, or slipped on wet ground or ice in attempts to avoid injuries. These veterinarians jumped off fences, twisting ankles or landing on nails, stepped on pitchforks, and were injured with chutes, speculums, lariats, norse tongs, halters, broken syringes, and an array of practice equipment. They were knocked over and through fences, squeezed against fences, and caught between bulls fighting. They were fallen on by horses while working cattle or else they twisted an ankle while getting off the horse.

Things did not improve much when the veterinarians returned to the hospital:

> In the clinics they were bitten, scratched, and knocked down by the animals. They were burned when steam valves burst, and slipped while reaching in a cage for an animal. They injured their backs picking up dogs and bumped their heads and legs on clinic equipment. They cut themselves during surgery and ran pinning equipment into their fingers and wrists.

Obviously, there is ample opportunity for injury within a veterinary environment. Basic safety precautions are listed in Table 36–1.

If a technician or other hospital employee is injured on the job, there are many unfortunate sequelae. The injury itself may result in pain, disability, and lost workdays for the affected person. In addition, both the employee and the hospital may be affected financially, or there may be legal and regulatory issues to face. Hospital morale may also suffer if staff are convinced that the hospital is not a safe work environment. Employees may be required to take on additional duties if a coworker is absent due to an injury or disease acquired at work. It is therefore in everyone's interest to learn about the hazards that are present in a veterinary environment and to take all reasonable steps to protect the hospital staff, patients, and clientele from injury and illness.

In all jurisdictions within the United States and Canada, the employer has the primary responsibility for hospital safety. The employer's duties include the following:

- To ensure that all employees are adequately trained to protect themselves from injury
- To provide employees with the facilities and protective equipment necessary to do their jobs safely
- To establish emergency procedures in case of accident or fire, and ensure that employees are familiar with these procedures
- To collect and make available mandatory forms and posters, including material safety data sheets for chemicals

• Table 36-1 •

BASIC SAFETY PRECAUTIONS FOR VETERINARY EMPLOYEES

Machinery and Equipment

1. Do not attempt to operate a machine unless you are familiar with its use.
2. Make sure all proper guards are in place before starting to work.
3. Tie long hair back to prevent it from getting caught in equipment. For the same reason, avoid loose-fitting clothing.
4. Vent all autoclaves before opening, and keep hands and face away from steam. Avoid handling autoclaved materials until they have cooled.
5. Use the insulated handle when picking up cautery or branding devices.
6. When using a centrifuge, ensure that the centrifuge is balanced with equal numbers of tubes and that the lid is securely bolted on. No attempt should be made to stop the centrifuge arm or remove samples until the arm has come to a complete stop.

Floors

1. Wear slip-proof shoes and avoid running.
2. Use nonslip mats or strips in areas that are frequently wet.

Housekeeping

1. Clean up spills as soon as possible.
2. Return equipment and chemicals to the proper storage area immediately after use.
3. Avoid clutter in drawers or counters.
4. Hallways, exits, and stairs should be free of obstructions. Equipment or chemicals should not be stored in these locations.
5. Store chemicals and heavy equipment on lower shelves to avoid injury or exposure to chemicals in case the container falls off the shelf.
6. Replace lids tightly on all containers.
7. Use a ladder or step stool to reach high places.
8. Follow a checklist for regular facility maintenance, including daily, weekly, monthly, semiannual, and annual procedures.

Hygiene

1. Food and beverages should not be stored with chemicals, drugs, vaccines, or patient samples. Human food can be stored with animal food.
2. Prepare and consume foods only in designated eating areas, away from chemicals, work surfaces, and patient handling areas.
3. Wash hands with a surgical soap after treating every patient, before and after using the bathroom, and before eating.

Laboratory

1. Wear a laboratory coat or uniform when working with chemicals or diagnostic specimens in a laboratory. In some circumstances, the use of additional protective equipment (gloves, face mask, face shield, or biological containment cabinet) may be advisable.
2. All persons should wash their hands after completing laboratory activities and should remove protective clothing before leaving the workplace.
3. Persons should not remove or insert contact lenses when working in a laboratory.
4. Work surfaces should be cleaned with a disinfectant at the end of the day and after any spill. Useful disinfectants include chlorhexidine, 70% isopropyl alcohol, and a 1:10 dilution of 5% bleach. Bleach is especially suitable for cleaning up blood spills, but is corrosive and will damage metal surfaces with prolonged use. If samples contain *Mycobacterium* or if the surface to be cleaned is metallic, glutaraldehyde is the recommended disinfectant. Gloves should be worn when using glutaraldehyde and care should be taken to avoid inhalation of glutaraldehyde vapors.

Chemicals
Storage

1. Corrosive chemicals should not be stored above shoulder height, as accidental dislodgment of the container could result in chemical splashing onto a person below. Storage in a closed cupboard at floor level is preferred.
2. Hazardous chemicals should not be stored in passageways, aisles, hallways, or next to emergency exits.
3. Separate storage areas should be used for each group of hazardous chemicals, including strong oxidizers (peroxides), flammable liquids, acids, alkalis, and compressed gases.
4. Flammable materials (ether, acetone) and compressed gases should not be stored where there is a possibility of exposure to heat, sunlight, or a source of combustion, including cigarettes. A fireproof cabinet is ideal.
5. For any hazardous chemical, it is advisable to purchase the smallest quantity that is needed, as there will be less material to spill or catch fire.
6. Storage areas should be tidy, with good access to all materials without climbing over bottles or reaching over boxes.
7. Some type of absorbing agent, such as kitty litter, should be kept in the storage area for use in cleaning up spills. If a spill occurs, it should be cleaned up immediately.
8. All containers should have a purchase and expiration date written on the label or box, and stocks should be reviewed at least annually. Expired or deteriorated chemicals should be discarded.

Use

1. Caps should be replaced on chemical bottles immediately after use.
2. Wear gloves, a laboratory coat or waterproof apron, and protective goggles when mixing or diluting chemicals.
3. Chemicals should not be mixed together unless the label or material safety data sheet (MSDS) states that the chemicals are compatible. One example of incompatible chemicals is bleach and ammonia-containing disinfectants. Mixtures of these two compounds may release clouds of extremely toxic chlorine gas.
4. If a material is to be diluted with water, start with the water and gradually add the chemical to it. That way, if the solution is spilled or reacts, it is the water or diluted chemical that is splashed, rather than the chemical in concentrated form.

• Table 36–1 •

BASIC SAFETY PRECAUTIONS FOR VETERINARY EMPLOYEES *(Continued)*

Disposal

1. Many chemicals cannot be safely (or legally) discarded with regular garbage. The MSDS should be consulted to determine correct disposal options for any particular chemical. Municipalities often have regulations that govern disposal of chemicals and should be consulted for further information.
2. Waste materials, including solvents, oils, grease, paints, and other flammable substances, should be placed in covered metal containers prior to disposal.
3. Broken glass must be clearly identified and placed in a puncture-proof container.
4. Although small amounts of some liquid chemicals may be discarded into the sewer system and flushed with copious amounts of water, this is not a good option for chemicals that can damage sewer pipes or chemicals that are an environmental hazard.

Electricity

1. Do not remove light switch or electrical outlet covers.
2. Keep circuit breaker boxes closed.
3. When using electrical equipment in wet areas (e.g., a portable dryer), it must be properly grounded and only plugged into a ground-fault circuit interruption outlet.
4. Extension cords must never be run across aisles or floors or through a window or door.
5. Appliances with defective plugs should not be used until repaired. Never alter or remove the ground terminals on plugs.

Ergonomics

1. When lifting a heavy object, whether an animal, equipment, or container, keep the back straight and use the leg muscles—not the back muscles—to lift. Bend at the knees, rather than at the waist.
2. Do not attempt to lift an object weighing more than 50 lb without assistance. Pregnant persons should not lift any heavy object.
3. Use portable or fixed steps for moving large dogs onto examination tables or into a bathing area. Some dogs can be readily led up the steps, avoiding lifting.
4. Use a walk-on weigh scale, rather than lifting an animal to be weighed.
5. When restraining an animal or working with a microscope or computer, avoid a fixed, static posture. Occasional stretching or movement is helpful in preventing fatigue.
6. When using a computer, adjust the monitor position, brightness, and contrast to the most comfortable level. To avoid glare, locate the monitor at right angles to windows and other light sources. Windows should have blinds or drapes to minimize glare. Characters on the screen should not have a visible flicker or waver.
7. Computer keyboards should be thin and detached from the screen, allowing the user to adjust the keyboard position.
8. A foam support placed under the wrist may help avoid strain during prolonged keyboard use.
9. Office chairs should be stable, with an adjustable seat height and angle and an adjustable backrest. The front edge of the seat should be contoured. The backrest should provide firm support to the lumbar region of the back and should extend up almost to the lower end of the shoulder blade. A woven fabric covering is more comfortable than plastic or wood.
10. Petite persons and pregnant women should use a footrest, especially if the table height is fixed.
11. Ensure adequate lighting in all workplaces.

Noise

1. Occupational Safety and Health Administration (OSHA) standards require a hearing conservation program if employees are exposed to noise levels above 85 decibels (dB) based on an 8-hour time-weighted average. This level may be exceeded in areas where dogs are housed. The noise level from a single barking dog may be 80 to 90 dB, and if several dogs are housed in one area, noise levels may be as high as 115 dB. At 115 dB, an employee can only work approximately 15 minutes in the area without hearing protection before the daily limit is exceeded.
2. The employer must identify a noise hazard area by means of signs placed at all entrances to the room, indicating that a noise hazard exists and hearing protection is required for prolonged exposure.
3. Noise levels can be reduced by acoustical tiles or sound-absorbing panels hung from the ceiling. Commercial panels are available for this purpose, or homemade baffles can be constructed.
4. If sound-absorbing panels cannot be installed, personal hearing protection is an alternative means of reducing exposure to noise. Several varieties of earphones or earplugs are available, but the protection method chosen must reduce noise by at least 20 dB. Personal hearing protection is not necessary for persons who enter and leave the room immediately.
5. Some attempt may be made to reduce barking noise through the use of citronella collars and by closing doors to the kennel area.

- To notify employees of impending inspections and special hazards
- To report accidents that result in serious injury
- To maintain a log of occupational illnesses and injuries (in the United States, businesses with 11 or more employees)
- To post warning signs at emergency exits, radiation areas, and areas in which hearing protection is required (in the United States)

✎ TECHNICIAN NOTE

In all jurisdictions within the United States and Canada, the employer has the primary responsibility for hospital safety.

The responsibilities of the employee are to learn the safety hazards and approved procedures for avoiding injury in the workplace, to wear the protective equipment provided, and to report incidents or conditions that could result in injury.

In the United States, the Occupational Safety and Health Administration (OSHA) has been established under the Department of Labor to ensure that health and safety standards are maintained in every workplace. Many states have developed their own OSHA plans, which may vary in some details from the federal standards. In Canada, workplace safety is a provincial responsibility. Regardless of the jurisdiction, safety regulations are enforced by means of inspections by government personnel, and noncompliance is subject to stiff penalties (in the United States, up to $70,000 for each infraction). Any hospital is subject to an unannounced inspection, although most visits arise from employee complaints or workers' compensation claims. During the visit, the compliance officer checks for unsafe conditions and procedures and inspects the hospital's written documentation regarding hospital safety hazards, emergency procedures, safe work procedures, and staff training. The inspector also ensures that required notices such as the OSHA Workplace Safety and Health Protection poster or the provincial Occupational Health and Safety Act are displayed in the workplace. Inspectors also ensure that all necessary personal protection equipment is available and in good repair. Persons seeking more information on regulatory requirements are advised to contact their local state or provincial veterinary association or consult the references listed in Table 36–2.

ANIMAL-RELATED INJURY

Veterinary technicians are constantly exposed to sick or fractious animals and their blood, urine, and feces, and the potential for animal-related injury or disease is always present. The most important animal-related hazards in the veterinary environment are:

- Animal kicks, bite wounds, scratches, squeeze injuries, and other physical trauma
- Parasites and zoonotic diseases (see Chapters 6 and 7)
- Allergy to animal dander or fleas
- Exposure to feces, urine, blood, and tissues that contain pathogenic microorganisms such as *Salmonella* and *Listeria*

• Table 36–2 •

REFERENCES FOR OCCUPATIONAL SAFETY AND HEALTH ADMINISTRATION (OSHA) REQUIREMENTS
1. The Complete Veterinary Practice Regulatory Compliance Manual Philip Seibert RR 1 Box 313, Calhoun, TN 37309   (423) 336-1925
2. AVMA Guide to Hazard Communication American Veterinary Medical Association 1931 N. Meacham Road, Suite 100 Schaumburg, IL 60173-4360   1-800-248-2862
3. Hazard Communication Compliance Kit and OSHA Compliance Guide for the Veterinary Practice American Animal Hospital Association PO Box 150899, Denver, CO 80215-0899   1-800-252-2242

- Handling contaminated needles, bacterial cultures, and other biomedical wastes.

Trauma

Animals are capable of inflicting serious injury to people that handle them. Dogs primarily defend themselves with their teeth, cats scratch as well as bite, rabbits can inflict deep scratches with the nails of their powerful hind legs, budgerigars can nip with their beaks, and larger birds can bite or scratch with their claws. Persons working with cattle are at risk of being kicked, squeezed, or trampled and those working with horses can be bitten, struck by the front hooves, squeezed, or kicked by the rear hooves (Fig. 36–1). Persons working with ratites, exotic pets, or captive wildlife such as deer or elk may also suffer an injury when handling or treating these patients. In fact, animals are the most common source of injury to veterinarians and their staff. Restraint and handling of animals is discussed in Chapter 1.

Surveys undertaken to investigate the incidence of animal-related trauma have shown the animal species most commonly

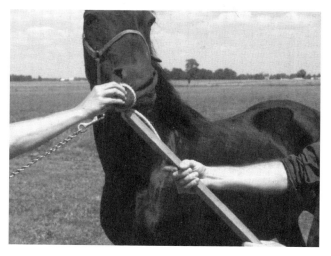

Figure 36-1. Horses are a common source of animal-related injury.

associated with injury to veterinarians are cattle, followed by horses and dogs (Landercasper et al., 1988). The most common injuries are lacerations and puncture wounds, followed by fractures (including facial fractures and dislodged teeth) and sprains and torn ligaments. One survey reported that 64.6% of veterinarians suffer a major animal-related injury sometime during their career, with 14% of the injuries being serious enough to require hospitalization (Landercasper et al., 1988).

TECHNICIAN NOTE

The animal species most commonly associated with injury to veterinarians are cattle, followed by horses and dogs.

Basic guidelines for avoiding animal-related injury are given in Table 36–3.

Bite Wounds

Veterinary technicians, veterinarians, and other hospital employees are frequently bitten by dogs, cats, and other animals. The most common location of canine bite wounds is the radius or ulna and the most common location for feline bite wounds is the hand.

Bite wounds are potentially more serious than other puncture wounds because of the amount of bruising and tissue

• Table 36–3 •

PREVENTING ANIMAL-RELATED INJURIES
1. When restraining an animal, pay attention to the animal and its reactions, not the procedure.
2. Learn proper restraint methods for all species of patients.
3. Obtain help from coworkers when lifting, restraining, or treating animals.
4. Use mechanical devices (chutes, stanchions, ropes) for restraint of large animal patients.
5. Use restraint equipment such as muzzles, leashes, capture poles, squeeze cages, and leather gloves for restraint of fractious small animal patients.
6. Do not put your face close to the hoof or mouth of an unsedated animal.
7. If you feel unsafe working around a potentially dangerous animal, discuss the need for tranquilization with the veterinarian.
8. Ensure that lighting is good and footing is not slippery before beginning to work.
9. Avoid working with a fractious animal when alone. A second person can provide diversion for the animal, apply first aid, and call for help if needed. If you must work alone, there should always be a means to summon immediate assistance if needed (whistle, alarm).
10. Plan a quick exit route in case an animal becomes aggressive.
11. Do not put any part of your body between a large animal and the side of its enclosure.
12. It is advisable to wear latex examination gloves, a surgical mask, and a gown when treating animals that are suffering from serious zoonotic diseases. If rabies is prevalent in the area, use particular caution when working with unvaccinated animals.

injury that occurs. This is not surprising, given that the jaws of a large dog can produce 150 to 450 psi of pressure, which is enough to bend steel bars and penetrate stainless steel feeding bowls.

TECHNICIAN NOTE

Bite wounds are potentially more serious than other puncture wounds because of the amount of bruising and tissue injury that occurs.

Bite wounds not only traumatize tissue but may also become infected. The risk of infection is estimated to be 2% to 5% for a dog bite and 30% to 50% for a cat bite. Usually, wounds are contaminated with the bacteria that reside in the dog's or cat's mouth, although occasionally human skin bacteria may invade the wound. Of the more than 64 species of bacteria that are found in the canine and feline mouth, the one most commonly associated with wound infections is *Pasteurella multocida*. This small gram-negative coccobacillus is present in 50% of canine mouths and 80% of feline mouths. Other bacteria, including *Capnocytophaga, Streptococcus, Staphylococcus, Klebsiella, Enterobacter*, and anaerobic bacteria, may also cause bite wound infections.

Typically, *P. multocida* infection causes rapid development of local swelling, erythema (redness), and pain, usually within a few hours of the bite. Shortly after the bite occurs, the wound may start to exude a blood-tinged fluid. After 24 to 48 hours, local swelling may resolve, or the bacteria may spread into other tissues, causing swelling and pain some distance away from the wound. In some cases, systemic signs, such as swollen lymph nodes, and flu-like symptoms, such as fever, chills, and muscle pain, may be present. Occasionally, even more severe complications may develop, including osteomyelitis, septic arthritis, tendon and joint infections, meningitis, brain abscess, and septicemia, as well as scar formation and disfigurement. Persons with underlying diseases or immune system dysfunction are at particularly high risk of serious wound complications. Victims of bite wounds may also go on to develop diseases transmitted by animal bites, including rabies and cat-scratch disease.

Capnocytophaga has recently been recognized as the causative agent of a distinctive illness that follows a scratch or bite. The incubation time is 3 to 6 days, followed by symptoms resembling influenza. These symptoms may be present even if there is no significant lesion at the site of trauma. As with other bacteria that invade bite wounds, *Capnocytophaga* infections are potentially most dangerous in persons who are immunocompromised or who have undergone a splenectomy.

The risk of complications from bite or scratch wounds can be substantially reduced by prompt first aid following a bite wound (Table 36–4).

Allergies

Allergies to animal dander, fur, and saliva are common among persons working in veterinary hospitals. Cats are frequently the allergen source, although allergies to dogs, horses, cows, and laboratory species (rabbits, rats, mice, hamsters, gerbils, and

• Table 36–4 •

TREATMENT OF CANINE OR FELINE BITE WOUNDS

1. Wash the wound thoroughly with a surgical preparation solution such as chlorhexidine or povidone-iodine. Surgical preparation solutions are preferred to soaps, which may contain detergents that cause pain and delay wound healing. A sterile gauze may be used to gently clean the wound, but vigorous scrubbing should be avoided. After washing, an open wound should be irrigated with up to 1 liter of normal saline using an 18-gauge blunted needle on a 35-ml syringe. The saline should be applied with maximum pressure, in order to flush out bacteria, devitalized tissue, and other materials.

2. If the wound is severe, seek medical attention within 24 hours. The infection potential of a bite wound is reduced if it is treated promptly with deep irrigation and debridement, which should only be administered by a physician. Some physicians advocate suturing but many do not unless the wound is on the face or is deep and hemorrhagic. If signs of infection are present, the physician will likely culture the wound and prescribe antibiotics.

3. Use of prophylactic antibiotics in persons with fresh, clean wounds is controversial. Studies show that the incidence of canine bite wound infections is not reduced when antibiotics are given prophylactically. Feline bite wounds have a higher risk of infection and most physicians routinely prescribe antibiotics for persons with deep cat bites. In the case of a bite wound that is already visibly infected, it is generally agreed that antibiotics should be administered. There is no single antibiotic that is effective against all of the aerobic and anaerobic bacteria that cause wound infections, and therefore culture and sensitivity testing are commonly required. Penicillin, tetracycline, or amoxicillin with clavulanic acid can be administered while awaiting culture results. Cephalosporins and aminoglycosides are not recommended, as they often are ineffective against *Pasteurella* infections in human bite wounds. Antibiotics should only be used if prescribed by a physician.

4. Soaking the affected region in hot water (or applying a hot, damp cloth) may give temporary pain relief. If purulent material accumulates, it may require drainage by a physician.

5. Tetanus is a potential (although uncommon) complication of any bite wound. There are two ways to prevent tetanus from occurring: use of tetanus toxoid (which causes the formation of antibodies and confers long-term immunity) and the use of human tetanus immune globulin (injection of preformed antibody—gives short-term protection only). It is advisable that all persons working in veterinary hospitals be vaccinated with tetanus toxoid every 5 years to develop active immunity to this disease. Tetanus toxoid must be administered before a bite wound occurs, to allow time for an immune response to develop. Persons who have not been previously immunized with tetanus toxoid should be given tetanus immune globulin immediately after a bite wound occurs.

6. If the biting animal is potentially rabid, the local health department and the victim's physician should be contacted, as rabies prophylaxis may be necessary.

Affected persons usually have a positive skin test to allergens from one or more animal species. Desensitization using repeated injection of allergen extracts is sometimes successful in reducing the severity of the allergic response. An experimental vaccine against feline allergies is currently being developed. Allergic persons are advised to avoid contact with the offending animal species, and to consult with an allergist regarding the use of antihistamines and other drugs to prevent or treat symptoms. If contact with the animal species cannot be avoided, use of gloves and a surgical mask is effective in reducing exposure to most allergens.

Vaccine Self-Inoculation

Veterinary hospital employees occasionally inject themselves with vaccines intended for use in animals. Adverse reactions including anaphylaxis and delayed hypersensitivity have been reported and are thought to be induced by the adjuvants (mineral oils, aluminum hydroxide) contained in the vaccines. Anaphylactic reactions occur shortly after inoculation and are characterized by dyspnea, skin eruptions, and shaking. Immediate administration of epinephrine is an effective treatment, but should be undertaken under the supervision of a physician.

Some vaccines, including brucellosis (strain 19) and *Mycobacterium paratuberculosis* (Johne's disease) are associated with a particularly high incidence of reactions following accidental self-inoculation. Delayed hypersensitivity reactions to these vaccines usually occur hours to days after inoculation, with clinical signs of swelling, redness, and pain at the injection site. Granuloma formation may also occur.

If self-inoculation occurs with any vaccine, the site should be immediately washed with soap and water. Bleeding should be encouraged to help drain injected material from the wound. Medical treatment should be sought at once. Tetanus prophylaxis is recommended following self-inoculation if the victim does not have a current tetanus toxoid immunization. Treatment with warm packs and immobilization of the area is helpful in reducing local pain and irritation.

TECHNICIAN NOTE

If self-inoculation occurs with any vaccine, the site should be immediately washed with soap and water.

Laboratory Hazards

Most technicians and other hospital employees are well aware of the potential for catching a zoonotic disease from a living patient (e.g., a dog with rabies). There are equally serious but less obvious hazards associated with handling diagnostic samples, including bacterial or fungal cultures, blood, feces, urine, and tissue specimens, which may contain the same viruses, bacteria, protozoa, or parasites that cause zoonotic diseases.

Infections are usually acquired by one of three routes: ingestion, direct contact, or inhalation.

Ingestion of contaminated materials may occur by eating or drinking, smoking, biting nails, chewing on pens, or otherwise

guinea pigs) are also commonly reported. The route of exposure to animal allergens is usually airborne, with common clinical signs including itchy and runny nose and eyes, conjunctivitis, or asthma. More serious symptoms include coughing, wheezing, and shortness of breath. Symptoms usually peak within 1 hour of exposure to the allergen, although delayed asthmatic reactions may be seen up to 12 hours after contact. Allergic symptoms may occur following a lick, scratch, or bite, but this is relatively rare.

placing articles in the mouth after handling contaminated specimens. Frequent, thorough handwashing is the best way to prevent ingestion of infective substances. It is also a good idea to avoid touching the face or eyes with the hands when doing laboratory work.

Ingestion may also occur when pipetting liquids by mouth. Mouth pipetting should NEVER be employed when working with urine, blood, serum, or other specimen from a veterinary patient.

Infections may also be acquired through *direct skin* or *mucous membrane contact* with contaminated materials. A few infectious agents are able to penetrate intact skin, and many can cross intact mucous membranes in the mouth, nose, and conjunctiva. Almost all agents can invade if there are cuts or abrasions present in the skin. Again, handwashing is the single best way to prevent infection by this route. In some circumstances the use of protective equipment such as gloves, goggles, a face shield, or biological safety cabinet may be advisable.

Infection by *inhalation* of microorganisms may occur whenever aerosols are produced, as when performing a dental prophylaxis using an ultrasonic scaler. Infective aerosols may also be inhaled when examining a fungal or bacterial culture that is producing spores or when flaming an inoculating loop or needle that has been used to culture bacteria. The risk of inhaling microorganisms is greatly reduced if a surgical mask is worn. Goggles are also recommended in some cases, particularly dental procedures.

Spills may occur when working with a diagnostic sample such as urine or blood, or when handling a broth or other liquid culture. Because of the potential for disease transmission, it is a good practice to treat all spills with disinfectant such as chlorhexidine or a 1:10 dilution of 5% bleach, followed by application of an absorbent material such as cat litter to absorb all liquid. Gloves should be worn for spill cleanup if a zoonotic agent is present or if a strong disinfectant such as bleach or glutaraldehyde is used. If spills are likely to occur, it may be helpful to place a paper towel on the work surface before starting.

Universal Precautions

Health care workers who treat human patients are very aware of the risks of disease transmission when working with human blood and other body fluids. This caution is justified because of the risk of acquiring the human immunodeficiency virus (HIV) or hepatitis B or C viruses from human specimens. The most common route of exposure to these agents in a health care setting is a needlestick injury, although infection may also occur after direct skin or mucous membrane contact with infected blood.

In response to this problem, the human health care professions have adopted "universal precautions" when handling blood, saliva, and other body fluids. Universal precautions specify that gloves should be worn when touching blood and body fluids, mucous membranes, or nonintact skin on all human patients. Gloves are also worn when handling items or surfaces soiled with blood or body fluids, and for performing venipuncture. Hands and other skin surfaces are washed immediately and thoroughly after contact with blood or other body fluids. Since it is impossible to reliably identify all patients infected with HIV or hepatitis viruses, precautions are used when handling blood and body fluid from ALL patients (hence the term "universal").

Although universal precautions are not routinely applied when working with veterinary patients or their body fluids and excretions, there are a few agents that may be transmitted from animal blood and fluids to humans (either directly, or by inhalation of aerosols) and universal precautions should be applied when working with samples containing these agents. Samples from patients diagnosed with anthrax, brucellosis, tularemia, *Erysipelothrix* infection, rabies, equine encephalitis, viral disease in monkeys, plague, Q fever, chlamydiosis, *Hantavirus* infection, and other readily transmissible zoonotic diseases should be handled only with universal precautions. Pregnant women should also use universal precautions when handling specimens that may contain toxoplasmosis oocysts or *Listeria* organisms.

Sharps

Caution is needed when handling sharps (needles and scalpel blades), particularly those that have been used for necropsy or surgical procedures. Not only are these materials often coated with infectious materials but they can cause a skin wound that will inoculate the infectious material into the wound site, vastly increasing the probability of infection.

All scalpel blades, needles, and other sharp disposable objects should be capped or discarded in a puncture-proof, sturdy container immediately after use. Needles and other sharps should never be thrown into regular trash containers, even if capped. Once filled, sharps containers should not be opened and the contents should not be transferred to another container.

> **TECHNICIAN NOTE**
>
> All scalpel blades, needles, and other sharp disposable objects should be capped or discarded in a puncture-proof, sturdy container immediately after use.

To prevent needlestick injuries, needles should not be purposely bent or broken or otherwise manipulated by hand. It is safer to dispose of a syringe and needle together, rather than to attempt to remove the needle and to reuse the syringe. Recapping needles is a common cause of needlestick injury, and capping is not advised before disposal. Capping should only be attempted by the "one-handed" method (the cap is placed on a flat surface, and the needle is threaded onto the syringe using only one hand).

RADIATION SAFETY

Persons working in veterinary hospitals may be exposed to electromagnetic radiation produced by x-ray machines, fluoroscopes, lasers, and ultraviolet lamps. Electromagnetic radiation consists of photons of energy traveling at the speed of light. Photons are identical, no matter what type of electromagnetic radiation is involved; however, different forms of radiation have different wavelengths.

Some forms of electromagnetic radiation such as light and heat cause few problems in humans or animals at normal exposures. Other forms of electromagnetic radiation, including x-rays, have a potential to damage cells even in relatively small doses. One factor that determines the risk associated with a given type of radiation is whether or not it is an *ionizing* or a *nonionizing* form of radiation. Ionizing radiation (such as x-rays) causes the formation of ions and free radicals as it passes through tissues. These ions may cause chromosomal damage and have other deleterious effects. Nonionizing radiation either does not penetrate very well through tissues (e.g., visible light) or it may penetrate tissues and pass through them with minimal harmful effects (e.g., radio waves). High doses of nonionizing radiation can damage tissue (e.g., too much infrared or ultraviolet radiation can cause a burn), but the potential for chromosomal damage is less than for ionizing radiation.

X-rays and other forms of ionizing radiation cannot be detected by human senses and a person may be bombarded with even a fatal dose of x-rays yet feel no unusual sensation. X-rays are able to penetrate human tissue in the same way that they penetrate through the chest or leg of an animal being radiographed and can therefore cause damage not only to the skin but to underlying organs. This also means that if the abdomen of a pregnant woman is irradiated with x-rays, the fetus is also exposed.

An individual's exposure to x-rays can come from a variety of sources: environmental, medical, and occupational. *Environmental sources* include cosmic rays produced by the sun, and building materials such as concrete, soil, and brick (which contain minute amounts of radioactive materials such as uranium and radon). In North America, the average environmental exposure is approximately 2 mSv (millisievert) per year.* *Medical exposure* results from x-rays ordered by a physician or dentist, including dental x-rays, chest or abdominal x-rays, and mammograms. The average dose of medical and dental x-rays has been calculated to be 0.5 to 0.7 mSv per person per year in the United States (DHHS, 1988). *Occupational exposure* refers to the radiation that is received when a person takes x-rays as part of his or her job. Veterinary hospital personnel have a potential occupational exposure whenever they are in a room where a radiograph is being taken, unless they are standing behind a lead screen. The extent of occupational exposure depends on many factors, including the number of x-rays taken, the use of shielding devices such as lead aprons and gloves, and the person's proximity to the x-ray beam. For any person who operates an x-ray machine in the United States, the maximum permissible whole-body dose is 50 mSv (5 rem) per year. In Canada, the maximum permissible dose is 20 mSv (2 rem) per year. Veterinary personnel using appropriate precautions are rarely exposed to more than a fraction of this. One survey of veterinarians reported a maximum exposure equivalent to 14.4 mSv (1.44 rem) per year.

The 50 mSv yearly limit applies only to nonpregnant adults who are required to take x-rays as part of their job. For persons under 18 (including student trainees) the allowable whole-body

exposure is only 5 mSv (0.5 rem) in the United States and 1 mSv (0.1 rem) in Canada. Canadian regulations also specify that the maximum permissible occupational exposure to a pregnant woman's abdomen during the 9 months of pregnancy is 2 mSv (0.2 rem).

Effect of Radiation on Adults

It has been well established that the risk of health problems rises as the amount of radiation exposure increases. In the case of a low-dosage exposure, cellular damage may result but is usually repaired and no permanent harm is likely. Higher levels of radiation can cause permanent damage to chromosomes and may injure the skin, gonads, bone marrow, and other tissues. Chromosomal damage may also lead to increased risk of cancer, particularly of the thyroid gland, bone, and lymphatic and hematopoietic systems. There is also some potential for development of lens cataracts following long-term exposure of the eyes to low levels of radiation.

TECHNICIAN NOTE

It has been well established that the risk of health problems rises as the amount of radiation exposure increases.

Veterinary staff using appropriate safety precautions are at very low risk for these problems provided their exposure is under the occupational limit, 50 mSv per year (Wiggins et al, 1989; Schenker et al, 1990).

Effect of Radiation on the Fetus

Pregnant woman who receive high doses of radiation are at increased risk of spontaneous abortion or congenital defects in the fetus. The effect on the fetus depends upon the amount of radiation received and the time during gestation that it occurs. If a woman is exposed to a large dose of radiation in the period *immediately before* pregnancy begins, there is an increased incidence of leukemia and Down's syndrome in the children conceived after exposure. Presumably these children are affected because the egg cell from which they arose was damaged by the radiation. If a woman is extensively exposed to radiation during the *first 2 weeks after conception,* there is no higher incidence of fetal malformations, but a very high incidence of embryo death is observed. If extensive radiation exposure is received *between 3 and 11 weeks after conception,* severe abnormalities may result, including brain abnormalities (epilepsy, retardation, microcephaly), and ocular, genital, and skeletal defects. If high doses of radiation are received *between 11 and 16 weeks after conception,* abnormalities such as stunted growth, mental retardation, and microcephaly are seen but are generally less severe than for fetuses affected in the 3- to 11-week period. Fetuses who receive high doses of radiation *after 16 weeks* have an even lower incidence of defects, and the defects reported are generally minor (including hair loss and skin lesions).

Given the potential for fetal loss or damage, many women are hesitant to undertake radiographic duties when pregnant.

---

*A sievert (Sv) is a metric unit that indicates the amount of biological damage that can occur from radiation. One sievert is equal to 100 rem, which is equal to the biological effect of 100 rad of x-rays being absorbed by the body. The higher the Sv, the higher the exposure to x-rays and the more potential for tissue damage. It is most common for low doses to be expressed in millisieverts (mSv), which is one thousandth of a sievert. 1 Sv = 1000 mSv = 100 rem. Similarly, 1 mSv = 0.1 rem = 100 mrem.

However, it is generally accepted that there is no increased risk of obvious birth defects or embryonic death for the children of mothers who are exposed to less than 50 mSv of x-ray radiation during pregnancy. Some investigators believe there is a possibility that lower doses of x-rays may have subtle effects on the fetus, including increased risk of leukemia and nervous system changes. The U.S. National Council on Radiation Protection and Measurements therefore recommends that the fetal radiation dose not exceed 5 mSv during pregnancy. There is some evidence of a slightly increased risk of spontaneous abortion among veterinarians and veterinary assistants who take more than four radiographs per week during pregnancy, even though the 5 mSv exposure limit is not exceeded (Johnson et al, 1987; Schenker et al, 1990). A pregnant employee should discuss this issue with her physician to determine the course of action with which she is most comfortable. If an employee continues to perform radiography duties while pregnant, she must wear a dosimeter and good-quality protective equipment (apron, gloves), and use care in avoiding unnecessary exposure to x-rays (in particular, avoid exposure to the primary x-ray beam).

TECHNICIAN NOTE

If an employee continues to perform radiographic duties while pregnant, she must wear a dosimeter and good-quality protective equipment (apron, gloves), and use care in avoiding unnecessary exposure to x-rays (in particular, avoid exposure to the primary x-ray beam).

Protecting Yourself from X-Ray Radiation

The basic principle of protection from x-ray radiation is simply to avoid unnecessary exposure to x-rays. The level of exposure should be ALARA (*as low as reasonably achievable*). This can be done in three ways:

1. Time—decreasing the time one is exposed to x-rays
2. Distance—increasing distance from the source
3. Shielding—use of protective clothing containing lead

Exposure to x-rays may occur in two ways. The first (and by far the most serious) is contact with the primary beam, which is the stream of x-rays that flows from the machine and passes through the animal, the photographic film, and the hands of any personnel that are "in the way" of the beam. It is a basic principle of veterinary radiography safety that no human hands or other body parts should be placed in the primary beam, even if lead gloves are worn. The other form of exposure, more common but less intense, is the x-rays that are bounced off (scattered) after contacting the x-ray table and the animal. This scattered radiation strikes persons who are standing nearby. The closer a person stands to an x-ray beam, the greater the amount of scattered radiation that strikes him or her. In the case of the primary beam, the strength of x-rays falls off as the square of the distance from the source. Thus, a person who is in the path of the primary beam, 2 feet away from the source of the beam, will receive only one-fourth the amount of radiation received by a person that is 1 foot away from the source of the beam.

To prevent unnecessary exposure to x-rays, the following precautions should be taken:

1. *Do not take any more x-rays than necessary.* Some practices rotate x-ray duties between staff members, so that no one employee receives the entire exposure to x-rays. It also makes sense to use the best technique possible to limit the number of retakes. Careful measurement of the animal, adequate sedation, proper positioning, use of a technique chart, and optimal film processing all help to reduce the frequency of retakes.
2. *When exposing a film, use the least amount of radiation possible.* Fast screens and film should be used to reduce the amount of radiation required to produce an image. Use of higher kilovoltage techniques allows the milliampere-seconds (mAs) setting to be reduced, which in turn decreases the dose of x-rays received by the animal and hospital employees. Obviously, only persons who are thoroughly familiar with the operation of the x-ray machine should adjust machine controls.
3. *Stay as far from the x-ray beam as possible when the radiograph is being taken.* The ideal solution is to be out of the room or behind a lead screen when the radiograph is taken, and in some states this is a legal requirement. Restraint of the animal can be achieved through the use of anesthetics or passive restraint devices such as sandbags and foam wedges. Walls composed of concrete block or double-thick dry wall provide some protection, and by leaving the room one increases the distance from the primary beam such that very little radiation exposure occurs anyway. If a person stays in the room to press the button, he or she can be effectively protected by a lead-lined screen placed between the control panel and the x-ray table. If no lead screen is available, protective equipment must be worn.
4. *Any person restraining an animal for radiography must keep the hands out of the primary beam.* Exposure to high doses of radiation occurs whenever hands are exposed to the primary beam, whether or not lead-lined gloves are worn. Gloves are not designed to protect the hands from these levels of radiation. If the outline of fingers or gloves appears on the developed image, the hands were exposed to the primary beam. This type of exposure usually arises when handling very small patients such as a bird or when photographing extremities. Small patients can be taped to the cassette and rope or gauze can be used to hold a leg that is being radiographed (Fig. 36–2).

   It is much easier to avoid exposure to the primary beam if it is collimated down to the bare minimum. Ideally, there should be a clear (nonexposed) border of ½ inch around the outside of the exposed film, which indicates that the beam size was reduced to cover less than the area of the photographic plate.

   If it is necessary to restrain animals for radiographic procedures, it is a good idea to stand as upright as possible. Persons who sit on or lean over the x-ray table are exposed to much greater amounts of scattered radiation.
5. *All persons in the room where an x-ray is being taken must wear protective clothing,* including lead-lined gloves and an apron unless standing behind a lead barrier or control booth.

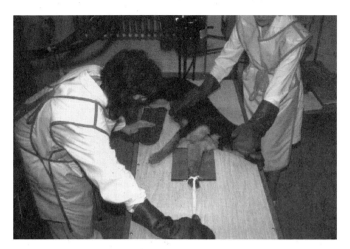

Figure 36-2. Use of gauze ties to restrain animals. The hands are kept well away from the direct x-ray beam.

a. *Gloves*. Bulky, full-hand gloves offer good protection from x-ray exposure. Seamless lead-vinyl gloves are available that are lighter and more flexible than conventional gloves, yet offer comparable protection. One-sided gloves (hand shields), are commercially available and have the advantage of allowing greater dexterity. However, one-sided gloves may not adequately protect the hands from scatter radiation and are not legal for use in some jurisdictions in the United States. Whatever type of glove is used, there should be enough gloves for every person in the room (usually, a minimum of two pairs per practice).

b. *Aprons*. Aprons used for x-ray voltages up to 150 kVp must contain 0.5 mm of lead sheet. The thickness of lead contained in an apron must be permanently marked on the outside of the apron. At 70 kVp, this amount of shielding reduces exposure by a factor of 800.

In addition to mandatory gloves and aprons, other protective equipment is available and its use is recommended. Thyroid collars protect the thyroid gland, which is a potential site of x-ray–induced cancer. Lead glasses protect the eyes from radiation and thus help to prevent the development of cataracts.

All equipment must be in good repair and tested yearly for leaks (more often, if damage is suspected). This testing can be done by placing the glove on a cassette and taking a radiograph using enough kilovolt peak and milliampere-seconds to slightly penetrate the lead.* Aprons can be examined in a similar manner, using masking tape to divide the apron into sections and radiographing each section separately. The test radiographs should be checked for signs of exposure (black), which indicate tears or cracks in the lead. Gloves and aprons can also be tested using fluoroscopic equipment, if available.

X-ray aprons and gloves should not be folded for storage, as creases may cause permanent weak lines and cracks. It is acceptable to leave the apron on the x-ray table between use, or it may be hung over a round

surface. Gloves should be stored in a vertical position to allow air circulation inside the glove. Equipment containing lead should never be machine-washed, but can be safely wiped with hospital disinfectants.

X-ray safety equipment is expensive and easily damaged and should never be used to restrain or capture fractious animals. A single bite can damage the lead and make the glove virtually useless.

6. *If a portable x-ray unit is used, special precautions must be taken to prevent exposure.* Persons in the vicinity should be warned that x-rays are about to be taken, and cautioned to put adequate distance between themselves and the x-ray beam. Persons near the x-ray source must wear protective gloves and aprons. No person should stand in the direct path of the beam, even at a distance. X-ray cassettes should never be held by hand, as any person who holds or stands behind the cassette when a radiograph is taken receives direct exposure to the primary beam. In addition, the portable x-ray machine should never be held by hand when the exposure is being made.

7. *Monitor x-ray exposure using a dosimeter (also called a "monitor" or "film badge").* A dosimeter is a small piece of thermoluminescent material or radiosensitive film that should be worn by each person taking radiographs. Badges used in veterinary radiography are usually worn on the outside collar of the apron, at the level of the thyroid gland, although wrist badges and waist-level monitors are also available. The dosimeter records the amount and type of radiation received by that person. After a period of use (1 to 3 months), the thermoluminescent plaque from the dosimeter is returned to the dosimeter service so that the exposure to x-rays can be measured. Exposure results are returned to the employer and must be made available to all employees.

Every person who is occupationally exposed to ionizing radiation (in other words, in the room when a radiograph is taken or assisting in a procedure using a portable x-ray machine) is required to wear a dosimeter. Staff members who assist in radiography should have their own dosimeters clearly marked with their names.

Dosimeters provide several types of useful information. They verify that the legal dose limit has not been exceeded, and give each employee an exact measure of occupational exposure. Comparison of dosimeter readings also allows the veterinarian or employee to detect changes in exposure levels, which may be due to poor technique, increased workload, or equipment problems. Dosimeters are sensitive to dosages as small as 0.2 mSv (20 mrem). Exposures smaller than this are indicated on the report as a dash (—).

8. Persons under 18 years of age should not be in the room when a radiograph is taken.

*The following are approximate settings that can be used to check protective clothing for leaks: aprons and thyroid shields: 90 kVp and 5 to 10 mAs; gloves: 90 kVp and 10 to 20 mAs. At the correct exposure, a gray image should result.

 TECHNICIAN NOTE

Persons under 18 years of age should not be in the room when a radiograph is taken.

Developing X-Ray Films

Strangely enough, poor darkroom procedures can lead to excessive exposure to x-rays. If incorrect developing times or temperatures are used, it will be necessary to retake numerous films, increasing employee exposure to radiation. A common problem is the use of developer that is over 1 month old, or which has not been mixed or replenished according to the manufacturer's recommendations. Another common mistake is failure to agitate the chemicals in hand tanks before use. Failure to use good darkroom technique may lead to underdevelopment of the films (films appear too light). In order to compensate, the x-ray machine operator may increase exposure settings, causing unnecessary exposure to radiation. When the developing problem is corrected, the radiographs often appear very dark, an indication that the settings on the x-ray machine have been set artificially high to overcome the poor developing performance.

Chemicals used to develop and fix x-ray film are corrosive. The chief hazards associated with exposure to these chemicals are:

- Severe eye irritation, including the potential for permanent corneal damage if the liquid is splashed in the eye.
- Respiratory tract irritation and burning if concentrated vapors are inhaled.
- Skin irritation if there is direct contact with unprotected skin. Allergic dermatitis has also been reported after chronic exposure to these chemicals.

Federal regulations in the United States and Canada require that hazard labels be present on or adjacent to developing tanks. Staff must be trained in safe handling techniques for pouring, mixing, or transporting chemicals. Protective equipment such as gloves and goggles must be provided for persons who hand-develop x-rays using tanks. Hands should be washed after hand-developing films, even if gloves are worn. The darkroom should be equipped with an eyewash fountain in case of eye exposure.

Ventilation of the darkroom by means of an exhaust fan or similar device is usually necessary to prevent the accumulation of toxic vapors. Tanks should be kept covered when not in use.

The use of automatic processors greatly reduces the potential exposure to developing chemicals. There is some risk of chemical exposure when cleaning or replenishing the automatic processor and employees should use appropriate protective clothing and equipment (gloves, protective eyewear, waterproof apron) for these procedures.

Developing chemicals may react dangerously with other chemicals, including liquid drain cleaners, and should never be poured into a sink or drain in which other chemicals may be present. Environmental regulations in many areas prohibit disposal of fixer solutions into sinks or drains. Silver recovery units are a responsible alternative method of disposal.

HAZARDS ASSOCIATED WITH ANESTHESIA

In recent years, concerns have been raised about the safety of operating room personnel exposed to high levels of waste anesthetic gas in human and veterinary hospitals. The term *waste anesthetic gas* refers to vapors of nitrous oxide, halothane, isoflurane, or methoxyflurane that are present in the

• Table 36–5 •

SOURCES OF WASTE ANESTHETIC GAS
• Anesthetic machines in use • Expired air from anesthetized patients (leaking around endotracheal tubes or masks) • Expired air from recovering patients • Anesthetic chambers • Liquid anesthetic spills • Anesthetic machine components such as rubber reservoir bags and rubber hoses (absorb anesthetic gases and release them into the air of the room in which they are stored)

room air of a veterinary hospital. Exposure to these agents can occur in several ways (Table 36–5).

Surveys of veterinary hospitals reveal a wide range in waste anesthetic gas levels, depending upon the location within the clinic and the anesthetic equipment and techniques used. The highest levels of contamination are associated with spills of anesthetic liquids. Liquid anesthetic rapidly evaporates when it is poured or spilled, producing a large amount of anesthetic vapor that rapidly mixes with room air. Accidental spillage of only 1 ml of liquid halothane, for example, will evaporate to form 200 ml of gas with a concentration of 1 million parts per million (ppm).* Liquid anesthetic can also penetrate intact skin and be absorbed into the circulation.

Even without a spill, considerable amounts of waste gas may be generated within the average veterinary hospital (Table 36–6). This is a silent danger, often undetected by the staff or veterinarian. It is sometimes erroneously believed that if the odor of anesthetic gas is not present, the room air is "safe." Unfortunately, the human nose can only detect halothane if the concentration is at least 30 ppm. This level is already 15 times higher than the maximum recommended level.

Significant levels of waste gas are commonly found in areas where anesthetic machines are in use, including surgery suites, surgical preparation rooms, and treatment rooms where den-

---

*The term *parts per million* is a measure of concentration. An atmosphere that is 100% composed of a certain gas has 1 million ppm of that gas. If the concentration of a gas is 1% in room air, this is equivalent to 10,000 ppm. Patients connected to an anesthetic machine delivering 1% halothane in oxygen are therefore breathing 10,000 ppm of halothane and 990,000 ppm of oxygen.

• Table 36–6 •

HALOTHANE CONCENTRATIONS WITHIN VETERINARY HOSPITALS	
LOCATION	**ppm**
Personnel breathing zone	
With scavenging	1.45
No scavenging	2.00
Air around unscavenged anesthetic chamber	>10
Nose and mouth of anesthetized patient	
Intubated, cuff inflated	3.25
Intubated, cuff not inflated	6.10
Air outside recovery cage door	1.07
Nose of patient in recovery cage	5.43

Modified from Short CE and Harvey RC: Anesthetic waste gases in veterinary medicine. Cornell Vet 73:363–374, 1983.

tistry or minor surgery is performed. Recovery rooms may also be contaminated by moderate levels of waste gas as it is exhaled by animals awakening from anesthesia.

During the anesthetic period itself, the level of waste gas is highest immediately adjacent to the anesthetic machine and the patient's mouth. The actual level depends upon several factors, including the duration of anesthesia (the longer the machine is in use, the higher the waste gas concentration in the room air), the flow rate of the carrier gas (higher flow rates may lead to more waste gas pollution), and whether an effective scavenging system is used. If no scavenging system is present, anesthetic gas mixed with oxygen is vented through an open pop-off valve at a rate approximately equal to the oxygen flow rate (usually 500 ml to 3 liters/minute). If a nonrebreathing system such as a Bain circuit is in use, the gas exits through the relief valve or reservoir bag outlet. Either way, all of the waste gas enters the room air when no scavenger is present.

Surveys of veterinary hospitals indicate that levels of waste anesthetic gas in *unscavenged* veterinary surgeries range from 1 to 34 ppm for halothane, 1 to 62 ppm for methoxyflurane, and 6 to 270 ppm for nitrous oxide. Levels for *scavenged* surgery rooms are usually between 0 and 10 ppm depending upon the sampling location (see Table 36–6).

Room ventilation also affects the waste gas level, and rooms with a ceiling fan, wall fan, or other ventilating device generally have lower levels of waste gas. It is advised that all rooms in which anesthetic gases are released have at least 15 air changes per hour.

What Are the Effects of Waste Anesthetic Gas?

Since the first study of waste anesthetic gas was published in 1967, many investigators have attempted to determine the toxicity of isoflurane, halothane, methoxyflurane, nitrous oxide, and other anesthetic agents used for medical and veterinary anesthesia. Although much of the evidence is contradictory, it is generally accepted that exposure to waste anesthetic gas is associated with a higher than normal incidence of both acute and chronic health problems. These problems appear to be dose-dependent (in other words, the greater the exposure, the greater the risk).

Short-term problems, such as those that occur during or immediately after exposure to waste anesthetic gas, include drowsiness, headache, fatigue, nausea, pruritus, depression, and irritability. These symptoms usually resolve spontaneously when the affected person leaves the area, but their frequent occurrence indicates that excessive levels of waste gas are present and a potential for long-term toxicity exists.

Long-term effects of anesthetic gas may include any of the following: reproductive disorders (including increased risk of spontaneous abortion and increased incidence of congenital defects), liver or kidney damage, and nervous system dysfunction (muscle weakness, tingling sensations, and numbness). It is thought that these effects are due to the action of metabolites produced by the breakdown of anesthetic agents within the body. These toxic metabolites include inorganic fluoride or bromide ions, oxalic acid, free radicals, and other substances known to have harmful effects on animal tissues. If this theory is correct, anesthetics that are retained by the body and metabolized (such as methoxyflurane and halothane) have greater potential for long-term toxicity than those that are rapidly eliminated through the lungs (such as isoflurane). Significant

amounts of methoxyflurane or halothane may linger in the liver, kidney, and body fat stores for long periods of time. For example, anesthetists have been shown to have traces of halothane in their breath as long as 64 hours after administering this gas to a patient.

All hospital staff (and in particular, pregnant women) should avoid exposure to high levels of waste anesthetic gas, particularly nitrous oxide, during pregnancy. Controls should be introduced to reduce waste gas levels to 2 ppm in room air. When volatile anesthetics are used with nitrous oxide, the maximum advisable concentration is 0.5 ppm for isoflurane, methoxyflurane, and halothane, and 25 ppm for nitrous oxide (8-hour time-weighted average). It is generally accepted that provided these limits are not exceeded, exposure to waste anesthetic gas is associated with minimal risk, even to pregnant women.

How Can Exposure to Waste Gas Be Minimized?

There are five important ways in which exposure to waste gas can be reduced to a minimum:

1. Install an effective scavenging system.
2. Test the anesthetic machine for gas leaks before it is used each day.
3. Utilize anesthetic techniques that reduce waste gas release.
4. Use and maintain anesthetic equipment with care.
5. Utilize protective equipment when exposure is unavoidable (e.g., when cleaning up liquid anesthetic spills) (Fig. 36–3).

Scavenging Systems

A scavenger (more properly termed a gas scavenging system) is an apparatus that collects waste gas from the pop-off valve of an anesthetic machine and conducts it to a disposal point outside the building. The installation and use of an effective scavenger is the single most important step in reducing the exposure of hospital employees to waste anesthetic gas. One survey of veterinary hospitals showed that scavengers reduced waste halothane concentrations by up to 94%.

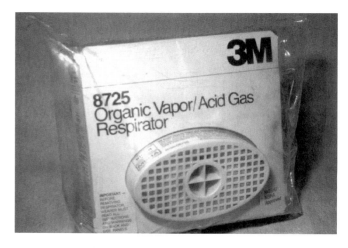

Figure 36–3. A cartridge respirator, suitable for cleaning up spills of anesthetic liquids and other organic chemicals.

TECHNICIAN NOTE

The installation and use of an effective scavenger is the single most important step in reducing the exposure of hospital employees to waste anesthetic gas.

Many types of scavengers are available, but all of them have the same basic design. Waste gas from the anesthetic machine is conveyed to a disposal point by a tube or hose connected to the pop-off valve of the anesthetic machine. In some systems (passive scavenging systems) the tube simply carries the waste gas to an open window or exhaust vent in the wall. The gas flows by gravity and because it is pushed by the pressure of gas in the anesthetic machine. Another type of system (active scavenging system) uses a vacuum pump or fan to draw the gas away from the anesthetic machine and discharges it through a vent to the outdoors. The vacuum system can be part of the hospital's central vacuum system or (preferably) it can be an independent system. Both active and passive scavenging systems are effective, provided they are correctly installed.

Modern anesthetic machines are equipped with pop-off valves that are designed to allow easy connection to scavenging systems. Adaptors for use with older equipment are also available from anesthetic equipment suppliers. It is important to choose the type of pop-off connection that matches the type of scavenging system used, whether high vacuum, low vacuum, or passive. Nonrebreathing systems (such as a Bain circuit or Ayre's T-piece) should also be connected to a scavenger or other exhaust system. This can be achieved by connecting the scavenger hose to the outlet of the reservoir bag or the circuit. "Bag tail valves" and other adaptors can be obtained from suppliers of anesthetic equipment.

No matter which type of scavenging system is chosen, the guidelines given in Table 36–7 should be followed.

Every anesthetic machine or anesthetic chamber in the hospital must be connected to a scavenger when in use. If it is not practical to install scavenging equipment in a specialized room (such as the radiography room), it is advised that either anesthesia be maintained with an injectable agent or that an anesthetic machine with an activated charcoal cartridge be used. These cartridges, available from safety supply firms, can effectively absorb isoflurane, halothane, and methoxyflurane vapors, (not nitrous oxide) but must be replaced after 12 hours of use.

Leak Testing

Leakage of gas from anesthetic machines is a significant source of operating room pollution. Contamination from this source is not reduced by a scavenging system, as the gas escapes before it can reach the scavenger. In some cases, the presence of a leak is obvious—there may be an audible hiss, the odor of anesthetic, or a jet of air coming out of the rebreathing bag or hose. Unfortunately, small leaks are often inaudible and the odor is undetectable and can only be found by leak-testing the machine. Leak-testing procedures should be performed at least daily, following a procedure similar to that outlined in Table 36–8. In addition, periodic inspection of the anesthetic machine

• Table 36–7 •

GUIDELINES FOR THE USE OF WASTE GAS SCAVENGING SYSTEMS
1. The anesthetic gas should be confined within the hose from the pop-off valve to the outlet, without passing through open air gaps.
2. Air from the scavenging system must be discharged outside the building, away from doors, windows, and air intakes. Scavengers which discharge gas onto the floor of the surgery room, into the attic or basement of the clinic, or into a recirculating central vacuum system will contaminate all building rooms with waste gas.
3. If a passive system is used, the hose should be as short as possible (maximum 10 feet in length) and should travel a downward course toward the exhaust. If possible, the hose should not travel on the floor, where it may be stepped on or trapped under equipment and occluded.
4. Scavenging systems may become blocked, leading to accumulation of gas in the anesthetic circuit. The obvious indication that this is occurring is an overdistended reservoir bag. Such a blockage must be immediately resolved (if necessary, by disconnecting the scavenger) or it may lead to circulatory problems or lung damage in the patient. Some anesthetic machines are equipped with pressure-releasing valves, which minimize this hazard.
5. If an active system is used, the vacuum should not be so strong that it draws too much air from the anesthetic machine. The reservoir bag should always contain sufficient amount of air to allow the patient to breathe comfortably. Anesthetic machines equipped with negative pressure-releasing valves will allow room air to enter the circuit if a vacuum inadvertently develops within the circuit.
6. Scavenging systems with exhaust fans should be explosion-proof and designed to handle waste gases that contain oxygen.

(including leak testing) should be undertaken by a qualified medical equipment repair technician.

Once it has been determined that a leak is present, its location can sometimes be found by listening carefully for the source, or it may be located using a solution of liquid soap (such as dishwashing detergent) mixed with water. This solu-

• Table 36–8 •

LEAK TESTING PROCEDURES
1. Assemble the anesthetic machine together with all hoses and connections.
2. Close the pop-off valve and place a hand or stopper over the Y-piece, closing off all avenues of gas escape from the machine.
3. Turn on the oxygen tank and adjust the flowmeter to supply at least 2 liters of oxygen per minute.
4. The reservoir bag is allowed to gradually fill with oxygen. The anesthetist should be able to squeeze the inflated bag with significant pressure without causing escape of air from the bag. Alternatively, the anesthetist can adjust the oxygen flow such that a circuit pressure of 30 cm H_2O is maintained for 30 seconds (this is indicated on the manometer). If the oxygen flow required to maintain this pressure is over 200 ml/minute, there is significant leakage from the machine.
5. If nitrous oxide is used, a high-pressure test should also be performed. The nitrous oxide cylinder is turned on and the tank pressure gauge reading is noted. The cylinder is then turned off. With the flowmeter set to zero, the pressure should be maintained in the system such that the tank pressure gauge reading is unchanged after 1 hour.

tion is gently squirted on all potential leakage points, and each location is observed for bubble formation, indicating the escape of gas. Common locations for gas leaks include the tank connection to the machine, carbon dioxide absorbers, unidirectional valves, and reservoir bags. Once the source of the leak is identified, it can often be fixed by tightening a connection or replacing a part. If the leak cannot be fixed, the machine should not be used until it is serviced by qualified personnel.

Anesthetic Techniques

The anesthetist, by his or her choice of anesthetic techniques, can considerably reduce the amount of waste gas released into the room air. The procedures outlined in the box below help to minimize waste gas release.

Equipment Concerns

Hoses, reservoir bags, masks, endotracheal tubes, and other rubber components of the anesthetic circuit should be washed with soap and water and air-dried after each procedure. Washing not only removes absorbed waste gas but also reduces the transfer of microorganisms between patients.

Anesthetic vaporizers should be filled or drained only in a well-ventilated area—ideally, outside the veterinary clinic. If

vaporizers are filled inside a building, the procedure should be done just before leaving work in the evening. When pouring liquid anesthetic into the machine it is a good idea to use a filling device (supplied by most anesthetic manufacturers) rather than a funnel. Care should be taken to avoid overfilling the vaporizer or spilling the anesthetic.

TECHNICIAN NOTE

Waste gas concentrations around the patient's head can be reduced by 50% if an endotracheal tube is used instead of a mask.

Because of the risk of exposure to significant levels of waste gas when emptying or filling anesthetic vaporizers, pregnant personnel should not be assigned to these tasks.

Empty anesthetic bottles should be capped before being discarded, as residual anesthetic may evaporate into the room air. Likewise, filling devices should be stored between uses in a sealed plastic bag.

If a bottle of anesthetic is accidentally broken or a spill

- Avoid the use of anesthetic chambers as much as possible. Anesthetic chambers were the greatest source of anesthetic pollution noted in a survey of veterinary facilities (Short and Harvey, 1983). Unless a scavenging system is connected to the chamber, large amounts of waste gas are released when the chamber is opened. In addition, the fur of the patient is saturated with anesthetic during the induction, and gives off significant waste gas vapor when the animal is removed from the chamber. If a chamber must be used, it should be connected to a scavenging device and the chamber should be washed with soap and water immediately after each use to remove residual anesthetic. Chambers should only be used where ventilation is excellent, and the use of an exhaust fan or other means of evacuating room air to the outside is recommended.
- Avoid the use of face masks to maintain anesthesia. Waste gas concentrations around the patient's head can be reduced by 50% if an endotracheal tube is used instead of a mask. The high contamination level associated with masks is probably due to the escape of anesthetic gas around the mask, particularly if it is not fitted tightly over the animal's face. If face mask inductions are required, the animal should be intubated as soon as it reaches an appropriate depth.
- Cuffed endotracheal tubes significantly reduce the escape of waste gas into room

air, compared to uncuffed tubes. To be effective, however, the tube must be of adequate size and the cuff must be inflated and in good repair.
- The vaporizer or nitrous oxide flowmeter should not be turned on until the anesthetic machine is connected to the endotracheal tube and the cuff is inflated. It is inadvisable to fill the reservoir bag with anesthetic gas before connecting the machine to the patient, as the gas is released directly into the room air. Once the procedure is under way, the patient should not be disconnected from the breathing circuit unless the vaporizer has first been turned to zero.
- The contents of the reservoir bag should not be released into the room air. Rather, the bag should be squeezed gently while still attached to the machine, to allow the scavenger to retrieve the waste gas.
- If possible, maintain the connection between the animal and the machine, with the animal breathing pure oxygen, for several minutes after the vaporizer is turned off. This allows expired anesthetic from the animal's lungs to enter the scavenging system rather than the room air. Obviously this is not always possible, for example, if the animal is awakening from anesthesia and is chewing on the endotracheal tube.
- Whenever possible, avoid being closer than 3 feet to the nose of a recovering or anesthetized animal.

occurs, the area should be immediately evacuated and cleanup procedures initiated as discussed under chemical spills.

TECHNICIAN NOTE

Because of the risk of exposure to significant levels of waste gas when emptying or filling anesthetic vaporizers, pregnant personnel should not be assigned to these tasks.

Measurement of Waste Gas Levels in a Veterinary Hospital

There are several ways in which a hospital can periodically monitor waste anesthetic gas levels to ensure that the 2 ppm limit is not exceeded. One method is to hire a professional monitoring service to visit the hospital to evaluate ventilation and scavenging techniques and to collect air samples to be analyzed for waste gas concentration. These monitoring services may be available through the companies which install and maintain anesthetic gas machines, or they may be listed under "Safety," "Industrial Hygiene," or "Air Sampling" in the yellow pages of the telephone book. It is also possible for clinic employees to monitor waste gas levels using detector tubes or dosimeter badges (similar to radiation badges) obtained from safety supply companies and monitoring services such as Assay Technology (800–833–1258). Some badges detect only one chemical, such as halothane or nitrous oxide, whereas others are sensitive to all organic vapors, including methoxyflurane, isoflurane, and halothane. The badges are worn for a timed period in a location where anesthetic gases are being used, then returned to the supplier for analysis. Results are given as time-weighted average in parts per million.

Compressed Gas Cylinders

Oxygen and nitrous oxide are purchased as compressed gases in metal cylinders. Several potential safety hazards associated with compressed gas cylinders are listed in Table 36–9.

CHEMICAL HAZARDS

Veterinary technicians frequently treat animals that have been poisoned or burned by chemicals such as pesticides, pharmaceuticals, and cleaning agents. These same chemicals are handled by veterinary hospital employees on a daily basis and may be as harmful to humans as they are to animals. Fortunately, it is possible to reduce the hazards significantly by taking commonsense safety precautions when storing, using, or disposing of chemicals (see Table 36–2).

How Do Chemicals Enter the Body?

No matter how a chemical enters the body, it can cause two types of problems: acute and chronic. Acute effects are those experienced after a single large dose or exposure (e.g., pesticide splashing into the eyes) and often result in a trip to a hospital emergency room. Chronic effects are more insidious, as they usually result from repeated small doses absorbed over a long period of time. Chronic effects may not be apparent for years after the chemical exposure, and are therefore difficult to

• Table 36–9 •

SAFETY PRECAUTIONS FOR COMPRESSED GAS CYLINDERS

1. Although oxygen and nitrous oxide are not flammable, they support combustion and should not be used in a room with an open flame. It is recommended that no sources of ignition (matches, Bunsen burners, and so forth) be present in any room in which oxygen or nitrous oxide cylinders are stored or used, and that smoking be prohibited in these areas. Cylinders should be stored in a dry, cool, place, away from furnaces, water heaters, and direct sunlight. The storage area should be identified by a sign indicating that compressed gases are present and that smoking is prohibited. Gas cylinders should be stored away from emergency exits or areas with heavy traffic.
2. Oxygen and nitrous oxide must not be stored or used near flammable chemicals such as ether, acetone, or gasoline.
3. Care should be taken to avoid dropping cylinders containing compressed air. Pressurized gas may be suddenly released if a cylinder is damaged or knocked over and the regulator (pressure-reducing valve) becomes detached from the tank. The force of the gas escaping from the tank may cause the tank to move like a rocket through walls and other objects. To prevent this occurrence, large cylinders should be chained or belted to a wall and should always be stored in an upright position. Transportation carts and floor-mounting collars are also acceptable means of securing compressed gas cylinders. Valve caps should be used on all large cylinders that are not connected to gas lines.
4. If a cylinder must be moved to another location, a handcart should be used, rather than rolling the cylinder.
5. Full tanks should be kept separate from empty tanks and should be labeled for quick identification. Cylinders should be used in the order in which they are received (first in, first out).
6. Supply tanks should be turned off when not in use. Supply lines from central gas supply systems should be identified with the gas they contain. All staff should know the location of the emergency shut-off valve for the central gas supply.
7. Impact-resistant protective goggles should be worn when connecting or disconnecting tanks, as air escaping from the tanks can potentially cause severe eye damage. Similarly, high-pressure leaks can cause severe injury to skin and underlying tissues and one should never attempt to stop such leaks by using hand pressure.

trace back to any particular chemical or other cause. Both the acute and chronic affects of any given chemical are listed on its material safety data sheet (MSDS).

Chemicals normally enter the body by one of three routes: *inhalation, mucous membrane* or *skin exposure,* and *ingestion.*

Inhalation

Hazardous vapors are given off by many substances used in veterinary hospitals, including ethylene oxide, pesticides, film-developing chemicals, and formaldehyde. Harmful vapors may also be given off by items that seem innocuous, including correction fluid such as Liquid Paper (the Gillette Company, Boston, MA), marker pens, and photocopy machine toner.

Hazardous vapors and dusts affect the body in several ways. Vapors such as formaldehyde may cause direct irritation of the eyes and respiratory tract. Vapors from chemicals such as ethylene oxide or ether may be absorbed from the lungs, enter the blood stream, and affect internal organs. A few gases (e.g., pure nitrous oxide) can cause asphyxiation if oxygen is unable to reach and bind to hemoglobin in the red blood cells.

There are two important ways to prevent inhalation of

injurious gases, vapors, and dusts: (1) increase ventilation and (2) wear protective equipment.

Ventilation. There is less likelihood of injury from chemical vapors if the vapor is immediately diluted with fresh air. Open doors or windows, or exhaust fans that direct exhaust outside of the room may be used to increase ventilation in critical areas such as a surgical preparation room where patients are masked with anesthetic gases, a bathing area where pesticides are in use, or a darkroom where tanks are used to develop x-rays. More sophisticated ventilation devices, such as biological containment cabinets, fume hoods, and ventilation systems, are available for special purposes, including preparation of cytotoxic drugs and sterilization using ethylene oxide.

Protective Equipment. If dangerous fumes or dusts are present and ventilation is not adequate, it is necessary to use protective equipment. Three types of equipment are commonly used: surgical masks, disposable respirators, and cartridge respirators. *Surgical masks* are an effective barrier against some dusts and bacterial spores. They are most useful when working with potentially harmful bacteria or fungal cultures, and when performing a dental prophylaxis. *Disposable respirators* are similar to surgical masks but are designed to screen out dust, nuisance odors, hot air, and hazardous mists. *Cartridge respirators* fit over the nose and mouth area so that the wearer breathes only air that has passed through the respirator filters. The most common use of cartridge respirators in veterinary clinics is for persons handling liquid anesthetics (as when filling vaporizers) and for cleaning up spills of toxic liquids such as x-ray fluids and ethylene oxide. Respirators can be obtained at a reasonable cost through safety supply catalogues, safety supply outlets, and some hardware stores. Use of respirators is only permitted where prevention or elimination of a hazardous condition is not reasonably practicable, or where the exposure results from temporary or emergency conditions only. Any person who uses a respirator must be given instruction on its proper use and its limitations.

TECHNICIAN NOTE

To prevent accidental ingestion of chemicals, food and drink should not be stored in proximity to chemicals or in a refrigerator that is used for chemical storage.

Ingestion

It is unlikely that a veterinary clinic employee would knowingly eat or drink a hazardous chemical, but there is a potential to ingest these materials by smoking, eating, or drinking while handling chemicals.* Ingestion of harmful materials not only irritates the gastrointestinal tract but may also lead to absorption of the material and resultant spread throughout the body. Nursing mothers who are exposed to toxic chemicals such as pesticides may excrete them in breast milk.

To prevent accidental ingestion of chemicals, food and drink should not be stored in proximity to chemicals, or in a refrigerator that is used for chemical storage. Food or other items that are suspected to have been contaminated by a chemical spill or splash should be discarded.

Hands should be washed immediately after handling chemicals, and both the hands and face should be washed again before eating. After handling toxic chemicals on the job, it is a good idea to shower and change clothes after arriving home from work.

Absorption Through Direct Contact

Absorption of chemicals such as pesticides through the eyes, mucous membranes, or skin is very common. Some chemicals may be absorbed through intact skin, or (more commonly) they can enter through a rash, skin puncture, or wound. One obvious effect of chemical absorption is local irritation and tissue damage. The eyes are particularly sensitive to chemicals, as is evident to anyone who has splashed formalin or x-ray fixer into the eyes. The skin, although less sensitive than the eyes, may also be irritated by chemicals, and the use of concentrated disinfectant solutions and other chemicals may lead to skin rashes and even allergic dermatitis.

Chemicals that are absorbed through the skin or mucous membranes may enter the blood and be distributed throughout the body. This phenomenon is familiar to anyone who has applied dimethyl sulfoxide (DMSO) without wearing gloves, and has shortly after perceived a garlic taste in the mouth. Once present in the tissues, chemicals may affect almost any organ, including the brain, heart, liver, kidney, reproductive tract, immune system, and bone marrow. Some chemicals are teratogenic (cause birth defects), carcinogenic (cause cancer), and/or mutagenic (cause chromosomal mutations, leading to increased risk of birth defects in future offspring and increased risk of cancer).* Some of the chemicals used in veterinary hospitals, including ethylene oxide, formaldehyde, and cytotoxic drugs, have the potential to cause multiple adverse effects, including local inflammation, internal organ damage, chromosomal changes, increased risk of miscarriage, and cancer.

Use of Protective Equipment

TECHNICIAN NOTE

To minimize exposure to hazardous chemicals, it is necessary to wear protective equipment when working with these substances.

To minimize exposure to hazardous chemicals, it is necessary to wear protective equipment when working with these substances. The employer must provide all personal protective equipment (including equipment used for handling chemicals and laboratory samples, preventing exposure to x-rays, and

---

*Smoking not only creates the risk of chemical ingestion but may also lead to fire or explosion. Smoking should not be permitted in areas where oxygen, nitrous oxide, flammable liquids, pesticides, ethylene oxide, and other chemicals are stored or used.

*Obviously, birth defects and cancer may arise from many causes other than exposure to chemicals. Birth defects most commonly occur if a teratogen is ingested between 25 and 35 days after conception, although some risk is present throughout the entire period from 21 days to 90 days of pregnancy. The most common teratogenic effects include low birth weight, mental retardation, and functional deficits.

restraining animals) and the employee must wear it as required by the employer. Protective equipment is readily accessible through safety supply companies and hardware stores. The employer must ensure that protective equipment is properly cleaned and maintained, and that sufficient equipment is available to fit each employee correctly.

OSHA regulations require that staff members be trained to recognize when use of the equipment is necessary, the type of equipment to use in each situation, how to wear and adjust the equipment, the limitations of the equipment, and the proper care of the equipment. In the United States, the employer must certify in writing that each employee has completed this training prior to working with the hazard.

Wherever possible, engineering controls are preferred over protective equipment. For example, it is better to install an exhaust fan in the darkroom than to require employees to wear a respirator when developing x-rays.

The type of protective equipment worn should reflect the hazards that are present. Simply wearing a laboratory coat or uniform over street clothes may be sufficient when working with chemicals that have low toxicity (e.g., diluted hospital disinfectants). Long-sleeved shirts and pants offer more protection than shorts or a skirt. Similarly, conventional shoes offer more protection than open-toed shoes and sandals. If significant exposure is expected (e.g., when cleaning up a chemical spill), rubber boots, coveralls, and a rubber or plastic apron should be worn.

Gloves

It is sometimes advisable to wear hand protection when using chemicals. This is particularly true when working with concentrated solutions, as they have more potential for harm than diluted solutions. Gloves should be worn when handling formalin and formaldehyde, carbon dioxide absorber (soda lime or barium hydroxide lime), concentrated pesticides and disinfectants, chemicals used to fix and develop x-ray films, and cytotoxic drugs.

Several types of gloves are available, and the MSDS for each chemical should be consulted to determine the appropriate type of glove to use. Latex surgical or examination gloves provide adequate protection against most infectious organisms and mild chemicals. Latex gloves are easily torn, and double gloving may be advisable in some situations. Nitrile gloves are comfortable and are more resistant to puncture and chemicals than latex, but fine detail work may be difficult if the gloves are bulky. Nitrile gloves are generally more expensive than latex. Vinyl gloves are inexpensive but only suitable for light duties such as dishwashing.

Unfortunately, gloves do not always provide full protection, as some chemicals (particularly acids and solvents) can penetrate gloves or may be splashed onto skin and clothing beyond the glove margins. Hands should always be washed after removing the gloves. Protective creams can be worn under gloves or on their own and are helpful in preventing skin contact with irritating substances.

Eye Protection

Almost all chemicals are harmful if splashed or sprayed into the eyes, and in situations where an eye splash may occur it is advisable to wear safety glasses, goggles, or a face shield. Protective eyewear should be worn when pouring or handling concentrated pesticides and disinfectants, corrosive or toxic chemicals (including chemicals used to develop x-rays), and cytotoxic drugs. Protective eyewear should also be worn when connecting or disconnecting compressed gas cylinders and when performing dentistries with ultrasonic equipment.

TECHNICIAN NOTE

Every practice must have at least one eyewash station available in case of accidental eye splash with a toxic chemical.

Every practice must have at least one eyewash available in case of accidental eye splash with a toxic chemical. Faucet-mounted eyewash devices are relatively inexpensive and provide copious amounts of fresh water, unlike hand-held eyewash bottles. Hand-held devices are used to remove foreign bodies but are not suitable for chemical splash injuries. Eyewash devices must be available within 100 feet (or 10 seconds) of any area where chemicals are used. Persons working with chemicals must know the location of the eyewash and be able to safely reach the eyewash in the event of eye exposure, even if they cannot see (as would be the case after a corrosive chemical was splashed into the eye).

Contact lenses may increase the damage caused by any chemical that is splashed into the eye by trapping the material next to the cornea. Contact lenses should be removed immediately after a chemical is splashed into the eye. Persons who wear contact lenses should notify their coworkers of this fact, so a co-worker giving first aid will know to remove the contact lens if the eye is injured. Once removed, contact lenses should not be replaced until a physician is consulted.

Regulatory Requirements

In the United States, employers must conduct a formal hazard assessment to determine the safety hazards present in the workplace, including chemicals. A complete list of hazardous chemicals used in the hospital must be prepared, and a written plan must list the protective equipment and procedures that are to be used when handling each chemical. This information is usually obtained by conducting a systematic inventory of all chemicals in the hospital, and by consulting the MSDS for each chemical. Details on preparation of the hazardous chemical list and other OSHA requirements are given in the references listed in Table 36–2. Generally, any chemical that has a label or MSDS warning that it is toxic, carcinogenic, an irritant or sensitizer, flammable or combustible, unstable, reactive, or corrosive is considered to be hazardous. Most veterinary practices have over 100 materials (injectable drugs, cleaning products, laboratory chemicals) in use at any given time that are considered to be hazardous by OSHA. Foods, drugs, or cosmetics intended for personal consumption by employees are exempt from listing and training requirements, as are many common consumer products when purchased and used in small quantities (e.g., laundry detergent). Pills or tablets are also exempt from these requirements.

In addition, OSHA regulations require that employees know specific details on what chemicals they are handling, the type of dangers associated with the material, and how to protect themselves from injury. In the United States, a written plan must be prepared giving details on the safety training program for staff members and the person responsible for ensuring that all training is received.

Labels

In order to work safely with a chemical, it is necessary that the container be clearly labeled with the identity of the substance and the potential hazards associated with it. If the chemical is unfamiliar, the employee should consult the label for information on protective equipment that should be worn. It is a wise practice to routinely double-check the label before using a chemical, in the same way that persons handling pharmaceuticals double-check the label before dispensing a drug. Labels should be replaced when they start to peel off or become illegible. If a container is difficult to label (e.g., a shampoo container) a color-coded system can be used instead of an adhesive label, provided all persons using that material are familiar with the identification system used.

Any chemical received by the practice should already have a supplier label when it is delivered. This label is produced by the manufacturer, and gives the name of the chemical and a brief description of the risks associated with handling it. Some labeling requirements are waived for common consumer chemicals, such as those purchased in small quantities from retail outlets and small quantities of laboratory chemicals.

When a chemical is diluted or transferred to another container (e.g., when transferring isopropyl alcohol from a large bottle to a dispensing bottle) the new container must be identified by a new label. This is particularly important if the new container is to be used by several people or over several days. If the chemical is hazardous, the label must also outline brief hazard warnings and handling precautions. These labels, called workplace labels or secondary labels, can be prepared by the practice or purchased from safety suppliers.

Material Safety Data Sheets

Every company that supplies chemicals to a veterinary practice must provide material safety data sheets (MSDS) for all hazardous chemicals. These sheets are valid for 3 years, after which time the supplier should send a new MSDS with the next shipment. The MSDS has detailed information on the chemical, including the following:

- A list of hazardous ingredients
- Information on normal use of the chemical
- Physical data such as the boiling point and vapor pressure
- Warning of fire or explosion hazard and how to extinguish fires
- List of incompatible materials and decomposition products
- Toxicological properties, including effects of short-term and long-term exposure, carcinogenicity, and teratogenicity
- First-aid measures in case of exposure
- Preventive measures when handling the product, including personal protective equipment that should be used

The MSDS is only useful as a reference if every person in the hospital has easy access to it. Regulations therefore require that the MSDS for all hazardous chemicals used by the hospital staff be gathered together and kept in a place that is readily accessible to all staff.

TECHNICIAN NOTE

Every company that supplies chemicals to a veterinary practice must provide material data safety sheets (MSDS) for all hazardous chemicals.

HAZARDOUS CHEMICALS USED IN VETERINARY HOSPITALS

Pesticides

Any chemical used to control pests can be described as a "pesticide." Most pesticides fall into into one of five classes: rodenticides, fungicides, herbicides, fumigants, and insecticides. Insecticides are the class most commonly used by veterinary hospital staff, in the form of flea and tick sprays and repellents, collars, shampoos, dips, foams, tablets, and similar products. These products may contain organophosphates, carbamates, chlorinated hydrocarbons, pyrethrins and other botanicals, insect growth regulators, amitraz, or DEET (diethyltoluamide). Human exposure may occur when handling or diluting insecticides or when applying them to animals.

TECHNICIAN NOTE

Of all the insecticides used in veterinary hospitals, the organophosphates and carbamates are most frequently associated with human toxicity.

Of all the insecticides used in veterinary hospitals, the organophosphates and carbamates are most frequently associated with human toxicity. These agents inhibit acetylcholinesterase, the enzyme that degrades the neurotransmitter acetylcholine. Persons suffering from acute organophosphate or carbamate poisoning may show a multitude of clinical signs which reflect overstimulation of the central nervous system, skeletal muscles, and the parasympathetic nervous system. Clinical signs include salivation, lacrimation, nausea, cramps, diarrhea, sweating, muscle weakness, twitching, blurred vision, restlessness, headache, dizziness, confusion, and slurred speech. One survey of large-animal veterinarians who used pour-on organophosphates to treat cattle grubs reported that many veterinarians experienced headache, nausea, dizziness, and irritation of the nose and throat, particularly when these products were used in a poorly ventilated location (Beat and Morgan, 1977). Treatment of affected persons includes washing the skin with mild soap and water in cases of skin exposure, removal of contaminated clothing, and administration of atropine and pralidoxime chloride (2-PAM).

Recently, attention has been focused on possible chronic toxicity of organophosphates and carbamates. Long-term exposure to organophosphates may cause subtle behavioral effects for weeks to months after exposure, including decreased mental alertness and intellectual functioning, poor neuromuscular control, sleep disorders, memory loss, and psychotic, schizoid, and paranoid reactions (Bukowski, 1990). One 1995 survey of sheep farmers who used sheep dip containing organophosphates found them to have slow reaction times, poor short-term memory, difficulty on reasoning tests, and an increased incidence of psychiatric problems compared with farmers who were not exposed to organophosphates. As with waste anesthetic gases, it is probably wise to minimize exposure to organophosphates as much as possible.

Pyrethroids and other botanicals such as limonene, pennyroyal, oil of citronella, *Melaleuca* oil ("tea tree"), and rotenone are derived from natural sources such as plant oils and flowers. The most commonly reported adverse effect associated with botanical agents is dermatitis due to a contact allergy. Rotenone is reported to cause reproductive problems in pregnant laboratory animals, including increased incidence of babies born dead, and reduced maternal and fetal weight gains.

Amitraz (Mitaban), a chemical used in the treatment of demodectic mange in dogs, can be absorbed through intact skin and may cause dizziness and fatigue in persons who bathe dogs without wearing gloves and other protective equipment. It is essential to use gloves and an apron when mixing amitraz with water or when treating dogs. Hands and arms should be washed with soap and water after treatment. There is also some danger of toxicity if amitraz vapors are inhaled, and the drug should only be applied in areas where ventilation is excellent. Because of the toxicity associated with inhalation of vapors or skin absorption of amitraz residues, it is a good idea to avoid close contact with dogs bathed with amitraz within the past 24 hours.

Insect growth regulators (methoprene, fenoxycarb, lufenuron) appear to have very low toxicity for humans, but are often combined with more toxic insecticides for quick kill of adult insects. For example, one commonly used insecticide contains chlorpyrifos (an organophosphate) as well as methoprene.

Despite this list of potential hazards, pesticides can be safely used in veterinary hospitals, provided a few common-sense rules are observed (Table 36–10). Although it is unlikely that a person will show signs of illness after giving a single flea bath, the risk of toxicity increases with exposure. Many of the signs of pesticide exposure are subtle and nonspecific (nausea, dizziness, headache, fatigue), and it is often difficult to know if a staff member is being exposed to toxic levels of these drugs. Any person who experiences symptoms suggestive of pesticide toxicity or observes these symptoms in others should immediately contact medical personnel or a poison control center for advice.

Disinfectants

Most disinfectants used in veterinary hospitals are relatively nontoxic, particularly when diluted with water. The most common health problem arising from the prolonged use of disinfectants is skin irritation. Disinfectants remove protective lipids and protein from the skin and after prolonged use may cause dehydration and death of superficial cells. Affected skin has a red, peeling, dry, and cracked appearance, and may be itchy. Dermatitis can be prevented by wearing gloves when handling disinfectants.

TECHNICIAN NOTE

The most common health problem arising from the prolonged use of disinfectants is skin irritation.

If persons with skin irritation continue to have contact with the offending disinfectant, they may develop an allergy to that disinfectant. Symptoms of a contact allergy to disinfectants (allergic contact dermatitis) are more severe than for simple irritation, and include blistering of the skin and extreme pruritus following contact with the offending substance. Fortunately, allergic dermatitis can usually be successfully treated by applying corticosteroid ointments and avoiding future skin contact with the offending agent.

Concentrated disinfectant solutions may be irritating to the hands, eyes, and respiratory tract. Gloves should be used when handling concentrated solutions, and safety goggles should be used if there is a possibility of splashing. Repeated exposure to vapors from concentrated bleach solutions may cause coughing, runny nose, wheezing, and other respiratory problems, and persons should ensure adequate ventilation when using this agent. Bleach should never be mixed with any disinfectant containing ammonia (e.g., quaternary ammonium compounds) as the combination of bleach and ammonia produces chlorine gas, which is extremely toxic.

Glutaraldehyde is somewhat toxic, particularly if used as a concentrated solution. Glutaraldehyde vapors may cause lung irritation, cough, and headaches. Glutaraldehyde is also known to be mutagenic and toxic to fetuses. For these reasons, it is wise to avoid breathing vapors from concentrated solutions, to wear goggles if there is any possibility of eye splash, to wear protective clothing including gloves when handling this agent, and to wash skin that has been exposed to this agent.

Latex Allergies

Persons who routinely wear latex gloves may eventually develop a contact allergy to latex. It is thought that proteins found in natural latex are responsible for the allergic reaction. Reactions to latex gloves include dermatitis (similar to a contact allergy to a pesticide or disinfectant), nasal congestion and sneezing, conjunctivitis, and swelling of the lips, eyelids, and throat. Severe reactions may involve the respiratory tract and include asthma, coughing, and dyspnea.

Persons with an allergy to latex should use plastic, vinyl, or nitrile gloves, or glove liners inside latex gloves. Barrier creams may also help reduce contact with latex. "Hypoallergenic" latex gloves are available, but may cause allergic reactions in some individuals.

• Table 36–10 •

SAFE USE OF PESTICIDES

1. All staff who handle or dispense pesticides must be familiar with the chemicals contained in the preparations used in the hospital, and the class of insecticide to which each chemical belongs (organophosphate, pyrethroid, insect growth regulator, and so forth). Consult the MSDS (material safety data sheet) for information on hazards and protective equipment that should be worn for a particular pesticide.
2. When treating an animal it is wise to use the least toxic chemical that is effective, for both human and animal safety. Follow the label directions, and avoid "extra label" use unless it is backed by an expert opinion. Agricultural insecticides and preparations intended for use in cattle should not be used on pets, as excessive exposure to both humans and animals may result. When dispensing a pesticide to an animal owner, advise him or her to read the label carefully before using the product, and to follow all label directions.
3. All pesticide containers must be clearly labeled with the name of the pesticide and brief hazard warnings. Pesticide solutions should not be stored in beverage containers such as empty bottles.
4. Many pesticides (pyrethrins, carbamates, any pour-on product) can be readily absorbed through intact skin. Skin exposure to pesticides can be avoided by wearing gloves. An apron or waterproof coveralls should also be worn when bathing an animal with insecticidal shampoos or dips. Gloves and coveralls must also be worn when applying insecticidal dips and spray to livestock. Protective gloves should not be reused indefinitely, as pesticides are absorbed into the rubber and will eventually penetrate through them. Laboratory coats, coveralls, and other protective clothing should be laundered between uses.
5. If gloves are not worn when handling an insecticide (e.g., when applying flea powder to an animal), hands should be washed as soon as possible after applying the pesticide. Persons whose hands have contacted a pesticide solution or dust should avoid putting their fingers near their mouth or eyes.
6. Protective eyewear should be worn when pouring or mixing concentrated pesticide solutions or when working around pesticide mists and sprays. Eyewashes should be available in case of accidental exposure. If an eye splash occurs, avoid rinsing the eyes using the spray attachment for a tub or sink, as the water stream from these devices may injure the cornea.
7. Rubber mats or nonslip flooring should be provided in bathing areas where splashes are likely to occur. Waterproof footwear is necessary if the bather is standing in excessively wet areas.
8. All pesticides (even shampoos) should be used only in areas with good ventilation. If the odor of insecticidal chemicals is strong in the area in which they are used, ventilation is inadequate. If this is the case, doors and windows should be opened, or portable fans used to increase air flow. Use of a pesticide filter mask or respirator may be necessary in some situations (e.g., when spraying a barn). The MSDS lists the respiratory protection required when working with a specific chemical.
9. Although it is unlikely that veterinary staff will deliberately drink insecticidal solutions, ingestion may occur if the chemical is present on the hands, eating utensils, or food. Open containers of food, beverages, cigarettes, and similar articles should not be left on the counter of a room in which insecticides are being used. Obviously, it is inadvisable to eat, drink, or smoke when using insecticides.
10. If possible, insecticide administration should not be assigned to only one person on the staff. Administration of baths and dips should be assigned to several staff members on a rotating basis. Pregnant employees may want to minimize their exposure to pesticides, as some authorities suggest that human fetuses and infants are particularly sensitive to the effects of pesticides.

Formalin and Formaldehyde

Formaldehyde and its derivatives (including formalin, which is a 37% solution of formaldehyde in methanol and water) are used in hospital disinfectants, some diagnostic test kits, and for preservation of tissue samples being sent to a laboratory for histopathologic study. Both liquid formaldehyde and formaldehyde vapors are toxic. *Liquid formaldehyde* is intensely irritating to eyes and skin, causing burning and tearing, and in severe cases, corneal damage. *Formaldehyde vapors* are irritating to the nose, throat, and respiratory tract. The eyes are particularly sensitive to formaldehyde vapors, and lacrimation (watery eyes) may occur even at low concentrations (0.1 to 3.0 ppm in room air). Chronic exposure to formaldehyde is known to cause cancer in hamsters and rats and formaldehyde is considered to be a potential human carcinogen.

OSHA has established a short-term formaldehyde exposure limit of 2 ppm, and an 8-hour time-weighted average limit of 8 ppm. If there is a chance that employees will be exposed to higher concentrations, the hospital must develop a written plan for safe storage and handling of formaldehyde and emergency procedures in case of spills. Exposure levels can be monitored using dosimeter badges.

To minimize the concentration of formaldehyde vapors in room air, formaldehyde and formalin should only be used in areas with excellent ventilation. Gloves should be worn when working with formaldehyde or tissues preserved in formalin. Goggles and an emergency eyewash station are recommended if there is a danger of splashing formaldehyde into the eyes.

Formalin should be ordered in small, prediluted containers to minimize handling of this agent.

TECHNICIAN NOTE

To minimize the concentration of formaldehyde vapors in room air, formaldehyde and formalin should only be used in areas with excellent ventilation.

Ethylene Oxide

Ethylene oxide is a gas sterilization agent, most commonly used in veterinary clinics for sterilizing materials that cannot withstand conventional autoclaving. Ethylene oxide for veterinary hospital use is usually purchased as a liquid in ampules, but is also available as a compressed gas in tanks.

In recent years, many concerns have been raised regarding the safety of this agent. Several hazards are associated with ethylene oxide use:

- Ethylene oxide is flammable and potentially explosive.
- Liquid ethylene oxide can cause severe burns if it is accidentally splashed onto the skin or eyes.
- Exposure to ethylene oxide vapors may irritate the eyes and respiratory system.
- Chronic exposure to moderate levels of ethylene oxide

(10 ppm) has been shown to cause chromosomal abnormalities in male and female laboratory animals and may cause similar problems in humans. It is therefore considered to be a "mutagenic" agent and has been classified as a potential human carcinogen.

Given the potential adverse health problems associated with ethylene oxide, OSHA has set an exposure limit of 1 ppm (8-hour time-weighted average), with a maximum level of 5 ppm (time-weighted average) for any 15-minute period. OSHA requires hospitals using ethylene oxide to prepare a detailed written plan for safe handling, storage, and use of ethylene oxide, if there is a chance that workers may be exposed to concentrations above this level.

Precautions for safe use of ethylene oxide are outlined in Table 36–11.

Cytotoxic Drugs

Probably the most hazardous pharmaceuticals the veterinary technician is likely to handle are the cytotoxic drugs used in

• Table 36–11 •

SAFE USE OF ETHYLENE OXIDE

1. Ethylene oxide ampules should be stored away from heat and sources of ignition. Smoking should be prohibited near the sterilizer when loading or unloading. Batteries should be removed from electrical instruments and sterilized separately to avoid the possibility of an electrical spark igniting the gas during the sterilization cycle.
2. All employees who handle ethylene oxide must be trained in safe handling techniques for this substance, and routine work and emergency procedures must be reviewed by the employer and employees at least annually. Written procedures should include procedures for loading and unloading the sterilizer and an emergency plan in case of ethylene oxide spill or gas release. All employees with potential exposure to ethylene oxide should read the MSDS (material safety data sheet) carefully.
3. Care should be taken to avoid accidental breakage of glass ampules, as the spilled liquid quickly evaporates, contaminating the room with ethylene oxide vapor. When preparing to sterilize a load, the ampule should be broken while still encased in its protective wrappings. A laboratory coat and neoprene rubber or butyl rubber gloves should be worn when breaking the ampule. If contact with liquid ethylene oxide occurs, all contaminated clothing should be removed, and the skin or eyes should be flushed with water for at least 15 minutes. The affected area should be covered with a dressing and the person transported immediately to medical care.
4. Only approved sterilizing boxes should be used, and provision must be made for ventilation of the box. Sterilizing boxes must be contained within a dedicated local exhaust system designed to suction escaping gas away from the sterilizing box.
5. The concentration of ethylene oxide in a sterilizing box may exceed 100,000 ppm during the sterilization process, and for this reason the box should never be opened until the sterilization period is over.
6. If ethylene oxide is used in a veterinary clinic, gas levels must be initially monitored using dosimeter badges. The hospital's supplier of ethylene oxide can usually recommend a badge supplier.

cancer chemotherapy (also called antineoplastic, chemotherapeutic, or anticancer agents). The agents most commonly used in veterinary medicine include cyclophosphamide (Cytoxan), vincristine (Oncovin), cisplatin (Platinol), azathioprine (Imuran), and doxorubicin (Adriamycin). If technicians and other hospital personnel are assigned to handle or administer cancer chemotherapeutic agents, or to dispose of materials contaminated with these drugs, they must receive special training in the toxicity of these agents and the techniques required for safe handling. Staff must also be familiar with spill cleanup procedures and first aid after acute exposure to these agents.

There is ample evidence that cytotoxic drugs can induce cancers in laboratory animals. Many anticancer agents can induce birth defects and miscarriage. Cytotoxic drugs are also extremely irritating to eyes, skin, and tissues, even in very low doses. A single needle prick to a finger with a syringe containing the cytotoxic drug mitomycin-C has caused the eventual loss of function of that hand.

Nurses working in cancer wards have shown a higher than expected incidence of liver damage, nausea, dizziness and lightheadedness, chronic headaches, hair loss, dermatitis (particularly after exposure to cisplatin, methotrexate, and vincristine), menstrual cycle irregularities, and miscarriage. Many of the side effects observed in nurses were the same as those noted by patients receiving antineoplastic drugs. Exposure was thought to arise from accidental contact through routine handling of the drug preparations.

It is suspected that inhalation of drug aerosols and skin absorption of powders and liquids are the chief routes by which cytotoxic drugs gain entry into the body. Skin exposure may occur when crushing or dividing a tablet or when handling urine or stool from an animal that has been treated with antineoplastic drugs. Inhalation of aerosols may occur when breaking an ampule, when withdrawing a syringe from a vial, when adjusting the amount of drug in a syringe, when expelling air from a partly filled syringe, or when liquid containing the drug leaks from tubing or a syringe.

The minimum necessary protective equipment when handling or administering cytotoxic drug tablets is a long-sleeved laboratory coat and disposable latex gloves. Whether intact or broken, cytotoxic drug capsules and tablets should never be manipulated with bare hands. Hands should be washed thoroughly after removing gloves. For procedures involving liquid cytotoxic drugs, it is recommended that personnel handling the drugs wear a disposable surgical gown (or other long-sleeved, back-closure, disposable protective garment with tight-fitting cuffs and neck) and disposable latex gloves. Special techniques are required to avoid generating aerosols when opening ampules, removing liquid from an ampule, reconstituting powders, and administering these agents to a patient.

TECHNICIAN NOTE

Persons who are pregnant, breast-feeding, or attempting to conceive are advised not to handle cytotoxic drugs.

Cytotoxic wastes (syringes, intravenous sets, gauzes, gloves) should be placed in a sealable plastic bag and disposed by incineration or held for biomedical waste pickup. Latex gloves should be worn when handling urine, feces, vomitus, and other body fluids from an animal that has received cytotoxic drugs within the previous 48 hours. Patient waste may be disposed of through the sewage system.

Persons who are pregnant, breast-feeding, or attempting to conceive are advised not to handle cytotoxic drugs.

If a veterinary hospital regularly prepares and administers injectable cytotoxic drugs, consideration should be given to the purchase of a glove box, biological safety cabinet, or a vertical laminar flow hood. This equipment has been shown to significantly reduce exposure to aerosols of cytotoxic drugs. Alternatively, preparation of cytotoxic agents may be contracted to a local pharmacy or hospital.

FIRST AID AND EMERGENCY RESPONSE

Despite the best of precautions, accidental exposure to chemicals may occur. Basic guidelines for handling chemical spills are given in Table 36–12, and guidelines for treatment of eye and skin exposure to chemicals are given in Tables 36–13 and 36–14. A written cleanup procedure for chemical spills should be posted in the clinic, giving details of cleanup procedures and protective equipment required. If an employee is unfamiliar with the procedure for cleaning up the spilled chemical, the MSDS should be consulted before cleaning up.

All veterinary hospitals should have a fire safety plan that includes specifics on safe storage of chemicals and garbage, a list of fire hazards and potential ignition sources, precautions when using portable heaters, location and type of fire extinguishers available, and identification of emergency exits and alarm systems. Hospitals with more than 10 employees must prepare written plans, but smaller hospitals may communicate the plan orally.

• Table 36–12 •

EMERGENCY PROCEDURES FOR CHEMICAL SPILLS

All veterinary hospitals should have a chemical spill kit prepared in advance and stored in an easily accessible location. The spill kit should contain an absorbent material such as cat litter, gloves, a dustpan and brush, and a plastic bag. Commercial spill kits can be purchased for cleanup of mercury, acids, and flammable solvents.

If the spill involves a relatively nontoxic liquid or solid (e.g., overturning a bottle of laboratory stain), the technician should immediately place a towel, newspaper, kitty litter, or other absorbent material on top of the spill. When the liquid is completely absorbed, the absorbent material should be swept up (or picked up using gloved hands) and placed in an airtight, sealed plastic bag for disposal outside the hospital.

If the spilled material gives off potentially hazardous vapors (formalin, anesthetic liquid, ethylene oxide, bleach), all adjacent doors and windows should be opened to increase ventilation. If a large amount of material is present and toxic fumes are being produced (e.g., a whole bottle of halothane is dropped and broken, or a vial of ethylene oxide is opened and exposed to the room air), all personnel should leave the area at once. A person who is trained in the use of a respirator and wearing protective clothing (apron, gloves) should reenter the room and clean up the mess by first increasing ventilation and then using cat litter or other absorbent as described above. If a respirator is not available or if staff are not trained in its use, the fire department should be contacted.

• Table 36–13 •

TREATMENT OF CHEMICAL SPLASH TO THE EYES

If a corrosive chemical is splashed into the eyes, the affected person should first call for help. Contact lenses, if worn, should be removed. Then both eyes must be continuously washed for 15 minutes with lukewarm or cold water, using an eyewash fountain or bottle. It is necessary to hold the eyelids open during the washing period; otherwise the natural inclination is to close the eyes which keeps water away from the cornea. The affected person should not rub or touch the eyes, as this is likely to introduce more chemical. After 15 minutes of continuous washing, the person should seek medical attention. Take the MSDS (material safety data sheet) from the chemical, or the labeled bottle, to the hospital with the injured person.

Emergency exits must be kept free from obstructions and at least two exits must be available for use so that persons within the building can escape without using a key.

Fire prevention also includes designation of duties in case of a fire and a fire response plan (Table 36–15). This plan should be posted at a central location within the clinic.

It is difficult for anyone to respond to an emergency such as a fire or chemical exposure in an effective manner if he or she has never had training or practice. All persons working in a veterinary hospital should undergo fire safety training annually. Responsibilities should be assigned to specific personnel (e.g., the receptionist calls the fire department; the technician locates all persons in the building and supervises evacuation of persons and animals). Some provision should be made for an evacuation plan (where are the exits, and what alternative exit should be used if one is blocked?) and a location should be designated where all personnel are to report after leaving the hospital. Emergency telephone numbers should be memorized by all staff members. Every employee must know the location of the fire extinguisher and protective equipment such as goggles, gloves, and a respirator. Every person should have some experi-

• Table 36–14 •

TREATMENT AFTER SKIN CONTACT WITH CHEMICALS

In case of splashing or other skin contact with a corrosive or toxic substance, all contaminated clothing should be removed and placed in a plastic bag. If the chemical is a powder or other dry material, brush away as much of the chemical as possible using gloved hands. The affected area should then be rinsed with water. For liquid chemicals, immediate water rinse is advisable. If the chemical is not corrosive (e.g., isopropyl alcohol) it is probably adequate to wash the exposed area with soap and water. If the chemical is toxic or corrosive (e.g., concentrated bleach or formaldehyde) the exposed skin should be flushed with cold water and soap for 15 minutes. If the exposure is extensive or the material is very toxic (e.g., ethylene oxide liquid) the person should be transported to medical attention immediately after the 15-minute flushing period. During transport, the affected area should be covered with a loose clean cloth. Cold packs or ice can be used as necessary to relieve pain.

• Table 36–15 •

FIRE RESPONSE
1. The first person to detect the fire calls for help immediately. Notify the fire department by calling 911 (or other applicable phone number for your area). Stay on the line and follow the dispatcher's instructions.
2. Alert all staff and clients that a fire has occurred. The veterinarian will report immediately to the site of the fire and decide if evacuation is necessary. If the fire is not contained, instruct all clients and staff not involved in fighting the fire to leave the hospital. All persons should meet in a preassigned location to determine if everyone has been evacuated. No person is to reenter the building unless directed to do so.
3. Once everyone is assembled outside and all personnel are accounted for, the veterinarian should decide if animals can be evacuated without endangering human safety. If so, they may be removed from the building and placed in vehicles or portable containers or tied with leads to stationary objects (fences, posts).
4. If possible to do so without endangering human safety: a. Close windows and doors. b. Turn off oxygen tanks and natural gas lines. c. Turn off fans. d. Use a fire extinguisher if the fire is small and the employee knows how to handle the fire extinguishing equipment. Do not attempt to fight a fire if it is spreading beyond the immediate area where it started, or if it could spread to block the escape route.

ence in operating the fire extinguisher, and know the types of fires that it can effectively extinguish.*

TECHNICIAN NOTE

All laboratories and veterinary clinics should be equipped with one or more fire extinguishers of a size easily manipulated by the employees.

All laboratories and veterinary clinics should be equipped with one or more fire extinguishers of a size easily manipulated by the employees. Different classes of fire extinguisher are designed to extinguish different types of fires (flammable solvents, paper, electrical). A veterinary hospital should have an extinguisher that is effective against a wide range of materials: a dry chemical (ABC) type is often recommended. Hospitals with computer equipment may prefer to use a carbon dioxide extinguisher, which has less potential for harming electrical equipment. Fire extinguishers should be placed no less than 75 feet apart. They should be inspected monthly by a hospital employee to ensure that they are properly charged, and a qualified person should inspect each fire extinguisher annually. Hospitals, like homes, should be equipped with smoke detectors on each floor, including the basement.

---

*A local fire marshall or fire station personnel will often conduct a courtesy fire safety inspection of a veterinary hospital and recommend improvements in fire safety. They may also be willing to train staff on fire safety and fire extinguisher operation.

References

Beat VB and Morgan DP: Evaluation of hazards involved in treating cattle with pour-on organophosphate insecticides. J Am Vet Med Assoc 170:812–814, 1977.

Bukowski J: Real and potential occupational health risks associated with insecticide use. Compendium Continuing Educ Small Anim Pract 12:1617–1623, 1990.

DHHS (US Department of Health and Human Services): Guidelines for Protecting the Safety and Health of Health Care Workers. National Institute for Occupational Safety and Health (NIOSH), Washington, DC, US Government Printing Office, 1988.

Johnson JA, Buchan RM, and Reif JS: Effect of waste anesthetic gas and vapor exposure on reproductive outcome in veterinary personnel. Am Ind Hyg Assoc J 48:62–66, 1987.

Landercasper MD, Cogbill TH, Strutt PJ, et al: Trauma and the veterinarian. J Trauma 28:1255–1259, 1988.

Schenker MB, Samuels SJ, Green RS, et al: Adverse reproductive outcomes among female veterinarians. Am J Epidemiol 132:96–106, 1990.

Short CE and Harvey RC: Anesthetic waste gases in veterinary medicine. Cornell Vet 73:363–374, 1983.

Thigpen CK and Dorn RC: Nonfatal accidents involving insured veterinarians in the United States 1967–1969. J Am Vet Med Assoc 163:369–374, 1973.

Wiggins P, Schenker MB, Green R, et al: Prevalence of hazardous exposures in veterinary practice. Am J Ind Med 16:55–66, 1989.

Recommended Reading

Animal-Related Injury
Barber JL and Ford RB: Animal bite wounds in humans. Anim Health Tech 3:277–279, 1982.

Ohman JL: Allergy in man caused by exposure to animals. J Am Vet Med Assoc 172:1403–1406, 1978.

Underman AE: Bite wounds inflicted by dogs and cats. Vet Clin North Am Small Anim Pract 17(1):195–207, 1987.

US Department of Health and Human Services: Guidelines for Protecting the Safety and Health of Health Care Workers. National Institute for Occupational Safety and Health (NIOSH), Washington, DC, US Government Printing Office, 1988.

Radiation
Brent RL: The effects of embryonic and fetal exposure to x-ray, microwave, and ultrasound. Clin Obstet Gynecol 26:484–511, 1983.

Dekaban AS: Abnormalities in children exposed to x-radiation during various stages of gestation. J Nucl Med 9:471–477, 1968.

Moore RM, Davis YM, and Kaczmarek RG: An overview of occupational hazards among veterinarians, with particular reference to pregnant women. Am Ind Hyg Assoc J 54:113–120, 1993.

Oppenheim BE, Griem ML, and Meier P: The effects of diagnostic x-ray exposure on the human fetus: An examination of the evidence. Radiology 114:529–534, 1975.

Rendano VT and Ryan G: Technical assistance in radiology. Part II Basic considerations and radiation safety. Vet Technician 9:547–551, 1988.

Seibert PJ: Radiation issue. Veterinary Safety and Health Digest 9, March-April 1995.

Waste Anesthetic Gas
Ad Hoc Committee of the American Society of Anesthesiologists: Occupational disease among O.R. personnel: A study. Anesthesiology 41:321–340, 1974.

Canadian Standards Association, Anaesthetic Gas Scavenging Systems (Publication CAN3-Z168.8-M82), Rexdale, Ontario, 1982.

Gross ME and Branson KR: Reducing exposure to waste anesthetic gas. Vet Technician 14:175–177, 1993.

Heath MM: Anesthesia: Hazards of the operating room. Vet Technician 7:24–28, 1986.

Lietzemayer DW: Current methods for removal of anesthetic gas. Vet Technician 11:213–220, 1990.

McKelvey D and Hollingshead KW: Small Animal Anesthesia. St Louis, Mosby-Year Book, 1994.

Paddleford RR: Manual of Small Animal Anesthesia. New York, 1988, Churchill Livingstone.

Potts DL and Craft BF: Occupational exposure of veterinarians to waste anesthetic gases. Appl Ind Hyg 3:132–138, 1988.

Purdham JT: Anaesthetic Gases and Vapours. Hamilton, Ontario. Canadian Center for Occupational Health and Safety, 1986.

Sass-Kortsak AM, Purdham JT, Bozek PR, et al: Exposure of hospital operating room personnel to potentially harmful environmental agents. Am Ind Hyg Assoc J 53:203–207, 1992.

Shenkar MB, Samuels SJ, Green RS, et al: Adverse reproductive outcomes among female veterinarians. Am J Epidemiol 132:96–106, 1990.

Short CE and Harvey RC: Anesthetic waste gases in veterinary medicine. Cornell Vet 73:363–374, 1983.

Spence AA: Environmental pollution by inhalation anaesthetics. Br J Anaesthesiol 59:96–103, 1987.

Pesticides

Wiggins P, Schenker MB, Green R, et al: Prevalence of hazardous exposures in veterinary practice: Am J Ind Med 16:55–66, 1989.

Disinfectants

Falk ES, Hektoen H, and Thune PO: Skin and respiratory tract symptoms in veterinary surgeons. Contact Dermatitis 12:274–278, 1985.

National Institute of Occupational Safety and Health: Guidelines for Protecting the Safety and Health of Health Care Workers. US Department of Health and Human Services, Washington, DC, 1988.

Vainio H: Inhalation anesthetics, anticancer drugs and sterilizants as chemical hazards in hospitals. Scand J Work Environ Health 8:94–107, 1982.

Ethylene Oxide

National Institute of Occupational Safety and Health: Ethylene Oxide Sterilizers in Health Care Facilities. Current Intelligence Bulletin 52. US Department of Health and Human Services, Cincinnati, 1989.

Seibert PJ: The Veterinary Safety and Health Digest 11, July-August 1995.

Steenland K, Styaner L, Greife A, et al: Mortality among workers exposed to ethylene oxide. N Engl J Med 324:1402–1407, 1991.

Vainio H: Inhalation anesthetics, anticancer drugs and sterilizants as chemical hazards in hospitals. Scand J Work Environ Health 8:94–107, 1982.

Cytotoxic Drugs

Bacovsky R: Guidelines for handling and disposal of hazardous pharmaceuticals. Can Soc Hosp Pharmacists 416:979–1049, 1991.

Dickinson KL and Ogilvie GK: Safe handling and administration of chemotherapeutic agents in veterinary medicine. *In* Kirk RW (editor): Current Veterinary Therapy 12, Philadelphia, WB Saunders, 1995, pp 475–478.

Falck K, Grohn P, and Sorsa M: Mutagenicity in urine of nurses handling cytotoxic drugs: Lancet 1:1250–1251, 1979.

Fox LE: Chemotherapy safety for the practicing veterinarian. Perspectives May/June 1995, pp 8–15.

Hahn KA and Morrison WB: Safety guidelines for handling chemotherapeutic drugs. Vet Med November, 1094–1099, 1991.

Hemminki K, Kyyronen P, and Lindbohm ML: Spontaneous abortions and malformations in the offspring of nurses exposed to anesthetic gases and cytostatic drugs. J Epidemio Community Health 39:141–147, 1985.

Holt L: Cytotoxic drugs. Vet Technician 16:675–678, 1995.

National Institute of Occupational Safety and Health: Guidelines for Protecting the Safety and Health of Health Care Workers. US Department of Health and Human Services, Washington, DC, 1988, sect 5, p. 13.

Nikula E, Kivinitty K, and Leisti J: Chromosomal abberations in lymphocytes of nurses handling cytostatic agents. Scand J Work Environ Health 10:71–74, 1984.

Selevan SG, Lindbohm MJ, Hornung RW, et al: A study of occupational exposure to antineoplastic drugs and fetal loss in nurses. N Engl J Med 313:1173–1178, 1985.

Swanson LV: Potential hazards associated with low-dose exposure to antineoplastic agents—Part I. Evidence for concern. Compendium Continuing Educ Small Anim Pract 10:290–298, 1988.

Swanson LV: Potential hazards associated with low-dose exposure to antineoplastic agents—Part II. Recommendations for minimizing exposure. Compendium Continuing Educ Small Anim Pract 10:615–623, 1988.

Vainio H: Inhalation anesthetics, anticancer drugs and sterilizants as chemical hazards in hospitals. Scand J Work Environ Health 8:94–107, 1982.

Vaughn MC and Christensen WD: Occupational exposure to cancer chemotherapeutic drugs: A literature review. Am Ind Hyg Assoc J 45:B8–B18, 1985.

Yodaiken RE and Bennett D: OSHA work-practice guidelines for personnel dealing with cytotoxic (antineoplastic) drugs. Am J Hosp Pharmacists 43:1193–1204, 1986.

See also *Cytotoxic Drug Safety,* a video by Wallace Morrison, distributed by the American Animal Hospital Association, PO Box 150899, Denver, CO 80215-0899.

Appendix

Common Abbreviations Used in Veterinary Medicine

a	Artery	BER	Basal energy requirement
aa	Of each	bid	Twice daily
AA	Amino acid	BLD	Blood
AAHA	American Animal Hospital Association	BLV	Bovine leukosis virus
Ab	Antibody; antibiotics	BM	Bowel movement
ABG	Arterial blood gas	BMR	Basal metabolic rate
ac	Before meals	BOL	Large pill (hora)
ACD	Acid-citrate-dextrose	BP	Blood pressure
ACE	Angiotensin converting enzyme	BRD	Bovine respiratory disease
ACTH	Adrenocorticotropic hormone	BRSV	Bovine respiratory syncytial virus
AD	Right ear	BSA	Body surface area
ADH	Antidiuretic hormone	BSP	Bromsulphalein
ad lib	Freely, as wanted	BT	Blue tongue
ADR	Active defense reflex; adverse drug reaction	BUN	Blood urea nitrogen
		BUTE	Phenylbutazone
A Fib	Atrial fibrillation	BV	Bronchovesicular
Ag	Antigen	BVD	Bovine virus diarrhea
A:G	Albumin-globulin ratio	BW	Body weight
AGID	Agar gel immunodiffusion	c̄	with
AL	Left ear	C & S	Culture and sensitivity
ALB	Albumin	C-S	Coughing-sneezing
ALK PHOS	Alkaline phosphatase	C-spine	Cervical spine
ALP	Alkaline phosphatase	Ca	Calcium
ALT	Alanine transaminase	CA	Carcinoma; coronary artery; cardiac arrest
AM	Antemortem		
AMA	Against medical advice; American Medical Association	CAE	Caprine arthritis-encephalitis
		caps	Capsules
AMI	Acute myocardial infarction	CAV-1	Canine adenovirus type 1
amp	Ampule	CBC	Complete blood count
ANA	Antinuclear antibody	cc	Cubic centimeter
ANS	Autonomic nervous system	CC	Chief complaint
AP	Anterior posterior; arterial pressure	CCM	Congestive cardiomyopathy
APC	Atrial premature contraction	CD	Canine distemper
APTT	Activated partial thromboplastin time	CEA	Canine erythrocyte antigen
ARF	Acute renal failure	CEM	Contagious equine metritis
ARR	Arrhythmia	CFJ	Coxofemoral joint
AS	Aortic stenosis; left ear	CGP	Circulating granulocyte pool
ASAP	As soon as possible	CHD	Canine hip dysplasia; coronary heart disease
ASD	Atrial septal defect		
ASIF	Association for the Study of Internal Fixation	CHF	Congestive heart failure
		CHOL	Cholesterol
AST	Aspartate aminotransferase	CHV	Canine hepatitis virus
AU	Each ear	CI	Cardiac insufficiency
AV	Atrioventricular	CID	Combined immunodeficiency
AV block	Atrioventricular as in first-, second-, third-degree AV block	CIN	Chronic interstitial nephritis
		CITE	Concentration immunoassay technology
BAR	Bright, alert, and responsive	Cl	Chloride
BAER	Brain stem auditory-evoked response	CM	Cardiomyopathy
BBB	Blood-brain barrier	CMT	California mastitis test
BE	Barium enema colon only	CNE	Canine distemper encephalitis

CNS	Central nervous system
COB	Care of body
CODE E	Used in emergency for cardiac arrest
CPA	Cardiopulmonary arrest
CPD	Citrate-phosphate-dextrose
CPK	Serum creatine phosphokinase
CPR	Cardiopulmonary resuscitation
CPU	Central processing unit
Creat	Creatinine
CRF	Chronic renal failure; corticotropin releasing factor
CRT	Capillary refill time; cathode-ray tube
CSF	Cerebrospinal fluid; colony-stimulating factor
CMS	Cervical stenotic myelopathy
CTZ	Chemoreceptor trigger zone
CVA	Cardiovascular accident; cerebrovascular accident
CVP	Central venous pressure
CVS	Cardiovascular system
cwt	Hundredweight
CXR	Chest x-ray
D BILI	Direct bilirubin
D/S	Dextrose in saline
D_5W	5% dextrose in water
Ddx	Differential diagnosis
DEC	Decrease; diethylcarbamazine
DES	Diethylstilbestrol
DHL	Canine distemper-hepatitis-leptospirosis vaccine
DIC	Disseminated intravascular coagulation
DJD	Degenerative joint disease
DLH	Domestic longhair
DM	Diabetes mellitus
DMSO	Dimethyl sulfoxide
DOA	Dead on arrival
DOS	Disk operating system
DRG	Diagnosis-related group
DS	Dose or days not acceptable
DSH	Domestic shorthair
DTM	Dermatophyte test medium
DV	Dorsal ventral
Dx	Diagnosis
EAE	Enzootic abortion of ewes
ECF	Extracellular fluid
ECG or EKG	Electrocardiogram
ECHO	Echocardiogram
EDTA	Ethylenediaminetetraacetic acid
EEE	Eastern equine encephalomyelitis
EEG	Electroencephalogram
EENT	Eyes, ears, nose, throat
EFA	Essential fatty acids
EHV	Equine herpesvirus
EIA	Equine infectious anemia
ELISA	Enzyme-linked immunosorbent assay
EM	Electron microscopy

EMD	Electromechanical dissociation
EMG	Electromyogram
ER	Emergency room
ERG	Electroretinogram
ESR	Erythrocyte sedimentation rate
F-A	Fecal analysis
FA	Fluorescent antibody; fatty acids
FB	Foreign body
FD	Feline distemper
FeLV	Feline leukemia virus
FeSV	Feline sarcoma virus
FIP	Feline infectious peritonitis
FIV	Feline immunodeficiency virus
FPV	Feline panleukopenia virus
FSH	Follicle-stimulating hormone
FUO	Fever of unknown origin
FUS	Feline urological syndrome
FVR	Feline viral rhinotracheitis
Fx	Fracture
g	Gram
gal	Gallon
GAS	General adaptation syndrome
GDV	Gastric dilation volvulus
GFR	Glomerular filtration rate
GGT	Gamma glutamyltransferase
GI	Gastrointestinal
gm	Gram
GnRH	Gonadotropin releasing hormone
gtt	Drops (guttae)
GU	Genitourinary
GUI	Graphical-user interface
h	Hour
Hb	Hemoglobin
HBC	Hit by car
HBs	Harsh bronchial sounds
HC	Health certificate
HCT	Hematocrit
HIS	Hospital information systems
HR	Heart rate
hs	At bedtime (hora somni)
HSA	Hemangiosarcoma
Hx	History
I BILI	Indirect bilirubin
IBK	Infectious bovine keratoconjunctivitis
IBR	Infectious bovine rhinotracheitis
IC	Intracardiac
ICF	Intracellular fluid
ICH	Infectious canine hepatitis
ICU	Intensive care unit
ID	Intradermal
IM	Intramuscular
IN	Intranasal
IOP	Intraocular pressure
IP	Intraperitoneal
ISE	Ion-selective electrode
IT	Intratracheal
IU	International unit

IV	Intravenous
IVD	Intervertebral disk disease
IVP	Intravenous pyelogram
K	Potassium
K-9	Canine
Kcal	Kilocalorie
KCS	Keratoconjunctivitis sicca
kg	Kilogram
L or LT	Left
LBBB	Left bundle branch block
LDA	Left displaced abomasum
LDH	Lactate dehydrogenase
LN	Lymph node
LRS	Lactated Ringer's solution
LSA	Lymphosarcoma
m²	Meter squared
MAC	Minimum alveolar concentration
MAOI	Monoamine oxidase inhibitor
MAP	Mean arterial pressure
μg	Microgram
μl	Microliter
mcg	Microgram
MCH	Mean corpuscular hemoglobin
MCHC	Mean corpuscular hemoglobin concentration
MCT	Mast cell tumor
MCV	Mean corpuscular volume
MEA	Mean electrical axis
mEq	Milliequivalents
MER	Maintenance energy requirements
Mg	Magnesium
MGP	Marginated granulocyte pool
MI	Mitral insufficiency or myocardial insufficiency; myocardial infarction
MIC	Minimal inhibitory concentration
MIP	Mare's immunological pregnancy test
ml	Milliliter
MLV	Modified live virus
MM	Mucous membrane
MRI	Magnetic resonance imaging
Na	Sodium
NC	No change
NCC	Nucleated cell count
NMR	Nuclear magnetic resonance
non rep	Do not repeat
NPL	No palpable lesions
NPO	Nothing per os (nothing by mouth)
NR	Not remarkable
NRBC	Nucleated red blood cell
NRC	National Research Council
NS	Normal saline
NSF	No significant findings
NSR	Normal sinus rhythm
NVL	No visible lesions
OB	Obstetrics
OCD	Osteochondritis dissecans
OD	Right eye (oculus dexter)

OFA	Orthopedic Foundation for Animals
OHE	Ovariohysterectomy (spay)
OL	Left eye
OPP	Ovine progressive pneumonia
OS	Left eye (oculus sinister)
OSA	Osteosarcoma
OTC	Over the counter
OU	Both eyes
P	Phosphorus
P3	Third phalanx or coffin bone
PAC	Premature atrial contraction
PAT	Paroxysmal atrial tachycardia
pc	After meals
PCV	Packed cell volume
PDA	Patent ductus arteriosus
PDQ	Pretty darned quick
PDR	Passive defense reflex
PE	Pulmonary edema; physical examination
PEA	Phenylethyl alcohol
PEG	Percutaneous endoscopic gastrostomy
per os	Orally, by mouth
PG	Prostaglandin
PGA	Polyglycolic acid
PI3	Parainfluenza-3
PK	Pigmentary keratitis
PM	Postmortem
PMSG	Pregnant mare serum gonadotropin
PNS	Parasympathetic nervous system
PO	Postoperative, per os
POVMR	Problem-oriented veterinary medicine record
PPH	Pertinent past history
ppm	Parts per million
PPM	Persistent pupillary membrane
PPN	Partial parenteral nutrition
PPV	Porcine parvovirus
PRA	Progressive retinal atrophy
PRAA	Persistent right aortic arch
prn	As necessary
PRRS	Porcine reproductive and respiratory syndrome
PRV	Pseudorabies virus
PS	Pulmonic stenosis
PSS	Physiologic saline
PTA	Prior to admission
PTH	Parathyroid hormone
PTS	Put to sleep
PTT	Partial thromboplastin time
PU	Penile urethrostomy
PVC	Premature ventricular contraction
PWD	Powder
q	Every
q2h	Every 2 hours
q6h	Every 6 hours
QBC	Quantitative buffy coat
qd	Every day
qh	Every hour

qid	Four times a day
qns	Quantity not sufficient
qod	Every other day
qs	Quantity sufficient
R or RT	Right
RACL	Ruptured anterior cruciate ligament
RADs	Radiographs
RAM	Random access memory
RAS	Reticular activating system
RBBB	Right bundle branch block
RBC	Red blood cell
RDA	Right displaced abomasum
RER	Resting energy requirement
Retic	Reticulocyte
RHF	Right heart failure
RID	Radical immunodiffusion
R/O	Rule out
RTG	Ready to go
RV	Rabies vaccination; residual volume
Rx	Take (prescription)
s̄	Without (sine)
SC or SQ	Subcutaneous
SCC	Squamous cell carcinoma
SDH	Sorbitol dehydrogenase
SGOT	Serum glutamic-oxaloacetic transaminase
SGPT	Serum glutamic-pyruvate transaminase
Sig	Label (prescription)
SIM	Sulfide-indole-motility (medium)
SMEDI	Stillbirths, mummified fetuses, embryonic death, and infertility
SNS	Sympathetic nervous system
SOAP	Subjective, objective, assessment, plan
SOB	Shortness of breath
S/P	Status post
sp.	Species
sp. gr.	Specific gravity
SR	Suture removal
ss	One half
stat	Statum (immediately)
Sx	Signs, symptoms
T BILI	Total bilirubin
tab	Tablet
TAT	Tetanus antitoxin
TBW	Total body water
TDN	Total digestible nutrients
TEME	Thromboembolic meningoencephalitis
TGC	Time gain compensation
TGE	Transmissible gastroenteritis
TGEV	Transmissible gastroenteritis virus
TI	Tricuspid insufficiency
tid	Thrice daily
T-L	Thoracolumbar vertebra
TLC	Tender loving care
TP	Total protein
TPN	Total parenteral nutrition
TPP	Total plasma protein
TPR	Temperature, pulse, respiration
TR	Trace
TRF	Thyrotropin-releasing factor
TRH	Thyrotropin-releasing hormone
TRIG	Triglycerides
TS-FIPV	Temperature-sensitive feline infectious peritonitis virus
TSH	Thyroid-stimulating hormone
TSI	Triple sugar iron
TT	Tetanus toxoid
Tx	Treatment
U	Unit
UA	Urinalysis
UG	Urogenital
UGI	Upper gastrointestinal tract (includes esophagus, stomach, and duodenum)
ung	Ointment
UO	Urinary obstruction
URI	Upper respiratory infection
US	Ultrasound
USG	Urine specific gravity
UT DICT	As directed (ut dictum)
UTI	Urinary tract infection
v.	Vein
V TACH	Ventricular tachycardia
vc	Vital capacity
VD	Ventral dorsal
V-D	Vomiting and diarrhea
VECCS	Veterinary Emergency and Critical Care Society
VEE	Venezuelan equine encephalomyelitis
VER	Visual evoked response
VES	Ventricular extrasystole
VMDB	Veterinary medical database
VPC	Ventricular premature contraction
VS	Vital signs
VSD	Ventricular septal defect
VSV	Vesicular stomatitis virus
WBC	White blood cell
WEE	Western equine encephalomyelitis
WNL	Within normal limits
XRT	Radiation therapy

Index

Note: Page numbers in *italics* refer to illustrations; page numbers followed by t refer to tables.